Edited by
Felix Kratz, Peter Senter,
and Henning Steinhagen

Drug Delivery in Oncology

Related Titles

Fialho, A., Chakrabarty, A. (eds.)

Emerging Cancer Therapy

Microbial Approaches and Biotechnological Tools

2010
ISBN: 978-0-470-44467-2

Jorgenson, L., Nielson, H. M. (eds.)

Delivery Technologies for Biopharmaceuticals

Peptides, Proteins, Nucleic Acids and Vaccines

2009
ISBN: 978-0-470-72338-8

Airley, R.

Cancer Chemotherapy

Basic Science to the Clinic

2009
ISBN: 978-0-470-09254-5

Missailidis, S.

Anticancer Therapeutics

2009
ISBN: 978-0-470-72303-6

Dübel, S. (ed.)

Handbook of Therapeutic Antibodies

2007
ISBN: 978-3-527-31453-9

Knäblein, J. (ed.)

Modern Biopharmaceuticals

Design, Development and Optimization

2005
ISBN: 978-3-527-31184-2

Edited by Felix Kratz, Peter Senter, and Henning Steinhagen

Drug Delivery in Oncology

From Basic Research to Cancer Therapy

Volume 2

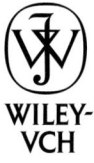

WILEY-VCH Verlag GmbH & Co. KGaA

The Editors

Dr. Felix Kratz
Head of the Division of
Macromolecular Prodrugs
Tumor Biology Center
Breisacherstrasse 117
D-79106 Freiburg
Germany

Dr. Peter Senter
Vice President Chemistry
Seattle Genetics, Inc.
218, Drive S.E. Bothell
Seattle, WA 98021
USA

Dr. Henning Steinhagen
Vice President
Head of Global Drug Discovery
Grünenthal GmbH
Zieglerstr. 6
52078 Aachen
Germany

All books published by **Wiley-VCH** are carefully produced. Nevertheless, authors, editors, and publisher do not warrant the information contained in these books, including this book, to be free of errors. Readers are advised to keep in mind that statements, data, illustrations, procedural details or other items may inadvertently be inaccurate.

Library of Congress Card No.: applied for

British Library Cataloguing-in-Publication Data
A catalogue record for this book is available from the British Library.

Bibliographic information published by the Deutsche Nationalbibliothek
The Deutsche Nationalbibliothek lists this publication in the Deutsche Nationalbibliografie; detailed bibliographic data are available on the Internet at <http://dnb.d-nb.de>.

© 2012 Wiley-VCH Verlag & Co. KGaA, Boschstr. 12, 69469 Weinheim, Germany

All rights reserved (including those of translation into other languages). No part of this book may be reproduced in any form – by photoprinting, microfilm, or any other means – nor transmitted or translated into a machine language without written permission from the publishers. Registered names, trademarks, etc. used in this book, even when not specifically marked as such, are not to be considered unprotected by law.

Composition   Laserwords Private Ltd., Chennai
Printing and Binding   betz-druck GmbH, Darmstadt
Cover Design   Schulz Grafik-Design, Fußgönheim

Printed in the Federal Republic of Germany
Printed on acid-free paper

ISBN: 978-3-527-32823-9
oBook ISBN: 978-3-527-63405-7

Foreword

It is highly likely that the reason our therapies so often fail our patients with cancer is that either (i) those therapies actually never get to their intended targets or (ii) those therapies are "intercepted" by similar targets on normal cells. If we want to understand why many of our therapies fail our patients, and what we can do to possibly remedy those failures, this book *Drug Delivery in Oncology* can help all of us achieve that understanding – and with this book it will be a state-of-the-art understanding.

Drs. Kratz, Senter, and Steinhagen have assembled a respectable breadth of both seasoned and precocious investigators to put together this very special treatise (49 chapters in all). The chapters are well written with basic science, preclinical, and clinical perspectives.

The book begins with a history and the limitations of conventional chemotherapy. Expert discussions of the vascular physiology of tumors that affect drug delivery (and how to defeat those issues) then follow. There are excellent discussions of the neonatal Fc receptor, development of cancer targeted ligands, and antibody-directed enzyme prodrug therapy (ADEPT).

A very special part of this book is the emphasis on tumor imaging. Again, the authors are major experts in this field, which undoubtedly will continue to mature to enable us to document whether or not our therapeutics actually make it to their intended target(s) – and if not, why not.

There are impressive chapters on macromolecular drug delivery systems, including biospecific antibodies, antibody–drug conjugates, and antibody–radionuclide conjugates. Up-to-date discussions of polymer-based drug delivery systems including PEGylation, thermoresponsive polysaccharide-based and even low-density lipoprotein–drug complexes are also presented.

Those with an interest in learning about nano- and microparticulate drug delivery systems can study liposomes to immunoliposomes, to hydrogels, micelles, albumin–drug nanoparticles, and even carbon nanotubes, which are all covered in this book.

Other special delivery systems covered include peptides–drug conjugates, vitamin–drug conjugates, and growth factor–drug conjugates, conjugates of drugs with fatty acids, RNA and RNA interference delivery, and specific targeted organ drug delivery.

As investigators who want to more effectively treat and indeed cure cancer we have many worries. The first of these is that many of our therapeutics just do not make it into the targets in the tumors. This book gives the reader a comprehensive insight into multiple ways to address this problem. A second major worry is that we are losing our pharmacologists who can solve those drug delivery issues. The editors and the authors of this incredible treatise give us comfort that these pharmacologists are alive and well, and thinking as to how they can contribute to getting control of this awful disease.

Daniel D. Von Hoff, MD, FACP
Physician in Chief and Distinguished Professor,
Translational Genomics Research Institute (TGen)
Professor of Medicine, Mayo Clinic
Chief Scientific Officer, Scottsdale Healthcare and US Oncology

Contents to Volume 1

Part I   Principles of Tumor Targeting   *1*

1   **Limits of Conventional Cancer Chemotherapy**   *3*
    Klaus Mross and Felix Kratz

2   **Pathophysiological and Vascular Characteristics of Solid Tumors in Relation to Drug Delivery**   *33*
    Peter Vaupel

3   **Enhanced Permeability and Retention Effect in Relation to Tumor Targeting**   *65*
    Hiroshi Maeda

4   **Pharmacokinetics of Immunoglobulin G and Serum Albumin: Impact of the Neonatal Fc Receptor on Drug Design**   *85*
    Jan Terje Andersen and Inger Sandlie

5   **Development of Cancer-Targeting Ligands and Ligand–Drug Conjugates**   *121*
    Ruiwu Liu, Kai Xiao, Juntao Luo, and Kit S. Lam

6   **Antibody-Directed Enzyme Prodrug Therapy (ADEPT) – Basic Principles and its Practice So Far**   *169*
    Kenneth D. Bagshawe

Part II   Tumor Imaging   *187*

7   **Imaging Techniques in Drug Development and Clinical Practice**   *189*
    John C. Chang, Sanjiv S. Gambhir, and Jürgen K. Willmann

| 8 | Magnetic Nanoparticles in Magnetic Resonance Imaging and Drug Delivery 225
Patrick D. Sutphin, Efrén J. Flores, and Mukesh Harisinghani

| 9 | Preclinical and Clinical Tumor Imaging with SPECT/CT and PET/CT 247
Andreas K. Buck, Florian Gärtner, Ambros Beer, Ken Herrmann, Sibylle Ziegler, and Markus Schwaiger

Contents to Volume 2

Foreword V
Preface XXIII

Part III   Macromolecular Drug Delivery Systems 289

Antibody-Based Systems 289

| 10 | **Empowered Antibodies for Cancer Therapy** 291
Stephen C. Alley, Simone Jeger, Robert P. Lyon, Django Sussman, and Peter D. Senter
| 10.1 | Introduction and Rationale for Approach 291
| 10.2 | Examples of Empowered Antibody Technologies 291
| 10.2.1 | ADCC 291
| 10.2.2 | Antibody–Drug Conjugates for Cancer Therapy 295
| 10.2.2.1 | Target Antigen Selection 295
| 10.2.2.2 | Conjugation Technologies 297
| 10.2.2.3 | Drug and Linker Selection 301
| 10.3 | Clinical Developments 307
| 10.3.1 | Gemtuzumab Ozogamicin (Mylotarg) and Other Calicheamicin-Based ADCs 307
| 10.3.2 | Brentuximab Vedotin and Other Auristatin-Based ADCs 309
| 10.3.3 | Trastuzumab–DM1 and Other Maytansinoid-Based ADCs 310
| 10.4 | Alternative Scaffolds 310
| 10.5 | Conclusions and Perspectives 311
References 311

| 11 | **Mapping Accessible Vascular Targets to Penetrate Organs and Solid Tumors** 325
Kerri A. Massey and Jan E. Schnitzer
| 11.1 | Introduction 325
| 11.2 | Current Approaches to Therapy 325
| 11.3 | Defining New Target Spaces 326
| 11.3.1 | Vascular Endothelium as an Accessible Target Space 327
| 11.3.2 | Pathways Across the Endothelium 328

11.3.3	Caveolae as a Transvascular Pumping Target Space	*329*
11.3.4	Applying the Concept of New Target Spaces to Solid Tumors	*330*
11.4	Difficulties in Studying Endothelial Cells	*332*
11.4.1	Endothelial Cells in Culture	*332*
11.4.2	Historic Approaches to Vascular Mapping	*333*
11.5	Methods to Identify Tissue-Specific Targets	*334*
11.5.1	Antibody-Based Approaches	*334*
11.5.2	Phage-Based Approaches	*335*
11.5.3	Large-Scale Approaches	*335*
11.6	MS-Based Approaches to Map the Vascular Endothelial Cell Proteome	*336*
11.6.1	Defining Analytical Completeness	*337*
11.6.2	Quantification and Normalization of MS Data	*338*
11.7	Means to Validation	*339*
11.8	*In vivo* Tissue Targeting: The Lungs as Proof of Principle	*341*
11.9	Targeting Lung Tumors	*343*
11.10	Future Directions	*346*
	References	*346*
12	**Considerations of Linker Technologies**	*355*
	Laurent Ducry	
12.1	Introduction	*355*
12.2	Linkage Site and Cross-Linking Chemistry	*355*
12.3	Linkers for Cytotoxic ADCs	*357*
12.3.1	Chemically Labile Linkers	*357*
12.3.2	Enzyme-Labile Linkers	*361*
12.3.3	Noncleavable Linkers	*367*
12.4	Linkers for Radioactive Immunoconjugates	*369*
12.5	Conclusions	*370*
	References	*371*
13	**Antibody–Maytansinoid Conjugates: From the Bench to the Clinic**	*375*
	Hans Erickson	
13.1	Introduction	*375*
13.2	Conjugation Strategies	*376*
13.3	Selecting the Optimal Linker	*381*
13.4	Clinical Candidates	*384*
13.5	Activation of AMCs by Targeted Cancer Cells	*385*
13.5.1	Isolation of Maytansinoid Metabolites	*385*
13.5.2	Target Cell Metabolites of AMCs with SMCC-DM1, SPP-DM1, and SPDB-DM4 Linker-Maytansinoid Combinations	*386*
13.5.3	Lysosomal Activation is Necessary for both Cleavable and Uncleavable Conjugates	*387*

13.5.4	Efficiency of Antigen-Mediated Processing 387
13.5.5	Efflux of Metabolites from Targeted Cancer Cells and Bystander Effects 388
13.5.6	Target Cell Activation of Cleavable and Uncleavable AMCs 389
13.6	*In Vivo* Tumor Delivery Studies 390
13.7	Conclusions 392
	References 392

14 Calicheamicin Antibody–Drug Conjugates and Beyond 395
Puja Sapra, John DiJoseph, and Hans-Peter Gerber
14.1	Introduction 395
14.2	Discovery of Calicheamicin and Mechanism of Action 397
14.3	Calicheamicin ADCs 399
14.3.1	Gemtuzumab Ozogamicin (Mylotarg) 399
14.3.2	Clinical Development of Gemtuzumab Ozogamicin (Mylotarg) 400
14.3.3	CMC-544 402
14.3.3.1	CD22 Expression and Function 402
14.3.4	Preclinical Activity of CMC-544, an Anti-CD22–Calicheamicin Conjugate, in Models of NHL 402
14.3.5	Effect of CMC-544 in a Model of ALL 403
14.4	Clinical Development of Calicheamicin Conjugates: CMC-544 404
14.5	Conclusions and Future Directions 405
	References 407

15 Antibodies for the Delivery of Radionuclides 411
Anna M. Wu
15.1	Introduction 411
15.2	Rationale for Using Antibodies for Radionuclide Delivery 413
15.2.1	Radionuclides for Imaging 415
15.2.1.1	γ Emitters 417
15.2.1.2	Positron Emitters 417
15.2.2	Radionuclides for Therapy 418
15.2.2.1	β Emitters 421
15.2.2.2	α Emitters 422
15.2.2.3	Auger Electron Emitters 423
15.2.3	Antibodies as Delivery Agents 423
15.2.3.1	Intact Antibodies 424
15.2.3.2	Engineered Antibody Fragments 424
15.2.3.3	Pretargeting 429
15.3	Clinical Development 431
15.3.1	Radioimmunoimaging 431
15.3.2	Radioimmunotherapy 434

15.4	Conclusions and Perspectives	434
	Acknowledgments	435
	References	435

16 Bispecific Antibodies and Immune Therapy Targeting 441
Sergej M. Kiprijanov
16.1 Introduction 441
16.2 Treatment Options in Cancer in the Pre-Antibody Era 442
16.3 Antibodies as Therapeutic Agents 443
16.4 Next Generation of Therapeutic Antibodies 449
16.5 Rationale for Immunotherapy with BsAbs 450
16.5.1 Retargeting BsAbs 450
16.5.2 BsAbs of Dual Action 452
16.5.3 BsAbs of Enhanced Selectivity 453
16.6 BsAb Formats 454
16.6.1 Hetero-Oligomeric Antibodies 455
16.6.2 Bispecific Single-Chain Antibodies 457
16.6.3 Recombinant IgG-Like BsAbs 460
16.6.4 Other Novel BsAb Constructs 463
16.7 BsAbs in the Clinic 463
16.7.1 Clinical Data for First-Generation BsAbs 464
16.7.2 Recombinant Bispecific Molecules Entering Clinical Trials 464
16.7.2.1 Bispecific T-Cell Engager Molecules 464
16.7.2.2 Other scFv–scFv Tandem Molecules 468
16.7.2.3 TandAbs 469
16.7.2.4 BsAbs of Dual Action 471
16.8 Conclusions and Future Prospects 472
References 473

Polymer-Based Systems 483

17 Design of Polymer–Drug Conjugates 485
Jindřich Kopeček and Pavla Kopečková
17.1 Introduction 485
17.2 Polymer Carriers 486
17.2.1 Impact of the Molecular Weight of the Polymer Carrier on its Fate and Efficiency 488
17.2.2 Structural Factors Influencing the Cellular Uptake and Subcellular Fate of Macromolecules 490
17.2.3 Other Design Factors 493
17.3 Binding Drugs to Polymer Carriers 496
17.4 Attachment of Targeting Moieties 498
17.4.1 Subcellular Targeting 500
17.4.1.1 Mitochondrial Targeting 501

17.4.1.2	Hormone-Mediated Nuclear Delivery *501*
17.5	Novel Designs of Polymer Therapeutics *503*
17.5.1	Design of Backbone Degradable, Long-Circulating Polymer Carriers *503*
17.5.2	Drug-Free Macromolecular Therapeutics *504*
17.6	Conclusions and Perspectives *506*
	Acknowledgments *506*
	References *507*

18	**Dendritic Polymers in Oncology: Facts, Features, and Applications** *513*
	Mohiuddin Abdul Quadir, Marcelo Calderón, and Rainer Haag
18.1	Introduction *513*
18.2	Chemistry and Architecture *515*
18.3	Dendritic Architectures and Oncology: Background and Application *517*
18.3.1	Complexation of Anticancer Agents by Dendritic Architectures *520*
18.3.2	Anticancer Agents can be Chemically Conjugated with Dendrimer Functional Groups *523*
18.3.3	Tumor Microenvironment and Attachment of Targeting Moiety to the Dendrimer *528*
18.4	Intracellular Trafficking, Cytotoxicity, and Pharmacokinetics of a Dendritic Architecture are Tunable *535*
18.5	Other Medical Applications of Dendritic Polymers *537*
18.5.1	Photodynamic Therapy *537*
18.5.2	Boron Neutron Capture Therapy *538*
18.5.3	Diagnostic Application of Dendrimers *539*
18.5.4	Gene Delivery with Dendrimers *542*
18.6	Novel Therapeutic Approaches with Dendrimers *545*
18.7	Conclusions *547*
	Acknowledgments *547*
	References *547*

19	**Site-Specific Prodrug Activation and the Concept of Self-Immolation** *553*
	André Warnecke
19.1	Introduction *553*
19.2	Rationale and Chemical Aspects of the Concept of Self-Immolation *554*
19.2.1	Cyclization Strategies *556*
19.2.2	Elimination Strategies *558*
19.2.3	Self-Immolative versus Classic Strategies – A Comparison *562*
19.3	Elimination-Based Trigger Groups for Tumor-Specific Activation *564*
19.3.1	Enzymatic and Related Biocatalytic Activation *564*
19.3.2	Reductive Activation *566*
19.3.3	Oxidative Activation *569*

19.3.4	pH-Dependent Activation	*569*
19.3.5	Other Methods of Activation	*571*
19.4	Branched Elimination Linkers–Chemical Adaptors or Building Blocks for More Complex Self-Immolative Architectures	*573*
19.5	Clinical Impact	*582*
19.6	Conclusion and Perspectives	*584*
	References	*585*

20 Ligand-Assisted Vascular Targeting of Polymer Therapeutics *591*
Anat Eldar-Boock, Dina Polyak, and Ronit Satchi-Fainaro

20.1	Overview of Tumor Angiogenesis	*591*
20.2	Potential Angiogenic Markers	*596*
20.2.1	Integrins	*596*
20.2.2	Selectins	*596*
20.2.3	APN (CD13)	*598*
20.2.4	Hyaluronic Acid Binding Receptor (CD44)	*598*
20.3	Drug Delivery Strategy: Targeted Polymer Therapeutics	*599*
20.4	Novel Targeted Polymeric Drug Delivery Systems Directed to Tumor Endothelial Cells	*601*
20.4.1	RGD-Based Polymer–Drug Conjugates	*601*
20.4.2	Selectin-Targeted Polymer–Drug Conjugates	*612*
20.4.3	APN-Targeted Polymer Therapeutics	*613*
20.4.4	HA-Based Polymer Therapeutics	*615*
20.5	Opportunity for Dual Targeting of Angiogenesis-Related Markers	*616*
20.6	Tumor Angiogenesis-Targeted Polymeric Drug Delivery Systems: Summary and Lessons Learnt	*617*
	References	*619*

21 Drug Conjugates with Poly(Ethylene Glycol) *627*
Hong Zhao, Lee M. Greenberger, and Ivan D. Horak

21.1	Introduction	*627*
21.2	Rationale for PEGylation and PEG-Drug Conjugates	*627*
21.3	Permanent PEGylation	*630*
21.3.1	First-Generation PEG Linker: SS-PEG	*630*
21.3.2	Second-Generation PEG Linkers	*631*
21.3.2.1	SC-PEG	*631*
21.3.2.2	PEG-Aldehyde	*632*
21.3.2.3	U-PEG	*633*
21.3.2.4	Other Permanent Linkers	*637*
21.4	Releasable PEGylation	*638*
21.4.1	Releasable PEG Linkers Based on Ester Linkage	*638*
21.4.1.1	PEG–Paclitaxel	*638*
21.4.1.2	PEG–Camptothecin Analogs	*641*

21.4.2	Releasable PEG Linkers Based on Amide or Other Amino-Derived Linkages 646
21.4.2.1	Releasable PEG Linkers Based on Aromatic Systems 646
21.4.2.2	Releasable PEG Linkers Based on an Aliphatic System 649
21.4.2.3	Aromatic Amides 651
21.4.2.4	Acid-Activated PEG–Drug Conjugates 651
21.4.2.5	Other Releasable Linkers 653
21.5	Summary of Clinical Status 653
21.6	Conclusions and Perspectives 655
	Acknowledgments 656
	References 657

22 Thermo-Responsive Polymers 667
Drazen Raucher and Shama Moktan

22.1	Introduction 667
22.2	Hyperthermia in Cancer Treatment 668
22.3	Synergistic Advantages of Combining Thermo-Responsive Polymers and Hyperthermia 670
22.4	Selected Thermo-Responsive Polymer Classes 671
22.4.1	Synthetic Polymers 671
22.4.2	*N*-Isopropylacrylamide-Based Polymers 671
22.4.3	PEO-Based Polymers 674
22.4.4	Poly(Organophosphazene)-Based Polymers 677
22.4.5	Miscellaneous 678
22.5	Elastin-Like Biopolymers 678
22.5.1	ELP Synthesis 678
22.5.2	Cell-Penetrating Peptides for Intracellular Delivery of ELPs 680
22.5.3	Efficiency and Mechanism of CPP-ELP Cellular Uptake 681
22.5.4	ELPs for Delivery of Peptides 682
22.5.5	Delivery of c-Myc Inhibitory Peptides by ELPs 684
22.5.6	ELP-Based Delivery of a Cell Cycle Inhibitory p21 Mimetic Peptide 685
22.5.7	ELP Delivery of Conventional Drugs 690
22.5.8	*In Vivo* Studies with Thermo-Responsive ELP Carriers 692
22.5.9	Optimizing *In Vivo* Delivery of ELP Carriers with CPPs 693
22.6	Conclusions and Perspectives 695
	Acknowledgements 696
	References 697

23 Polysaccharide-Based Drug Conjugates for Tumor Targeting 701
Gurusamy Saravanakumar, Jae Hyung Park, Kwangmeyung Kim, and Ick Chan Kwon

23.1	Introduction 701
23.2	Chemistry of Polysaccharide–Drug Conjugation 707
23.3	Polysaccharide-Drug Conjugates 711

23.3.1	Dex-Based Drug Conjugates	711
23.3.2	Chitin– and Chitosan–Drug Conjugates	717
23.3.3	HA–Drug Conjugates	724
23.3.4	Heparin–Drug Conjugates	727
23.3.5	Pullulan–Drug Conjugates	730
23.3.6	Other Natural Polymer–Drug Conjugates	730
23.3.6.1	Alginate–Drug Conjugates	730
23.3.6.2	Arabinogalactan–Drug Conjugates	732
23.3.6.3	Pectin–Drug Conjugates	732
23.3.6.4	Xyloglucan–Drug Conjugates	734
23.3.6.5	Polygalactosamine–Drug Conjugates	735
23.4	Cyclodextrin–Drug Conjugates	735
23.5	Conclusions and Perspectives	738
	References	739

24   Serum Proteins as Drug Carriers of Anticancer Agents   747
Felix Kratz, Andreas Wunder, and Bakheet Elsadek

24.1	Introduction	747
24.2	Rationale for Exploiting Albumin, Transferrin, and LDL as Carriers for Drug Delivery to Solid Tumors	752
24.3	Examples of Drug Delivery Systems with Serum Proteins	759
24.3.1	Synthetic Approaches for Realizing Drug Conjugates, Drug Complexes, and Drug Nanoparticles with Albumin, Transferrin, or LDL	759
24.3.2	Drug Complexes and Conjugates with Albumin, Transferrin, and LDL	762
24.3.2.1	Drug Conjugates with Transferrin and Albumin	772
24.3.2.2	LDL–Drug Complexes	786
24.4	Clinical Development	788
24.5	Conclusions and Perspectives	791
	References	793

25   Future Trends, Challenges, and Opportunities with Polymer-Based Combination Therapy in Cancer   805
Coralie Deladriere, Rut Lucas, and María J. Vicent

25.1	Introduction	805
25.1.1	Combination Therapy in Cancer	805
25.2	Concept of Polymer–Drug Conjugates for Combination Therapy	810
25.3	Challenges and Opportunities Associated with the Use of Polymer-Based Combination Therapy	812
25.3.1	Identification of Appropriate Drug Combinations and Drug Ratios	812
25.3.2	Kinetics of Drug Release	814
25.3.3	Loading Capacity	815
25.3.4	Correlation of *In Vitro* Studies with Behavior *In Vivo*	815
25.3.5	Physicochemical Characterization	816

25.3.6	Clinical Development	816
25.4	Representative Examples of Polymer–Drug Conjugates for Combination Therapy	817
25.4.1	Preclinical Development	817
25.4.1.1	*In Vitro* Status	817
25.4.1.2	*In Vivo* Status	821
25.4.2	Clinical Development	829
25.4.2.1	Family I: Polymer–Drug Conjugate plus Free Drug	829
25.5	Conclusions and Perspectives	830
	Acknowledgments	831
	References	831

26	**Clinical Experience with Drug–Polymer Conjugates**	**839**
	Khalid Abu Ajaj and Felix Kratz	
26.1	Introduction	839
26.2	Rationale for Developing Drug–Polymer Conjugates	840
26.3	Clinical Development	846
26.4	Conclusions and Perspectives	874
	References	878

Part IV Nano- and Microparticulate Drug Delivery Systems 885

Lipid-Based Systems 885

27	**Overview on Nanocarriers as Delivery Systems**	**887**
	Haifa Shen, Elvin Blanco, Biana Godin, Rita E. Serda, Agathe K. Streiff, and Mauro Ferrari	
27.1	Introduction	887
27.2	Overview on Liposome-Based Systems	889
27.3	Overview on Polymer Micelle-Based Systems	892
27.4	Other Nanoparticulate Drug Delivery Systems	894
27.4.1	Chitosan and Chitosan-Coated Nanoparticles	894
27.4.2	Albumin Nanoparticles	895
27.4.3	Carbon Nanotubes	896
27.5	MSV Drug Delivery Systems	896
27.6	Conclusions and Perspectives	900
	References	901

28	**Development of PEGylated Liposomes**	**907**
	I. Craig Henderson	
28.1	Introduction and Rationale	907
28.2	Structure, Formation, and Characteristics of Liposomes	907
28.2.1	Non-PEGylated Liposomes	907
28.2.2	Sterically Stabilized or "Stealth" Liposomes	910
28.2.3	Tumor Targeting	910

28.2.4	Implication of Tumor Targeting for Dosing PLD	912
28.3	Pharmacokinetics of Stealth Liposomes	913
28.4	Clinical Development	915
28.4.1	Toxicity Profile	915
28.4.1.1	PPE	916
28.4.1.2	Infusion Reactions	918
28.4.1.3	Cardiotoxicity	918
28.4.2	First Clinical Indication: AIDS-Related Kaposi's Sarcoma	919
28.4.3	Activity in Solid Tumors and Hematological Malignancies	924
28.4.3.1	Ovarian Cancer	925
28.4.3.2	Breast Cancer	929
28.4.3.3	Multiple Myeloma	933
28.4.3.4	Soft-Tissue Sarcomas	937
28.4.3.5	Other Tumors	938
28.4.4	Optimal Dose Schedule for PLD	938
28.5	Newer Applications of PEGylated Liposomes	939
28.6	Conclusions and Perspective	941
	References	941
29	**Immunoliposomes**	**951**
	Vladimir P. Torchilin	
29.1	Introduction: Drug Targeting and Liposomes as Drug Carriers	951
29.1.1	Drug Targeting	951
29.1.2	Longevity of Pharmaceutical Nanocarriers in the Blood and the Enhanced Permeability and Retention Effect	952
29.1.3	Liposomes	953
29.2	Tumor-Targeted Liposomes in Cancer Chemotherapy	955
29.2.1	Derivatization of PEGylated Liposomes	955
29.2.2	Antibody-Targeted Liposomes	956
29.2.3	Liposomes Modified with Nucleosome-Specific Antibodies	961
29.2.4	Other Targeting Ligands	966
29.3	Preparation and Administration of Antibody-Targeted Liposomal Drugs	968
29.4	Conclusions	971
	References	971
30	**Responsive Liposomes (for Solid Tumor Therapy)**	**989**
	Stavroula Sofou	
30.1	Introduction	989
30.2	Rationale: Uniformity in Delivery and Actual Delivery	989
30.2.1	Rationale for Responsive Targeting	993
30.2.2	Rationale for Responsive Release	994
30.3	Examples	994
30.3.1	Preclinical Development	994

30.3.1.1	Activation by Tumor-Intrinsic Stimuli	994
30.3.1.2	Activation at the Tumor by External Stimuli	1000
30.3.2	Clinical Development	1006
30.4	Conclusions and Perspectives	1007
	Acknowledgments	1008
	References	1008

31 Nanoscale Delivery Systems for Combination Chemotherapy 1013
Barry D. Liboiron, Paul G. Tardi, Troy O. Harasym, and Lawrence, D. Mayer

31.1	Introduction	1013
31.2	Rationale for Fixed Ratio Anticancer Combination Therapy	1014
31.2.1	Biological Basis for the Importance of Drug Ratios	1014
31.3	Application of Drug Delivery Systems to Develop Fixed-Ratio Drug Combination Formulations	1022
31.3.1	Formulation Strategies for Multiagent Drug Delivery Vehicles	1022
31.3.2	Examples of Dual-Drug Delivery Systems	1026
31.4	Liposome-Based CombiPlex® Formulations	1029
31.4.1	Preclinical Development of CombiPlex Formulations	1030
31.4.1.1	CPX-351 (Cytarabine/Daunorubicin) Liposome Injection	1030
31.4.1.2	CPX-1 (Floxuridine/Irinotecan) Liposome Injection	1032
31.4.1.3	CombiPlex Systems for Reactive Agents: CPX-571	1033
31.5	Clinical Studies of CombiPlex Formulations	1036
31.5.1	Clinical Activity of CPX-351	1036
31.5.2	Clinical Activity of CPX-1	1038
31.5.2.1	Phase I Clinical Trial of CPX-1	1038
31.5.2.2	Phase II Clinical Trials of CPX-1	1039
31.6	CombiPlex Formulations of Hydrophobic Agents	1040
31.6.1	Nanoparticle CombiPlex Formulations for Delivering Drug Combinations Containing Hydrophobic Agents	1040
31.7	Conclusions	1043
	References	1044

Polymer-Based Systems 1051

32 Micellar Structures as Drug Delivery Systems 1053
Nobuhiro Nishiyama, Horacio Cabral, and Kazunori Kataoka

32.1	Introduction	1053
32.2	Rationale and Recent Advances in Micellar Structures as Drug Delivery Systems	1054
32.2.1	Smart Polymeric Micelles for Site-Specific Drug Delivery	1054
32.2.2	Polyion Complex Micelles for Gene and siRNA Delivery	1058
32.2.3	Other Block Copolymer Assemblies	1060

32.2.4	Theranostic Nanodevices *1062*
32.3	Conclusions and Perspectives *1063*
	References *1064*

33 Tailor-Made Hydrogels for Tumor Delivery *1071*
Sungwon Kim and Kinam Park

33.1	Introduction *1071*
33.2	Rationale for Hydrogel-Based Cancer Therapy *1071*
33.3	Examples *1072*
33.3.1	Materials and Biodegradability *1072*
33.3.2	Injectable Formulations *1076*
33.3.2.1	*In Situ* Gelation *1077*
33.3.2.2	Nanogels *1078*
33.3.3	Therapeutic Mechanisms *1079*
33.3.3.1	Small-Molecule Drugs *1079*
33.3.3.2	Protein and Peptide Drugs *1082*
33.3.3.3	Gene and siRNA Delivery *1085*
33.3.3.4	Cell Delivery *1087*
33.3.3.5	Photodynamic Therapy *1087*
33.3.3.6	Radiotherapy *1088*
33.3.3.7	Thermotherapy *1088*
33.3.3.8	Embolization *1089*
33.4	Conclusions and Perspectives *1090*
	References *1091*

34 pH-Triggered Micelles for Tumor Delivery *1099*
Haiqing Yin and You Han Bae

34.1	Introduction *1099*
34.2	Tumor Extracellular Acidity *1100*
34.3	General Approaches to Construct pH-Sensitive Polymeric Micelles for Tumor Delivery *1103*
34.4	Recent Development in pH-Sensitive Micelles for Tumor-Targeted Drug Delivery *1104*
34.4.1	pH-Triggered Drug Release *1104*
34.4.1.1	Tumor Extracellular pH (pH_e)-Triggered Drug Release *1104*
34.4.1.2	Endocytic pH-Triggered Drug Release *1106*
34.4.2	Tumor pH_e-Triggered Modulation of Micelle Surface Functionality *1113*
34.4.2.1	pH_e-Triggered Conversion of Micelle Surface Charge *1113*
34.4.2.2	pH_e-Triggered Exposure of Cell Penetrating Peptide (TAT) *1113*
34.4.3	Beyond pH-Triggered Drug Release – Multifunctional pH-Sensitive Micelles *1114*
34.4.3.1	Synergy of Receptor-Mediated Endocytosis and Endocytic pH-Triggered Drug Release *1115*
34.4.3.2	Overcoming Multidrug Resistance *1117*

34.4.3.3	TAT-Functionalized Micelles with a Pop-Up Mechanism for Versatile Tumor Targeting *1121*	
34.4.3.4	Virus-Mimetic Cross-Linked Micelles (Nanogels) for Maximal Drug Efficacy *1122*	
34.5	Conclusions and Perspective *1125*	
	References *1126*	

35 Albumin–Drug Nanoparticles *1133*
Neil Desai

35.1	Introduction *1133*
35.2	Rationale for Using Albumin Nanoparticles for Drug Delivery *1133*
35.3	Examples of Albumin-Based Nanoparticles *1135*
35.3.1	*In Vitro* and Animal Studies with Albumin-Based Nanoparticles *1139*
35.3.1.1	Delivery of Hydrophobic Small-Molecule Drugs Using *nab* Technology *1139*
35.3.1.2	Other Albumin Nanoparticles Carrying Small Molecules *1145*
35.3.1.3	Albumin Nanoparticle Delivery of Oligonucleotides and Proteins *1150*
35.3.2	Clinical Studies with Albumin-Based Nanoparticles *1152*
35.4	Conclusions and Perspectives *1156*
	Acknowledgments *1156*
	References *1156*

36 Carbon Nanotubes *1163*
David A. Scheinberg, Carlos H. Villa, Freddy Escorcia, and Michael R. McDevitt

36.1	Introduction *1163*
36.1.1	Chemistry of CNTs for Biologic Applications *1164*
36.1.2	Covalent Modifications of Nanotubes *1166*
36.1.3	Noncovalent Modifications *1167*
36.2	Arming of CNTs *1167*
36.2.1	Interactions with Cells and Tissues *1168*
36.2.2	Immunologic Responses *1169*
36.2.3	Biodegradability and Biologic Persistence *1169*
36.3	Toxicity of CNTs *1170*
36.3.1	Pharmacokinetic Issues *1173*
36.3.1.1	Absorption *1174*
36.3.1.2	Distribution *1175*
36.3.1.3	Metabolism *1177*
36.3.1.4	Excretion *1178*

36.3.2	Imaging Modalities	*1178*
36.4	Conclusions	*1180*
	References	*1181*

Contents to Volume 3

Part V   Ligand-Based Drug Delivery Systems   *1187*

37 **Cell-Penetrating Peptides in Cancer Targeting**   *1189*
Kaido Kurrikoff, Julia Suhorutšenko, and Ülo Langel

38 **Targeting to Peptide Receptors**   *1219*
Andrew V. Schally and Gabor Halmos

39 **Aptamer Conjugates: Emerging Delivery Platforms for Targeted Cancer Therapy**   *1263*
Zeyu Xiao, Jillian Frieder, Benjamin A. Teply, and Omid C. Farokhzad

40 **Design and Synthesis of Drug Conjugates of Vitamins and Growth Factors**   *1283*
Iontcho R. Vlahov, Paul J. Kleindl, and Fei You

41 **Drug Conjugates with Polyunsaturated Fatty Acids**   *1323*
Joshua Seitz and Iwao Ojima

Part VI   Special Topics   *1359*

42 **RNA Drug Delivery Approaches**   *1361*
Yuan Zhang and Leaf Huang

43 **Local Gene Delivery for Therapy of Solid Tumors**   *1391*
Wolfgang Walther, Peter M. Schlag, and Ulrike Stein

44 **Viral Vectors for RNA Interference Applications in Cancer Research and Therapy**   *1415*
Henry Fechner and Jens Kurreck

45 **Design of Targeted Protein Toxins**   *1443*
Hendrik Fuchs and Christopher Bachran

46 **Drug Targeting to the Central Nervous System**   *1489*
Gert Fricker, Anne Mahringer, Melanie Ott, and Valeska Reichel

47 Liver Tumor Targeting *1519*
Katrin Hochdörffer, Giuseppina Di Stefano, Hiroshi Maeda, and Felix Kratz

48 Photodynamic Therapy: Photosensitizer Targeting and Delivery *1569*
Pawel Mroz, Sulbha K. Sharma, Timur Zhiyentayev, Ying-Ying Huang, and Michael R. Hamblin

49 Tumor-Targeting Strategies with Anticancer Platinum Complexes *1605*
Markus Galanski and Bernhard K. Keppler

Index *1631*

Preface

Modern oncology research is highly multidisciplinary, involving scientists from a wide array of specialties focused on both basic and applied areas of research. While significant therapeutic advancements have been made, there remains a great need for further progress in treating almost all of the most prevalent forms of cancer. Unlike many other diseases, cancer is commonly characterized by barriers to penetration, heterogeneity, genetic instability, and drug resistance. Coupled with the fact that successful treatment requires elimination of malignant cells that are very closely related to normal cells within the body, cancer therapy remains one of the greatest challenges in modern medicine.

Early on, chemotherapeutic drugs were renowned for their systemic toxicities, since they poorly distinguished tumor cells from normal cells. It became apparent to scientists within the field that further advancements in cancer medicine would require new-generation drugs that ideally targeted critical pathways, unique markers, and distinguishing physiological traits that were selectively found within the malignant cells and solid tumor masses. Several new areas of research evolved from this realization, including macromolecular-based therapies that exploit impaired lymphatic drainage often associated with solid tumors, antiangiogenesis research to cut the blood supply off from growing tumors, antibody-based strategies that allow for selective targeting to tumor-associated antigens, and new drug classes that attack uniquely critical pathways that promote and sustain tumor growth. A large proportion of both recently approved and clinically advanced anticancer drugs fall within these categories.

Beyond the generation of such drug classes, it has also been recognized that approved cancer drugs could be made more effective and less toxic through delivery and transport technologies that maximize tumor exposure while sparing normal tissues from chemotherapeutic damage. By doing so, existing or highly potent cytotoxic drugs may display improved therapeutic indices. This has attracted considerable attention and has spawned the area of macromolecular-based delivery strategies.

There are few places where those actively engaged in drug delivery or who may wish to enter the field can find the major advancements consolidated in one place. This prompted us to organize the series of books entitled *Drug Delivery in Oncology* comprised of 49 chapters written by 121 internationally recognized leaders in the field. The work within the book series overviews many of the major breakthroughs in cancer medicine made in the last 10–15 years and features many of the chemotherapeutics of the future. Included among them are recombinant antibodies, antibody fragments, and antibody fusion proteins as well as tumor-seeking ligands for selective drug delivery and tumor imaging, and passive targeting strategies using macromolecules and nano- and microparticulate systems.

One of the special distinguishing features of this series is that the chapters are written for novices and experts alike. Each chapter is written in a style that allows interested readers to not only to find out about the most recent advancements within the field being discussed, but to actually see the data in numerous illustrations, photos, graphs, and tables that accompany each chapter.

None of this would have been possible without the devoted efforts of the contributing authors, all of whom shared the common goal of creating a new series of books that would provide an important cornerstone in the modern chemotherapeutic treatment of cancer. We are all very thankful for their efforts.

We also wish to thank the publishing team at Wiley-VCH in Weinheim, Germany. In particular, we want to give our wholehearted thanks and kind acknowledgments to Frank Weinreich, Gudrun Walter, Bernadette Gmeiner, Claudia Nußbeck, Hans-Jochen Schmitt, and Ina Wiedemann, who were always helpful and supportive during the 2 years it took to put all this together. It is our hope that this series will provide readers with inspired ideas and new directions for research in drug delivery in oncology.

July 2011

Felix Kratz
Peter Senter
Henning Steinhagen

Part III
Macromolecular Drug Delivery Systems

Antibody-Based Systems

10
Empowered Antibodies for Cancer Therapy

Stephen C. Alley, Simone Jeger, Robert P. Lyon, Django Sussman, and Peter D. Senter

10.1
Introduction and Rationale for Approach

Multiple studies have demonstrated the clinical activities of monoclonal antibodies (mAbs) in the forms of monotherapy or when combined with chemotherapeutic drugs [1, 2]. These mAbs recognize antigens that are preferentially expressed on tumor cell surfaces or on nontumor cells within the tumor mass, and elicit activities through such mechanisms as cell signaling, antibody-dependent cellular cytotoxicity (ADCC), antibody-dependent cellular phagocytosis (ADCP), and complement-dependent cytotoxicity (CDC). While these mechanisms are applicable to clinically approved mAbs such as trastuzumab (Herceptin®), cetuximab (Erbitux®), bevacizumab (Avastin®), and rituximab (Rituxan®), there are many examples of mAbs that recognize tumor-associated antigens, but are devoid of significant activities in preclinical and clinical studies. As a result, there has been considerable research focused on ways to improve effector function activities on antitumor mAbs by increasing their affinities for the Fcγ receptor (FcγR) on neutrophils, macrophages, and natural killer cells [3, 4]. Another method to increase the activities of mAbs is to append potent cancer drugs to them in a manner that allows for specific release of the drug at the tumor target site [5]. In the past few years this area has advanced significantly, with agents that have been designed for potency, stability, and safety. This chapter will discuss progress in these areas of cancer drug development, with an emphasis on important parameters that have been addressed in developing innovative new agents with promising activity profiles.

10.2
Examples of Empowered Antibody Technologies

10.2.1
ADCC

ADCC (Figure 10.1), ADCP, and CDC, are forms of antibody effector functions that are often responsible for antibody activity [6–8]. At a molecular level, ADCC

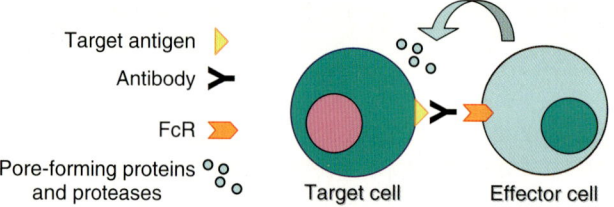

Figure 10.1 ADCC mechanism. Cells expressing the target antigen (yellow) bind to a therapeutic antibody (black) and recruit effector cells, which bind to the antibody via FcγRs (orange). The effector cells (natural killer and monocytes) release pore-forming proteases (blue) that lyse the target cells.

and ADCP activities are due to the interactions between the Fc region of a therapeutic antibody and FcγRI, II, and III on immune cells such as neutrophils, macrophages, and natural killer cells. CDC is mediated through the interactions between the antibody Fc portion with one of the components of complement. A great deal of research has focused on optimizing effector function by increasing the binding affinity between the antibody with the cognate FcγR.

The antibody-binding sites for FcγRs have been determined using scanning alanine mutagenesis, in which solvent-exposed amino acids were individually mutated to alanine and the resulting molecules were tested for FcγR binding [3]. Residues were identified that were involved in binding to all or each particular FcγRs, which led to the development of IgG variants with greatly enhanced ADCC activities. An extension of this work used structure-based computational design to rationally introduce amino acid mutations into human IgG1 Fc regions for affinity improvement [9]. The optimized Fc–FcγR interaction translated into a 100-fold enhancement of *in vitro* effector functions and a 50-fold increased *in vivo* B-cell depletion in cynomolgus monkeys using an engineered anti-CD20 mutant compared to the wild-type antibody. Specifically, native rituximab required a dose of nearly 10 µg/kg/day to achieve 50% B-cell depletion, while a dose of 0.2 µg/kg/day of the effector function-enhanced variant was sufficient. An anti-CD30 antibody variant based on this technology is now in a clinical phase I trial (XmAb2513, Table 10.1).

Another approach that has been used to increase antibody ADCC activity involves engineering the carbohydrate structures bound to Asn297 on the antibody heavy chains. Although these branched sugars are not directly involved in Fc–FcγR interactions, they can affect binding affinity by changing the conformation of the Fc portion of the antibody [10, 11]. The structure of the carbohydrate attached to the C_H2 domain of IgGs is shown in Figure 10.2a.

One of the first indications that carbohydrate structure influenced effector functions involved the chimeric anti-CD52 antibody alemtuzumab (Campath-1H®). This antibody had a different carbohydrate structure and higher efficacy when produced in the rat myeloma line YB2/0 than when expressed in Chinese hamster ovary (CHO) cells [15]. Analysis of the glycosylation pattern revealed the presence

10.2 Examples of Empowered Antibody Technologies

Table 10.1 Representative effector function-enhanced antibodies in clinical trials.

Agent	Antibody format	Target	Indication	Clinical status	Developer
XmAb2513	Fc mutations	CD30	Hodgkin's lymphoma, anaplastic large cell lymphoma	phase I	Xencor
GA-101	glyco-mAb	CD20	NHL	phase II/II	Roche
GA-201	glyco-mAb	EGFR	solid tumors	phase I	Roche
MDX-1401	afucosylated	CD30	relapsed or refractory Hodgkin's lymphoma	phase I	Bristol-Myers Squibb
BIW-8962	afucosylated	GM2 ganglioside	multiple myeloma	phase I/II	Kyowa Hakko Kirin Pharma
KW-0761	afucosylated	CCR4	adult T-cell leukemia-lymphoma	phase II	Kyowa Hakko Kirin Pharma
MEDI-563	afucosylated	interleukin-5 receptor	asthma	phase IIa	MedImmune

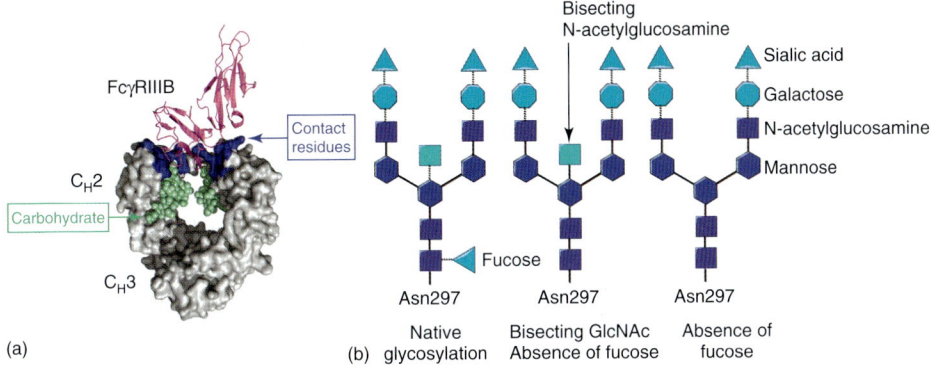

Figure 10.2 X-ray crystal structure of the Fc portion of an antibody bound to FcγRIIIB and diagram of carbohydrate structure. (a) Crystal structure of the Fc region of a human IgG1 antibody (gray) in complex with FcγRIIIB (magenta) [12]. The N-linked carbohydrates attached at Asn297 in each of the two C_H2 domains are highlighted in green. The residues in contact with FcγRIIIB (blue) have been the subject of intensive mutational studies in order to find antibody variants with differential FcγRIIIB binding affinity [3]. (b) The presence and composition of the N-linked glycans play an important role for the recognition of antibodies by FcγRs [13]. As a result, glycoengineering became a powerful tool to modulate antibody–FcR interaction. For example, the presence of a bisecting GlcNAc in combination with the absence of fucose was found to increase FcγR-mediated therapeutic efficacy of mAbs [4]. Further studies revealed that the absence of fucose is sufficient to produce highly effector function enhanced antibodies [14].

of bisecting N-acetylglucosamine (GlcNAc) and the absence of fucose in antibodies produced in the rat cell line. In contrast, CHO cells are not able to incorporate bisecting GlcNAc into the antibody structure. This prompted investigators to establish an efficient system to produce antibodies in CHO cells that were transfected with N-acetylglucosaminetransferase III to achieve increased amounts of bisected nonfucosylated oligosaccharides (Figure 10.2b) [4, 16]. The resulting mAbs had higher affinities for FcγRIIIa and improved ADCC activities. However, the glycoengineered antibodies were comprised of heterogeneous mixtures of N-linked oligosaccharides.

More detailed investigation on the influence of the glycosylation pattern on FcγR binding revealed that the absence of fucose rather than the presence of GlcNAc played a more pronounced role of ADCC enhancement [14, 17]. To exploit this, mAb expression in rat myeloma YB2/0 cells lines that are deficient in α1,6-fucosyltransferase provides nonfucosylated mAbs that exhibit 50-fold greater ADCC activity than fucosylated variants produced in CHO cells [14]. In contrast, only a slight increase of ADCC could be observed by the addition of GlcNAc to highly fucosylated IgG1. Based on these findings, CHO cells that lacked α1,6-fucosyltransferase were established in order to produce mAbs that were fully devoid of fucose, but had an otherwise normal glycosylation pattern [18].

The potential advantage of amplified ADCC activity of defucosylated therapeutic antibodies has been demonstrated in various preclinical *in vivo* models [19–21]. Defucosylated chimeric anti-CCR4 IgG1 antibody had significantly higher antitumor activity compared with the highly fucosylated parent antibody in a CCR4-positive T-cell leukemia model with human peripheral blood mononuclear cell-engrafted mice [19]. Recently, afucosylated trastuzumab has been reported to more than double the median progression-free survival compared with conventional trastuzumab in mice with HER2/*neu*-positive breast cancer [22].

Several ADCC-enhanced antibodies have now entered clinical evaluation (Table 10.1) [23, 24]. Anti-CD20 (GA-101) and anti-epidermal growth factor receptor (EGFR) (GA-201) glycoengineered antibodies are produced using N-acetylglucosaminetransferase III-transfected CHO cells [4]. In a phase I/II trial in patients with relapsed/refractory CD20-positive non-Hodgkin's lymphoma (NHL), GA-101 had a similar safety profile to rituximab and showed promising efficacy. GA-201 is being tested in a phase I clinical trial in heavily pretreated patients with metastatic solid tumors. Preliminary data showed that the drug was safe and had clinical activity [25]. MDX-1401, a defucosylated fully human antibody targeting human CD30, is currently in a phase I trial in relapsed/refractory CD30-positive Hodgkin's lymphoma patients [26, 27]. Evidence of activity in the form of stable disease and 40% or more tumor reduction was obtained in several of the patients treated. The results suggest that the defucosylated mAb is more active than the parent antibody tested earlier. The clinical potential of the anti-ganglioside GM2 humanized defucosylated antibody BIW-8962 is being tested in a phase I/II study in patients with multiple myeloma [28]. The preclinical activities of this engineered mAb were pronounced. A phase I/II study of KW-0761, a defucosylated humanized anti-CCR4 antibody, in relapsed patients with adult T-cell leukemia/lymphoma and peripheral T-cell lymphoma showed good tolerability and potential efficacy [29]. Interestingly, the drug appeared active at much lower doses than other therapeutic antibodies used to treat malignant lymphoma. In a phase I dose escalation study, a clinical response was observed in one of three patients at the lowest dose of 0.01 mg/kg, which is approximately 1/1000 of the rituximab dose [30, 31]. This finding might be a result of the markedly enhanced effector functions of KW-0761. Another clinical stage antibody includes defucosylated humanized anti-interleukin-5 receptor MEDI-563 [32]. The drug has proven safe and effective in a phase I trial of patients with mild asthma and is now progressing to a phase II study. As these trials proceed, the activities of ADCC-enhanced mAbs will become apparent, particularly in systems where the parental fucosylated mAbs have been subject to previous clinical evaluation.

10.2.2
Antibody–Drug Conjugates for Cancer Therapy

A powerful approach to conscript the specificities of mAbs for therapeutic activity is to append drugs to them that exert their effects when they are delivered to the target site. This is an area of research that began long before the advent of mAb technology, but only came to fruition in the past few years with insights generated from earlier studies with antibody–drug conjugates (ADCs) composed of conventional chemotherapeutics, unstable linkers, and mAbs that were unsuitable for prolonged use. In developing new generation ADCs with highly promising activities, attention has focused on all aspects of the technology, from choice of an appropriate target, generation of potent and stable ADCs that can be administered repeatedly, to methods for reproducibly generating the therapeutics in ways that preserve both the characteristics of the mAb carriers and the drug payloads.

10.2.2.1 Target Antigen Selection
The criteria for selection of an appropriate antigen for drug delivery are empirical. Under ideal circumstances, the antigen should be homogeneously expressed in high copy number on tumor cells, with no expression elsewhere. Once the ADC binds to the antigen, the complex should rapidly internalize, allowing drug release within the target cell to rapidly take place (Figure 10.3). While many of these criteria are met with ADCs in clinical development, most of them fall short in one aspect or another. For example, ADC approaches have been extended even to targets that are not present on the tumor cells, but on noninternalizing extracellular matrix proteins that surround tumor cells, such as the extradomain B of fibronectin and the long isoform of tenascin C [33, 34]. These proteins are present in the stroma surrounding proliferating tumor cells and tumor neovasculature, and provide a means for drug delivery in the tumor vicinity, rather than directly within the target cells of interest. Significant effects in preclinical models have been obtained with a variety of drugs attached to antibodies directed against these antigens. Another example includes ADCs directed against prostate-specific membrane antigen (PSMA), which may

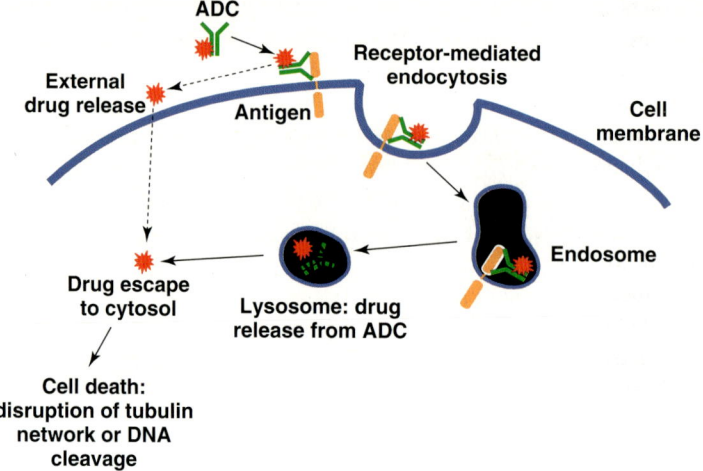

Figure 10.3 Mechanism of drug delivery for an ADC. An antibody (green) conjugated to a drug (red) binds to a target antigen (orange) on the surface of a cell. Upon internalization, the ADC traffics via endosomes to lysosomes, where the antibody is degraded and drug released. The drug must then traffic to the site where it exerts its cytotoxic effect, such as tubulin in the cytosol or DNA in the nucleus. For antigens that are noninternalizing and linkers that provide a mechanism for drug release outside the cell, the drug can in principle be released from the ADC extracellularly and then enter the cell.

exhibit activities on both the target tumor cells as well as on neovascular cells that are also PSMA-positive [35, 36].

ADC technologies are applicable to tumor models with a wide spectrum of antigen expression. Multiple ADC approaches have been utilized for the treatment of CD33-positive acute myelogenous leukemia (AML) [37, 38], a disease that typically expresses between 5000 and 10 000 receptors per cell. Successful treatment of tumors with such low antigen expression likely requires that the drug be highly potent, the tumor be easily accessed, and that there be a minimal degree of targeting to nontumor cells. The other extreme is exemplified by the HER2 antigen on metastatic breast cancer, which is greatly overexpressed in very high copy numbers on a subpopulation of patients with metastatic breast cancer [39]. Pronounced activities have been reported for an anti-HER2–DM1 conjugate at well-tolerated doses [40–42]. In a study designed to gain insight on the importance of tumor antigen expression, investigators measured the activity of an anti-EphB2–auristatin ADC on cell lines that had 71 000 or 308 000 EphB2 antigens per cell [43]. Although the difference in antigen expression was 4.3-fold, the difference in ADC potency in cell culture was approximately 100-fold. However, there was no difference in the *in vivo* activities of the ADC on subcutaneously implanted cell lines. Taken together, these results point to a multifactorial basis for ADC activity, in which parameters such as antigen density, binding affinity, internalization, subcellular localization, efficiency of drug release, and sensitivity of the target cells to released drug can impact activity [44–46].

All of the targets that have been used for ADCs are present on normal tissues to varying degrees. The ability to utilize such antigens for drug delivery depends on the extent of normal tissue expression and the sensitivity of normal cells to the targeted drug. A clinical trial of bivatuzumab mertansine (anti-CD44v6–DM1) was carried out in patients with incurable squamous cell carcinoma of the head and neck or esophagus, although the antigen was known to be present on normal skin keratinocytes [47]. At the highest dose used in the trial (140 mg/m^2) a patient died from epidermal necrolysis, a target-related toxicity, and the trial was discontinued due to a negative risk–benefit assessment. An additional example of an ADC hampered by normal tissue cross-reactivity was BR96–doxorubicin, which was targeted to the Lewis-Y antigen on carcinoma cells [48]. Patients with breast cancer treated with high doses of the ADC experienced gastrointestinal toxicities, consistent with Lewis-Y expression on normal gut epithelial cells [49]. In cases where significant normal tissue cross-reactivities are known, it has become a standard practice to utilize relevant preclinical models to understand how they may affect toxicity in the clinic [50].

It is noteworthy that two recent ADCs with very promising clinical activities have favorable expression profiles on tumor versus normal tissues. One such agent, brentuximab vedotin, recognizes the CD30 antigen on Hodgkin's and anaplastic large cell lymphomas, and is minimally expressed on normal cells [51, 52]. Another is trastuzumab–DM1, which is against the HER2/*neu* protooncogene that is highly overexpressed in subpopulations of patients with metastatic breast cancer [42]. As will be discussed, both ADCs exhibit pronounced clinical activities at tolerated doses.

The requirement for antigen internalization for ADC activity is an area that is currently receiving significant attention. The rate and extent of internalization can influence not only intratumoral uptake and distribution of antibody-based reagents [53], but may also impact the amount of drug released within the tumor and normal cells [54]. The fact that inefficiently internalized antigens such as CD20 have been targeted by ADCs with promising preclinical *in vivo* activities [55, 56] suggests that rapid internalization is not required. Further insight into the necessity of internalization was provided in a study of several cell surface receptors on NHL [57]. It was shown that poorly internalized antigens such as CD20, CD21, and CD72 were suitable for drug delivery, providing that the drug was attached through a readily cleavable linker [57]. Corresponding noncleavable linkers that required mAb degradation for drug release were much less effective. Thus, it is possible that extracellular drug release may play a role in ADC activity, particularly with ADCs that are poorly internalized. This mechanism would be consistent with the activities of ADCs against the stromal antigens mentioned earlier [33, 34].

10.2.2.2 Conjugation Technologies

Several methods are currently in use to reproducibly produce ADC, albeit with varying degrees of product heterogeneity (Figure 10.4). The original method to produce Mylotarg® (anti-CD33–calicheamicin, Figure 10.5) involved reacting the *N*-hydroxysuccinimide ester of a calicheamicin derivative directly with lysine

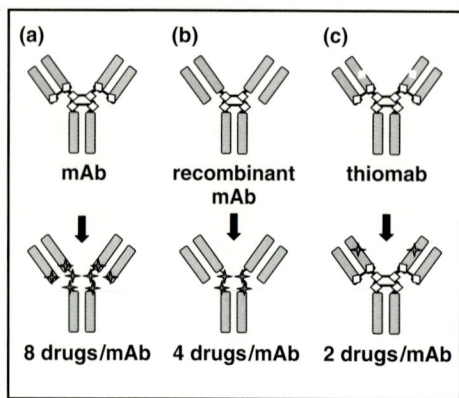
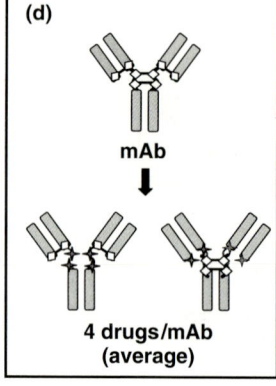
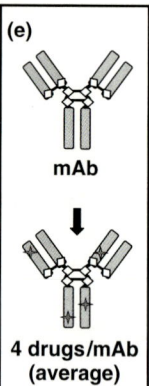

Figure 10.4 Drug conjugation strategies. ADCs can be homogenous products when (a) mAbs are fully reduced and eight drugs are added to the eight reduced interchain cysteines [48, 51, 61]. (b) Alternatively, a recombinant mAb with four interchain cysteines mutated to alanine yields an ADC with four drugs/mAb after full reduction and conjugation [62]. (c) Finally, additional unpaired cysteines can be genetically introduced into the mAb, requiring full reduction and reoxidation of the interchain disulfides, followed by drug conjugation to yield two drugs/mAb [63]. (d) ADC mixtures containing a small number of drug-loaded species can be formed by partial reduction of mAb disulfides followed by conjugation to yield an average of four drugs/mAb. There will be zero, two, four, six, and eight drugs on each mAb conjugated to the eight interchain cysteines [64]. (e) ADCs with the greatest structural complexity are formed by alkylating lysines with a drug-linker [37] or alkylating lysines with a maleimide-containing linker followed by conjugation to a thiol-containing drug yielding an average two to four drugs/mAb. These ADCs will be composed of zero to nine drugs on each mAb conjugated to the approximately 100 mAb lysines [65–67]. (Adapted from [62].)

residues distributed on an anti-CD33 antibody [58, 59]. The drawback of this particular approach was that on order to generate nonaggregated ADCs with two to three drug molecules attached per mAb, approximately 50% of the mAb component contained no drug at all. The process for making such ADCs has since been improved through the use of propylene glycol and octanoic acid in the conjugation process, which lowered aggregation levels and allowed for more uniform drug loading [60]. mAb–maytansine conjugates (Figure 10.5) are also generated through lysine acylation [45], but given the relative hydrophilicity of the drug component, issues with ADC aggregation have not apparently been an issue. In both of these examples, the ADCs contain drug to mAb molar ratios in the range of 2–4, presumably involving an array of lysine residues distributed throughout the antibody structure. The precise points of attachment have not been reported.

An alternative strategy for drug attachment involves the use of internal antibody disulfides. IgGs contain reducible disulfide bonds that covalently link the heavy and light chains together. It was found that all four interchain disulfide bonds in

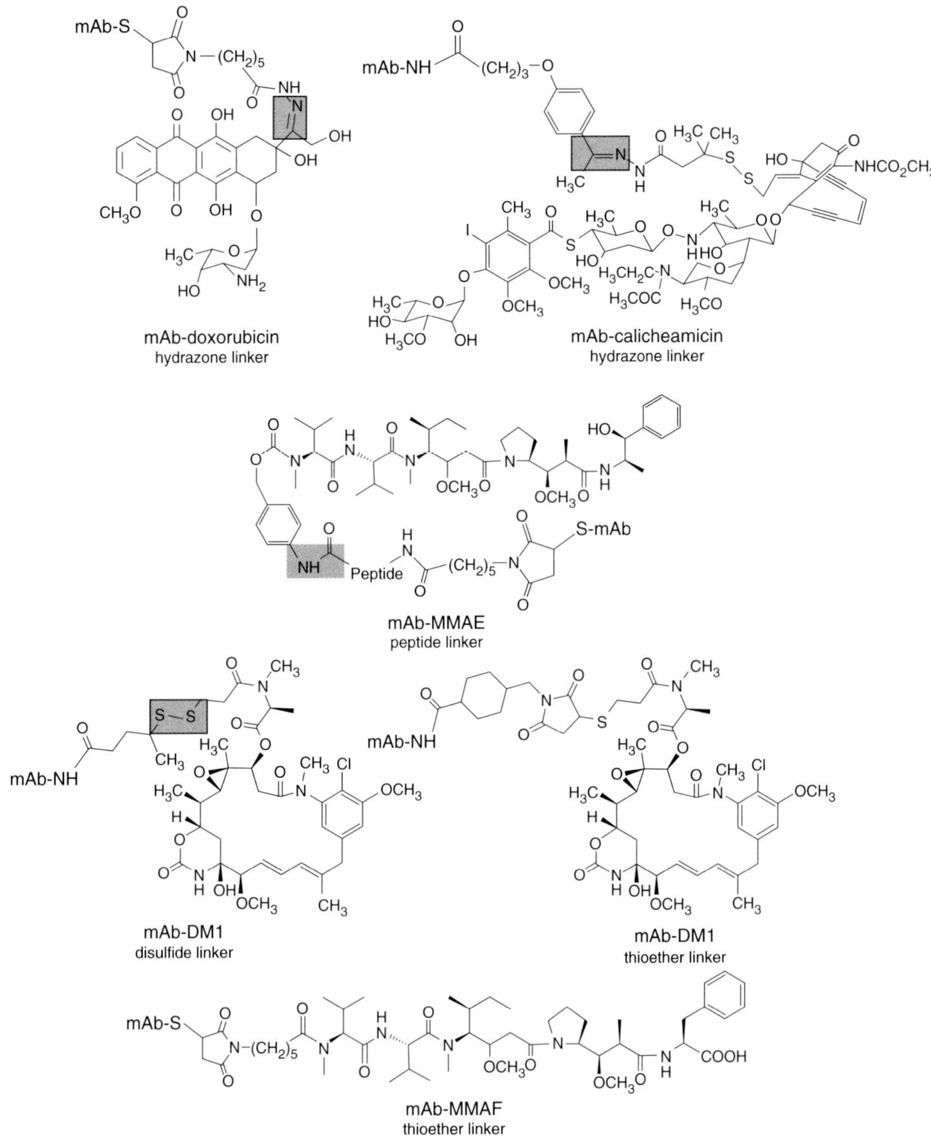

Figure 10.5 Structures of ADCs for cancer therapy. The drugs used to prepare the conjugates range from doxorubicin to highly potent agents like the auristatin analog MMAE and MMAF. Cleavable linkers (shaded) include hydrazones, disulfides, and peptides. Noncleavable linkers include thioethers, in which drug release is mediated by intracellular antibody degradation and the released drug contains the residue to which it was attached.

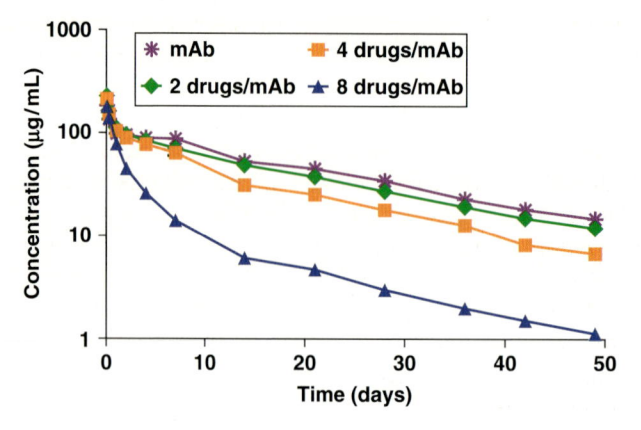

Figure 10.6 Pharmacokinetics of ADCs with different drug loads. Unconjugated cAC10 as well as purified cAC10–Val–Cit–MMAE with two, four, or eight drugs/mAb were injected into mice and the mAb concentration measured by enzyme-linked immunosorbent assay. (Adapted from [69].)

an IgG1 mAb could be reduced and modified with drug, leading to highly uniform ADCs with eight drugs/mAb [61]. The ADC remained intact in the absence of the disulfides, which is consistent with previous reports of fully active mAbs devoid of interchain disulfide bonds [68]. Since the drugs were distal to the antigen-binding sites, there was no impact on antigen binding. However, subsequent studies [69] demonstrated that such heavily loaded antibodies underwent accelerated clearance from the circulation (Figure 10.6). Reducing the drug load to two or four drugs/mAb circumvented this problem and led to ADCs with equal activities as those with eight drugs/mAb, but with significantly less toxicity. This was an early demonstration of the impact that drug loading could have on ADC pharmacokinetics and tolerability.

As with the lysine-based ADCs, partially loaded cysteine adducts are heterogeneous. Analytical studies on an ADC having an average of 4 drugs/mAb demonstrated that species with zero, two, four, six, and eight drugs/mAb were present, although the predominant species had four drugs/mAb [64]. The drugs were attached to both heavy–heavy and heavy–light chain disulfides. Thus, several species are present in ADCs derived from native mAb disulfides, although there are far fewer than those obtained through lysine modification.

In order to address the issue of ADC heterogeneity, significant attention has been directed toward the use of recombinant technologies for site-specific drug attachment (Figure 10.4). The first method reported was to mutate some of the cysteines involved in interchain disulfide formation, allowing all of the nonmutated disulfides to be modified with drug [62]. It was therefore possible to generate ADCs with two or four drugs/mAb, all of which were attached at predetermined sites. The engineered ADCs were compared to the nonrecombinant mixtures, and it was shown that the drug/mAb ratio played a more pronounced role in ADC activity, potency, and tolerability than the position of drug substitution. This work was followed up with an alternative strategy in which cysteine residues were introduced through site-specific mutagenesis and highly uniform ADCs were produced with approximately two drugs/mAb [63]. Consistent with the previous approach, the resulting conjugates were active and well-tolerated. There were indications that the ADC derived from a cysteine-mutated mAb exhibited less neutropenia than an ADC formed using the interchain disulfides, but the comparison was compromised since drug-loading levels differed by approximately 50%. The use of a cysteine-modified mAb construct was extended to thio-trastuzumab–DM1, which was active in preclinical models and displayed a favorable tolerability profile in rats and monkeys [41]. A comparison with similarly substituted ADCs derived from interchain cysteine modification was not made.

To summarize, several methods are available for the production of ADCs. The advantage of using nonrecombinant approaches is that they can be applied to almost any mAb without having to generate a novel construct together with a new production cell line. Since the resulting product is comprised of a mixture of species, the process for generating ADCs in this manner needs to be robust and highly reproducible. Recombinant methods may eventually assume a greater role in the production of ADCs, since high yields of nearly homogeneous products can be generated, and site-specific placement of the drug may impact research that could lead to further improvements in ADC technology.

10.2.2.3 Drug and Linker Selection

Much of the early work in antibody-mediated drug delivery relied on cytotoxic agents that were clinically approved such as doxorubicin, methotrexate, mitomycin, 5-fluorouracil, and vinca alkaloids, since they were readily available, and much was known about their chemical and stability characteristics [70]. The drugs had relatively low potency, requiring generally more than 10^6 drug molecules/cell to achieve cell kill [46, 71]. This proved to be a major limitation, since many tumor antigens are expressed at levels that would not allow such high concentrations of drugs to accumulate within target cells of interest. BR96–doxorubicin (Figure 10.5) is an example of an early-generation ADC that was studied extensively in clinical trials. The antibody is directed against the Lewis-Y tetrasaccharide antigen on human carcinomas and, as previously indicated, is also found in normal tissues including epithelial cells in the gastrointestinal tract [48, 49]. Doxorubicin was attached through an acid-labile hydrazone linker, which was designed to release the drug once the ADC internalized into acidic endosomal and lysosomal vesicles. The ADC was highly uniform in composition, since all four of the interchain disulfides were modified with drug, leading to an ADC with eight drug molecules/mAb [72].

Treatment of tumor-bearing mice and rats with BR96–doxorubicin led to immunologically specific tumor cures. However, the doses required for efficacy were in the range of 500 mg/kg, reflecting the low potency of the doxorubicin component. In a phase I clinical trial, the maximum tolerated dose (MTD) of BR96–doxorubicin was approximately 700 mg/m^2 (approximately 17 mg/kg), with gastrointestinal dose-limiting toxicities [73]. A subsequent phase II trial associated

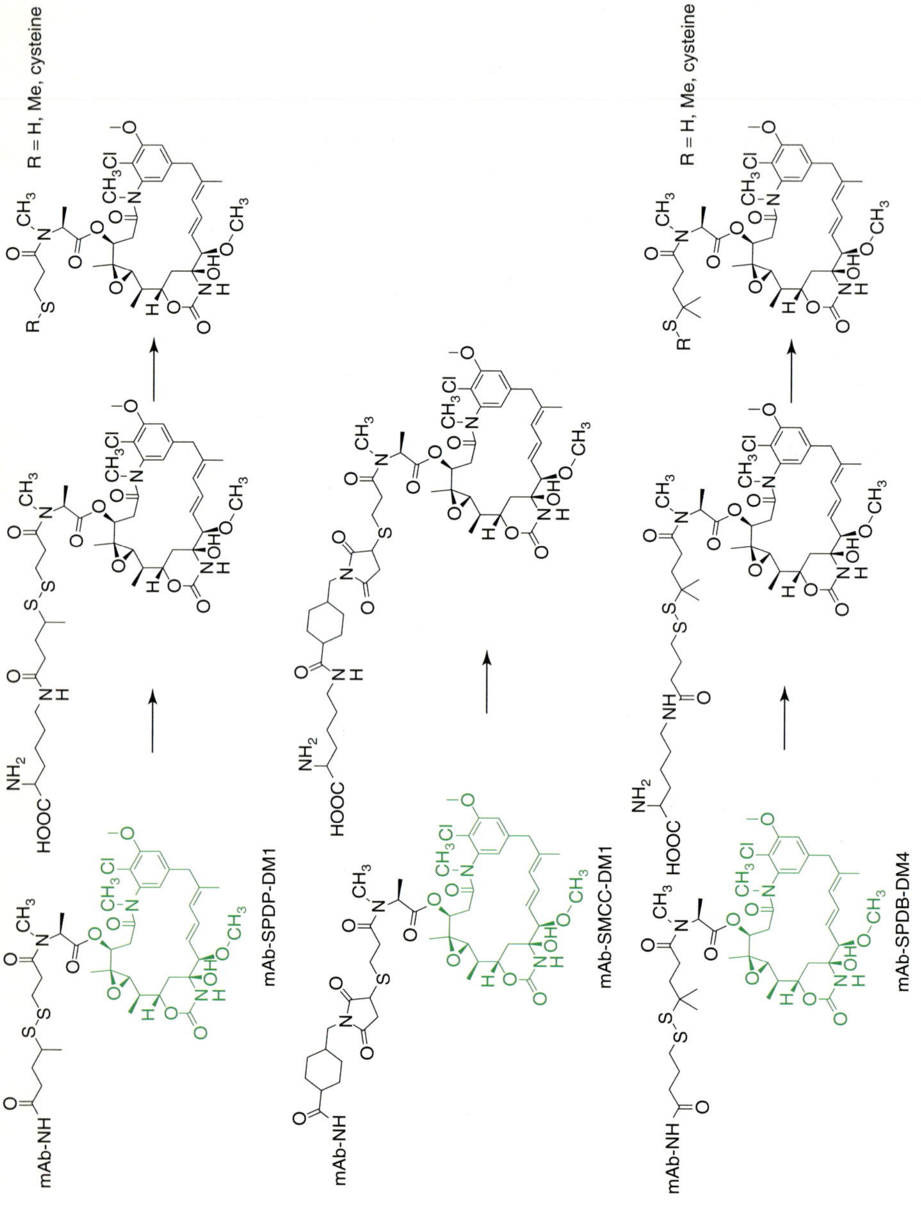
mAb-SPDP-DM1
mAb-SMCC-DM1
mAb-SPDB-DM4
R = H, Me, cysteine
R = H, Me, cysteine

toxicity with normal gut expression of Lewis-Y [49]. The lack of promising activities of BR96–doxorubicin were likely due to the low potency of the drug component, the unstable linker used (half-life to drug release was 43 h), and the presence of target antigen on highly sensitive nontumor tissues. The results with low potency ADCs such as BR96–doxorubicin prompted significant efforts toward utilizing drugs that were too toxic to use in an untargeted manner.

Until recently, the most advanced ADC was Mylotarg (Figure 10.5), consisting of a highly potent derivative of the natural product calicheamicin attached to an anti-CD33 antibody through an acid-labile hydrazone linker [74, 75]. As with BR96–doxorubicin, the half-life for drug release from the ADC was in the range of 48–72 h, reflecting the inherent instability of hydrazones at neutral pH [76]. Due to the highly potent nature of the drug component, pronounced antitumor activities were obtained at doses as low as approximately 2 mg (mAb component)/kg [58, 59, 77–79]. *In vitro* assays indicate that ADCs of calicheamicin may be as much as 1000-fold more potent than doxorubicin conjugates, which is consistent with their relative *in vivo* potencies [48, 77, 80]. Other promising ADCs using calicheamicin are directed against the CD22 [81–83] and 5T4 [78] antigens, recognizing B-cell lymphomas and epithelial tumors, respectively. Interestingly, it has been reported that Mylotarg was active in $CD33^-$ *in vivo* tumor models [84]. The effects appeared to be due to non-antigen-mediated ADC uptake and were dependent on the acid-labile hydrazone linker. It is therefore possible that some of the activity of Mylotarg may be due to non-antigen-mediated uptake of the ADC or to free drug that falls off the antibody. It is noteworthy that Mylotarg has shown activity in some patients with malignancies that appear to be $CD33^-$ [84, 85]. In summary, while Mylotarg has been shown to have clinical activity, it contains an unstable hydrazone linker, significant amounts of unconjugated mAb, and considerable heterogeneity.

Another drug class that has been the subject of considerable research and clinical development is the maytansinoids. As with calicheamicin, the drugs are derived from a mixture of natural products. The linker technologies for the maytansinoids utilize either disulfides or thioethers (Figure 10.5). The rationale for using disulfide linkers is that the concentration of thiols such as glutathione and cysteine are much higher in tumor cells than in the blood. However, disulfides tend to be unstable and the original mAb–DM1 conjugates had a half-life for drug release of approximately 24–48 h *in vivo* [45, 86, 87]. For that reason, a series of maytansinoid disulfide linker derivatives with varying degrees of steric hindrance were developed, from which DM4 was selected as a lead agent for antibody conjugation [88]. The hindered disulfide ADC was considerably more stable than the unhindered disulfide, with a

Figure 10.7 Catabolism of maytansine ADCs. DM1-SPDP (N-succinimidyl 3-(2-pyridyldithio)propionate) and DM4-SPDB (N-succinimidyl 4-(2-pyridyldithio)butyrate) disulfide ADCs are first degraded to lysine-linked disulfides, which are then reduced to thiols and may be subsequently S-methylated or cysteineylated. DM1-SMCC (N-succinimidyl 4-(N-maleimidomethyl)cyclohexane-1-carboxylate) thioether ADCs are degraded to lysine-linked DM1. Maytansinol, the parent drug, is shown in blue. (Adapted from [95].)

half-life for drug release of 102 h [45]. The anti-CanAg ADC huC242–DM4 showed improved efficacy over huC242–DM1 in xenograft models, reflecting advantages in a more stable linker technology [45, 89]. Similar results were obtained with an anti-integrin–DM4 ADC [90], and the technology has been applied to an array of antigen targets [44–46].

The necessity of having a cleavable bond within the linker to facilitate maytansinoid drug release was called into question based on data obtained with thioether-linked maytansinoid ADCs (Figure 10.5). While examples of thioether-linked maytansinoids were inactive or significantly less active *in vitro* and *in vivo* than the corresponding disulfide conjugates [65, 89], active thioether-linked maytansinoid conjugates have been reported [40, 91]. The mechanism for drug release involves antibody degradation, leading to a new form of the drug that contains the appended linker and the antibody lysine residue to which it was attached (Figure 10.7) [89, 92]. One of the potential limitations of releasing drugs in this manner is that bystander activity on antigen-negative tumor cells or sections within a tumor that do not bind sufficient amounts of the ADC is minimal [92]. The most advanced maytansinoid ADC, trastuzumab–DM1 [40], contains the thioether linkage. Several maytansinoid ADCs have shown promising preclinical activities [35, 45, 93, 94].

High stability of the drug-linker in circulation is important not only to protect nontarget tissues from chemotherapeutic damage, but also because it helps maximize total tumor exposure to the targeted drug. Protease-cleavable linkers may be advantageous compared to those that are acid or reductively labile, since hydrolysis is enzymatic and controllable through the selection of linker peptides that are cleaved by intracellular or tumor-associated enzymes. One enzyme that has been extensively studied for drug release is cathepsin B, which is present both within the lysosomes of tumor cells and also in the stroma of solid tumors [96–98]. To utilize this enzyme for drug release, drugs such as doxorubicin [99], mitomycin C [96], camptothecin [100], talisomycin [101], and auristatin family members were linked to mAbs through dipeptide sequences that were stable in circulation, but highly susceptible to cathepsin-mediated cleavage [51, 61, 102]. Rather than attaching the linkers directly to the drug, a spacer was used that allowed drug release to take place without any chemical modification.

The most extensively studied drug class to which the peptide linker technology has been applied is the auristatins, which are comprised of totally synthetic pentapeptides that kill cells through the inhibition of tubulin polymerization [44, 46]. Initially, an auristatin derivative, monomethyl auristatin E (MMAE), was modified with various dipeptide linkers and the resulting drug derivatives were linked to mAb cysteines, generating ADCs with eight drugs/mAb (Figure 10.5) [51, 61, 102]. The antibodies used were directed against the CD30 antigen on Hodgkin's lymphoma and the Lewis-Y antigen on carcinomas. *In vitro* studies demonstrated that peptide-linked ADCs were highly potent with 10- to 100-fold greater immunologically dependent cell-killing activity compared to corresponding conjugates of mAb–auristatin conjugates containing an acid-labile hydrazone linker [61]. The *in vivo* half-lives of drug release from the peptide-based ADCs were

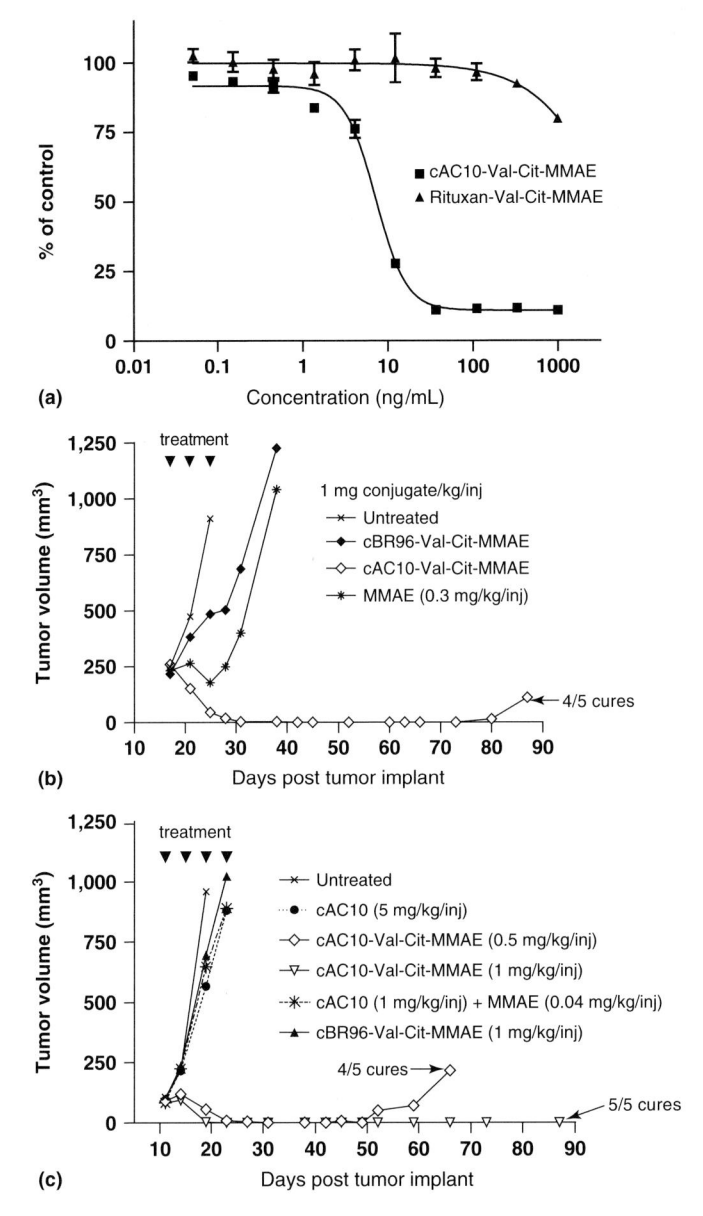

Figure 10.8 In vitro and in vivo activity of auristatin ADCs. (a) In vitro ADC cytotoxicity was evaluated by treating CD30+ Karpas 299 cells with CD30-binding cAC10–Val–Cit–MMAE and control nonbinding Rituxan–Val–Cit–MMAE for 96 h. (b) In vivo ADC activity was evaluated by treating CD30+ Karpas 299 xenografts in SCID mice with CD30-binding cAC10–Val–Cit–MMAE and nonbinding cBR96–Val-Cit-MMAE. (c) In vivo ADC activity was evaluated by treating CD30+ Karpas 299 xenografts in SCID mice with CD30-binding cAC10–Val–Cit–MMAE and a molar equivalent mixture of cAC10 and unconjugated MMAE. (Adapted from [51, 61].)

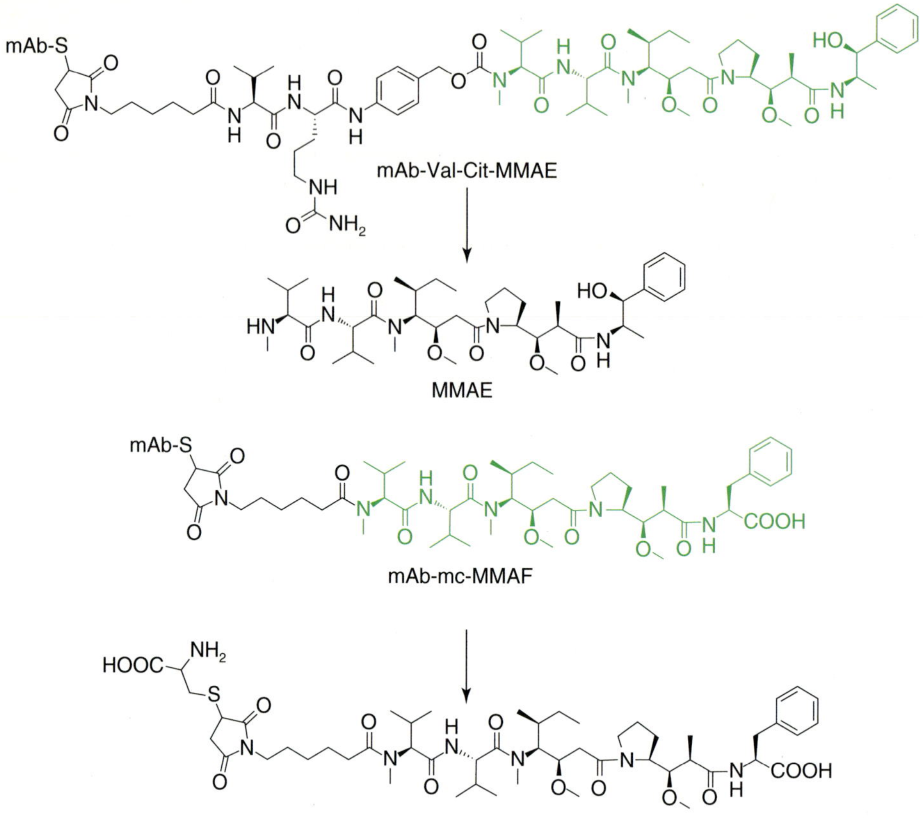

Figure 10.9 Catabolism of auristatin ADCs. Val–Cit–MMAE and mc-MMAF ADCs are degraded to MMAE and Cys-mc-MMAF, respectively. The parent drugs MMAE and MMAF are shown in blue. (Adapted from [95].)

6 and 10 days in mice and cynomolgus monkeys, respectively [103], which was a great deal longer than previously described linker technologies. The more stable peptide-linked MMAE ADCs were less toxic than corresponding hydrazone-linked ADCs, most likely owing to this enhanced stability. The peptide that was selected for further studies was comprised of valine–citrulline (Val–Cit), since it was shown to be stable in plasma, but rapidly cleaved within target cells.

mAb–Val–Cit–MMAE ADCs were highly active *in vivo* at doses that were as low as 1/200 the MTD (Figure 10.8) [51, 61]. The unprecedented therapeutic was most likely due to a combination of effective ADC delivery, stability of the linker in the circulation, and efficient intratumoral release of a highly potent drug. The technology has since been extended to several antigens, including CD30 [51, 61], Lewis-Y [51, 61], BCMA [104], CD19 [57, 105], CD20 [56], CD70 [106], CD79b [57], CD22 [57], E selectin [107], EphB2 [43], glycoprotein NMB [108], melanotransferrin/p97 [109], MUC16 [110], PSMA [36], and TMEFF2 [111].

Further advancements in the auristatin technology involved the generation of noncleavable thioether linkers for drug attachment (Figure 10.5). Upon intracellular degradation of the antibody, the released drug was comprised of the cysteine-adduct of the linker-monomethyl auristatin F (MMAF) derivative, a degradation reaction that took place rapidly upon ADC internalization (Figure 10.9) [102]. ADCs with a thioether or a peptide linkage had similar half-lives of 7 days for drug release *in vivo* [103, 112]. It was possible to increase the stability by simply substituting a haloacetamide for the maleimide in the drug-linker complex used to make an ADC [112]. The resulting acetamide adducts did not lose any detectable drug over 2 weeks when injected into mice. However, the tolerability, efficacy, and intratumoral drug concentrations resulting from ADCs that were indefinitely stable *in vivo* were no different from the corresponding maleimido-thioether adducts. This suggested that extending ADC stability half-life significantly beyond the ADC clearance half-life minimally impacts biological activity.

10.3
Clinical Developments

As indicated earlier, a large number of clinical trials have been undertaken with ADCs starting with mouse antibodies and low-potency clinically approved drugs. As technology developed, the ADCs that have emerged as being clinically promising are now comprised of chimeric and humanized antibodies with highly potent drugs and advanced linker technologies. The most advanced ADCs are shown in Table 10.2.

10.3.1
Gemtuzumab Ozogamicin (Mylotarg) and Other Calicheamicin-Based ADCs

Up until just recently, Mylotarg was the only clinically approved ADC, receiving an accelerated approval in the United States in 2000 for AML patients over 60 years in first relapse who are not candidates for chemotherapy [37]. The accelerated approval was based on the results of three open-label, single-arm phase II trials with 277 patients [127, 131, 132]. Since then, blinded randomized trials have failed to demonstrate clinical benefit. In a phase III trial in AML patients older than 60 years who achieved a complete response after their first round of induction chemotherapy, 232 patients were randomized to receive three cycles of 6 mg/m^2 of Mylotarg or no additional therapy. There was no significant difference in overall survival, disease-free survival, relapse probability, or nonrelapse mortality [133]. Preliminary analysis of a phase III trial in AML patients who were mostly younger than 60 years and receiving their first round of induction chemotherapy, 1115 patients were randomized to three treatment arms with and without 3 mg/m^2 Mylotarg. There was no difference in the overall remission rates and treatment deaths with and without Mylotarg, but there was a statistically significant improvement in relapse rate and disease-free survival after 3 years for

Table 10.2 ADCs in the clinic.

Agent	Clinical status	Target	Indication	Drug class	Leading references
Brentuximab vedotin (SGN-35)	phase III	CD30	Hodgkin's lymphoma, anaplastic large cell lymphoma	auristatin	[113–115]
CDX-011 (CRO11–Val–Cit–MMAE)	phase II	GPNMB (novel glycoprotein)	melanoma, breast cancer	auristatin	[108, 116–118]
SGN-75	phase I	CD70	NHL, RCC	auristatin	[119]
PSMA ADC	phase I	PSMA	prostate cancer	auristatin	[36]
MEDI-547	phase I	EphA2	solid tumors	auristatin	[120]
MN immunoconjugate	phase I	MN	cancer	auristatin	[121]
Trastuzumab–DM1	phase III	HER2/*neu*	breast cancer	maytansinoid	[42, 122]
AVE9633	phase I	CD33	AML	maytansinoid	[123]
HuN901–DM1	phase I and II	CD56	small cell lung cancer, multiple myeloma	maytansinoid	[94, 124, 125]
HuC242–DM4	phase I	CanAg	colorectal cancer	maytansinoid	[126]
Gemtuzumab ozogamicin	withdrawn	CD33	AML	calicheamicin	[37, 127]
Inotuzumab ozogamicin	phase III	CD22	NHL	calicheamicin	[82, 128, 129]
MEDX-1203	phase I	CD70	NHL, RCC	duocarmycin	[130]

Data from the listed references, http://www.clinicaltrials.gov, and sponsor web sites.

those patients receiving Mylotarg [134]. A final phase III trial in 627 previously untreated AML patients under 60 evaluated the addition of 6 mg/m^2 Mylotarg to standard induction chemotherapy [135]. Patients with a complete response following induction therapy and additional consolidation therapy were further randomized to receive three doses of 5 mg/m^2 of Mylotarg or no additional therapy [13]. Preliminary results show that there was no significant difference in complete response rates or relapse-free survival following a complete response between standard induction chemotherapy with and without Mylotarg nor was there a significant difference in disease-free survival for postconsolidation Mylotarg versus no treatment. There was a statistically significant increase in adverse events for the Mylotarg plus chemotherapy arm. The lack of improvement in disease treatment with Mylotarg coupled with safety concerns prompted the drug safety monitoring committee to recommend early closure of the entire trial. In June 2010, Pfizer announced the voluntary withdrawal of Mylotarg from the US market due to concerns about drug safety and the failure to demonstrate clinical benefit to patients (http://www.fda.gov/NewsEvents/Newsroom/PressAnnouncements/ucm216448.htm).

Inotuzumab ozogamicin is comprised of the same calicheamicin drug-linker derivative as Mylotarg, but recognizes the CD22 antigen on NHL. It is currently in a phase III trial in combination with rituximab. In a phase I/II dose escalation trial, the MTD was found to be $1.8\,mg/m^2$ when dosed every 4 weeks and an expansion cohort was enrolled at this dose. In this expansion cohort, the objective response rate was 88% (14/16) for follicular lymphoma and 71% (10/14) for diffuse large B-cell lymphoma (10/14) [128].

10.3.2
Brentuximab Vedotin and Other Auristatin-Based ADCs

Brentuximab vedotin (SGN-35) is comprised of the chimeric anti-CD30 mAb cAC10 with an average of four MMAE molecules/mAb conjugated through a dipeptide linker. CD30 is a member of the tumor necrosis factor receptor family and is expressed quite sparingly in normal tissues, with some expression in activated, but not resting, T- and B-cells. The ADC is currently in several clinical trials for the treatment of Hodgkin's lymphoma and anaplastic large cell lymphoma. The pivotal trial for relapsed or refractory Hodgkin's lymphoma following an autologous stem cell transplant utilized a dose of 1.8 mg/kg every 3 weeks. This dose was based on data from a phase I trial that included both Hodgkin's lymphoma and systemic anaplastic large cell lymphoma (sALCL) patients, where those treated with 1.2 mg/kg of SGN-35 or higher provided an objective response rate of 54% (15/28), with nine complete responses. Nearly all (93%) of the patients experienced tumor regression during the course of therapy [136]. In contrast, the unconjugated anti-CD30 mAb provided no clinical responses in Hodgkin's lymphoma at doses as high as 12 mg/kg given weekly. These results demonstrate that ADCs can greatly enhance the activities of the mAbs from which they were derived. In a second phase I trial with weekly dosing, patients receiving 0.4–1.4 mg/kg had an objective response rate of 56% (22/39). Among the five sALCL patients treated in the phase I clinical trials, four had complete responses [113]. This conjugate has provided among the most pronounced activities of any ADC yet tested, underscoring the technological advancements that have been made in target selection, drug and linker design, and conjugation methodology.

Another auristatin-based conjugate in an early stage clinical trial includes CDX-011 (CRO11–Val–Cit–MMAE), an antiglycoprotein NMB mAb conjugated to Val–Cit–MMAE. The drug is being evaluated in patients with melanoma and breast cancer in phase I/II studies. For both indications, 1.88 mg/kg dosed every 3 weeks was found to be the MTD. In 37 melanoma patients at all dose levels there were two partial responses [116], while in 32 breast cancer patients treated at 1.88 mg/kg there were four partial responses [117]. SGN-75, an anti-CD70 mAb directly conjugated to the drug-linker mc (maleimidocaproyl)-MMAF, is being tested in both NHL and renal cell carcinoma (RCC), where CD70 expression has been demonstrated [119]. Other auristatin ADCs in the clinic target PSMA [36], EphA2 [120], and MN (carbonic anhydrase IX) [121].

10.3.3
Trastuzumab–DM1 and Other Maytansinoid-Based ADCs

The most advanced maytansinoid ADC is trastuzumab–DM1, which consists of the anti-HER2 mAb trastuzumab (Herceptin) with DM1 linked to lysine residues through a noncleavable linker technology. This ADC was designed to release the drug upon lysosomal antibody degradation inside target cells, and the released drug consists of DM1 with a linker and lysine attached to it. A phase I clinical trial was carried out in patients with HER2-positive metastatic breast cancer with escalating doses of trastuzumab–DM1 starting at 0.3 mg/kg and going up to 4.8 mg/kg every 3 weeks [137, 138]. Partial responses were obtained in 25% of the patients, with dose-limiting toxicities of thrombocytopenia. In a subsequent phase II trial in third-line metastatic breast cancer with 3.6 mg/kg, trastuzumab–DM1 dosed every 3 weeks, a 33% objective response rate in 110 patients was observed demonstrating single-agent activity in a population heavily pretreated with agents including trastuzumab [122]. A phase III trial investigating trastuzumab–DM1 versus capecitabine and lapatinib in second-line metastatic breast cancer and a phase II trial investigating trastuzumab–DM1 versus trastuzumab and docetaxel in front-line therapy are currently ongoing.

Several other maytansine ADCs are currently being clinically evaluated. Phase I dose escalation and MTD expansion cohort data have recently been reported, including the anti-CD56 IMGN901 (a disulfide-linked DM1 ADC for multiple myeloma and solid tumors), the anti-CD19 SAR3419 (a disulfide-linked DM4 ADC for NHL), and the anti-CD138 BT-062 (a disulfide-linked DM4 ADC for multiple myeloma). Treatment with IMGN901 provided one partial response in the first 26 multiple myeloma patients [124] and five objective responses in 113 patients with a variety of solid tumors [139]. Objective responses from SAR3419 treatment were obtained in five of 27 patients [140], while two of 25 patients treated with BT-062 had objective responses [141].

10.4
Alternative Scaffolds

There are a large number of recombinant scaffolds that have been developed as antibody alternatives [142–144]. Examples include designed ankyrin repeat proteins (DARPins, MW 14.5 kDa, $t_{1/2}$ in mice less than 3 min [145]), anticalins (MW ~20 kDa, $t_{1/2}$ less than 60 min [146, 147], aptamers (MW 5–15 kDa, $t_{1/2}$ in mice 5–10 min [148]), affibodies (MW 7 kDa, $t_{1/2}$ in mice 15 min [149]), Kunitz domain protein (7 kDa, $t_{1/2}$ in mice 27 min [150]), and many others. While these molecules are of interest, they are rapidly cleared from the body and provide exposure times that are probably too short to have effective therapeutic efficacy. Mathematical modeling in support of this assumption has shown that fast clearing molecules with molecular weights in the range of 25 kDa should be very poor at accumulating within solid tumors, in contrast to mAbs that compensate for poor penetration rates by having circulation half-lives in excess of 1 week [151]. To address this issue, many of the scaffolds have been modified with polyethylene glycol to generate molecules that circulate for longer time periods. An example of this is a 14.5-kDa DARPin, whose $t_{1/2\beta}$ was increased to approximately 50 h through conjugation to 40- or 60-kDa poly(ethylene glycol) [152]. The resulting conjugate displayed superior intratumoral uptake compared to the unmodified DARPin, confirming that increased exposure correlates with increased intratumoral uptake. Further work is needed to determine if these pharmacokinetic-extended scaffolds present advantages over IgGs for therapeutic drug delivery.

10.5
Conclusions and Perspectives

In the past few years, the progress made in antibody therapeutics has been considerable. Detailed information about how IgGs interact with Fc receptors has led to the generation of several new mAbs with greatly increased effector function potencies. Clinical studies with these ADCC-enhanced mAbs are currently underway and there are positive indications of activity. One of the challenges in this field will be to demonstrate that these engineered mAbs outperform their native counterparts and can be used safely over extended time periods.

The advancements that have recently been made with ADCs are encouraging. Based on an understanding of how the antigen target, drug potency, linker stability, drug stoichiometry, and conjugation technology influence ADC activity, many new conjugates have been developed and are moving through clinical development. Brentuximab vedotin and trastuzumab–DM1 are leading the way, based on the pronounced clinical activities in settings where the patients are resistant to conventional chemotherapy. Future advancements in the field are likely to stem from novel recombinant carriers for drug delivery, combined with innovations in drug and linker design. Given the progress over the past few years, it is likely that ADCs will assume a significant role in the clinical treatment of cancer.

References

1. Carter, P.J. (2006) Potent antibody therapeutics by design. *Nat. Rev. Immunol.*, **6**, 343–357.
2. Reichert, J.M. and Valge-Archer, V.E. (2007) Development trends for monoclonal antibody cancer therapeutics. *Nat. Rev. Drug Discov.*, **6**, 349–356.
3. Shields, R.L., Namenuk, A.K., Hong, K., Meng, Y.G., Rae, J., Briggs, J., Xie, D., Lai, J., Stadlen, A., Li, B., Fox, J.A., and Presta, L.G. (2001) High resolution mapping of the binding site on human IgG1 for FcγRI, FcγRII, FcγRIII, and FcRn and design of IgG1 variants with

improved binding to the FcγR. *J. Biol. Chem.*, **276**, 6591–6604.

4. Umana, P., Jean-Mairet, J., Moudry, R., Amstutz, H., and Bailey, J.E. (1999) Engineered glycoforms of an antineuroblastoma IgG1 with optimized antibody-dependent cellular cytotoxic activity. *Nat. Biotechnol.*, **17**, 176–180.

5. Wu, A.M. and Senter, P.D. (2005) Arming antibodies: prospects and challenges for immunoconjugates. *Nat. Biotechnol.*, **23**, 1137–1146.

6. Carter, P. (2001) Improving the efficacy of antibody-based cancer therapies. *Nat. Rev. Cancer*, **1**, 118–129.

7. Cartron, G., Dacheux, L., Salles, G., Solal-Celigny, P., Bardos, P., Colombat, P., and Watier, H. (2002) Therapeutic activity of humanized anti-CD20 monoclonal antibody and polymorphism in IgG Fc receptor FcgammaRIIIa gene. *Blood*, **99**, 754–758.

8. Clynes, R.A., Towers, T.L., Presta, L.G., and Ravetch, J.V. (2000) Inhibitory Fc receptors modulate *in vivo* cytotoxicity against tumor targets. *Nat. Med.*, **6**, 443–446.

9. Lazar, G.A., Dang, W., Karki, S., Vafa, O., Peng, J.S., Hyun, L., Chan, C., Chung, H.S., Eivazi, A., Yoder, S.C., Vielmetter, J., Carmichael, D.F., Hayes, R.J., and Dahiyat, B.I. (2006) Engineered antibody Fc variants with enhanced effector function. *Proc. Natl. Acad. Sci. USA*, **103**, 4005–4010.

10. Arnold, J.N., Wormald, M.R., Sim, R.B., Rudd, P.M., and Dwek, R.A. (2007) The impact of glycosylation on the biological function and structure of human immunoglobulins. *Annu. Rev. Immunol.*, **25**, 21–50.

11. Radaev, S., Motyka, S., Fridman, W.H., Sautes-Fridman, C., and Sun, P.D. (2001) The structure of a human type III Fc gamma receptor in complex with Fc. *J. Biol. Chem.*, **276**, 16469–16477.

12. Sondermann, P., Huber, R., Oosthuizen, V., and Jacob, U. (2000) The 3.2-Å crystal structure of the human IgG1 Fc fragment–FcγRIII complex. *Nature*, **406**, 267–273.

13. Radaev, S. and Sun, P. (2002) Recognition of immunoglobulins by Fcgamma receptors. *Mol. Immunol.*, **38**, 1073–1083.

14. Shinkawa, T., Nakamura, K., Yamane, N., Shoji-Hosaka, E., Kanda, Y., Sakurada, M., Uchida, K., Anazawa, H., Satoh, M., Yamasaki, M., Hanai, N., and Shitara, K. (2003) The absence of fucose but not the presence of galactose or bisecting N-acetylglucosamine of human IgG1 complex-type oligosaccharides shows the critical role of enhancing antibody-dependent cellular cytotoxicity. *J. Biol. Chem.*, **278**, 3466–3473.

15. Lifely, M.R., Hale, C., Boyce, S., Keen, M.J., and Phillips, J. (1995) Glycosylation and biological activity of CAMPATH-1H expressed in different cell lines and grown under different culture conditions. *Glycobiology*, **5**, 813–822.

16. Mossner, E., Brunker, P., Moser, S., Puntener, U., Schmidt, C., Herter, S., Grau, R., Gerdes, C., Nopora, A., van Puijenbroek, E., Ferrara, C., Sondermann, P., Jager, C., Strein, P., Fertig, G., Friess, T., Schull, C., Bauer, S., Dal Porto, J., Del Nagro, C., Dabbagh, K., Dyer, M.J., Poppema, S., Klein, C., and Umana, P. (2010) Increasing the efficacy of CD20 antibody therapy through the engineering of a new type II anti-CD20 antibody with enhanced direct and immune effector cell-mediated B-cell cytotoxicity. *Blood*, **115**, 4393–4402.

17. Shields, R.L., Lai, J., Keck, R., O'Connell, L.Y., Hong, K., Meng, Y.G., Weikert, S.H.A., and Presta, L.G. (2002) Lack of fucose on human IgG1 N-linked oligosaccharide improves binding to human Fc gamma RIII and antibody-dependent cellular toxicity. *J. Biol. Chem.*, **277**, 26733–26740.

18. Yamane-Ohnuki, N., Kinoshita, S., Inoue-Urakubo, M., Kusunoki, M., Iida, S., Nakano, R., Wakitani, M., Niwa, R., Sakurada, M., Uchida, K., Shitara, K., and Satoh, M. (2004) Establishment of FUT8 knockout Chinese hamster ovary cells: an ideal host cell line for producing completely defucosylated antibodies with enhanced

antibody-dependent cellular cytotoxicity. *Biotechnol. Bioeng.*, **87**, 614–622.
19. Niwa, R., Shoji-Hosaka, E., Sakurada, M., Shinkawa, T., Uchida, K., Nakamura, K., Matsushima, K., Ueda, R., Hanai, N., and Shitara, K. (2004) Defucosylated chimeric anti-CC chemokine receptor 4 IgG1 with enhanced antibody-dependent cellular cytotoxicity shows potent therapeutic activity to T-cell leukemia and lymphoma. *Cancer Res.*, **64**, 2127–2133.
20. Iida, S., Misaka, H., Inoue, M., Shibata, M., Nakano, R., Yamane-Ohnuki, N., Wakitani, M., Yano, K., Shitara, K., and Satoh, M. (2006) Nonfucosylated therapeutic IgG1 antibody can evade the inhibitory effect of serum immunoglobulin G on antibody-dependent cellular cytotoxicity through its high binding to FcgammaRIIIa. *Clin. Cancer Res.*, **12**, 2879–2887.
21. Niwa, R., Sakurada, M., Kobayashi, Y., Uehara, A., Matsushima, K., Ueda, R., Nakamura, K., and Shitara, K. (2005) Enhanced natural killer cell binding and activation by low-fucose IgG1 antibody results in potent antibody-dependent cellular cytotoxicity induction at lower antigen density. *Clin. Cancer Res.*, **11**, 2327–2336.
22. Junttila, T.T., Parsons, K., Olsson, C., Lu, Y., Xin, Y., Theriault, J., Crocker, L., Pabonan, O., Baginski, T., Meng, G., Totpal, K., Kelley, R.F., and Sliwkowski, M.X. (2010) Superior *in vivo* efficacy of afucosylated trastuzumab in the treatment of HER2-amplified breast cancer. *Cancer Res.*, **70**, 4481–4489.
23. Griggs, J. and Zinkewich-Peotti, K. (2009) The state of the art: immune-mediated mechanisms of monoclonal antibodies in cancer therapy. *Br. J. Cancer*, **101**, 1807–1812.
24. Kubota, T., Niwa, R., Satoh, M., Akinaga, S., Shitara, K., and Hanai, N. (2009) Engineered therapeutic antibodies with improved effector functions. *Cancer Sci.*, **100**, 1566–1572.
25. Markman, B., Gomez-Roca, C., Cervantes-Ruiperez, A., Delord, J., Paz Ares, L., Soria, J., Corral, J., Hollingsworth, S., Manenti, L., and Tabernero, J. (2010) Phase I PK/PD study of RO5083945 (GA201), the first glycoengineered anti-EGFR monoclonal antibody (mAb) with optimized antibody dependent cellular cytotoxicity (ADCC). *J. Clin. Oncol.*, **28**, 2522.
26. Cardarelli, P.M., Moldovan-Loomis, M.C., Preston, B., Black, A., Passmore, D., Chen, T.H., Chen, S., Liu, J., Kuhne, M.R., Srinivasan, M., Assad, A., Witte, A., Graziano, R.F., and King, D.J. (2009) *In vitro* and *in vivo* characterization of MDX-1401 for therapy of malignant lymphoma. *Clin. Cancer Res.*, **15**, 3376–3383.
27. Thertulien, R., Frankel, A.E., Evens, A.M., Kaufman, J., Horwitz, S., Assad, A., Cardelli, P.M., Tian, J., Zhang, Z., and MacDowall, M.C. (2009) A phase I, open-label, dose-escalation, multidose study of MDX-1401 (defucosylated human antiCD30 monoclonal antibody) in patients with CD30-positive refractory/relapsed Hodgkin's lymphoma. Annual Meeting of the American Association for Cancer Research, Denver, CO, abstract 1227.
28. Ishii, T., Chanan-Khan, A.A., Jafferjee, J., Ersing, N., Takahashi, T., Mizutani, M., Shiotsu, Y., and Hanai, N. (2009) A humanized anti-ganglioside GM2 antibody, BIW-8962, exhibits ADCC/CDC activity against multiple myeloma cells and potent anti-tumor activity in mouse xenograft models. American Society of Hematology Annual Meeting, San Francisco, CA, abstract 1718.
29. Yamamoto, K., Utsunomiya, A., Tobinai, K., Tsukasaki, K., Uike, N., Uozumi, K., Yamaguchi, K., Yamada, Y., Hanada, S., Tamura, K., Nakamura, S., Inagaki, H., Ohshima, K., Kiyoi, H., Ishida, T., Matsushima, K., Akinaga, S., Ogura, M., Tomonaga, M., and Ueda, R. (2010) Phase I study of KW-0761, a defucosylated humanized anti-CCR4 antibody, in relapsed patients with adult T-cell leukemia-lymphoma and peripheral T-cell lymphoma. *J. Clin. Oncol.*, **28**, 1591–1598.
30. Yamamoto, K., Tobinai, K., Akinaga, S., and Ueda, R. (2010) Reply to R. Suzuki. *J. Clin. Oncol.*, **28**, e406.

31. Suzuki, R. (2010) Dosing of a phase I study of KW-0761, an anti-CCR4 antibody, for adult T-Cell leukemia-lymphoma and peripheral T-cell lymphoma. *J. Clin. Oncol.*, **28**, e404–e405.
32. Busse, W.W., Katial, R., Gossage, D., Sari, S., Wang, B., Kolbeck, R., Coyle, A.J., Koike, M., Spitalny, G.L., Kiener, P.A., Geba, G.P., and Molfino, N.A. (2010) Safety profile, pharmacokinetics, and biologic activity of MEDI-563, an anti-IL-5 receptor alpha antibody, in a phase I study of subjects with mild asthma. *J. Allergy Clin. Immunol.*, **125**, 1237–1244.
33. Schliemann, C. and Neri, D. (2007) Antibody-based targeting of the tumor vasculature. *Biochim. Biophys. Acta*, **1776**, 175–192.
34. Schliemann, C. and Neri, D. (2010) Antibody-based vascular tumor targeting. *Recent Results Cancer Res.*, **180**, 201–216.
35. Henry, M.D., Wen, S., Silva, M.D., Chandra, S., Milton, M., and Worland, P.J. (2004) A prostate-specific membrane antigen-targeted monoclonal antibody–chemotherapeutic conjugate designed for the treatment of prostate cancer. *Cancer Res.*, **64**, 7995–8001.
36. Ma, D., Hopf, C.E., Malewicz, A.D., Donovan, G.P., Senter, P.D., Goeckeler, W.F., Maddon, P.J., and Olson, W.C. (2006) Potent antitumor activity of an auristatin-conjugated, fully human monoclonal antibody to prostate-specific membrane antigen. *Clin. Cancer Res.*, **12**, 2591–2596.
37. Bross, P.F., Beitz, J., Chen, G., Chen, X.H., Duffy, E., Kieffer, L., Roy, S., Sridhara, R., Rahman, A., Williams, G., and Pazdur, R. (2001) Approval summary: gemtuzumab ozogamicin in relapsed acute myeloid leukemia. *Clin. Cancer Res.*, **7**, 1490–1496.
38. Sievers, E.L. (2003) Antibody-targeted chemotherapy of acute myeloid leukemia using gemtuzumab ozogamicin (Mylotarg). *Blood Cells Mol. Dis.*, **31**, 7–10.
39. Slamon, D.J., Leyland-Jones, B., Shak, S., Fuchs, H., Paton, V., Bajamonde, A., Fleming, T., Eiermann, W., Wolter, J., Pegram, M., Baselga, J., and Norton, L. (2001) Use of chemotherapy plus a monoclonal antibody against HER2 for metastatic breast cancer that overexpresses HER2. *N. Engl. J. Med.*, **344**, 783–792.
40. Junttila, T.T., Li, G., Parsons, K., Phillips, G.L., and Sliwkowski, M.X. (2010) Trastuzumab–DM1 (T–DM1) retains all the mechanisms of action of trastuzumab and efficiently inhibits growth of lapatinib insensitive breast cancer. *Breast Cancer Res. Treat.* DOI:10.1007/s10549-010-1090-x.
41. Junutula, J.R., Flagella, K.M., Graham, R.A., Parsons, K.L., Ha, E., Raab, H., Bhakta, S., Nguyen, T., Dugger, D.L., Li, G., Mai, E., Lewis Phillips, G.D., Hirairagi, H., Fuji, R.N., Tibbitts, J., Vandlen, R., Spencer, S.D., Scheller, R.H., Polakis, P., and Sliwkowski, M.X. (2010) Engineered thio-trastuzumab–DM1 conjugate with an improved therapeutic index to target HER2-positive breast cancer. *Clin. Cancer Res.*, **16**, 4769–4778.
42. Lewis Phillips, G.D., Li, G., Dugger, D.L., Crocker, L.M., Parsons, K.L., Mai, E., Blattler, W.A., Lambert, J.M., Chari, R.V., Lutz, R.J., Wong, W.L., Jacobson, F.S., Koeppen, H., Schwall, R.H., Kenkare-Mitra, S.R., Spencer, S.D., and Sliwkowski, M.X. (2008) Targeting HER2-positive breast cancer with trastuzumab–DM1, an antibody–cytotoxic drug conjugate. *Cancer Res.*, **68**, 9280–9290.
43. Mao, W., Luis, E., Ross, S., Silva, J., Tan, C., Crowley, C., Chui, C., Franz, G., Senter, P., Koeppen, H., and Polakis, P. (2004) EphB2 as a therapeutic antibody drug target for the treatment of colorectal cancer. *Cancer Res.*, **64**, 781–788.
44. Carter, P.J. and Senter, P.D. (2008) Antibody–drug conjugates for cancer therapy. *Cancer J.*, **14**, 154–169.
45. Chari, R.V. (2008) Targeted cancer therapy: conferring specificity to cytotoxic drugs. *Acc. Chem. Res.*, **41**, 98–107.
46. Senter, P.D. (2009) Potent antibody drug conjugates for cancer therapy. *Curr. Opin. Chem. Biol.*, **13**, 235–244.

47. Tijink, B.M., Buter, J., de Bree, R., Giaccone, G., Lang, M.S., Staab, A., Leemans, C.R., and van Dongen, G.A. (2006) A phase I dose escalation study with anti-CD44v6 bivatuzumab mertansine in patients with incurable squamous cell carcinoma of the head and neck or esophagus. *Clin. Cancer Res.*, **12**, 6064–6072.
48. Trail, P.A., Willner, D., Lasch, S.J., Henderson, A.J., Hofstead, S., Casazza, A.M., Firestone, R.A., Hellström, I., and Hellström, K.E. (1993) Cure of xenografted human carcinomas by BR96-doxorubicin immunoconjugates. *Science*, **261**, 212–215.
49. Tolcher, A.W., Sugarman, S., Gelmon, K.A., Cohen, R., Saleh, M., Isaacs, C., Young, L., Healey, D., Onetto, N., and Slichenmyer, W. (1999) Randomized phase II study of BR96-doxorubicin conjugate in patients with metastatic breast cancer. *J. Clin. Oncol.*, **17**, 478–484.
50. Dixit, R. and Coats, S. (2009) Preclinical efficacy and safety models for mAbs: the challenge of developing effective model systems. *IDrugs*, **12**, 103–108.
51. Francisco, J.A., Cerveny, C.G., Meyer, D.L., Mixan, B.J., Klussman, K., Chace, D.F., Rejniak, S.X., Gordon, K.A., DeBlanc, R., Toki, B.E., Law, C.L., Doronina, S.O., Siegall, C.B., Senter, P.D., and Wahl, A.F. (2003) cAC10-vcMMAE, an anti-CD30-monomethyl auristatin E conjugate with potent and selective antitumor activity. *Blood*, **102**, 1458–1465.
52. Oflazoglu, E., Kissler, K.M., Sievers, E.L., Grewal, I.S., and Gerber, H.P. (2008) Combination of the anti-CD30-auristatin-E antibody-drug conjugate (SGN-35) with chemotherapy improves antitumour activity in Hodgkin lymphoma. *Br. J. Haematol.*, **142**, 69–73.
53. Thurber, G.M., Schmidt, M.M., and Wittrup, K.D. (2008) Antibody tumor penetration: transport opposed by systemic and antigen-mediated clearance. *Adv. Drug Deliv. Rev.*, **60**, 1421–1434.
54. Alley, S.C., Zhang, X., Okeley, N.M., Anderson, M., Law, C.L., Senter, P.D., and Benjamin, D.R. (2009) The pharmacologic basis for antibody–auristatin conjugate activity. *J. Pharmacol. Exp. Ther.*, **330**, 932–938.
55. Dijoseph, J.F., Dougher, M.M., Armellino, D.C., Kalyandrug, L., Kunz, A., Boghaert, E.R., Hamann, P.R., and Damle, N.K. (2007) CD20-specific antibody-targeted chemotherapy of non-Hodgkin's B-cell lymphoma using calicheamicin-conjugated rituximab. *Cancer Immunol. Immunother.*, **56**, 1107–1117.
56. Law, C.L., Cerveny, C.G., Gordon, K.A., Klussman, K., Mixan, B.J., Chace, D.F., Meyer, D.L., Doronina, S.O., Siegall, C.B., Francisco, J.A., Senter, P.D., and Wahl, A.F. (2004) Efficient elimination of B-lineage lymphomas by anti-CD20–auristatin conjugates. *Clin. Cancer Res.*, **10**, 7842–7851.
57. Polson, A.G., Calemine-Fenaux, J., Chan, P., Chang, W., Christensen, E., Clark, S., de Sauvage, F.J., Eaton, D., Elkins, K., Elliott, J.M., Frantz, G., Fuji, R.N., Gray, A., Harden, K., Ingle, G.S., Kljavin, N.M., Koeppen, H., Nelson, C., Prabhu, S., Raab, H., Ross, S., Stephan, J.P., Scales, S.J., Spencer, S.D., Vandlen, R., Wranik, B., Yu, S.F., Zheng, B., and Ebens, A. (2009) Antibody-drug conjugates for the treatment of non-Hodgkin's lymphoma: target and linker-drug selection. *Cancer Res.*, **69**, 2358–2364.
58. Hamann, P.R., Hinman, L.M., Beyer, C.F., Lindh, D., Upeslacis, J., Flowers, D.A., and Bernstein, I. (2002) An anti-CD33 antibody–calicheamicin conjugate for treatment of acute myeloid leukemia. Choice of linker. *Bioconjug. Chem.*, **13**, 40–46.
59. Hamann, P.R., Hinman, L.M., Hollander, I., Beyer, C.F., Lindh, D., Holcomb, R., Hallett, W., Tsou, H.R., Upeslacis, J., Shochat, D., Mountain, A., Flowers, D.A., and Bernstein, I. (2002) Gemtuzumab ozogamicin, a potent and selective anti-CD33 antibody–calicheamicin conjugate for treatment of acute myeloid leukemia. *Bioconjug. Chem.*, **13**, 47–58.

60. Hollander, I., Kunz, A., and Hamann, P.R. (2008) Selection of reaction additives used in the preparation of monomeric antibody–calicheamicin conjugates. *Bioconjug. Chem.*, **19**, 358–361.
61. Doronina, S.O., Toki, B.E., Torgov, M.Y., Mendelsohn, B.A., Cerveny, C.G., Chace, D.F., DeBlanc, R.L., Gearing, R.P., Bovee, T.D., Siegall, C.B., Francisco, J.A., Wahl, A.F., Meyer, D.L., and Senter, P.D. (2003) Development of potent monoclonal antibody auristatin conjugates for cancer therapy. *Nat. Biotechnol.*, **21**, 778–784.
62. McDonagh, C.F., Turcott, E., Westendorf, L., Webster, J.B., Alley, S.C., Kim, K., Andreyka, J., Stone, I., Hamblett, K.J., Francisco, J.A., and Carter, P. (2006) Engineered antibody–drug conjugates with defined sites and stoichiometries of drug attachment. *Protein Eng. Des. Sel.*, **19**, 299–307.
63. Junutula, J.R., Raab, H., Clark, S., Bhakta, S., Leipold, D.D., Weir, S., Chen, Y., Simpson, M., Tsai, S.P., Dennis, M.S., Lu, Y., Meng, Y.G., Ng, C., Yang, J., Lee, C.C., Duenas, E., Gorrell, J., Katta, V., Kim, A., McDorman, K., Flagella, K., Venook, R., Ross, S., Spencer, S.D., Lee Wong, W., Lowman, H.B., Vandlen, R., Sliwkowski, M.X., Scheller, R.H., Polakis, P., and Mallet, W. (2008) Site-specific conjugation of a cytotoxic drug to an antibody improves the therapeutic index. *Nat. Biotechnol.*, **26**, 925–932.
64. Sun, M.M., Beam, K.S., Cerveny, C.G., Hamblett, K.J., Blackmore, R.S., Torgov, M.Y., Handley, F.G., Ihle, N.C., Senter, P.D., and Alley, S.C. (2005) Reduction-alkylation strategies for the modification of specific monoclonal antibody disulfides. *Bioconjug. Chem.*, **16**, 1282–1290.
65. Chari, R.V., Martell, B.A., Gross, J.L., Cook, S.B., Shah, S.A., Blättler, W.A., McKenzie, S.J., and Goldmacher, V.S. (1992) Immunoconjugates containing novel maytansinoids: promising anticancer drugs. *Cancer Res.*, **52**, 127–131.
66. Lu, S.X., Takach, E.J., Solomon, M., Zhu, Q., Law, S.J., and Hsieh, F.Y. (2005) Mass spectral analyses of labile DOTA-NHS and heterogeneity determination of DOTA or DM1 conjugated anti-PSMA antibody for prostate cancer therapy. *J. Pharm. Sci.*, **94**, 788–797.
67. Wang, L., Amphlett, G., Blättler, W.A., Lambert, J.M., and Zhang, W. (2005) Structural characterization of the maytansinoid-monoclonal antibody immunoconjugate, huN901–DM1, by mass spectrometry. *Protein Sci.*, **14**, 2436–2446.
68. Andersen, D.C. and Reilly, D.E. (2004) Production technologies for monoclonal antibodies and their fragments. *Curr. Opin. Biotechnol.*, **15**, 456–462.
69. Hamblett, K.J., Senter, P.D., Chace, D.F., Sun, M.M., Lenox, J., Cerveny, C.G., Kissler, K.M., Bernhardt, S.X., Kopcha, A.K., Zabinski, R.F., Meyer, D.L., and Francisco, J.A. (2004) Effects of drug loading on the antitumor activity of a monoclonal antibody drug conjugate. *Clin. Cancer Res.*, **10**, 7063–7070.
70. Pietersz, G.A., Rowland, A., Smyth, M.J., and McKenzie, I.F. (1994) Chemoimmunoconjugates for the treatment of cancer. *Adv. Immunol.*, **56**, 301–387.
71. Alley, S.C., Zhang, X., Okeley, N.M., Anderson, M., Law, C.L., Senter, P.D., and Benjamin, D.R. (2009) The pharmacologic basis for antibody-auristatin conjugate activity. *J. Pharmacol. Exp. Ther.*, **330**, 932–938.
72. Firestone, R.A., Willner, D., Hofstead, S.J., King, H.D., Kaneko, T., Braslawsky, G.R., Greenfield, R.S., Trail, P.A., Lasch, S.J., Henderson, A.J., Casazza, A.M., and Hellström, I. (1996) Synthesis and antitumor activity of the immunoconjugate BR96–Dox. *J. Control. Release*, **39**, 251–259.
73. Saleh, M.N., Sugarman, S., Murray, J., Ostroff, J.B., Healey, D., Jones, D., Daniel, C.R., LeBherz, D., Brewer, H., Onetto, N., and LoBuglio, A.F. (2000) Phase I trial of the anti-Lewis Y drug immunoconjugate BR96–doxorubicin in patients with lewis Y-expressing

epithelial tumors. *J. Clin. Oncol.*, **18**, 2282–2292.

74. Damle, N.K. (2004) Tumour-targeted chemotherapy with immunoconjugates of calicheamicin. *Expert Opin. Biol. Ther.*, **4**, 1445–1452.

75. Damle, N.K. and Frost, P. (2003) Antibody-targeted chemotherapy with immunoconjugates of calicheamicin. *Curr. Opin. Pharmacol.*, **3**, 386–390.

76. Boghaert, E.R., Khandke, K.M., Sridharan, L., Dougher, M., Dijoseph, J.F., Kunz, A., Hamann, P.R., Moran, J., Chaudhary, I., and Damle, N.K. (2007) Determination of pharmacokinetic values of calicheamicin-antibody conjugates in mice by plasmon resonance analysis of small (5 µl) blood samples. *Cancer Chemother. Pharmacol.*, **61**, 1027–1035.

77. Boghaert, E.R., Sridharan, L., Armellino, D.C., Khandke, K.M., DiJoseph, J.F., Kunz, A., Dougher, M.M., Jiang, F., Kalyandrug, L.B., Hamann, P.R., Frost, P., and Damle, N.K. (2004) Antibody-targeted chemotherapy with the calicheamicin conjugate hu3S193-N-acetyl γ calicheamicin dimethyl hydrazide targets Lewis^Y and eliminates Lewis^Y-positive human carcinoma cells and xenografts. *Clin. Cancer Res.*, **10**, 4538–4549.

78. Boghaert, E.R., Sridharan, L., Khandke, K.M., Armellino, D., Ryan, M.G., Myers, K., Harrop, R., Kunz, A., Hamann, P.R., Marquette, K., Dougher, M., Dijoseph, J.F., and Damle, N.K. (2008) The oncofetal protein, 5T4, is a suitable target for antibody-guided anti-cancer chemotherapy with calicheamicin. *Int. J. Oncol.*, **32**, 221–234.

79. Hamann, P.R., Hinman, L.M., Beyer, C.F., Greenberger, L.M., Lin, C., Lindh, D., Menendez, A.T., Wallace, R., Durr, F.E., and Upeslacis, J. (2005) An anti-MUC1 antibody–calicheamicin conjugate for treatment of solid tumors. Choice of linker and overcoming drug resistance. *Bioconjug. Chem.*, **16**, 346–353.

80. Trail, P.A., King, H.D., and Dubowchik, G.M. (2003) Monoclonal antibody drug immunoconjugates for targeted treatment of cancer. *Cancer Immunol. Immunother.*, **52**, 328–337.

81. DiJoseph, J.F., Armellino, D.C., Boghaert, E.R., Khandke, K., Dougher, M.M., Sridharan, L., Kunz, A., Hamann, P.R., Gorovits, B., Udata, C., Moran, J.K., Popplewell, A.G., Stephens, S., Frost, P., and Damle, N.K. (2004) Antibody-targeted chemotherapy with CMC-544: a CD22-targeted immunoconjugate of calicheamicin for the treatment of B-lymphoid malignancies. *Blood*, **103**, 1807–1814.

82. DiJoseph, J.F., Goad, M.E., Dougher, M.M., Boghaert, E.R., Kunz, A., Hamann, P.R., and Damle, N.K. (2004) Potent and specific antitumor efficacy of CMC-544, a CD22-targeted immunoconjugate of calicheamicin, against systemically disseminated B-cell lymphoma. *Clin. Cancer Res.*, **10**, 8620–8629.

83. DiJoseph, J.F., Popplewell, A., Tickle, S., Ladyman, H., Lawson, A., Kunz, A., Khandke, K., Armellino, D.C., Boghaert, E.R., Hamann, P., Zinkewich-Peotti, K., Stephens, S., Weir, N., and Damle, N.K. (2005) Antibody-targeted chemotherapy of B-cell lymphoma using calicheamicin conjugated to murine or humanized antibody against CD22. *Cancer Immunol. Immunother.*, **54**, 11–24.

84. Boghaert, E.R., Khandke, K., Sridharan, L., Armellino, D., Dougher, M., Dijoseph, J.F., Kunz, A., Hamann, P.R., Sridharan, A., Jones, S., Discafani, C., and Damle, N.K. (2006) Tumoricidal effect of calicheamicin immuno-conjugates using a passive targeting strategy. *Int. J. Oncol.*, **28**, 675–684.

85. Jedema, I., Barge, R.M., van der Velden, V.H., Nijmeijer, B.A., vanDongen, J.J., Willemze, R., and Falkenburg, J.H. (2004) Internalization and cell cycle-dependent killing of leukemic cells by gemtuzumab ozogamicin: rationale for efficacy in CD33-negative malignancies with endocytic capacity. *Leukemia*, **18**, 316–325.

86. Liu, C., Tadayoni, B.M., Bourret, L.A., Mattocks, K.M., Derr, S.M., Widdison, W.C., Kedersha, N.L., Ariniello, P.D., Goldmacher, V.S., Lambert, J.M., Blättler, W.A., and Chari, R.V. (1996) Eradication of large colon tumor xenografts by targeted delivery of maytansinoids. *Proc. Natl. Acad. Sci. USA*, **93**, 8618–8623.

87. Tolcher, A.W., Ochoa, L., Hammond, L.A., Patnaik, A., Edwards, T., Takimoto, C., Smith, L., de Bono, J., Schwartz, G., Mays, T., Jonak, Z.L., Johnson, R., DeWitte, M., Martino, H., Audette, C., Maes, K., Chari, R.V., Lambert, J.M., and Rowinsky, E.K. (2003) Cantuzumab mertansine, a maytansinoid immunoconjugate directed to the CanAg antigen: a phase I, pharmacokinetic, and biologic correlative study. *J. Clin. Oncol.*, **21**, 211–222.

88. Widdison, W.C., Wilhelm, S.D., Cavanagh, E.E., Whiteman, K.R., Leece, B.A., Kovtun, Y., Goldmacher, V.S., Xie, H., Steeves, R.M., Lutz, R.J., Zhao, R., Wang, L., Blättler, W.A., and Chari, R.V. (2006) Semisynthetic maytansine analogues for the targeted treatment of cancer. *J. Med. Chem.*, **49**, 4392–4408.

89. Erickson, H.K., Widdison, W.C., Mayo, M.F., Whiteman, K., Audette, C., Wilhelm, S.D., and Singh, R. (2010) Tumor delivery and *in vivo* processing of disulfide-linked and thioether-linked antibody–maytansinoid conjugates. *Bioconjug. Chem.*, **21**, 84–92.

90. Chen, Q., Millar, H.J., McCabe, F.L., Manning, C.D., Steeves, R., Lai, K., Kellogg, B., Lutz, R.J., Trikha, M., Nakada, M.T., and Anderson, G.M. (2007) α_v Integrin-targeted immunoconjugates regress established human tumors in xenograft models. *Clin. Cancer Res.*, **13**, 3689–3695.

91. Kovtun, Y.V., Audette, C.A., Ye, Y., Xie, H., Ruberti, M.F., Phinney, S.J., Leece, B.A., Chittenden, T., Blättler, W.A., and Goldmacher, V.S. (2006) Antibody–drug conjugates designed to eradicate tumors with homogeneous and heterogeneous expression of the target antigen. *Cancer Res.*, **66**, 3214–3221.

92. Erickson, H.K., Park, P.U., Widdison, W.C., Kovtun, Y.V., Garrett, L.M., Hoffman, K., Lutz, R.J., Goldmacher, V.S., and Blättler, W.A. (2006) Antibody–maytansinoid conjugates are activated in targeted cancer cells by lysosomal degradation and linker-dependent intracellular processing. *Cancer Res.*, **66**, 4426–4433.

93. Tassone, P., Goldmacher, V.S., Neri, P., Gozzini, A., Shammas, M.A., Whiteman, K.R., Hylander-Gans, L.L., Carrasco, D.R., Hideshima, T., Shringarpure, R., Shi, J., Allam, C.K., Wijdenes, J., Venuta, S., Munshi, N.C., and Anderson, K.C. (2004) Cytotoxic activity of the maytansinoid immunoconjugate B-B4–DM1 against CD138$^+$ multiple myeloma cells. *Blood*, **104**, 3688–3696.

94. Tassone, P., Gozzini, A., Goldmacher, V., Shammas, M.A., Whiteman, K.R., Carrasco, D.R., Li, C., Allam, C.K., Venuta, S., Anderson, K.C., and Munshi, N.C. (2004) *In vitro* and *in vivo* activity of the maytansinoid immunoconjugate huN901–N2'-deacetyl-N2'-(3-mercapto-1-oxopropyl)–maytansine against CD56$^+$ multiple myeloma cells. *Cancer Res.*, **64**, 4629–4636.

95. Alley, S.C., Okeley, N.M., and Senter, P.D. (2010) Antibody–drug conjugates: targeted drug delivery for cancer. *Curr. Opin. Chem. Biol.*, **14**, 529–537.

96. Dubowchik, G.M., Mosure, K., Knipe, J.O., and Firestone, R.A. (1998) Cathepsin B-sensitive dipeptide prodrugs. 2. Models of anticancer drugs paclitaxel (Taxol), mitomycin C and doxorubicin. *Bioorg. Med. Chem. Lett.*, **8**, 3347–3352.

97. Dubowchik, G.M., Radia, S., Mastalerz, H., Walker, M.A., Firestone, R.A., Dalton King, H., Hofstead, S.J., Willner, D., Lasch, S.J., and Trail, P.A. (2002) Doxorubicin immunoconjugates containing bivalent, lysosomally-cleavable dipeptide linkages. *Bioorg. Med. Chem. Lett.*, **12**, 1529–1532.

98. Sloane, B.F., Yan, S., Podgorski, I., Linebaugh, B.E., Cher, M.L., Mai, J., Cavallo-Medved, D., Sameni, M., Dosescu, J., and Moin, K. (2005)

Cathepsin B and tumor proteolysis: contribution of the tumor microenvironment. *Semin. Cancer Biol.*, **15**, 149–157.
99. Dubowchik, G.M. and Firestone, R.A. (1998) Cathepsin B-sensitive dipeptide prodrugs. 1. A model study of structural requirements for efficient release of doxorubicin. *Bioorg. Med. Chem. Lett.*, **8**, 3341–3346.
100. Walker, M.A., Dubowchik, G.M., Hofstead, S.J., Trail, P.A., and Firestone, R.A. (2002) Synthesis of an immunoconjugate of camptothecin. *Bioorg. Med. Chem. Lett.*, **12**, 217–219.
101. Walker, M.A., King, H.D., Dalterio, R.A., Trail, P., Firestone, R., and Dubowchik, G.M. (2004) Monoclonal antibody mediated intracellular targeting of tallysomycin S(10b). *Bioorg. Med. Chem. Lett.*, **14**, 4323–4327.
102. Doronina, S.O., Mendelsohn, B.A., Bovee, T.D., Cerveny, C.G., Alley, S.C., Meyer, D.L., Oflazoglu, E., Toki, B.E., Sanderson, R.J., Zabinski, R.F., Wahl, A.F., and Senter, P.D. (2006) Enhanced activity of monomethylauristatin F through monoclonal antibody delivery: effects of linker technology on efficacy and toxicity. *Bioconjug. Chem.*, **17**, 114–124.
103. Sanderson, R.J., Hering, M.A., James, S.F., Sun, M.M., Doronina, S.O., Siadak, A.W., Senter, P.D., and Wahl, A.F. (2005) In vivo drug-linker stability of an anti-CD30 dipeptide-linked auristatin immunoconjugate. *Clin. Cancer Res.*, **11**, 843–852.
104. Ryan, M.C., Hering, M., Peckham, D., McDonagh, C.F., Brown, L., Kim, K.M., Meyer, D.L., Zabinski, R.F., Grewal, I.S., and Carter, P.J. (2007) Antibody targeting of B-cell maturation antigen on malignant plasma cells. *Mol. Cancer Ther.*, **6**, 3009–3018.
105. Gerber, H.P., Kung-Sutherland, M., Stone, I., Morris-Tilden, C., Miyamoto, J., McCormick, R., Alley, S.C., Okeley, N., Hayes, B., Hernandez-Ilizaliturri, F.J., McDonagh, C.F., Carter, P.J., Benjamin, D., and Grewal, I.S. (2009) Potent antitumor activity of the anti-CD19 auristatin antibody drug conjugate hBU12–vcMMAE against rituximab-sensitive and -resistant lymphomas. *Blood*, **113**, 4352–4361.
106. Law, C.L., Gordon, K.A., Toki, B.E., Yamane, A.K., Hering, M.A., Cerveny, C.G., Petroziello, J.M., Ryan, M.C., Smith, L., Simon, R., Sauter, G., Oflazoglu, E., Doronina, S.O., Meyer, D.L., Francisco, J.A., Carter, P., Senter, P.D., Copland, J.A., Wood, C.G., and Wahl, A.F. (2006) Lymphocyte activation antigen CD70 expressed by renal cell carcinoma is a potential therapeutic target for anti-CD70 antibody–drug conjugates. *Cancer Res.*, **66**, 2328–2337.
107. Bhaskar, V., Law, D.A., Ibsen, E., Breinberg, D., Cass, K.M., DuBridge, R.B., Evangelista, F., Henshall, S.M., Hevezi, P., Miller, J.C., Pong, M., Powers, R., Senter, P., Stockett, D., Sutherland, R.L., von Freeden-Jeffry, U., Willhite, D., Murray, R., Afar, D.E., and Ramakrishnan, V. (2003) E-selectin up-regulation allows for targeted drug delivery in prostate cancer. *Cancer Res.*, **63**, 6387–6394.
108. Tse, K.F., Jeffers, M., Pollack, V.A., McCabe, D.A., Shadish, M.L., Khramtsov, N.V., Hackett, C.S., Shenoy, S.G., Kuang, B., Boldog, F.L., MacDougall, J.R., Rastelli, L., Herrmann, J., Gallo, M., Gazit-Bornstein, G., Senter, P.D., Meyer, D.L., Lichenstein, H.S., and LaRochelle, W.J. (2006) CR011, a fully human monoclonal antibody–auristatin E conjugate, for the treatment of melanoma. *Clin. Cancer Res.*, **12**, 1373–1382.
109. Smith, L.M., Nesterova, A., Alley, S.C., Torgov, M.Y., and Carter, P.J. (2006) Potent cytotoxicity of an auristatin-containing antibody–drug conjugate targeting melanoma cells expressing melanotransferrin/p97. *Mol. Cancer. Ther.*, **5**, 1474–1482.
110. Chen, Y., Clark, S., Wong, T., Dennis, M.S., Luis, E., Zhong, F., Bheddah, S., Koeppen, H., Gogineni, A., Ross, S., Polakis, P., and Mallet, W. (2007) Armed antibodies targeting the mucin repeats of the ovarian cancer antigen,

111. Afar, D.E., Bhaskar, V., Ibsen, E., Breinberg, D., Henshall, S.M., Kench, J.G., Drobnjak, M., Powers, R., Wong, M., Evangelista, F., O'Hara, C., Powers, D., DuBridge, R.B., Caras, I., Winter, R., Anderson, T., Solvason, N., Stricker, P.D., Cordon-Cardo, C., Scher, H.I., Grygiel, J.J., Sutherland, R.L., Murray, R., Ramakrishnan, V., and Law, D.A. (2004) Preclinical validation of anti-TMEFF2-auristatin E-conjugated antibodies in the treatment of prostate cancer. *Mol. Cancer Ther.*, **3**, 921–932.

112. Alley, S.C., Benjamin, D.R., Jeffrey, S.C., Okeley, N.M., Meyer, D.L., Sanderson, R.J., and Senter, P.D. (2008) Contribution of linker stability to the activities of anticancer immunoconjugates. *Bioconjug. Chem.*, **19**, 759–765.

113. Fanale, M., Bartlett, N.L., Forero-Torres, A., Rosenblatt, J.D., Horning, S.J., Franklin, A.R., Lynch, C., Sievers, E.L., and Kennedy, D.A. (2009) The antibody–drug conjugate brentuximab vedotin (SGN-35) induced multiple objective responses in patients with relapsed or refractory CD30-positive lymphomas in a phase 1 weekly dosing study. *Blood*, **214**, 2731.

114. Chen, R., Gopal, A.K., Smith, S.E., Ansell, S.M., Rosenblatt, J.D., Klasa, R., Conners, J.M., Engert, A., Larson, E.K., Kennedy, D.A., Sievers, E.L., and Younes, A. (2010) Results of a pivotal phase II study of brentuximab vedotin (SGN-35) in patients with relapsed or refractory Hodgkin lymphoma. *Blood*, **116**, abstract 283.

115. Forero-Torres, A., Leonard, J.P., Younes, A., Rosenblatt, J.D., Brice, P., Bartlett, N.L., Bosly, A., Pinter-Brown, L., Kennedy, D., Sievers, E.L., and Gopal, A.K. (2009) A Phase II study of SGN-30 (anti-CD30 mAb) in Hodgkin lymphoma or systemic anaplastic large cell lymphoma. *Br. J. Haematol.*, **146**, 171–179.

116. Hwu, P., Sznol, M., Pavlick, A., Kluger, H., Kim, K.B., Boasberg, P., Sanders, D., Simantov, R., Crowley, E., and Hamid, O. (2009) A phase I/II study of CR011-vcMMAE, an antibody–drug conjugate (ADC) targeting glycoprotein NMB (GPNMB) in patients (pts) with advanced melanoma. *J. Clin. Oncol.*, **27** (15S), abstract 9032.

117. Burris, H., Saleh, M., Bendell, J., Hart, L., Rose, A.A.N., Dong, Z., Siegel, P.M., Crane, M.F., Donovan, D., Crowley, E., Simantov, R., and Vahdat, L. (2009) A phase (Ph) I/II study of CR011-VcMMAE, an antibody-drug conjugate, in patients (Pts) with locally advanced or metastatic breast cancer (MBC), 32nd Annual San Antonio Breast Cancer Symposium, San Antonio, TX, abstract 6096.

118. Pollack, V.A., Alvarez, E., Tse, K.F., Torgov, M.Y., Xie, S., Shenoy, S.G., MacDougall, J.R., Arrol, S., Zhong, H., Gerwien, R.W., Hahne, W.F., Senter, P.D., Jeffers, M.E., Lichenstein, H.S., and LaRochelle, W.J. (2007) Treatment parameters modulating regression of human melanoma xenografts by an antibody–drug conjugate (CR011–vcMMAE) targeting GPNMB. *Cancer Chemother. Pharmacol.*, **60**, 423–435.

119. Oflazoglu, E., Stone, I.J., Gordon, K., Wood, C.G., Repasky, E.A., Grewal, I.S., Law, C.L., and Gerber, H.P. (2008) Potent anticarcinoma activity of the humanized anti-CD70 antibody h1F6 conjugated to the tubulin inhibitor auristatin via an uncleavable linker. *Clin. Cancer Res.*, **14**, 6171–6180.

120. Lee, J.W., Han, H.D., Shahzad, M.M., Kim, S.W., Mangala, L.S., Nick, A.M., Lu, C., Langley, R.R., Schmandt, R., Kim, H.S., Mao, S., Gooya, J., Fazenbaker, C., Jackson, D., Tice, D.A., Landen, C.N., Coleman, R.L., and Sood, A.K. (2009) EphA2 immunoconjugate as molecularly targeted chemotherapy for ovarian carcinoma. *J. Natl. Cancer Inst.*, **101**, 1193–1205.

121. Al-Ahmadie, H.A., Alden, D., Qin, L.X., Olgac, S., Fine, S.W., Gopalan, A., Russo, P., Motzer, R.J., Reuter, V.E., and Tickoo, S.K. (2008) Carbonic anhydrase IX expression in clear cell

MUC16, are highly efficacious in animal tumor models. *Cancer Res.*, **67**, 4924–4932.

renal cell carcinoma: an immunohistochemical study comparing 2 antibodies. *Am. J. Surg. Pathol.*, **32**, 377–382.

122. Krop, I., LoRusso, P., Miller, K.D., Modi, S., Yardley, D., Rodriguez, G., Zheng, M., Amler, L., and Rugo, H. (2009) A phase II study of trastuzumab-DM1 (T-DM1), a novel HER2 antibody-drug conjugate, in patients previously treated with lapatinib, trastuzumab, and chemotherapy, 32nd Annual San Antonio Breast Cancer Symposium, San Antonio, TX, abstract 5090.

123. Legrand, O., Vidriales, M.B., Thomas, X., Dumontet, C., Vekhoff, A., Morariu-Zamfir, R., Lambert, J., San Miguel, J.F., and Marie, J.-P. (2007) An open label, dose escalation study of AVE9633 administered as a single agent by intravenous (IV) infusion weekly for 2 weeks in 4-week cycle to patients with relapsed or refractory CD33-positive acute myeloid leukemia (AML). *Blood*, **110**, 1850.

124. Chanan-Khan, A.A., Jagannath, S., Munshi, N.C., Schlossman, R.L., Anderson, K.C., Lee, K., DePaolo, D., Miller, K.C., Zildjian, S., Fram, R.J., and Qin, A. (2007) Phase I study of huN901–DM1 (BB-10901) in patients with relapsed and relapsed/refractory CD56-positive multiple myeloma. *Blood*, **110**, 1174.

125. McCann, J., Fossella, F.V., Villalona-Calero, M.A., Tolcher, A.W., Fidias, P., Raju, R., Zildjian, S., Guild, R., and Fram, R. (2007) Phase II trial of huN901–DM1 in patients with relapsed small cell lung cancer (SCLC) and CD56-positive small cell carcinoma. *J. Clin. Oncol.*, **25**, 18084.

126. Mita, M.M., Ricart, A.D., Mita, A.C., Patnaik, A., Sarantopoulos, J., Sankhala, K., Fram, R.J., Qin, A., Watermill, J., and Tolcher, A.W. (2007) A phase I study of a CanAg-targeted immunoconjugate, huC242–DM4, in patients with Can Ag-expressing solid tumors. *J. Clin. Oncol.*, **25**, 3062.

127. Sievers, E.L. (2001) Efficacy and safety of gemtuzumab ozogamicin in patients with CD33-positive acute myeloid leukaemia in first relapse. *Expert Opin. Biol. Ther.*, **1**, 893–901.

128. Fayad, L., Patel, H., Verhoef, G., Smith, M.R., Johnson, P.W.M., Czuczman, M.S., Coiffier, B., Hess, G., Gine, E., Advani, A., Offner, F., Vanderdries, E.R., Shapiro, M., and Dang, N.H. (2008) Safety and clinical activity of the anti-CD22 immunoconjugate inotuzumab ozogamicin (CMC-544) in combination with rituximab in follicular lymphoma or diffuse large B-cell lymphoma: preliminary report of a phase 1/2 study. *Blood*, **112**, 266.

129. Dijoseph, J.F., Dougher, M.M., Armellino, D.C., Evans, D.Y., and Damle, N.K. (2007) Therapeutic potential of CD22-specific antibody-targeted chemotherapy using inotuzumab ozogamicin (CMC-544) for the treatment of acute lymphoblastic leukemia. *Leukemia*, **21**, 2240–2245.

130. Zhang, Q., Derwin, D., Sufi, B., Chen, L., Guerlavais, V., Green, L., Passmore, D., Sung, J., Rangan, V., Dai, R., Kwok, E., Chong, C., Pan, C., Huber, M., Rao, C., Deshpande, S., Cardarelli, P., King, D., Terrett, J.A., and Gangwar, S. (2009) The critical role of cleavable linkers for efficacy and low toxicity with minor groove binding alkylating agent (MGBA) based antibody–drug conjugates. Annual Meeting of the American Association for Cancer Research, Denver, CO, abstract 1722.

131. Larson, R.A., Boogaerts, M., Estey, E., Karanes, C., Stadtmauer, E.A., Sievers, E.L., Mineur, P., Bennett, J.M., Berger, M.S., Eten, C.B., Munteanu, M., Loken, M.R., Van Dongen, J.J., Bernstein, I.D., and Appelbaum, F.R. (2002) Antibody-targeted chemotherapy of older patients with acute myeloid leukemia in first relapse using Mylotarg (gemtuzumab ozogamicin). *Leukemia*, **16**, 1627–1636.

132. Larson, R.A., Sievers, E.L., Stadtmauer, E.A., Lowenberg, B., Estey, E.H., Dombret, H., Theobald, M., Voliotis, D., Bennett, J.M., Richie, M., Leopold, L.H., Berger, M.S., Sherman, M.L., Loken, M.R., van Dongen, J.J., Bernstein, I.D., and Appelbaum, F.R.

(2005) Final report of the efficacy and safety of gemtuzumab ozogamicin (Mylotarg) in patients with CD33-positive acute myeloid leukemia in first recurrence. *Cancer*, **104**, 1442–1452.

133. Lowenberg, B., Beck, J., Graux, C., van Putten, W., Schouten, H.C., Verdonck, L.F., Ferrant, A., Sonneveld, P., Jongen-Lavrencic, M., von Lilienfeld-Toal, M., Biemond, B.J., Vellenga, E., Breems, D., de Muijnck, H., Schaafsma, R., Verhoef, G., Dohner, H., Gratwohl, A., Pabst, T., Ossenkoppele, G.J., and Maertens, J. (2010) Gemtuzumab ozogamicin as postremission treatment in AML at 60 years of age or more: results of a multicenter phase 3 study. *Blood*, **115**, 2586–2591.

134. Burnett, A.K., Kell, W.J., Goldstone, A.H., Milligan, D., Ann Hunter, A., Prentice, A.G., Russell, N.H., Gibson, B., Wheatley, K., and Hills, R.K. (2006) The addition of gemtuzumab ozogamicin to induction chemotherapy for AML improves disease free survival without extra toxicity: preliminary analysis of 1115 patients in the MRC AML15 trial. *Blood*, **108**, 13.

135. Petersdorf, S., Kopecky, K., Stuart, R.K., Larson, R.A., Nevill, T.J., Stenke, L., Slovak, M.L., Tallman, M.S., Willman, C.L., Erba, H., and Appelbaum, F.R. (2009) Preliminary results of Southwest Oncology Group Study S0106: an international intergroup phase 3 randomized trial comparing the addition of gemtuzumab ozogamicin to standard induction therapy versus standard induction therapy followed by a second randomization to post-consolidation gemtuzumab ozogamicin versus no additional therapy for previously untreated acute myeloid leukemia. American Society of Hematology Annual Meeting, San Francisco, CA, abstract 790.

136. Younes, A., Forero-Torres, A., Bartlett, N., Leonard, J.P., Lynch, C., Kennedy, D.A., and Sievers, E.L. (2008) Multiple complete responses in a phase 1 dose-escalation study of the antibody–drug conjugate SGN-35 in patients with relapsed or refractory CD30-positive lymphomas. American Society of Hematology National Meeting, New Orleans, LO, abstract 1006.

137. Beeram, M., Krop, I., Modi, S., Tolcher, A., Rabbee, N., Girish, S., Tibbitts, J., Holden, S., Lutzker, S., and Burris, H. (2007) A phase I study of trastuzumab-MCC–DM1 (T–DM1), a first-in-class HER2 antibody–drug conjugate (ADC), in patients (pts) with HER2$^+$ metastatic breast cancer (BC). *J. Clin. Oncol.*, **25**, 1042.

138. Krop, I.E., Beeram, M., Modi, S., Rabbee, N., Girish, S., Tibbitts, J., Holden, S.N., Lutzker, S.G., and Burris, H.A. (2007) A phase I study of trastuzumab–DM1, a first-in-class HER2 antibody–drug conjugate, in patients with advanced HER2$^+$ breast cancer. 30th Annual Breast Cancer Symposium, San Antonio, TX, abstract 310.

139. Fossella, F., Woll, P.J., Lorigan, P., Tolcher, A., O'Brien, M., O'Keeffe, J., Zildijan, S., Qin, A., O'Leary, J., and Villalona-Calero, M. (2009) Investigation of IMGN901 in CD56$^+$ solid tumors: results from a phase I/II trial (study 001) and a phase I trial (study 002). 13th World Conference on Lung Cancer, Vancouver, http://www.immunogen.com/pdf/IMGN901%20solid%20tumor%20eposter%20WCLC%207-09.pdf.

140. Younes, A., Gordon, L., Kim, S., Romaguera, J., Copeland, A.R., de Castro Farial, S., Kwak, L., Fayad, L., Hagemeister, F., Fanale, M., Lambert, J., Bagulho, T., and Morariu-Zamfir, R. (2009) Phase 1 multi-dose escalation study of the anti-CD19 maytansinoid immunoconjugate SAR3419 administered by IV infusion every 3 weeks to patients with relapsed/refractory B-cell NHL. *Blood*, **114**, 585.

141. Chanan-Khan, A., Jagannath, S., Heffner, T., Avigan, D., Lee, K., Lutz, R.J., Haeder, T., Ruehle, M., Uherek, C., Wartenberg-Demand, A., Munshi, N., and Anderson, K. (2009) Phase 1 Study of BT062 given as repeated single dose once every 3 weeks in patients

with relapsed or relapsed/refractory multiple myeloma. *Blood*, **114**, 1862.

142. Binz, H.K., Amstutz, P., and Plückthun, A. (2005) Engineering novel binding proteins from non-immunoglobulin domains. *Nat. Biotechnol.*, **23**, 1257–1268.

143. Friedman, M. and Stahl, S. (2009) Engineered affinity proteins for tumour-targeting applications. *Biotechnol. Appl. Biochem.*, **53**, 1–29.

144. Low, P.S. and Kularatne, S.A. (2009) Folate-targeted therapeutic and imaging agents for cancer. *Curr. Opin. Chem. Biol.*, **13**, 256–262.

145. Zahnd, C., Kawe, M., Stumpp, M.T., de Pasquale, C., Tamaskovic, R., Nagy-Davidescu, G., Dreier, B., Schibli, R., Binz, H.K., Waibel, R., and Pluckthun, A. (2010) Efficient tumor targeting with high-affinity designed ankyrin repeat proteins: effects of affinity and molecular size. *Cancer Res.*, **70**, 1595–1605.

146. Schlehuber, S. and Skerra, A. (2005) Lipocalins in drug discovery: from natural ligand-binding proteins to "anticalins". *Drug Discov. Today*, **10**, 23–33.

147. Skerra, A. (2008) Alternative binding proteins: anticalins – harnessing the structural plasticity of the lipocalin ligand pocket to engineer novel binding activities. *FEBS J.*, **275**, 2677–2683.

148. Keefe, A.D., Pai, S., and Ellington, A. (2010) Aptamers as therapeutics. *Nat. Rev. Drug Discov.*, **9**, 537–550.

149. Wikman, M., Steffen, A.C., Gunneriusson, E., Tolmachev, V., Adams, G.P., Carlsson, J., and Stahl, S. (2004) Selection and characterization of HER2/neu-binding affibody ligands. *Protein Eng. Des. Sel.*, **17**, 455–462.

150. Devy, L., Rabbani, S.A., Stochl, M., Ruskowski, M., Mackie, I., Naa, L., Toews, M., van Gool, R., Chen, J., Ley, A., Ladner, R.C., Dransfield, D.T., and Henderikx, P. (2007) PEGylated DX-1000: pharmacokinetics and anti-neoplastic activity of a specific plasmin inhibitor. *Neoplasia*, **9**, 927–937.

151. Schmidt, M.M. and Wittrup, K.D. (2009) A modeling analysis of the effects of molecular size and binding affinity on tumor targeting. *Mol. Cancer Ther.*, **8**, 2861–2871.

152. Zahnd, C., Kawe, M., Stumpp, M.T., de Pasquale, C., Tamaskovic, R., Nagy-Davidescu, G., Dreier, B., Schibli, R., Binz, H.K., Waibel, R., and Pluckthun, A. Efficient tumor targeting with high-affinity designed ankyrin repeat proteins: effects of affinity and molecular size. *Cancer Res.* **70**, 1595–1605.

11
Mapping Accessible Vascular Targets to Penetrate Organs and Solid Tumors

Kerri A. Massey and Jan E. Schnitzer

11.1
Introduction

The ultimate goal of molecular medicine is to create cures for disease without causing unwanted side-effects. Antibodies were put forward as a "magic bullet" that could target specific proteins with exquisite sensitivity over 100 years ago [1], but the vast majorities of therapeutic targets developed to date are within the tumor. Even the most specific antibodies have little access to the tumor due to poor delivery. Poor delivery is a major problem for treating many diseases, including solid tumors, and has been recognized as a key clinical challenge for nearly a century. To achieve any efficacy, doses must be increased, resulting in unnecessary exposure to the rest of the body. Eventually, the required escalated dose leads to serious adverse side-effects and even cessation of treatment, leaving patients with few therapeutic options.

Clearly, specificity for a therapeutic target is not sufficient to create effective therapies, and better delivery strategies must be explored to overcome current limitations. Ideal delivery would rapidly concentrate the entire dose of a therapeutic agent into the tumor where it can be most effective, thereby sparing off-target normal tissue and reducing or eliminating toxic side-effects. Unfortunately, little is understood about key *in vivo* biological interfaces, and how they naturally mediate and control selective transport *in vivo* [2]. Here, we will discuss the key biological and technical barriers that must be overcome to enable targeted delivery *in vivo*.

11.2
Current Approaches to Therapy

Chemotherapeutics are small drugs designed to inhibit key cellular processes necessary for tumor growth and progression. As these drugs are small, they can more readily enter most tissues. Lipophilic chemotherapies can even enter the most restrictive tissues, including retina, testes, and brain. This pervasive access

Drug Delivery in Oncology: From Basic Research to Cancer Therapy, First Edition.
Edited by Felix Kratz, Peter Senter, and Henning Steinhagen.
© 2012 Wiley-VCH Verlag GmbH & Co. KGaA. Published 2012 by Wiley-VCH Verlag GmbH & Co. KGaA.

is not specific to tumors and, consequently, most organs in the body are exposed to the chemotherapeutic unnecessarily. Most chemotherapeutics act by killing cells that rapidly divide. They are effective against cancer cells, as well as other healthy, rapidly dividing cells, such as those in bone marrow, the digestive tract, and hair follicles, which leads to many of the well-known side-effects of these drugs.

To improve upon chemotherapeutics, much modern cancer research has been focused on the development of tumor cell-targeted drug therapies, usually in the form of monoclonal antibodies (mAbs), sometimes even linked to cytotoxic agents. Antibodies are very specific for a single target, when they have access to their target site. Under *in vitro* conditions, individual tumor cells are in direct contact with cell culture media; therefore, therapeutic antibodies have unfettered access to cells and the opportunity to bind their targets. Most current targeted drugs are directed against specific proteins expressed by cells located deep within the solid tumor, where access to target sites is often restricted. The vast majority of these treatments have failed *in vivo*, where drug targeting is much more complex. For example, less than 0.01% of tumor-specific antibodies injected intravenously will reach and bind to target tissues *in vivo* because the vascular endothelium that lines blood vessels severely limits movement of circulating antibodies out of the blood and into the underlying tissue [3].

Most tumor-targeting strategies rely on intrinsic passive vascular leakiness to bypass the endothelium and penetrate into tumors. However, reliance on the "enhanced permeability and retention (EPR) effect" has had limited efficacy in humans. Although tumor vasculature may be leakier than normal vasculature, this is clearly insufficient to yield enough access inside tumors to completely benefit patients with cancer. Regardless of size, only a small proportion of the injected dose of all current targeted molecular therapies ever reaches the inside of the tumor where they can be most effective. High dosages (above milligrams per kilogram) with peak blood levels (above micromolar) far in excess of the affinity a compound has for its target (nanomolar) are required to deliver only a small fraction of the injected dose to the tumor, often leading to severe systemic side-effects [4, 5]. Without a means to cross the blood–tissue interface formed by the vascular endothelium, therapies will remain circulating in the blood until degraded and removed, ultimately unable to interact with and destroy tumor cells [3, 6]. To bypass these problems, accessible new targets and ways to penetrate into a specific tissue such as a solid tumor *in vivo* are needed.

11.3
Defining New Target Spaces

Traditionally, therapeutic targets were identified by comparing tumors to normal tissue to identify genes and proteins that were altered with tumor progression. The "therapeutic target space" is extremely broad in scope. Genomic and proteomic technologies have rapidly advanced large-scale expression analysis to identify thousands of potential tumor targets [7, 8]. The proteins constituting the therapeutic target space are usually identified from the majority of cells residing within the tumor that form the solid mass, rendering them mostly inaccessible to compounds injected into the blood. The sheer number of "hits" can overwhelm the necessary, but time-consuming, *in vivo* validation process [9–14]. Some researchers have even questioned whether "omics" will ever provide clinically useful targets [13]. The challenge in target discovery today clearly has become identifying which few of the many potential targets are readily accessible to agents circulating in the blood and, thus, form an "accessible target space."

11.3.1
Vascular Endothelium as an Accessible Target Space

All blood vessels are lined by a layer of endothelial cells that form a barrier between the blood and tissue. Endothelial cells play an important role in blood vessel permeability, vasoregulation, tissue metabolism and growth, and overall organ homeostasis. Endothelial cells also play a key role in many pathological events, such as coagulation, inflammation, tissue edema, hypoxia, and even tumor metastasis [15, 16].

The vascular endothelium offers a promising, alternative target to tumor cells sequestered inside the cancerous tissue [3, 17–20]. The vascular endothelium is in direct contact with the blood and is, therefore, accessible to antibodies, probes, or other agents that are injected intravenously. Additionally, endothelial cells are highly adapted to meet the needs of the underlying tissue. When endothelial cells are transplanted into a new microenvironment, they rapidly adapt to take on the phenotype and function of the local vasculature [21–27]. Defining the proteins present in the accessible target space may uncover tissue- or tumor-specific molecules that may be useful as targets for site-directed delivery of drugs, genes, or imaging agents (Figure 11.1).

Tumor vascular targeting is likely to be very powerful as a means to deliver therapeutic agents directly to diseased tissue. Primarily, endothelial cell targets are directly accessible to intravenously injected antibodies, while tumor cell targets require delivery into the tumor to be effective. Vascular targeting of antibodies conjugated to imaging agents may provide useful diagnostic and prognostic tools for detection and assessment of primary tumors, and even metastatic lesions whose vasculatures appear to be quite similar to that of the primary tumor. Site-specific vascular targeting of antibodies linked to cytotoxic agents could also prevent tumor growth. Damage to only one endothelial cell is sufficient to initiate coagulation and occlusion of a microvessel serving hundreds and even thousands of tumor cells. Several mAbs that target tumor vasculature have been developed and are in clinical trials [28]. Although large-scale identification and quantification of tumor vascular targets has only just begun, the results are promising [28–31].

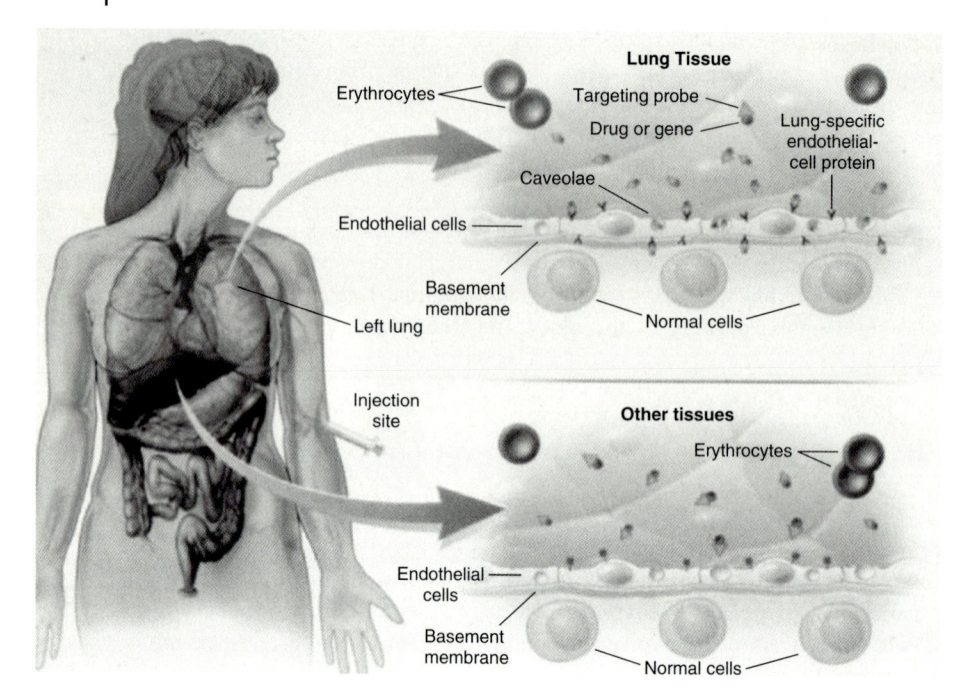

Figure 11.1 Schematic overview of the accessible target space. Intravenously injected agents can bind proteins expressed at the luminal surface of endothelial cells and exposed to the blood. If those proteins are only exposed to the blood in a specific tissue, *in vivo* single-organ targeting is possible.

11.3.2
Pathways Across the Endothelium

Vascular targeting is a significant advance over simple systemic delivery of drugs; however, penetration into target tissue or tumors is still necessary to access many therapeutic targets. Sinusoidal endothelium, found in liver, spleen, and bone marrow, and fenestrated endothelium, found in kidneys, endocrine glands, and intestines, are relatively permissive barriers with large intracellular gaps or transcellular openings that allow the relatively rapid exchange of molecules from the blood into and out of tissue. However, continuous endothelium forms a tight barrier that is far more restrictive.

Although endothelial cells form a barrier between blood and tissue, transport across the endothelial cell barrier is essential to support the underlying tissue. Therefore, endothelial cells must have transport pathways to move blood-borne nutrients into the tissue. It may be possible to exploit these transport mechanisms to target therapies into tissue and tumors. Although diffusion and convection provide access for small molecules, water, and solutes [32], larger molecules may require active transport to move into or across endothelial cells.

11.3.3
Caveolae as a Transvascular Pumping Target Space

Caveolae are one form of active transport present in endothelial cells. Caveolae are abundant, 60-nm flask-shaped invaginations found at the plasma membrane in most continuous endothelia that may be involved in endocytosis and transcytosis [33–39]. *In vivo*, caveolae can occupy up to 50–70% of the endothelial cell plasma membrane [40–42].

The possible role of caveolae in transport has been vigorously debated since caveolae were first discovered and described in 1953 [39, 43]. Over 50 years of *in vitro* and *in vivo* evidence has accumulated to suggest that caveolae can indeed function as active transport vesicles. As shown in Figure 11.2, caveolae form an important subdomain of the accessible target space and may indeed function as a "transvascular pumping target space."

Caveolae contain much of the classic machinery needed for vesicular budding and fusion, including NSF (N-ethylmaleimide-sensitive factor), SNAP (soluble NSF attachment protein), v-SNARES (SNAP receptors), and several GTPases known to play roles in vesicle budding [44]. Much like other vesicular pathways, caveolae-mediated endocytosis is sensitive to N-ethylmaleimide, a thioalkylating agent that inhibits the fusion of vesicles to target membranes [45, 46].

Isolated endothelial cell membranes with caveolae attached allow the final stages of caveolae budding to be studied in relative isolation. When GTP and ATP are added to isolated plasma membranes, caveolae budding is induced. Free caveolae can be isolated and verified by Western analysis and electron microscopy. This

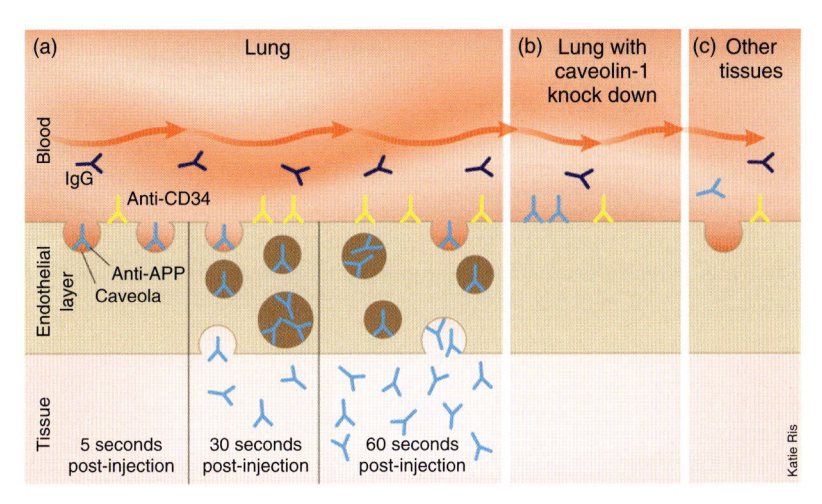

Figure 11.2 Overview of caveolae-dependent trafficking of antibodies. (a) Antibodies that target caveolae (anti-APP, light blue) are rapidly transcytosed. Antibodies that bind outside of caveolae (anti-CD34, yellow) bind the endothelial cell surface but are not transcytosed. Nonspecific IgG molecules (dark blue) stayed in the blood. (b) Transcytosis does not occur in the absence of caveolae. (c) Anti-APP does not accumulate in other organs that express little to no APP, even if these tissues have caveolae.

reconstituted, cell-free, in vitro assay was used to identify dynamin as the GTPase mediating this fission. Dynamin forms a ring around the neck of caveolae, likely acting as a pinchase to form free vesicles [47, 48]. This was subsequently confirmed in hepatocytes [49], which have readily apparent caveolae in cell culture, but interestingly have very few to no caveolae natively in liver tissue in vivo. Thus, caveolae can bud to form free vesicles in an energy-dependent manner.

Cultured endothelial cells have been used to show that caveolae can endocytose select ligands, such as cholera toxin and albumin–gold complexes [50–52]. Caveolae may also provide a route of entry for many viruses, including SV40 [53, 54], ebolavirus [55], and polyomavirus [56, 57]. Transport is dependent on caveolae; when cholesterol-binding agents, such as filipin, are used to reduce caveolae number, transport is significantly decreased [58, 59].

Caveolin-1 knockout mice provide needed insight into the role of caveolae in vivo. Caveolins are structural coat proteins that oligomerize around the bulb of caveolae, and appear necessary for caveolae formation in vitro and in vivo [60–66]. Although viable, these animals lack all caveolae in microvascular endothelium. Albumin and albumin–gold particles interact with caveolae proteins in vivo and can be endo- or transcytosed by caveolae [33, 35, 67, 68]. In caveolin-1 knockout mice, albumin–gold particles still bound to the endothelial cell surface in vivo, but were not transported into or across endothelial cells [69]. As often happens with knockout mice, compensatory pathways likely mediate transport of essential nutrients and other molecules to underlying tissue cells. Indeed, these animals demonstrate increased paracellular transport and overall microvascular permeability [62, 69, 70].

More recent studies have explored the in vivo function of caveolae using lung tissue engrafted into the dorsal skinfold window chamber. Here as well, caveolae have been shown to pump targeted antibodies out of the blood and into underlying tissue. Antibodies targeted to caveolae were rapidly pumped into lung tissue and quickly spread throughout the tissue (Figure 11.3). When short hairpin RNA was used to acutely knockout down caveolin-1 expression in the engrafted tissue, all rapid transport was lost (Figure 11.3) [71]. Additionally, control IgG and antibodies that bound outside of caveolae were not pumped into tissue (Figure 11.3), strongly indicating that rapid transendothelial movement of antibodies was dependent on caveolae. Thus, caveolae clearly form an important target space that merits further exploration.

11.3.4
Applying the Concept of New Target Spaces to Solid Tumors

Solid tumors interact in a complex manner with the surrounding microenvironment. Tumor cells alter, and are altered by, their surrounding microenvironment, including the stroma, vasculature, extracellular matrix, and circulating immune cells. Most tumors depend heavily on sufficient vascularization for nutrition, growth, and metastasis. Without the ability to recruit new blood vessels rapidly, most tumors would remain quite small with a diameter of 1–2 mm (passive diffusion-limited size) and localized to their primary site [72–74]. Many tumors,

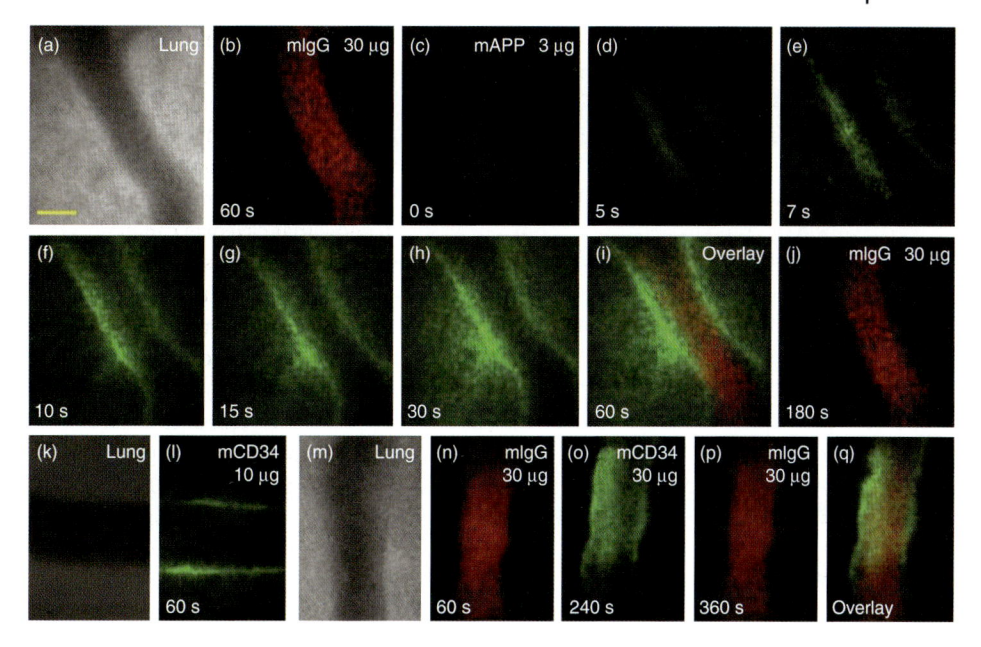

Figure 11.3 Trafficking of fluorescently labeled antibodies. (a–j) Mice with engrafted lung tissue were intravenously injected with fluorescent control mIgG (red) followed by lung-specific antibodies (T3.883, green) 60 s later. Fluorescent images were recorded at the given times after injection. (k–q) Mice with engrafted lung tissue were intravenously injected with fluorescent antibodies against CD34 (J120, green) and/or mIgG (red) and imaged at the given times.

especially malignant ones, are highly vascularized [21, 25, 26], and the microcirculatory blood supply limits tumor growth, size, and metastatic potential [9, 11–14, 17].

Tumor microvessels are originally derived from normal vessels, but their morphology differs significantly [3]. Tumor vessels form a chaotic network of dilated vessels that lack the strict organization of the vasculature of normal organs. The capillaries of neoplastic tissues also show increased permeability for macromolecules [75, 76], reduced basement membrane development with altered composition [11, 12], increased proliferation rate of the endothelial cells [77], and altered cellular composition of the blood vessels themselves [73, 74]. These abnormalities of the tumor vasculature are accompanied by phenotypic changes where some normal endothelial intracellular and surface markers appear to be absent [78]. Since tumors depend on neovascularization for growth and metastasis, and marked changes occur in both the phenotype and function of tumor vasculature, many investigators have suggested that both the process of angiogenesis and the vasculature itself are potential targets for tumor therapy [9, 10, 13, 74, 75, 79]. Defining the accessible target space in tumors will likely yield targets that can mediate *in vivo* delivery as well as identify new therapeutic targets that can inhibit tumor progression.

The tumor endothelium, along with the fibrous stroma and high interstitial pressures in tumors, form substantial barriers that can limit transport from the circulatory blood directly into the tumor, thereby preventing the therapy from reaching its intended target to be effective [3, 6]. Thus, even with a specific probe, crossing the vascular wall to penetrate deeply throughout solid tumors can be a significant problem and may severely limit targeted anticancer therapies *in vivo*.

Tumor vascular endothelium also has caveolae, but little is known about their molecular architecture, function, and possible clinical utility, in part because tumor-induced caveolar targets have yet to be discovered. Understanding caveolae function and defining the proteins present in the transvascular pumping target space is essential to both target and penetrate into solid tumors *in vivo*.

11.4
Difficulties in Studying Endothelial Cells

Although the endothelial cell surface and its caveolae form important target spaces, endothelial cells are only a small fraction of any whole-tissue homogenate. Even highly enriched endothelial cell proteins can be missed when the total organ homogenate is analyzed [80]. Studying endothelial cells requires a reliable method to isolate these cells from the entire tissue.

11.4.1
Endothelial Cells in Culture

Isolating a specific cell type and growing cells *in vitro* allows direct access and manipulation of cultured cells. In the late 1970s, two groups independently isolated and successfully cultured endothelial cells [81, 82]. These studies provided vital insight into the molecular components and functions of endothelial cells, and revealed how sensitive the cells are to changes in the environment, including alteration in cell morphology and protein expression when exposed to different vasoactive compounds, cytokines, shear stress, or inflammatory compounds. This enabled the discovery of novel adhesion molecules and receptors [83–86].

As studies of endothelial cells advanced, it became apparent that endothelial cells in culture differ significantly from those *in vivo*. Once in culture, endothelial cells isolated from unique vascular beds de-differentiate into a more common phenotype [87–89]. They lose many of their distinctive characteristics found *in vivo* including expression of tissue-specific proteins as well as the usual abundance of caveolae which decreases 30- to 100-fold in cultured endothelial cells [88]. More recent mass spectrometry (MS) analysis shows a profound change in protein expression *in vitro* versus *in vivo*. Approximately 40% of the proteins expressed *in vivo* are not found *in vitro* [90]; thus, endothelial cells and their caveolae should be studied *in vivo* to best maintain their protein functions and phenotype.

11.4.2
Historic Approaches to Vascular Mapping

Numerous techniques have been developed to focus on proteins expressed at the luminal surface of endothelial cells, including lectin analysis, iodination, biotinylation, and silica-coating techniques. These techniques were first applied *in vitro* and have since been adapted for use *in vivo* as it became apparent that cultured endothelial cells are quite different from endothelial cells retained in their *in vivo* environment. As proteins at the surface of endothelial cells *in vitro* and *in vivo* are directly exposed to the media or circulating blood, they also can be labeled by reagents added directly to the media of cultured cells, perfused through the vasculature, or injected intravenously in the intact animal [91–94]. Different lectins can bind to different sets of surface glycoproteins. Lectin analysis has been used to identify changes between different segments of vasculature [95], different organs [92], different species [96], and *in vitro* versus *in situ* protein expression [94]. *In vitro* radioiodination of surface compounds identified albumin-binding proteins [51, 97]. However, *in situ* radiolabeling requires high amounts of ^{125}I in excess of 10 mCi, which makes this process difficult [94]. Additionally, small radionuclides can readily enter the underlying tissue and radiolabel nonendothelial cells. As there is no simple way to separate and identify radiolabeled proteins, radiolabeling is most often used to verify the presence of known proteins in a sample.

Biotinylation of surface proteins is a significant advance for vascular mapping because the strong interaction between biotin and avidin can be used to purify the biotinylated proteins, which can then be identified with MS [98, 99] or antibodies [100–104]. Surface biotinylation has been used to identify proteins at the endothelial cell surface [98, 105] and components of cell junctions [100], to determine differences between luminal and abluminal cell surfaces [103, 106], to identify signaling molecules present at the cell surface [104], and to determine the protein composition of different membrane subdomains [101]. Importantly, *in vivo* biotinylation of the endothelial cell surface identifies a unique pattern of proteins from the whole-tissue homogenate, showing that this method isolates a subset of proteins [98, 99, 105, 107]. Unfortunately, it is difficult to control the degree and specificity of biotinylation *in vivo*. Biotin may not have equal access to all parts of the cell surface and all proteins may not be biotinylated similarly. Biotinylation reagents are quite small and can readily enter almost all tissues to label perivascular proteins in the surrounding tissue [98]. They can even cross lipid membranes and label intracellular components. Using polar or charged biotinylation reagents can reduce entry inside cells, but access into tissue remains and greatly complicates identification of tissue-specific endothelial cell surface proteins useful for direct targeting of antibodies, proteins, nanoparticles, and gene vectors.

In contrast to iodination and biotinylation, colloidal silica particles offer a strategy to specifically label proteins at the endothelial cell surface (Figure 11.4). When perfused through the vasculature *in vivo*, colloidal silica nanoparticles coat the exposed

Multiple methods exist to identify the proteins present in a sample, including two-dimensional gels, proteins arrays, and MS. In two-dimensional gels, mixtures of proteins are separated by two distinct properties such as molecular weight and isoelectric point, providing better separation between proteins [121]. Tissue-specific spots are easily identified, and can be excised and identified by MS [29, 30]. Successful identification of proteins requires that the proteins migrate onto the gel. Many proteins simply do not separate well on such gels and can be under-represented or lost altogether. Protein arrays use antibodies or peptides to identify the proteins present in the sample, but are limited by affinity of the probes and the complexity of the sample [122]. MS offers a high-throughput method to rapidly identify large numbers of proteins based on the presence of digested peptides; however, highly complex samples are difficult to separate and low abundance proteins can be lost [123].

11.6
MS-Based Approaches to Map the Vascular Endothelial Cell Proteome

Although far simpler than total tissue homogenate, isolated endothelial cell membranes and their caveolae are still a highly complex mixture of proteins. Additionally, integral membrane proteins present a special challenge for MS-based identifications. Plasma membrane proteins, regardless of the cell or tissue of origin, have generally been under-represented in proteomics analysis mainly due to their low abundance. In addition, the inherent insolubility of membrane proteins due to their hydrophobic nature have rendered them difficult to isolate and identify compared to cytosolic and nuclear proteins. In many high-throughput protein identification approaches, soluble proteomes are readily characterized. It is not uncommon for thousands of proteins to be identified in such samples. However, when more challenging proteomes are analyzed, the numbers of proteins identified are significantly lower [29, 31, 124]. Poor identification of integral membrane proteins can significantly impact characterization of key target spaces, such as the accessible target space and the transvascular pumping target space.

Recent reports show that an additional gel-based preparation step can greatly enhance protein identification, especially for integral membrane proteins [31]. To create a three-dimensional MS approach, proteins were first separated by size on sodium dodecyl sulfate polyacrylamide gel electrophoresis gels and digested in gel, before being used in traditional two-dimensional MS methods such as MudPIT [31], as shown schematically in Figure 11.5. These experiments showed that gel prefractionation dramatically increased sensitivity, identified greater numbers of proteins, provided better protein coverage, and identified proteins across a broad dynamic range. While previous analysis of the lung vascular plasma membranes identified 450 proteins [29], these three-dimensional MS/MS approaches identified 1834 proteins [123].

11.6 MS-Based Approaches to Map the Vascular Endothelial Cell Proteome

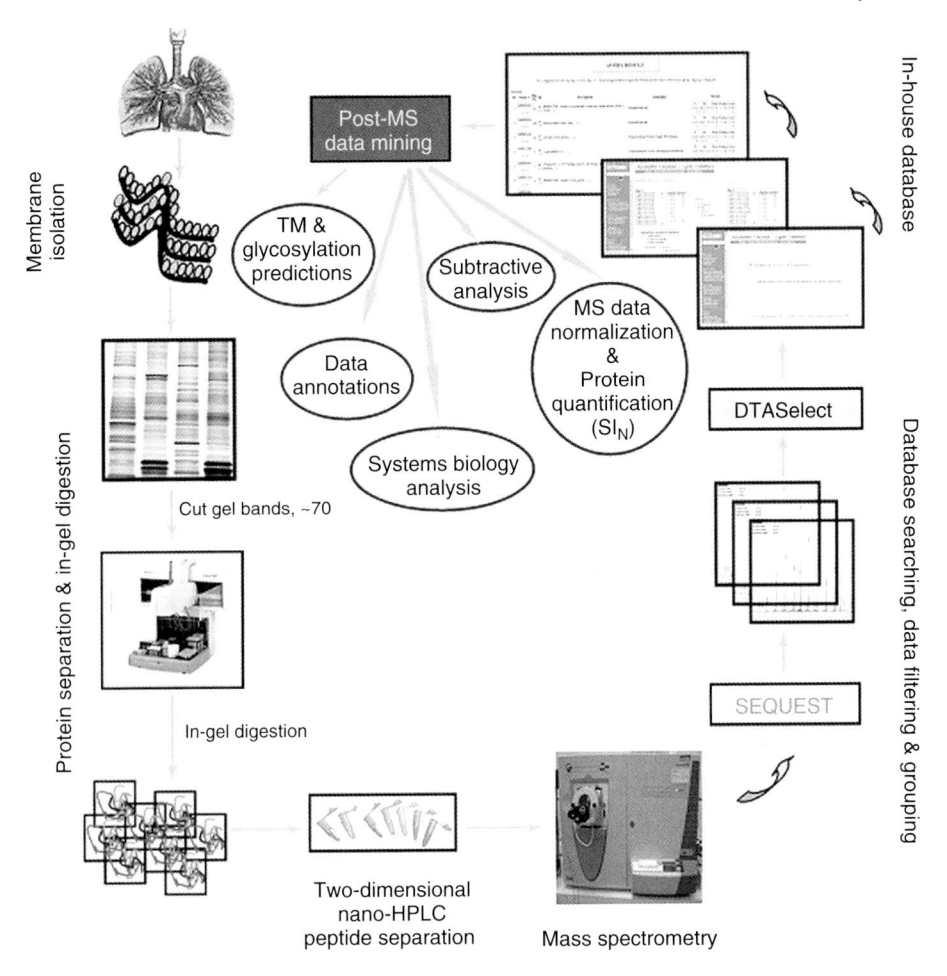

Figure 11.5 Schematic illustration of the proteomics approach developed to more comprehensively map complex proteomes. Shown is the workflow from sample submission, sample separation, sample digestion, peptide separations, MS analysis, database searching, quantification, and data mining that cumulates in the quantitative mapping of a given proteome.

11.6.1
Defining Analytical Completeness

Current large-scale MS-based approaches cannot identify all proteins in a complex sample. Although subfractionation helps reduce the complexity for membrane proteomes, it is still not possible to identify every protein and its modifications in a complex sample. Therefore, replicate measurements are absolutely necessary to maximize the ability of a single method to identify proteins. When a sample of endothelial cell plasma membrane was repeatedly analyzed, seven to 10 replicates were needed to reach 95% analytical completeness (Figure 11.6) [29]. After this

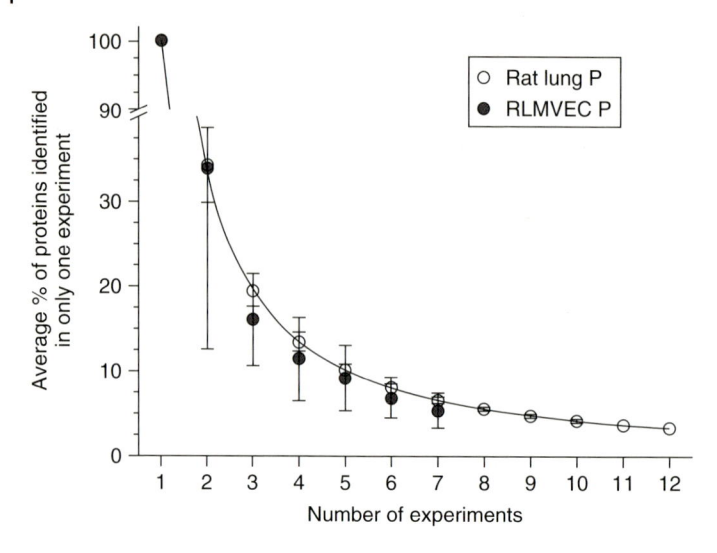

Figure 11.6 Confidence of analytical completeness is calculated as a function of the number of analytical runs. Each point represents the percentage of proteins identified only in an individual run compared to all preceding experiments. RLMVC, rat lung microvascular endothelial cell.

point, additional replicates failed to identify significant amounts of new proteins. Comprehensive measurement is clearly necessary to define the endothelial cell proteins within a given tissue and to identify differences between tissues.

11.6.2
Quantification and Normalization of MS Data

Multiple replicate measurements and even multiple MS-based approaches are likely necessary to comprehensively define the proteins present in a sample. MS measurements contain inherent biases and variations. Replicate samples, regardless of the abundance feature used, will usually show variation in protein abundance that is likely not a reflection of biological change. Proper quantification and normalization is needed to minimize inherent experimental bias and variability so that real changes between distinct samples can be reliably detected.

Currently, MS experiments rely on chemically [125] or biosynthetically tagged proteins [126] in order to quantify relative differences in protein expression [127]. Although these methods are valuable, comparisons between multiple datasets and with previously existing data are impossible. Additionally, labeling agents are expensive, add extra analytical complexity, and require additional MS/MS spectra interpretation. To overcome these limitations, there has been much interest in developing new, label-free methods to normalize and quantify MS data [128–133]. Most label-free methods are based on using one MS output feature of abundance, such as spectral or peptide counts [130, 131, 134, 135] to determine relative protein abundance of a target protein in several samples. Other measures, such as chromatographic peak intensity and peak area have also been shown to correlate with protein abundance [136–141], but these measures require complex algorithms to integrate the area under the curve or total elution curve for each isotope pattern.

Recent studies suggest that combining measures of MS abundance may provide more accurate normalization and quantification of MS data. We have recently developed and validated a novel label-free method of MS quantification and normalization that we call SI_N [142]. By normalizing data around a Spectral Index that takes peptide number, spectral count, peak precursor ion intensities, and protein length into account, this method reduces variance between replicates and across a dynamic range of protein loads. In addition, SI_N can accurately determine the correct amount of each protein standard in a mixture better than other tested methods, thus allowing the quantitative comparison of biologically distinct datasets with high confidence and relative ease [142].

11.7
Means to Validation

A single organ or tumor likely contains more than 100 000 distinct proteins. Tissue prefractionation reduces the number of potential targets to around 2000 proteins identified in the accessible target space [29, 31]. Subtractive proteomics and bioinformatic interrogation reduces proteins further to those few endothelial cell surface proteins (less than 100) that are accessible and exhibit apparent specificity for a single tissue [29–31]. Currently, detailed proteomic characterization of major organs has not been completed for any organism, especially humans. Thus, we cannot rely on MS-based analyses to validate tissue-specific protein expression. Instead, Western analysis, tissue immunostaining, and *in vivo* dynamic imaging of antibody targeting can be used to provide the necessary validation that protein targets are both accessible and sufficiently specific to enable tumor targeting *in vivo*.

Western analysis is a straightforward technique to test tissue specificity of a target protein. To verify restricted tissue expression, the probe can be tested against proteins isolated from many different organs [30]. Additionally, the localization of the target protein can be assessed by analyzing whole-tissue homogenates as well as different subfractions [71]. Further localization of the probe to a specific cell type or even subcellular domain such as caveolae can be further verified in tissue slices by using immunohistochemistry, immunofluorescence, and electron microscopy [71].

Western analysis and tissue staining can localize a protein to the endothelial cell plasma membrane, but true accessibility of the protein to antibodies in the blood must be verified. The classic way to determine protein accessibility is to inject radiolabeled probes. At various times following intravenous injection, major tissue types can be dissected and analyzed for biodistribution analysis, which quantifies the amount of radioactivity in each dissected organ. Biodistribution analysis allows a quantitative assessment of the tissue distribution of the probe. By extracting tissue at different time points after injection, an approximate time course can also be created [143]. Biodistribution analyses are robust and quantitative, but also invasive and static, requiring the killing of many animals at each time point.

Numerous *in vivo* imaging systems have been developed to provide a more dynamic analysis of *in vivo* events. γ-Scintigraphic [144], positron emission tomography [145], and luminescence imaging [146] are noninvasive methods that provide visual as well as quantitative analysis of probe targeting. Importantly, these methods can be used over time in the same animal, reducing the number of animals needed and increasing statistical power. Moreover, minor tissues that are difficult to isolate can also be studied with *in vivo* imaging. The methods can provide important quantitative data for assessing targeting at the whole-body and organ level, but unfortunately, do not have the resolution required to image probe processing at the cellular level.

Intravital microscopy (IVM) is rapidly becoming a powerful method to obtain analysis of cellular events *in vivo*. Especially when paired with tissue or tumors growing in dorsal skinfold window chambers, IVM is a noninvasive method to image and quantify many cellular events, such as immune cell migration, mitosis, pyknosis and apoptosis, and the growth and connectivity of blood vessels. IVM is especially powerful for visualizing and quantifying targeting, processing and efficacy of candidate antibody probes (e.g., transendothelial transport by caveolae with interstitial accumulation). Thus, IVM can present a high-resolution, dynamic view of endothelial cell targeting as well as the movement of probes into tissue, ultimately to better assess tissue and tumor targeting, uptake and accumulation in live animals [71].

To obtain even more detailed analysis of cellular events, probes can be intravenously injected and at set times following injection, tissue can be excised. The probe can then be localized with immunohistochemistry, immunofluorescence, and/or electron microscopy. This provides valuable confirmation of the ability of antibody to target the endothelial cell surface, to be transcytosed across the endothelial cell barrier, and to penetrate deep into the tissue. This is especially important to determine subcellular organelles such as caveolae are involved in probe transport. However, these are static methods and can only provide "snapshots" over time. Combining multiple imaging modalities is likely necessary to create an accurate picture of protein targeting and processing *in vivo*.

Ultimately, targeting and penetration of probes into human tissue and tumors are the most clinically relevant experiments. However, few methods exist to directly study human tissue and tumors to assess experimental therapies. Therefore, relevant animal models must be developed and studied. Almost all new therapies progress to human clinical trials largely justified by their efficacy in subcutaneous tumor models [147–149]. However, the vast majority of these treatments fail in humans for unknown reasons. Indeed, tumors are often treated as a "black box" where treatment is injected and outcome observed without knowledge of the dynamic events and interplay that occurred *in vivo*. Clearly, new techniques are needed to bridge the gap between rodent and human studies and speed clinical translation of new therapies. Enhancing the ability to image the cellular responses to therapy in real time may indeed be the first step in understanding how therapies work and devising better treatments for human disease.

11.8
In vivo Tissue Targeting: The Lungs as Proof of Principle

Several proteins, including angiotensin-converting enzyme [150], and the cell adhesion molecules PECAM [151, 152] and ICAM [152], have been used to specifically target the lung and to deliver therapeutic compounds *in vivo*. A partial list of endothelial cell proteins found in lung and tumor vasculature can be found in Table 11.1. Although these probes have great utility to target the vasculature and even deliver therapies to vascular endothelial cells, without a means to bypass the endothelial barrier, many of these antibodies and their cargo will remain bound at the endothelial cell surface and unable to reach cells within the underlying tissue, which is often the therapeutic target.

Our ability to quantitatively map protein expression at the blood–tissue barrier led to the identification of key target proteins in lung and solid tumors that are

Table 11.1 Endothelial cell proteins found in lung and tumor vasculature (partial list).

Markers	Lung	Tumor	Other tissue
Lung endothelial markers			
ACE	highly enriched	present	heart, kidney, and liver
APP2	highly enriched	not expressed	none
Aquaporin 1	present	present	heart and kidney
Carbonic anhydrase	highly enriched	not expressed	heart, kidney, and liver
DDPIV	enriched	enriched	liver
ECE	present	present	heart, kidney, and liver
OX-45	highly enriched	not expressed	none
PV-1	highly enriched	highly enriched	heart, kidney, and liver
RAGE	present	present	heart and liver
STR	present	present	heart, kidney, and liver
TM	present	present	heart, kidney, and liver
Tumor endothelial markers			
AnnA1	none	highly enriched	none
AnnA8	low	highly enriched	none
APN	present	enriched	heart
C-CAM	enriched	present	liver
Endoglin	present	present	heart and liver
EphrinA5	present	present	heart, kidney, and liver
EphrinA7	low	present	heart, kidney, and liver
MPO	low	enriched	heart
Neuropilin	low	present	heart and liver
Nucleolin	present	enriched	heart
TfR	present	enriched	heart and liver
Tie2	low	enriched	kidney and liver
VEGFR1	low	highly enriched	kidney
VEGFR2	low	present	heart, kidney, and liver
VitDBP	none	enriched	liver

sufficiently specific to mediate *in vivo* targeting (see Figure 11.7 for an example of lung targeting). These studies are presented here as proof of principle of the power of focusing global identification strategies on key target spaces.

We have identified aminopeptidase P2 (APP2) as uniquely enriched in lung endothelial cells. APP2 is highly abundant and concentrated in endothelial cell caveolae. Indeed, APP2 is one of the most caveolae-specific proteins, making it an attractive target for further work [71]. Electron microscopy showed that APP2 antibodies specifically immunolabel caveolae in vascular lung endothelium and can target colloidal gold nanoparticles to caveolae after pulmonary artery perfusion *in situ* (Figure 11.8) [18, 71]. Little to no labeling of caveolae was seen with control antibodies.

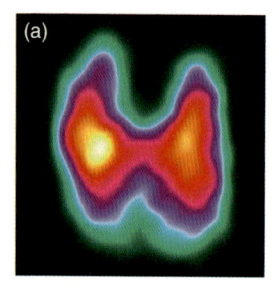

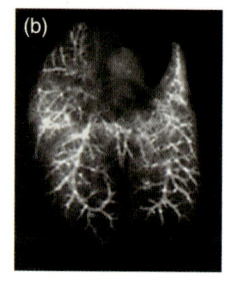

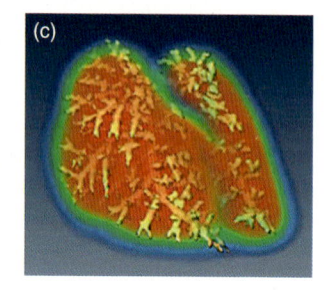

Figure 11.7 APP2 antibodies specifically target the lungs. ^{125}I-labeled antibodies to APP2 were injected intravenously. After 24 h, lungs were isolated, perfused with an X-ray contrast agent via the pulmonary artery and imaged with planar γ-scintigraphic (a), X-ray (b), and tomographic SPECT/CT (c). X-ray and CT scans showed the pulmonary arterial tree. Three-dimensional visualization after CT and SPECT data sets were acquired is shown in overlap (c).

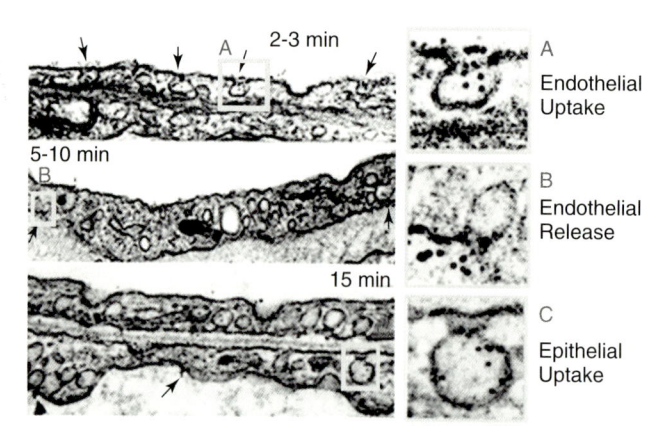

Figure 11.8 Sequential transcytosis of APP2-specific antibodies by caveolae. The rat lung was perfused *in situ* with APP2 antibodies linked to 5- to 10-nm gold nanoparticles and processed for electron microscopy at the indicated times. Gold nanoparticles could be readily found within endothelial caveolae. Some gold nanoparticles were also taken up by epithelial caveolae and even delivered into the airspace.

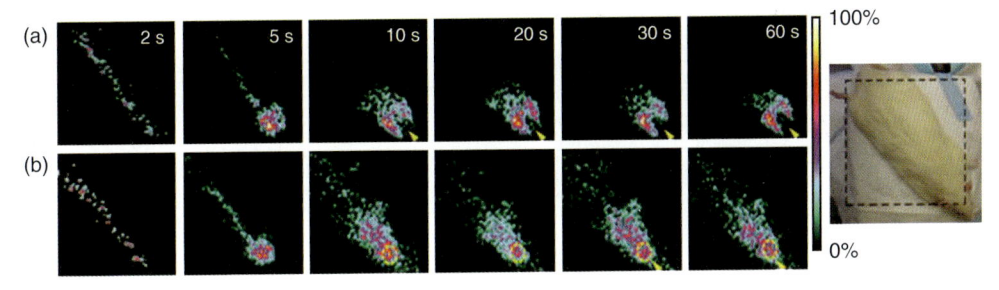

Figure 11.9 Dynamic and planar γ-scintigraphic live imaging of rapid lung immunotargeting *in vivo*. Rats were imaged at 1-s intervals immediately following tail vein injection with (a) ^{125}I-labeled lung-specific antibodies or (b) ^{125}I-labeled mIgG. Arrowheads (a) and dotted yellow line (b) denote the heart. Photo, right panel, shows orientation of the rat during imaging.

To dynamically follow antibody targeting in real-time at high resolution, we performed IVM by engrafting rat lung tissue into dorsal skinfold window chambers on nude mice [71]. Fluorescently conjugated APP2 antibodies bound to the lung endothelial cells within seconds of intravenous injection and quickly penetrated throughout the lung tissue in less than 2 min (see Figure 11.3) [71]. At all times, the signal inside blood vessels remained negligible [71]. Thus, by definition, this transendothelial transport is an active process because it occurred against an appreciable concentration gradient. Targeting caveolae was necessary for active pumping. Control IgG did not leak into tissue; other antibodies that bound the endothelial cell surface outside of caveolae were not pumped into lung; APP2 antibodies could bind, but were not pumped into lung tissue that lacked caveolae due to caveolin-1 knockdown (see Figure 11.3) [71].

Dynamic γ-scintigraphy verified the speed and specificity of lung targeting by intravenous injected radiolabeled APP2 antibodies. The lung silhouette was first evident within 10 s postinjection (Figure 11.9) [71]. The lung signal was specific by 1 min and reached a maximum within 2 min [71, 153]. In contrast, control IgG was detected throughout the entire rat without any lung targeting [71]. The strong, specific lung signal seen with APP2 antibodies was maintained essentially unchanged from 1 to 24 h, as shown by biodistribution analysis and hybrid single photon emission computed tomography/computed tomography (SPECT/CT) [71]. Quite significant levels were detected specifically in the lung for up to 30 days [71, 153]. Our most recent analysis showed that more than 80% of APP2 antibody bound on the first pass through isolated, perfused lungs [153].

11.9 Targeting Lung Tumors

When injected into rats bearing lung tumors, APP2 antibodies did not traffic to the tumors, but instead concentrated in surrounding, tumor-free lung tissue

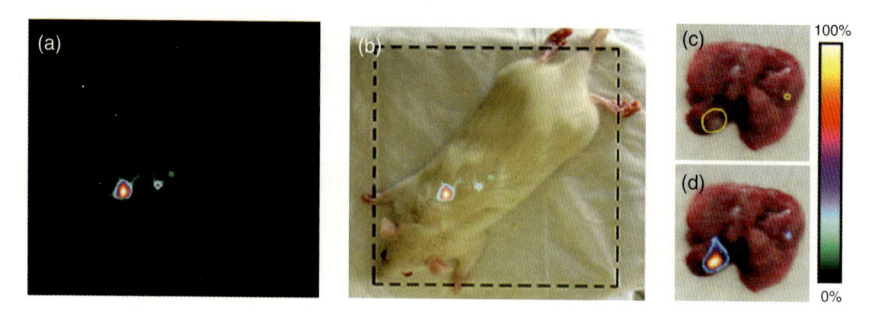

Figure 11.10 Tumor-bearing rats were intravenously injected with ^{125}I-labeled TC1 antibodies and imaged 4 h later (a) and (b). Tumor-bearing lungs were excised for imaging. Tumors, circled in yellow (c), could be seen to overlap with hotspots from planar imaging (d).

[30]. When the luminal endothelial surface of vasculature from lung tumors was isolated and run on a two-dimensional blot, a distinct pattern of proteins was seen, suggesting that the solid tumors might form a distinct type of tissue. When this extract was further analyzed with MS and Western analysis, APP2 expression was lost. As expected, several known tumor angiogenesis markers were upregulated. One surprising result was the apparent induced expression of Annexin-A1 (AnnA1) specifically at the endothelial cell surface of vasculature in solid tumors; AnnA1 did not appear at the surface of vascular endothelial cells in normal organs. Immunohistochemistry showed that AnnA1 was also found in diverse human solid tumors (prostate, liver, breast, lung), but not matched normal tissue. AnnA1 was indeed accessible to the blood. Intravenously injected AnnA1 antibodies specifically targeted tumor vasculature, but did not accumulate in normal lung tissues (Figure 11.10). Although tumor-bearing mice treated with radiolabeled, isotype-matched control IgG died, injections of radiolabeled AnnA1 antibodies drastically increased animal survival and led to the virtual elimination of the tumors even many times after just one injection [30]. This increased survival is striking because in this model, many animals die within 2–4 days of treatment and thus may lack sufficient time to benefit from the treatment.

Although AnnA1 has been studied for decades, no clear function for this protein has been established [154]. We have recently used AnnA1 knockout mice to show that this protein plays an important role in angiogenesis [155], namely significant retardation of vessel growth as compared to control mice. As a likely consequence, tumor growth and metastasis are significantly decreased (Figure 11.11), while rodent survival and tumor necrosis are greatly increased when tumors are grown in AnnA1 knockout mice [155]. Thus, our quantitative proteomic studies have revealed key targets that can mediate *in vivo* tumor targeting as well as new therapeutic targets.

11.9 Targeting Lung Tumors | **345**

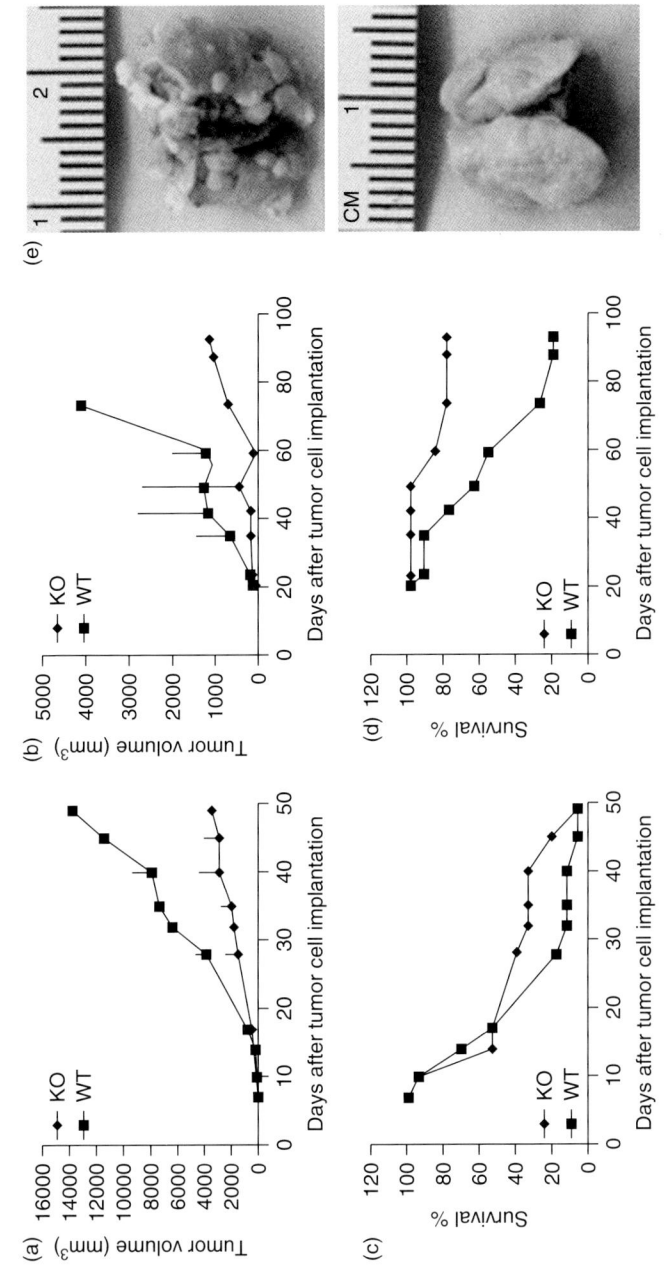

Figure 11.11 Impaired tumor growth and spontaneous metastasis in AnnA1 knockout mice. Subcutaneous tumors in AnnA1 knockout mice grew slower (a, b) and metastasized slower (C, D) than tumors in wild wild-type mice, regardless of tumor type (B16 tumors: A, C; LLC tumors: B, D). Lungs of mice with primary subcutaneous LLC tumors were excised at day 38 (wild-type (WT) animals) and day 59 (knockout (KO) mice) after tumor cell implantation. Large numbers of metastases were found in wild-type mice (e, top) but not in AnnA1 knockout mice (e, bottom).

11.10
Future Directions

Specific delivery to the tumors could profoundly alter common treatment for many human cancers, enabling powerful new approaches including *in vivo* functional imaging, viral delivery of gene vectors, and nanoparticle-based delivery of drugs or effector molecules. Additionally, old therapies that have been abandoned due to toxicity could be engineered to specifically target the tumor.

If therapeutic agents can be specifically pumped into tissue, this may increase efficacy because a larger effective dose is delivered to the tumor. Once concentrated in tumors, targeted radionuclides may also destroy the local microvasculature, essentially trapping radiolabeled mAbs within tumors where they can continue to destroy tumor cells. Systemic side-effects are also likely to decrease because far less drug will be systemically available. Many types of tumors are often aggressive and can metastasize to the bones, liver, lungs, and brain; endothelial surface antigens associated with one type of tumor appear to be expressed in many different neoplastic and metastatic lesions [30, 156], which may facilitate the development of targeted therapies. Early diagnostic therapies are focused on physical exams. By targeting mAbs conjugated to imaging agents, it may also be possible to diagnose tumors at earlier stages and thereby increase survival rates.

Pumping functional and molecular imaging agents into tumors could provide a high signal/noise ratio and allow the *in vivo* state of diseased tissue to be interrogated in real time. Additionally, expression changes of proteins or biomarkers deep inside tumor tissue could be readily imaged noninvasively during development or physiological perturbations, as well as during disease onset and progression. Finally, the function of key pathways could be specifically tested, for instance, through the rapid delivery of inhibitory antibodies, peptides, DNA, or RNA into lung tissue for direct access to cells, allowing noninvasive analysis of complex protein interactions and signaling pathways *in vivo* with far greater control than is currently possible.

References

1. Strebhardt, K. and Ullrich, A. (2008) Paul Ehrlich's magic bullet concept: 100 years of progress. *Nat. Rev. Cancer*, **8**, 473–480.
2. Minchinton, A.I. and Tannock, I.F. (2006) Drug penetration in solid tumours. *Nat. Rev. Cancer*, **6**, 583–592.
3. Dvorak, H.F., Nagy, J.A., and Dvorak, A.M. (1991) Structure of solid tumors and their vasculature: implications for therapy with monoclonal antibodies. *Cancer Cells*, **3**, 77–85.
4. Baluna, R. and Vitetta, E.S. (1997) Vascular leak syndrome: a side effect of immunotherapy. *Immunopharmacology*, **37**, 117–132.
5. Vitetta, E.S. (2000) Immunotoxins and vascular leak syndrome. *Cancer J.*, **6** (Suppl. 3), S218–S224.
6. Huang, X. *et al.* (1997) Tumor infarction in mice by antibody-directed targeting of tissue factor to tumor vasculature. *Science*, **275**, 547–550.
7. Hanash, S. (2003) Disease proteomics. *Nature*, **422**, 226–232.
8. Stratton, M.R., Campbell, P.J., and Futreal, P.A. (2009) The cancer genome. *Nature*, **458**, 719–724.

9. Drews, J. (2000) Drug discovery: a historical perspective. *Science*, **287**, 1960–1964.
10. Lindsay, M.A. (2003) Target discovery. *Nat. Rev. Drug Discov.*, **2**, 831–838.
11. Workman, P. (2001) New drug targets for genomic cancer therapy: successes, limitations, opportunities and future challenges. *Curr. Cancer Drug Targets*, **1**, 33–47.
12. Anzick, S.L. and Trent, J.M. (2002) Role of genomics in identifying new targets for cancer therapy. *Oncology*, **16** (Suppl. 4), 7–13.
13. Huber, L.A. (2003) Is proteomics heading in the wrong direction? *Nat. Rev. Mol. Cell Biol.*, **4**, 74–80.
14. Perou, C.M. et al. (2000) Molecular portraits of human breast tumours. *Nature*, **406**, 747–752.
15. Fajardo, L.F. (1989) The complexity of endothelial cells. *Am. J. Clin. Pathol.*, **92**, 241–250.
16. Jaffe, E.A. (1987) Cell biology of endothelial cells. *Hum. Pathol.*, **18**, 234–239.
17. Carver, L.A. and Schnitzer, J.E. (2003) Caveolae: mining little caves for new cancer targets. *Nat. Rev. Cancer*, **3**, 571–581.
18. McIntosh, D.P. et al. (2002) Targeting endothelium and its dynamic caveolae for tissue-specific transcytosis in vivo: a pathway to overcome cell barriers to drug and gene delivery. *Proc. Natl. Acad. Sci. USA*, **99**, 1996–2001.
19. Burrows, F.J. and Thorpe, P.E. (1993) Eradication of large solid tumors in mice with an immunotoxin directed against tumor vasculature. *Proc. Natl. Acad. Sci. USA*, **90**, 8996–9000.
20. Schnitzer, J.E. (1998) Vascular targeting as a strategy for cancer therapy. *N. Engl. J. Med.*, **339**, 472–474.
21. Madri, J.A. and Williams, S.K. (1983) Capillary endothelial cell culture: phenotype modulation by matrix components. *J. Cell Biol.*, **97**, 153–165.
22. Goerdt, S. et al. (1989) Characterization and differential expression of an endothelial cell-specific surface antigen in continuous and sinusoidal endothelial, in skin vascular lesions and in vitro. *Exp. Cell Biol.*, **57**, 185–192.
23. Gumkowski, F. et al. (1987) Heterogeneity of mouse vascular endothelium. *Blood Vessels*, **24**, 11–23.
24. Hagemeier, H.H. et al. (1986) A monoclonal antibody reacting with endothelial cells of budding vessels in tumors and inflammatory tissues, and non-reactive with normal adult tissues. *Int. J. Cancer*, **38**, 481–488.
25. Aird, W.C. et al. (1997) Vascular bed-specific expression of an endothelial cell gene is programmed by the tissue microenvironment. *J. Cell Biol.*, **138**, 1117–1124.
26. Janzer, R.C. and Raff, M.C. (1987) Astrocytes induce blood–brain barrier properties in endothelial cells. *Nature*, **325**, 253–257.
27. Stewart, P.A. and Wiley, M.J. (1981) Developing nervous tissue induces formation of blood–brain barrier characteristics in invading endothelial cells: a study using quail-chick transplantation chimeras. *Dev. Biol.*, **84**, 183–192.
28. Schliemann, C. and Neri, D. (2010) Antibody-based vascular tumor targeting. *Recent Results Cancer Res.*, **180**, 201–216.
29. Durr, E. et al. (2004) Direct proteomic mapping of the lung microvascular endothelial cell surface in vivo and in cell culture. *Nat. Biotechnol.*, **22**, 985–992.
30. Oh, P. et al. (2004) Subtractive proteomic mapping of the endothelial surface in lung and solid tumours for tissue-specific therapy. *Nature*, **429**, 629–635.
31. Li, Y. et al. (2009) Enhancing identifications of lipid-embedded proteins by mass spectrometry for improved mapping of endothelial plasma membranes in vivo. *Mol. Cell Proteomics*, **8**, 1219–1235.
32. Wagner, R.C. and Chen, S.-C. (1991) Transcapillary transport of solute by the endothelial vesicular system: Evidence from thin serial section analysis. *Microvasc. Res.*, **42**, 139–150.
33. Milici, A.J. et al. (1987) Transcytosis of albumin in capillary endothelium. *J. Cell Biol.*, **105**, 2603–2612.
34. Ghitescu, L. and Bendayan, M. (1992) Transendothelial transport

of serum albumin: a quantitative immunocytochemical study. *J. Cell Biol.*, **117**, 745–755.

35. Ghitescu, L. et al. (1986) Specific binding sites for albumin restricted to plasmalemmal vesicles of continuous capillary endothelium: receptor-mediated transcytosis. *J. Cell Biol.*, **102**, 1304–1311.

36. Ghinea, N. et al. (1994) How protein hormones reach their target cells. Receptor-mediated transcytosis of hCG through endothelial cells. *J. Cell Biol.*, **125**, 87–97.

37. Schnitzer, J.E. et al. (1994) Caveolin-enriched caveolae purified from endothelium in situ are transport vesicles for albondin-mediated transcytosis of albumin. *Mol. Biol. Cell*, **5**, A75.

38. Jacobson, B.S., Stolz, D.B., and Schnitzer, J.E. (1996) Identification of endothelial cell-surface proteins as targets for diagnosis and treatment of disease. *Nat. Med.*, **2**, 482–484.

39. Palade, G.E. (1953) Fine structure of blood capillaries. *J. Appl. Phys.*, **24**, 1424.

40. Bruns, R.R. and Palade, G.E. (1968) Studies on blood capillaries. I. General organization of blood capillaries in muscle. *J. Cell Biol.*, **37**, 244–276.

41. Johansson, B.R. (1979) Size and distribution of endothelial plasmalemmal vesicles in consecutive segments of the microvasculature in cat skeletal muscle. *Microvasc. Res.*, **17**, 107–117.

42. Simionescu, M., Simionescu, N., and Palade, G.E. (1974) Morphometric data on the endothelium of blood capillaries. *J. Cell Biol.*, **60**, 128–152.

43. Severs, N.J. (1988) Caveolae: static in-pocketings of the plasma membrane, dynamic vesicles or plain artifact? *J. Cell Sci.*, **90**, 341–348.

44. Schnitzer, J.E., Liu, J., and Oh, P. (1995) Endothelial caveolae have the molecular transport machinery for vesicle budding, docking, and fusion including VAMP, NSF, SNAP, annexins, and GTPases. *J. Biol. Chem.*, **270**, 14399–14404.

45. Goda, Y. and Pfeffer, S.R. (1991) Identification of a novel, N-ethylmaleimide-sensitive cytosolic factor required for vesicular transport from endosomes to the trans-Golgi network in vitro. *J. Cell Biol.*, **112**, 823–831.

46. Schnitzer, J.E., Allard, J., and Oh, P. (1995) NEM inhibits transcytosis, endocytosis, and capillary permeability: implication of caveolae fusion in endothelia. *Am. J. Physiol.*, **268**, H48–H55.

47. Oh, P., McIntosh, D.P., and Schnitzer, J.E. (1998) Dynamin at the neck of caveolae mediates their budding to form transport vesicles by GTP-driven fission from the plasma membrane of endothelium. *J. Cell Biol.*, **141**, 101–114.

48. Oh, P. and Schnitzer, J.E. (1996) Dynamin-mediated fission of caveolae from plasma membranes. *Mol. Biol. Cell*, **7**, 83a.

49. Henley, J.R. et al. (1998) Dynamin-mediated internalization of caveolae. *J. Cell Biol.*, **141**, 85–99.

50. Parton, R.G., Joggerst, B., and Simons, K. (1994) Regulated internalization of caveolae. *J. Cell Biol.*, **127**, 1199–1215.

51. Schnitzer, J.E., Carley, W.W., and Palade, G.E. (1988) Specific albumin binding to microvascular endothelium in culture. *Am. J. Physiol.*, **254**, H425–H437.

52. Tran, D. et al. (1987) Ligands internalized through coated or noncoated invaginations follow a common intracellular pathway. *Proc. Natl. Acad. Sci. USA*, **84**, 7957–7961.

53. Pelkmans, L., Kartenback, J., and Helenius, A. (2001) Caveolar endocytosis of Simian virus 40 reveals a novel two-step vesicular transport pathway to the ER. *Nat. Cell Biol.*, **3**, 473–483.

54. Norkin, L.C. (1999) Simian virus 40 infection via MHC class I molecules and caveolae. *Immunol. Rev.*, **168**, 13–22.

55. Empig, C.J. and Goldsmith, M.A. (2002) Association of the caveola vesicular system with cellular entry by filoviruses. *J. Virol.*, **76**, 5266–5270.

56. Mackay, R.L. and Consigli, R.A. (1976) Early events in polyoma virus infection: attachment, penetration, and nuclear entry. *J. Virol.*, **19**, 620–636.

57. Richterova, Z. et al. (2001) Caveolae are involved in the trafficking of mouse polyomavirus virions and artificial VP1 pseudocapsids toward cell nuclei. *J. Virol.*, **75**, 10880–10891.
58. Schnitzer, J.E. and Oh, P. (1994) Albondin-mediated capillary permeability to albumin. Differential role of receptors in endothelial transcytosis and endocytosis of native and modified albumins. *J. Biol. Chem.*, **269**, 6072–6082.
59. Orlandi, P.A. and Fishman, P.H. (1998) Filipin-dependent inhibition of cholera toxin: evidence for toxin internalization and activation through caveolae-like domains. *J. Cell Biol.*, **141**, 905–915.
60. Fra, A.M. et al. (1994) Detergent-insoluble glycolipid microdomains in lymphocytes in the absence of caveolae. *J. Biol. Chem.*, **269**, 30745–30748.
61. Parolini, I. et al. (1999) Phorbol ester-induced disruption of the CD4–Lck complex occurs within a detergent-resistant microdomain of the plasma membrane. Involvement of the translocation of activated protein kinase C isoforms. *J. Biol. Chem.*, **274**, 14176–14187.
62. Drab, M. et al. (2001) Loss of caveolae, vascular dysfunction, and pulmonary defects in caveolin-1 gene-disrupted mice. *Science*, **293**, 2449–2452.
63. Razani, B., Woodman, S.E., and Lisanti, M.P. (2002) Caveolae: from cell biology to animal physiology. *Pharmacol. Rev.*, **54**, 431–467.
64. Peters, K.R., Carley, W.W., and Palade, G.E. (1985) Endothelial plasmalemmal vesicles have a characteristic striped bipolar surface structure. *J. Cell Biol.*, **101**, 2233–2238.
65. Rothberg, K.G. et al. (1992) Caveolin, a protein component of caveolae membrane coats. *Cell*, **68**, 673–682.
66. Griffoni, C. et al. (2000) Knockdown of caveolin-1 by antisense oligonucleotides impairs angiogenesis *in vitro* and *in vivo*. *Biochem. Biophys. Res. Commun.*, **276**, 756–761.
67. Schnitzer, J.E., Carley, W.W., and Palade, G.E. (1988) Albumin interacts specifically with a 60-kDa microvascular endothelial glycoprotein. *Proc. Natl. Acad. Sci. USA*, **85**, 6773–6777.
68. Schnitzer, J.E. et al. (1992) Non-coated caveolae-mediated endocytosis of modified proteins via novel scavenger receptors, gp30 and gp18. *Mol. Biol. Cell.*, **3**, 59a.
69. Razani, B. et al. (2001) Caveolin-1 null mice are viable but show evidence of hyperproliferative and vascular abnormalities. *J. Biol. Chem.*, **276**, 38121–38138.
70. Schubert, W. et al. (2002) Microvascular hyperpermeability in caveolin-1$^{-/-}$ knock-out mice. Treatment with a specific nitric-oxide synthase inhibitor, L-NAME, restores normal microvascular permeability in Cav-1 null mice. *J. Biol. Chem.*, **277**, 40091–40098.
71. Oh, P. et al. (2007) Live dynamic imaging of caveolae pumping targeted antibody rapidly and specifically across endothelium in the lung. *Nat. Biotechnol.*, **25**, 327–337.
72. Nicolson, G.L. (1988) Cancer metastasis: tumor cell and host organ properties important in metastasis to specific secondary sites. *Biochim. Biophys. Acta*, **948**, 175–224.
73. Blood, C.H. and Zetter, B.R. (1990) Tumor interactions with the vasculature: angiogenesis and tumor metastasis. *Biochim. Biophys. Acta*, **1032**, 89–118.
74. Zetter, B.R. (1990) The cellular basis of site-specific tumor metastasis. *N. Engl. J. Med.*, **322**, 605–612.
75. Dvorak, H.F. et al. (1988) Identification and characterization of the blood vessels of solid tumors that are leaky to circulating macromolecules. *Am. J. Pathol.*, **133**, 95–109.
76. Abell, R.G. (1946) The permeability of blood capillary sprouts and newly formed blood capillaries as compared to that of older blood capillaries. *Am. J. Physiol.*, **147**, 237–241.
77. Hobson, B. and Denekamp, J. (1984) Endothelial proliferation in tumours and normal tissues: continuous labelling studies. *Br. J. Cancer*, **49**, 405–413.
78. Schlingemann, R.O. et al. (1991) Differential expression of markers for

endothelial cells, pericytes, and basal lamina in the microvasculature of tumors and granulation tissue. *Am. J. Pathol.*, **138**, 1335–1347.
79. Jain, R.K. (1998) The next frontier of molecular medicine: delivery of therapeutics. *Nat. Med.*, **4**, 655–657.
80. Schnitzer, J.E. (2001) Caveolae: from basic trafficking mechanisms to targeting transcytosis for tissue-specific drug and gene delivery *in vivo*. *Adv. Drug Deliv. Rev.*, **49**, 265–280.
81. Gimbrone, M.A. Jr., Cotran, R.S., and Folkman, J. (1973) Endothelial regeneration: studies with human endothelial cells in culture. *Ser. Haematol.*, **6**, 453–455.
82. Jaffe, E.A. et al. (1973) Culture of human endothelial cells derived from umbilical veins. Identification by morphologic and immunologic criteria. *J. Clin. Invest.*, **52**, 2745–2756.
83. Jaffe, E.A. (1987) Cell biology of endothelial cells. *Hum. Pathol.*, **18**, 234–239.
84. Nagel, T. et al. (1994) Shear stress selectively upregulates intercellular adhesion molecule-1 expression in cultured human vascular endothelial cells. *J. Clin. Invest.*, **94**, 885–891.
85. Resnick, N. and Gimbrone, M.A. Jr. (1995) Hemodynamic forces are complex regulators of endothelial gene expression. *FASEB J.*, **9**, 874–882.
86. Topper, J.N. and Gimbrone, M.A. Jr. (1999) Blood flow and vascular gene expression: fluid shear stress as a modulator of endothelial phenotype. *Mol. Med. Today*, **5**, 40–46.
87. Madri, J.A. and Williams, S.K. (1983) Capillary endothelial cell cultures: phenotypic modulation by matrix components. *J. Cell Biol.*, **97**, 153–165.
88. Schnitzer, J.E. (1997) The endothelial cell surface and caveolae in health and disease in *Vascular Endothelium: Physiology, Pathology and Therapeutic Opportunities* (eds G.V.R. Born and C.J. Schwartz), Schattauer, Stuttgart, pp. 77–95.
89. Thum, T., Haverich, A., and Borlak, J. (2000) Cellular dedifferentiation of endothelium is linked to activation and silencing of certain nuclear transcription factors: implications for endothelial dysfunction and vascular biology. *FASEB J.*, **14**, 740–751.
90. Durr, E. et al. (2004) Direct proteomic mapping of the lung microvascular endothelial cell surface *in vivo* and in cell culture. *Nat. Biotechnol.*, **22**, 985–992.
91. Cole, S.R., Ashman, L.K., and Ey, P.L. (1987) Biotinylation: an alternative to radioiodination for the identification of cell surface antigens in immunoprecipitates. *Mol. Immunol.*, **24**, 699–705.
92. Belloni, P.N. and Nicolson, G.L. (1988) Differential expression of cell surface glycoproteins on various organ-derived microvascular endothelia and endothelial cell cultures. *J. Cell Physiol.*, **136**, 398–410.
93. Merker, M.P., Carley, W.W., and Gillis, C.N. (1990) Molecular mapping of pulmonary endothelial membrane glycoproteins of the intact rabbit lung. *FASEB J.*, **4**, 3040–3048.
94. Schnitzer, J.E., Shen, C.P., and Palade, G.E. (1990) Lectin analysis of common glycoproteins detected on the surface of continuous microvascular endothelium *in situ* and in culture: identification of sialoglycoproteins. *Eur. J. Cell. Biol.*, **52**, 241–251.
95. Schnitzer, J.E. et al. (1994) Segmental differentiation of permeability, protein glycosylation, and morphology of cultured bovine lung vascular endothelium. *Biochem. Biophys. Res. Commun.*, **199**, 11–19.
96. Schulte, B.A. and Spicer, S.S. (1983) Histochemical evaluation of mouse and rat kidneys with lectin–horseradish peroxidase conjugates. *Am. J. Anat.*, **168**, 345–362.
97. Ghinea, N. et al. (1989) Endothelial albumin binding proteins are membrane-associated components exposed on the cell surface. *J. Biol. Chem.*, **264**, 4755–4758.
98. Rybak, J.N. et al. (2005) In vivo protein biotinylation for identification of organ-specific antigens accessible from the vasculature. *Nat. Methods.*, **2**, 291–298.
99. Scheurer, S.B. et al. (2005) A comparison of different biotinylation reagents, tryptic digestion procedures, and mass

spectrometric techniques for 2-D peptide mapping of membrane proteins. *Proteomics*, **5**, 3035–3039.
100. Alexander, J.S., Blaschuk, O.W., and Haselton, F.R. (1993) An N-cadherin-like protein contributes to solute barrier maintenance in cultured endothelium. *J. Cell Physiol.*, **156**, 610–618.
101. Fridlich, R., David, A., and Aviram, I. (2006) Membrane proteinase 3 and its interactions within microdomains of neutrophil membranes. *J. Cell Biochem.*, **99**, 117–125.
102. Fujimoto, T. et al. (1992) Localization of inositol 1,4,5-trisphosphate receptor-like protein in plasmalemmal caveolae. *J. Cell Biol.*, **119**, 1507–1513.
103. Sargiacomo, M. et al. (1989) Integral and peripheral protein composition of the apical and basolateral membrane domains in MDCK cells. *J. Membr. Biol.*, **107**, 277–286.
104. Walker, J. et al. (1993) The adenosine 5′,5‴,P1,P4-tetraphosphate receptor is at the cell surface of heart cells. *Biochemistry*, **32**, 14009–14014.
105. Scheurer, S.B. et al. (2005) Identification and relative quantification of membrane proteins by surface biotinylation and two-dimensional peptide mapping. *Proteomics*, **5**, 2718–2728.
106. Roberts, L.M. et al. (2008) Subcellular localization of transporters along the rat blood–brain barrier and blood–cerebral-spinal fluid barrier by *in vivo* biotinylation. *Neuroscience*, **155**, 423–438.
107. De La Fuente, E.K. et al. (1997) Biotinylation of membrane proteins accessible via the pulmonary circulation in normal and hyperoxic rats. *Am. J. Physiol.*, **272**, L461–L470.
108. Schnitzer, J.E. et al. (1995) Separation of caveolae from associated microdomains of GPI-anchored proteins. *Science*, **269**, 1435–1439.
109. Oh, P. and Schnitzer, J.E. (1999) Immunoisolation of caveolae with high affinity antibody binding to the oligomeric caveolin cage. Toward understanding the basis of purification. *J. Biol. Chem.*, **274**, 23144–23154.
110. Kaplan, K.L. et al. (1983) Monoclonal antibodies to E92, an endothelial cell surface antigen. *Arteriosclerosis*, **3**, 403–412.
111. Kohler, G. and Milstein, C. (1975) Continuous cultures of fused cells secreting antibody of predefined specificity. *Nature*, **256**, 495–497.
112. Parks, W.M. et al. (1985) Identification and characterization of an endothelial, cell-specific antigen with a monoclonal antibody. *Blood*, **66**, 816–823.
113. Testa, J.E. et al. (2009) Ubiquitous yet distinct expression of podocalyxin on vascular surfaces in normal and tumor tissues in the rat. *J. Vasc. Res.*, **46**, 311–324.
114. Smith, G.P. (1985) Filamentous fusion phage: novel expression vectors that display cloned antigens on the virion surface. *Science*, **228**, 1315–1317.
115. Pasqualini, R. and Ruoslahti, E. (1996) Organ targeting *in vivo* using phage display peptide libraries. *Nature*, **380**, 364–366.
116. Rajotte, D. et al. (1998) Molecular heterogeneity of the vascular endothelium revealed by *in vivo* phage display. *J. Clin. Invest.*, **102**, 430–437.
117. Valadon, P. et al. (2006) Screening phage display libraries for organ-specific vascular immunotargeting *in vivo*. *Proc. Natl. Acad. Sci. USA*, **103**, 407–412.
118. Valadon, P. et al. (1998) Aspects of antigen mimicry revealed by immunization with a peptide mimetic of *Cryptococcus neoformans* polysaccharide. *J. Immunol.*, **161**, 1829–1836.
119. Seaman, S. et al. (2007) Genes that distinguish physiological and pathological angiogenesis. *Cancer Cell.*, **11**, 539–554.
120. St Croix, B. et al. (2000) Genes expressed in human tumor endothelium. *Science*, **289**, 1197–1202.
121. Righetti, P.G. (2005) Electrophoresis: the march of pennies, the march of dimes. *J. Chromatogr. A*, **1079**, 24–40.
122. Templin, M.F. et al. (2002) Protein microarray technology. *Drug Discov. Today*, **7**, 815–822.
123. Li, Y. et al. (2009) Enhancing identifications of lipid-embedded proteins

by mass spectrometry for improved mapping of endothelial plasma membranes *in vivo*. *Mol. Cell Proteomics*, **8**, 1219–1235.
124. Griffin, N.M. and Schnitzer, J.E. (2011) Overcoming key technological challenges in using mass spectrometry for mapping cell surfaces in tissues. *Mol. Cell Proteomics*, **10**, R110.000935.
125. Shiio, Y. *et al.* (2002) Quantitative proteomic analysis of Myc oncoprotein function. *EMBO J.*, **21**, 5088–5096.
126. Ong, S.E. *et al.* (2002) Stable isotope labeling by amino acids in cell culture, SILAC, as a simple and accurate approach to expression proteomics. *Mol. Cell Proteomics*, **1**, 376–386.
127. Chen, X. *et al.* (2007) Amino acid-coded tagging approaches in quantitative proteomics. *Expert Rev. Proteomics*, **4**, 25–37.
128. Old, W.M. *et al.* (2005) Comparison of label-free methods for quantifying human proteins by shotgun proteomics. *Mol. Cell Proteomics*, **4**, 1487–1502.
129. Zhang, B. *et al.* (2006) Detecting differential and correlated protein expression in label-free shotgun proteomics. *J. Proteome Res.*, **5**, 2909–2918.
130. Andersen, J.S. *et al.* (2003) Proteomic characterization of the human centrosome by protein correlation profiling. *Nature*, **426**, 570–574.
131. Gilchrist, A. *et al.* (2006) Quantitative proteomics analysis of the secretory pathway. *Cell*, **127**, 1265–1281.
132. Takamori, S. *et al.* (2006) Molecular anatomy of a trafficking organelle. *Cell*, **127**, 831–846.
133. Kislinger, T. *et al.* (2006) Global survey of organ and organelle protein expression in mouse: combined proteomic and transcriptomic profiling. *Cell*, **125**, 173–186.
134. Liu, H., Sadygov, R.G., and Yates, J.R. III (2004) A model for random sampling and estimation of relative protein abundance in shotgun proteomics. *Anal. Chem.*, **76**, 4193–4201.
135. Ishihama, Y. *et al.* (2005) Exponentially modified protein abundance index (emPAI) for estimation of absolute protein amount in proteomics by the number of sequenced peptides per protein. *Mol. Cell Proteomics*, **4**, 1265–1272.
136. Cutillas, P.R. and Vanhaesebroeck, B. (2007) Quantitative profile of five murine core proteomes using label-free functional proteomics. *Mol. Cell Proteomics*, **6**, 1560–1573.
137. Bondarenko, P.V., Chelius, D., and Shaler, T.A. (2002) Identification and relative quantitation of protein mixtures by enzymatic digestion followed by capillary reversed-phase liquid chromatography-tandem mass spectrometry. *Anal. Chem.*, **74**, 4741–4749.
138. Silva, J.C. *et al.* (2006) Simultaneous qualitative and quantitative analysis of the *Escherichia coli* proteome: a sweet tale. *Mol. Cell Proteomics*, **5**, 589–607.
139. Silva, J.C. *et al.* (2006) Absolute quantification of proteins by LCMSE: a virtue of parallel MS acquisition. *Mol. Cell Proteomics*, **5**, 144–156.
140. Gao, B.B., Stuart, L., and Feener, E.P. (2008) Label-free quantitative analysis of one-dimensional PAGE LC/MS/MS proteome: application on angiotensin II stimulated smooth muscle cells secretome. *Mol. Cell Proteomics*, **7**, 2399–2409.
141. Chelius, D. and Bondarenko, P.V. (2002) Quantitative profiling of proteins in complex mixtures using liquid chromatography and mass spectrometry. *J. Proteome Res.*, **1**, 317–323.
142. Griffin, N.M. *et al.* (2010) Label-free, normalized quantification of complex mass spectrometry data for proteomic analysis. *Nat. Biotechnol.*, **28**, 83–89.
143. Muzykantov, V.R. *et al.* (1991) Endotoxin reduces specific pulmonary uptake of radiolabeled monoclonal antibody to angiotensin-converting enzyme. *J. Nucl. Med.*, **32**, 453–460.
144. Wirrwar, A. *et al.* (2001) High resolution SPECT in small animal research. *Rev. Neurosci.*, **12**, 187–193.
145. Rossin, R. *et al.* (2008) *In vivo* imaging of ^{64}Cu-labeled polymer nanoparticles targeted to the lung endothelium. *J. Nucl. Med.*, **49**, 103–111.
146. Weissleder, R. and Ntziachristos, V. (2003) Shedding light onto live molecular targets. *Nat. Med.*, **9**, 123–128.

147. Jain, R.K., Munn, L.L., and Fukumura, D. (2002) Dissecting tumour pathophysiology using intravital microscopy. *Nat. Rev. Cancer*, **2**, 266–276.
148. Tozer, G.M. et al. (2005) Intravital imaging of tumour vascular networks using multi-photon fluorescence microscopy. *Adv. Drug Deliv. Rev.*, **57**, 135–152.
149. Vajkoczy, P., Ullrich, A., and Menger, M.D. (2000) Intravital fluorescence videomicroscopy to study tumor angiogenesis and microcirculation. *Neoplasia*, **2**, 53–61.
150. Danilov, S.M. et al. (1989) Radioimmunoimaging of lung vessels: an approach using indium-111-labeled monoclonal antibody to angiotensin-converting enzyme. *J. Nucl. Med.*, **30**, 1686–1692.
151. Garnacho, C. et al. (2008) RhoA activation and actin reorganization involved in endothelial CAM-mediated endocytosis of anti-PECAM carriers: critical role for tyrosine 686 in the cytoplasmic tail of PECAM-1. *Blood*, **111**, 3024–3033.
152. Kozower, B.D. et al. (2003) Immunotargeting of catalase to the pulmonary endothelium alleviates oxidative stress and reduces acute lung transplantation injury. *Nat. Biotechnol.*, **21**, 392–398.
153. Chrastina, A. et al. (2010) lung vascular targeting using antibody to aminopeptidase P: CT-SPECT imaging, biodistribution and pharmacokinetic analysis. *J. Vasc. Res.*, **47**, 531–543.
154. Gerke, V. and Moss, S.E. (2002) Annexins: from structure to function. *Physiol. Rev.*, **82**, 331–371.
155. Yi, M. and Schnitzer, J.E. (2009) Impaired tumor growth, metastasis, angiogenesis and wound healing in annexin A1-null mice. *Proc. Natl. Acad. Sci. USA*, **106**, 17886–17891.
156. de Vries, C. et al. (1992) The fms-like tyrosine kinase, a receptor for vascular endothelial growth factor. *Science*, **255**, 989–991.

12
Considerations of Linker Technologies

Laurent Ducry

12.1
Introduction

The widespread interest in antibody–drug conjugates (ADCs) stems from their selective delivery of drug molecules within the human body. ADC-based cancer treatments exploit monoclonal antibodies (mAbs) to bind cancer cell-specific antigens, thereby enabling selective release of potent cytotoxic drugs in diseased tissues [1–6]. Several drugs per antibody, typically two to four, are needed to achieve the desired potency and pharmacokinetic profile [7, 8]. Importantly, linking multiple payloads to a single mAb must not alter its antigen-binding specificity (Figure 12.1).

The ideal linker should also confer ADC stability during both storage and in the bloodstream, so as to avoid undesired release of the payload, while facilitating release of the payload at the tumor site. Achieving this delicate balance is of paramount importance and illustrates the central role of linkers in ADC pharmacokinetics [9].

12.2
Linkage Site and Cross-Linking Chemistry

mAbs, which are comprised of globular proteins, have an array of amino acids that can be potential linkage sites for payloads [10]. However, due to their tertiary and

Biotechnology + Chemistry = Antibody-Drug Conjugates

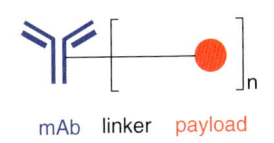

mAb   linker   payload

Figure 12.1 Schematic representation of an ADC.

Drug Delivery in Oncology: From Basic Research to Cancer Therapy, First Edition.
Edited by Felix Kratz, Peter Senter, and Henning Steinhagen.
© 2012 Wiley-VCH Verlag GmbH & Co. KGaA. Published 2012 by Wiley-VCH Verlag GmbH & Co. KGaA.

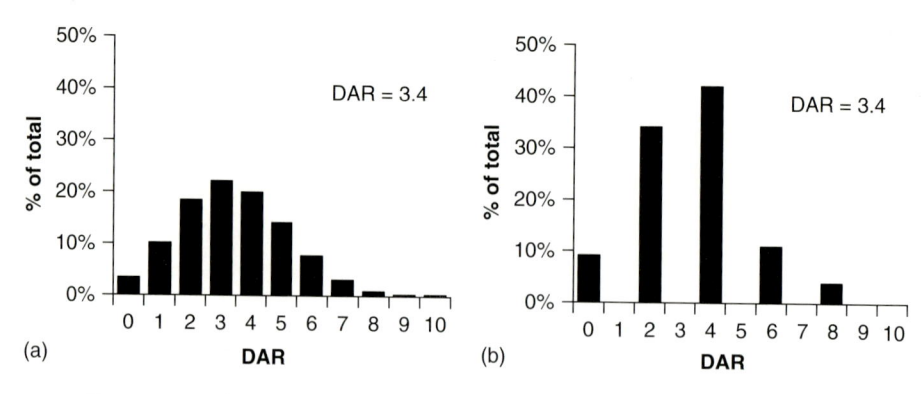

Figure 12.2 Schematic representation and prevalence of the different ADC subpopulations of (a) lysine and (b) cysteine conjugation [12].

quaternary structure, only solvent-accessible amino acids will be available for conjugation. In practice, high-yielding conjugations to mAbs occur through the ε-amino group of lysine residues or through the sulfhydryl group of cysteine residues.

The abundance of hydrophilic lysine side-chains at the protein surface gives multiple linkage sites for payload conjugation. Not surprisingly, conjugation affords a mixture of ADC species, each with distinct therapeutic properties. This heterogeneity is 2-fold: (i) varying drug-to-antibody ratios (DARs) ranging from 0 to 10 (Figure 12.2) and (ii) ADC species with the same number of drugs may have different linkage sites on the mAb. For example, 20 different sites of modification were identified for huN901–DM1 [11]. As ADCs generated through conjugation to solvent-accessible lysines are highly heterogeneous, a potential pitfall is sterically or conformationally induced interference by payloads bound at or near the antigen-binding site. Thus, it is essential to have a well-developed process that affords consistent subpopulations of compounds.

In contrast, conjugation through cysteine residues leads to less heterogeneous ADC species than its lysine counterpart, on account of the lower abundance of cysteine in proteins (e.g., IgG1 molecules contain only four interchain disulfide bonds). Interestingly, conjugation takes place on the disulfide bonds positioned between heavy and light chains or on the hinge disulfide bonds themselves, but not near the antigen-binding site. A prerequisite for cysteine conjugation is reduction of the interchain disulfide bonds to nucleophilic thiol groups. Consequently, even-numbered DARs are typically observed (Figure 12.2).

The reduction of interchain disulfide bonds prior to conjugation may adversely disrupt the quaternary structure of the mAb, and hence affect its immunoaffinity and/or stability *in vivo*. This risk can be mitigated by using recombinant antibodies with predetermined sites for drug attachment. A proof-of-concept was illustrated by engineered forms of cAC10, in which specific cysteine residues were replaced with serine to reduce potential conjugation sites, affording ADCs with unprecedented levels of uniformity [8]. More recently, cysteine residues have been spliced into the amino acid sequence, allowing site-specific conjugation with preservation of native

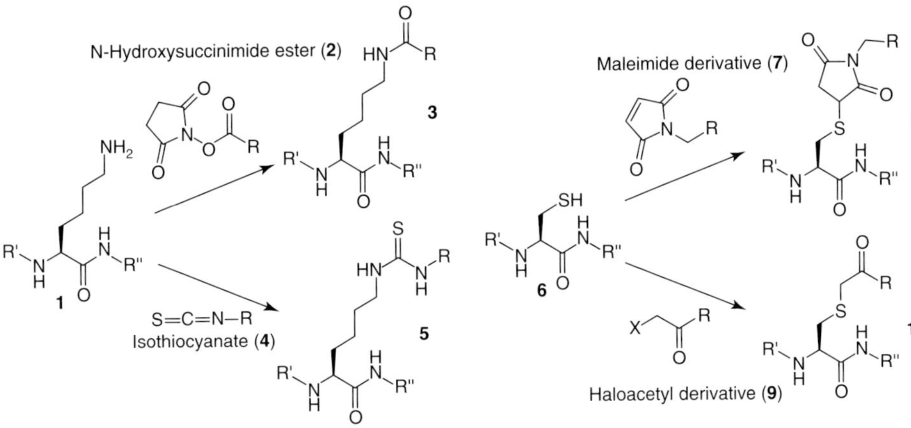

Scheme 12.1 Typical examples of reactions used to conjugate lysine (**1**) and cysteine (**6**) residues.

structural disulfide bonds; this bioengineering method affords nearly homogeneous THIOMAB drug conjugates (TDCs) with an improved therapeutic index [13].

Cross-linking the mAb to the drug requires a heterobifunctional reagent. In the case of lysine residues (**1**), acylating reagents such as succinimidyl esters (**2**) or the water-soluble sulfo-succidinyl esters, as well as isothiocyanates (**3**), which combine sufficient reactivity and stability in water, are typically used (Scheme 12.1). It is worth mentioning that the N-terminus of the protein is a potential conjugation site, and that tyrosine [14] and histidine residues may react with succinimide esters. The more reactive isocyanates and sulfonyl chlorides can also be used to functionalize lysine side-chains, despite their limited stability in water. For cysteine residues (**6**), conjugation is often achieved via a Michael-type addition to maleimide derivatives (**7**), affording stable thioether linkages. Alternatively, thiol groups can react selectively with activated alkylating groups such as haloacetyl derivatives (**9**) or vinyl sulfones, although the latter has not been applied so frequently in an ADC context.

Alternatively, sulfhydryl functionalities can be tethered to the ε-amino group of lysine residues (**1**) with 2-iminothiolane (Traut's reagent, **11**), or N-succinimidyl-S-acetylthioacetate (SATA, **13**) followed by hydrolysis of the protected sulfhydryl group (Scheme 12.2).

12.3
Linkers for Cytotoxic ADCs

12.3.1
Chemically Labile Linkers

In the case of ADCs with highly potent drugs, the linker must allow release of the cytotoxic payload once it has entered the target cell. By exploiting biological

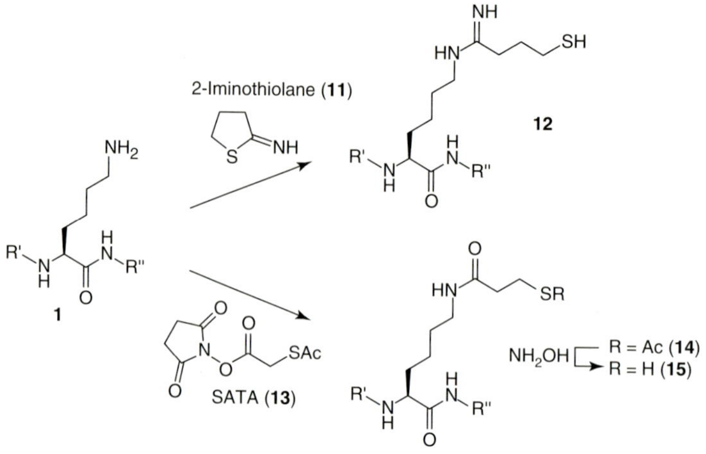

Scheme 12.2 Possible thiolation reagents.

differences between plasma and cytoplasmic compartments, various chemically labile linkers were developed. For example, hydrazone-based linkers are stable at neutral pH (bloodstream, pH 7.3–7.5), but are prone to cleavage once the ADC enters the acidic pH environment found within a cell (endosomes, pH 5.0–6.5; lysosomes, pH 4.5–5.0).

Conjugation of doxorubicin, an intercalating agent that blocks DNA replication, to the humanized mAb BR96 is a prominent example of an ADC featuring an acid-labile hydrazone linker [15]. Here, doxorubicin was first condensed with the semicarbazide group of the (6-maleimidocaproyl)hydrazone linker followed by conjugation to the cysteine residues of the mAb. BR96-doxorubicin (**16**) exhibits a relatively short half-life in the blood (43 h versus several days to weeks of native BR96 mAb) and low potency, requiring high DAR (about eight drugs per mAb molecule) and high dosage (above 100 mg/kg) to achieve a therapeutic effect. Despite promising preclinical results, this compound later failed to show sufficient clinical efficacy.

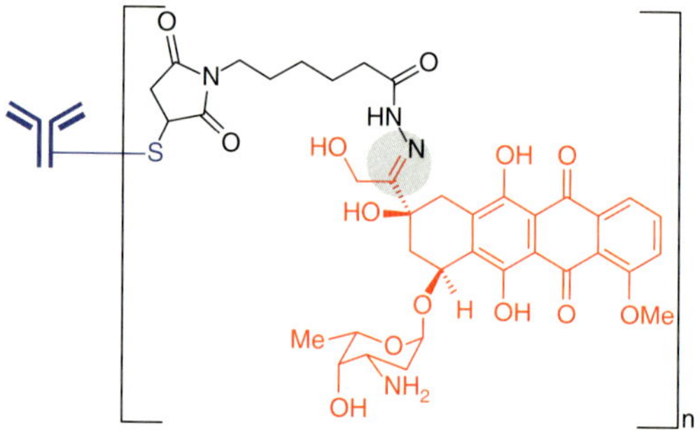

12.3 Linkers for Cytotoxic ADCs

Gemtuzumab ozogamicin (Mylotarg®, **17**) also uses a hydrazone linker, but with a more potent drug than doxorubicin. It consists of the DNA disruptor N-acetyl-γ-calicheamicin covalently attached to a humanized anti-CD33 mAb [16, 17]. Here, 4-(4-acetylphenoxy)butanoic acid links surface-exposed lysines of the mAb to N-acetyl-γ-calicheamicin dimethyl hydrazide via an amide and acyl hydrazone bond, respectively. In 2000, Mylotarg (**17**) was approved for the treatment of acute myeloid leukemia. Interestingly, this ADC is prepared with an average of two to three drugs/mAb, but half of the antibodies in the preparation contain no drug at all [17]. More recently, the heterogeneity of calicheamicin-containing ADCs has been suppressed by using additives in the process, further illustrating the importance of the conjugation conditions [18].

17

Upon internalization of the ADC, the calicheamicin prodrug is released by hydrolysis of the hydrazone moiety in the lysosomes of $CD33^+$ target cells; in control studies, the hydrolysis of an unconjugated intermediate at 37 °C over 24 h increased from 6% at pH 7.4 to 97% at pH 4.5 [19]. Incidentally, this linker is only moderately stable in Mylotarg (mean a half-life for drug release of 72 h) [20, 21], resulting in a narrow therapeutic window. In contrast, an unexpectedly high stability in both human plasma and serum (rate of hydrolysis of 1.5–2%/day over 4 days) was reported for CMC-544 (inotuzumab ozogamicin), an ADC consisting of a humanized anti-CD22 mAb attached to N-acetyl-γ-calicheamicin via the same acid-labile 4-(4′-acetylphenoxy)butanoic acid linker; however, a recent pharmacokinetic study revealed a lower stability in mice plasma for this ADC (half-life of 22–29 h) compared to Mylotarg (half-life of 47–54 h) [22].

Transformation of the calicheamicin prodrug into the active payload requires reductive cleavage of the disulfide bond. These S–S bonds are chemically labile in the presence of sulfhydryl groups, undergoing disulfide exchange reactions. Glutathione – a thiol-containing tripeptide – is present in 1000-fold higher concentration in the cytoplasm than in the bloodstream; this sulfhydryl gradient serves to activate prodrugs delivered into the cytoplasm while minimizing prodrug activation in the bloodstream. In the current example, Mylotarg (**17**) is significantly more potent than its corresponding amide-bearing conjugate **18**, indicating the hydrazone linker accounts for the release of the drug in the target cell [16]. However, upon switching the mAb, apparently conflicting results can be obtained. In the case of murine mAb CTM01 with the corresponding amide conjugate **18**, enhanced activities were observed in several *in vitro* and *in vivo* tumor models, suggesting cleavage of the S–S linkage was responsible for drug release [23].

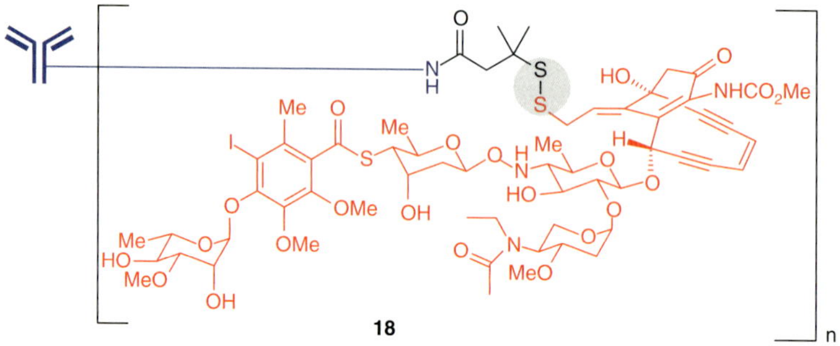

18

ADC **19** is another example of the use of disulfide linkers. It is composed of a mAb directed against the epidermal growth factor receptor, conjugated via a disulfide-bearing 4-mercaptopentanoate linker to a second-generation taxoid payload [24, 25].

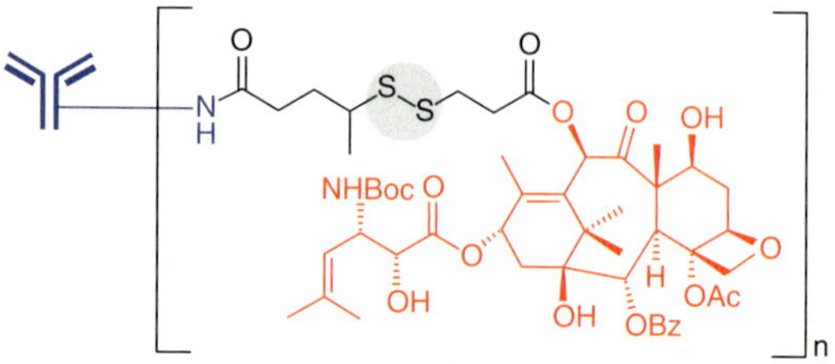

19

The most prominent examples of intracellularly cleavable disulfide-based linkers are ADCs using DM1 or DM4 as cytotoxic payloads [26–28]. These potent semisynthetic maytansine analogs are antimicrotubular cytotoxic agents. The mAb is first reacted with N-succinimidyl 4-(2′-pyridyldithio)pentanoate (SPP) or N-succinimidyl 4-(2′-pyridyldithio)butyrate (SPDB), followed by disulfide exchange reaction of the 2′-pyridyldithio moiety with DM1 or DM4, affording the ADCs **20** and **21**, respectively. *In vivo*, the ADC is believed to be internalized via antigen-mediated endocytosis followed by complete hydrolysis of the peptidic backbone, affording lysine residues linked to the toxin [28]. Further intracellular processing involving sequential cleavage of the disulfide linker through a disulfide exchange and thiol methylation (presumably catalyzed by intracellular methyltransferases) release the potent drugs DM1 or DM4, or the *S*-methyl analog of DM4 [29].

These cytotoxins are uncharged, enabling them to diffuse out of the target cells and knockout adjacent cells within the tumor that are not targeted by the antibody [30].

Despite its potent activity, the linker of DM1-containing ADC **20** is only moderately stable *in vivo* (half-life of 47 h in mice) [31]. The stability was ameliorated by introduction of sterically hindered *gem*-dimethyl groups adjacent to the disulfide bond, affording DM4-conjugate **21** with a improved half-life of 102 h in mice.

12.3.2
Enzyme-Labile Linkers

The ubiquity of proteases within the cell renders peptidic linkers an obvious choice for ADCs. The limited extracellular activity of proteases, due to the unfavorable pH and serum protease inhibitors, confers improved plasma stability for peptidic linkers relative to chemically labile linkers. In combination with protease's high specificity, drug release from the peptidic linker is efficiently controlled and, in some cases, enhanced by accumulation of lysosomal proteases, such as cathepsin or plasmin, in certain tumor tissues [32, 33].

The ADCs **22a** and **22b**, where BR96 is conjugated to doxorubicin via dipeptide linkers, showed improved immunological specificity compared to that of the corresponding hydrazone-based conjugate **16** [34]. The amide linkage that eliminates the positively charged amino group of doxorubicin may, however, decrease the water solubility of the ADC. Thus, for compounds with high DARs, the attachment of poly(ethylene glycol) (PEG) side-chains to the drug via a cleavable hydrazone bond was investigated [35]. Dipeptide-based ADCs releasing a highly potent cyclic derivative of doxorubicin has also been reported [36].

22a R' = Bn, R" = CH$_2$NH$_2$
22b R' = iPr, R" = NHCONH$_2$

Peptidic linkers are currently best exploited to conjugate cysteine residues of mAbs with monomethyl auristatin E (MMAE) and monomethyl auristatin F (MMAF), two tubulin inhibitors. Efficient hydrolysis of the dipeptide linker by cathepsin B has been established *in vitro* [37]. Following enzymatic cleavage, 1,6-elimination of the strongly electron-donating *p*-aminobenzyl oxycarbonyl (PABC) spacer occurs, releasing CO$_2$ and the drug in its active form; this self-eliminating spacer is necessary to separate the bulky payload from the site of enzymatic cleavage.

Compared to ADC **23** using a chemically labile hydrazone linker, ADC **24** bearing a phenylalanine–lysine linker and ADC **25a** bearing a valine–citrulline (vc) linker have a high stability (Table 12.1) [38]. In an alternative *in vitro* stability study, cAC10–vcMMAE showed less than 2% of the total drug was released in human and drug plasma over 10 days, and less than 5% in mouse plasma [39]. The superior *in vitro* stability of the valine–citrulline linker corroborates with *in vivo* results, affording a half-life of 6.0 days in mice (compared to 2 days for the hydrazone linker) and of 9.6 days in monkey [40]. For CR011–vcMMAE, pharmacokinetic data showed a half-life of 10.3 days in mice [41]. A kinetic study with radiolabeled ADC **25a**, prepared using ^{14}C-MMAE, demonstrated that after internalization and processing, high intracellular concentrations of MMAE (above 400 nmol/l) are reached within 24 h [42]. Slow diffusion of the released MMAE out of cells was observed, showing a bystander activity on neighboring, antigen-negative cells in culture. Interestingly, reversal of the conjugation site on the mAb to the C-terminus of auristatin drugs resulted in a different drug release profile, suggesting potential room to improve the current therapeutic window [43].

23

25a R' = Me, R" = OH
25b R' = CO$_2$H, R" = H

Table 12.1 In vitro stabilities of cBR96–MMAE conjugates at 37 °C [38].

ADC	Projected half-live mouse plasma (days)	Projected half-live human plasma (days)
23	2.1	2.6
24	12.5	80
25a	30	230

In an effort to extend the use of dipeptide linkers to other classes of cytotoxic drugs, the conjugation of streptonigrin was investigated [44]. However, in contrast to payloads containing primary or secondary aliphatic amines, the electron-deficient aryl amine of streptonigrin did not react with the *p*-nitrophenyl carbonate reagent usually employed to form the PABC-based linker system. In this case, linkage of the payload to the linker required the use of the corresponding benzylic bromide, affording ADC **26**. Following enzymatic cleavage, the benzyl amine spacer was shown to undergo quantitative 1,6-elimination within 30 min in analogy with the PABC spacer. However, despite encouraging *in vitro* data, ADC **26** was not as well tolerated as the analogous auristatin immunoconjugates **25a** and **25b**.

CC-1065, duocarmycins, and synthetic cyclopropabenzindol-4-one (CBI) derivatives are potent minor-groove-binding DNA alkylating agents that can potentially be used as ADC payloads. *seco*-CBI precursors, such as ADC **27**, are prodrugs bearing a phenolic hydroxyl group protected by an enzyme-labile carbamate [45]. Following enzymatic cleavage of the carbamate, the *seco*-structure undergoes spontaneous Winstein-cyclization with loss of HCl, revealing its active payload as a DNA-alkylating CBI moiety. In fact, ADC **27** incorporates double pro-drug properties: (i) it improves the drug's therapeutic efficacy by conjugating it to a tumor-specific mAb via an enzyme-cleavable valine–citrulline dipeptide linker and (ii) the prodrug of the cytotoxic agent requires intracellular carboxyesterases to unleash the payload [46, 47]. The two activating steps needed to trigger the release of the active drug may lead to an enlarged therapeutic window. In ADC **28**, the valine–citrulline linkage is used in conjunction with two consecutive self-immolative spacers. Following the enzymatic cleavage of the dipeptide, a domino-like mechanism will trigger elimination of the PABC spacer via 1,6-elimination, decarboxylation, elimination of the methylated ethylenediamine (MED) spacer by spontaneous cyclization reaction with concomitant release of the corresponding pentacyclic urea, and finally release of the prodrug [48]. The CBI prodrug used in **28** has potentially lower toxicities due to the reduced reactivity of the secondary chloride compared to the primary chloride in **27**.

Cleavable dipeptide linkers have also been used to conjugate 7-ethyl-10-hydroxy-camptothecin (SN-38), a potent topoisomerase I inhibitor [49, 50]. Labet-uzumab-CL2-SN-38(Et) (**29**) showed good *in vitro* stability (half-life of 41 and 66 h in mouse and human serum, respectively) as well as promising tumor reduction in animal models. Here, the PABC self-immolative spacer is connected to the 20-hydroxyl group of the drug. To improve water solubility, a defined PEG moiety as well as a triazoline group, resulting from an azide–acetylene click cycloaddition, were introduced in the linker structure.

ADCs **30** and **31** feature an amino-CBI and a hydroxy aza-CBI payload, respectively [51]. Due to the inherent hydrophobicity of this drug class, hydrophilic peptide-based linkers were incorporated to prevent aggregation. This was achieved by using a more hydrophilic dipeptide (valine–lysine instead of valine–citrulline) and incorporating a tetraethyleneglycol unit. In ADC **30**, the linker is directly attached to the amine of the CBI prodrug, whereas in ADC **31**, a self-eliminating PABC spacer was introduced between the dipeptide and the hydroxyl group of the aza-CBI toxin to ensure access of cathepsin B or other proteases to the site of cleavage.

Apart from proteases, glycosidase-based cleavage has also been developed using β-glucuronide linkers. ADCs **32a** and **32b**, which incorporate MMAE and MMAF payloads, utilize a similar self-eliminating spacer mechanism [52]. Interestingly, the cleavage site does not directly link the mAb to the payload. In terms of efficacy, high stability was observed in rat plasma (extrapolated half-life of 81 days) with low *in vivo* toxicity (comparable to the corresponding peptide-linked ADCs **25**). This carbohydrate motif has also been applied to ADCs bearing alternative payloads such as a doxorubicin derivative [52], a CBI minor-groove binder [53], and camptothecin analogs [54].

32a R' = Me, R" = OH
32b R' = CO$_2$H, R" = H

12.3.3
Noncleavable Linkers

Given the mechanistic proposals for chemical- and enzyme-labile linkers, it seemed unlikely that noncleavable linkers could release active payloads from ADCs. In a control experiment, ADC **33**, where the heterobifunctional linker N-succinimidyl-4-(N-maleimidomethyl)cyclohexane-1-carboxylate (SMCC) was used to covalently attach DM1 payloads to the mAb via noncleavable thioether bonds, was shown to be very potent [28, 55].

This fortuitous discovery suggested that a different release mechanism than those discussed thus far may account for the therapeutic effect. Indeed, after internalization of the ADC and proteolytic degradation of the mAb component, a maytansinoid metabolite (still attached via the SMCC linker to a lysine residue) is released. This modified drug was found to retain its cytotoxic properties despite the functionalization of the sulfhydryl group. The *in vivo* stability of the thioether-linked ADC **33** (half-life of 134 h in mice) was superior to that of disulfide linker-based compounds **20** and **21** (47 and 102 h, respectively).

This novel drug release mechanism is also operative in the maleimidocaproyl-MMAF (mcMMAF)-based ADC. Here, *in vivo* activity was observed for ADC **34**, despite the use of a noncleavable thioether linker *in lieu* of a dipeptide one (*cf.* ADC **25**) [56]. MMAE, although structurally similar, was not active when attached in this manner. As confirmed by mass spectrometry, the released drug was a cysteine-adduct of MMAF, in agreement with the mode of action proposed for the maytansinoid conjugate **33**. Furthermore, a biodistribution study in a mouse xenograft model using a ^{3}H-labeled mAb tethered to ^{14}C-labeled MMAF via a maleimidocaproyl linker showed that delivery of the ADC and retention of its degradation product Cys-mcMMAF is substantially greater in the tumor (peak concentration reached 2 days after dose) than in normal tissue (peak concentration reached after 2–4 h) [57]. Consequently, exposure of the payload was tens to hundreds times higher in tumors than in normal tissue.

It was recently shown that undesired drug release from the ADC to albumin cysteines in the plasma occurs with alkyl-maleimide ADCs [58]. To counteract this effect, the linker stability was enhanced by replacing the maleimide with an acetamide functionality (as in ADC **35**). This type of ADC led to no apparent degradation in the bloodstream for up to 14 days.

An interesting variant of this technology incorporates hydrophilic linkers, which allows ADCs to have higher DAR without compromising their solubility or pharmacokinetics [59]. These noncleavable thioether linkers employ sulfonate (36) or PEG functionalities (37) to promote water solubility, in analogy to branched PEG linkers used in antibody–paclitaxel conjugates [60]. This improved water solubility should limit aggregation, increase the efficiency of the conjugation step and simplify ADC purification.

In general, ADCs with noncleavable linkers were found to be better tolerated [61] and, in some cases, resulted in an improved therapeutic index. However, the mechanism by which ADCs with noncleavable linkers deliver their payload invokes several important considerations. Since ADC internalization followed by complete hydrolysis of the polypeptide backbone of the mAb is required for payload release, reduced efficacy may be encountered when ADC internalization is poor [61]. Thus,

ADCs bearing noncleavable linkers are highly dependent on the biology of the target cell. If the intention of the ADC is to deliver the payload to the tumor cells and its adjacent antigen-negative cells (i.e., bystander effect), the released payload should be a neutral molecule that can readily diffuse through hydrophobic cell membranes [30], whereas ADCs with noncleavable linkers release payloads bearing a zwitterionic amino acid residue (positively charged ammonium and negatively charged carboxylate). Finally, not all payloads retain their biological activity after mAb degradation, as evidenced by the rather innocuous MMAE metabolite, despite its structural similarity to MMAF.

12.4
Linkers for Radioactive Immunoconjugates

The impetus for the development of radioimmunoconjugates is to selectively deliver radiation to tumor cells without global tissue exposure. In this way, the radiation dose occurs at a much lower dose rate than external beam irradiation, but it is continually present for a defined period of time. Whereas cytotoxin-based ADCs kill individual target cells, the therapeutic advantage of radioimmunoconjugates is the ability to reach multiple cancer cells. For example β-emitters (e.g., ^{67}Cu, ^{90}Y, ^{131}I, ^{177}Lu, ^{186}Re) can penetrate up to about 1 cm, imposing their effect across several hundreds of cells, whereas α-emitters (e.g., ^{211}At, ^{213}Bi) have relatively short emission ranges (up to about 0.1 mm), but high decay energies. By judicious loading of the radionuclide on the mAb, the delicate balance of dose delivery to the tumor against exposure of healthy tissues to radiation can be realized. Current applications of this technology include selective delivery of radioactive isotopes to malignant tissue (e.g., lymphoma, leukemia) [62, 63] and in radioimmunoimaging [63, 64].

38

Another key distinction between cytotoxic immunoconjugates (ADCs) and radioactive immunoconjugates is that the latter do not have to release their payload for a biological effect to occur. Due to their inherent nature, metallic radionuclides are effectively bound to bifunctional chelating agents (BCAs) via chelating heteroatoms. Selecting a suitable BCA depends on the characteristics of the radionuclide (coordination number, radius, metal-binding character). Common chelators include DOTA **38** (1,4,7,10-tetraazacyclododecane-N,N',N'',N'''-tetraacetic acid) and DTPA

39 (diethylenetriamine pentaacetic acid); acyclic BCAs like DTPA derivatives exhibit a faster chelation rate, whereas macrocyclic BCAs like DOTA form more stable complexes. Interestingly, the preorganized CHX-A″-DTPA chelator **40** (cyclohexyl diethylenetriamine pentaacetic acid) exhibits rapid complexation kinetics with high *in vivo* stability. A variety of conjugation methods can then be employed to join the chelating linker to the mAb; however, they must not alter the antigen-binding domain. The most common method involves lysine conjugation with a 4-isothiocyanatobenzyl group, affording a stable thiourea linkage.

In 2002, ^{90}Y-ibritumomab tiuxetan (Zevalin®) became the first radioimmunoconjugate to be approved for marketing. It is an anti-CD20 mAb labeled with ^{90}Y via a DTPA chelator, aimed at the treatment of non-Hodgkin's lymphoma (NHL) [65]. ^{131}I-tositumomab (Bexxar®), which is also active against NHL, was approved a year later, but does not include a chelating linker since it is obtained by direct radioiodination of the mAb [66]. Both of these immunoconjugates improve the objective response rate compared with the unlabeled mAbs used to deliver the radionuclides [67], paving the way to more effective cancer treatments using radiolabeled antibodies.

12.5
Conclusions

Most cytotoxic agents, whether used for chemo- or radiation therapy, have severe side-effects that limit their efficacy and use. In recent years, the progress in linking such payloads to mAbs has been considerable, affording novel immunoconjugates for cancer therapy. Tissue specificity is typically governed by the mAb component, while the cytotoxic or radioactive drug provides the therapeutic effect. The efficiency and tolerability of immunoconjugates has been vastly improved in recent years, primarily due to an increased understanding of the interplay between the target antigen, drug potency, and conjugation technology. In particular, linker chemistry, which strongly influences the ADC specificity and safety, has been a major area of development. Compared to hydrazone- and disulfide-based linkers that are often labile in circulation, peptidic linkers as well as noncleavable linkers are remarkably stable *in vivo*, giving access to ADCs with improved therapeutic windows. Using these promising linkers to attach potent cytotoxic drugs or radionuclides to humanized or chimeric mAbs targeting cancer-specific antigens, should allow immunoconjugates to reach their full potential as targeted cancer therapies. Note, however, that no single linker or chelator is compatible with the full spectrum of available payloads, mAbs, and clinical applications. Consequently, several conjugation technologies will most likely be used in parallel or in combination in order to arm the numerous mAbs that are available as effective targeting agents but often lack the necessary potency to be curative on their own. Considering the various mAbs, linkers, and payloads that are already available, and knowing that each has an impact on the ADC safety and efficacy, the number of possible permutations and combinations is substantial, offering a large area to be explored.

References

1. Zangemeister-Wittke, U. (2005) *Pathobiology*, **72**, 279–286.
2. Wu, A.M. and Senter, P.D. (2005) *Nat. Biotechnol.*, **23**, 1137–1146.
3. Ricart, A.D. and Tolcher, A.W. (2007) *Nat. Clin. Pract. Oncol.*, **4**, 245–255.
4. Carter, P.J. and Senter, P.D. (2008) *Cancer J.*, **14**, 154–169.
5. Kratz, F., Müller, I.A., Ryppa, C., and Warnecke, A. (2008) *ChemMedChem*, **3**, 20–53.
6. Senter, P.D. (2009) *Curr. Opin. Chem. Biol.*, **13**, 235–244.
7. Hamblett, K.J., Senter, P.D., Chace, D.F., Sun, M.M.C., Lenox, J., Cerveny, C.G., Kissler, K.M., Bernhardt, S.X., Kopcha, A.K., Zabinski, R.F., Meyer, D.L., and Francisco, J.A. (2004) *Clin. Cancer Res.*, **10**, 7063–7070.
8. McDonagh, C.F., Turcott, E., Westendorf, L., Webster, J.B., Alley, S.C., Kim, K., Andreyka, J., Stone, I., Hamblett, K.J., Francisco, J.A., and Carter, P. (2006) *Protein Eng. Des. Sel.*, **19**, 299–307.
9. Ducry, L. and Stump, B. (2010) *Bioconjug. Chem.*, **21**, 5–13.
10. Sletten, E.M. and Bertozzi, C.R. (2009) *Angew. Chem. Int. Ed.*, **48**, 6974–6998 and references cited therein.
11. Wang, L., Amphlett, G., Blättler, W.A., Lambert, J.M., and Zhang, W. (2005) *Protein Sci.*, **14**, 2436–2446.
12. Stephan, J.-P., Chan, P., Lee, C., Nelson, C., Elliott, J.M., Bechtel, C., Raab, H., Xie, D., Akutagawa, J., Baudys, J., Saad, O., Prabhu, S., Wong, W.L.T., Vandlen, R., Jacobson, F., and Ebens, A. (2008) *Bioconjug. Chem.*, **19**, 1673–1683.
13. Junutula, J.R., Raab, H., Clark, S., Bhakta, S., Leipold, D.D., Weir, S., Chen, Y., Simpson, M., Tsai, S.P., Dennis, M.S., Lu, Y., Meng, Y.G., Ng, C., Yang, J., Lee, C.C., Duenas, E., Gorrell, J., Katta, V., Kim, A., McDorman, K., Flagella, K., Venook, R., Ross, S., Spencer, S.D., Wong, W.L., Lowman, H.B., Vandlen, R., Sliwkowski, M.X., Scheller, R.H., Polakis, P., and Mallet, W. (2008) *Nat. Biotechnol.*, **26**, 925–932.
14. Leavell, M.D., Novak, P., Behrens, C.R., Schoeniger, J.S., and Kruppa, G.H. (2004) *J. Am. Soc. Mass Spectrom.*, **15**, 1604–1611.
15. Trail, P.A., Willner, D., Lasch, S.J., Henderson, A.J., Hofstead, S., Casazza, A.M., Firestone, R.A., Hellström, I., and Hellström, K.E. (1993) *Science*, **261**, 212–215.
16. Hamann, P.R., Hinman, L.M., Beyer, C.F., Lindh, D., Upeslacis, J., Flowers, D.A., and Bernstein, I. (2002) *Bioconjug. Chem.*, **13**, 40–46.
17. Hamann, P.R., Hinman, L.M., Hollander, I., Beyer, C.F., Lindh, D., Holcomb, R., Hallett, W., Tsou, H.-R., Upeslacis, J., Shochat, D., Mountain, A., Flowers, D.A., and Bernstein, I. (2002) *Bioconjug. Chem.*, **13**, 47–58.
18. Hollander, I., Kunz, A., and Hamann, P.R. (2008) *Bioconjug. Chem.*, **19**, 358–361.
19. van der Velden, V.H.J., te Marvelde, J.G., Hoogeveen, P.G., Bernstein, I.D., Houtsmuller, A.B., Berger, M.S., and van Dongen, J.J.M. (2001) *Blood*, **97**, 3197–3204.

20. DiJoseph, J.F., Dougher, M.M., Kalyandrug, L.B., Armellino, D.C., Boghaert, E.R., Hamann, P.R., Moran, J.K., and Damle, N.K. (2006) *Clin. Cancer Res.*, **12**, 242–249.
21. DiJoseph, J.F., Khandke, K., Dougher, M.M., Evans, D.Y., Armellino, D.C., Hamann, P.R., and Damle, N.K. (2008) *Hematol. Meet. Rep.*, **5**, 74–77.
22. Boghaert, E.R., Khandke, K.M., Sridharan, L., Dougher, M., DiJoseph, J.F., Kunz, A., Hamann, P.R., Moran, J., Chaudhary, I., and Damle, N.K. (2008) *Cancer Chemother. Pharmacol.*, **61**, 1027–1035.
23. (a) Hamann, P.R., Hinman, L.M., Beyer, C.F., Greenberger, L.M., Lin, C., Lindh, D., Menendez, A.T., Wallace, R., Durr, F.E., and Upeslacis, J. (2005) *Bioconjug. Chem.*, **16**, 346–353; (b) Hamann, P.R., Hinman, L.M., Beyer, C.F., Lindh, D., Upeslacis, J., Shochat, D., and Mountain, A. (2005) *Bioconjug. Chem.*, **16**, 354–360.
24. Ojima, I., Geng, X., Wu, X., Qu, C., Borella, C.P., Xie, H., Wilhelm, S.D., Leece, B.A., Bartle, L.M., Goldmacher, V.S., and Chari, R.V.J. (2002) *J. Med. Chem.*, **45**, 5620–5623.
25. Wu, X. and Ojima, I. (2004) *Curr. Med. Chem.*, **11**, 429–438.
26. Ranson, M. and Sliwkowski, M.X. (2002) *Oncology*, **63** (Suppl. 1), 17–24.
27. Widdison, W.C., Wilhelm, S.D., Cavanagh, E.E., Whiteman, K.R., Leece, B.A., Kovtun, Y., Goldmacher, V.S., Xie, H., Steeves, R.M., Lutz, R.J., Zhao, R., Wang, L., Blättler, W.A., and Chari, R.V.J. (2006) *J. Med. Chem.*, **49**, 4392–4408.
28. Erickson, H.K., Park, P.U., Widdison, W.C., Kovtun, Y.V., Garrett, L.M., Hoffman, K., Lutz, R.J., Goldmacher, V.S., and Blättler, W.A. (2006) *Cancer Res.*, **66**, 4426–4433.
29. Erickson, H.K., Widdison, W.C., Mayo, M.F., Whiteman, K., Audette, C., Wilhelm, S.D., and Singh, R. (2010) *Bioconjug. Chem.*, **21**, 84–92.
30. Kovtun, Y.V., Audette, C.A., Ye, Y., Xie, H., Ruberti, M.F., Phinney, S.J., Leece, B.A., Chittenden, T., Blättler, W.A., and Goldmacher, V.S. (2006) *Cancer Res.*, **66**, 3214–3221.
31. Xie, H., Audette, C., Hoffee, M., Lambert, J.M., and Blättler, W.A. (2004) *J. Pharmacol. Exp. Ther.*, **308**, 1073–1082.
32. Koblinski, J.E., Ahram, M., and Sloane, B.F. (2000) *Clin. Chim. Acta*, **291**, 113–135.
33. Law, B. and Tung, C.-H. (2009) *Bioconjug. Chem.*, **20**, 1683–1695.
34. Dubowchik, G.M., Firestone, R.A., Padilla, L., Willner, D., Hofstead, S.J., Mosure, K., Knipe, J.O., Lasch, S.J., and Trail, P.A. (2002) *Bioconjug. Chem.*, **13**, 855–869.
35. King, H.D., Dubowchik, G.M., Mastalerz, H., Willner, D., Hofstead, S.J., Firestone, R.A., Lasch, S.J., and Trail, P.A. (2002) *J. Med. Chem.*, **45**, 4336–4343.
36. Jeffrey, S.C., Nguyen, M.T., Andreyka, J.B., Meyer, D.L., Doronina, S.O., and Senter, P.D. (2006) *Bioorg. Med. Chem. Lett.*, **16**, 358–362.
37. Toki, B.E., Cerveny, C.G., Wahl, A.F., and Senter, P.D. (2002) *J. Org. Chem.*, **67**, 1866–1872.
38. Doronina, S.O., Toki, B.E., Torgov, M.Y., Mendelsohn, B.A., Cerveny, C.G., Chace, D.F., DeBlanc, R.L., Gearing, R.P., Bovee, T.D., Siegall, C.B., Francisco, J.A., Wahl, A.F., Meyer, D.L., and Senter, P.D. (2003) *Nat. Biotechnol.*, **21**, 778–784.
39. Francisco, J.A., Cerveny, C.G., Meyer, D.L., Mixan, B.J., Klussman, K., Chace, D.F., Rejniak, S.X., Gordon, K.A., DeBlanc, R., Toki, B.E., Law, C.-L., Doronina, S.O., Siegall, C.B., Senter, P.D., and Wahl, A.F. (2003) *Blood*, **102**, 1458–1465.
40. Sanderson, R.J., Hering, M.A., James, S.F., Sun, M.M.C., Doronina, S.O., Siadak, A.W., Senter, P.D., and Wahl, A.F. (2005) *Clin. Cancer Res.*, **11**, 843–852.
41. Pollack, V.A., Alvarez, E., Tse, K.F., Torgov, M.Y., Xie, S., Shenoy, S.G., MacDougall, J.R., Arrol, S., Zhong, H., Gerwien, R.W., Hahne, W.F., Senter, P.D., Jeffers, M.E., Lichenstein, H.S., and LaRochelle, W.J. (2007) *Cancer Chemother. Pharmacol.*, **60**, 423–435.
42. Okeley, N.M., Miyamoto, J.B., Zhang, X., Sanderson, R.J., Benjamin, D.R.,

Sievers, E.L., Senter, P.D., and Alley, S.C. (2010) *Clin. Cancer Res.*, **16**, 888–897.

43. Doronina, S.O., Bovee, T.D., Meyer, D.W., Miyamoto, J.B., Anderson, M.E., Morris-Tilden, C.A., and Senter, P.D. (2008) *Bioconjug. Chem.*, **19**, 1960–1963.

44. Burke, P.J., Toki, B.E., Meyer, D.W., Miyamoto, J.B., Kissler, K.M., Anderson, M., Senter, P.D., and Jeffrey, S.C. (2009) *Bioorg. Med. Chem. Lett.*, **19**, 2650–2653.

45. Wang, Y., Li, L., Tian, Z., Jiang, W., and Larrick, J.W. (2006) *Bioorg. Med. Chem.*, **14**, 7854–7861.

46. Chen, L., Gangwar, S., Guerlavais, V., Lonberg, N., and Zhang, Q. (2008) International Patent Application WO 2008/103693 A2.

47. Sufi, B., Guerlavais, V., Chen, L., Gangwar, S., Zhang, Q., and Passmore, D.B. (2008) International Patent Application WO 2008/083312 A2.

48. Beusker, P.H., de Groot, F.M.H., Tietze, L.F., Major, F., and Joosten, J.A.F. Spijker, H.J. (2007) International Patent Application WO 2007/089149 A2.

49. Moon, S.-J., Govindan, S.V., Cardillo, T.M., D'Souza, C.A., Hansen, H.J., and Goldenberg, D.M. (2008) *J. Med. Chem.*, **51**, 6916–6926.

50. Govindan, S.V., Cardillo, T.M., Moon, S.-J., Hansen, H.J., and Goldenberg, D.M. (2009) *Clin. Cancer Res.*, **15**, 6052–6061.

51. Jeffrey, S.C., Torgov, M.Y., Andreyka, J.B., Boddington, L., Cerveny, C.G., Denny, W.A., Gordon, K.A., Gustin, D., Haugen, J., Kline, T., Nguyen, M.T., and Senter, P.D. (2005) *J. Med. Chem.*, **48**, 1344–1358.

52. Jeffrey, S.C., Andreyka, J.B., Bernhardt, S.X., Kissler, K.M., Kline, T., Lenox, J.S., Moser, R.F., Nguyen, M.T., Okeley, N.M., Stone, I.J., Zhang, X., and Senter, P.D. (2006) *Bioconjug. Chem.*, **17**, 831–840.

53. Jeffrey, S.C., Nguyen, M.T., Moser, R.F., Meyer, D.L., Miyamoto, J.B., and Senter, P.D. (2007) *Bioorg. Med. Chem. Lett.*, **17**, 2278–2280.

54. Burke, P.J., Senter, P.D., Meyer, D.W., Miyamoto, J.B., Anderson, M., Toki, B.E., Manikumar, G., Wani, M.C., Kroll, D.J., and Jeffrey, S.C. (2009) *Bioconjug. Chem.*, **20**, 1242–1250.

55. Chari, R.V.J. (2008) *Acc. Chem. Res.*, **41**, 98–107.

56. Doronina, S.O., Mendelsohn, B.A., Bovee, T.D., Cerveny, C.G., Alley, S.C., Meyer, D.L., Oflazoglu, E., Toki, B.E., Sanderson, R.J., Zabinski, R.F., Wahl, A.F., and Senter, P.D. (2006) *Bioconjug. Chem.*, **17**, 114–124.

57. Alley, S.C., Zhang, X., Okeley, N.M., Anderson, M., Law, C.-L., Senter, P.D., and Benjamin, D.R. (2009) *J. Pharmacol. Exp. Ther.*, **330**, 932–938.

58. Alley, S.C., Benjamin, D.R., Jeffrey, S.C., Okeley, N.M., Meyer, D.L., Sanderson, R.J., and Senter, P.D. (2008) *Bioconjug. Chem.*, **19**, 759–765.

59. Kellogg, B., Audette, C., Clancy, L., Emrich, S., Erickson, H., Fishkin, N., Jones, G., Kovtun, Y., Maloney, E., Mastico, R., Mayo, M., Okamoto, M., Pinkas, J., Singh, R., Sun, X., Wilhelm, S., and Zao, R. (2009) Annual Meeting of the American Association for Cancer Research, Denver, CO, abstract 5480.

60. Quiles, S., Raisch, K.P., Sanford, L.L., Bonner, J.A., and Safavy, A. (2010) *J. Med. Chem.*, **53**, 586–594.

61. Polson, A.G., Calemine-Fenaux, J., Chan, P., Chang, W., Christensen, E., Clark, S., de Sauvage, F.J., Eaton, D., Elkins, K., Elliott, J.M., Frantz, G., Fuji, R.N., Gray, A., Harden, K., Ingle, G.S., Kljavin, N.M., Koeppen, H., Nelson, C., Prabhu, S., Raab, H., Ross, S., Stephan, J.-P., Scales, S.J., Spencer, S.D., Vandlen, R., Wranik, B., Yu, S.-F., Zheng, B., and Ebens, A. (2009) *Cancer Res.*, **69**, 2358–2364.

62. Milenic, D.E., Brady, E.D., and Brechbiel, M.W. (2004) *Nat. Rev. Drug Discov.*, **3**, 488–498.

63. Boswell, C.A. and Brechbiel, M.W. (2007) *Nucl. Med. Biol.*, **34**, 757–778.

64. Nayak, T.K. and Brechbiel, M.W. (2009) *Bioconjug. Chem.*, **20**, 825–841.

65. (a) Wiseman, G.A., White, C.A., Witzig, T.E., Gordon, L.I., Emmanouilides, C., Raubitschek, A., Janakiraman, N., Gutheil, J., Schilder, R.J., Spies, S., Silverman, D.H.S., and Grillo-López, A.J. (1999) *Clin. Cancer Res.*, **5**,

3281s–3286s; (b) Witzig, T.E., Gordon, L.I., Cabanillas, F., Czuczman, M.S., Emmanouilides, C., Joyce, R., Pohlman, B.L., Bartlett, N.L., Wiseman, G.A., Padre, N., Grillo-López, A.J., Multani, P., and White, C.A. (2002) *J. Clin. Oncol.*, **20**, 2453–2463.

66. Davis, T.A., Kaminski, M.S., Leonard, J.P., Hsu, F.J., Wilkinson, M., Zelenetz, A., Wahl, R.L., Kroll, S., Coleman, M., Goris, M., Levy, R., and Knox, S.J. (2004) *Clin. Cancer Res.*, **10**, 7792–7798.

67. Sharkey, R.M., Burton, J., and Goldenberg, D.M. (2005) *Expert. Rev. Clin. Immunol.*, **1**, 47–62.

13
Antibody–Maytansinoid Conjugates: From the Bench to the Clinic

Hans Erickson

13.1
Introduction

Antibody–maytansinoid conjugates (AMCs) are targeted chemotherapeutic agents that utilize the specificity of monoclonal antibodies (mAbs) to deliver potent cell-killing maytansinoids to cancer cells that express the target antigen [1, 2]. Maytansinoids are potent antimitotic agents that inhibit tubulin polymerization by binding to the vinca alkaloid site on tubulin. They display significantly more potency toward human carcinoma cells than the vinca alkaloid drugs currently used in the clinic [3]. The first isolated maytansinoid, maytansine, was purified from the Ethiopian shrub *Maytenus seratta* [4]. Clinical development of maytansine as a chemotherapeutic agent for treating cancer was discontinued due to lack of efficacy, and significant dose-limiting neurotoxicity and gastrointestinal toxicity [3]. AMCs offer a means of maintaining the high potency to targeted cells while lowering systemic toxicity. Indeed, AMCs have been found to be well tolerated in patients and several have shown promising activity in clinical trials [5–10].

Several of the attributes believed important for an effective AMC include high levels of the target antigen on the surface of the cancer cells, minimal expression of the target antigen on healthy tissues, efficient internalization and drug release at the tumor, and known sensitivity of the cancer cell to antimitotic agents [1, 11]. AMCs utilize nonimmunogenic humanized (or fully human) antibodies with good specificity for their cancer antigen. A key component of an AMC is the linker that connects the maytansinoid to the antibody. The optimal linker appears to depend on several characteristics associated with the target antigen and on the biology of the cancer. The precise factors that dictate which linker will be optimal for a given target remain unclear. The linker should limit release of the cytotoxic agent from the conjugate during circulation while at the same time maximize release of the most active cytotoxic metabolite within the tumor [11]. Ultimately, linkers that balance plasma stability and efficient tumor release of the active cytotoxic metabolites are the most effective.

13.2
Conjugation Strategies

To improve the likelihood that the best possible linker is selected, conjugation chemistries have been developed to enable maytansinoid thiols to be linked to the antibody via uncleavable thioether-based linkers and cleavable disulfide-based linkers. Linkable maytansinoid thiols are structurally similar to maytansine with the N-acyl-N-methyl-L-alanyl ester groups at the C3 position of the macrocycle containing thiol groups that allow for conjugation (Figure 13.1). Disulfide-based linkers offer the unique advantage that the disulfide bond strength can be fine-tuned by introducing methyl substituents adjacent to the disulfide bond. A panel of such linkers with variable bond strengths has been developed [12]. Conjugates that utilize disulfide-based linkers are designated "cleavable" because their linkers may be cleaved within the tumor and to a much lesser extent in plasma, depending on the strength of their disulfide bond. The thioether-based linkers are designated as "uncleavable" because they generally cannot be cleaved by chemical or enzymatic processes in biological systems. Uncleavable conjugates release their payload following proteolytic cleavage of the polypeptide backbone of the antibody within the targeted cancer cells [13]. Conjugates described in this chapter are named according to the linker and maytansinoid used in the conjugation. Similar two-step conjugation strategies are employed for the synthesis of both cleavable and uncleavable conjugates using heterobifunctional linkers containing an N-hydroxy succinimidyl group for reaction with lysine residues from the antibody at one end, and a maleimide or a pyridyl disulfide group for reaction with the maytansinoid thiol at the other end of the linker. Each conjugate has an average of three to four maytansinoids linked per antibody molecule. Examples of reaction schemes utilized in the preparation of the uncleavable mAb-SMCC-DM1 (SMCC = N-succinimidyl-4-(N-maleimidomethyl)cyclohexane-1-carboxylate) and cleavable mAb-SPDB-DM4 (SPDB = N-succinimidyl-4-(2-pyridyldithio)butanoate) are shown in Figure 13.2. The structures of the AMCs currently undergoing clinical evaluations are shown in Figure 13.3.

Disulfide-linked AMCs with different bond strengths may be prepared by using different combinations of linkers and maytansinoid thiols in the conjugation [15, 16]. The SPDB-DM4 and SPP-DM1 (SPP = N-succinimidyl-4-(2-pyridyldithio) pentanoate) linker-maytansinoid combinations have been selected for the

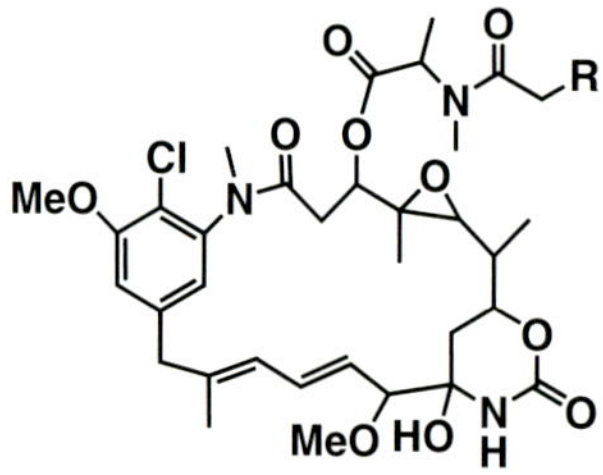

Figure 13.1 Structures of maytansine and the linkable maytansinoid thiols DM1 and DM4. R = H: maytansine; R = CH_2SH: DM1; R = $CH_2C(CH_3)_2SH$: DM4.

13.2 Conjugation Strategies | 377

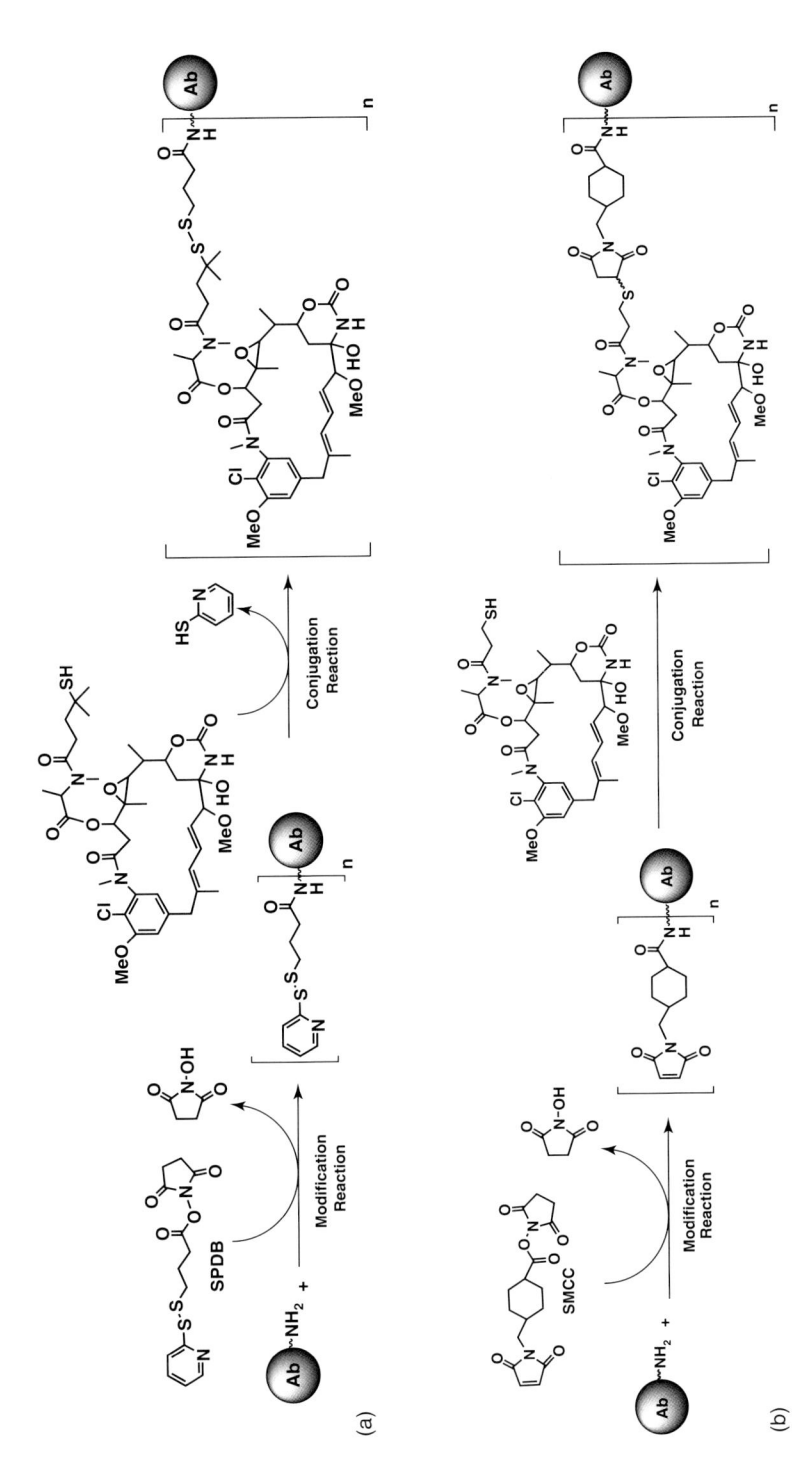

Figure 13.2 Conjugation strategy for the preparation of (a) cleavable and (b) uncleavable AMCs. (Adapted from [14].)

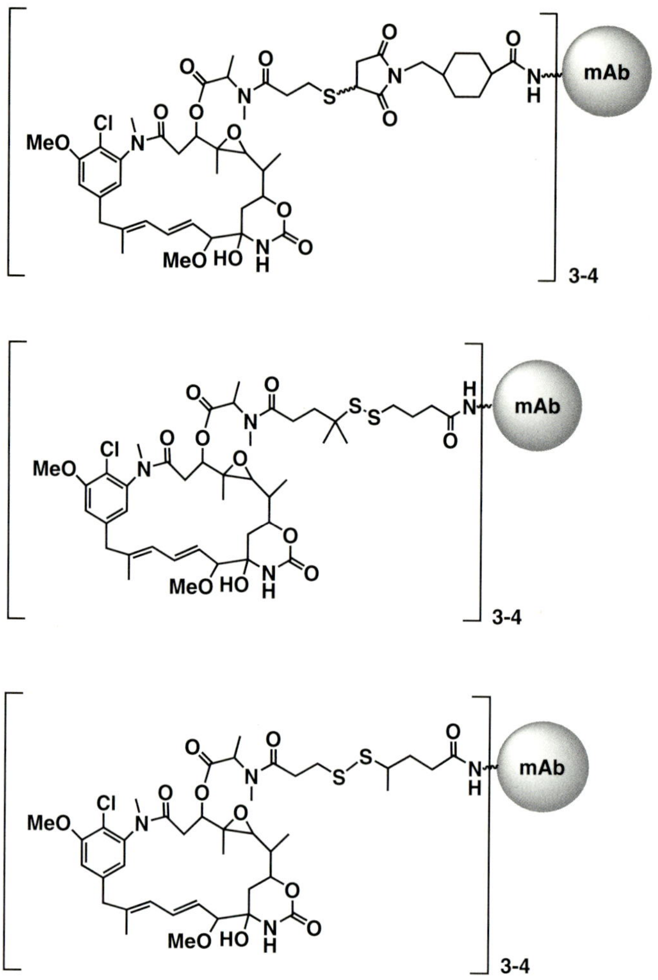

Figure 13.3 Structural representation of AMC conjugates currently in the clinic.

disulfide-linked AMCs currently in the clinic (Figure 13.3). The humAb-SPDB-DM4 conjugate is prepared by modifying with SPDB and then reacted with the DM4 maytansinoid thiol as shown in Figure 13.2. An analogous strategy is employed for the preparation of mAb-SPP-DM1 with SPP and DM1 in place of SDPB and DM4. The mAb-SPDB-DM4 conjugate is more resistant to cleavage via thiol–disulfide exchange than the mAb-SPP-DM1 conjugate due to increased steric hindrance provided by the presence of two methyl groups on the carbon adjacent to the maytansinoid side of the disulfide bond versus one methyl group on the carbon adjacent to the linker side of the disulfide bond in the case of SPP-DM1. The clearance of the anti-CanAg AMC, huC242-SPDB-DM4 ($t_{1/2}$ = 102 h, Figure 13.4), from mouse plasma resembles that of the uncleavable

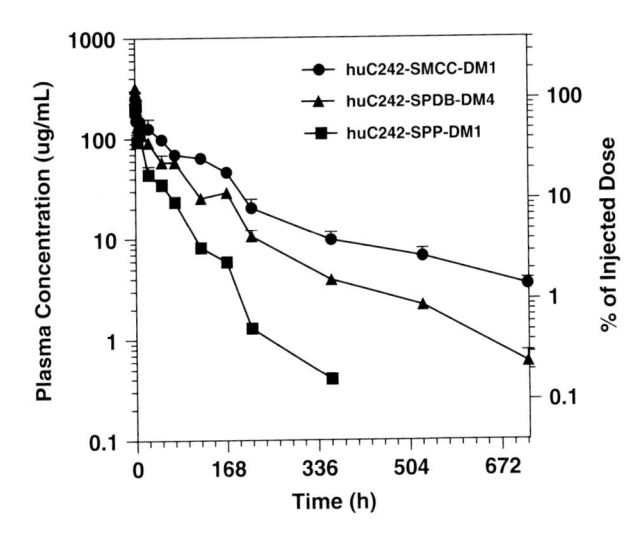

Figure 13.4 Plasma clearance of huC242-SMCC-DM1, huC242-SPDB-DM4, and huC242-SPP-DM1 in mice [1]. Female CD-1 mice were administered a single 10 mg/kg (based on antibody) intravenous dose of the conjugates. Plasma concentrations of the conjugates were determined using an enzyme-linked immunosorbent assay (ELISA)-based assay [18].

huC242-SMCC-DM1 conjugate ($t_{1/2} = 134$ h, Figure 13.4). Importantly, a similar long elimination half-life of 4–6 days was observed in patients treated with SAR3419 an anti-CD19 AMC that utilizes the SPDB-DM4 linker [9]. By contrast, the less-hindered huC242-SPP-DM1 conjugate ($t_{1/2} = 47$ h, Figure 13.4) was cleared more readily from plasma in mice than the mAb-SPDB-DM4 conjugates [1] and also exhibited a shorter half-life (40 h) in patients [17]. Several additional combinations of linkers and maytansinoids were combined to prepare a panel anti-HER2 conjugates with a broad range of disulfide bond sensitivities to thiol–disulfide exchange cleavage (Figure 13.5) [16]. A pharmacokinetic analysis of the conjugates along with the uncleavable trastuzumab-SMCC-DM1 is shown in Figure 13.5b where the concentration of conjugate and total antibody in plasma were measured in mice to determine the percentage of conjugated antibody in plasma following intravenous administration of the conjugates. A correlation was observed between the degree of steric hindrance and the percentage of the antibody that retained the maytansinoid load. The most hindered disulfide-linked conjugate, trastuzumab-SSNPP-DM4, displayed pharmacokinetics similar to trastuzumab-SMCC-DM1 with a conjugate concentration that was 70% of the total antibody concentration at day 7. Conjugates with incrementally lower levels of methyl group substitutions resulted in concomitantly lower percentages with no detectable amount of the completely unhindered trastuzumab-SPDP-DM1 observed at 7 days. These results demonstrate how the two-step conjugation strategy may be employed to fine-tune the disulfide bond of an AMC.

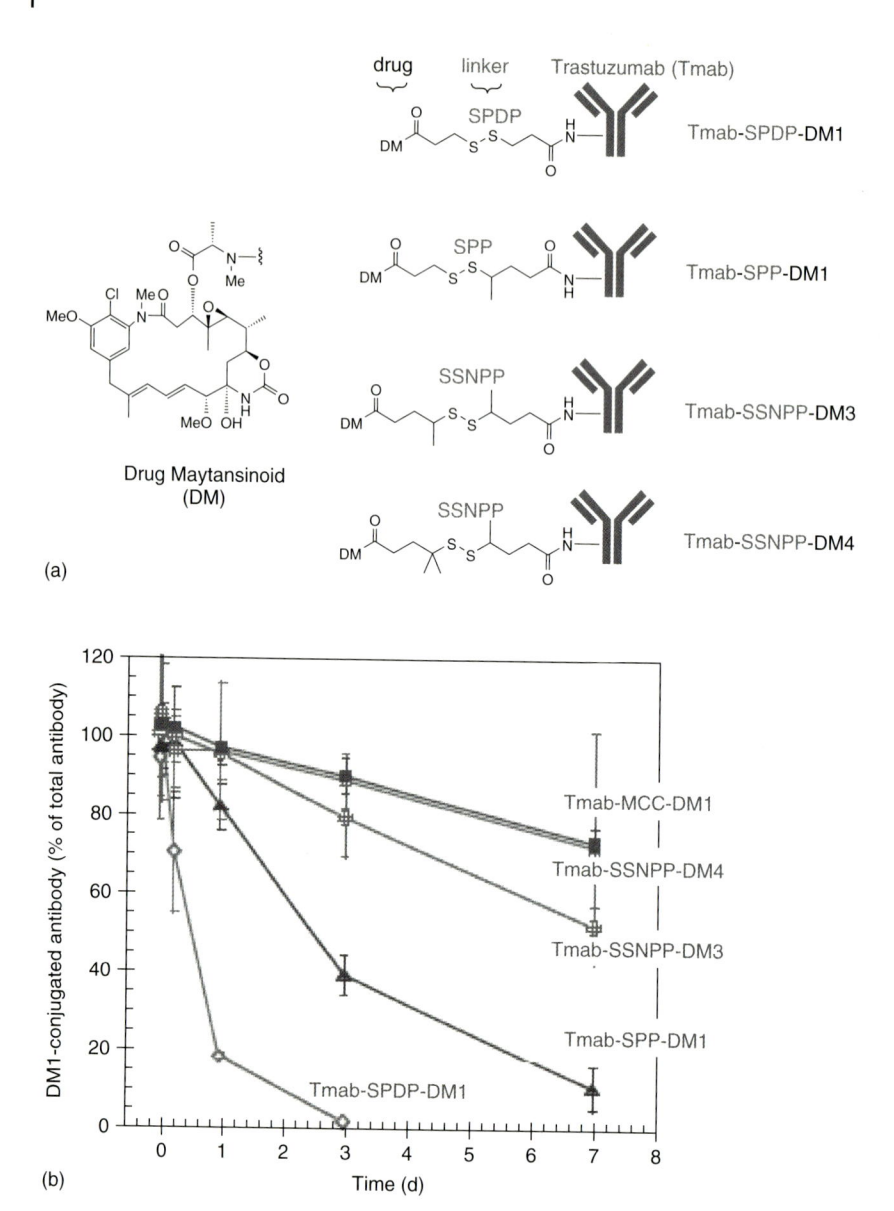

Figure 13.5 Structures of disulfide-linked trastuzumab maytansinoid conjugates with different bond strengths (a) and their pharmacokinetic properties (b). Female beige nude mice were given a single intravenous dose of 2 mg/kg (antibody dose) of the conjugates, and serum samples were collected and analyzed for total and conjugated trastuzumab using ELISA-based assays. The concentration of conjugated trastuzumab was divided by the total antibody concentration to determine the percent of total antibody that was conjugated to maytansinoid at each time point. Tmab-MCC-DM1 and trastuzumab-SMCC-DM1 represent the same uncleavable conjugate. From [16].

The effect of altering the linker cleavability in an AMC is not intuitive. A more labile linker may result in premature release of the payload that would potentially serve to increase the systemic toxicity and decrease the efficacy by limiting the amount of payload delivered to the tumor. Conversely, a highly stable linker may slow the rate of release of the active payload at the tumor, which may offset (or more than offset) the fact that more of the conjugate reaches the tumor with the payload intact. With regard to possible systemic toxicity, disulfide-linked conjugates – including those that utilize the relatively cleavable SPP-DM1 linker – have been shown to be very well tolerated in patients. In fact, the maximum tolerated doses (MTDs) reported for several disulfide-linked conjugates are higher than the established MTD of the uncleavable trastuzumab–DM1 [2]. With regard to the release of active payload at the tumor, in preclinical mouse studies, the exposure of tumors to the maytansinoid metabolites of trastuzumab-SPP-DM1 and trastuzumab-SMCC-DM1 was found to be similar, despite the nearly 3-fold faster clearance of the SPP-DM1 conjugate, suggesting that linker selections that decrease the cleavability of the SPP-DM1 linker-maytansinoid do not significantly increase the exposure of the tumor to the activated maytansinoid metabolites, at least in the case of AMCs targeting HER2 [19]. In addition, the disulfide linkers lead to the formation of maytansinoid metabolites that, for several targets, appear to offer a significant advantage over the metabolites of the more stable uncleavable conjugates [20]. A more thorough description of the metabolites formed with different linkers will be described in the metabolism sections below.

13.3
Selecting the Optimal Linker

The optimal linker for an AMC depends on the properties of the target antigen and possibly the biology of the tumor. The lead clinical candidates were selected empirically by preparing conjugates with several different combinations of linker and maytansinoid, as described in Figure 13.2, and testing to see which conjugate provided the greatest therapeutic window – the difference between the minimally effective dose in mouse xenografts models and the MTD. Ideally, multiple mouse (or rat) xenograft models are available that approximate the levels of the target antigen on the cancer to be treated. The lead candidate should display efficacy in those models at doses below the expected MTD in humans. The tolerated dose in humans may often be extrapolated from existing clinical data with AMCs that utilize the same linker provided there is little expression of the target on healthy tissue [21]. For AMCs targeting CD138, α_v integrin, CD19, and CanAg, the DM4 maytansinoid and the SPDB linker combination was selected [15, 22–24], and for targeting CD56, the DM1 maytansinoid and the SPP linker combination was selected [2]. The studies that led to the selection of SPDB-DM4 for an AMC targeting CD138, which is expressed on multiple myeloma, provide an example of how the optimal linker and maytansinoids are selected [24]. The efficacy of anti-CD138 conjugates prepared

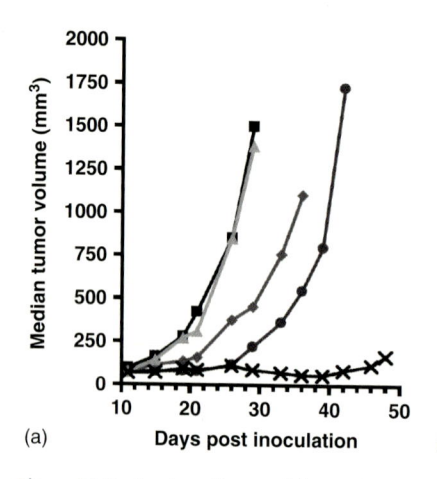

Figure 13.6 In vivo efficacy of the uncleavable and cleavable anti-CD138–maytansinoid conjugates. (a) Mice bearing MOLP-8 tumor xenografts were treated with a single intravenous administration of PBS (■), or nBT062-SMCC-DM1 at a dose of 100 (▲), 250 (♦), and 450(●) μg/kg, or (×) weekly dosing at 250 μg/kg (six doses). Dosages are based on the amount of linked DM1. (b) Mice bearing MOLP-8 tumor xenografts were treated with a single intravenous administration of PBS (■), or 250 μg/kg (linked maytansinoid) of nBT062-SPP-DM1 (♦), nBT062-SPDB-DM4 (●), nontargeting mAb-SPDB-DM4 (▼), and free DM4 (×). Unmodified antibody, nBT062 (▲) was administered at 13.8 mg/kg (equivalent to the amount of antibody in the conjugate dose of 250 μg/kg). PBS, phosphate-buffered saline. From [24].

using three different linker-maytansinoid constructs (SPDB-DM4, SPP-DM1, and SMCC-DM1) was evaluated in SCID mice bearing CD138$^+$ MOLP-8 tumors and is shown in Figure 13.6. The uncleavable anti-CD138-SMCC-DM1 conjugate was found to arrest tumor growth when administered weekly at 13.8 mg/kg. The disulfide-linked anti-CD138-SPDB-DM4 was considerably more active with similar efficacy observed with just a single 13.8 mg/kg dose. A single 13.8 mg/kg dose of the less-hindered anti-CD138-SPP-DM1 resulted in significant, but less-sustained, tumor growth delay. Based on these observations, the SPDB-DM4 conjugate was selected for this target.

Changes to the linker component of the conjugates targeting the CanAg antigen were found to impact their antitumor activity in ways that were similar to the anti-CD138 AMCs. Antitumor activities of the three anti-CanAg conjugates huC242-SPP-DM1, huC242-SPDB-DM4, and huC242-SMCC-DM1 were evaluated in mice bearing relatively large size (300 mm^3) COLO205 tumors. A single administration of around 15 mg/kg based on antibody dose (300 μg/kg based on DM1 or DM4 dose) of the disulfide-linked huC242-SPDB-DM4 conjugate was more active than the corresponding huC242-SPP-DM1, while the uncleavable huC242-SMCC-DM1 conjugate was found to be inactive [23]. The huC242-SPDB-DM4 was also found to be active in the HT-29 xenograft model where the expression of the CanAg antigen is heterogeneous (Figure 13.7b) [13]. While the uncleavable

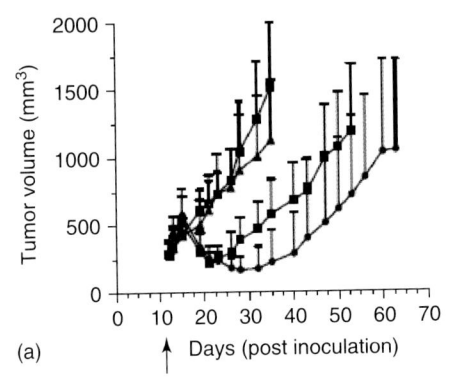

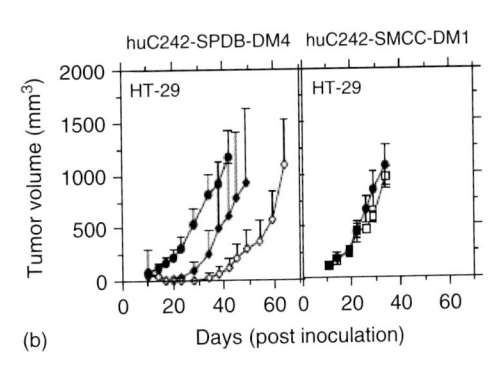

Figure 13.7 Antitumor activity of the anti-CanAg AMCs with SMCC-DM1, SPDB-DM4, and SPP-DM1 linkers in the (a) COLO205 and (b) HT-29 human colon tumor xenografts models. (a) Vehicle control (□), huC242-SMCC-DM1 (▲), huC242-SPP-DM1 (■), and huC242-SPDB-DM4 (●), and each administered at a dose of 300 μg/kg (approximately 15 mg/kg based on antibody dose). (Adapted from [23].) (b) Vehicle control (●), a single dose of 50 μg/kg huC242-SPDB-DM4 (♦), 150 μg/kg huC242-SPDB-DM4 (◊), or five daily injections of huC242-SMCC-DM1 at a dose of 150 μg/kg (□). Doses are based on the amount of conjugated DM4 or DM1. (Adapted from [13].)

huC242-SMCC-DM1 displayed no activity in either of these models, previous studies have demonstrated significant antitumor activity when smaller established COLO205 xenografts of 100 mm³ were treated with a greater total dose of around 38 mg/kg (based on antibody dose) administered as five daily injections [20].

In contrast to these two examples, the disulfide-linked trastuzumab conjugates shown in Figure 13.3 and the uncleavable trastuzumab-SMCC-DM1 conjugate were all found to exhibit similar activity in mouse xenografts models, with the trastuzumab-SMCC-DM1 conjugate displaying slightly more activity than the tested disulfide-linked versions (Figure 13.8) [16]. The trastuzumab-SMCC-DM1 was found to be better tolerated in rats than the cleavable trastuzumab-SPP-DM1 conjugate. Given its superior therapeutic window, trastuzumab-SMCC-DM1 was selected for clinical development. Recently AMCs to several antigen targets for the treatment for non-Hodgkin's lymphoma were evaluated, including CD19, CD20, CD21, CD22, CD72, CD79, and CD180 [25]. Cleavable conjugates prepared with the DM1 and SPP linker were found to be effective for all targets, including the poorly internalizing CD20, CD21, and CD72 antigens, while only CD22 and CD79 were effective targets for AMCs with the uncleavable SMCC-DM1 linker. The authors concluded that the cleavable SPP-DM1 linker may be the optimal choice for "poor" targets such as those with low or heterogeneous expression and poor internalization, and that the SMCC-DM1 linker and maytansinoid may be optimal for "good" targets. Unfortunately, the efficacy of the SPP-DM1 versions of the CD79 and CD22 targeting antibodies were not shown. It is possible that the cleavable conjugates of CD22 and CD79 were also more active than their uncleavable versions because other studies have shown that cleavable conjugates

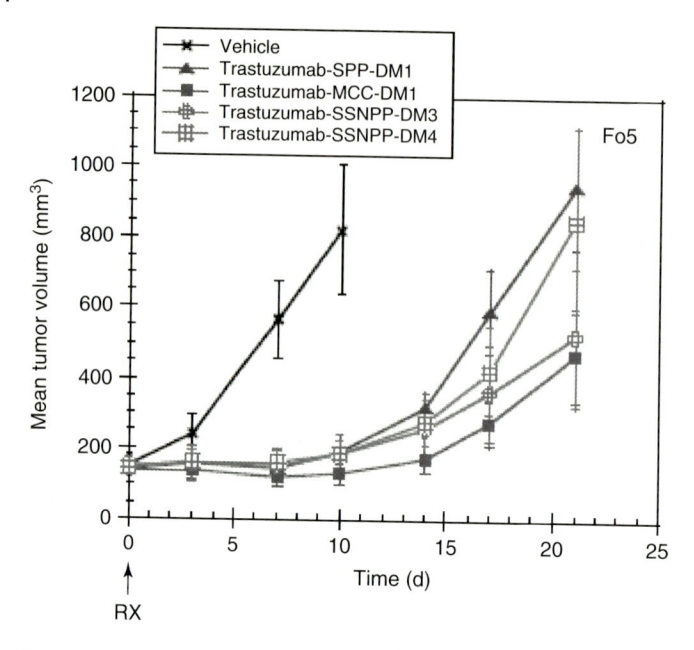

Figure 13.8 Antitumor activity of 10 mg/kg (based on antibody dose) of trastuzumab–maytansinoid conjugates prepared with SMCC-DM1 and cleavable disulfide-based linkers in mice bearing mammary tumor transplants from the MMTV-HER2 Fo5 line. (From [16].)

were more active than the uncleavable conjugate even for well-internalized and highly expressed or "good" targets [15, 22–24] – possibly by overcoming tumor barriers to antibody penetration [26].

13.4
Clinical Candidates

The most advanced AMC, trastuzumab emtansine (trastuzumab–DM1), utilizes the anti-HER2 antibody, trastuzumab (Herceptin®), which is itself approved in combination with chemotherapy for the treatment of HER2-positive metastatic breast cancer. While trastuzumab itself has only modest single-agent activity [27], trastuzumab–DM1 shows an objective response rate of about 33% in a phase II clinical trial where breast cancer patients that had received, on average, seven prior therapeutic agents for their metastatic disease were given 3.6 mg/kg trastuzumab–DM1 every 3 weeks [8]. Based on these favorable findings, a phase III trial for patients with second-line metastatic HER2-positive breast cancer and a phase III trial for first-line therapy were initiated and are ongoing.

In earlier clinical trials are AMCs targeting CD56, CD19, CD138, α_v integrin, and Cripto [2]. The disulfide-linked, anti-CD56 targeting, lorvotuzumab mertansine (huN901-SPP-DM1, IMGN901) has shown promising results in early clinical trials for the treatment of solid and liquid tumors that express the neural cell adhesion molecule (CD56) [6, 7]. CD56 is expressed on multiple myeloma and tumor cells of neuroendocrine origin, including Merkel cell carcinomas and small-cell lung carcinoma, and lorvotuzumab mertansine demonstrated activity in all these indications [6, 7, 28]. The CD19-targeting huB4-SPDB-DM4 (SAR3419) has also shown promising activity and tolerability in a phase I study for the treatment of B-cell malignancies [9]. Other AMCs are too early in their clinical development programs for their activity to be reported.

13.5
Activation of AMCs by Targeted Cancer Cells

13.5.1
Isolation of Maytansinoid Metabolites

Incorporation of a stable tritium isotope at the C20 methoxy group of DM1 or DM4 of the AMCs allows for the detection of maytansinoid metabolites formed within targeted cancer cells [23]. For *in vitro* studies, cultures of antigen-positive cells are exposed to the ^{3}H-conjugates, and any resulting ^{3}H-maytansinoid metabolites associated with acetone extracts of the cells and conditioned medium are separated by reversed-phase high-performance liquid chromatography (HPLC). The effluent from the column is monitored for tritium using an in-line flow scintillation analyzer [13]. Alternatively, if more sensitivity is required, the effluent is collected in fractions and the tritium can be monitored by liquid scintillation counting [23]. Metabolites are identified by liquid chromatography/mass spectroscopy and their coelution on reversed-phase HPLC with synthetically prepared standards. For *in vivo* studies, tumor tissues are isolated from tumor-bearing mice following treatment with the tritium-labeled conjugate and homogenized before extracting with acetone. *In vitro* and *in vivo* studies both offer unique advantages. *In vitro* studies allow for the estimation of both the maytansinoid metabolites generated by the target cells as well as the amount of unprocessed conjugate, thereby allowing the rate of antigen-mediated processing to be measured. Active or passive efflux of the metabolites from the targeted cancer cells can be assessed by monitoring the culture medium for metabolites and *in vitro* studies allow cellular functions such as lysosomal activation or inhibition of multidrug resistance (MDR) transporters to be probed [13, 26]. Unfortunately, the cytotoxic potency of an AMC measured *in vitro* does not always reflect its antitumor activity in mouse xenografts models, necessitating the need for *in vivo* metabolism studies. The concentration of metabolites in the tumor is affected by several additional factors beyond those of the target cell metabolism described *in vitro*. For example, the amount of conjugate that ultimately binds to the tumor cell *in vivo* is limited by several factors, such as barriers that limit antibody penetration into solid tumors [29, 30]. Therefore, direct measurements of the concentrations of maytansinoid metabolites within solid tumors *in vivo* provide important information distinct from that obtained *in vitro*.

13.5.2
Target Cell Metabolites of AMCs with SMCC-DM1, SPP-DM1, and SPDB-DM4 Linker-Maytansinoid Combinations

The metabolites identified from anti-CanAg-targeting AMCs typify what has been observed with AMCs targeting other antigens such as EpCAM, CD19, and HER2. The cellular metabolites of mAb-SMCC-³H-DM1, mAb-SPDB-³H-DM4 and mAb-SPP-³H-DM1 are shown in Figure 13.9. Lysine-SMCC-DM1 has been

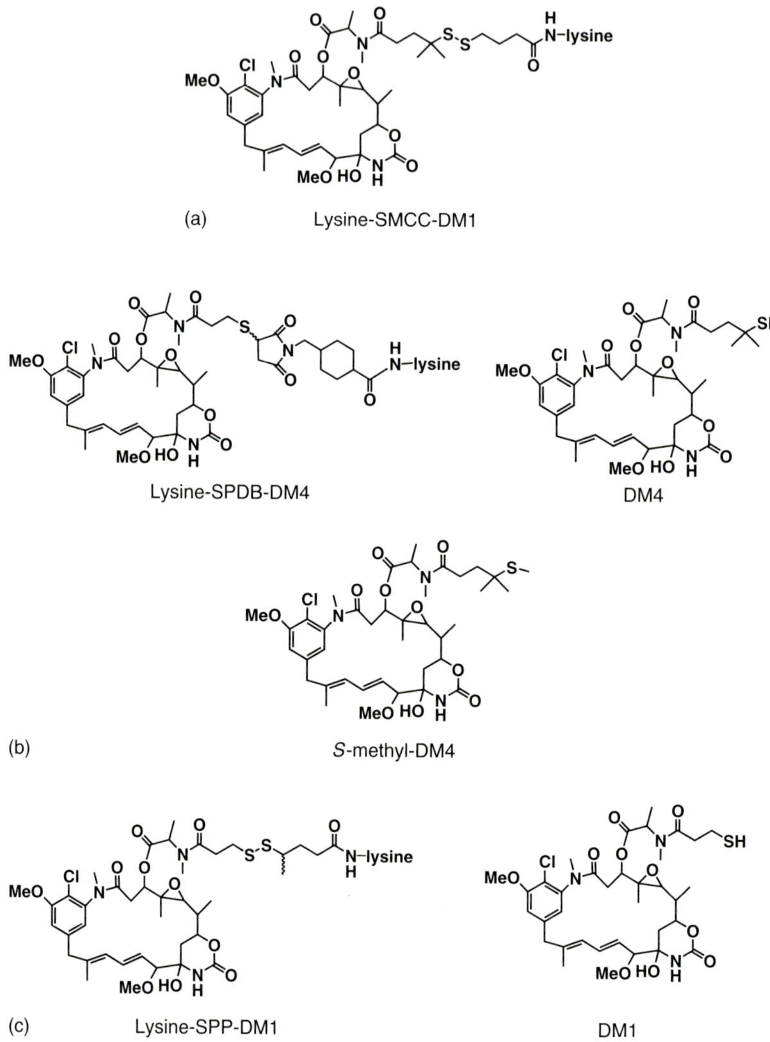

Figure 13.9 Target cell maytansinoid metabolites of (a) mAb-SMCC-DM1, (b) mAb-SPDB-DM4, and (c) mAb-SPP-DM1.

the only metabolite observed of several AMCs that utilize SMCC-DM1. The observed lysyl metabolite indicates that the polypeptide backbone of the conjugate is efficiently degraded in the lysosomes of the target cells to free the lysine to which the maytansinoids were originally linked. Lysine-SPDB-DM4, DM4, and S-methyl-DM4 are the major metabolites observed for AMCs that utilize SPDB-DM4, and lysine-SPP-DM1 and DM1 are the two major metabolites observed for the less-hindered disulfide-linked mAb-SPP-DM1. The observation that unconjugated DM4 was more efficiently methylated than unconjugated DM1 by the S-methyl transferase enzyme(s) endogenous to human carcinoma cells explains why S-methyl-DM1 is not an readily observed in tumor cells as a metabolite of conjugates that utilize SPP-DM1 [31].

13.5.3
Lysosomal Activation is Necessary for both Cleavable and Uncleavable Conjugates

The formation of all metabolites of both huC242-SPDB-DM4 and the huC242-SMCC-DM1 within targeted COLO205 cells and the G_2/M arrest induced by the conjugates were found to be blocked with the lysosomal inhibitor bafilomycin A1. The results suggest that the processing of both conjugates through the lysosomes was necessary for activity. Thus, cleavage to the disulfide bond to produce the DM4 metabolite must have occurred after formation of lysine-SPDB-DM4 [13]. Consistent with this, the rate of processing for the two conjugates to their respective metabolites was found to be the same. The rate of processing of the two anti-HER2 conjugates, trastuzumab-SPP-DM1 and trastuzumab-SMCC-DM1 to their respective metabolites (Figure 13.10) was also found to be the same, indicating a similar requirement for lysosomal processing of both cleavable and uncleavable conjugates. This is consistent with the finding that the anti-HER2 conjugate, trastuzumab-SPP-Rhodamine red was not reduced in the recycling endosomes, late endosomes, and lysosomes of HER2-positive SKBR3 cells [32]. Similar processing rates for the anti-EpCAM conjugates with SPP-DM1 and SMCC-DM1 by target cells were also observed [33], suggesting that lysosomal processing may generally be required for the activation of both cleavable and uncleavable AMCs. However, some exceptions have been reported, including the efficient reduction of disulfide-linked folate conjugates in endosomes [34] and the prelysosomal reduction of disulfide-linked AMCs targeting the epidermal growth factor receptor antigen in some cell lines [35].

13.5.4
Efficiency of Antigen-Mediated Processing

Binding of an AMC to the antigen on the cell surface results in internalization that ultimately leads to the release of the cytotoxic maytansinoid within the cell. The rate at which the bound AMC is processed to the active metabolites may be measured *in vitro* by measuring the total amount of conjugate bound to the cells and the total amount of processed metabolites produced by the cells as described for the

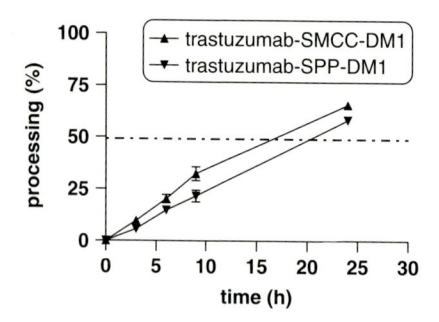

Figure 13.10 Target cell metabolism of trastuzumab-SMCC-DM1 and trastuzumab-SPP-DM1. The rate for the HER2-mediated processing of trastuzumab-SMCC-DM1 (▲) and trastuzumab-SPP-DM1 (▼) was calculated by dividing the metabolites of each conjugate formed at each time by the corresponding total maytansinoid levels at saturation. Cultures of BT474EEI breast carcinoma cells were exposed to a saturating concentration of the ^{3}H-conjugate for 2–3 h on ice. Cells were then washed and incubated in fresh medium at 37 °C. Cells were harvested at the indicated timepoints and precipitated with acetone. The acetone precipitate was solubilized and measured for residual radioactivity by liquid scintillation counting. Maytansinoid metabolites in the acetone extract were quantified using reversed-phase HPLC liquid scintillation counting. The chromatograms show the fraction number on the on the abscissa and the counts per minute on the ordinate. (Adapted from [19].)

trastuzumab–DM1 conjugates in Figure 13.10. The half-life for the HER2-mediated processing of the cleavable and uncleavable trastuzumab–DM1 conjugates was found to be about 18 h, similar to the value reported for ^{125}I-trastuzumab [36]. The half-life for the CD19-mediated processing of SAR3419 by Ramos cells was also found to be similar to the trastuzumab conjugates with a half-life for processing of 24 h [37]. The half-life for the anti-CD30 antibody–auristatin conjugate SGN-35 – a conjugate that utilizes a peptide linkage that also requires lysosomal processing – was recently reported to be 24 h using similar assays [38]. SGN-35 is currently in a pivotal trial for relapsed or refractory Hodgkin's lymphoma based on encouraging data from a phase I study with both Hodgkin's lymphoma and systemic anaplastic large-cell lymphoma patients [39].

13.5.5
Efflux of Metabolites from Targeted Cancer Cells and Bystander Effects

The efflux of metabolites from COLO205 cells exposed to huC242-SPDB-DM4 was found to depend on the intracellular concentration of the metabolites as shown in Table 13.1 [23]. Effluxed DM4 was converted to the S-cysteinyl-DM4 derivatives via thiol–disulfide exchange with cystine in the cell culture medium. We speculated that these effluxed metabolites could possibly enhance the effectiveness of cleavable AMCs via bystander effects. To test whether the metabolites were cytotoxic, their potencies were measured in cell-based viability assays [23]. The cytotoxic potency of DM4 is difficult to determine accurately *in vitro* because it reacts with cystine in the medium through thiol–disulfide exchange to yield a

Table 13.1 Dose-dependent efflux of maytansinoid metabolites from COLO205 cells following exposure to huC242-SPDB-^{3}H-DM4.

huC242-SPDB-^{3}H-DM4 (nM)	Sample	Lysine N$^\varepsilon$-SPDB-DM4 (pmol)	DM4-NEM/S-cysteinyl-DM4 (pmol)^a	S-Methyl-DM4 (pmol)	Total (pmol)	Number of molecules per cell
50	cell	7.2	17.6	147	172	5 100 000
	medium	64.9	19.0	20.1	104	3 080 000
5	cell	0.58	4.7	14.4	19.6	590 000
	medium	7.4	2.3	1.42	11.1	334 000
0.5	cell	0.87	0.25	0.16	1.28	39 000
	medium	ND	ND	ND	ND	ND

^{a}Sum of both metabolites. DM4 having a free thiol was trapped by reaction with N-ethyl maleimide (NEM); some DM4 reacted with cystine in growth medium to form the mixed disulfide S-cysteinyl-DM4.

charged S-cysteinyl-DM4 product that has a much lower cytotoxic potency. The S-methyl-DM4 metabolite was found to be the most potent with IC$_{50}$ values in the range of 0.01–0.03 nM (2- to 3-fold more cytotoxic than maytansine). Diffusion of the DM4 and S-methyl-DM4 metabolites from the targeted cancer cell *in vivo* to a neighboring cell would be expected to enhance the activity of the disulfide-linked conjugate via bystander killing. The lysine-SMCC-DM1 metabolite and the related lysine-SPDB-DM4 and lysine-SPP-DM1 metabolites were found to be much less cytotoxic than S-methyl-DM4, with IC$_{50}$ values between 2 and 20 nM, presumably because they have poor permeability across the cell membranes. The cytotoxic potencies of the huC242-SPDB-DM4, huC242-SPP-DM1, and huC242-SMCC-DM1 were similar toward COLO205 cells in spite of the large differences in the potencies of their metabolites as measured using cell-based viability assays, suggesting that when produced intracellularly, the maytansinoid metabolites all have similar high potencies [23]. Likewise, linker-independent cytotoxic potency *in vitro* was observed with AMCs targeting HER2 [16].

13.5.6
Target Cell Activation of Cleavable and Uncleavable AMCs

The metabolism studies conducted with several different AMCs and linkers suggest a model for the activation of an AMC where antigen-mediated endocytosis and trafficking to the lysosome results in the formation of the corresponding lysine-linker-maytansinoid via proteolytic degradation as shown in Figure 13.11. Diffusion of the lysine-linker-maytansinoid out of the lysosomes and into the cytoplasm allows for the disruption of mitosis via tubulin binding [33]. The uncleavable lysine-linker-maytansinoid undergoes no additional metabolism, whereas the cleavable lysine-linker-maytansinoid is cleaved in the reducing environment

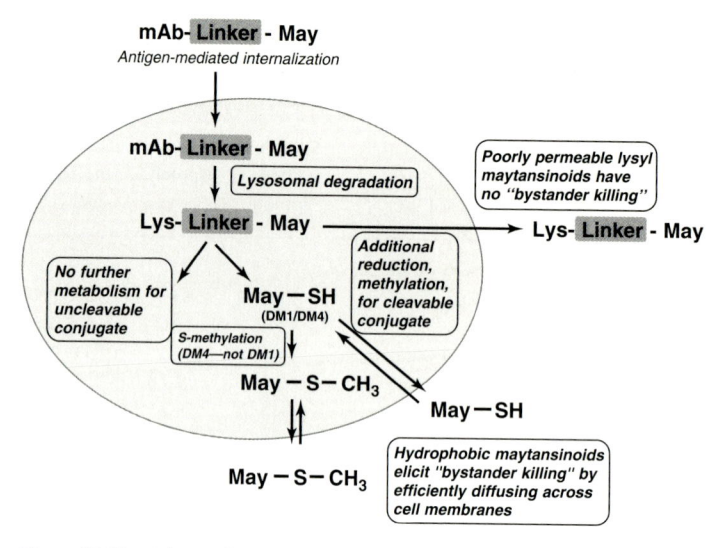

Figure 13.11 Scheme for the activation of cleavable and uncleavable AMCs.

of the cytoplasm to yield the free maytansinoid thiols DM1 and DM4. Further S-methylation of DM4 (but not DM1) by an endogenous S-methyl-transferase yields the additional S-methyl-DM4 metabolite of the mAb-SPDB-DM4 conjugate. All of the maytansinoid metabolites are effluxed from the target cell provided sufficient intracellular concentrations are achieved. The hydrophobic metabolites of the disulfide-linked conjugates readily diffuse across the cell membrane, allowing for the killing of neighboring bystander cells. In contrast, the poorly membrane-permeable lysine-linker-maytansinoids inefficiently diffuse across the membranes and have no bystander activity.

13.6
In Vivo Tumor Delivery Studies

The accumulation of maytansinoid metabolites in targeted tumor tissues following treatment of tumor-bearing mice with AMCs targeting several antigens including CanAg, CD19, and HER2 has been described [19, 23, 37]. The tumor metabolites for each of the conjugates were found to be the same as those shown in Figure 13.9 with the exception that the S-cysteinyl metabolites of the disulfide-linked conjugates that were formed by reaction with cystine in the cell culture medium following release of the maytansinoid thiol from the cell were not observed in extracts of tumor tissue – possibly because low pH of the tumor environment or low cystine concentrations lowers the reactivity of thiols via thiol–disulfide exchange [40], or since such species would only be formed outside the cell, they may diffuse away very quickly and thus be below the level of detection. The levels of the metabolites were measured in COLO205 tumor tissues of mice following a single intravenous administration of the tritium-labeled conjugates described in Figure 13.4. The area

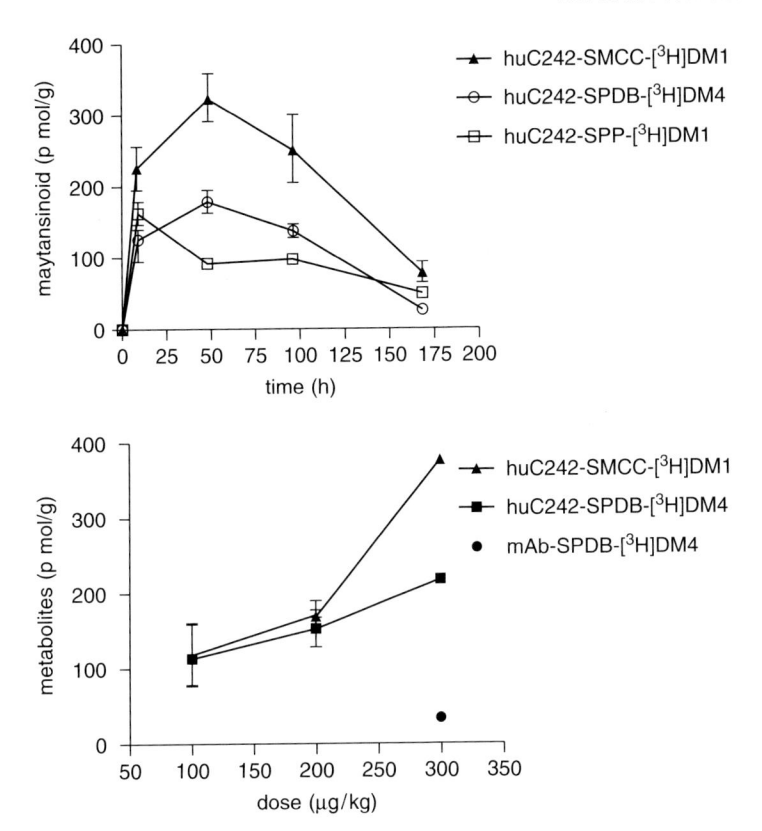

Figure 13.12 Accumulation of maytansinoid metabolites in tumor tissue following treatment of mice with the anti-CanAg AMCs. Mice were treated with a single administration of the tritium labeled anti-CanAg conjugates as described in Figure 13.4. Tumor tissues were harvested and analyzed for maytansinoid metabolites by extraction and reversed-phase HPLC with liquid scintillation counting. (Adapted from [23].)

under the curve (AUC) values over 7 days for the metabolites of the three anti-CanAg conjugates are shown in Figure 13.12. The AUC for the tumor metabolites of the uncleavable conjugate was about 2-fold greater than the corresponding AUC of the metabolite of the disulfide-linked conjugates at the 15 mg/kg dose. The levels were estimated to be high enough to allow for efficient diffusion from the targeted cancer cells (Table 13.1) [23]. We proposed that the diffusion of the metabolites of the disulfide-linked conjugate from the target cells may reduce the measured levels of metabolites of cleavable conjugates relative to the metabolites of the uncleavable conjugate. When the huC242-SMCC-DM1 and huC242-SPDB-DM4 conjugates were administered at lower doses of 200 and 100 µg/kg, the metabolite levels in the tumor were found to be the same for the two conjugates – possibly a consequence of less diffusion of metabolites from the targeted cells (Figure 13.12). One might speculate that at lower doses, the intracellular binding sites (tubulin) were not saturated, thus leading to little or no efflux, as observed *in vitro* at lower concentrations of the AMC (Table 13.1).

13.7
Conclusions

Promising data from several recent clinical trials have validated the potential of AMCs for cancer therapy. Once the antibody component of an AMC has been selected, optimization of the linker component is conducted by testing the antitumor activity of several conjugates prepared with cleavable disulfide-based linkers and uncleavable thioether-based linkers in mouse xenografts models. Much progress has been made to understand the mechanisms for their activation within cancer cells. In particular, the influence that the linker component has on the nature of the target cell metabolites is well understood. Reduction of the lysine-linker-maytansinoid metabolite of disulfide-linked conjugates generates highly active metabolites that can enhance the activity of the disulfide-linked conjugates via bystander killing. For AMCs targeting HER2, the disulfide-linked conjugates were not found to be more active in mouse models than the uncleavable trastuzumab-SMCC-DM1 conjugate, indicating that the optimal linker for an AMC depends on the characteristics of the target antigen and/or the biology of the tumor. The interchangeable linkers and maytansinoid thiols used to prepare AMCs allows for the linker component to be "fine-tuned" to achieve the conjugate with the best therapeutic index. Several new linkers are being developed that may allow for further optimizations by this flexible modular approach to AMC synthesis. For example, uncleavable conjugates prepared with a maleimidyl-based hydrophilic linker PEG4Mal were recently found to be more active toward targeted cancer cells that express the MDR-1 transporter than conjugates prepared with the SMCC-DM1 linker [26]. With this flexible technology and promising results emerging from clinical trials, AMCs are truly "poised to deliver" [41].

References

1. Chari, R.V. (2008) Targeted cancer therapy: conferring specificity to cytotoxic drugs. *Acc. Chem. Res.*, **41**, 98–107.
2. Lambert, J.M. (2010) Antibody–maytansinoid conjugates; a new strategy for the treatment of cancer. *Drugs Future*, **35**, 471–480.
3. Issell, B.F. and Crooke, S.T. (1978) Maytansine. *Cancer Treat. Rev.*, **5**, 199–207.
4. Kupchan, S.M., Komoda, Y., Branfman, A.R., Sneden, A.T., Court, W.A., Thomas, G.J. et al. (1977) The maytansinoids. Isolation, structural elucidation, and chemical interrelation of novel ansa macrolides. *J. Org. Chem.*, **42**, 2349–2357.
5. Chanan-Khan, A., Jagannath, S., Heffner, T., Avigan, D., Lee, K., Lutz, R.J. et al. (2009) Phase I study of BT062 given as repeated single dose once every 3 weeks in patients with relapsed or relapsed/refractory multiple myeloma. 51st Annu Meet Am Soc Hematol (Dec 5–8, New Orleans) 2008, Abst 1862.
6. Chanan-Khan, A., Wolf, J., Gharibo, M., Jagannath, S., Munshi, N., Anderson, K.C. et al. (2009) Phase 1 study of IMGN901, used as a monotherapy, in patients with heavily pre-treated CD56-positive multiple myeloma. A preliminary safety and efficacy analysis. 51st Annu Meet Am Soc Hematol (Dec 5–8, New Orleans) 2009, Abst 2883.
7. Fossella, F., Woll, P.J., Lorigan, P., Tolcher, A., O'Brien, M., O'Keeffe, J. et al. (2009) Investigation of IMGN901 in CD56[+] solid tumors: results from a phase I/II trial (study 001) and a phase I

trial (study 002). 13th World Conference on Lung Cancer, San Francisco, CA.

8. Krop, I.E., Beeram, M., Modi, S., Jones, S.F., Holden, S.N., Yu, W. et al. (2010) Phase I study of trastuzumab–DM1, an HER2 antibody–drug conjugate, given every 3 weeks to patients with HER2-positive metastatic breast cancer. J. Clin. Oncol., 28, 2698–2704.

9. Younes, A., Gordon, L., Kim, S., Romaguera, J., Copeland, A.R., de Castro Farial, S. et al. (2009) Phase I multi-dose escalation study of the anti-CD19 maytansinoid immunoconjugate SAR3419 administered by IV infusion every 3 weeks to patients with relapsed/refractory B-cell NHL. 51st Annu Meet Am Soc Hematol (Dec 5–8, New Orleans) 2009, Abst 585.

10. Galsky, M.D., Eisenberger, M., Moore-Cooper, S., Kelly, W.K., Slovin, S.F., DeLaCruz, A. et al. (2008) Phase I trial of the prostate-specific membrane antigen-directed immunoconjugate MLN2704 in patients with progressive metastatic castration-resistant prostate cancer. J. Clin. Oncol., 26, 2147–2154.

11. Alley, S.C., Okeley, N.M., and Senter, P.D. (2010) Antibody–drug conjugates: targeted drug delivery for cancer. Curr. Opin. Chem. Biol., 14, 529–537.

12. Widdison, W.C., Wilhelm, S.D., Cavanagh, E.E., Whiteman, K.R., Leece, B.A., Kovtun, Y. et al. (2006) Semisynthetic maytansine analogues for the targeted treatment of cancer. J. Med. Chem., 49, 4392–4408.

13. Erickson, H.K., Park, P.U., Widdison, W.C., Kovtun, Y.V., Garrett, L.M., Hoffman, K. et al. (2006) Antibody–maytansinoid conjugates are activated in targeted cancer cells by lysosomal degradation and linker-dependent intracellular processing. Cancer Res., 66, 4426–4433.

14. Singh, R. and Erickson, H.K. (2009) Antibody–cytotoxic agent conjugates: preparation and characterization. Methods Mol. Biol., 525, 445–467, xiv.

15. Chen, Q., Millar, H.J., McCabe, F.L., Manning, C.D., Steeves, R., Lai, K. et al. (2007) Alphav integrin-targeted immunoconjugates regress established human tumors in xenograft models. Clin. Cancer Res., 13, 3689–3695.

16. Lewis Phillips, G.D., Li, G., Dugger, D.L., Crocker, L.M., Parsons, K.L., Mai, E. et al. (2008) Targeting HER2-positive breast cancer with trastuzumab–DM1, an antibody–cytotoxic drug conjugate. Cancer Res., 68, 9280–9290.

17. Helft, P.R., Schilsky, R.L., Hoke, F.J., Williams, D., Kindler, H.L., Sprague, E. et al. (2004) A phase I study of cantuzumab mertansine administered as a single intravenous infusion once weekly in patients with advanced solid tumors. Clin. Cancer Res., 10, 4363–4368.

18. Xie, H. and Blattler, W.A. (2006) In vivo behaviour of antibody–drug conjugates for the targeted treatment of cancer. Expert Opin. Biol. Ther., 6, 281–291.

19. Erickson, H.K., Lewis Phillips, G.D., Provenzano, C., Leipold, D., Pinkas, J., Mai, E. et al. (2010) The effect of linker on target cell catabolism and PK/PD of trastuzumab–maytansinoid conjugates. AACR–NCI–EORTC Conference, Berlin, abstract A149.

20. Kovtun, Y.V., Audette, C.A., Ye, Y., Xie, H., Ruberti, M.F., Phinney, S.J. et al. (2006) Antibody–drug conjugates designed to eradicate tumors with homogeneous and heterogeneous expression of the target antigen. Cancer Res., 66, 3214–3221.

21. Polson, A.G. and Sliwkowski, M.X. (2009) Toward an effective targeted chemotherapy for multiple myeloma. Clin. Cancer Res., 15, 3906–3907.

22. Al-Katib, A.M., Aboukameel, A., Mohammad, R., Bissery, M.C., and Zuany-Amorim, C. (2009) Superior antitumor activity of SAR3419 to rituximab in xenograft models for non-Hodgkin's lymphoma. Clin. Cancer Res., 15, 4038–4045.

23. Erickson, H.K., Widdison, W.C., Mayo, M.F., Whiteman, K., Audette, C., Wilhelm, S.D. et al. (2010) Tumor delivery and in vivo processing of disulfide-linked and thioether-linked antibody–maytansinoid conjugates. Bioconjug. Chem., 21, 84–92.

24. Ikeda, H., Hideshima, T., Fulciniti, M., Lutz, R.J., Yasui, H., Okawa, Y.

et al. (2009) The monoclonal antibody nBT062 conjugated to cytotoxic maytansinoids has selective cytotoxicity against CD138-positive multiple myeloma cells *in vitro* and *in vivo*. *Clin. Cancer Res.*, **15**, 4028–4037.

25. Polson, A.G., Calemine-Fenaux, J., Chan, P., Chang, W., Christensen, E., Clark, S. et al. (2009) Antibody–drug conjugates for the treatment of non-Hodgkin's lymphoma: target and linker-drug selection. *Cancer Res.*, **69**, 2358–2364.

26. Kovtun, Y.V., Audette, C.A., Mayo, M.F., Jones, G.E., Doherty, H., Maloney, E.K. et al. (2010) Antibody–maytansinoid conjugates designed to bypass multidrug resistance. *Cancer Res.*, **70**, 2528–2537.

27. Smith, I., Procter, M., Gelber, R.D., Guillaume, S., Feyereislova, A., Dowsett, M. et al. (2007) 2-year follow-up of trastuzumab after adjuvant chemotherapy in HER2-positive breast cancer: a randomised controlled trial. *Lancet*, **369**, 29–36.

28. Lambert, J.M. (2005) Drug-conjugated monoclonal antibodies for the treatment of cancer. *Curr. Opin. Pharmacol.*, **5**, 543–549.

29. Jain, R.K. (1999) Transport of molecules, particles, and cells in solid tumors. *Annu. Rev. Biomed. Eng.*, **1**, 241–263.

30. Thurber, G.M., Schmidt, M.M., and Wittrup, K.D. (2008) Antibody tumor penetration: transport opposed by systemic and antigen-mediated clearance. *Adv. Drug Deliv. Rev.*, **60**, 1421–1434.

31. Erickson, H.K., Mayo, M., Widdison, W., Audette, C., Kovtun, Y., Chari, R. et al. (2007) Linker selection in antibody–maytansinoid conjugates impacts bystander killing in tumor xenograft mouse models. AACR–NCI–EORTC Conference, San Francisco, CA, abstract A86.

32. Austin, C.D., Wen, X., Gazzard, L., Nelson, C., Scheller, R.H., and Scales, S.J. (2005) Oxidizing potential of endosomes and lysosomes limits intracellular cleavage of disulfide-based antibody–drug conjugates. *Proc. Natl. Acad. Sci. USA*, **102**, 17987–17992.

33. Oroudjev, E., Lopus, M., Wilson, L., Audette, C., Provenzano, C., Erickson, H. et al. (2010) Maytansinoid–antibody conjugates induce mitotic arrest by suppressing microtubule dynamic instability. *Mol. Cancer Ther.*, **9**, 2700–2713

34. Yang, J., Chen, H., Vlahov, I.R., Cheng, J.X., and Low, P.S. (2006) Evaluation of disulfide reduction during receptor-mediated endocytosis by using FRET imaging. *Proc. Natl. Acad. Sci. USA*, **103**, 13872–13877.

35. Maloney, E., Fishkin, N., Audette, C., Clancy, L., Sun, X., Chari, R., and Singh, R. (2009) Designing potent antibody–maytansinoid conjugates (AMCs): the impact of lysosomal processing efficiency and conjugate linker selection on anticancer activity. AACR–NCI–EORTC Conference, Boston, MA, abstract B120.

36. Austin, C.D., De Maziere, A.M., Pisacane, P.I., van Dijk, S.M., Eigenbrot, C., Sliwkowski, M.X. et al. (2004) Endocytosis and sorting of ErbB2 and the site of action of cancer therapeutics trastuzumab and geldanamycin. *Mol. Biol. Cell*, **15**, 5268–5282.

37. Erickson, H.K., Mayo, M.F., Widdison, W.C., Audette, C. et al. (2009) Target-cell processing of the anti-CD19 antibody maytansinoid conjugate SAR3419 in preclinical models. AACR Annual Conference Denver, CO, abstract 5473.

38. Alley, S.C., Zhang, X., Okeley, N.M., Anderson, M., Law, C.L., Senter, P.D. et al. (2009) The pharmacologic basis for antibody–auristatin conjugate activity. *J. Pharmacol. Exp. Ther.*, **330**, 932–938.

39. Younes, A., Forero-Torres, A., Bartlett, N.L., Leonard, J.P., Lynch, C., Kennedy, D.A. et al. (2008) Multiple complete responses in a phase 1 dose-escalation study of the antibody–drug conjugate SGN-35 in patients with relapsed or refractory CD30-positive lymphomas. ASH Annual Meetings Abstracts 2008:112:1006.

40. Gatenby, R.A. and Gillies, R.J. (2004) Why do cancers have high aerobic glycolysis? *Nat. Rev. Cancer*, **4**, 891–899.

41. Hughes, B. Antibody–drug conjugates for cancer: poised to deliver? *Nat. Rev. Drug Discov.*, **9**, 665–667.

14
Calicheamicin Antibody–Drug Conjugates and Beyond

Puja Sapra, John DiJoseph, and Hans-Peter Gerber

14.1
Introduction

Cancer chemotherapy is fraught with systemic toxicities resulting from cytotoxicity to normal cells. Cancer cells share many common features with the normal host cells from which they originate, so finding unique targets against which anticancer drugs can be selectively directed is difficult. Invariably, the toxic side-effects often limit optimal dosing of anticancer drugs, leading to disease relapse and the development of drug resistance, and also poor quality of life for patients. One possible approach to improve the selective toxicity of anticancer drugs is by targeting anticancer drugs via monoclonal antibodies (mAbs) or ligands, against antigens or receptors that are uniquely or selectively overexpressed on cancer cells. In this regard, a number of mAb-based therapies, including immunotoxins, radioimmunotherapeutics, mAb–drug conjugates, and immunoliposomes, have received considerable attention.

Antibody-targeted chemotherapy relies on the specific binding of the targeting mAb–drug conjugate to the tumor antigen followed by internalization of the antigen–mAb–drug complex in order to ensure delivery of the cytotoxic agent inside the tumor cells. Targeted delivery of cytotoxic agents not only maximizes antitumor efficacy, but also significantly reduces exposure of cytotoxics to normal tissues, thereby improving the therapeutic index of the antibody-targeted chemotherapy agent. This concept has been successfully translated into commercial and clinical reality by the launch of Mylotarg®. Mylotarg (gemtuzumab ozogamicin, CMA-676) is an immunoconjugate of calicheamicin in which a calicheamicin derivative, N-acetyl-γ-calicheamicin dimethyl hydrazide (DMH), is covalently linked via an acid-hydrolyzable AcBut linker to a humanized IgG4 anti-CD33 antibody (gemtuzumab) [1, 2]. In addition to Mylotarg that gained US Food and Drug Administration (FDA) approval in 2000 for the treatment of acute myeloid leukemia (AML) patients, several other calicheamicin-based conjugates have also undergone preclinical and clinical development, including CMC-544. CMC-544 is similar to Mylotarg in that they both contain the same linker and calicheamicin derivative combination (ozogamicin). However, unlike Mylotarg targeting CD33 expressed

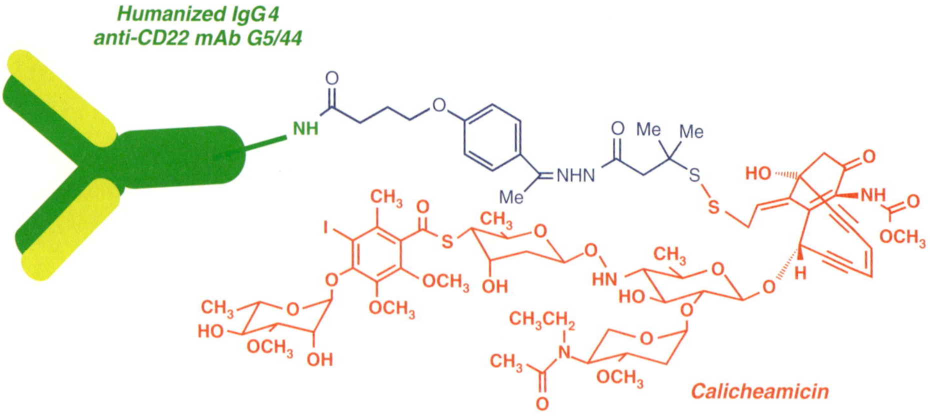

Figure 14.1 Calicheamicin conjugates consist on average of four loaded antibodies, conjugated to lysines. All linkers, shown here in red and blue, are based on an acid-labile AcBut hydrazone linker that is cleaved in the acid environment of late endosomes. The hydrazone linker is conjugated to the antibody via a disulfide linkage that has been stabilized by two methyl groups to prevent premature release of calicheamicin.

on myeloid cells and AML, CMC-544 is targeted to CD22 and used for the treatment of $CD22^+$ non-Hodgkin's lymphoma (NHL) [3] (Figure 14.1).

Calicheamicin is a DNA-damaging agent that, following intracellular activation, binds to DNA in the minor groove and introduces double-strand DNA breaks, leading to G_2/M arrest and subsequent cell death [4]. Importantly, the mechanism of action of calicheamicin is fundamentally different from the tubulin-binding class of cytotoxics, which represents the second class of payloads for antibody–drug conjugates (ADCs) currently undergoing advanced clinical testing. In contrast to spindle poisons like the auristatins or maytansines, which are most effective against rapidly proliferating cells, calicheamicin induces DNA double-strand breaks and apoptosis independent of cell cycle progression [1, 5–8]. Such properties may be advantageous when targeting malignant cells that are not markedly different in their proliferation status compared to normal cells. More recently, cancer stem cells (CSCs) were identified as promising therapeutic targets in oncology, as they may represent the "root problem" of cancer due to their self-renewal capabilities and their resistance toward conventional anticancer therapeutics (reviewed in [9]). CSC eradication is thought to be crucial for successful anticancer therapy. CSCs frequently display lower levels of steady-state proliferation compared to the more rapidly proliferating, fully differentiated cancer cells, which comprise the majority of malignant cells within tumors. The relative low proliferation rates of CSCs combined with the abundance of drug efflux mechanisms may account for the frequent relapse of cancer patients treated with conventional cytotoxics, which are most effective against rapidly proliferating tumor cells. Thus, for targeting of CSCs and other cells within tumors that contribute to malignancy, but which do not proliferate rapidly, the use of non-cell-cycle-dependent cytotoxics such as calicheamicin may be advantageous. In this chapter, we review the preclinical and clinical data generated with calicheamicin conjugates, and highlight some of the key differences between the pharmacological and physicochemical properties of DNA double-strand breakers and tubulin inhibitor-based conjugates. Finally, we discuss future trends in ADC development, aimed at the improvement of ADCs in oncology indications.

14.2
Discovery of Calicheamicin and Mechanism of Action

The calicheamicin story began in the early 1980s when a bacterium, *Micromonospora echinospora* ssp. *calichensis*, was isolated from a sample of caliche clay collected near Kerrville, TX, in August of 1981 [4, 10]. This study was part of a screening program aimed at identifying new classes of fermentation-derived antitumor antibiotics using a very sensitive biochemical induction assay [11]. This assay used a genetically engineered strain of *Escherichia coli* i-lysogen containing the *lacZ* reporter gene, which encodes the enzyme α-galactosidase. DNA-damaging agents result in the induction of the α-galactosidase gene and, in the presence of a suitable chromogenic substrate. The assay was used to assay bacterial colonies on agar plugs, and to follow the isolation and purification of the various calicheamicin metabolites. The calicheamicins identified in this *in vitro* screen turned out to be more potent than other cytotoxic antitumor compounds when tested against tumor models in mice [12].

Calicheamicin is a very potent tumoricidal agent that functions by efficiently cutting DNA. This is carried out by the enediyne aglycone functionality (the "warhead") of calicheamicin upon progression to a highly reactive diradical species [13]. This activated calicheamicin γ1 form consists of a diradical that causes a hydrogen abstraction in the phosphodiester sugar backbone of the DNA, thereby inducing DNA double-strand breaks (Figure 14.2). Calicheamicin γ1 binds DNA in the minor groove, with a preference for the d(TCCT)·d(AGGA) sequence, and inhibits the formation of a transcription complex [14].

In order for calicheamicin to become activated within cells, the presence of a cytoplasmic thiol cofactor, such as glutathione, is required (Figures 14.2 and 14.3). The activation of calicheamicin to calicheamicin γ1 is attributed to the high intracellular concentration of glutathione. Glutathione is a thiol-containing tripeptide that is present in micromolar concentrations in the blood, whereas its concentration in the cytoplasm is in the millimolar range (up to 1000-fold higher, reviewed in [15]). This is particularly the case in tumor cells, where irregular blood flow leads to a hypoxic state (decreased oxygen level), resulting in enhanced activity of reductive enzymes and therefore even higher glutathione concentrations [16].

Several metabolites of calicheamicin have been identified and described [17]. When comparing the *in vitro* potency of these metabolites, there is an about 20-fold lower potency of the γ-calicheamicin DMH derivative, compared to the activated, diradical form of calicheamicin (γ1 form). Compared to some of the most commonly use cytotoxic compounds, including cisplatin or doxorubicin,

N-Acetyl gamma Calicheamicin DMH
Binds DNA in minor groove

enediyne

−S-S-Reduction

Hydrogen abstraction from phosphodiester backbone of DNA

di-radical generation

Double-strand DNA Breaks

p-Phenylene Diradical

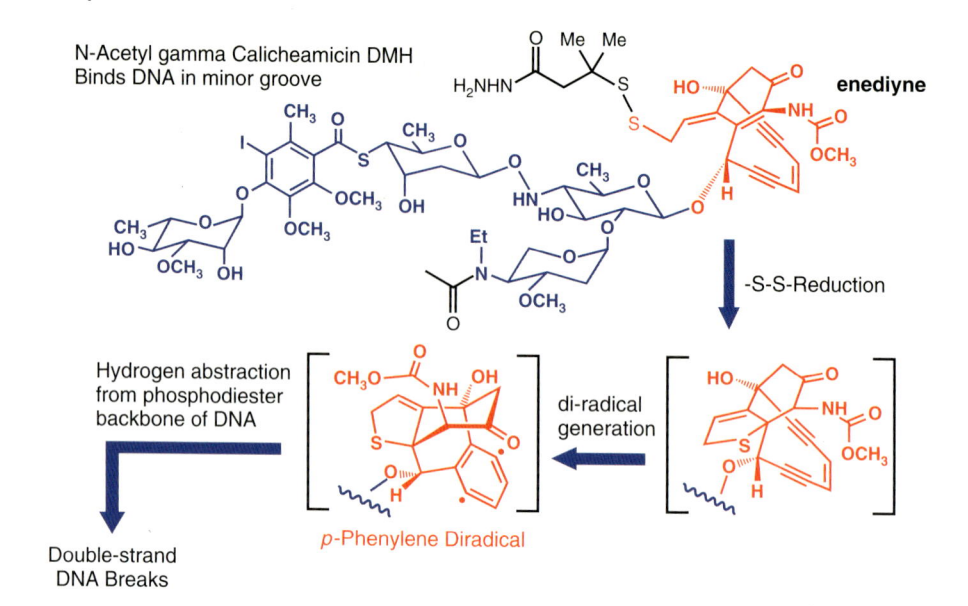

Figure 14.2 Calicheamicin is inactive before becoming activated or "triggered" by intracellular thiol groups, generating the highly active biradical form. The activation step requires glutathione (GSH), which triggers a disulfide reduction leading to the active enediyne form. Once activated, calicheamicin enters the nucleus and induces DNA double-strand breaks.

calicheamicin appears much more potent [3]. Calicheamicin γ1 is the metabolite to which several mAbs were eventually conjugated, forming the calicheamicin DMH derivative [12, 18]. Upon internalization of the ADC, the calicheamicin prodrug is released by hydrolysis of the hydrazone in lysosomes of antigen-positive target cells (Figure 14.3). The enediyne drug then becomes activated following reductive cleavage of the disulfide bond. Selective linker cleavage and calicheamicin release is based upon the differential properties between the plasma and some cytoplasmic compartments. Linkers were chosen that were stable in the blood's neutral pH environment, but become susceptible to cleavage once the ADC has entered the lower pH environment inside a cell. The focus during these early days of ADC development was on acid-cleavable hydrazone linkers, which are relatively stable at neutral pH (bloodstream pH 7.3–7.5), but undergo hydrolysis once internalized into the mildly acidic endosomes (pH 5.0–6.5) and lysosomes (pH 4.5–5.0). The disulfide linkage connecting the calicheamicin moiety with the hydrazone linker is stabilized by two methyl groups to prevent premature release of calicheamicin [18]. Most of the calicheamicin conjugates tested in preclinical and clinical settings consisted of this bifunctional linker, composed of an azide-labile, hydrazone-based linker and a stabilized disulfide linker, to allow for release of the prodrug calicheamicin in the reductive, intracellular environment. In preclinical models, the hydrazone linkage produced ADCs with higher potency than the corresponding amide-bearing conjugates, which still contained the stabilized

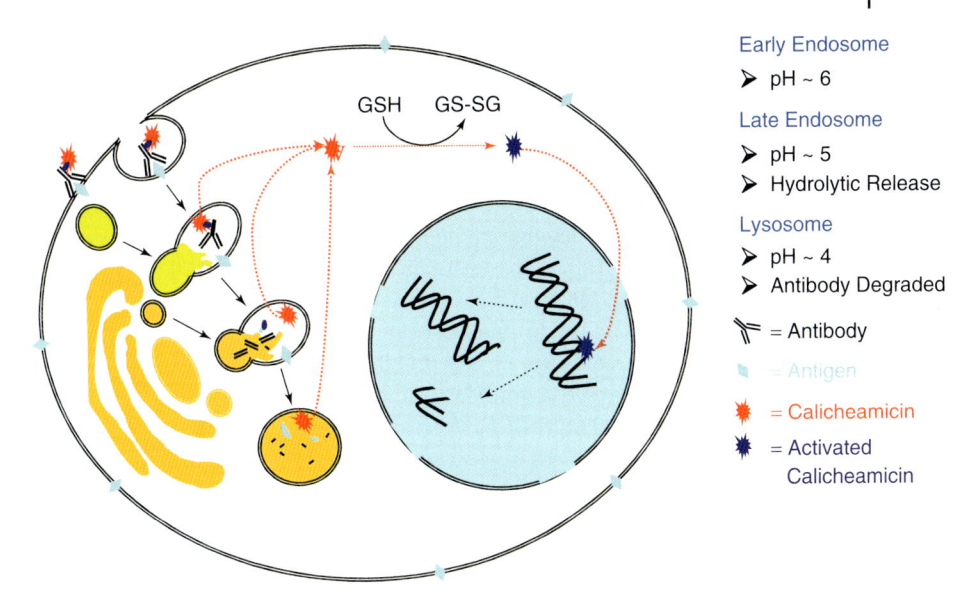

Figure 14.3 Mechanism of action associated with linker cleavage included the intracellular trafficking of the ADC from early to late lysosomes, with a concomitant change in pH from 6.5 to approximately 4.5, leading to progressive linker cleavage and intracellular drug release.

disulfide linkage, but lacked the hydrazone functionality [18]. These findings provided evidence that the stabilized disulfide bond alone is insufficient for efficient release of the drug in the target cell and that the hydrazone group is required to maximize potency.

14.3 Calicheamicin ADCs

14.3.1 Gemtuzumab Ozogamicin (Mylotarg)

Mylotarg is a conjugate of a derivative of calicheamicin, N-acetyl-γ-calicheamicin DMH, linked to a recombinant humanized antibody (hP67.6) against the hematopoietic antigen, CD33. The antibody component of Mylotarg, hP67.6, was produced by humanization of the mP67.6 by complementarity-determining region grafting. The IgG4 isotype was chosen in part because it is the least likely to participate in immune-mediated mechanisms such as complement fixation and antibody-dependent cellular cytotoxicity (ADCC). The linker used in Mylotarg is a bifunctional linker referred to as the AcBut linker. This linker is attached to the lysines of the antibody and also forms a hydrazone with the hydrazide of the N-acetyl-γ-calicheamicin DMH. The hydrazone linkage is hydrolyzed in the acidic environment of the endosomes/lysosomes through which the antibody is routed after internalization. However, approximately 50% of the hP67.6 molecules are not linked to calicheamicin.

The CD33 antigen is a 67-kDa type I transmembrane sialoglycoprotein, a founding member of the immunoglobulin superfamily subset of sialic acid binding immunoglobulin-related lectins (siglec-3) [19]. Functionally, CD33 is involved in cell–cell interactions and signaling in the hematopoietic and the immune system. Also, cross-linking of CD33 with mAbs in the context of normal $CD34^+$ cells cultured with stem cell factor and granulocyte macrophage colony-stimulating factor has been associated with inhibition of cell growth, suggesting a role for CD33 in the negative regulation of cell proliferation [20]. The CD33 antigen is expressed on the surface of leukemic blasts in more than 90% of patients with AML [21, 22]. The antigen is also expressed by immature myeloid cells and megakaryocyte precursors, and to a lesser degree by mature myeloid cells, but not by pluripotent stem cells [23].

In vitro, binding of Mylotarg to leukemic cells results in cellular internalization of Mylotarg; internalization and catabolism of 38% of the CD33–antibody complex occurred within 4 h [24]. Inside the cell, the low pH in endosomes and lysosomes causes the calicheamicin to be released from the antibody followed by conversion of calicheamicin to a reactive intermediate (as described above) that damages DNA, causing cell death. Mylotarg has been shown to be cytotoxic to the human leukemia cell line that expresses CD33 (HL-60), with both high potency and high selectivity relative to cell lines that do not express CD33. Mylotarg was 1000-fold more cytotoxic to HL-60 cells than a comparable, nontargeting conjugate and unconjugated hP67.6 antibody.

14.3.2
Clinical Development of Gemtuzumab Ozogamicin (Mylotarg)

AML is characterized by proliferation of leukemic blasts in the bone marrow and other tissues and, if untreated, is a rapidly fatal disease. Disappearance of red blood cells, platelets, and mature white blood cells leads to progressively more severe fatigue, infection, and hemorrhage during the disease course. To favorably affect the disease course, intensive chemotherapy must be supplemented with substantial supportive care (infection prevention and treatment, red blood cell and platelet transfusions, and growth factor administration). Chemotherapy in AML generally involves one to two courses of cytarabine and an anthracycline. Current combination chemotherapy regimens result in remission rates ranging from 50 to 80% [25–27]. mAb-based therapies are ideally suited for the treatment of AML because of the accessibility of neoplastic cells in the blood, bone marrow, spleen, and lymph nodes. Such neoplastic cells can be rapidly and efficiently targeted by specific mAbs [28].

Mylotarg was approved by the FDA in 2000 for treatment of patients aged 60 or over who have $CD33^+$ AML in first relapse and who are not otherwise candidates for cytotoxic chemotherapy. The clinically recommended dose of Mylotarg is

9 mg/m^2 administered as a 2- to 4-h intravenous infusion and repeated in two weeks. Three independent, noncomparative clinical trials of Mylotarg in patients with relapsed AML showed that Mylotarg induced a complete response (total absence of peripheral blasts and less than 5% leukemic blasts in the bone marrow) in 30% of the relapsed AML patients. Approximately a half of the responders demonstrated full hematopoietic recovery (absolute neutrophil count of 1500/µl or higher, hemoglobin above 9 g/dl, and platelet count of 100 000/µl or higher), whereas the remaining half of the responder population exhibited incomplete platelet recovery [29, 30]. The overall relapsed-free survival time of all patients who attained remission was greater than 6 months. The relapse-free survival of Mylotarg-treated elderly patients was still shorter (less than 6 months) than that of younger patients (under 16 months). The overall response rate of Mylotarg therapy is similar in elderly (60 years and above) and younger (under 60 years) patients with relapsed AML and similar in magnitude to that seen with combination chemotherapy. However, elderly patients, unlike their younger counterparts, cannot tolerate additional rounds of combination chemotherapy. In the absence of any other therapeutic alternative, Mylotarg represented the only therapeutic option for these elderly patients with relapsed AML.

No antibody response to any component within Mylotarg was detected in Mylotarg-treated patients in phase II studies. Infusion-related symptoms including fever, chills, and hypotension occurred in most patients receiving Mylotarg despite prophylactic treatment with antihistamine and acetaminophen. In addition, grade 3 or 4 hematological toxicity with neutropenia and thrombocytopenia was quite apparent in almost all patients treated with Mylotarg, which is consistent with the myeloid lineage-targeted cytotoxicity of Mylotarg. Approximately one quarter of the patients treated with Mylotarg exhibited National Cancer Institute grade 3 or 4 elevation of serum bilirubin and transaminases, indicative of liver toxicity that was transient and reversible. The most striking manifestation of the hepatic toxicity of Mylotarg is the development in 10% or less of the treated patients of often-fatal hepatic veno-occlusive disease, also known as hepatic sinusoidal obstruction syndrome, characterized by hepatomegaly, hepatic portal hypertension, hepatic necrosis, subendothelial edema, sinusoidal fibrosis, and occasionally, fibrous venular occlusion [31, 32].

Recently, Pfizer announced that, based on discussions with the FDA, the company would be discontinuing commercial availability of Mylotarg and voluntarily withdrawing the New Drug Application (NDA) for Mylotarg. This decision reflects the result from a postapproval study (SWOG S0106), combining chemotherapy and Mylotarg. The study did not demonstrate improved survival compared with chemotherapy alone in patients with previously untreated AML. Additionally, among all patients evaluable for early toxicity, the fatal induction toxicity rate was significantly higher in patients given the combination of standard induction chemotherapy and Mylotarg than in those treated with chemotherapy alone. Although the SWOG S0106 study did not confirm the clinical benefit of Mylotarg in combination, the results do not directly impact the risk/benefit of Mylotarg in its approved indication as a single agent. The approval of single agent Mylotarg in the

United States was granted under FDA's accelerated approval regulations based on overall response rate in three noncomparative studies of Mylotarg as a single agent and required submission of additional data to confirm clinical benefit.

14.3.3
CMC-544

14.3.3.1 CD22 Expression and Function

CD22 is a 135-kDa B-cell-restricted sialoglycoprotein expressed in the cytoplasm of early pre-B-cells and on the surface of mature B-cells [33–35]. It is lost prior to differentiation to plasma cells [36]. Although the precise function of CD22 is unclear, it is suggested to regulate signal transduction of the surface immunoglobulin receptors on B cells [37–41].

CD22 has been chosen as a target for conjugate delivery for a number of reasons. CD22 is expressed on the malignant cells of the majority of B-lymphocyte malignancies. Consistent with this notion, most patients newly diagnosed with indolent, intermediate-grade, or aggressive NHL expressed CD22 [42, 43]. CD22 is expressed on both normal and malignant cells of the mature B-lymphocyte lineage; however, as stated above, lymphocyte precursor cells and memory B-cells do not express CD22. Thus, the impact of treatment with CMC-544 on long-term immune functions is expected to be minimal. Moreover, based on *in vitro* testing of human NHL cell lines, CD22 is one of the better internalizing molecules among several B-lymphoid lineagespecific surface antigens and is not shed in the extracellular environment [43].

$CD22^+$ B-cell malignancies include indolent NHL, intermediate-grade and aggressive NHL, chronic lymphocytic leukemia, multiple myeloma, acute lymphocytic leukemia (ALL), and others [44]. NHL represents the fifth most common malignancy in adults and the incidence of NHL continues to increase. The majority (more than 90%) of NHL cases represents malignancies of the B-lymphocyte lineage and express CD22. NHL is the sixth leading cause of cancer deaths in the United States and Europe [45].

14.3.4
Preclinical Activity of CMC-544, an Anti-CD22–Calicheamicin Conjugate, in Models of NHL

CMC-544 is an antibody-targeted, intravenous chemotherapy agent composed of an antibody, targeting the CD22 antigen, which is linked to calicheamicin [46] (Figure 14.1). The targeting agent in CMC-544 is a humanized IgG4 antibody, G544, that specifically recognizes human CD22. Being an IgG4 isotype antibody, G544 is not expected to mediate effector functions such as complement-dependent cytotoxicity or ADCC.

CMC-544 binds to CD22 with high affinity ($K_D \sim 150$ pM) and exhibits a potent dose-dependent cytotoxicity against $CD22^+$ B-lymphoma cells *in vitro*. CMC-544 was between 7- and 100-fold more potent than an isotype-matched nonbinding conjugate (CMA-676), when tested against CD22$^+$ B-lymphoma cells [47]. CMC-544 was between 3- and 400-fold more potent against CD22$^+$ B-lymphoma cells than CD22$^-$ leukemic cells. CMC-544 ranged between being equivalent up to 38-fold higher in potency than unconjugated calicheamicin when tested *in vitro*. Unconjugated anti-CD22 antibody G544 had no effect on the growth of various B-cell lymphoma lines *in vitro*. CMC-544 caused dose-dependent regression of B-lymphoma xenografts grown as subcutaneous solid tumors in athymic nude mice [46]. Unconjugated anti-CD22 mAb G544 (the CD22-targeting antibody in CMC-544) had no effect on the growth of B-lymphoma cells *in vivo* [47]. This lack of antitumor efficacy of unconjugated G544 (humanized IgG4) is consistent with the lack of ability of IgG4 antibodies to fix complement or mediate ADCC.

CMC-544 administered at 120 µg or more of conjugated calicheamicin/kg q4d × 3 not only caused complete regression of B-lymphomas, but these treated mice remained tumor-free for at least 100 days and were considered cured [48]. This dose (120 µg/kg q4d × 3) was the minimum curative dose of CMC-544. The antitumor efficacy of CMC-544 was evident regardless of the size of the tumor before the initiation of therapy. CMC-544 is capable of causing regression of tumor masses as large as 10% of the body weight [49].

When evaluated simultaneously in the same RL B-cell lymphoma model, the antitumor effect of CMC-544 was longer lasting than that of the CHOP (cyclophosphamide, doxorubicin, vincristine, and prednisone) combination chemotherapy [3]. Similar findings were reported for the auristatin-based ADC SGN-35, when administered in combination with standard chemotherapy in models of Hodgkin's lymphoma [50]. There was evidence of synergistic or additive antitumor therapeutic effect of a combination of CMC-544 and rituximab at their respective doses studied. Additionally, the antitumor efficacy of CMC-544 was not inhibited by either prior or concurrent administration of rituximab [49].

In a model of systemically disseminated B-cell lymphomas grown in severe combined immunodeficient (SCID) mice, CMC-544 at dosages of 40 or 80 µg of conjugated calicheamicin/kg conferred almost complete protection against the disseminated B-cell lymphoma-induced hind-limb paralysis leading to death [48]. However, at a higher dose (160 µg of conjugated calicheamicin/kg), CMC-544 was less efficacious in protecting against the disease-associated hind-limb paralysis. SCID mice are more sensitive to the toxic effects of DNA-damaging agents, including calicheamicin. The same dose of CMC-544 has been proven to be curative with no lethality in subcutaneous B-cell lymphoma models in nude mice.

14.3.5
Effect of CMC-544 in a Model of ALL

ALL is primarily a B-cell or pre-B-cell malignancy. ALL blasts differentially express a number of B-lymphoid-specific antigens including CD22. The CD22 expressed on these blasts may allow preferential targeting by CMC-544. In order to investigate the effects of CMC-544 in ALL, mice were injected with Reh cells (a CD22$^+$ ALL-derived cell line) in the lateral tail vein and monitored for disease symptoms. All of the vehicle-treated mice succumbed to the disseminated disease by day 77. The average survival time for the group was 55 days. CMC-544, administered at a dose of 80 µg/kg of calicheamicin DMH produced 100% survival of the treated mice over the 127 day observation period. At the dose of 4 µg/kg calicheamicin DMH, 20-fold lower than the curative dose of 80 µg/kg, 90% of the mice still survived throughout the observation period. Flow cytometric analysis of bone marrow cells collected from the femur of these vehicle-treated mice demonstrated the presence of human $CD45^+$ leukemic cells. CMC-544 (80 µg/kg) inhibited by 75% the engraftment of the human $CD45^+$ cells [51].

Safety pharmacology assessment after a single intravenous dose of CMC-544 showed no toxicologically significant effects on the cardiovascular system in cynomolgus monkeys and on the central nervous system in rats. Thus, the non-clinical studies conducted with CMC-544 strongly supported its evaluation in subjects with B-cell malignancies, particularly NHL.

14.4
Clinical Development of Calicheamicin Conjugates: CMC-544

An open-label phase 1 study was conducted to test the safety, tolerability, and pharmacokinetics of CMC-544 administered as a single agent to subjects with $CD22^+$ B-cell NHL. CMC-544 was given intravenously approximately once every 21 days (±2 days) for at least four doses unless there was evidence of progressive disease or an unacceptable toxicity, or the subject refused [52]. These studies established the maximum tolerated dose (MTD; 1.8 mg/m^2) of inotuzumab ozogamicin administered every 28 days. Inotuzumab ozogamicin was tested either as a single agent or in combination with rituximab The MTD of inotuzumab ozogamicin was then determined in combination with rituximab in a phase I/II open-label, dose-escalation study in subjects with follicular NHL, or aggressive NHL (predominantly diffuse large B-cell lymphoma (DLBCL)). The inotuzumab ozogamicin plus rituximab combination is being further evaluated in a phase II study in subjects with relapsed/refractory $CD22^+$ DLBCL who are eligible for autologous stem cell transplant (aSCT). An additional phase I study is being planned to determine the tolerability, the initial safety profile, and the MTD of regimens R-CVP (rituximab in combination with cyclophosphamide, vincristine, and prednisone) or R-GDP (rituximab in combination with gemcitabine, dexamethasone, and cisplatinum) given in combination with inotuzumab ozogamicin in subjects with $CD22^+$ NHL. A phase III study of inotuzumab ozogamicin in combination with rituximab in subjects with relapsed DLBCL who are eligible for consolidation with aSCT and a phase III study in subjects with relapsed or refractory aggressive NHL who are not eligible for consolidation with aSCT are also planned.

The clinical data indicate that inotuzumab ozogamicin has an acceptable safety profile both as a single agent and in combination with rituximab, and has demonstrated promising preliminary clinical antitumor activity in subjects with NHL, including subjects with DLBCL.

14.5
Conclusions and Future Directions

A total of about 60 ADCs are currently being developed in oncology indications. Among them, close to 20 are undergoing clinical testing and the majority of these are tubulin inhibitor-based conjugates. When comparing some of the key characteristics of the three leading ADC compounds currently being developed in the clinic (Table 14.1), some early trends can be noticed.

First, the potencies of the three leading ADC platforms, when tested against standard tumor cell lines, are subnanomolar and similar activities were found when the free drugs were tested against tumor cells grown in culture. Such requirement for subnanomolar potencies of ADCs may represent the consequence of their limited uptake to tumor cells. The factors determining the uptake of

Table 14.1 Properties of the most successful ADCs developed in the clinic.

	CMC-544	SGN-35	Herceptin®–DM1
mAb	hIgG4, nonblocking, 0.1 nM	hIgG1, blocking, 2 nM	hIgG1, blocking, 1 nM
Loading	Lys/~7.2-load	Cys/ ~ 4–load	Lys/ ~ 4–load
Payload	DNA double-strand breaker, subnanomolar	tubulin inhibitor, subnanomolar	tubulin inhibitor, subnanomolar
Linker	hydrazone (acid labile)	peptide (stable)	thioether, noncleavable
Target copy number	CD22: ~10e4–10e5	CD30: ~10e4–10e5	HER2: ~2×10e5–10e6
Target internal	high ($t_{1/2}$ ~ 60 min)	high ($t_{1/2}$ = 30–60 min)	medium ($t_{1/2}$ ~ 4 h)
Activity/indication	ORR 80% in RR follicular lymphoma, 47% in RR DLBCL (NDA ~2015)	ORR >50% in RR Hodgkin's lymphoma (phase II, NDA ~2011)	ORR >40% in RR breast (phase III, NDA ~2011)
Target expression	clean normal B-cells	clean: tumor (high), some hematological cells	dirty: tumor (+++), normal tissues (+ heart)
Pharmacokinetics, $t_{1/2}$	12–30 h, increasing	3–8 days	3.5–3.7 days
Cellular trafficking	endo/lysosomal	endo/lysosomal	endo/lysosomal
DLT	thrombocytopenia, neutropenia, liver enzymes	neutropenia, liver enzymes (off-target)	thrombocytopenia (off-target)
MTD humans	~0.048 mg/kg, q4wk, i.v.	1.9 mg/kg, q3wk, i.v.	3.6 mg/kg, q3wk, i.v.

CMC-544 is an anti-CD22–calicheamicin conjugate developed in phase II in patients with NHL. Herceptin–DM1 is a HER2-directed, maytansine-based ADC currently being developed in phase II trials in patients with refractory metastatic breast cancer (reviewed in [53]). SGN-35 is an anti-CD30-directed ADC consisting of the tubulin-binding auristatin (monomethyl auristatin EMMAE) linked via a cleavable linker peptide (valine–citrulline), forming vc-MMAE (reviewed in [54]). ORR, overall response rate; RR, relapsing/remitting.

ADC to tumor cells include target antigen copy numbers on the surface of tumor cells, their internalization kinetics, and the subcellular trafficking to the lysosomal compartment following binding of the antibody to their respective targets. Thus, the target antigen biology is a critical parameter determining the pharmacological properties of ADCs. Cell surface antigens expressed on liquid tumors frequently display both rapid internalization kinetics and high copy numbers, exceeding 10 000 copies or more. The increased sensitivity of liquid tumors toward cytotoxic compounds relative to solid tumors, combined with the frequent absence of target antigen expression on normal tissues, may explain why two of the three most successful ADCs target lymphomas and leukemias. In contrast, solid tumors frequently express lower levels of antigens with slower internalization kinetics. It is worth noting that most of the targets selected for ADC development were identified based on their relative expression levels on tumors versus normal cells, but not based on their internalization kinetics. Therefore, target identification strategies with the goal to select for tumor antigens with rapid internalization kinetics and favorable intracellular trafficking may help to further improve the success of the ADC approach. However, in contrast to most antigens expressed on hematopoietic tumors, such as CD22 and CD33, antigens expressed on solid tumors are also present on cells within normal tissues. Thus, in the absence of targeting modalities with improved selectivity toward the most malignant cell types, including bispecific antibodies, the development of ADCs utilizing non-cell-cycle-dependent payloads may be impacted by their potential side effects on normal, nonproliferating tissues expressing the target antigen [16, 55].

In addition to the limited intracellular uptake of ADCs, the solid tumor environment poses unique challenges with regard to the numbers of ADC molecules that extravasate the tumors blood vessels and translocate via the tumor interstitium toward the cell surface of tumor cells. Several levels of biological barriers within tumors account for the low intratumoral uptake of therapeutic antibodies [56], which amounts to less than 0.01% of the injected dose in human tumors [57]. Furthermore, solid tumors have a heterogeneous blood supply and high interstitial fluid pressures, especially in necrotic zones, which may limit the diffusion of drugs or ADCs to poorly perfused areas [58]. Finally, the "binding site barrier" hypothesis suggests that antibodies (and presumably ADCs) with high binding affinities to their cell surface antigens bind tightly to the most proximal target cells relative to the tumor vasculature, preventing rapid diffusion and limiting their therapeutic effects [59]. In contrast, targets located within the tumor vasculature are readily accessible and none of the biological barriers present within soluble tumors may apply. Thus, targeting of tumor vasculature with ADCs represents an alternative approach that shows great promise to improve the utility of ADCs for the treatment of solid tumors.

Another key observation when reviewing the clinical data of ADC (Table 14.1) is that the dose-limiting toxicities (DLTs) found for tubulin inhibitors and DNA binders are surprisingly similar, including thrombocytopenia, neutropenia, and elevation in liver enzymes. Given the differences in the mechanism of action between both chemotypes and the molecular targets of the different ADCs, these findings indirectly suggest that the DLTs observed in clinical studies may be caused by off-target activities, such as FcRn- or pinocytosis-mediated cellular uptake to liver cells, including endothelial cells and hepatocytes. Recent improvements in drug-linker conjugations, in particular site-specific conjugation methods, reduced the off-target toxicity and potentially increased therapeutic indexes of conjugates in preclinical studies [60].

Finally, CSCs/tumor-initiating cells (TICs) represent a small population of cancer cells with tumor-initiating ability, self-renewal, and differentiation properties. In general, it was proposed that elimination of CSCs/TICs may be crucial to achieve cures for neoplastic diseases. There are several studies reporting that CSCs/TICs are more resistant to standard anticancer therapies compared to the more differentiated, non-CSC/TIC subpopulations. Recent advances in the development of targeting vehicles with the aim to improve selectivity toward malignant cells, including the development of bispecific targeting modalities, may help to avoid targeting normal tissues. The utility of bispecific targeting modalities for ADCs remains to be demonstrated. However, at least conceptually, bispecific targeting vehicles may provide fertile grounds for next-generation conjugates, reducing target toxicity in normal tissues expressing the target antigen. Furthermore, the use of highly potent, non-cell-cycle-dependent payloads such as calicheamicin for the targeting of CSCs may enable successful targeting of the "root problem" of cancer, contributing to the frequent relapse of solid tumors after treatment with cytotoxic compounds. The development of ADCs targeting these most malignant cell populations within tumors shows great promise to improve the therapeutic benefit of ADCs for patients with solid tumors.

References

1. Bernstein, I.D. (2000) Monoclonal antibodies to the myeloid stem cells: therapeutic implications of CMA-676, a humanized anti-CD33 antibody calicheamicin conjugate. *Leukemia*, **14**, 474–475.
2. Voutsadakis, I.A. (2002) Gemtuzumab ozogamicin (CMA-676, Mylotarg) for the treatment of CD33$^+$ acute myeloid leukemia. *Anti-Cancer Drugs*, **13**, 685–692.
3. DiJoseph, J.F., Dougher, M.M., Evans, D.Y., Zhou, B.B., and Damle, N.K. (2010) Preclinical anti-tumor activity of antibody-targeted chemotherapy with CMC-544 (inotuzumab ozogamicin), a CD22-specific immunoconjugate of calicheamicin, compared with non-targeted combination chemotherapy with CVP or CHOP. *Cancer Chemother. Pharmacol.*, **67**, 741–749.
4. Zein, N., Sinha, A.M., McGahren, W.J., and Ellestad, G.A. (1988) Calicheamicin gamma 1I: an antitumor antibiotic that cleaves double-stranded DNA site specifically. *Science*, **240**, 1198–1201.
5. Damle, N.K. (2004) Tumour-targeted chemotherapy with immunoconjugates of calicheamicin. *Expert Opin. Biol. Ther.*, **4**, 1445–1452.
6. Damle, N.K. and Frost, P. (2003) Antibody-targeted chemotherapy with immunoconjugates of calicheamicin. *Curr. Opin. Pharmacol.*, **3**, 386–390.
7. Dedon, P.C. and Goldberg, I.H. (1992) Free-radical mechanisms involved in the formation of sequence-dependent bistranded DNA lesions by the antitumor antibiotics bleomycin, neocarzinostatin,

and calicheamicin. *Chem. Res. Toxicol.*, **5**, 311–332.
8. Thorson, J.S. et al. (2000) Understanding and exploiting nature's chemical arsenal: the past, present and future of calicheamicin research. *Curr. Pharm. Des.*, **6**, 1841–1879.
9. Gupta, P.B., Chaffer, C.L., and Weinberg, R.A. (2009) Cancer stem cells: mirage or reality? *Nat. Med.*, **15**, 1010–1012.
10. Zein, N., Poncin, M., Nilakantan, R., and Ellestad, G.A. (1989) Calicheamicin gamma 1I and DNA: molecular recognition process responsible for site-specificity. *Science*, **244**, 697–699.
11. Greenstein, M., Wildey, M.J., and Maiese, W.M. (1995) The biochemical induction assay and its application in the detection of calicheamicins in *Enediyne Antibiotics as Antitumor Agents* (eds D.B. Borders and T.W. Doyle), Dekker, New York, pp. 29–47.
12. Hamann, P.R. et al. (2002) An anti-CD33 antibody–calicheamicin conjugate for treatment of acute myeloid leukemia. Choice of linker. *Bioconjug. Chem.*, **13**, 40–46.
13. Walker, S., Landovitz, R., Ding, W.D., Ellestad, G.A., and Kahne, D. (1992) Cleavage behavior of calicheamicin gamma 1 and calicheamicin T. *Proc. Natl. Acad. Sci. USA*, **89**, 4608–4612.
14. Ikemoto, N. et al. (1995) Calicheamicin–DNA complexes: warhead alignment and saccharide recognition of the minor groove. *Proc. Natl. Acad. Sci. USA*, **92**, 10506–10510.
15. Ellestad, G.A. (2006) From natural products to bioorganic chemistry. What's next? *J. Med. Chem.*, **49**, 6627–6634.
16. Senter, P.D. (2009) Potent antibody drug conjugates for cancer therapy. *Curr. Opin. Chem. Biol.*, **13**, 235–244.
17. Lee, M.D. et al. (1989) Calicheamicins, a novel family of antitumor antibiotics. 3. Isolation, purification and characterization of calicheamicins beta 1Br, gamma 1Br, alpha 2I, alpha 3I, beta 1I, gamma 1I and delta 1I. *J. Antibiot.*, **42**, 1070–1087.
18. Hamann, P.R. et al. (2002) Gemtuzumab ozogamicin, a potent and selective anti-CD33 antibody–calicheamicin conjugate for treatment of acute myeloid leukemia. *Bioconjug. Chem.*, **13**, 47–58.
19. Crocker, P.R. and Zhang, J. (2002) New I-type lectins of the CD33-related siglec subgroup identified through genomics. *Biochem. Soc. Symp.*, 83–94.
20. Vitale, C. et al. (2001) Surface expression and function of p75/AIRM-1 or CD33 in acute myeloid leukemias: engagement of CD33 induces apoptosis of leukemic cells. *Proc. Natl. Acad. Sci. USA*, **98**, 5764–5769.
21. Griffin, J.D., Linch, D., Sabbath, K., Larcom, P., and Schlossman, S.F. (1984) A monoclonal antibody reactive with normal and leukemic human myeloid progenitor cells. *Leuk. Res.*, **8**, 521–534.
22. Legrand, O. et al. (2000) The immunophenotype of 177 adults with acute myeloid leukemia: proposal of a prognostic score. *Blood*, **96**, 870–877.
23. Bernstein, I.D. et al. (1987) Treatment of acute myeloid leukemia cells *in vitro* with a monoclonal antibody recognizing a myeloid differentiation antigen allows normal progenitor cells to be expressed. *J. Clin. Invest.*, **79**, 1153–1159.
24. Bernstein, I.D. et al. (1992) Differences in the frequency of normal and clonal precursors of colony-forming cells in chronic myelogenous leukemia and acute myelogenous leukemia. *Blood*, **79**, 1811–1816.
25. Clarkson, B.D. and Berman, E. (1990) Clinical trials of chemotherapy and bone marrow transplantation in acute myelogenous leukemia in *Acute Myelogenous Leukemia: Progress and Controversies* (ed. R.P. Gale), Wiley-Liss, New York, pp. 239–272.
26. Rowe, J.M. et al. (1990) Clinical trials modules with acute myelogenous leukemia: the ECOG experience in *Acute Myelogenous Leukemia: Progress and Controversies* (ed. R.P. Gale), Wiley-Liss, New York, pp. 87–115.
27. Vogler, W.R. et al. (1990) New approaches in the treatment of acute myeloblastic leukemia: results of recent Southeastern Study Group trials in *Acute Myelogenous Leukemia: Progress and Controversies* (ed. R.P. Gale), Wiley-Liss, New York, pp. 303–312.

28. Scheinberg, D.A. et al. (1991) A phase I trial of monoclonal antibody M195 in acute myelogenous leukemia: specific bone marrow targeting and internalization of radionuclide. *J. Clin. Oncol.*, **9**, 478–490.
29. Larson, R.A. et al. (2002) Antibody-targeted chemotherapy of older patients with acute myeloid leukemia in first relapse using Mylotarg (gemtuzumab ozogamicin). *Leukemia*, **16**, 1627–1636.
30. Sievers, E.L. et al. (2001) Efficacy and safety of gemtuzumab ozogamicin in patients with CD33-positive acute myeloid leukemia in first relapse. *J. Clin. Oncol.*, **19**, 3244–3254.
31. Giles, F.J. et al. (2001) Mylotarg (gemtuzumab ozogamicin) therapy is associated with hepatic venoocclusive disease in patients who have not received stem cell transplantation. *Cancer*, **92**, 406–413.
32. Rajvanshi, P., Shulman, H.M., Sievers, E.L., and McDonald, G.B. (2002) Hepatic sinusoidal obstruction after gemtuzumab ozogamicin (Mylotarg) therapy. *Blood*, **99**, 2310–2314.
33. Boue, D.R. and Lebien, T.W. (1988) Structural characterization of the human B lymphocyte-restricted differentiation antigen CD22. Comparison with CD21 (complement receptor type 2/Epstein–Barr virus receptor). *J. Immunol.*, **140**, 192–199.
34. Bofill, M. et al. (1985) Human B cell development. II. Subpopulations in the human fetus. *J. Immunol.*, **134**, 1531–1538.
35. Schwartz-Albiez, R., Dorken, B., Monner, D.A., and Moldenhauer, G. (1991) CD22 antigen: biosynthesis, glycosylation and surface expression of a B lymphocyte protein involved in cell activation and adhesion. *Int. Immunol.*, **3**, 623–633.
36. Dorken, B. et al. (1986) HD39 (B3), a B lineage-restricted antigen whose cell surface expression is limited to resting and activated human B lymphocytes. *J. Immunol.*, **136**, 4470–4479.
37. Crocker, P.R. and Varki, A. (2001) Siglecs, sialic acids and innate immunity. *Trends Immunol.*, **22**, 337–342.
38. Doody, G.M. et al. (1995) A role in B cell activation for CD22 and the protein tyrosine phosphatase SHP. *Science*, **269**, 242–244.
39. Nitschke, L., Carsetti, R., Ocker, B., Kohler, G., and Lamers, M.C. (1997) CD22 is a negative regulator of B-cell receptor signalling. *Curr. Biol.*, **7**, 133–143.
40. Nitschke, L., Floyd, H., and Crocker, P.R. (2001) New functions for the sialic acid-binding adhesion molecule CD22, a member of the growing family of Siglecs. *Scand. J. Immunol.*, **53**, 227–234.
41. Tedder, T.F., Tuscano, J., Sato, S., and Kehrl, J.H. (1997) CD22, a B lymphocyte-specific adhesion molecule that regulates antigen receptor signaling. *Annu. Rev. Immunol.*, **15**, 481–504.
42. Hanna, R., Ong, G.L., and Mattes, M.J. (1996) Processing of antibodies bound to B-cell lymphomas and other hematological malignancies. *Cancer Res.*, **56**, 3062–3068.
43. Shan, D. and Press, O.W. (1995) Constitutive endocytosis and degradation of CD22 by human B cells. *J. Immunol.*, **154**, 4466–4475.
44. Vaickus, L., Ball, E.D., and Foon, K.A. (1991) Immune markers in hematologic malignancies. *Crit. Rev. Oncol. Hematol.*, **11**, 267–297.
45. Amercian Cancer Society (2006) *Cancer Facts and Figures 2006*, American Cancer Society, Atlanta, GA.
46. DiJoseph, J.F. et al. (2005) Antibody-targeted chemotherapy of B-cell lymphoma using calicheamicin conjugated to murine or humanized antibody against CD22. *Cancer Immunol. Immunother.*, **54**, 11–24.
47. DiJoseph, J.F. et al. (2004) Antibody-targeted chemotherapy with CMC-544: a CD22-targeted immunoconjugate of calicheamicin for the treatment of B-lymphoid malignancies. *Blood*, **103**, 1807–1814.
48. DiJoseph, J.F. et al. (2004) Potent and specific antitumor efficacy of CMC-544, a CD22-targeted immunoconjugate of calicheamicin, against systemically disseminated B-cell lymphoma. *Clin. Cancer Res.*, **10**, 8620–8629.

49. DiJoseph, J.F. et al. (2006) Antitumor efficacy of a combination of CMC-544 (inotuzumab ozogamicin), a CD22-targeted cytotoxic immunoconjugate of calicheamicin, and rituximab against non-Hodgkin's B-cell lymphoma. *Clin. Cancer Res.*, **12**, 242–249.
50. Oflazoglu, E., Kissler, K.M., Sievers, E.L., Grewal, I.S., and Gerber, H.P. (2008) Combination of the anti-CD30–auristatin-E antibody–drug conjugate (SGN-35) with chemotherapy improves antitumour activity in Hodgkin lymphoma. *Br. J. Haematol.* **142**, 69–73.
51. DiJoseph, J.F., Dougher, M.M., Armellino, D.C., Evans, D.Y., and Damle, N.K. (2007) Therapeutic potential of CD22-specific antibody-targeted chemotherapy using inotuzumab ozogamicin (CMC-544) for the treatment of acute lymphoblastic leukemia. *Leukemia*, **21**, 2240–2245.
52. Advani, A. et al. (2010) Safety, pharmacokinetics, and preliminary clinical activity of inotuzumab ozogamicin, a novel immunoconjugate for the treatment of B-cell non-Hodgkin's lymphoma: results of a phase I study. *J. Clin. Oncol.*, **28**, 2085–2093.
53. Krop, I.E. et al. (2010) Phase I study of trastuzumab–DM1, an HER2 antibody–drug conjugate, given every 3 weeks to patients with HER2-positive metastatic breast cancer. *J. Clin. Oncol.*, **28**, 2698–2704.
54. Gerber, H.P. (2010) Emerging immunotherapies targeting CD30 in Hodgkin's lymphoma. *Biochem. Pharmacol.*, **79**, 1544–1552.
55. Carter, P.J. and Senter, P.D. (2008) Antibody–drug conjugates for cancer therapy. *Cancer J.*, **14**, 154–169.
56. Rybak, J.N., Trachsel, E., Scheuermann, J., and Neri, D. (2007) Ligand-based vascular targeting of disease. *ChemMedChem*, **2**, 22–40.
57. Scott, A.M. et al. (2007) A phase I clinical trial with monoclonal antibody ch806 targeting transitional state and mutant epidermal growth factor receptors. *Proc. Natl. Acad. Sci. USA*, **104**, 4071–4076.
58. Stohrer, M., Boucher, Y., Stangassinger, M., and Jain, R.K. (2000) Oncotic pressure in solid tumors is elevated. *Cancer Res.*, **60**, 4251–4255.
59. Weinstein, J.N. and van Osdol, W. (1992) The macroscopic and microscopic pharmacology of monoclonal antibodies. *Int. J. Immunopharmacol.*, **14**, 457–463.
60. Junutula, J.R. et al. (2008) Site-specific conjugation of a cytotoxic drug to an antibody improves the therapeutic index. *Nat. Biotechnol.*, **26**, 925–932.

15
Antibodies for the Delivery of Radionuclides
Anna M. Wu

15.1
Introduction

The initial development of monoclonal antibodies (mAbs) was quickly followed by the realization that mAbs could be employed as delivery vehicles for a variety of cargoes for detection and treatment of disease. Radionuclides provide a particularly versatile class of agents for targeted delivery *in vivo*. A key feature of the radioactive decay of unstable isotopes is the generation of emissions that can be detected by well counting or scintillation counting *in vitro*, and visualized using planar, single photon emission computed tomography (SPECT), or positron emission tomography (PET) imaging *in vivo*. Equally important is the availability of radionuclides that, on decay, emit high-energy particles that can damage neighboring tissues and cells, opening the possibility of highly localized radiation therapy.

Over the ensuing years, the potential of radiolabeled antibodies has steadily been realized, with extensive preclinical and clinical evaluation ultimately leading to the registration of several antibody-based imaging agents in the 1990s, and more recently, approvals of two labeled antibodies for radioimmunotherapy (RIT) of non-Hodgkin's lymphoma (Table 15.1). However, the process of developing agents that combine defined biologicals with radioactive materials has not been without its challenges. All of the original antibody imaging agents in Table 15.1 are based on murine antibodies, evoking genuine concerns with regard to immunogenicity in human patients and precluding repeat administration. These concerns have largely been alleviated over the last decade by the widespread transition to humanized and fully human antibodies for clinical use.

Another major challenge in implementing radiolabeled antibodies for imaging or therapy has been the suboptimal pharmacokinetics of intact antibodies. Native antibodies typically exhibit a long biological half-life *in vivo* (days to weeks). This is generally advantageous if the antibody is a biologically active therapeutic, since the intervals between administration can be extended and lower proteins amounts are required overall. However, when antibodies are employed for delivery of radionuclides, additional concerns arise. Prolonged blood activity of a therapeutic

Drug Delivery in Oncology: From Basic Research to Cancer Therapy, First Edition.
Edited by Felix Kratz, Peter Senter, and Henning Steinhagen.
© 2012 Wiley-VCH Verlag GmbH & Co. KGaA. Published 2012 by Wiley-VCH Verlag GmbH & Co. KGaA.

Table 15.1 Radiolabeled antibodies for clinical use in cancer.

Generic name (trade name)	Company	FDA approval	Antibody, format	Target	Radiolabel	Approved indications
Satumomab pendetide[a] (OncoScint®)	Cytogen	1992	B72.3 mouse IgG1	TAG-72	^{111}In	colorectal and ovarian carcinoma
Arcitumomab (CEA-Scan®)	Immunomedics	1996	IMMU-4, mouse IgG1 Fab'	CEA	^{99m}Tc	colorectal, breast, and small-cell lung carcinoma
Nofetumomab merpentan (Verluma®)	Boehringer Ingelheim	1996	NR-LU-10, mouse IgG2b Fab	40-kDa glycoprotein	^{99m}Tc	small-cell and non-small-cell lung carcinoma
Capromab pendetide (ProstaScint®)	Cytogen	1996	7E11-C5.3, mouse IgG1	100-kDa glycoprotein	^{111}In	prostate carcinoma
Bectumomab (LymphoScan®)	Immunomedics	not in US	LL2, mouse IgG2a Fab'	CD22	^{99m}Tc	non-Hodgkin's lymphoma
Votumumab (HumaSPECT®)	Intracel	not in US	88BV59, human IgG3	altered cytokeratins	^{99m}Tc	colorectal, ovarian, and breast carcinoma
Igovomab[a] (Indimacis-125®)	CIS Bio International	not in US	OC125, mouse IgG1 F(ab')2	CA-125	^{111}In	ovarian cancer
Ibritumomab tiuxetan (Zevalin®)	Spectrum Pharma	2002	2B8, mouse IgG1	CD20	^{111}In/^{90}Y	non-Hodgkin's lymphoma, RIT
Tositumomab (Bexxar®)	SmithKline Beecham	2003	B1, mouse IgG2a	CD20	^{131}I	non-Hodgkin's lymphoma, RIT

[a] Not marketed in the United States.

radioisotope attached to an intact antibody can result in significant radiation exposure to normal organs and tissues, with the bone marrow being a primary concern. In a similar fashion, the extended circulation time of an imaging radionuclide conjugated to an intact antibody requires a significant delay (often days) following administration to allow background activity to clear and enable visualization of targeted tissues. Advances in antibody technology have addressed this issue by providing recombinant antibody derivatives with a spectrum of pharmacokinetic properties (extended or accelerated kinetics *in vivo*) to match the requirements of a particular imaging or therapeutic application. Pretargeting approaches also provide a strategy for optimizing target tissue uptake and contrast for imaging and therapeutic purposes, and new technologies for producing bispecific or otherwise engineered reagents now form the basis of effective pretargeting protocols.

Additional areas of progress include wider research and commercial availability of radionuclides, including nonstandard isotopes, for SPECT, PET, and RIT. Progress in radiolabeling chemistry includes general as well as site-specific conjugation approaches and applications using novel chemistries, such as "click" chemistry [1]. Finally, developments in molecular imaging instrumentation, in particular PET, have renewed interest in the potential of antibodies as imaging agents. This includes broad adoption of clinical PET, particularly in oncology and neurosciences, due to the widespread availability and demonstrated utility of 2-deoxy-2-^{18}F-fluoro-D-glucose (^{18}F-FDG) as a metabolic imaging probe. In parallel, development of small-animal imaging instrumentation (SPECT, PET, optical, magnetic resonance imaging (MRI), ultrasound, etc.) has expanded interest in imaging in preclinical disease models. Above all, advances in molecular therapeutics (including therapeutic antibodies) has spurred demand for molecular imaging biomarkers to facilitate the development and implementation of patient-specific medicine, and has rekindled interest in radiolabeled antibodies for imaging and therapeutic use.

15.2
Rationale for Using Antibodies for Radionuclide Delivery

Applications of radiolabeled antibodies in oncology have recently been driven by advances in several main areas. First and foremost has been the ease of generation of antibody-based reagents with virtually any specificity. The mammalian immune system is highly evolved to generate immunoglobulins through a process based on the innate diversity of antibodies expressed by naïve B lymphocytes, superimposed upon by a powerful selection, amplification, and somatic hypermutation system, and resulting in highly specific, high-affinity antibodies. Production of classic hybridomas by immunization of mice, followed by retrieval and fusion of mature B lymphocytes to myeloma cells, provides a method of permanent production of the antibodies of interest. Molecular cloning can be used to retrieve the genes encoding the antibody with the desired specificity and these genes can be further manipulated to produced engineered antibodies through recombinant DNA technology.

As the demand for humanized and human antibodies for clinical use has increased, parallel developments in antibody technology have emerged to provide more direct isolation or generation of suitable binders. Display technologies have allowed the generation of large libraries of human antibodies in bacterial, yeast, or mammalian systems. For example, in phage display, human antibodies are fused to a bacteriophage coat protein and displayed on the surface of phage particles to generate highly diverse libraries; powerful selection methods allow rapid isolation of phage with the desired binding specificity and affinity, and recovery of the DNA that encodes the antibody variable region genes for further development. Fully *in vitro* display techniques, such as ribosome display or *in vitro* compartmentalization, eliminate the need for microbial or mammalian cell culture. New techniques for reproducible cloning of individual human B cells provide an alternative approach for rapid generation of high-affinity human mAbs [2]. Finally, transgenic mice carrying germline human immunoglobulin loci can be immunized and subjected to conventional hybridoma production, except that the resultant antibodies are fully human.

In parallel, interest in antibodies as a delivery modality has been spurred by the dramatic increase in identification of candidate molecules that define disease states, as an outgrowth of broad-based research efforts in genomics, proteomics, and systems biology. Antibodies provide a robust path for generating reagents capable of highly specific recognition of candidate proteins. In many cases, biologically active antibodies can lead directly to therapeutics; alternatively, new antibodies recognizing novel cell surface targets in disease can be tagged with radiolabel for imaging or targeted radiotherapy. One potential limitation is that *in vivo* applications would be limited to antibodies recognizing cell surface targets. Nonetheless, there are numerous classes of cell surface biomarkers, such as growth factor receptors, adhesion molecules, proteases, and differentiation and activation markers, that have already served as targets for antibody therapeutics.

A third key element is, of course, the radionuclide. The spectrum of physical properties presented by radionuclides is both tantalizing and frustrating, since selection of the ideal isotope for a given application invariably requires compromises. Fortunately, the field of radiolabeling of proteins for imaging or therapeutic applications continues to expand on several fronts. For example, recent years have seen broader interest and availability of nonstandard radionuclides, particularly for PET imaging. In parallel, improved methodologies for conjugation and radiolabeling proteins allow great control over the extent and location of protein modification, as well as the chemical nature and stability of any linkers used for attaching the label.

Finally, developments on several fronts have led to an increased focus on molecular imaging – a growing field particularly suited for adoption of radiolabeled antibodies. Antibodies typically have affinities in the nanomolar range, allowing one to probe and detect target molecules at nanomolar concentrations when combined with radioactive detection and imaging systems. Nuclear medical imaging approaches (SPECT and PET) are also of interest because the technology is highly applicable in the clinic – photons emitted by nuclear decay or positron annihilation can escape the human body and be detected by external scanners. In fact, the field has benefitted in recent years from a form of "reverse translation" – the production of scaled-down "microSPECT" and "microPET" imaging systems designed specifically for small-animal imaging and preclinical investigations. Finally, widespread adoption of multimodality imaging is accelerating the development of molecularly targeted agents, including antibodies. Fusion of nuclear medicine (SPECT or PET) with CT allows the clinician to associate specific biological or biochemical changes with an anatomical location, greatly enhancing interpretation of images. In summary, all these factors have contributed to ongoing, fertile investigations in the development and implementation of radiolabeled antibodies for *in vivo* detection and treatment.

15.2.1
Radionuclides for Imaging

External detection of radioactive isotopes requires the emission of a high-energy photon that can escape the body and interact with a detector in a scanner. Currently used imaging nuclides fall into two general classes: γ-ray emitters and positron emitters. The γ-rays (photons) are detected and imaged using planar γ-cameras, or SPECT, which enables three-dimensional reconstruction of the radioactivity in the body. A overall limitation of using single-photon emitters is that there is no directional information associated with the decay. Collimators are required for better localization of the source of the signal and these result in a loss of sensitivity. On the other hand, a potential advantage of using γ-cameras and/or SPECT is the ability to simultaneously distinguish photons of different energies. As a result two (or more) different tracers can be detected at the same time through energy windowing. Both γ-camera and SPECT imaging have been widely implemented for decades, and several standard γ-emitting radionuclides are widely and inexpensively available.

In recent years, PET has evolved to become a mainstay in medical imaging, particularly in oncology and neurology. Ejection of a positron during nuclear decay is followed by scattering in surrounding tissue until the β^+ particle interacts with a ordinary electron and the particles annihilate. The resultant 511-keV photons, emitted in coincidence at approximately 180°, interact with a ring of detectors in the PET scanner and mathematical reconstruction results in a three-dimensional map of the activity concentration (Figure 15.1). Due to the higher information content of the decay (production of two photons with a defined geometrical relationship between the emissions), PET imaging is more sensitive, has higher resolution, and offers absolute quantitation compared to single-photon imaging modalities.

Regardless of the general imaging approach employed, there are several broad issues that need to be considered when selecting a radionuclide for antibody-based delivery. The inherent physical properties of the radioisotope will define its application. These properties include physical half-life, type of decay, and decay energy. Common sense indicates that an attempt should be made to match physical half-life of the selected radionuclide to the biological half-life of the antibody/probe, in order

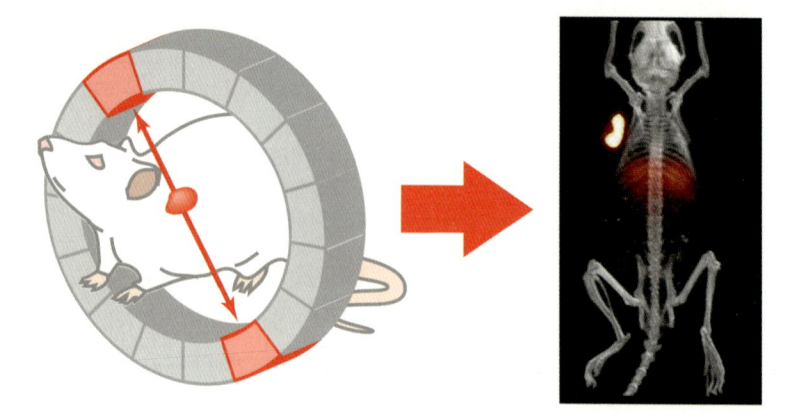

Figure 15.1 Generation of a PET image. Following injection of the radiotracer (e.g., an engineered antibody fragment labeled with a positron-emitting nuclide), sufficient time is allowed to elapse for blood and normal tissue clearance to occur. The subject is placed in the PET scanner, which contains a ring of detectors. Decay of the radionuclide results in ejection of a positron that will annihilate with a nearby electron, releasing two 511-keV photons at an angle of approximately 180° (red arrows, left). Detection of these two emissions in coincidence enables reconstruction of a fully three-dimensional activity map, which can be displayed as PET images.

to maximize the information gained from each dose. For example, combining ^{18}F (110 min) with an intact antibody would not be an efficient approach, since by the time an antibody distributes, targets, and clears *in vivo*, many decay half-lives will have passed. Photon energy will impact the detection of γ-emitting radionuclides, since most γ/SPECT cameras have been optimized for imaging ^{99m}Tc (140 keV). PET scanners are optimized to detect the emission of a positron which always results in a pair of 511-keV photons; however, the energy of the ejected positron can impact image resolution, since higher-energy positrons will scatter over longer distances before annihilating. In addition, many positron-emitting radionuclides also emit γ particles in cascade, which can further complicate detection of the "true" annihilation signal.

Production and availability also dictates which radionuclides are developed in conjunction with antibodies as imaging agents. A small number of radionuclides have been amenable to generator production, whereby a longer-lived mother radionuclide (e.g., ^{99}Mo, 66 h) is used as the source of a shorter half-life daughter isotope (e.g., ^{99m}Tc, 6 h). Generators containing ^{99}Mo can be constructed, transported to nuclear medicine facilities, and used for several days as a source of ^{99m}Tc, which is recovered as pertechnetate by elution with saline. Other radionuclides (e.g., ^{131}I, ^{111}In, etc.) are typically produced centrally in reactors or accelerators, and must have half-lives compatible with shipping. Finally, very short-half-life positron-emitting nuclides (^{15}O, 2 min; ^{13}N, 10 min; ^{11}C, 20 min), require the availability of a biomedical cyclotron and radiochemistry facilities on-site.

Table 15.2 Radionuclides commonly used for γ imaging alone or in combination with RIT.

Radionuclide	$t_{1/2}$ (h)	Eγ (keV)	Additional considerations
^{99m}Tc	6.0	140	generator-produced
^{123}I	13.1	159	–
^{111}In	67.3	171, 245	–
^{67}Cu	62	90, 184	also RIT
^{131}I	193	365	also RIT
^{177}Lu	161	133	also RIT
^{186}Re	90	122, 137	also RIT
^{188}Re	17	155, 633	generator-produced; also RIT

15.2.1.1 γ Emitters

A comprehensive listing of radionuclides that have been incorporated into diagnostic antibodies is provided by Boswell and Brechbiel [3]. Table 15.2 summarizes the physical properties of a smaller set of radionuclides that are more commonly used in conjunction with antibodies for cancer diagnosis. ^{99m}Tc is produced via a ^{99}Mo/^{99m}Tc generator, leading to its broad availability in nuclear medicine departments and widespread incorporation into SPECT imaging agents. This is reflected in the use of ^{99m}Tc in the radioimmunoscintigraphy agents arcitumomab (CEA-Scan) and nofetumomab merpentan (Verluma) (Table 15.1), although its physical half-life of 6 h has necessitated the use of antibody fragments, rather than intact antibodies, as the vehicle. Antibodies and fragments labeled with ^{99m}Tc for SPECT imaging continue to be the focus of many preclinical and clinical studies, although periodic severe shortages of reactor-produced ^{99}Mo needed for generator production has strained routine use as well as research in general using ^{99m}Tc (see, e.g., [4]). ^{123}I and ^{111}In are essentially pure γ emitters (although associated Auger electrons can be utilized for RIT; see below). Since both emit photons with energies similar to that of ^{99m}Tc, they are readily detectable with standard preclinical and clinical γ and SPECT cameras. In addition, several β-emitting radionuclides in various stages of development as components of targeted RIT agents (including the approved drug, tositumomab), also emit an imageable γ component (Table 15.2). These enable concurrent imaging of the radioimmunotherapeutic agent to confirm targeting and evaluate dosimetry, and provide an elegant example of the use of a "companion imaging biomarker" to tailor administration of drugs to individual patients.

15.2.1.2 Positron Emitters

The positron-emitting isotopes of the naturally occurring elements oxygen, nitrogen, and carbon (^{15}O, 2 min; ^{13}N, 10 min; ^{11}C, 20 min) have half-lives too short for labeling biologicals, including antibodies, for imaging purposes. Rather, they are more suited for incorporation into small-molecule tracers using simple, fast radiochemistry. Above all, use of very short half-life radionuclides requires that

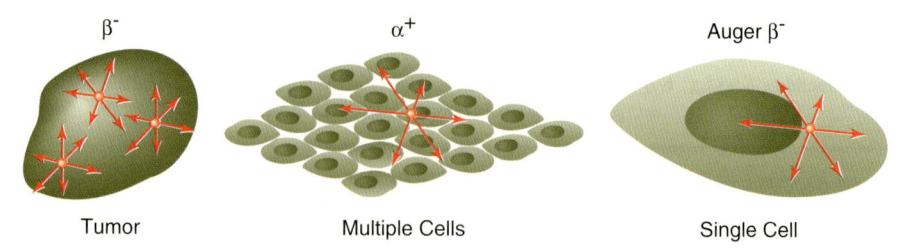

Figure 15.2 Radioactive decay products and effective therapeutic range. The β emitters release high-energy electrons that can penetrate up to several millimeters while depositing energy in surrounding tissue. Thus, they can irradiate and kill cells in a nearby "field" without the necessity of targeting every cells. The α particles have a much higher LET due to their high mass, but travel much shorter distances – a few cell diameters at the maximum. Auger electrons are very low energy and must be deposited intracellularly, ideally in or adjacent to the cell nucleus, in order to kill the target cell.

As is the case for selecting an imaging radionuclide, multiple factors must be considered when choosing a therapeutic radionuclide for conjugation to an antibody for targeted delivery. Selection ultimately must be driven by the final clinical application. The overall goal must be specific delivery to targeted tumor tissues, at levels that deposit sufficiently high radiation doses (above 50 Gy) to kill tumor cells, while minimizing dose to sensitive normal tissues and organs such as the bone marrow and kidneys. Furthermore, an important consideration is serum persistence, since blood-borne activity contributes significantly to whole-body dose. The use of a therapeutic moiety that is always "on" requires that a balance must be found between exposure and clearance; the radiolabeled antibody must persist in the circulation long enough to perfuse and localize to target tissues, while simultaneously clearing from the blood and normal tissues. Thus, the speed as well as specificity of localization to tumor versus normal tissues and blood are key concerns.

Assuming that appropriately specific localization is achieved, the energy deposition and range of an isotope's emissions determine whether it can be effectively be employed in micrometastases, small tumors, or bulky disease, or when target expression or delivery is heterogeneous. Indeed, one can envision that in the future, a cocktail of radionuclides (or even an antibody cocktail) might be employed in RIT in order to ensure that sufficient dose is delivered to all areas of disease. It is also important to consider the relationship between the physical half-life of a radionuclide and the biological half-life of the carrier. For example, combining a short-lived radionuclide with an intact antibody would result in significant radiodecay by the time good target tissue uptake and whole-body clearance is achieved, thus "wasting" the radioactive dose. Instead, it is often desirable to match the physical and biological half-lives of the RIT agent.

Selection of conjugation chemistry is critical, since radioactive metabolites will retain cytotoxic activity until physical decay or biological elimination are complete [3, 7]. Availability of radioisotopes at high specific activity is essential and remains challenging as the field continues to grow.

15.2.2.1 β Emitters

Most efforts in developing radioimmunotherapeutic agents have focused on high-energy β-emitting radionuclides as the cytotoxic moiety. In general, the energy and range of the emitted electrons ensures a homogeneous dose distribution over millimeter ranges. The radioactive iodine isotope ^{131}I ($t_{1/2} = 8.0$ days) features in many early as well as current studies, in part due to practical factors including reactor-based production and a long physical half-life, enabling shipping from central production sites. Early adoption of ^{131}I was facilitated by the ease of attaching radioiodine to proteins (by direct reaction with exposed tyrosine residues). Radioiodinated antibodies deposit the bulk of the radioactive dose within 1–2 mm of the localization site. However, the associated γ emissions of ^{131}I and long half-life (8 days) can result in significant whole-body dose in addition. Furthermore, organs such as thyroid, and to a lesser extent stomach, scavenge the free iodide that is released following internalization and metabolism of radioiodinated proteins. As a result, steps may need to be taken (such as pretreatment of the subject with potassium iodide) to block unwanted uptake and concentration of radioiodide. Another consequence of the metabolism of radioiodinated proteins is that the radioiodine can also be lost from the targeted tumor tissue if the antibody is internalized after binding cell-surface antigen. In that case, stable iodination procedures may need to be utilized [9].

Radiometals, including ^{90}Y and ^{67}Cu (Table 15.4), comprise a second class of high-energy β emitters utilized in RIT [7, 10]. As a class, radiometals offer a broad range of half-lives, emissions, and path lengths (Table 15.4). The presence of concomitant γ emissions enables detection by planar or SPECT imaging, and can provide useful, patient-specific information on targeting, normal tissue distribution and clearance, and dosimetry. The radiometals also possess a range of coordination chemistries, which dictates the labeling strategy [7]. In some cases, radiometals such as $^{186/188}$Re and ^{99m}Tc can be directly attached to antibodies following reduction of internal disulfide bridges. More often a chelator is employed, consisting of a multidentate ligand. Simple metals such as yttrium and copper can be effectively captured by linear chelators such as DTPA (diethylenetriaminepentaacetic anhydride) and its derivatives, or macrocyclic compounds such as TETA (1,4,8,11-tetraazacyclotetradecane-1,4,8,11-tetraacetic acid) or DOTA (1,4,7,10-tetraazacyclododecane-1,4,7,10-tetraacetic acid). Metals such as rhenium and technetium, with more complex oxidation states, can be effectively chelated by MAG3 or N_2S_4 ligands [7]. These chelators must also be rendered bifunctional, with reactive groups that can interact covalently with the chosen antibody vehicle. Most currently used chemistries react with ε-amino groups on surface lysine residues; alternatively, maleimide and alternate chemistries are available for conjugation to free thiol groups that can be exposed after mild reduction of disulfide bridges within antibodies. A Tc(I)-carbonyl complex has been developed that efficiently labels hexahistidine-tagged recombinant proteins, producing a particularly facile approach for radiolabeling [11]. The choice of the chelator and chemical linkage to the protein vehicle is critical, since in most cases metabolism of radiometal-labeled antibodies results in intracellular trapping of radioactive metabolites, not only in the target tumor, but also in the organs of primary clearance (typically liver and/or kidney). Continued development of effective chelating moieties and linker strategies that would facilitate subsequent metabolism and excretion remains critical for improving the overall performance of β-emitting radiometals in radioimmunoconjugates.

15.2.2.2 α Emitters

The α emitters are heavy hitters, depositing high energy within a very short distance from the decay site. It has been suggested that only a few α particles are required to kill a cell through efficient production of DNA double-strand breaks. Three of the most commonly studied α emitters are listed in Table 15.4, although many additional radionuclides have been explored [3]. Several challenges have delayed the implementation of α particle emitters in RIT. The very short path length of α particles is both an advantage and disadvantage. High LET over short distances ensures that only the targeted cells are killed, with little dose deposited in adjacent normal tissues. However, as noted above, this limits α particle RIT to easily accessible disease such as leukemias/lymphomas, small-volume disease states (micrometastases, minimal residual disease), or disease that is reachable through intracavitary (e.g., intraperitoneal, intrathecal) delivery.

The α-emitting radiometals ^{212}Bi and ^{213}Bi, which are rather short-lived (around 1 h half-life), can be used directly, or by using an "*in vivo* generator" – employing the parent radionuclide ^{212}Pb or ^{225}Ac in the immunoconjugate. An additional challenge can be conjugation/chelation of the radionuclide, particularly when the parental radiometals ^{212}Pb or ^{225}Ac are used. For example, the 10-day half-life of ^{225}Ac requires stringent chelation in order to ensure that the radiometal remains attached to the antibody vehicle for days. The decay of ^{225}Ac releases four daughter nuclei, which in turn are α emitters that can impart additional radiation dose, increasing the overall therapeutic impact. However, the physical recoil experienced by daughter nuclei following ejection of an α particle can also cause the radioactive daughters to break free of the chelator and subsequent retention of the daughter nuclides at the target site becomes an issue. Current supplies of the α-emitting radiometal series associated with ^{225}Ac and ^{224}Ra (source of ^{212}Pb and ^{212}Bi) are also limited as they are derived from byproducts of weapons development programs [8].

^{211}At provides an interesting alternative for α particle therapy, with a longer half-life (7.2 h) more appropriate for use with antibody vehicles, which also enables local/regional shipping of the radionuclide, labeling group, or the labeled product itself. ^{211}At generally reacts chemically as a halogen and can be used in direct labeling of protein tyrosine residues. Careful studies have demonstrated that even though the At–C bond is weaker than the I–C bond, radioastatinated antibodies exhibit comparable stability to that of radioiodinated antibodies and are suitable for clinical studies [12, 13]. However, similar to the case for radioiodine, following internalization, metabolism of astatinated proteins can result in release and elimination of the radiolabel, including radioastatine attached to antibodies specifically bound and internalized in targeted tumor tissue. In addition, progress in developing ^{211}At-labeled antibodies for RIT have been hampered by supply limitations. Clinically relevant amounts can be produced in cyclotrons; however, energies of 28–29 MeV are needed, well beyond the reach of standard medical cyclotrons.

15.2.2.3 Auger Electron Emitters

Auger electrons are extremely low-energy orbital electrons that can be emitted after electron capture or internal conversion events. They are characterized by highly localized energy deposition (within several cubic nanometers) and are associated with the radiodecay of many commonly used imaging radionuclides, including ^{99m}Tc, ^{123}I, ^{111}In, ^{67}Ga, and ^{201}Tl [3]. However, highest effectiveness requires that the radionuclide be delivered to the nucleus of the cell. Rapidly internalizing antibodies and peptides have been employed to facilitate cytoplasmic and perinuclear localization. More recently, addition of subcellular trafficking signals, such as nuclear localization signals (NLSs), has appeared as a promising strategy to redirect antibodies carrying Auger emitters to the cellular nucleus for increased killing effect [14, 15].

15.2.3
Antibodies as Delivery Agents

As noted above, antibodies can be readily generated with high affinity and essentially any desired specificity. Conventional hybridoma technologies (which yield murine mAbs, or human antibodies when humanized transgenic mice are used) take advantage of the mammalian immune system's highly optimized mechanisms for generation of diversity, biological selection and amplification, and affinity maturation. Microbial (bacteriophage, bacterial, yeast) and *in vitro* (ribosomal) display technologies offer additional advantages of speed and the ability to isolate antibodies that recognize challenging targets, such as self-antigens, small molecules, toxic agents, and anything that cannot be used as a standard immunogen.

There are several concerns that must be weighed when selecting an antibody as an *in vivo* delivery agent, particularly when the cargo is a radionuclide. As is the case in all antibody applications, the targeted antigen must be representative of the disease in question. High expression in the target tissue, and low normal tissue expression, are essential to achieve sufficient contrast for successful imaging, or sufficient discrimination to enable effective deposition of cytotoxic radiation doses while sparing normal tissues in RIT applications. At first glance, it would seem that targeted antigens must be on the cell surface in order to be useful. However, cells are dynamic entities and many examples are emerging where proteins assumed to be intracellular (mitochondrial, lysosomal) often end up exposed on the cell surface in disease states. Thus, classes of proteins that might initially be dismissed based on intracellular localization, may yield suitable cell surface markers on closer examination.

A key consideration in selection of an antibody as a delivery agent for radionuclides is the fate of the antibody, and radiolabel, following administration. In particular, whether or not an antibody is internalized after engaging its target on the cell surface will have a dramatic impact on subsequent processing, degradation, and elimination of radioactive metabolites. This information is important to ascertain at an early stage, since selection of a radiolabeling approach is dependent on it.

15.2.3.1 Intact Antibodies

For imaging applications, ideally the targeting agent should localize at a high level in the target tissue, and clear rapidly from the normal tissues and circulation. Intact antibodies exhibit long residence times in the circulation (1–3 weeks), which allows ample time for accumulation in the tumor. However, days are required for background activity levels to drop in the blood and normal organs, making them unsuitable as radiolabeled imaging agents. Despite their prolonged circulation time, intact mAbs have been employed in radioimmunoimaging studies by numerous groups over the years. As noted above, a series of radiolabeled antibodies labeled with SPECT radionuclides (^{99m}Tc, ^{111}In) were approved by the US Food and Drug Administration (FDA) for imaging in the 1990s, but did not achieve widespread adoption. Recent activity (reviewed in Ref. [16]) has shifted to PET as the preferred imaging modality, spurred by broader availability of clinical PET scanners and small-animal imagers in combination with improved availability of longer-lived positron emitters, including ^{64}Cu, ^{89}Zr, and ^{124}I.

Development of radioimmunotherapeutics continues to focus on intact antibodies, due to their ability to achieve high absolute levels of uptake in targeted tissues over extended periods of time and thus high area under the curve values. However, this must be balanced with higher radiation exposure to sensitive normal tissues, in particular the bone marrow, placing limits on the levels of activity that can be administered. Engineered fragments (see Section 15.2.3.2), such as minibodies, small immunoproteins (SIPs) [17], or scFv–Fc [18, 19], may provide a better balance between target tissue uptake and blood clearance, resulting in lower marrow doses. Alternatively, pretargeting strategies, described below, provide an elegant approach for separating the targeting function of the antibody from the delivery of the radionuclide itself.

15.2.3.2 Engineered Antibody Fragments

One strategy for improving and optimizing the targeting and clearance properties of antitumor antibodies is to produce smaller antibody fragments. Early imaging studies of ^{18}F-, ^{64}Cu-, or ^{124}I-labeled Fab and F(ab')$_2$ demonstrated their feasibility as PET tracers [20–23]. Subsequently, protein engineering has been employed to produce recombinant antibody fragments optimized for radiolabeled applications (Figure 15.3) [24]. scFv fragments (25 kDa) clear rapidly from the blood ($t_{1/2\beta} = 0.5$–2 h), but only reach low activity levels in tumors as a result. Diabodies (scFv dimers, 55 kDa) exhibit slightly longer residence time in the blood ($t_{1/2\beta} = 3$–7 h) and significantly improved tumor retention due to bivalency. Larger fragments have been produced by fusing the immunoglobulin $C_H 3$ domain or Fc region ($C_H 2$–$C_H 3$ domains) to make minibodies (scFv–$C_H 3$ dimers, 80 kDa) and scFv–Fc fragments (105 kDa), respectively. Figure 15.4 illustrates a comparison between an intact

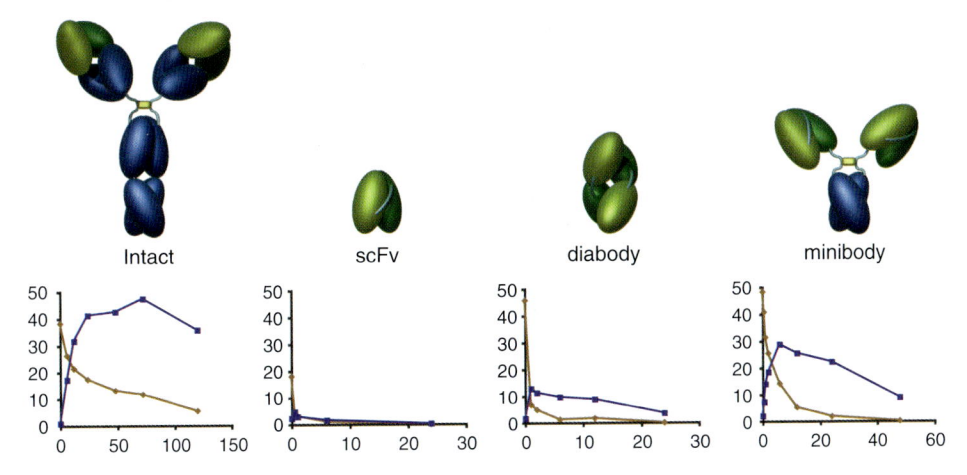

Figure 15.3 Intact antibodies, engineered antibody fragments, and targeting and clearance properties. Diagrams of the intact antibody (150 kDa), scFv (25 kDa), diabody (55 kDa), and minibody (80 kDa) illustrate the components of each. Variable regions are shown in green (V_L, light green; V_H, dark green). Linkers and hinges are shown in aqua, and the interchain disulfide bridges in intact antibody and minibody are shown in yellow. Below each are examples of blood clearance curves (red) and tumor uptake curves (blue) from biodistribution studies conducted using anti-CEA intact antibodies and engineered fragments. Time (in hours) is shown on the x-axis and percent injected dose per gram (%ID/g) on the y-axis. (Reproduced with permission from [25].)

antibody and its corresponding minibody, radiolabeled with ^{124}I for microPET imaging studies in tumor-bearing mice. Essentially identical targeting and image contrast is achieved, but requiring only 1 day for the minibody, compared to 1 week for the intact antibody.

As a result, employing antibody engineering for the development of vehicles for radionuclide delivery enables generation and selection of agents with optimal target tissue uptake and blood clearance for the desired application, from very rapid imaging through RIT. A further advantage of engineered antibody fragments is the ability to direct clearance either via hepatic or renal routes, by selecting formats that are above or below the threshold for first pass renal clearance (about 60 kDa). For example, one could select a small fragment (e.g., diabody) to direct clearance to the kidneys if the goal is to image in the liver or upper abdominal region, or a larger fragment (e.g., minibody) if clear visualization in the pelvic region is desired. For RIT, fragments could provide highly favorable overall biodistribution and clearance kinetics. Rapid blood clearance will minimize exposure to the bone marrow, which is often the root of dose-limiting toxicity in RIT. The kidneys should also be avoided to their susceptibility to delayed toxicity following radiation damage. For these applications, minibodies or larger scFv–Fc fragments with appropriate clearance kinetics directed to the liver would be preferable.

Carcinoembryonic antigen (CEA)-specific T84.66 diabody and minibody labeled with ^{123}I were initially evaluated by γ-camera imaging in athymic mice bearing LS174T colon cancer xenografts [28, 29]. The larger minibody fragment persists

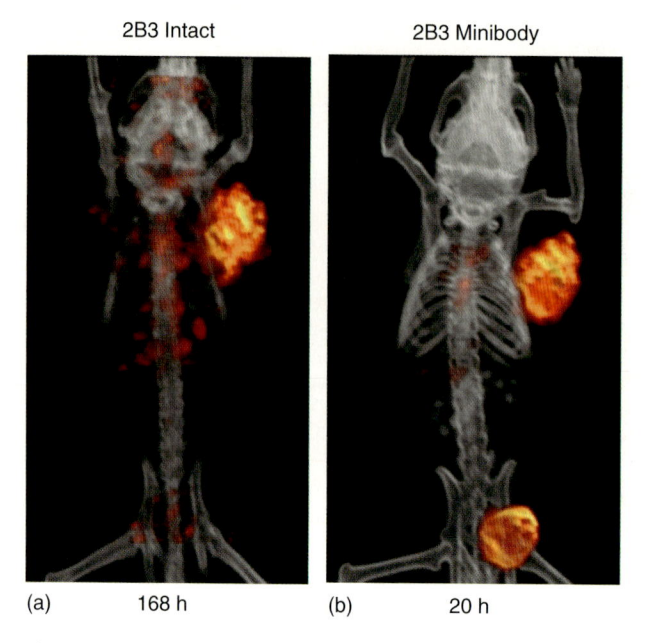

Figure 15.4 MicroPET/CT imaging comparison of intact antibody and minibody. Humanized intact 2B3 anti-PSCA antibody and humanized 2B3 minibody were radiolabeled with ^{124}I. MicroPET studies were performed on athymic mice bearing LAPC-9 PSCA-positive human prostate cancer xenografts. Images were scaled the same. There is blood pool activity remaining from the intact antibody at 168 h (a) and elimination of radioiodine via the bladder is apparent in the minibody image at 20 h (b). (Reproduced with permission from [26, 27].)

longer than diabodies in serum ($t_{1/2} = 6 - 11$ h), allowing higher accumulation of activity in tumors [28, 30, 31]. Labeling of the anti-CEA minibody fragment with ^{64}Cu, using DOTA as chelator, enabled evaluation by microPET imaging [30]. Tumors could be readily detected at 2–24 h postinjection. However, significant nonspecific uptake was seen in the kidney and liver region, which would hamper detection of lesions in these regions. The CEA-specific T84.66 diabody and minibody were also radiolabeled with ^{124}I and evaluated by microPET in mice bearing LS174T xenografts [31]. Both diabody and minibody demonstrated excellent uptake in the tumors and little activity in normal tissues, enhancing the overall images.

An elegant approach for engineering antibody fragments for RIT capitalizes on the role of the neonatal Fc receptor (FcRn), which binds to the IgG Fc region and is responsible for the prolonged serum half-life of intact antibodies. Clearance can

Figure 15.5 Serial microPET images of scFv–Fc fragments with FcRn binding site mutations. Mice carried LS174T (CEA-positive) xenografts on the left shoulder and negative control C6 tumors on the right shoulder. Anti-CEA scFv–Fc fragments carrying the indicated mutations were radiolabeled with ^{124}I for microPET imaging at the timepoints shown: (a) wild-type scFv-Fc, (b) H435Q, (c) I123A, (d) H310A, and (e) H310A/H345Q double mutant. (Reproduced with permission from [18].)

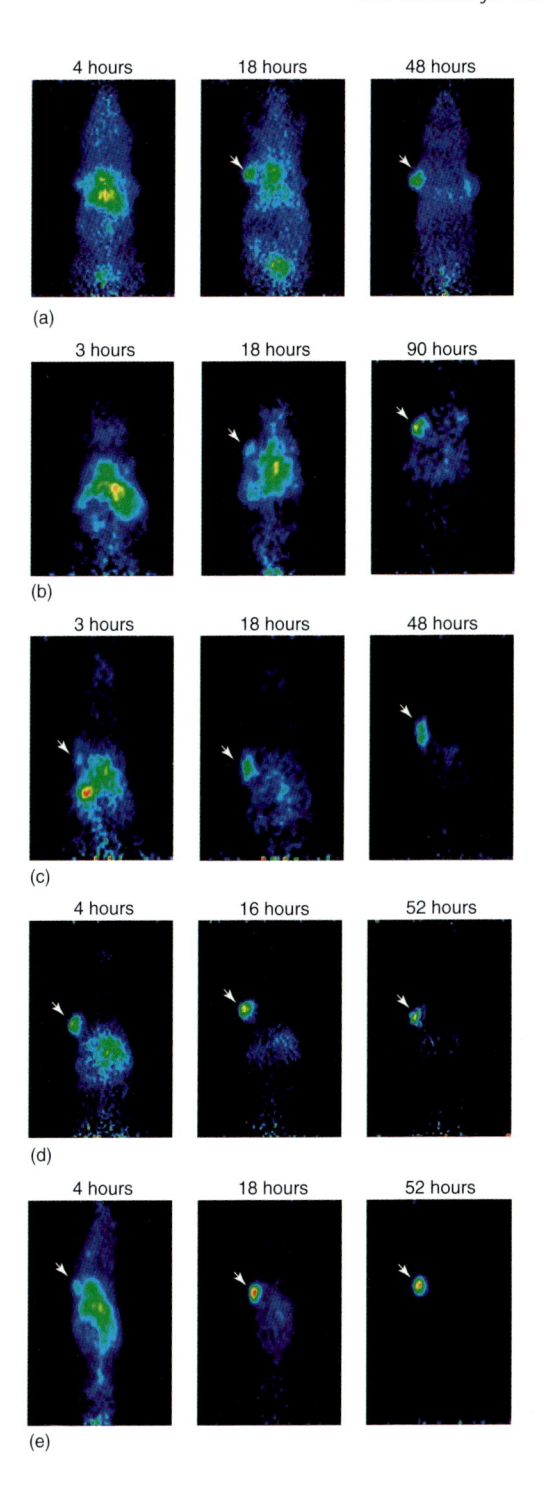

15.2 Rationale for Using Antibodies for Radionuclide Delivery | 427

(a) 4 hours | 18 hours | 48 hours

(b) 3 hours | 18 hours | 90 hours

(c) 3 hours | 18 hours | 48 hours

(d) 4 hours | 16 hours | 52 hours

(e) 4 hours | 18 hours | 52 hours

be tailored by introducing mutations into the Fc region at sites involved with FcRn binding, as was shown in a study with anti-CEA T84.66 scFv–Fc fragments [18]. Site-specific mutations of the IgG1 Fc residues involved in this interaction resulted in five variants (I253A, H310A, H435Q, H435R, and H310A/H435Q) that exhibited distinct blood clearances in mice that ranged from 83.4 to 7.96 h, which was much faster than that of the wild-type (around 12 days). These differences in clearance kinetics can be clearly visualized by serial microPET imaging (Figure 15.5). The pharmacokinetics of radioiodinated versus radiometal-labeled I253A, H310A, and H310A/H435Q scFv–Fc variants were further evaluated in xenografted mice in order to predict their therapeutic potential. Tumor uptakes were inversely related to blood clearance and hepatic radiometal activity correlated with the blood clearance rate of the fragment (i.e., faster clearance resulted in higher activity). Based on the biodistribution data with ^{125}I and ^{111}In, it was predicted that the fast-clearing scFv–Fc double mutant would be able to deliver more than 7000 cGy to the tumor with favorable tumor to liver and kidney ratios when radiolabeled with ^{131}I, whereas as for ^{90}Y therapy a slow clearing antibody would be the protein of choice as the liver/kidney activities would be lower [19].

Engineered antibody fragments provide a general strategy for *in vivo* targeting of cell surface biomarkers, as has been demonstrated in a growing number of antibody–antigen systems by preclinical PET imaging. For example, the C6.5 diabody has demonstrated efficient targeting to HER2-positive tumors [32]. Excellent tumor uptake was achieved when the C6.5 diabody was radiolabeled with ^{124}I and evaluated by PET in SCID mice bearing HER2-positive human ovarian carcinoma (SKOV-3) xenografts [33]. High-contrast images have also been obtained with ^{124}I-anti-CD20 minibodies [34]. Humanized minibodies specific for prostate stem cell antigen (PSCA) have been employed for detection of prostate cancer xenografts [27, 35]. In addition, imaging tumor neoangiogenesis in mice bearing solid F9 tumor was accomplished using ^{76}Br-labeled L19-SIP – an engineered scFv – $C_{H}4_{e-S2}$ fragment that binds the fibronectin ED-B domain [17, 36]. Although tumors were clearly visible from 5 to 46 h after injection, long retention of the radioactivity in the blood and very slow renal excretion resulted in low target to nontarget ratios that were explained to be partially due to debromination. Figure 15.6 demonstrates the broad applicability of imaging tumors by immunoPET based on cancer cell surface marker expression, summarizing examples using minibodies specific for CEA, CD20, HER2, and PSCA, and radiolabeled with either ^{124}I or ^{64}Cu [25]. The necessity of using a residualizing label such as a radiometal chelate with internalizing antibodies (trastuzumab/Herceptin) is clearly illustrated, along with accompanying normal tissue uptake (primarily hepatic) when this approach is taken. Antibody imaging can also be employed as an indirect, cell surface readout of intracellular events. For example, Smith-Jones *et al.* elegantly probed the inhibition of hsp90 by 17-(allylamino)-17-demethoxygeldanamycin, by utilizing ^{68}Ga-labeled trastuzumab F(ab')$_2$ imaging to quantify expression of HER2 *in vivo* [37].

A particularly promising combination for radioimmunoimaging would be a rapidly clearing engineered antibody fragment in combination with ^{18}F. The anti-CEA T84.66 diabody was labeled with ^{18}F and evaluated by PET in

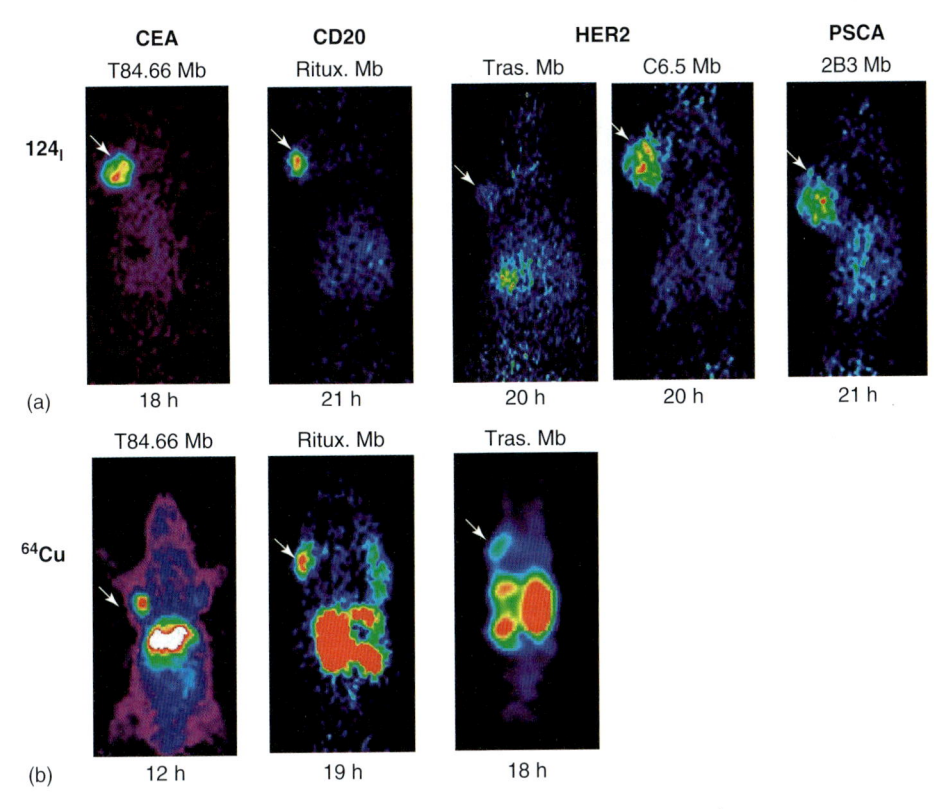

Figure 15.6 MicroPET imaging applied to several cancer cell surface targets. Mice were injected with ^{124}I-labeled (a) or ^{64}Cu-DOTA-labeled (b) minibodies directed against the cell surface targets shown. The T84.66, rituximab (Ritux.), C6.5, and 2B3 minibodies do not internalize, and provide excellent images when labeled with ^{124}I. However, trastuzumab (Tras.) does internalize and ^{124}I signal is lost, necessitating the use of the residualizing ^{64}Cu-DOTA complex as the radiolabel. Hepatic clearance is evident in the bottom row of images, with trapping of the radioactive metabolites in the liver. (Reproduced with permission from [25].).

tumor-bearing mice [38]. Tumors were visible from 1 to 6 h postinjection. Liu et al. adapted ^{18}F labeling of proteins using N-succinimidyl-4-^{18}F-fluorobenzoate to a microfluidic chip platform and demonstrated rapid immunoPET detection of HER2- and PSCA-expressing tumor xenografts in mouse models (Figure 15.7) [39].

15.2.3.3 Pretargeting

Pretargeting approaches, in which the antibody targeting and radioactive detection functions are separated, have been employed to facilitate antibody imaging. Typically, a cancer-specific antibody is administered and allowed to localize in target tissues. A clearing step is often included to remove nonbound antibody that is still in the circulation, followed by administration of a radiolabeled hapten that

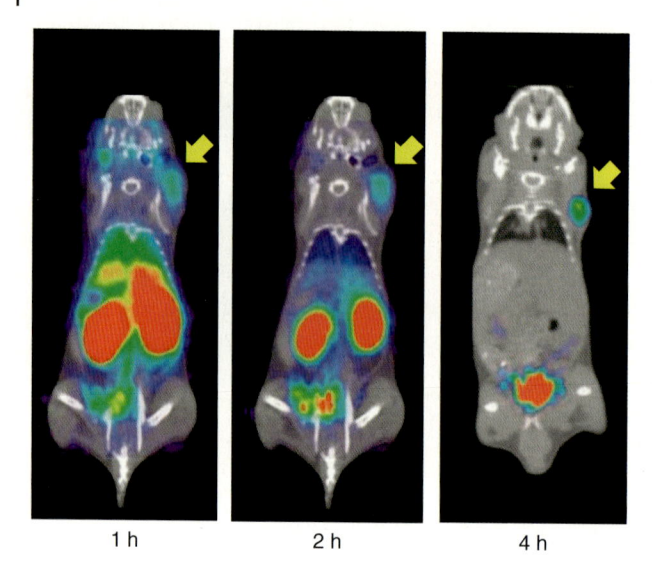

Figure 15.7 Same-day imaging using ^{18}F-labeled diabodies. PSCA-specific diabodies were radiolabeled with ^{18}F for imaging of LAPC-9 tumor-bearing mice. Serial microPET/CT images were acquired at 1, 2, and 4 h, demonstrating the rapid tumor localization of these engineered fragments in conjunction with fast blood clearance. (Reproduced with permission from [39].)

quickly binds to the prelocalized antibody. Strategies involving streptavidin- or avidin-based pretargeting approaches have been developed for RIT. For PET and RIT applications, the biodistribution, clearance, and tumor targeting of a directly labeled mAb and mAb–streptavidin pretargeting were compared in mice bearing human colorectal carcinoma xenografts using ^{64}Cu as tracer [40]. The antibody pretargeting strategy with ^{64}Cu-DOTA-biotin displayed more rapid tumor uptake, substantially faster clearance, and superior tumor to normal tissue ratios. However, a major limitation of using streptavidin is that it is highly immunogenic which limits repeated administration of therapeutic doses.

Bispecific antibodies (BsAbs), where one arm binds to the tumor antigen and the other captures a radiolabeled hapten (see Chapter 16), are an attractive alternative, and can be applied to antibody-based imaging as well as RIT. For example, the use of different antitumor mAbs for BsAb preparation and ^{68}Ga-labeled chelate enhanced the sensitivity of tumor detection in mice with rat pancreatic carcinoma or human colon carcinoma xenografts [41, 42]. A clinical PET imaging pretargeting study using ^{68}Ga-chelate and BsAbs targeting MUC1 was carried out in 10 patients with primary breast cancer [43]. Fourteen of 17 known lesions were clearly visualized at 60–90 min after injection of ^{68}Ga-chelate in patients pretreated with BsAb and a clearing agent. A bispecific anti-*CEA* × anti-*di-DTPAF*(*ab'*)$_2$ antibody was evaluated as a pretargeted radioimmunoscintigraphy agent in 11 patients with colorectal carcinoma. The best imaging results were obtained using a 4-day interval between administration of the BsAb and the hapten (an ^{111}In-DTPA-labeled peptide), with images acquired 24 h after injection of the peptide. [44]. A series of clinical studies using this system of pretargeted RIT, with ^{131}I-labeled hapten as the therapeutic agent, has been conducted in patients with medullary thyroid carcinoma, with promising results with regard to efficacy and survival benefit [45].

A flexible BsAb pretargeting system based on an antihapten antibody specific for a synthetic compound, histamine-succinyl-glycine (HSG), which can be labeled with any radionuclide, has also been developed [46, 47]. When evaluated by PET imaging in mice bearing colon cancer xenografts, tumor activity was about 3-old higher in the pretargeted mice (15% ID/g) compared of those injected with ^{18}F-FDG (5% ID/g) at 1 h and the background in normal tissues was lower [47].

A modular approach for producing multivalent, multifunctional antibody-based targeting molecules has recently been developed. Using the "dock-and-lock" system [48], a bispecific complex consisting of three Fab' fragments (bivalent for CEA and monovalent for HSG) was recently evaluated for pretargeting in conjunction with ^{124}I-labeled bivalent HSG [49, 50]. Tumors smaller than 0.3 mm in diameter were detected by pretargeting using the bivalent ^{124}I-HSG peptide, but not by using ^{18}F-FDG [50]. Thus, pretargeting appears to be highly applicable for antibody-based imaging (SPECT or PET) and RIT. One should note, however, that a target that rapidly internalizes upon binding of BsAb would not be a good candidate for pretargeting applications.

15.3
Clinical Development

15.3.1
Radioimmunoimaging

ImmunoPET has sparked new interest, in particular due to improved availability of positron emitters with longer physical half-lives, such as ^{124}I and ^{89}Zr. In a 1991 study, nine patients with ductal breast carcinoma were imaged with ^{124}I-labeled mAbs for quantitative measurement of tumor uptake [51]. Subsequently, one patient with neuroblastoma was scanned with ^{124}I-labeled 3F9 mAb for estimating tumor dosimetry during treatment planning for RIT [52]. These early studies illustrated the potential of using ^{124}I-labeled mAbs in PET. With ^{124}I now being commercially available, interest in ^{124}I-labeled mAbs has been renewed. In a phase I study, ^{124}I-HuMV833 (anti-vascular endothelial growth factor) was evaluated for tissue distribution and clearance in patients with a variety of progressive tumors [53]. ImmunoPET has also been investigated in patients with renal cancers since ^{18}F-FDG-PET was less effective than CT [54, 55]. In a recent pilot clinical study ^{124}I-chimeric G250 (cG250), specific for carbonic anhydrase IX (overexpressed in clear-cell renal carcinoma), was evaluated in 26 patients with renal masses. The ^{124}I-cG250 mAb was able to identify 15 of 16 clear-cell carcinomas accurately, and was negative for less aggressive, non-clear-cell renal masses (Figure 15.8) [56]. This

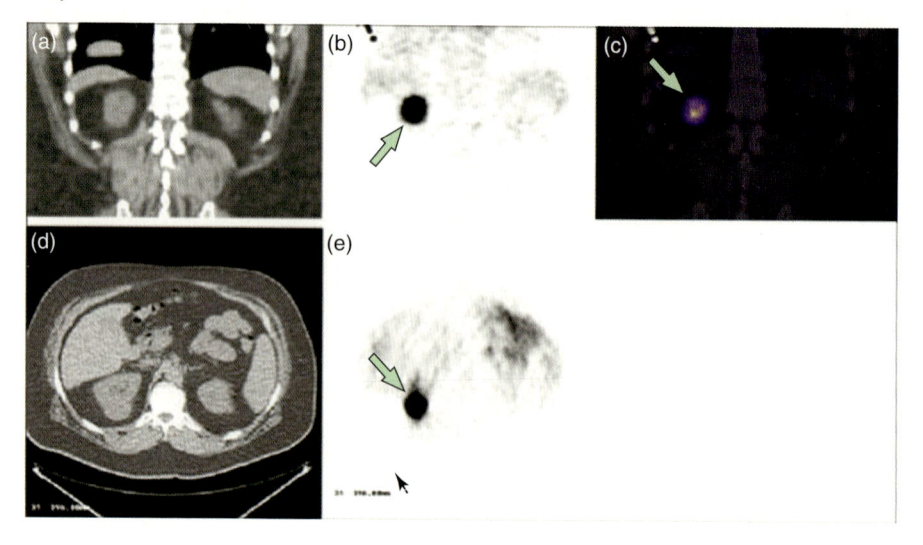

Figure 15.8 ImmunoPET imaging of a patient with clear-cell carcinoma using ^{124}I-labeled intact cG250 antibody. CT, PET, and fused PET/CT images; coronal (a)–(c) and transaxial (d) and (e) images. (Reproduced with permission from [56].)

study illustrates the potential of antibody-based molecular imaging for applications such as identification of aggressive tumors or as an aid in patient stratification.

Clinical translation using ^{89}Zr in immunoPET has recently been achieved [57, 58]. Chimeric U36, which binds to CD44v6, was radiolabeled with ^{86}Zr and administered to 20 patients with head and neck squamous cell carcinoma (HNSCC) scheduled to undergo neck dissection with or without resection of the primary tumor [57]. ImmunoPET was performed up to 6 days after injection of ^{89}Z-cU36 mAb. All 17 primary tumors as well as lymph node metastases in 18 of 25 positive neck regions were detected. It was concluded that the sensitivity and accuracy of immunoPET was at least as good as CT/MRI with optimal tumor uptakes at later imaging times. Trastuzumab has likewise been radiolabeled with ^{89}Zr for immunoPET imaging in patients with metastatic breast cancer [59]. Of interest, lesions in the brain were imageable, consistent with the notion that the blood–brain barrier is disrupted at the site of brain metastases.

Engineered antibody fragments are transitioning to clinical evaluation as tracers using a γ-camera and SPECT imaging. An anti-TAG-72 CC49 ^{123}I-scFv fragment (25 kDa) was evaluated in a presurgical study of colorectal carcinoma in five patients with metastatic lesions in the liver [60], demonstrating that early, same-day imaging of both primary and metastatic tumors was feasible. An anti-CEA scFv, also labeled with ^{123}I, demonstrated targeting and detection as early as 1 h after injection by immunoscintigraphy in patients with colon or breast carcinoma [61]. Furthermore, the ^{123}I-CEA-specific scFv was effective for localizing lesions in a radioimmunoguided surgery protocol [62]. A presurgical imaging study was

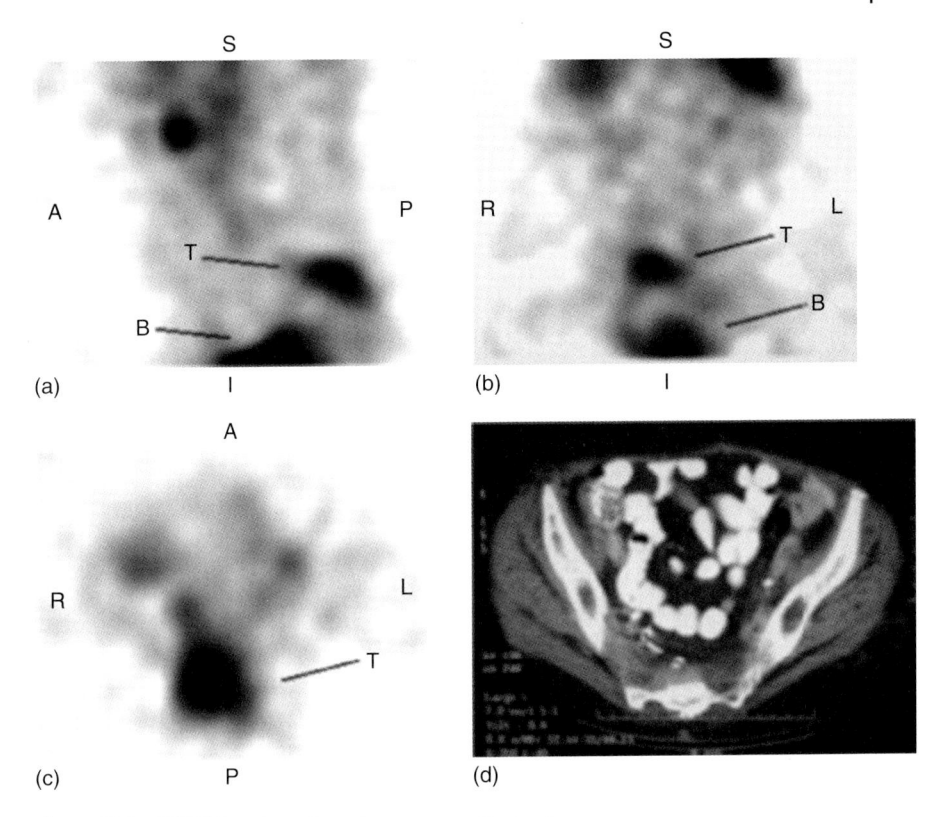

Figure 15.9 SPECT imaging of a colon cancer patient using ^{123}I-labeled anti-CEA minibody. Sagittal (a), coronal (b), and axial (c) SPECT views are shown, with targeting to a presacral recurrence (T). Bladder (B) activity is also apparent. No obvious tumor recurrence was visible in the CT image (d). (Reproduced with permission from [63].)

conducted using the T84.66 anti-CEA ^{123}I-minibody in 10 patients with colorectal carcinoma. In seven of the eight patients with no prior chemotherapy, the minibody imaged eight of 10 lesions that were 1.0 cm or larger in size (Figure 15.9) [63]. The study demonstrated the sensitivity and specificity of the minibody in detecting infiltrative and diffuse lesions that could not be detected by CT. Santimaria et al. evaluated a L19 (scFv)$_2$ fragment labeled with ^{123}I as an imaging marker of angiogenesis in 20 patients with cancer [64]. Selective localization to aggressive lung or colon cancer was observed. In a subsequent phase I/II clinical study, ^{123}I-L19 (scFv)$_2$ was evaluated in five patients with HNSCC. Successful imaging comparable to ^{18}F-FDG-PET was achieved in four of five patients. Imaging of three lymphoma patients using the larger L19-SIP fragment labeled with ^{131}I demonstrated excellent localization to disease sites, favorable dosimetry, and partial responses to treatment [65].

15.3.2
Radioimmunotherapy

Early work by the DeNardos demonstrated that Lym-1 anti-DR antibody radiolabeled with ^{131}I or ^{67}Cu induced remissions in lymphoma patients that had failed multiple prior chemotherapy regimens [66, 67]. A high initial response rate was observed, although the majority of patients eventually relapsed. Nonetheless, these encouraging results spurred further investigations of radiolabeled antibodies targeting a different target on B-cells – the integral membrane protein CD20. Since then, numerous studies have evaluated RIT using ^{131}I-tositumomab and ^{90}Y-ibritumomab tiuxetan in recurrent or refractory lymphomas, with an excellent initial overall response rate (60–80%) and a significant proportion of patients achieving durable remissions [68, 69] Ultimately, FDA approval of ^{90}Y-ibritumomab tiuxetan (Zevalin), in 2002, and ^{131}I tositumomab (Bexxar), in 2003, for relapsed, refractory, or transformed CD20$^+$ B-cell non-Hodgkin's lymphoma marked the realization of many years of effort in the field.

Progress continues, albeit more slowly, on development of RIT for solid tumors. In addition to the clinical examples described above (using an ^{131}I-labeled SIP fragment in lymphoma or CEA-directed pretargeted therapy in conjunction with an ^{131}I-labeled hapten in medullary thyroid carcinoma), studies of radiolabeled intact antibodies also remain an area of active interest. The J591 antibody recognizing prostate-specific membrane antigen has been radiolabeled with a variety of radionuclides for imaging and therapeutic purposes [70]. Phase I RIT studies using ^{90}Y- or ^{177}Lu-DOTA-J591 confirmed targeting, established the maximum tolerated dose, and demonstrated biological activity in a subset of patients, and a phase II trial is in progress [70]. A pretherapy biodistribution and dosimetry study using ^{111}In-MxDTPA-trastuzumab has been conducted in HER2-positive breast cancer patients, laying the groundwork for future RIT studies [71].

15.4
Conclusions and Perspectives

Tumor-specific antibodies, particularly in the current era of antibody engineering, represent an ideal class of vehicles for the delivery of radionuclides, either for detection (radioimmunoimaging) or treatment (RIT) purposes. The panel of potential cell surface markers that can serve as targets is rapidly expanding, and methods for the generation of human or humanized antibodies for recognition of these targets are robust and routine. Protein engineering allows broad control of the format, and biochemical and biological properties of antibody derivatives. Broad experience in preclinical models and the continued expansion of clinical studies builds confidence to our ability to use these reagents in a predictable and efficacious fashion.

Promising areas for future research include extension to applications beyond lymphoma and current studies on solid tumors. For example, with a few exceptions, the application of radiolabeled antibodies for detection and treatment of brain tumors remains largely unexplored. This area has been largely ignored due to the common perception that antibodies and antibody-like molecules cannot cross the blood–brain barrier. However, it is increasingly apparent that tumor vasculature provides unique access (although not without its own set of challenges) and disruption of normal endothelial structures may provide a route for delivery to primary or metastatic brain lesions. An additional complementary area for further development is inflammation and immune responses. As the significance of the host's surveillance and initial reaction to malignant cells, and the role of immune responses in cancer progression becomes better defined, and in parallel as advances in cancer immunotherapy progress into clinical studies, antibodies can provide highly specific tools for evaluation of and intervention in these processes.

Finally, use of antibodies as delivery agents for radionuclides is particularly appealing due to their innate potential as "theranostics." The combination of imageable radionuclides and antibody specificity has provided an obvious approach for visualizing highly specific molecular targets *in vivo*. The resulting knowledge regarding target expression and accessibility can translate directly into targeted treatments, employing therapeutic radionuclides or other biologically active cargoes, including drugs, toxins, enzymes, cytokines, and other biologicals. Particularly in combination with advances and widespread adoption of PET, antibody-based imaging opens a door to quantitative and longitudinal visualization of biological processes in living organisms. Clearly, antibody-targeted delivery of radionuclides stands to play an expanding role in the detection, characterization, and targeted treatment of cancer.

Acknowledgments

The author wishes to thank not only present and past members of her laboratory, but also the many collaborators and colleagues in the field of antibody-targeted imaging and therapeutics who have shared their efforts, struggles, and successes over the years. Work in the author's laboratory was supported by National Institutes of Health grants CA 49304, CA107399, CA 86306, CA 92131, DoE DE-SC0001220, and DoD W81WXH-08-1-0442. The author is a member of the UCLA Jonsson Comprehensive Cancer Center (CA16042).

References

1. Nwe, K. and Brechbiel, M.W. (2009) Growing applications of "click chemistry" for bioconjugation in contemporary biomedical research. *Cancer Biother. Radiopharm.*, **24**, 289–302.
2. Kwakkenbos, M.J., Diehl, S.A. *et al.* (2009) Generation of stable monoclonal antibody-producing B cell receptor-positive human memory B cells by genetic programming. *Nat. Med.* **16**, 123–128.
3. Boswell, C.A. and Brechbiel, M.W. (2007) Development of radioimmunotherapeutic and diagnostic antibodies: an inside-out view. *Nucl. Med. Biol.*, **34**, 757–778.

4. Mohmood, U., (2009) MICoE Task Force looks to the future. *J. Nucl. Med.*, **50**, 15N.
5. Pagani, M., Stone-Elander, S. et al. (1997) Alternative positron emission tomography with non-conventional positron emitters: effects of their physical properties on image quality and potential clinical applications. *Eur. J. Nucl. Med.*, **24**, 1301–1327.
6. Nayak, T.K. and Brechbiel, M.W. (2009) Radioimmunoimaging with longer-lived positron-emitting radionuclides: potentials and challenges. *Bioconjug. Chem.*, **20**, 825–841.
7. Schubiger, P.A., Alberto, R. et al. (1996) Vehicles, chelators, and radionuclides: choosing the "building blocks" of an effective therapeutic radioimmunoconjugate. *Bioconjug. Chem.*, **7**, 165–179.
8. Brechbeil, M.W. (2007) Targeted alpha-therapy: past, present, future?. *Dalton Trans.*, 4918–4928.
9. Wilbur, D.S. (1992) Radiohalogenation of proteins: an overview of radionuclides, labeling methods, and reagents for conjugate labeling. *Bioconjug. Chem.*, **3**, 433–470.
10. Volkert, W.A., Goeckeler, W.F. et al. (1991) Therapeutic radionuclides: production and decay property considerations. *J. Nucl. Med.*, **32**, 174–185.
11. Waibel, R., Alberto, R. et al. (1999) Stable one-step technetium-99m labeling of His-tagged recombinant proteins with a novel Tc(I)-carbonyl complex. *Nat. Biotechnol.*, **17**, 897–901.
12. Vaidyanathan, G. and Zalutsky, M.R. (2008) Astatine radiopharmaceuticals: prospects and problems. *Curr. Radiopharm.*, **1**, 177.
13. Zalutsky, M.R., Reardon, D.A. et al. (2008) Clinical experience with alpha-particle emitting ^{211}At: treatment of recurrent brain tumor patients with ^{211}At-labeled chimeric antitenascin monoclonal antibody 81C6. *J. Nucl. Med.*, **49**, 30–38.
14. Costantini, D.L., Bateman, K. et al. (2008) Trastuzumab-resistant breast cancer cells remain sensitive to the auger electron-emitting radiotherapeutic agent ^{111}In-NLS-trastuzumab and are radiosensitized by methotrexate. *J. Nucl. Med.*, **49**, 1498–1505.
15. Costantini, D.L., Hu, M. et al. (2008) Peptide motifs for insertion of radiolabeled biomolecules into cells and routing to the nucleus for cancer imaging or radiotherapeutic applications. *Cancer Biother. Radiopharm.*, **23**, 3–24.
16. McCabe, K.E., Wu, A.M. (2010) Positive progress in ImmunoPET – not just a coincidence. *Cancer Biother. Radiopharm.*, **25**, 253–261.
17. Borsi, L., Balza, E. et al. (2002) Selective targeting of tumoral vasculature: comparison of different formats of an antibody (L19) to the ED-B domain of fibronectin. *Int. J. Cancer*, **102**, 75–85.
18. Kenanova, V., Olafsen, T. et al. (2005) Tailoring the pharmacokinetics and positron emission tomography imaging properties of anti-carcinoembryonic antigen single-chain Fv–Fc antibody fragments. *Cancer Res.*, **65**, 622–631.
19. Kenanova, V., Olafsen, T. et al. (2007) Radioiodinated versus radiometal-labeled anti-carcinoembryonic antigen single-chain Fv–Fc antibody fragments: optimal pharmacokinetics for therapy. *Cancer Res.*, **67**, 718–726.
20. Westera, G., Reist, H.W. et al. (1991) Radioimmuno positron emission tomography with monoclonal antibodies: a new approach to quantifying *in vivo* tumour concentration and biodistribution for radioimmunotherapy. *Nucl. Med. Commun.*, **12**, 429–437.
21. Garg, P.K., Garg, S. et al. (1991) Fluorine-18 labeling of monoclonal antibodies and fragments with preservation of immunoreactivity. *Bioconjug. Chem.*, **2**, 44–49.
22. Anderson, C.J., Connett, J.M. et al. (1992) Copper-64-labeled antibodies for PET imaging. *J. Nucl. Med.*, **33**, 1685–1691.
23. Page, R.L., Garg, P.K. et al. (1994) PET imaging of osteosarcoma in dogs using a fluorine-18-labeled monoclonal antibody Fab fragment. *J. Nucl. Med.*, **35**, 1506–1513.

24. Wu, A.M. and Senter, P.D. (2005) Arming antibodies: prospects and challenges for immunoconjugates. *Nat. Biotechnol.*, **23**, 1137–1146.
25. Olafsen, T. and Wu, A.M. (2010) Antibody vectors for imaging. *Semin. Nucl. Med.*, **40**, 167–181.
26. Olafsen, T., Gu, Z. et al. (2007) Targeting, imaging, and therapy using a humanized antiprostate stem cell antigen (PSCA) antibody. *J. Immunother.*, **30**, 396–405.
27. Leyton, J.V., Olafsen, T. et al. (2008) Humanized radioiodinated minibody for imaging of prostate stem cell antigen-expressing tumors. *Clin. Cancer Res.*, **14**, 7488–7496.
28. Hu, S., Shively, L. et al. (1996) Minibody: a novel engineered anti-carcinoembryonic antigen antibody fragment (single-chain Fv–C_H3) which exhibits rapid, high-level targeting of xenografts. *Cancer Res.*, **56**, 3055–3061.
29. Wu, A.M., Williams, L.E. et al. (1999) Anti-carcinoembryonic antigen (CEA) diabody for rapid tumor targeting and imaging. *Tumor Target.*, **4**, 47–58.
30. Wu, A.M., Yazaki, P.J. et al. (2000) High-resolution microPET imaging of carcinoembryonic antigen-positive xenografts by using a copper-64-labeled engineered antibody fragment. *Proc. Natl. Acad. Sci. USA*, **97**, 8495–8500.
31. Sundaresan, G., Yazaki, P.J. et al. (2003) ^{124}I-labeled engineered anti-CEA minibodies and diabodies allow high-contrast, antigen-specific small-animal PET imaging of xenografts in athymic mice. *J. Nucl. Med.*, **44**, 1962–1969.
32. Adams, G.P., Schier, R. et al. (1998) Prolonged *in vivo* tumour retention of a human diabody targeting the extracellular domain of human HER2/neu. *Br. J. Cancer*, **77**, 1405–1412.
33. Gonzalez Trotter, D.E., Manjeshwar, R.M. et al. (2004) Quantitation of small-animal ^{124}I activity distributions using a clinical PET/CT scanner. *J. Nucl. Med.*, **45**, 1237–1244.
34. Olafsen, T., Betting, D. et al. (2006) MicroPET imaging of CD20 lymphoma xenografts using engineered antibody fragments. *J. Nucl. Med.*, **47**, 33P.
35. Lepin, E.J., Leyton, J.V. et al. (2010) An affinity matured minibody for PET imaging of prostate stem cell antigen (PSCA)-expressing tumors. *Eur. J. Nucl. Med. Mol. Imaging*, **37**, 1529–1538.
36. Rossin, R., Berndorff, D. et al. (2007) Small-animal PET of tumor angiogenesis using a ^{76}Br-labeled human recombinant antibody fragment to the ED-B domain of fibronectin. *J. Nucl. Med.*, **48**, 1172–1179.
37. Smith-Jones, P.M., Solit, D. et al. (2006) Early tumor response to Hsp90 therapy using HER2 PET: comparison with ^{18}F-FDG PET. *J. Nucl. Med.*, **47**, 793–796.
38. Cai, W., Olafsen, T. et al. (2007) PET imaging of colorectal cancer in xenograft-bearing mice by use of an ^{18}F-labeled T84.66 anti-carcinoembryonic antigen diabody. *J. Nucl. Med.*, **48**, 304–310.
39. Liu, K., Lepin, E.J. et al. (2011) Microfluidic-based biomolecule radiolabeling for immunoPET. *Mol. Imaging*, **10**, 168–176.
40. Lewis, M.R., Wang, M. et al. (2003) In vivo evaluation of pretargeted ^{64}Cu for tumor imaging and therapy. *J. Nucl. Med.*, **44**, 1284–1292.
41. Schuhmacher, J., Klivenyi, G. et al. (1995) Multistep tumor targeting in nude mice using bispecific antibodies and a gallium chelate suitable for immunoscintigraphy with positron emission tomography. *Cancer Res.*, **55**, 115–123.
42. Klivenyi, G., Schuhmacher, J. et al. (1998) Gallium-68 chelate imaging of human colon carcinoma xenografts pretargeted with bispecific anti-CD44V6/anti-gallium chelate antibodies. *J. Nucl. Med.*, **39**, 1769–1776.
43. Schuhmacher, J., Kaul, S. et al. (2001) Immunoscintigraphy with positron emission tomography: gallium-68 chelate imaging of breast cancer pretargeted with bispecific anti-MUC1/anti-Ga chelate antibodies. *Cancer Res.*, **61**, 3712–3717.

44. Aarts, F., Boerman, O.C. et al. (2010) Pretargeted radioimmunoscintigraphy in patients with primary colorectal cancer using a bispecific anticarcinoembryonic antigen CEA X anti-di-diethylenetriaminepentaacetic acid F(ab′)$_2$ antibody. *Cancer*, **116** (Suppl. 4), 1111–1117.

45. Kraeber-Bodere, F., Salaun, P.Y. et al. (2010) Pretargeted radioimmunotherapy in rapidly progressing, metastatic, medullary thyroid cancer. *Cancer*, **116** (Suppl. 4), 1118–1125.

46. Rossi, E.A., Sharkey, R.M. et al. (2003) Development of new multivalent-bispecific agents for pretargeting tumor localization and therapy. *Clin. Cancer Res.*, **9**, 3886S–3896S.

47. McBride, W.J., Zanzonico, P. et al. (2006) Bispecific antibody pretargeting PET (immunoPET) with an ^{124}I-labeled hapten-peptide. *J. Nucl. Med.*, **47**, 1678–1688.

48. Goldenberg, D.M., Rossi, E.A. et al. (2008) Multifunctional antibodies by the dock-and-lock method for improved cancer imaging and therapy by pretargeting. *J. Nucl. Med.*, **49**, 158–163.

49. Sharkey, R.M., Karacay, H. et al. (2007) Bispecific antibody pretargeting of radionuclides for immuno single-photon emission computed tomography and immuno positron emission tomography molecular imaging: an update. *Clin. Cancer Res.*, **13**, 5577s–5585s.

50. Sharkey, R.M., Karacay, H. et al. (2008) Metastatic human colonic carcinoma: molecular imaging with pretargeted SPECT and PET in a mouse model. *Radiology*, **246**, 497–507.

51. Wilson, C.B., Snook, D.E. et al. (1991) Quantitative measurement of monoclonal antibody distribution and blood flow using positron emission tomography and ^{124}iodine in patients with breast cancer. *Int. J. Cancer*, **47**, 344–347.

52. Larson, S.M., Pentlow, K.S. et al. (1992) PET scanning of iodine-124-3F9 as an approach to tumor dosimetry during treatment planning for radioimmunotherapy in a child with neuroblastoma. *J. Nucl. Med.*, **33**, 2020–2023.

53. Jayson, G.C., Zweit, J. et al. (2002) Molecular imaging and biological evaluation of HuMV833 anti-VEGF antibody: implications for trial design of antiangiogenic antibodies. *J. Natl. Cancer Inst.*, **94**, 1484–1493.

54. Aide, N., Cappele, O. et al. (2003) Efficiency of [^{18}F]FDG PET in characterising renal cancer and detecting distant metastases: a comparison with CT. *Eur. J. Nucl. Med. Mol. Imaging*, **30**, 1236–1245.

55. Kang, D.E., White, R.L. Jr. et al. (2004) Clinical use of fluorodeoxyglucose F 18 positron emission tomography for detection of renal cell carcinoma. *J. Urol.*, **171**, 1806–1809.

56. Divgi, C.R., Pandit-Taskar, N. et al. (2007) Preoperative characterisation of clear-cell renal carcinoma using iodine-124-labelled antibody chimeric G250 (^{124}I-cG250) and PET in patients with renal masses: a phase I trial. *Lancet Oncol.*, **8**, 304–310.

57. Borjesson, P.K., Jauw, Y.W. et al. (2006) Performance of immuno-positron emission tomography with zirconium-89-labeled chimeric monoclonal antibody U36 in the detection of lymph node metastases in head and neck cancer patients. *Clin. Cancer Res.*, **12**, 2133–2140.

58. Zalutsky, M.R. (2006) Potential of immuno-positron emission tomography for tumor imaging and immunotherapy planning. *Clin. Cancer. Res.*, **12**, 1958–1960.

59. Dijkers, E.C., Oude Munnink, T.H. et al. (2010) Biodistribution of ^{89}Zr-trastuzumab and PET imaging of HER2-positive lesions in patients with metastatic breast cancer. *Clin. Pharmacol. Ther.*, **87**, 586–592.

60. Larson, S.M., El-Shirbiny, A.M. et al. (1997) Single chain antigen binding protein (sFv CC49). First human studies in colorectal carcinoma metastatic to liver. *Cancer*, **80**, 2458–2468.

61. Begent, R.H., Verhaar, M.J. et al. (1996) Clinical evidence of efficient tumor

targeting based on single-chain Fv antibody selected from a combinatorial library. *Nat. Med.*, **2**, 979–984.

62. Mayer, A., Tsiompanou, E. et al. (2000) Radioimmunoguided surgery in colorectal cancer using a genetically engineered anti-CEA single-chain Fv antibody. *Clin. Cancer Res.*, **6**, 1711–1719.

63. Wong, J.Y., Chu, D.Z. et al. (2004) Pilot trial evaluating an ^{123}I-labeled 80-kilodalton engineered anticarcinoembryonic antigen antibody fragment (cT84.66 minibody) in patients with colorectal cancer. *Clin. Cancer Res.*, **10**, 5014–5021.

64. Santimaria, M., Moscatelli, G. et al. (2003) Immunoscintigraphic detection of the ED-B domain of fibronectin, a marker of angiogenesis, in patients with cancer. *Clin. Cancer Res.*, **9**, 571–579.

65. Sauer, S., Erba, P.A. et al. (2009) Expression of the oncofetal ED-B-containing fibronectin isoform in hematologic tumors enables ED-B-targeted ^{131}I-L19SIP radioimmunotherapy in Hodgkin lymphoma patients. *Blood*, **113**, 2265–2274.

66. DeNardo, S.J., DeNardo, G.L. et al. (1988) Treatment of B cell malignancies with ^{131}I Lym-1 monoclonal antibodies. *Int. J. Cancer Suppl.*, **3**, 96–101.

67. Deshpande, S.F., DeNardo, S.J. et al. (1988) Copper-67-labeled monoclonal antibody Lym-1, a potential radiopharmaceutical for cancer therapy: labeling and biodistribution in RAJI tumored mice. *J. Nucl. Med.*, **29**, 217–225.

68. Palanca-Wessels, M.C. and Press, O.W. (2010) Improving the efficacy of radioimmunotherapy for non-Hodgkin lymphomas. *Cancer* **116** (Suppl. 4), 1126–1133.

69. Macklis, R.M. (2007) Radioimmunotherapy as a therapeutic option for non-Hodgkin's lymphoma. *Semin. Radiat. Oncol.*, **17**, 176–183.

70. Tagawa, S.T., Beltran, H. et al. (2010) Anti-prostate-specific membrane antigen-based radioimmunotherapy for prostate cancer. *Cancer*, **116** (Suppl. 4), 1075–1083.

71. Wong, J.Y., Raubitschek, A. et al. (2010) A pretherapy biodistribution and dosimetry study of indium-111-radiolabeled trastuzumab in patients with human epidermal growth factor receptor 2-overexpressing breast cancer. *Cancer Biother. Radiopharm.*, **25**, 387–394.

16
Bispecific Antibodies and Immune Therapy Targeting
Sergej M. Kiprijanov

16.1
Introduction

The recent clinical and commercial success of therapeutic antibodies has generated great interest in antibody-based therapeutics for hematological malignancies, solid tumors, autoimmune, and inflammatory diseases. Being highly specific, naturally evolved molecules, the antibodies are able to bind to primary and metastatic cancer cells with high affinity and cause the destruction of tumor cells by complement-dependent cytolysis (CDC), by antibody-dependent cellular cytotoxicity (ADCC), and/or by delivering an apoptotic signal to a target cell. Although therapeutic monoclonal antibodies (mAbs) have become a major, often well-tolerated treatment modality for many cancer patients [1], their efficacy needs further improvement. Malfunction of naked immunoglobulins in some therapeutic settings is accounted for by interaction of antitumor antibodies with the inhibitory constant fragment of antibody (Fc) receptors (e.g., FcγRIIb) on myeloid cells [2] and by different escape mechanisms developed by cancer cells to evade mortality [3]. One alternative immunotherapeutic strategies is based on the activation of host immune mechanisms using bispecific antibodies (BsAbs) [4]. The quest for bispecific proteins that can bind to and act on two different therapeutic targets has engaged scientists for more than two decades. Although first clinical experience with BsAbs was discouraging due to immunogenicity and severe side-effects caused by mass release of inflammatory cytokines, a new second generation of bispecific molecules has now been produced by using DNA recombinant technology. In parallel, interest in bispecifics is growing not only among the scientific community, but also from biotech and big pharma drug developers. The motivation behind this interest is simple: "two are better than one" and "two products for the price of one." These expectations apply to a variety of biomedical applications that have been pursued with bispecific molecules, but mainly to immunotherapy.

Drug Delivery in Oncology: From Basic Research to Cancer Therapy, First Edition.
Edited by Felix Kratz, Peter Senter, and Henning Steinhagen.
© 2012 Wiley-VCH Verlag GmbH & Co. KGaA. Published 2012 by Wiley-VCH Verlag GmbH & Co. KGaA.

16.2
Treatment Options in Cancer in the Pre-Antibody Era

The first effective anticancer drugs were brought to clinical trials in the early 1940s. The promising results arose from the efforts to assess the therapeutic value of a series of toxins developed for chemical warfare [5]. Although impressive regressions of acute lymphoblastic leukemia (ALL) and adult lymphomas have been observed with single agents, such as nitrogen mustard, antifolates, corticosteroids, and the vinca alkaloids, the responses were only partial and not long lasting. When complete remissions were obtained, as in ALL, they lasted less than 9 months and relapse was associated with resistance to the original drug [6]. Nevertheless, the principle was established that tumors might be more susceptible to toxins than normal tissues and that drugs could be administered systemically to induce tumor regression.

A second enduring principle that soon became obvious was that human tumors, when they do respond, contain subclones that become drug resistant. Under the selective pressure of a toxic therapy, the genetic diversity within most human tumors leads to rapid outgrowth of the drug-resistant cells. A vast array of resistance mechanisms, involving mutations or amplification of the target enzyme, overexpression of drug transporters, or mutations in cell death pathways, can defeat single agents, no matter how well designed and targeted. Therefore, the current chemotherapeutic regimes include multidrug combinations that hit cancer cells at different stages and/or via different mechanisms. For example, the CHOP regime used for the treatment of non-Hodgkin's lymphoma (NHL) comprises cyclophosphamide (alkylating agent; DNA cross-linking), hydroxydaunorubicin (doxorubicin; intercalating agent; DNA damage), Oncovin® (vincristine; tubulin binding; cell division), and prednisone (prednisolone; immunomodulation). Accordingly, the FOLFIRI/FOLFOX regime used in colorectal cancer (CRC) comprises folinic acid (leucovorin; enhancer of 5-fluorouracil (5-FU); thymidylate synthase), 5-FU (antimetabolite; inhibition of DNA and RNA synthesis), and irinotecan (Camptosar®) or oxaliplatin (Eloxatin®; topoisomerase inhibitor/DNA cross-linking). In some clinical settings, chemotherapy is used in combination with radiation.

However, patients with metastatic breast cancer (MBC), hormone-refractory prostate cancer, and some other cancers have limited clinical options. High-dose chemotherapy or irradiation has become dose limiting due to severe toxicities to normal tissues and organs. Only a small fraction of chemical drug reaches the tumor and the vast majority of the applied drug dose is taken up by normal tissues [7], thus resulting in unfavorable side-effects. Therefore, new nontoxic targeted therapies were needed to provide an antitumor effect without enhancing treatment toxicities. To some extent, this problem has been solved after the appearance of antibody-based drug products.

16.3
Antibodies as Therapeutic Agents

Antibodies are capable of highly specific interactions with a wide variety of ligands, including small chemical molecules, peptides, carbohydrates, and protein structures. More than three decades ago, Georges Köhler and César Milstein invented a means of cloning individual antibodies, thus opening up the way for tremendous advances in the fields of cell biology, clinical diagnostics, and therapy [8]. However, in spite of their early promise, the mouse mAbs appeared to be largely unsuccessful as therapeutic reagents due to insufficient activation of the human effector functions and to immune reactions against proteins of rodent origin. These problems have been overcome to a large extent using genetic engineering techniques to produce chimeric mouse/human, humanized, and fully human antibodies (for review, see [9]). This approach appeared to be particularly suitable due to the domain structure of the antibody molecule, where functional domains carrying antigen-binding activities (antibody-binding fragments (Fabs) or variable fragments (Fvs)) or effector functions (constant fragment (Fc)) can be exchanged between antibodies (Figure 16.1). The genetic engineering techniques also allow

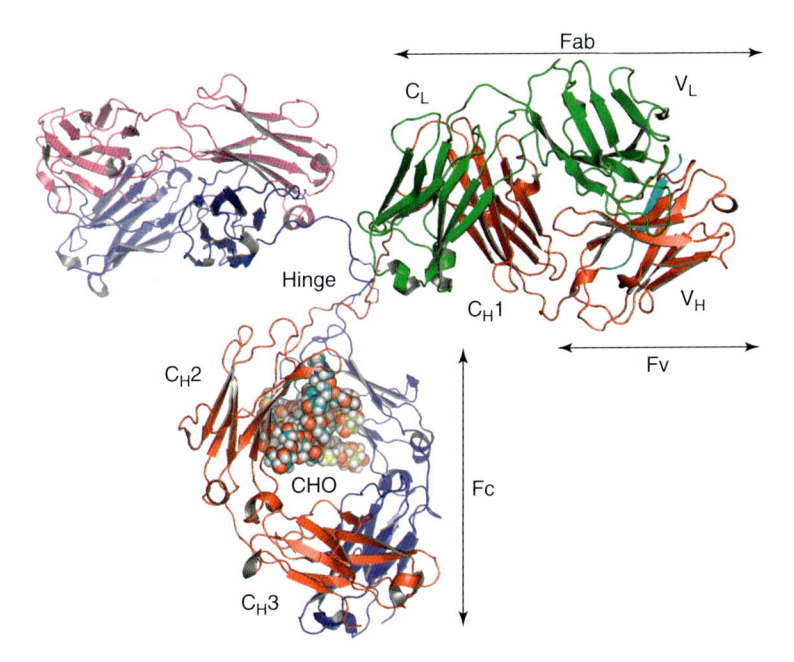

Figure 16.1 Domain organization of an IgG molecule. The antigen-binding surface is formed by variable domains of the heavy (V_H) and light (V_L) chains. Effector functions are determined by the constant C_H2 and C_H3 domains. The carbohydrate moiety is indicated as CHO. The figure was prepared using the program PyMOL (www.pymol.org) on the basis of crystal structure of an intact, murine monoclonal IgG2a anti-canine lymphoma antibody, MAb231 (Protein Data Bank entry 1IGT).

the generation of even smaller than Fv stable antigen-binding domain antibodies (dAbs) derived from the variable domains of the antibody heavy chain (HC) or light chain (LC) (V_H and V_L, respectively) and ranging from 11 to 15 kDa [10].

On the basis of sequence variation, the residues in the variable domains (V-region) are assigned either to the hypervariable complementarity-determining regions (CDRs) or to framework regions (FRs). It is possible to replace much of the rodent-derived sequence of an antibody with sequences derived from human immunoglobulins without loss of function. This new generation of "chimeric" and "humanized" antibodies represents an alternative to human hybridoma-derived antibodies, and should be less immunogenic than their rodent counterparts. Furthermore, genetically truncated versions of the antibody may be produced ranging in size from the smallest antigen-binding unit or Fv through Fab' to $F(ab')_2$ fragments. Somewhat later it became possible to produce fully human recombinant antibodies derived either from antibody libraries [11] or single immune B-cells [12], or from transgenic mice bearing human immunoglobulin loci [13, 14].

The research and development of mAbs is a rapidly progressing field. Currently, the antibodies are a well-established therapeutic modality. More than 30 immunoglobulins and their derivatives have been approved for different clinical indications over the last 20 years (Table 16.1). A total of 14 therapeutic antibodies have been approved for use in oncology; 11 in the United States and/or Europe. Both in liquid and solid tumors, antibodies have become an integral component of treatment regimens that have improved and extended the lives of cancer patients [15]. In hematologic cancers, rituximab (Rituxan/MabThera) has become a component of the standard care in many NHL subtypes due to the improved efficacy that it adds to chemotherapy regimens. In solid tumors, an anti-angiogenic antibody drug Avastin is becoming a standard of care in metastatic CRC (mCRC), nonsquamous non-small-cell lung cancer (NSCLC), MBC, metastatic renal cell carcinoma, and glioblastoma as a first- or second-line therapy. Despite these advances, however, there remains significant unmet need in cancer treatment. For example, clinical trials demonstrated that Avastin is ineffective for treatment of freshly operated colon cancer, and in advanced gastric cancer and advanced pancreatic cancer [16]. There are also well-documented severe side-effects associated with Avastin treatment, such as gastrointestinal perforation (often fatal), high blood pressure, bleeding, and wound healing complications, developing venous thromboembolism [17]. In addition, therapeutic effect is often seen only in subsets of patients. For example, only about 25% of women with breast cancer respond to treatment with the blockbuster breast cancer drug Herceptin. Similarly, only 48% of NHL patients respond to Rituxan, which targets CD20. No antibody therapies are currently available for the treatment of many other cancer types, including gastric, pancreas, liver, bladder, or prostate cancers.

Table 16.1 List of marketed therapeutic antibodies.

Year of approval	Product name	Species/isotype	Indication	Molecular target/mechanism of action	Developer/marketer
1986	Orthoclone OKT3® (muromonab-CD3)	murine IgG2a, κ	acute kidney transplant rejection	anti-CD3	Ortho Biotech/J&J
1994	ReoPro® (abciximab)	chimeric Fab, κ	coronary intervention and angioplasty	GPIIa/IIIb antagonist	Centocor/Eli Lilly/J&J
1995 (withdrawn in 2000 due to lack of efficacy)	Panorex® (edrecolomab)	murine IgG2a, κ	colon cancer (Germany)	anti-EpCAM	GSK/Centocor
1997	Rituxan®/MabThera® (rituximab)	chimeric IgG1, κ	CD20+ NHL; rheumatoid arthritis; CLL	anti-CD20	Biogen Idec/Genentech/Roche
1997 (in 2009 discontinued in the EU for commercial reasons)	Zenapax® (daclizumab)	humanized IgG1, κ	kidney transplant rejection	anti-CD25 (IL-2 receptor), inhibits T-cell activation	Protein Design Labs/Roche
1998	Synagis® (palivizumab)	humanized IgG1, κ	human RSV	anti-RSV F protein	MedImmune/Abbott
1998	Simulect® (basiliximab)	chimeric IgG1, κ	kidney transplant rejection	anti-CD25 (inhibits T-cell activation)	Novartis
1998	Herceptin® (trastuzumab)	humanized IgG1, κ	HER2-positive MBC; HER2-positive metastatic stomach cancer (2010)	anti-HER2 (c-erbB2)	Genentech/Roche
1998	Remicade® (infliximab)	chimeric IgG1, κ	Crohn's disease; ulcerative colitis	anti-TNF-α	Centocor/J&J

(continued overleaf)

Table 16.1 (continued)

Year of approval	Product name	Species/isotype	Indication	Molecular target/mechanism of action	Developer/marketer
2000/2010 (voluntarily withdrawn)	Mylotarg® (gemtuzumab ozogamicin)	humanized IgG4, κ	CD33⁺ AML	anti-CD33 ADC	UCB Celltech/Wyeth/Pfizer
2001	Campath® (alemtuzumab)	humanized IgG1, κ	B-CLL	anti-CD52	Millennium/Ilex/Berlex
2002	Zevalin™ (ibritumomab tiuxetan)	murine IgG1, κ	relapsed or refractory low-grade, follicular, or transformed NHL	anti-CD20 with ^{90}Y	Biogen Idec
2002	Humira™ (adalimumab)	human IgG1, λ	rheumatoid arthritis; Crohn's disease	anti-TNF-α	MedImmune/Abbott
2003	Bexxar® (tositumomab and ^{131}I-tositumomab)	murine IgG2a, λ	NHL, CLL	anti-CD20 labeled with ^{131}I	Corixa/GSK
2003/2004 (FDA)	Xolair™ (omalizumab)	humanized IgG1, κ	allergic asthma	anti-IgE	Tanox/Genentech/Roche
2003/2009 (voluntarily withdrawn)	Raptiva™ (efalizumab)	humanized IgG1, κ	psoriasis	anti-CD11a (prevention of T-cell activation)	XOMA/Genentech
2004	Avastin® (bevacizumab)	humanized IgG1, κ	CRC; lung cancer; MBC; glioblastoma multiforme metastatic renal cancer	anti-VEGF	Genentech/Roche
2004	Erbitux™ (cetuximab)	chimeric IgG1, κ	CRC; head and neck cancer	anti-EGFR	ImClone/BMS/Merck
2004 (withdrawn from the market in 2006–2008)	Tysabri® (natalizumab)	humanized IgG4, κ	relapsing form of multiple sclerosis; Crohn's disease	anti-α$_4$ integrins (α$_4$β$_7$ and α$_4$β$_1$ = VLA-4 on lymphocytes and monocytes)	Biogen Idec/Elan

2005/2010 FDA	Actemra™ (tocilizumab)	humanized IgG1, κ	Castleman's disease; rheumatoid arthritis	anti-IL-6 receptor	Chugai/Roche
2006	Lucentis™ (ranibizumab)	humanized Fab, κ	wet form of age-related macular degeneration	anti-VEGF	Genentech/Novartis
2006	Vectibix™ (panitumumab)	human IgG2, κ	CRC	anti-EGFR	Amgen
2007	Soliris® (eculizumab)	humanized IgG2/4, κ	paroxysmal nocturnal hemoglobinuria	anti-complement protein C5	Alexion
2008	Cimzia® (certolizumab pegol)	humanized PEGylated Fab, κ	Crohn's disease; rheumatoid arthritis	anti-TNF-α	UCB Celltech
2008/2009 FDA	Stelara™ (ustekinumab)	human IgG1, κ	Psoriasis	anti-IL-12/IL-23	Centocor/J&J
2008	Theraloc® (nimotuzumab)	humanized IgG1, κ	glioma (approved in India, Philippines, and Indonesia)	anti-EGFR	Oncoscience/Kalbe Farme/YM BioSciences
2008	Licartin (metuximab)	murine ^{131}I-labeled F(ab')$_2$ fragment, κ	liver cancer (hepatocellular carcinoma), approved in China	anti-HAb18G/CD147	Chengdu Hoist Hi-tech (Chengdu, China)
2009	Removab® (catumaxomab)	mouse/rat trifunctional IgG, mouse κ, rat λ	malignant ascites at ovarian cancer, approved in the European Union	BsAb EpCAM × CD3 to attract T-cells via CD3 and NK cells via Fc	Fresenius/Trion Pharma
2009	Simponi™ (golimumab)	human IgG1, κ	rheumatoid arthritis; psoriatic arthritis; ankylosing spondylitis	anti-TNF-α	J&J Centocor/Schering-Plough
2009	Ilaris™ (canakinumab)	human IgG1, κ	cryopyrin-associated periodic syndrome	anti-IL-1β	Novartis/Medarex

(continued overleaf)

Table 16.1 (continued)

Year of approval	Product name	Species/isotype	Indication	Molecular target/mechanism of action	Developer/marketer
2009 FDA/2010 EMEA	Arzerra™ (ofatumumab)	human IgG1, κ	CLL	anti-CD20	Genmab/GSK
2010	Prolia™ (denosumab)	human IgG2, κ	osteoporosis; bone loss	anti-RANKL	Amgen
2011	Xgeva™ (denosumab)	human IgG2, κ	bone metastases from solid tumors	anti-RANKL	Amgen
BLA under review	Abthrax™ (raxibacumab)	human IgG1, λ	inhalation anthrax	against protective antigen of *Bacillus anthracis*	Human Genome Sciences
BLA under review (positive decision of FDA advisory panel)	Benlysta™ (belimumab (LymphoStat-B))	human IgG1, λ	systemic lupus erythematosus	anti-BlyS (B-lymphocyte stimulator)	Human Genome Sciences /GSK
BLA under review (rejected by FDA advisory panel; discontinued in development)	Numax™ (motavizumab)	humanized IgG1, κ	human RSV	anti-RSV F protein	MedImmune/AstraZeneca
2011	Yervoy™ ipilimumab	human IgG1, κ	advanced metastatic melanoma	CD152/CTLA-4 (cytotoxic T-lymphocyte-associated antigen 4)	BMS

Compilation made using publicly available internet resources. BLA, Biologics License Application; RSV, respiratory syncytial virus.

16.4
Next Generation of Therapeutic Antibodies

The vast majority of approved antibody drugs are made on the basis of naked immunoglobulins of the IgG class. Therapeutic activity of naked antibodies is determined by their specificity (antigen recognition) and by the ability to trigger deleterious effects on tumor cells either by direct killing via ADCC and/or CDC; or by cross-linking the receptor followed by its internalization and apoptosis induction; or by deprivation of tumorigenic stimuli provided by the certain growth factors [15]. However, the antibodies are not generally effective as single agents against solid tumors and need to be administered in combination with chemo- and/or radiotherapy. Quite often, therapeutic efficacy is observed only in subsets of patients. Malfunction of naked immunoglobulins in some therapeutic settings is accounted for by FcγRIIIa (CD16a) polymorphism [18], interaction of antitumor antibodies with inhibitory Fc receptors (FcRs) (e.g., FcγRIIb) on myeloid cells [2], and by different escape mechanisms developed by cancer cells to evade mortality [3]. To generate more potent antibodies that work better in combination or possibly as single-agent therapy, different enhancement approaches have been designed [19]. For example, inefficient recruitment of natural killer (NK) cells in patients having the low-affinity FcγRIIIa-158F allotype [20] can be successfully addressed either by producing antibodies with low fucose content in the cells with natural aberrant fucosylation pathways [21, 22] or by targeted glycoform engineering [23, 24]. A recent example of an antibody with a glycoengineered Fc portion is GA101 (obinutuzumab) from GlycArt and Roche [25]. GA101 is a humanized anti-CD20 mAb engineered to increase target cell death. The adapted Fc region exhibits 50-fold higher binding affinity to FcγRIII that results in a 10- to 100-fold increase in ADCC against CD20$^+$ NHL cell lines. In addition, it possesses a modified elbow hinge that may contribute to reduced CDC activity [26]. In human lymphoma xenograft models, GA101 exhibited superior antitumor activity in comparison with approved chimeric anti-CD20 antibody rituximab, resulting in the induction of complete tumor remission and increased overall survival of treated animals [25, 27]. Phase I clinical trials demonstrated that GA101 produced a 43% overall response rate (9/21) in relapsed/refractory NHL patients [28, 29] and 62% (8/13) in relapsed/refractory chronic lymphocytic leukemia (CLL) patients [30]. The compound is currently being explored as a single agent in phase II in relapsed/refractory indolent/aggressive NHL and B-CLL, and in combination with chemotherapy in a phase Ib study [29, 31].

Fine tuning of the Fc region affinity to activating (e.g., FcγRIIIa/CD16a) or inhibitory (e.g., FcγRIIb/CD32b) receptors can be achieved by Fc engineering using either random or rational mutagenesis approaches [32–34]. Fc engineering and Fc isotype chimerism also allow generation of antibodies with enhanced complement recruitment [35, 36], and extend antibody half-life in circulation by increasing the binding to the neonatal FcR (FcRn) [37, 38].

Conjugated antibodies are another approach to antibody enhancement currently being explored in oncology. Conjugated antibodies contain cancer-killing payloads such as chemical drug, toxins, or radioisotopes. The rationale for this approach is that the antibody can bring the cancer-killing agent directly to the cancer cell with minimal damage of the bystander healthy cells. Examples of conjugated antibodies include the radioimmunotherapeutic drugs Bexxar and Zevalin, and the drug-conjugated antibody Mylotarg (Table 16.1). However, the conjugated antibodies have experienced limited success thus far as a result of toxicity issues and complicated methods of administration. For example, Mylotarg has been recently withdrawn from the US market and is no longer commercially available to new patients *(http://www.fda.gov/NewsEvents/Newsroom/PressAnnouncements/ ucm216448.htm)*. At initial approval, Mylotarg was associated with a serious liver condition called veno-occlusive disease, which can be fatal. This rate has increased in the postmarket setting. The later approaches in the generation of the antibody–drug conjugates (ADCs) appear to largely avoid the unwanted side-effects. The recent advances include site-specific coupling with highly cytotoxic drugs [39, 40] and optimized linkers that are hydrolyzable in the cytoplasm, resistant or susceptible to proteases, or resistant to multidrug-resistance efflux pumps [41]. IgGs have also been engineered to contain unique drug conjugation positions for generating homogeneous drug conjugates with a defined antibody/drug stoichiometry [42, 43]. A number of ADCs are now being studied in clinical trials for different cancer indications. The most advanced are brentuximab vedotin (SGN-35; Seattle Genetics/Takeda), trastuzumab–DM1 (Genentech/Immunogen), and inotuzumab ozogamicin (Wyeth/Pfizer), which are in pivotal phase II or in phase III clinical trials for Hodgkin's lymphoma, breast cancer, and NHL, respectively [41].

16.5
Rationale for Immunotherapy with BsAbs

The third approach to address limitations of mAbs is the generation of BsAbs. A BsAb is a man-made antibody that is able to bind two targets simultaneously (Figure 16.2). BsAbs do not exist in nature, besides the rare cases of the formation bispecific IgG4 (BsIgG) via Fab arm exchange [44, 45], and must be made in the laboratory. BsAbs are designed either (i) to recruit the effector cells of the immune system (retargeting BsAb), (ii) to block two or more targets simultaneously (BsAb of dual action), or (iii) to provide higher selectivity of targeting cancer cells by simultaneous binding of two tumor-associated antigens (BsAb of enhanced selectivity).

16.5.1
Retargeting BsAbs

Retargeting BsAb (Figure 16.3) can override the natural specificity of an immunological effector cell for its target and redirect lysis toward a cell population it would otherwise ignore. Immunological effector cells that can potentially be recruited by BsAbs include granulocytes, monocytes, macrophages, NK cells, and T-cells. In contrast, human IgG1, which is the most widely used antibody isotype for tumor therapy, cannot recruit T-cells (the majority of which do not express FcRs), nor

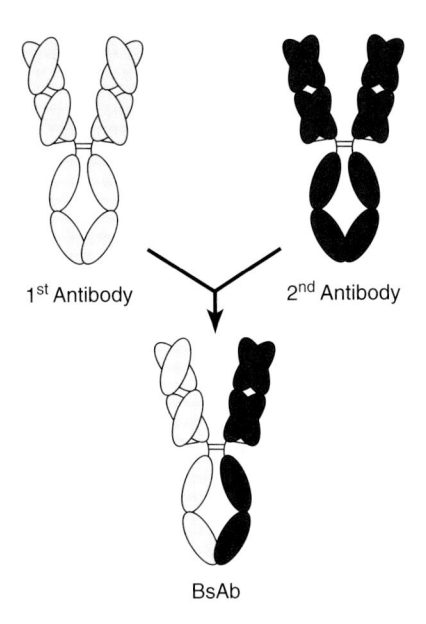

Figure 16.2 BsAb consists of two mAbs produced by chemical, genetic, or hybridoma technology with two different antigen specificities.

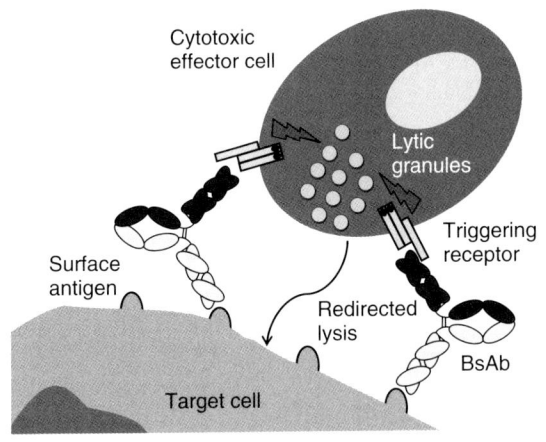

Figure 16.3 Redirected lysis of target cell by a cytotoxic effector cell mediated by a BsAb. The simultaneous binding of the BsAb to both a surface antigen on the target cell and to a triggering receptor on the effector cell induces the effector cell to kill the target cell by delivering a cytotoxic payload.

does it effectively trigger ADCC by polymorphonuclear neutrophils (PMNs), the most numerous cytotoxic effector cell population in humans [46]. For cancer immunotherapy, the most desired effector cell populations are professional cell killers, such as $CD56^{dim}CD16^+$ NK cells [47] and $CD8^+$ cytotoxic T-lymphocytes (CTLs) [3]. Both CTLs and NK cells contain preformed lytic granules comprising proteases of the granzyme family (especially granzyme A and B), perforin, and granulysin [48], and can kill several target cells in succession without killing themselves via the formation of the secretory synapses [49]. Although the mechanism of apoptosis induction by granulocytes remains elusive, PMNs are also increasingly recognized as an important effector cell population for rejection of malignant tumors [50]. Recruited PMNs produce several cytotoxic mediators, including reactive oxygen species, proteases, membrane-perforating agents, and soluble mediators of cell killing, such as tumor necrosis factor (TNF)-α, interleukin (IL)-1β, interferons, and antimicrobial peptides defensins, which are highly toxic against tumors [51]. Myeloid cells infiltrate tumors engineered to secrete ILs or chemokines in their microenvironment and play a key role in all of these cytokine-induced tumor rejections, often in cooperation with CD8$^+$ T-lymphocytes [51].

To mediate redirected lysis, a BsAb must bind a target cell directly to a triggering molecule on the effector cell. The best-studied cytotoxic triggering receptors are multi-chain signaling complexes such as: (i) T-cell receptor/CD3 complex on T-cells; (ii) CD2 on T-cells and NK cells; (iii) FcRs, such as low-affinity FcγRIIIa (CD16a) on NK cells, and high-affinity FcγRI (CD64) and FcαRI (CD89) expressed by monocytes, macrophages, and granulocytes [4, 50]; and (iv) activating NK cell receptors, such as NKp46, NKp44, NKp30, NKp80 (KLR-F1) [52], and NKG2D, which is also expressed on CD8$^+$ T-cells [53]. Due to the high affinity for IgG, all CD64 receptors appear to be occupied by serum IgGs. Therefore, a BsAb targeting CD64 should bind to the outside of the Fc-binding domain of CD64. It has been demonstrated that BsAbs can operate at lower concentrations than conventional antibodies and require lower target antigen expression. For example, a comparison of recombinant CD19 × CD3 BsAb comprising two single-chain Fvs (scFvs) of antibody molecules connected in tandem by a peptide linker ((scFv)$_2$) with anti-CD20 chimeric mAb, rituximab, demonstrated 10^5-fold difference in their cytotoxic efficacy (ED$_{50}$) *in vitro* [54]. Furthermore, combinations of BsAbs with effector cell-activating cytokines allow the increase of effector cell numbers and their functional state [55, 56].

16.5.2
BsAbs of Dual Action

For most diseases, several mediators contribute to overall pathogenesis by either unique or overlapping mechanisms. The simultaneous blockade of several targets or targeting different pathogenic cell pools might therefore yield better therapeutic efficacy than inhibition of a single target (Figure 16.4). Designing of dual-action antibodies could help solve a major problem associated with monotherapy: cancer cells can become resistant to a single agent, mutating in ways that allow them to dodge the action of the drug. Having a single drug that can hit the cancer from multiple directions would simplify treatment and make it more efficient. A single antibody that could do the work of two is also attractive from a business perspective. It might cost half as much to manufacture as two separate antibodies, and the path to regulatory approval might also be shorter and less expensive, involving one set of clinical trials instead of multiple trials for two separate drugs in various dosage combinations. Proof of concept for this approach has been demonstrated in experimental models, such as for BsAbs cotargeting the epidermal growth factor receptor (EGFR) and the insulin-like growth factor receptor (IGFR) [57], and for the "two-in-one" antibody targeting the human EGFR2 (ErbB2, p185^{neu}, HER2/*neu*, HER2) on cancer cells and inhibiting tumor angiogenesis via trapping the vascular endothelial growth factor (VEGF) [58].

Figure 16.4 Comparison of traditional immunotherapy using a combination of two monospecific antibodies (a) with an approach with BsAb of dual action (b). The following antitumor activities are indicated: (1) induction of apoptosis upon receptor cross-linking, (2) CDC, (3) ADCC, and (4) blocking growth factor (GF), which triggers tumor cell growth and proliferation or angiogenesis. As outlined in the figure, the higher antitumor effect can be achieved by using tetravalent bispecific constructs or "two-in-one" antibodies that allow bivalent binding to each antigen.

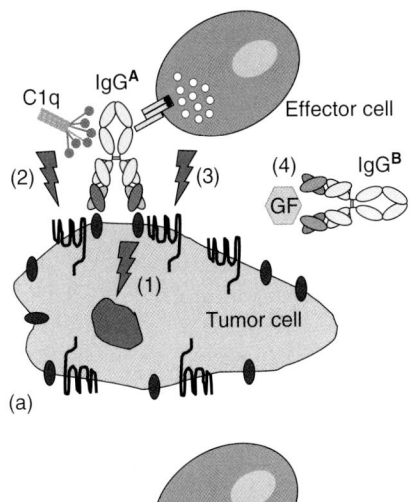

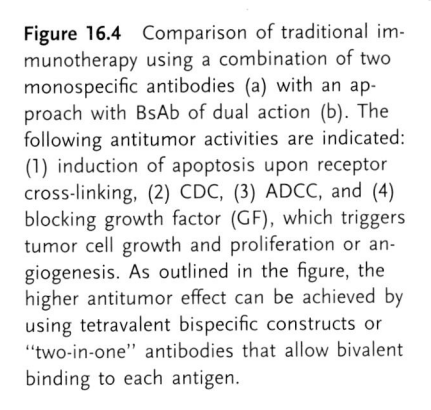

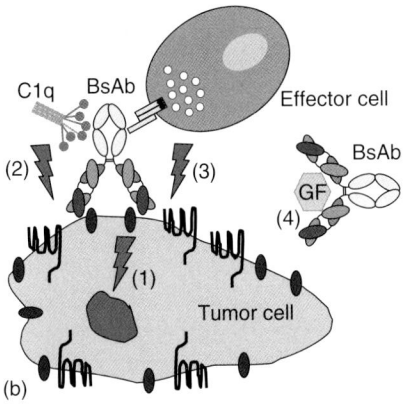

16.5.3
BsAbs of Enhanced Selectivity

The vast majority of tumor antigens are not really "tumor specific" (expressed exclusively on cancer cells); they are rather "tumor associated." Although they are quite often overexpressed on tumor cells, these molecules are also present on normal cells and healthy tissues. For example, CD20, a target for the antilymphoma blockbuster rituximab, is expressed on all B cells; the human EGFR (ErbB1, HER1), a target for cetuximab (Erbitux) and panitumumab (Vectibix) approved for treatment of CRC, is expressed on all epithelial tissues; HER2, a target for another bestseller, antibody trastuzumab (Herceptin), which is approved for treatment of HER2-positive MBC, is also present on heart and muscle cells. Lack of tumor specificity is a main reason for the adverse side-effects associated with antibody therapy, such as acne-like skin rash in the case of Erbitux and Vectibix, and cardiotoxicity observed in some patients treated with Herceptin. However, there are combinations of tumor-associated antigens that can be found only on tumor cells and never on healthy tissues. For example, coexpression of CD38 and CD138 is thought to be exquisitely specific for myeloma cells [59], while CD38 alone is

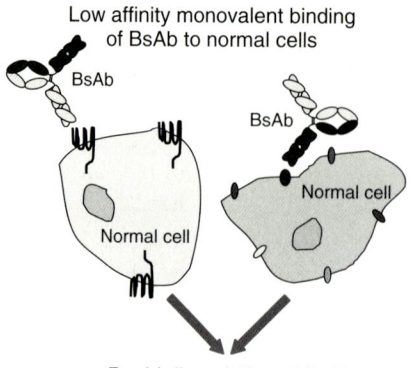

Figure 16.5 BsAbs of enhanced selectivity. Combining two low- or moderate-affinity antibodies against two different tumor-associated antigens that bind weakly to cells expressing only one antigen (a) can generate a dual-targeting bispecific molecule with high avidity for cancer cells expressing both antigens (b). The following antitumor activities are indicated: (1) induction of apoptosis upon receptor cross-linking, (2) CDC, and (3) ADCC.

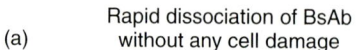

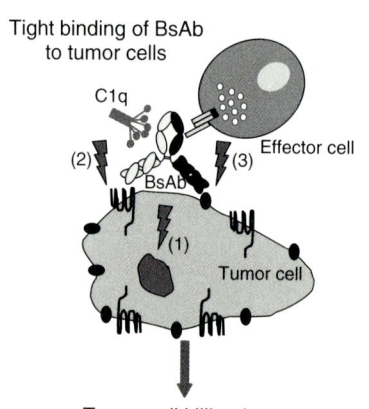

present on the surface of many immune cells (white blood cells), including CD4$^+$ and CD8$^+$ T-cells, and NK cells. Accordingly, CD138 is widely expressed on plasma cells. Combining two low/moderate-affinity antibodies (or antibody fragments) against each antigen can generate a dual-targeting bispecific molecule with high avidity for myeloma cells expressing both antigens, while binding weakly to cells expressing only one antigen (Figure 16.5). A similar approach has been proposed for targeting tumor cells coexpressing two members of the epidermal growth factor family of receptor tyrosine kinases, HER2 (ErbB2) and HER3 (ErbB3) [60]. Another example includes cotargeting CD5 (T-cell marker) and one of the B-cell markers, such as CD19, CD20, or CD23, that are coexpressed in most CLLs [61].

16.6
BsAb Formats

Various strategies have been used to prepare BsAbs. In one approach, bispecific molecules are generated by two or more different polypeptide chains capable of heterodimerization, resulting in bivalent or multivalent proteins. For example, the traditional IgG molecule is a heterotetramer comprising two HCs and two LCs linked together via disulfide bridges. Production of such hetero-oligomeric BsAbs requires: (i) the simultaneous expression of two or more antibody chains, in equal amounts and in the same bacterial or eukaryotic cell, or (ii) laborious refolding from inclusion bodies containing individually expressed polypeptides. In contrast, the second approach embodies the principle of "one gene–one product." In this case, the individual protein domains, such as HC and LC antibody variable domains (V_H and V_L, respectively) from two antibodies of different specificity, are fused together as a single polypeptide chain, and the functional antigen-binding modules (Fv) are either formed from the complementary domains of the same polypeptide chain or are generated by homodimerization of the single-chain molecule.

16.6.1
Hetero-Oligomeric Antibodies

Early approaches to the formation of hetero-oligomeric antibodies exploited chemical random cross-linking of polyclonal antibodies [62] and mAbs [63], or by site-specific conjugation of antibody fragments (Fab′) derived from pepsin-digested antibodies of different specificity [64, 65]. Alternatively, monoclonal BsAbs were produced by fusion of two hybridoma lines, generating hybrid hybridomas (quadromas) [66] or using a trioma (cross-species hybridoma) technology [67]. The resulting functional BsAb is a heterotetramer composed of two different HCs and two different LCs. A major limitation of quadroma technology is the production of inactive antibodies due to the random LC–HC and HC–HC associations resulting in up to 10 different combinations; only around 10% of the antibodies produced by this method are of the desired specificity [66]. The correct BsAb must then be separated in a costly procedure from a large quantity of other similar molecules. This limitation has been partly overcome by using hybridomas from different species (e.g., rat and mouse) as fusion partners, due to preferential species-restricted HC/LC pairing [68].

A further limitation of quadroma BsAb from rodent cell lines is their immunogenicity. Repeated doses of rodent antibodies elicit an anti-immunoglobulin response, referred to as the human anti-murine antibody (HAMA) response. Generally, the HAMA response compromises BsAb therapy, although there are indications that it can be beneficial for patient outcome in some cases [69].

Recent advances in recombinant antibody technology [9, 70–72] provide an opportunity to develop alternative methods for engineering and producing BsAb molecules from the antibody fragments (Figure 16.6). In analogy to natural antibody Fv modules, which are stably associated through the constant domain interactions of the LCs and HCs, bispecific Fab- or scFv-based fusion proteins may be constructed to include domains with known multimerization properties. For example, bispecific Fabs have been generated by heterodimerization through leucine zippers [73] or through pairing of complementary oligonucleotides covalently linked to Fab′ fragments [74]. Similarly, scFv fragments have been genetically fused either with

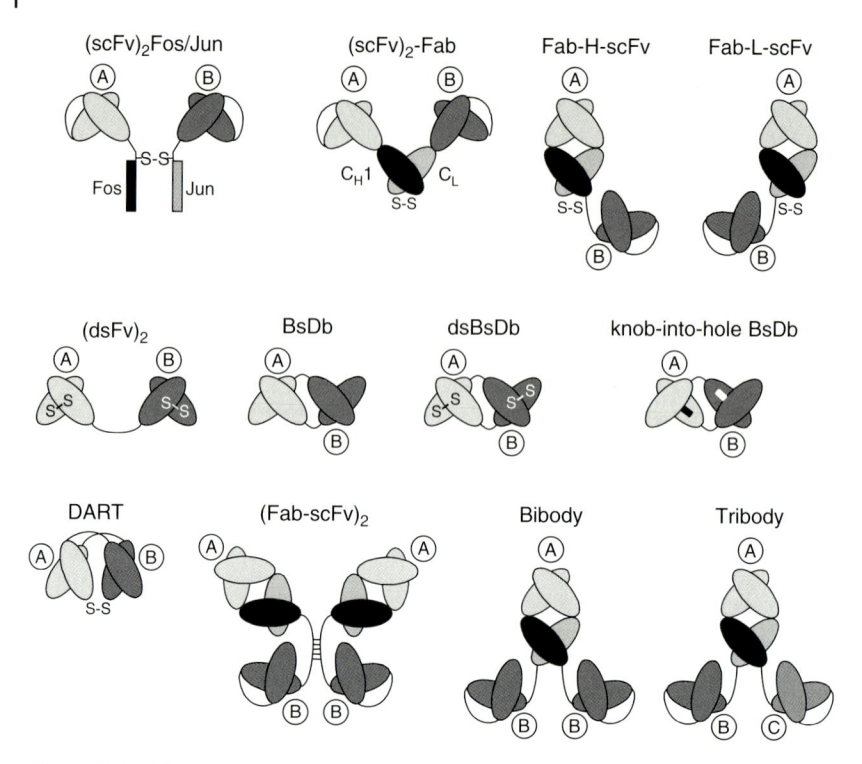

Figure 16.6 Schematic representation of recombinant hetero-oligomeric bispecific molecules. Double scFvs can be formed either by interaction of Fos and Jun leucine zippers ((scFv)$_2$Fos/Jun) or C_H1 and C_L domains ((scFv)$_2$–Fab). Fab-H–scFv and Fab-L–scFv are generated by fusion of a scFv to the C-terminus of the C_H1 or C_L domain, respectively, of an antibody Fab fragment. A dsFv–dsFv′ tandem ((dsFv)$_2$) can be formed by coexpression of three gene products (V_H^A, V_L^B, and $V_H^B - V_L^A$ fusion) encoding variable domains with an extra cysteine residue. Noncovalent association of two hybrid scFv fragments comprising V_H and V_L domains of different specificity leads to the formation of a BsDb. The noncovalent associations of the diabody chains can be further stabilized by artificially introduced disulfide bonds either in the V_H/V_L interface (dsBsDb) or at the C-terminus of each diabody chain (DART), or by the "knob-into-hole" mutations (knob-into-hole BsDb). In tetravalent (Fab-scFv)$_2$, the scFv fragments are fused to the antibody hinge region. Bispecific and even trispecific molecules can be formed by fusion of scFv to an Fd fragment and a light chain of Fab (bibody and tribody). The antigen-binding sites of different specificity (A, B, and C) are indicated.

Fos and Jun leucine zippers [75] ((scFv)$_2$Fos/Jun; Figure 16.6) or with the first constant domain of human HC (C_H1) and the constant domain of human κ chain (C_L) ((scFv)$_2$–Fab; Figure 16.6) to facilitate the formation of heterodimers [76, 77]. Bispecific disulfide-stabilized Fv (dsFv) tandem molecules, (dsFv)$_2$, could be formed by connecting two dsFv modules with a peptide linker, in which the V_H/V_L interface is stabilized by a disulfide bridge (Figure 16.6). Formation of such molecules can be achieved only by coexpression of three separate gene constructs

(V_H^A, V_L^B, and V_H^B–V_L^A fusion) in the same cell and usually results in a very low yield of functional product [78]. Bispecific Fab–scFv fragments have been generated by genetically fusing a scFv to the C-terminus of either the HC or the LC of a Fab fragment of different antigen-binding specificity (Fab-H–scFv and Fab-L–scFv, respectively; Figure 16.6) [79, 80].

The recombinant bispecific molecules can also be formed by noncovalent association of two single-chain fusion products consisting of V_H and V_L domains of different specificity, separated by a short linker (less than 12 amino acids) that prevents intramolecular V_H/V_L pairing, giving a four-domain heterodimer bispecific diabody (BsDb; Figure 16.6) [81, 82]. Crystallographic analysis has demonstrated that two antigen binding sites are located on opposite sides of the diabody, assembled both in V_H-to-V_L [83] and in V_L-to-V_H [84] orientation, such that they are able to cross-link two cells. BsDbs are potentially less immunogenic than the quadroma-derived BsAbs and can easily be produced in bacteria in relatively high yields [85, 86]. However, cosecretion of two hybrid scFv fragments forming a BsDb can give rise to two types of dimer: active heterodimers and inactive homodimers. Another problem is that two chains of diabodies are held together by noncovalent associations of the V_H and V_L domains, and can diffuse away from one another [87]. The stability of BsDbs could be enhanced by introduction of a disulfide bridge or "knob-into-hole" mutations into the V_H/V_L interface (dsBsDb and "knob-into-hole" BsDb, respectively; Figure 16.6) [88, 89]. Alternatively, the diabody can be stabilized by a covalent disulfide bond formation through the cysteine residues artificially placed at the C-terminus of each diabody chain [90]. This Cys-diabody format was used by MacroGenics to develop the dual-affinity retargeting (DART) bispecific molecules, which could be easily produced in mammalian cells, and demonstrated high stability and biological activity both *in vitro* and *in vivo* (DART, Figure 16.6) [91, 92].

Unlike native antibodies, there is only one binding domain for each specificity in all of the BsAb formats mentioned above. Bivalent binding is an important means of increasing the functional affinity, and possibly the selectivity, of antibodies and antibody fragments for particular cell types carrying densely clustered antigens. Therefore, a number of multivalent BsAb-like molecules of different molecular weight have been developed. For example, a scFv fragment can be genetically fused to a Fab fragment through a hinge region thus resulting in a bispecific tetravalent molecule ((Fab–scFv)$_2$; Figure 16.6) [93]. Somewhat smaller bispecific (bibody; Figure 16.6) and even trispecific (tribody; Figure 16.6) trivalent molecules could be generated by the fusion of scFvs to Fd (V_H + C_H1 of an antibody) and LCs of a Fab fragment [79].

16.6.2
Bispecific Single-Chain Antibodies

The smallest functional single-chain BsAbs of molecular weight around 25–30 kDa can be generated by connecting two dAbs with the peptide linker to form dimeric dAbs (di-dAbs, Figure 16.7) [94]. Larger bispecific molecules can be generated

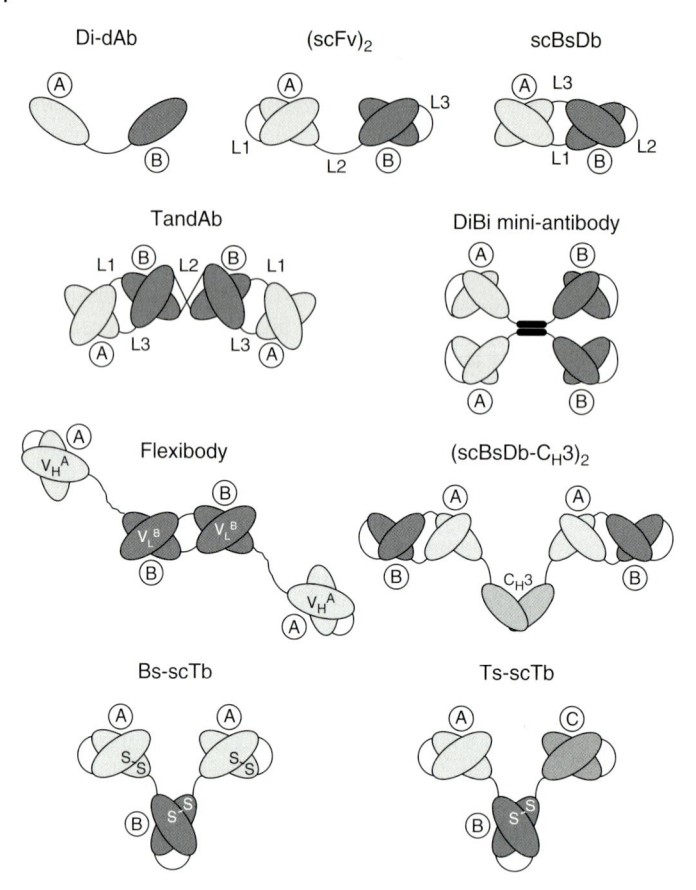

Figure 16.7 Schematic representation of recombinant single-chain bispecific molecules. di-dAbs are formed by connecting two dAbs of different specificity with the peptide linker. In (scFv)₂, the adjacent V_H and V_L domains of the same specificity are separated by long linkers allowing the independent formation of functional Fv modules. In contrast, another order of the V_H and V_L domains forces the whole molecule either to fold head-to-tail to form a scBsDb or to homodimerize, resulting in a tetravalent TandAb. A dimeric bispecific mini-antibody (DiBi miniantibody) is formed by dimerization of scFv–scFv tandem through the linker between two scFv moieties. In a tetravalent flexibody, the intermolecular pairing (with formation of a diabody-like structure in the middle of the molecule) is preceded by intramolecular pairing of two adjacent N- or C-terminal V_H and V_L domains, leading to the formation of functional Fv module in the same polypeptide chain. An also tetravalent (scBsDb–C_H3)₂ molecule is obtained by joining scBsDb to C_H3 antibody domain that dimerizes spontaneously. The antigen-binding sites of different specificity (A and B) are indicated.

using scFv antibody fragments as building blocks. There are two basic strategies for generation of scFv-based bispecifics. Depending on the order of the antibody variable domains and on the length of peptides separating them, the single-chain molecule either forms a (scFv)₂, a tandem of two scFv modules composed of two adjacent V_H and V_L of the same specificity ((scFv)₂; Figure 16.7) [95], or folds head-to-tail with the formation of a diabody-like structure, a single-chain bispecific diabody (scBsDb; Figure 16.7) [87, 96, 97]. In the case of (scFv)$_2$, each scFv comprises V_H and V_L domains of the same specificity separated by a peptide linker of at least 12 amino acids (L1 and L3; Figure 16.7). The linker in the middle of the molecule does not greatly influence the structure as a whole, and can vary in length as long as the antigen-binding sites remain intact (L2; Figure 16.7) [98]. In contrast, two halves of the bispecific scBsDb molecule are represented by nonfunctional hybrid scFvs, that are composed of the V_H and V_L derived from antibodies of different specificity. Each hybrid scFv has a fairly rigid structure determined by a short linker connecting the variable domains, which precludes specific V_H/V_L interaction within the same scFv (L1 and L3; Figure 16.7). Unlike (scFv)$_2$, the linker in the middle of scBsDb is critical for the structure of the whole molecule (L2; Figure 16.7). If the linker is long (15 or more amino acids) and flexible, the molecule can fold head-to-tail into a diabody-like structure, which has two antigen-binding sites on different sides of the molecule (scBsDb; Figure 16.7). It has been demonstrated that, at least in *Escherichia coli*, the head-to-tail folding and formation of functional diabody-like molecules is favored [87]. Moreover, the scBsDb format facilitates the production of relatively stable bispecific constructs from weakly associated Fv fragments [87]. If the linker in the middle of the scBsDb molecules is short and rigid, the molecule cannot fold head-to-tail and dimerizes to a tetravalent homodimer, known as a tandem diabody (TandAb; Figure 16.7) [96, 99].

The distinct structural geometry of (scFv)$_2$ and scBsDb also determines the potential difference in their biological properties. Due to the rigid scBsDb structure, the estimated distance between its antigen-binding sites is almost always 60–65 Å, as deduced from the scBsDb model deposited at the Research Collaboratory for Structural Bioinformatics of the Protein Data Bank under entry code 1OSQ [87]. In contrast, (scFv)$_2$ can span distances of between 50 Å, with a five-amino-acid middle linker, similar to that in diabody and scBsDb, and up to 100–120 Å, with a 20-amino-acid linker, which is similar to the distance between Fv modules in IgG and F(ab')$_2$. Even much larger polypeptide chains, such as human serum albumin (HSA), have been successfully used as linkers connecting two scFv fragments of different specificity [100]. The linker in the middle of the scFv–scFv tandem molecule can also be designed to contain a dimerization motif (e.g., helix–loop–helix) to form tetravalent dimeric bispecific (DiBi) mini-antibodies (DiBi mini-antibody; Figure 16.7) [101]. Tetravalent bispecific molecules have also been created by the fusion of scBsDb to the C_H3 domain of an antibody ((scBsDb–C_H3)$_2$; Figure 16.7) [102].

Unlike many other BsAb formats, TandAb is a homodimer comprising only antibody variable domains, and its formation is determined by the association of complementary V_H and V_L domains located on different polypeptide chains (TandAb; Figure 16.7). The TandAb is twice the size of the diabody and (scFv)$_2$, is able to bind bivalently to both effector and target cells, and possesses improved pharmacokinetic characteristics, greater stability, and enhanced biological activity both *in vitro* and *in vivo* relative to diabody [96, 103, 104]. Interchain pairing of cognate V_H

and V_L domains of the same specificity can also be used for the formation of bispecific scFv^A–diabody^B–scFv^A tandem molecules, called "flexibodies" (Figure 16.7) [70]. Depending on the association strength of complementary domains involved in the interchain pairing and on the length of the linker separating them, dimers, trimers, and even tetramers of bispecific single-chain molecules could be formed. The generated bispecific CD19 × CD3 flexibodies appear to possess higher avidity and enhanced activity in mediating T-cell cytotoxicity against CD19$^+$ leukemia cells relative to bivalent diabody and scBsDb [105]. Also, spontaneous swapping of N-terminal V_L and V_H domains and formation of tetravalent homodimers of a bispecific anti-melanoma-associated proteoglycan NG2 (MAPG)/anti-CD28 (scFv)$_2$, rM28, has been demonstrated, and such dimerization of a "subagonistic" (scFv)$_2$ molecule has resulted in a dimer with "supra-agonistic" properties in inducing vigorous T-cell activation and killing melanoma cell lines [106]. The supra-agonistic effect was attributed to dimerization of the (scFv)$_2$ molecule and retained after substitution of the anti-MAPG scFv by a scFv targeting CD20 [107].

A trivalent single-chain molecule comprising three functional scFv modules connected in a tandem (triple body (scTb)) can also be generated and successfully expressed in mammalian cells [108]. The distal (N-terminal and C-terminal) scFv modules were specific for tumor antigen and the scFv in the middle of the molecule was to recruit the effector NK cells via binding to CD16. Similar to normal IgG1, the scFv organization of the bispecific scTb (Bs-scTb)) allows bivalent binding to the target tumor cells and monovalent binding to the effector cells (Figure 16.7). Each Fv module of the scTb was additionally stabilized by a disulfide bond artificially introduced into V_H/V_L interface. Comparison of the trivalent Bs-scTb of two different antitumor specificities, CD19 × CD16 and CD33 × CD16, with the corresponding bivalent (scFv)$_2$ molecules demonstrated superior properties of the triple bodies, such as greater cell-binding activity, higher tumor cell-killing potency, and favorable pharmacokinetics [108, 109]. Generation of the dual targeting trispecific scTb (Ts-scTb)) has also been demonstrated (Ts-scTb; Figure 16.7). The described CD123 × CD16 × CD33 Ts-scTb molecule possessed enhanced selectivity to the leukemia stem cells coexpressing CD123 and CD33, and was very efficient in mediating ADCC of primary leukemia cells isolated from patients with acute myeloid leukemia (AML) [110].

16.6.3
Recombinant IgG-Like BsAbs

Although small recombinant BsAbs, such as diabodies and (scFv)$_2$, may have an advantage in terms of tumor penetration, their size below kidney clearance threshold (around 60 kDa) leads to rapid elimination from the bloodstream by extravasation and glomerular filtration. This limitation could be overcome by generation of IgG-like bispecific molecules, which are too large to be easily filtered by the kidneys and comprise an Fc region binding to the FcRn that is responsible for antibody recycling and long serum half-life [111]. In addition, IgG-like BsAb are capable of supporting secondary immune functions, such as ADCC and CDC. However, production of BsIgG by coexpressing two different antibodies is inefficient due to mispairing of the HCs and LCs. To avoid HC homodimerization, a solution was to re-engineer the C_H3 domain of the Fc to favor HC heterodimerization over homodimerization. Remodeling C_H3 domains using "knobs-into-holes" mutations in conjunction with engineered disulfide bonds led to nearly quantitative formation of stable HC heterodimers [112]. The LC mispairing could be circumvented by using an identical LC for each arm of the BsIgG (Figure 16.8a) or by fusing the V_L, V_H, and Fc in a single-chain format ((scFv)$_2$–Fc, Figure 16.8a). The bispecific scFv–Fc knobs-into-holes molecules were able to bind and cross-link both target antigens [113]. One could hypothesize that this format, which is slightly smaller (120 kDa) than a normal IgG (150 kDa), might provide some gains in tumor penetration, while maintaining the long circulation half-life and effector functions provided by the intact Fc region.

To completely circumvent the HC homodimerization and HC–LC mispairing issues, a number of BsAb formats have been developed by direct addition of a new antigen-binding specificity to a fully functional antibody or to an Fc-containing antibody-like molecule. In one approach, a scFv fragment specific for one antigen can be genetically fused to the C-terminus of the IgG HC or scFv–Fc specific for another antigen (IgG-H–(scFv)$_2$ and scFv–Fc–scFv, respectively; Figure 16.8b) [93, 114]. A tetravalent IgG-H–(scFv)$_2$ antibody produced by this technique was reported to be bispecific, retained Fc-associated effector functions, and had a half-life *in vivo* equal to that of human IgG [93]. To decrease aggregation propensity of the BsIgG-H–(scFv)$_2$, the molecule can be stabilized by introduction of an additional disulfide bridge into V_H/V_L interface of the scFv moiety [115]. A functional tetravalent molecule can also be formed by fusion of the disulfide-stabilized scFv to C-terminus of the antibody LC (IgG-L–(scFv)$_2$; Figure 16.8b) [116].

In an alternative approach, two scFvs of different specificity were fused to N-termini of C_H1 and C_L, to form two polypeptides, scFv^A–C_H1–C_H2–C_H3 and scFv^B–C_L, respectively [77]. Coexpression of these polypeptides in mammalian cells resulted in the formation of a covalently linked bispecific heterotetramer, (scFv)$_4$–IgG (Figure 16.8c). It has been demonstrated that fully human (scFv)$_4$–IgG construct directed against both EGFR and IGFR could be successfully used for inhibiting tumor cell proliferation *in vitro* [117]. A drawback of this format is its low expression level in mammalian cells, probably because of both its large size (around 200 kDa) and structural complexity. Interestingly, these difficulties have been overcome in a recently described dual-variable-domain immunoglobulins (DVD-Igs) (Figure 16.8c) [118]. Also tetravalent and similar in size with (scFv)$_4$–IgG, the DVD-Ig has more "natural" domain organization, $V_H^A - V_H^B - C_H1 - C_H2 - C_H3$ and $V_L^A - V_L^B - C_L$, in its HC and LC, respectively. Coexpression of these extended HCs and LCs in mammalian cells resulted in efficient formation of antigen-binding Fv modules and good production yields of DVD-Ig on the level of normal IgG [118, 119].

In another group of molecules, Fc region preceded by the hinge was used as a C-terminal extension of already bispecific smaller constructs, such as diabodies, single-chain diabodies, and scFv–scFv tandems (di-diabody, (scBsDb)$_2$–Fc, and

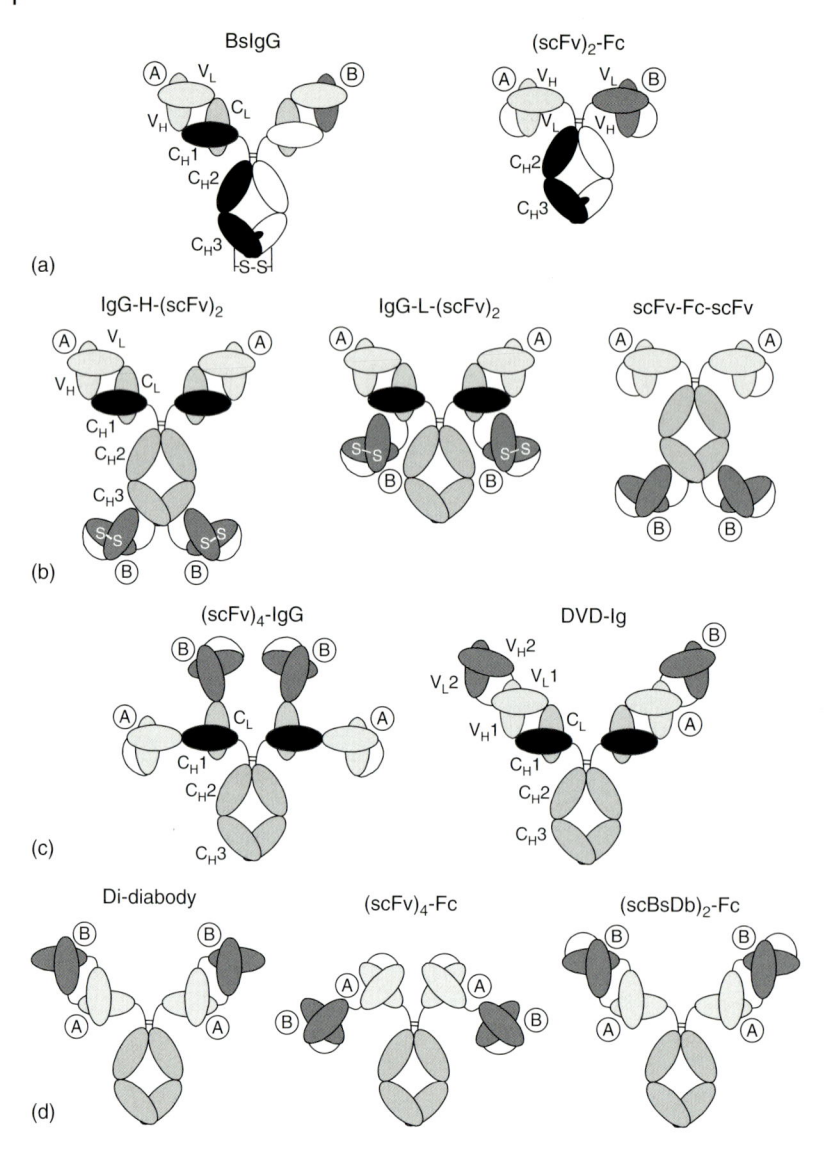

Figure 16.8 Recombinant IgG-like BsAb formats. (a) Use of "knobs-into-holes" approach for heterodimerization to form BsIgG and (scFv)$_2$–Fc bivalent bispecific molecules. In the BsIgG molecule, both specificities share the same light chain. (b) C-terminal scFv fusion approach. In IgG-H–scFv$_2$, scFv–Fc–scFv, and IgG-L–scFv$_2$, the scFv (or disulfide-stabilized scFv) fragments are fused either to the C-terminus of Fc region or of the C$_L$ domain. (c) N-terminal scFv or V-domain fusion approach. In (scFv)$_4$–IgG, the V$_H$ and V$_L$ domains of a human IgG1 molecule are replaced by two scFv fragments of different specificity. In DVD-Ig, the IgG HCs and LCs are expanded by adding an additional V$_H$ or V$_L$ domain of another specificity to the N-terminus of the HC or LC, respectively. (d) Fc fusion approach to form tetravalent molecules from the bispecific small constructs composed of the antibody variable domains. The antigen-binding sites of different specificity (A and B) are indicated.

(scFv)$_4$–Fc; Figure 16.8d) [102, 120, 121]. In a di-diabody format, one half of the diabody, the hybrid scFv comprising the V$_H$ and V$_L$ domains of different specificity, was fused to the Fc region, thus generating the "heavier chain" (V$_L^A$ – V$_H^B$ – C$_H$2 – C$_H$3) and the other hybrid scFv noncovalently associates with it as a "lighter chain" (V$_L^B$ – V$_H^A$) [120]. Although bispecific di-diabody construct can be expressed in mammalian cells at much higher levels (above 400 mg/l in nonoptimized conditions) than, for example, (scFv)$_4$–IgG, it has a tendency to form inactive molecules *in vivo* due to dissociation of the noncovalently bound lighter chains followed by the rapid clearance of the lighter chains from circulation [122]. This drawback can be circumvented by using scBsDb as a fusion partner for Fc [102]. The derived tetravalent (scBsDb)$_2$–Fc molecule appeared to be produced with reasonable yields, was stable and more active biologically than the bivalent diabodies, and was able to mediate ADCC [123].

Feasibility of constructing oligospecific IgG-like molecules by fusion of scFv or (scFv)$_2$ to the N- or C-termini of intact IgG has also been demonstrated [124].

16.6.4
Other Novel BsAb Constructs

The aforementioned methods and constructs utilized Fv modules comprising the V$_H$ and V$_L$ domains as antigen-binding units. Using single dAbs from camelids (V$_{HH}$ or nanobody) or of human origin (dAb) instead of scFv allowed generation of smaller and more stable bispecific molecules that can also be produced at higher yields [125, 126]. An absolutely different "two-in-one" antibody engineering concept has recently been described in which the binding site on an antibody was engineered to recognize two different antigens [58]. The authors of this study observed that the anti-HER2 antibody trastuzumab recognizes its antigen primarily via the contacts in CDRs of the HC. They constructed therefore a library of mutant LC CDRs, and selected antibody variants that bound both HER2 and VEGF-A, both with high affinity. However, the structural studies showed that both antigen-binding sites overlap and, therefore, the "two-in-one" antibody cannot bind two antigens simultaneously [58].

16.7
BsAbs in the Clinic

There are numerous challenges in the development of BsAb therapeutics, especially in the production of homogeneous functional material of sufficient quantity and purity to meet clinical needs. At least 20 different BsAbs have been tested in small-scale cancer therapy trials, with antitumor responses in a few cases [50, 127, 128]. Most of the clinically tested BsAbs have been generated either by quadroma technology or by chemical coupling of Fab′ fragments derived from fully murine or humanized mAbs.

16.7.1
Clinical Data for First-Generation BsAbs

Results from the early clinical trials suggested that the purity of BsAb (i.e., the absence of contamination with monospecific mAbs), target antigen selection, HAMA response, preactivation of effector cells, and the function of cytokines are all critical issues in this therapeutic approach. The BsAb fragments, such as F(ab')$_2$, demonstrated lower toxicity, caused by massive cytokine release, than BsAbs containing an Fc portion. In addition, correct selection of the effector cell population is also crucial issue for retargeting BsAbs. Chemically cross-linked BsAbs from Medarex that are recruiting the myeloid effector cells, MDX-H210 (specific for HER2 × CD64) and MDX-447 (specific for EGFR × CD64), underwent phase I clinical trials in patients with advanced breast cancer [129] or head and neck cancer [130], respectively (Table 16.2). These trials led to somewhat disappointing results, probably due to the low concentrations of antibodies and low effector/target cell ratios used. For example, testing MDX-447 in 64 patients with advanced solid tumors as monotherapy ($n = 41$) or combined with granulocyte colony stimulating factor (G-CSF; $n = 23$) demonstrated no objective complete responses (CRs) or partial responses (PRs) in either group [130]. No objective responses were also seen in a single dose study in 30 advanced breast cancer patients treated with MDX-H210 in combination with G-CSF. A total of 11 patients had stable disease (SD) and 19 patients progressive disease (PD) at the end of the study period [129].

Strategy of T-cell retargeting appeared to be more successful. In April 2009, the first BsAb, catumaxomab (Removab; Fresenius Biotech/TRION Pharma), specific for both epithelial cell adhesion molecule (EpCAM) on tumor cells and CD3 on T-cells, was approved by the European Medicines Agency (EMEA) for the intraperitoneal treatment of malignant ascites in patients with EpCAM-positive carcinomas (Table 16.1) [131]. Catumaxomab is a trioma made half mouse/half rat full-length IgG whose antitumor activity results from T-cell-mediated lysis, ADCC, and phagocytosis via activation of FcγR-positive accessory cells. Another trioma-derived antibody that targets HER2 and CD3 (ertumaxomab) has completed phase I trials in 17 patients with MBC (Table 16.2) [132]. The antibody was administered intravenously and the observed toxicity was mostly related to the cytokine release. Three patients out of 17 responded to treatment with ertumaxomab (1 CR/2 PR); roughly one-third of the treated patients developed immune reaction to mouse or rat protein (HAMA/human anti-rat antibody response) [132].

16.7.2
Recombinant Bispecific Molecules Entering Clinical Trials

16.7.2.1 Bispecific T-Cell Engager Molecules
The bispecific T-cell engager (BiTE) antibodies are generated from two scFv fragments (one of which had a specificity against human CD3), arranged in tandem with a five-amino-acid linker, on a single polypeptide ((scFv)$_2$; Figure 16.7) [133, 134]. The most advanced product, CD19 × CD3 BiTE blinatumomab (MT103;

Table 16.2 BsAbs in recent clinical trials.

Name	Species	Specificity	Format	Clinical stage/indication (number of patients)	Developer
MDX-H210	murine × humanized	HER2 × CD64	F(ab')₂ chemical conjugate	phase I completed/advanced breast cancer (n = 30)	Medarex/BMS
MDX-447	humanized × humanized	EGFR × CD64	F(ab')₂ chemical conjugate	phase I/II completed/head and neck cancer (n = 64)	Medarex/BMS
Ertumaxomab	murine × rat	HER2 × CD3	intact IgG (trioma)	phase II ongoing/MBC (n = 19)	Fresenius/Trion
Blinatumomab (MT103)	murine × murine	CD19 × CD3	BiTE (scFv)₂	phase I completed/NHL (n = 38); phase II/ALL ongoing (up to 130)	Micromet
MT110	human × deimmunized	EpCAM × CD3	BiTE (scFv)₂	phase I ongoing/lung and gastrointestinal cancer (up to 50)	Micromet
MT111/MEDI-565	human × deimmunized	CEA × CD3	BiTE (scFv)₂	phase I ongoing/advanced gastrointestinal cancer	MedImmune/Astra Zeneca
rM28	murine × murine	MAPG × CD28	(scFv)₂/flexibody	phase I/II completed/metastatic melanoma (n = 14)	University of Tübingen
MM-111	human × human	HER2 × HER3	scFv–HSA–scFv	phase I/II ongoing/HER2-positive breast and gastric cancers (n = 12)	Merrimack
DT2219ARL	murine × murine	CD22 × CD19	DT390–(scFv)₂ immunotoxin	phase I ongoing/B-cell leukemia or lymphoma (up to 36)	Scott and White Cancer Institute
AFM13	murine × human	CD30 × CD16a	TandAb	phase I ongoing/Hodgkin's lymphoma (up to 40)	Affimed Therapeutics
CVX-241	humanized	Tie2 × VEGFR	mAb–peptide conjugate	phase I ongoing/advanced solid tumors (up to 45)	Pfizer

Micromet) was highly efficient in redirecting unstimulated primary T-cells against $CD19^+$ lymphoma cells *in vitro*, demonstrated high antitumor activity in animal models [135], and was the first genetically engineered BsAb to entered clinical trials [136]. Due to its small size (50 kDa), blinatumomab has a relatively short biological half-life of 2–3 h. To obtain steady-state serum levels, the studies were using continuous intravenous infusion of the BiTE antibody over 4–8 weeks per cycle. Phase I trial in patients ($n = 38$) with NHL demonstrated that blinatumomab induced partial and complete tumor regression in 11 patients (4 CR/7 PR) at much lower doses than are required for the therapeutic mAb rituximab [137]. The first results from an ongoing phase II trial in patients with B-cell precursor ALL indicate that T-cells recruited by blinatumomab are able to locate and eradicate rare disseminated tumor cells in the bone marrow that can only be detected by quantitative polymerase chain reaction assays detecting tumor cell-specific genomic aberrations. Residual tumor cells in the bone marrow of B-ALL patients (referred to as minimal residual disease (MRD)), as can be found after extensive chemotherapy, pose a very high risk of relapse and reduced survival when compared with MRD-negative patients. Of 20 evaluable patients treated, 16 (80%) achieved a complete MRD response [138]. As of June 2010, seven out of 11 evaluable patients without bone marrow transplantation were in hematological remission with a median of nearly 18 months and ranging up to 23 months. Overall, the side-effect profile of blinatumomab in B-ALL patients appeared to be very favorable.

Another BiTE antibody, anti-EpCAM/anti-CD3 MT110, entered clinical trials in April 2008 in patients with EpCAM-positive advanced, recurrent, or metastatic solid tumors (Table 16.2). Unlike fully murine blinatumomab, MT110 comprises human anti-EpCAM and deimmunized anti-CD3 scFv modules [139]. In preclinical development, MT110 demonstrated clear antitumor activity in animal models of human colon carcinoma, metastatic ovarian cancer, and established pancreatic cancer (Figure 16.9) [139, 140]. As of May 2010, 28 patients with locally advanced, recurrent or mCRC, gastric, and lung cancer had been treated with MT110 at dose levels ranging from 1 to 24 µg/day, in 4-week treatment cycles. Out of 22 patients evaluable for response, disease stabilization was observed in nine patients, with a median duration of 91 days. Consistent with the BiTE mode of action, investigators observed redistribution and expansion of T-cells in blood, and infiltration of T-cells into tumor tissue. None of the patients developed antibodies against MT110. To date, no maximum tolerated dose has been reached and dose escalation continues (www.micromet.de).

The third product candidate of the BiTE class, anti-carcinoembryonic antigen (CEA, CD66e, CEACAM5)/anti-CD3 MT111/MEDI-565, has recently received acceptance of an Investigational New Drug application from the US Food and Drug Administration (FDA) and entered clinical trials in patients with advanced gastrointestinal cancers (http://phx.corporate-ir.net/phoenix.zhtml?c=197259&p=irol-newsArticle&ID=1515442&highlight=). The product has been developed by Micromet together with MedImmune (now part of Astra Zeneca). MT111 is composed of a human anti-CEA scFv and a deimmunized human $CD3\varepsilon$-specific antibody fragment [141]. The antibody was capable in mediating killing of CEA-positive

(a)

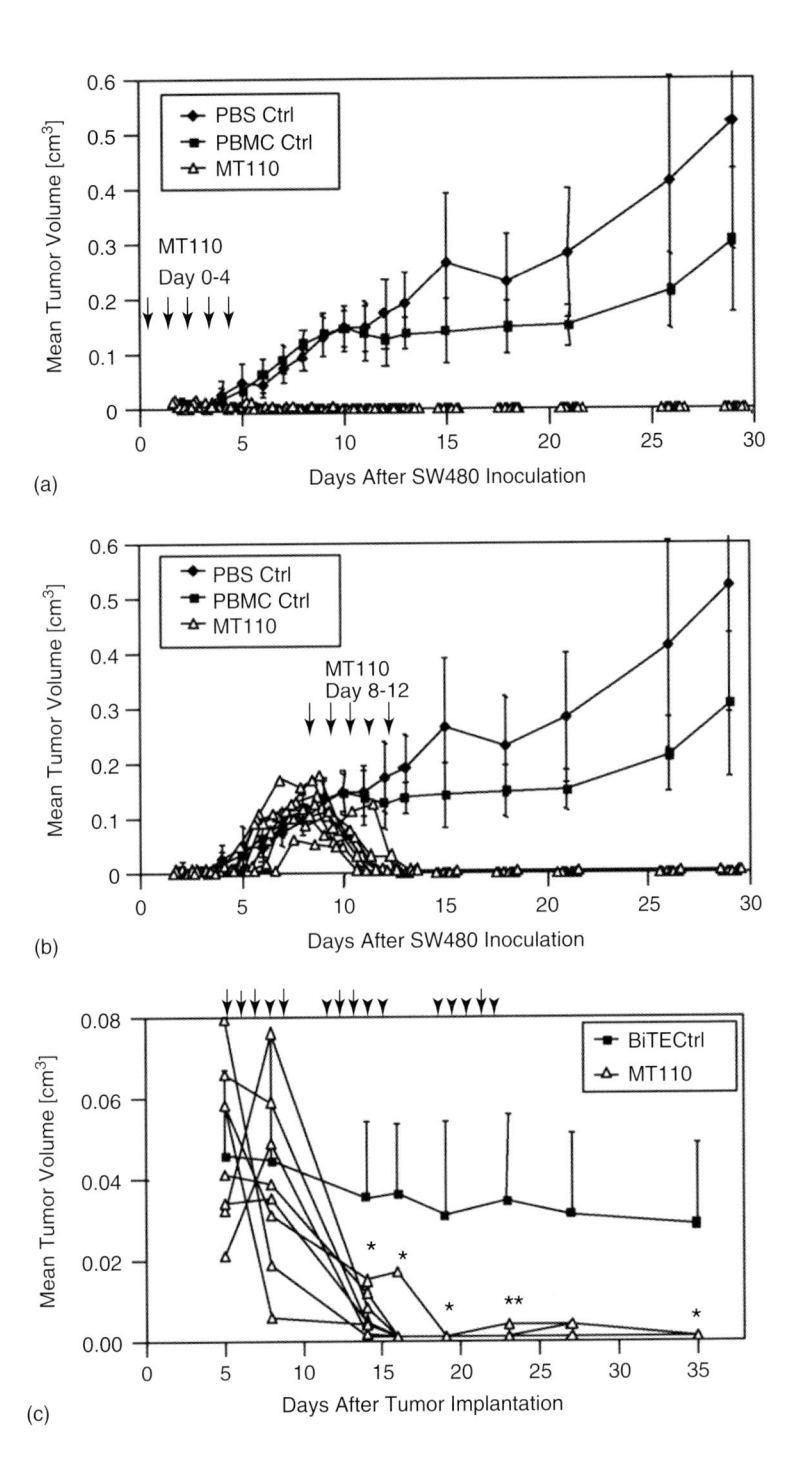

(b)

(c)

Figure 16.9 Antitumor activity of anti-EpCAM/anti-CD3 BiTE MT110 in animal models of human colon carcinoma and metastatic ovarian cancer. In each experiments, cohorts of eight NOD/SCID mice were used. In colon carcinoma models (a) and (b), the mice were inoculated subcutaneously with 5×10^6 SW480 human colon cancer cells in the absence or presence of 5×10^6 unstimulated human PBMCs from the healthy donors. Animals were either treated via the tail vein injection with phosphate-buffered saline vehicle control (PBS) or 1 μg MT110 per mouse per day. In the early disease model (a), treatment was started 1 h after SW480 inoculation and continued on days 1–4. In the established tumor model (b), treatment was delayed to days 8–12. Mean values of tumor growth curves are shown for mice treated with phosphate-buffered saline vehicle control in the absence (♦) or presence (■) of human PBMCs. For MT110-treated animals (△), individual tumor growth curves are shown. In the ovarian tumor model (c), patient tumor samples freshly dissected during primary surgery of ovarian cancer peritoneal metastasis were cut into pieces of 50–100 mm^3 and single pieces subcutaneously implanted into the right flank of NOD/SCID mice. Cohorts of eight animals were treated via tail vein injection with a bispecific control antibody (●) or 5 μg MT110 (△) per mouse per day on days 5–9, 12–16, and 19–23. Mean values of tumor growth curves are shown for mice treated with the bispecific control antibody, whereas individual tumor growth curves are shown for the MT110-treated animals. Error bars indicate standard deviation calculated for the mean value of tumor growth curves. Arrows indicate treatment timepoints. Asterisks label readings that were statistically significant ($P < 0.05$) from readings of the control group [139].

metastatic colorectal cells by autologous T-cells from patients previously treated with chemotherapy [141] and caused significant tumor growth retardation in animal models of CRC [142].

16.7.2.2 Other scFv–scFv Tandem Molecules

The recombinant supra-agonistic (scFv)$_2$ dimer (tetravalent flexibody; Figure 16.7), anti-MAPG/anti-CD28 rM28 [106], has also been tested in clinical trials in patients with malignant melanoma (Table 16.2). By targeting both CD28 and MAPG, recombinant bispecific single-chain antibody rM28 enhances cytotoxic T-cell recognition of melanoma cells, which may result in immune effector cell-mediated tumor cell death and a decrease in distant metastases. Due to formation of dimers, this agent appears to have a longer serum half-life in comparison with monomeric (scFv)$_2$ molecules, such as BiTEs. When activated, CD28 facilitates interactions between T-cells and other immune effector cells resulting in CTL responses; MAPG is a surface antigen expressed on the majority of melanomas, including primary cutaneous, ocular, and metastatic melanomas. As of September 2010, the trials had been completed; the results are not yet available (http://clinicaltrials.gov/show/NCT00204594).

As the aforementioned examples show, most of the BsAbs tested so far in the clinic have been molecules that bind a tumor marker and a receptor that recruits effector cells of the immune system (retargeting BsAbs). However, bispecific molecules directed against multiple tumor receptor targets are just starting to enter clinical trials and it will be exciting to monitor their progress. A BsAb of dual action, MM-111 from Merrimack Pharmaceuticals, specific for both HER2 and HER3, has entered clinical trials in HER2-positive cancers (Table 16.2) (http://www.merrimack

pharma.com/pipeline/MM-111%20Posters/ASCO_2010_MM-111_TrialsInProgress. pdf). MM-111 is a bispecific scFv–scFv tandem molecule ((scFv)$_2$) where a high-affinity scFv against HER2 ($K_D = 0.3$ nM) is linked to a low-affinity scFv against HER3 ($K_D = 16$ nM) via a modified HSA linker to enhance serum half-life of the construct (*http://www.merrimackpharma.com/pipeline/MM-111%20Posters/ IBC2008_MM-111_Poster_FINAL.pdf*). MM-111 targets the HER2/HER3 heterodimer and blocks ligand binding to HER3, thus inhibiting HER3 phosphorylation and signaling downstream from this receptor; this results in attenuation of tumor proliferation. Inhibition of tumor growth by MM-111 has been observed in several murine xenograft models of human breast, lung, gastric, and ovarian cancers that overexpress HER2. Combination of MM-111 with approved anti-HER2 mAb trastuzumab (Herceptin; Table 16.1) resulted in complete eradication of tumors in an animal model of human breast cancer [143]. MM-111 offers a novel approach for the treatment of HER2-positive breast cancers that are resistant to Herceptin or Tykerb® (lapatinib), and it is the first antibody binding two different receptors on the same cell to enter clinical development.

Another example of BsAb of enhanced selectivity is DT2219ARL immunotoxin which recently entered clinical development (Table 16.2). The single-chain molecule comprises two scFv modules recognizing human B-cell markers CD22 and CD19 linked to the C-terminus of the truncated form of diphtheria toxin, DT$_{390}$, with potential antineoplastic activity [144]. The V_L and V_H domains of anti-CD22 and anti-CD19 scFvs are linked together by an aggregation stabilizing linker (ARL) consisting of a 20-amino-acid segment of human muscle aldolase; the CDR3 region of the anti-CD22 V_H derived from murine hybridoma RFB4 was mutated to enhance its affinity. The anti-CD19 (derived from hybridoma HD37) and anti-CD22 portions of the immunotoxin specifically bind to CD19 and CD22 receptors on tumor B cells and induce their internalization. Upon internalization, DT$_{390}$ catalyzes ADP ribosylation of elongation factor-2, which results in the irreversible inhibition of protein synthesis and cell death. The molecule appeared to be very active in killing CD22$^+$CD19$^+$ lymphoma and leukemia cells, and was able to eradicate systemic cancer in highly aggressive human B-cell malignancy models in SCID mice (Figure 16.10). *In vitro* and *in vivo* studies demonstrated that the bispecific DT2219ARL had greater activity than its two monospecific counterparts targeting either CD22 or CD19, and that the presence of both ligands on the same molecule is responsible for the superior activity of the bispecific immunotoxin [144].

16.7.2.3 TandAbs
The first TandAb antibody that entered clinical trials in October 2010, AFM13, is a bispecific, CD30 × CD16a tetravalent molecule (Figure 16.7) specifically designed to treat Hodgkin's lymphoma (Table 16.2) (*http://affimed.com/press-releases/14/2010-11-15-Affimed-enrolls-first-patients-in-Phase-I-Hodgkin-s-Lymphoma-Study-*). The molecule comprises murine hybridoma-derived anti-CD30 V_H and V_L domains, and fully human anti-CD16 moiety, which specifically interacts only with activating FcγRIIIa isoform on NK cells and does not bind to glycosylphosphatidylinositol-anchored FcγRIIIb on granulocytes. Preclinical data

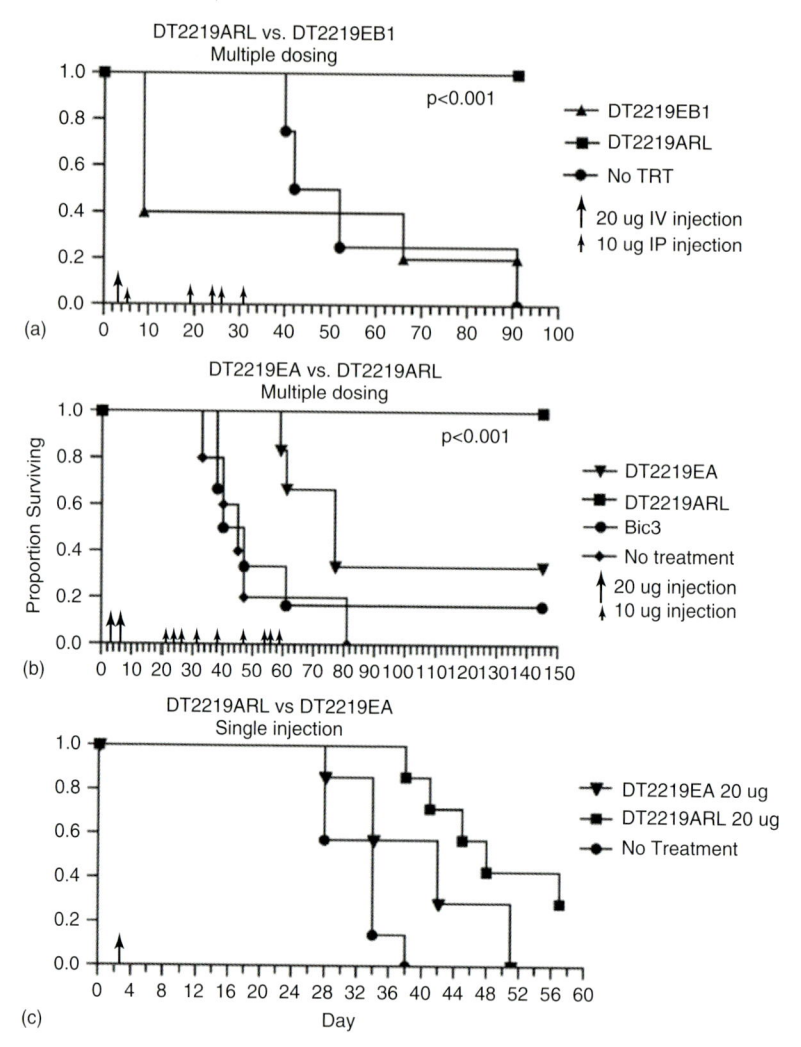

Figure 16.10 Antileukemia activity *in vivo* of anti-CD22/anti-CD19 bispecific immunotoxin DT2219ARL. Groups of SCID mice were given 10^6 Daudi cells (human Burkitt's lymphoma cell line) intravenously to induce systemic leukemia disease. (a) Three days following Daudi injection, mice were treated with multiple intraperitoneal injections of either DT2219ARL or DT2219EB1 immunotoxins in order to compare them to no treatment controls. Data were graphed as proportion surviving versus time. Statistical analysis was performed using the log-rank test and the DT2219ARL group significantly differed from the no treatment group ($P < 0.001$). (b) Three days following Daudi injection, mice were treated with either DT2219EA or DT2219ARL in comparison to no treatment controls and to Bic3 immunotoxin control treated mice. The DT2219ARL group significantly differed from the DT2219EA group, the Bic3 group, and the no treatment group ($P < 0.001$). (c) Three days following Daudi injection, mice were given a single intraperitoneal injection of DT2219EA and DT2219ARL in comparison to no treatment controls. Only the DT2219ARL group significantly differed from the no treatment group [144].

indicate a specific and very effective engagement of human NK cells by AFM13 for killing CD30$^+$ Reed-Sternberg cells causing Hodgkin's disease (*http://affimed.com/afm13*). The product has received Orphan Drug designation from both FDA and EMEA. The rational for development of AFM13 was based on positive results of two small-scale phase I/II studies (15 and 16 patients, respectively) performed by an academic group using quadroma-derived CD30 × CD16 BsAb [145–147]. One CR and one PR (lasting 6 and 3 months, respectively), three minor responses (lasting 1–15 months), two SDs (for 2 and 17 months, respectively), and one mixed response were achieved in first study [146, 147]. A second randomized pilot study in 16 patients with refractory HD resulted in one CR and three PRs lasting 5–9 months (three of four of these responses occurred after continuous BsAb infusion) and four cases of SD for 3 to more than 6 months [145]. In both studies, the BsAb treatment was well tolerated.

The second rationale for AMF13 came from the studies with CD30 × CD16 recombinant BsDbs (Figure 16.6) that demonstrated that BsDbs were more effective than quadroma-derived BsAb in mediating NK cell cytotoxicity against tumor cells [148]. Although the BsDbs were relatively rapidly cleared from the bloodstream through the kidneys, their antitumor activity in animal tumor models was similar to that of the quadroma-derived BsAb. The CD30 × CD16 BsDb could markedly reduce subcutaneous growth of Hodgkin's lymphoma [148]. The rapid clearance of the BsDb was probably compensated for by better tumor penetration and a more efficient induction of cell lysis.

The third rationale for AFM13 development derived from impressive experimental data demonstrating superiority of the tetravalent TandAb format over the bivalent BsAbs. In a preclinical study, treatment of SCID mice bearing an established Burkitt's lymphoma (5 mm in diameter) with human peripheral blood mononuclear cells (PBMCs), CD19 × CD3 TandAb, and anti-CD28 costimulation resulted in the complete elimination of tumors in all animals within 10 days (Figure 16.11) [103]. In contrast, mice receiving human PBMCs in combination with either bivalent CD19 × CD3 BsDb alone or with anti-CD28 mAb showed only partial tumor regression [103]. These findings suggest a future trend in the development of multivalent BsAbs.

16.7.2.4 BsAbs of Dual Action

The first bispecific molecule of dual action that recently entered clinical trials is an antibody–peptide conjugate CVX-241 (Table 16.2) (*http://clinicaltrials.gov/ct2/show/NCT01004822*). CVX-241 is a fusion protein containing angiopoietin-2 (Ang2) and VEGF-derived peptides covalently attached, via a proprietary diketone linker, to a humanized catalytic aldolase mAb. The Ang2/VEGF peptide moieties of the fusion protein CVX-241 block both Ang2 and VEGF receptors (Tie2 and VEGFR, respectively), thus inhibiting tumor angiogenesis and tumor cell proliferation. Both VEGF and Ang2 are upregulated in a variety of cancer cell types, and trigger different signaling pathways playing crucial roles in tumor angiogenesis.

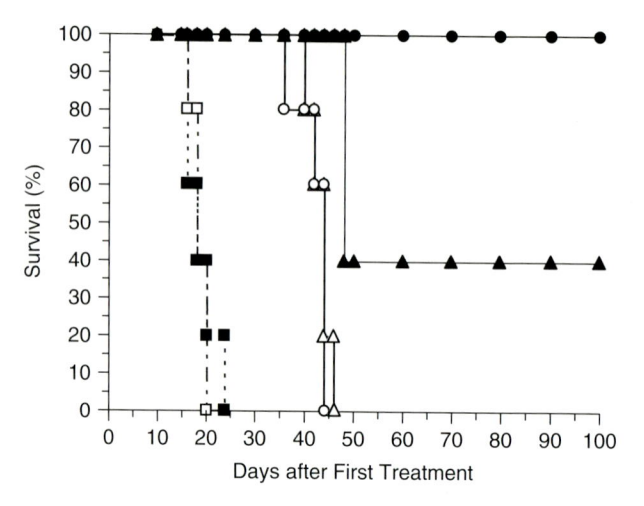

Figure 16.11 Survival of SCID mice bearing human Burkitt's lymphoma xenografts. The mice received either phosphate-buffered saline (□), preactivated human PBMCs alone (■), or preactivated human PBMCs followed 4–6 h later by the administration of CD3 × CD19 BsDb (△), TandAb (○), CD3 × CD19 BsDb plus anti-CD28 mAb 15E8 (▲), or TandAb in combination with mAb 15E8 (●) [103].

16.8
Conclusions and Future Prospects

A great deal of knowledge has come from the clinical successes and failures of the first generation of antibody therapeutics. The recent technological advances have allowed circumventing numerous developmental challenges and clinical problems, such as immunogenicity of mouse mAbs, lack of therapeutic efficacy, toxicity associated with cytokine storms, and unfavorable pharmacokinetics. Much has also been done in the field of BsAbs and new more potent molecules are on the way to meet patient needs. The formulation of an ideal bispecific construct depends on future results of comparative animal and clinical studies of various designs. The results of clinical trials with the antibody therapeutics of the next generation, including new recombinant BsAbs, should offer important data regarding side-effects and responses observed in treated patients. In addition, continued progress in cellular and molecular immunology should allow for the design of more rational treatment models, through the development of methods that use the activation of the effector cells responsible for the antitumor activity of BsAbs. Analysis of the immunosuppressed status and stage of disease in patients must also be taken into account before the application of BsAb therapeutics. Depending on the presence and activation status of the human effector cells in a tumor environment, combinations of BsAb attracting T-cells, NK cells, and/or myeloid cells to the same tumor site might be useful. The therapies using retargeting BsAbs appear to be more efficient in cases where tumor cells are easily accessible to the effector cells, such as in hematologic malignancies or MRD.

A lesson learned during recent years is that the new biological entities, particularly naked mAbs, are more effective when used in combination with other therapeutic agents, including perhaps other antibodies. Since not all patients are responsive, presumably due to the differences in the receptors being targeted, molecular testing will become a paradigm of biological therapy to choose drugs on an individual patient basis. However, these considerations can have stunning financial implications. If the average monthly price is US$3478 for Herceptin and US$7735 for Avastin (Genentech pricing of April 2009), combinations of these together with drugs in breast cancer treatment can exceed US$11000 monthly along with pharmacy and dispensing costs. Since these can be prescribed over several months, the costs can challenge the healthcare system and third-party payers. These financial hurdles can theoretically be circumvented by bispecific agents. However, although clinical data are starting to emerge, it is not yet clear whether BsAbs of dual action will have enhanced clinical benefits over combination therapy with multiple single-targeted agents or if dual targeting might be counterproductive (e.g., in activating a system by receptor cross-linking or modulating a separate pathway in an unexpected manner). These studies are highly anticipated, especially in light of recent results showing that coadministration of an anti-VEGF antibody bevacizumab and an anti-EGFR antibody cetuximab plus chemotherapy worsened clinical outcomes in mCRC patients [149, 150], despite promising results in preclinical models and early clinical studies. It is likely that varied results will be observed depending on the bispecific construct used and the particular combination of therapeutic targets; however, both successes and failures will add important insights for researchers in this emerging field.

References

1. Ross, J.S., Gray, K., Gray, G.S., Worland, P.J., and Rolfe, M. (2003) Anticancer antibodies. *Am. J. Clin. Pathol.*, **119**, 472–485.
2. Clynes, R.A., Towers, T.L., Presta, L.G., and Ravetch, J.V. (2000) Inhibitory Fc receptors modulate *in vivo* cytoxicity against tumor targets. *Nat. Med.*, **6**, 443–446.
3. Baeuerle, P.A., Kufer, P., and Lutterbüse, R. (2003) Bispecific antibodies for polyclonal T-cell engagement. *Curr. Opin. Mol. Ther.*, **5**, 413–419.
4. van Spriel, A.B., van Ojik, H.H., and van De Winkel, J.G. (2000) Immunotherapeutic perspective for bispecific antibodies. *Immunol. Today*, **21**, 391–397.
5. Chabner, B.A. and Roberts, T.G. Jr. (2005) Timeline: chemotherapy and the war on cancer. *Nat. Rev. Cancer*, **5**, 65–72.
6. Chabner, B.A. (2006) Clinical strategies for cancer treatment: the role of drugs, in *Cancer Chemotherapy and Biotherapy: Principles and Practice* (eds B.A. Chabner and D.L. Longo), Lippincott Williams & Wilkins, Baltimore, MD, pp. 1–14.
7. Bosslet, K., Straub, R., Blumrich, M., Czech, J., Gerken, M., Sperker, B., Kroemer, H.K., Gesson, J.P., Koch, M., and Monneret, C. (1998) Elucidation of the mechanism enabling tumor selective prodrug monotherapy. *Cancer Res.*, **58**, 1195–1201.
8. Köhler, G. and Milstein, C. (1975) Continuous cultures of fused cells secreting antibody of predefined specificity. *Nature*, **256**, 495–497.

9. Kipriyanov, S.M. and Le Gall, F. (2004) Generation and production of engineered antibodies. *Mol. Biotechnol.*, **26**, 39–60.
10. Holt, L.J., Herring, C., Jespers, L.S., Woolven, B.P., and Tomlinson, I.M. (2003) Domain antibodies: proteins for therapy. *Trends Biotechnol.*, **21**, 484–490.
11. Welschof, M., Terness, P., Kipriyanov, S.M., Stanescu, D., Breitling, F., Dörsam, H., Dübel, S., Little, M., and Opelz, G. (1997) The antigen-binding domain of a human IgG-anti-F(ab')$_2$ autoantibody. *Proc. Natl. Acad. Sci. USA*, **94**, 1902–1907.
12. Terness, P., Welschof, M., Moldenhauer, G., Jung, M., Moroder, L., Kirchhoff, F., Kipriyanov, S., Little, M., and Opelz, G. (1997) Idiotypic vaccine for treatment of human B-cell lymphoma. Construction of IgG variable regions from single malignant B cells. *Hum. Immunol.*, **56**, 17–27.
13. Green, L.L. (1999) Antibody engineering via genetic engineering of the mouse: XenoMouse strains are a vehicle for the facile generation of therapeutic human monoclonal antibodies. *J. Immunol. Methods*, **231**, 11–23.
14. Tomizuka, K., Shinohara, T., Yoshida, H., Uejima, H., Ohguma, A., Tanaka, S., Sato, K., Oshimura, M., and Ishida, I. (2000) Double trans-chromosomic mice: maintenance of two individual human chromosome fragments containing Ig heavy and kappa loci and expression of fully human antibodies. *Proc. Natl. Acad. Sci. USA*, **97**, 722–727.
15. Argyriou, A.A. and Kalofonos, H.P. (2009) Recent advances relating to the clinical application of naked monoclonal antibodies in solid tumors. *Mol. Med.*, **15**, 183–191.
16. Kindler, H.L., Niedzwiecki, D., Hollis, D., Sutherland, S., Schrag, D., Hurwitz, H., Innocenti, F., Mulcahy, M.F., O'Reilly, E., Wozniak, T.F. et al. (2010) Gemcitabine plus bevacizumab compared with gemcitabine plus placebo in patients with advanced pancreatic cancer: phase III trial of the Cancer and Leukemia Group B (CALGB 80303). *J. Clin. Oncol.*, **28**, 3617–3622.
17. Nalluri, S.R., Chu, D., Keresztes, R., Zhu, X., and Wu, S. (2008) Risk of venous thromboembolism with the angiogenesis inhibitor bevacizumab in cancer patients: a meta-analysis. *J. Am. Med. Assoc.*, **300**, 2277–2285.
18. Presta, L.G., Shields, R.L., Namenuk, A.K., Hong, K., and Meng, Y.G. (2002) Engineering therapeutic antibodies for improved function. *Biochem. Soc. Trans.*, **30**, 487–490.
19. Beck, A., Wurch, T., Bailly, C., and Corvaia, N. (2010) Strategies and challenges for the next generation of therapeutic antibodies. *Nat. Rev. Immunol.*, **10**, 345–352.
20. Cartron, G. (2009) FCGR3A polymorphism story: a new piece of the puzzle. *Leuk. Lymphoma*, **50**, 1401–1402.
21. Olivier, S., Jacoby, M., Brillon, C., Bouletreau, S., Mollet, T., Nerriere, O., Angel, A., Danet, S., Souttou, B., Guehenneux, F. et al. (2010) EB66 cell line, a duck embryonic stem cell-derived substrate for the industrial production of therapeutic monoclonal antibodies with enhanced ADCC activity. *mAbs*, **2**, 405–415.
22. Shinkawa, T., Nakamura, K., Yamane, N., Shoji-Hosaka, E., Kanda, Y., Sakurada, M., Uchida, K., Anazawa, H., Satoh, M., Yamasaki, M. et al. (2003) The absence of fucose but not the presence of galactose or bisecting N-acetylglucosamine of human IgG1 complex-type oligosaccharides shows the critical role of enhancing antibody-dependent cellular cytotoxicity. *J. Biol. Chem.*, **278**, 3466–3473.
23. Schuster, M., Umana, P., Ferrara, C., Brunker, P., Gerdes, C., Waxenecker, G., Wiederkum, S., Schwager, C., Loibner, H., Himmler, G. et al. (2005) Improved effector functions of a therapeutic monoclonal Lewis Y-specific antibody by glycoform engineering. *Cancer Res.*, **65**, 7934–7941.
24. Yamane-Ohnuki, N., Kinoshita, S., Inoue-Urakubo, M., Kusunoki, M., Iida, S., Nakano, R., Wakitani, M., Niwa, R., Sakurada, M., Uchida, K. et al. (2004) Establishment of FUT8

knockout Chinese hamster ovary cells: an ideal host cell line for producing completely defucosylated antibodies with enhanced antibody-dependent cellular cytotoxicity. *Biotechnol. Bioeng.*, **87**, 614–622.

25. Mössner, E., Brunker, P., Moser, S., Püntener, U., Schmidt, C., Herter, S., Grau, R., Gerdes, C., Nopora, A., van Puijenbroek, E. et al. (2010) Increasing the efficacy of CD20 antibody therapy through the engineering of a new type II anti-CD20 antibody with enhanced direct and immune effector cell-mediated B-cell cytotoxicity. *Blood*, **115**, 4393–4402.

26. Czuczman, M.S. and Gregory, S.A. (2010) The future of CD20 monoclonal antibody therapy in B-cell malignancies. *Leuk. Lymphoma*, **51**, 983–994.

27. Dalle, S., Reslan, L., Manquat, S.B., Herting, F., Klein, C., Umana, P., and Dumontet, C. (2008) Compared antitumor activity of GA101 and Rituximab against the human RL follicular lymphoma xenografts in SCID beige mice. *Blood*, **112**, 1585.

28. Salles, G.A., Morschhauser, F., Cartron, G., Lamy, T., Milpied, N.J., Thieblemont, C., Tilly, H., Birkett, J., and Burgess, M. (2008) A phase I/II study of RO5072759 (GA101) in patients with relapsed/refractory CD20$^+$ malignant disease. *Blood*, **112**, 234.

29. Salles, G., Morschhauser, F., Lamy, T., Milpied, N., Thieblemont, C., Tilly, H., Bieska, G., Carlile, D., and Cartron, G. (2009) Phase I study of RO5072759 (GA101) in patients with relapsed/refractory CD20$^+$ non-Hodgkin lymphoma (NHL). *Blood*, **114**, 1704.

30. Morschhauser, F., Cartron, G., Lamy, T., Milpied, N.-J., Thieblemont, C., Tilly, H., Weisser, M., Birkett, J., and Salles, G.A. (2009) Phase I study of RO5072759 (GA101) in relapsed/refractory chronic lymphocytic leukemia. *Blood*, **114**, 884.

31. Oflazoglu, E. and Audoly, L.P. (2010) Evolution of anti-CD20 monoclonal antibody therapeutics in oncology. *mAbs*, **2**, 14–19.

32. Stavenhagen, J.B., Gorlatov, S., Tuaillon, N., Rankin, C.T., Li, H., Burke, S., Huang, L., Vijh, S., Johnson, S., Bonvini, E. et al. (2007) Fc optimization of therapeutic antibodies enhances their ability to kill tumor cells *in vitro* and controls tumor expansion *in vivo* via low-affinity activating Fcgamma receptors. *Cancer Res.*, **67**, 8882–8890.

33. Lazar, G.A., Dang, W., Karki, S., Vafa, O., Peng, J.S., Hyun, L., Chan, C., Chung, H.S., Eivazi, A., Yoder, S.C. et al. (2006) Engineered antibody Fc variants with enhanced effector function. *Proc. Natl. Acad. Sci. USA*, **103**, 4005–4010.

34. Stavenhagen, J.B., Gorlatov, S., Tuaillon, N., Rankin, C.T., Li, H., Burke, S., Huang, L., Johnson, S., Koenig, S., and Bonvini, E. (2008) Enhancing the potency of therapeutic monoclonal antibodies via Fc optimization. *Adv. Enzyme Regul.*, **48**, 152–164.

35. Idusogie, E.E., Wong, P.Y., Presta, L.G., Gazzano-Santoro, H., Totpal, K., Ultsch, M., and Mulkerrin, M.G. (2001) Engineered antibodies with increased activity to recruit complement. *J. Immunol.*, **166**, 2571–2575.

36. Natsume, A., In, M., Takamura, H., Nakagawa, T., Shimizu, Y., Kitajima, K., Wakitani, M., Ohta, S., Satoh, M., Shitara, K. et al. (2008) Engineered antibodies of IgG1/IgG3 mixed isotype with enhanced cytotoxic activities. *Cancer Res.*, **68**, 3863–3872.

37. Vaccaro, C., Zhou, J., Ober, R.J., and Ward, E.S. (2005) Engineering the Fc region of immunoglobulin G to modulate *in vivo* antibody levels. *Nat. Biotechnol.*, **23**, 1283–1288.

38. Zalevsky, J., Chamberlain, A.K., Horton, H.M., Karki, S., Leung, I.W., Sproule, T.J., Lazar, G.A., Roopenian, D.C., and Desjarlais, J.R. (2010) Enhanced antibody half-life improves *in vivo* activity. *Nat. Biotechnol.*, **28**, 157–159.

39. Doronina, S.O., Toki, B.E., Torgov, M.Y., Mendelsohn, B.A., Cerveny, C.G., Chace, D.F., DeBlanc, R.L., Gearing, R.P., Bovee, T.D., Siegall, C.B. et al.

(2003) Development of potent monoclonal antibody auristatin conjugates for cancer therapy. *Nat. Biotechnol.*, **21**, 778–784.

40. McDonagh, C.F., Turcott, E., Westendorf, L., Webster, J.B., Alley, S.C., Kim, K., Andreyka, J., Stone, I., Hamblett, K.J., Francisco, J.A. et al. (2006) Engineered antibody–drug conjugates with defined sites and stoichiometries of drug attachment. *Protein Eng. Des. Sel.*, **19**, 299–307.

41. Alley, S.C., Okeley, N.M., and Senter, P.D. (2010) Antibody–drug conjugates: targeted drug delivery for cancer. *Curr. Opin. Chem. Biol.*, **14**, 529–537.

42. Junutula, J.R., Raab, H., Clark, S., Bhakta, S., Leipold, D.D., Weir, S., Chen, Y., Simpson, M., Tsai, S.P., Dennis, M.S. et al. (2008) Site-specific conjugation of a cytotoxic drug to an antibody improves the therapeutic index. *Nat. Biotechnol.*, **26**, 925–932.

43. Junutula, J.R., Flagella, K.M., Graham, R.A., Parsons, K.L., Ha, E., Raab, H., Bhakta, S., Nguyen, T., Dugger, D.L., Li, G. et al. (2010) Engineered thio-trastuzumab–DM1 conjugate with an improved therapeutic index to target HER2-positive breast cancer. *Clin. Cancer Res.*, **16**, 4769–4778.

44. Labrijn, A.F., Buijsse, A.O., van den Bremer, E.T., Verwilligen, A.Y., Bleeker, W.K., Thorpe, S.J., Killestein, J., Polman, C.H., Aalberse, R.C., Schuurman, J. et al. (2009) Therapeutic IgG4 antibodies engage in Fab-arm exchange with endogenous human IgG4 in vivo. *Nat. Biotechnol.*, **27**, 767–771.

45. van der Neut Kolfschoten, M., Schuurman, J., Losen, M., Bleeker, W.K., Martinez-Martinez, P., Vermeulen, E., den Bleker, T.H., Wiegman, L., Vink, T., Aarden, L.A. et al. (2007) Anti-inflammatory activity of human IgG4 antibodies by dynamic Fab arm exchange. *Science*, **317**, 1554–1557.

46. Peipp, M. and Valerius, T. (2002) Bispecific antibodies targeting cancer cells. *Biochem. Soc. Trans.*, **30**, 507–511.

47. Cooper, M.A., Fehniger, T.A., and Caligiuri, M.A. (2001) The biology of human natural killer-cell subsets. *Trends Immunol.*, **22**, 633–640.

48. Clayberger, C. and Krensky, A.M. (2003) Granulysin. *Curr. Opin. Immunol.*, **15**, 560–565.

49. Trambas, C.M. and Griffiths, G.M. (2003) Delivering the kiss of death. *Nat. Immunol.*, **4**, 399–403.

50. van Ojik, H.H. and Valerius, T. (2001) Preclinical and clinical data with bispecific antibodies recruiting myeloid effector cells for tumor therapy. *Crit. Rev. Oncol. Hematol.*, **38**, 47–61.

51. Di Carlo, E., Forni, G., Lollini, P., Colombo, M.P., Modesti, A., and Musiani, P. (2001) The intriguing role of polymorphonuclear neutrophils in antitumor reactions. *Blood*, **97**, 339–345.

52. McQueen, K.L. and Parham, P. (2002) Variable receptors controlling activation and inhibition of NK cells. *Curr. Opin. Immunol.*, **14**, 615–621.

53. Raulet, D.H. (2003) Roles of the NKG2D immunoreceptor and its ligands. *Nat. Rev. Immunol.*, **3**, 781–790.

54. Dreier, T., Lorenczewski, G., Brandl, C., Hoffmann, P., Syring, U., Hanakam, F., Kufer, P., Riethmüller, G., Bargou, R., and Baeuerle, P.A. (2002) Extremely potent, rapid and costimulation-independent cytotoxic T-cell response against lymphoma cells catalyzed by a single-chain bispecific antibody. *Int. J. Cancer*, **100**, 690–697.

55. Sahin, U., Kraft Bauer, S., Ohnesorge, S., Pfreundschuh, M., and Renner, C. (1996) Interleukin-12 increases bispecific-antibody-mediated natural killer cell cytotoxicity against human tumors. *Cancer Immunol. Immunother.*, **42**, 9–14.

56. Albertsson, P.A., Basse, P.H., Hokland, M., Goldfarb, R.H., Nagelkerke, J.F., Nannmark, U., and Kuppen, P.J. (2003) NK cells and the tumour microenvironment: implications for NK-cell function and anti-tumour activity. *Trends Immunol.*, **24**, 603–609.

57. Lu, D., Zhang, H., Ludwig, D., Persaud, A., Jimenez, X., Burtrum, D., Balderes, P., Liu, M., Bohlen, P., Witte, L. et al. (2004) Simultaneous blockade of both the epidermal growth

factor receptor and the insulin-like growth factor receptor signaling pathways in cancer cells with a fully human recombinant bispecific antibody. *J. Biol. Chem.*, **279**, 2856–2865.

58. Bostrom, J., Yu, S.F., Kan, D., Appleton, B.A., Lee, C.V., Billeci, K., Man, W., Peale, F., Ross, S., Wiesmann, C. *et al.* (2009) Variants of the antibody herceptin that interact with HER2 and VEGF at the antigen binding site. *Science*, **323**, 1610–1614.

59. Stevenson, G.T. (2006) CD38 as a therapeutic target. *Mol. Med.*, **12**, 345–346.

60. Robinson, M.K., Hodge, K.M., Horak, E., Sundberg, A.L., Russeva, M., Shaller, C.C., von Mehren, M., Shchaveleva, I., Simmons, H.H., Marks, J.D. *et al.* (2008) Targeting ErbB2 and ErbB3 with a bispecific single-chain Fv enhances targeting selectivity and induces a therapeutic effect *in vitro*. *Br. J. Cancer*, **99**, 1415–1425.

61. Ahmadi, T., Maniar, T., Schuster, S., and Stadtmauer, E. (2009) Chronic lymphocytic leukemia: new concepts and emerging therapies. *Curr. Treat. Options Oncol.*, **10**, 16–32.

62. Nisonoff, A. and Rivers, M.M. (1961) Recombination of a mixture of univalent antibody fragments of different specificity. *Arch. Biochem. Biophys.*, **93**, 460–462.

63. Anderson, P.M., Crist, W., Hasz, D., Carroll, A.J., Myers, D.E., and Uckun, F.M. (1992) G19.4(αCD3) × B43(αCD19) monoclonal antibody heteroconjugate triggers CD19 antigen-specific lysis of t(4;11) acute lymphoblastic leukemia cells by activated CD3 antigen-positive cytotoxic T cells. *Blood*, **80**, 2826–2834.

64. Brennan, M., Davison, P.F., and Paulus, H. (1985) Preparation of bispecific antibodies by chemical recombination of monoclonal immunoglobulin G1 fragments. *Science*, **229**, 81–83.

65. Glennie, M.J., McBride, H.M., Worth, A.T., and Stevenson, G.T. (1987) Preparation and performance of bispecific F(ab'γ)$_2$ antibody containing thioether-linked Fab'γ fragments. *J. Immunol.*, **139**, 2367–2375.

66. Milstein, C. and Cuello, A.C. (1983) Hybrid hybridomas and their use in immunohistochemistry. *Nature*, **305**, 537–540.

67. Mocikat, R., Selmayr, M., Thierfelder, S., and Lindhofer, H. (1997) Trioma-based vaccination against B-cell lymphoma confers long-lasting tumor immunity. *Cancer Res.*, **57**, 2346–2349.

68. Lindhofer, H., Mocikat, R., Steipe, B., and Thierfelder, S. (1995) Preferential species-restricted heavy/light chain pairing in rat/mouse quadromas. Implications for a single-step purification of bispecific antibodies. *J. Immunol.*, **155**, 219–225.

69. Marme, A., Strauss, G., Bastert, G., Grischke, E.M., and Moldenhauer, G. (2002) Intraperitoneal bispecific antibody (HEA125 × OKT3) therapy inhibits malignant ascites production in advanced ovarian carcinoma. *Int. J. Cancer*, **101**, 183–189.

70. Kipriyanov, S.M. and Le Gall, F. (2004) Recent advances in the generation of bispecific antibodies for tumor immunotherapy. *Curr. Opin. Drug Discov. Dev.*, **7**, 233–242.

71. Carter, P.J. (2006) Potent antibody therapeutics by design. *Nat. Rev. Immunol.*, **6**, 343–357.

72. Kipriyanov, S.M. (2003) Generation of antibody molecules through antibody engineering. *Methods Mol. Biol.*, **207**, 3–25.

73. Kostelny, S.A., Cole, M.S., and Tso, J.Y. (1992) Formation of a bispecific antibody by the use of leucine zippers. *J. Immunol.*, **148**, 1547–1553.

74. Chaudri, Z.N., Bartlet-Jones, M., Panayotou, G., Klonisch, T., Roitt, I.M., Lund, T., and Delves, P.J. (1999) Dual specificity antibodies using a double-stranded oligonucleotide bridge. *FEBS Lett.*, **450**, 23–26.

75. de Kruif, J. and Logtenberg, T. (1996) Leucine zipper dimerized bivalent and bispecific scFv antibodies from a semi-synthetic antibody phage display library. *J. Biol. Chem.*, **271**, 7630–7634.

76. Müller, K.M., Arndt, K.M., Strittmatter, W., and Plückthun, A. (1998) The first

constant domain (C_H1 and C_L) of an antibody used as heterodimerization domain for bispecific miniantibodies. *FEBS Lett.*, **422**, 259–264.
77. Zuo, Z., Jimenez, X., Witte, L., and Zhu, Z. (2000) An efficient route to the production of an IgG-like bispecific antibody. *Protein Eng.*, **13**, 361–367.
78. Schmiedl, A., Breitling, F., and Dübel, S. (2000) Expression of a bispecific dsFv–dsFv' antibody fragment in *Escherichia coli*. *Protein Eng.*, **13**, 725–734.
79. Schoonjans, R., Willems, A., Schoonooghe, S., Fiers, W., Grooten, J., and Mertens, N. (2000) Fab chains as an efficient heterodimerization scaffold for the production of recombinant bispecific and trispecific antibody derivatives. *J. Immunol.*, **165**, 7050–7057.
80. Lu, D., Jimenez, X., Zhang, H., Bohlen, P., Witte, L., and Zhu, Z. (2002) Fab–scFv fusion protein: an efficient approach to production of bispecific antibody fragments. *J. Immunol. Methods*, **267**, 213–226.
81. Holliger, P., Prospero, T., and Winter, G. (1993) "Diabodies": small bivalent and bispecific antibody fragments. *Proc. Natl. Acad. Sci. USA*, **90**, 6444–6448.
82. Kipriyanov, S.M., Moldenhauer, G., Strauss, G., and Little, M. (1998) Bispecific CD3 × CD19 diabody for T cell-mediated lysis of malignant human B cells. *Int. J. Cancer*, **77**, 763–772.
83. Perisic, O., Webb, P.A., Holliger, P., Winter, G., and Williams, R.L. (1994) Crystal structure of a diabody, a bivalent antibody fragment. *Structure*, **2**, 1217–1226.
84. Carmichael, J.A., Power, B.E., Garrett, T.P., Yazaki, P.J., Shively, J.E., Raubischek, A.A., Wu, A.M., and Hudson, P.J. (2003) The crystal structure of an anti-CEA scFv diabody assembled from T84.66 scFvs in V_L-to-V_H orientation: implications for diabody flexibility. *J. Mol. Biol.*, **326**, 341–351.
85. Zhu, Z., Zapata, G., Shalaby, R., Snedecor, B., Chen, H., and Carter, P. (1996) High level secretion of a humanized bispecific diabody from *Escherichia coli*. *Biotechnology*, **14**, 192–196.
86. Cochlovius, B., Kipriyanov, S.M., Stassar, M.J., Christ, O., Schuhmacher, J., Strauss, G., Moldenhauer, G., and Little, M. (2000) Treatment of human B cell lymphoma xenografts with a CD3 × CD19 diabody and T cells. *J. Immunol.*, **165**, 888–895.
87. Kipriyanov, S.M., Moldenhauer, G., Braunagel, M., Reusch, U., Cochlovius, B., Le Gall, F., Kouprianova, O.A., Von der Lieth, C.W., and Little, M. (2003) Effect of domain order on the activity of bacterially produced bispecific single-chain Fv antibodies. *J. Mol. Biol.*, **330**, 99–111.
88. FitzGerald, K., Holliger, P., and Winter, G. (1997) Improved tumour targeting by disulphide stabilized diabodies expressed in *Pichia pastoris*. *Protein Eng.*, **10**, 1221–1225.
89. Zhu, Z., Presta, L.G., Zapata, G., and Carter, P. (1997) Remodeling domain interfaces to enhance heterodimer formation. *Protein Sci.*, **6**, 781–788.
90. Olafsen, T., Cheung, C.W., Yazaki, P.J., Li, L., Sundaresan, G., Gambhir, S.S., Sherman, M.A., Williams, L.E., Shively, J.E., Raubitschek, A.A. et al. (2004) Covalent disulfide-linked anti-CEA diabody allows site-specific conjugation and radiolabeling for tumor targeting applications. *Protein Eng. Des. Sel.*, **17**, 21–27.
91. Johnson, S., Burke, S., Huang, L., Gorlatov, S., Li, H., Wang, W., Zhang, W., Tuaillon, N., Rainey, J., Barat, B. et al. (2010) Effector cell recruitment with novel Fv-based dual-affinity re-targeting protein leads to potent tumor cytolysis and *in vivo* B-cell depletion. *J. Mol. Biol.*, **399**, 436–449.
92. Veri, M.C., Burke, S., Huang, L., Li, H., Gorlatov, S., Tuaillon, N., Rainey, G.J., Ciccarone, V., Zhang, T., Shah, K. et al. (2010) Therapeutic control of B cell activation via recruitment of Fcγ receptor IIb (CD32B) inhibitory function with a novel bispecific antibody scaffold. *Arthritis Rheum.*, **62**, 1933–1943.
93. Coloma, M.J. and Morrison, S.L. (1997) Design and production of novel

tetravalent bispecific antibodies. *Nat. Biotechnol.*, **15**, 159–163.
94. Els Conrath, K., Lauwereys, M., Wyns, L., and Muyldermans, S. (2001) Camel single-domain antibodies as modular building units in bispecific and bivalent antibody constructs. *J. Biol. Chem.*, **276**, 7346–7350.
95. Löffler, A., Kufer, P., Lutterbuse, R., Zettl, F., Daniel, P.T., Schwenkenbecher, J.M., Riethmuller, G., Dörken, B., and Bargou, R.C. (2000) A recombinant bispecific single-chain antibody, CD19 × CD3, induces rapid and high lymphoma-directed cytotoxicity by unstimulated T lymphocytes. *Blood*, **95**, 2098–2103.
96. Kipriyanov, S.M., Moldenhauer, G., Schuhmacher, J., Cochlovius, B., Von der Lieth, C.W., Matys, E.R., and Little, M. (1999) Bispecific tandem diabody for tumor therapy with improved antigen binding and pharmacokinetics. *J. Mol. Biol.*, **293**, 41–56.
97. Kontermann, R.E. and Muller, R. (1999) Intracellular and cell surface displayed single-chain diabodies. *J. Immunol. Methods*, **226**, 179–188.
98. Mack, M., Riethmuller, G., and Kufer, P. (1995) A small bispecific antibody construct expressed as a functional single-chain molecule with high tumor cell cytotoxicity. *Proc. Natl. Acad. Sci. USA*, **92**, 7021–7025.
99. Völkel, T., Korn, T., Bach, M., Müller, R., and Kontermann, R.E. (2001) Optimized linker sequences for the expression of monomeric and dimeric bispecific single-chain diabodies. *Protein Eng.*, **14**, 815–823.
100. Müller, D., Karle, A., Meissburger, B., Höfig, I., Stork, R., and Kontermann, R.E. (2007) Improved pharmacokinetics of recombinant bispecific antibody molecules by fusion to human serum albumin. *J. Biol. Chem.*, **282**, 12650–12660.
101. Müller, K.M., Arndt, K.M., and Plückthun, A. (1998) A dimeric bispecific miniantibody combines two specificities with avidity. *FEBS Lett.*, **432**, 45–49.
102. Alt, M., Müller, R., and Kontermann, R.E. (1999) Novel tetravalent and bispecific IgG-like antibody molecules combining single-chain diabodies with the immunoglobulin $\gamma 1$ Fc or $C_H 3$ region. *FEBS Lett.*, **454**, 90–94.
103. Cochlovius, B., Kipriyanov, S.M., Stassar, M.J., Schuhmacher, J., Benner, A., Moldenhauer, G., and Little, M. (2000) Cure of Burkitt's lymphoma in severe combined immunodeficiency mice by T cells, tetravalent CD3 × CD19 tandem diabody, and CD28 costimulation. *Cancer Res.*, **60**, 4336–4341.
104. Reusch, U., Le Gall, F., Hensel, M., Moldenhauer, G., Ho, A.D., Little, M., and Kipriyanov, S.M. (2004) Effect of tetravalent bispecific CD19 × CD3 recombinant antibody construct and CD28 costimulation on lysis of malignant B cells from patients with chronic lymphocytic leukemia by autologous T cells. *Int. J. Cancer*, **112**, 509–518.
105. Le Gall, F., Kipriyanov, S., Reusch, U., Moldenhauer, G., and Little, M. (2006) Multimeric single chain tandem Fv-antibodies. European Patent EP1293514 (B1).
106. Grosse-Hovest, L., Hartlapp, I., Marwan, W., Brem, G., Rammensee, H.G., and Jung, G. (2003) A recombinant bispecific single-chain antibody induces targeted, supra-agonistic CD28-stimulation and tumor cell killing. *Eur. J. Immunol.*, **33**, 1334–1340.
107. Otz, T., Grosse-Hovest, L., Hofmann, M., Rammensee, H.G., and Jung, G. (2009) A bispecific single-chain antibody that mediates target cell-restricted, supra-agonistic CD28 stimulation and killing of lymphoma cells. *Leukemia*, **23**, 71–77.
108. Kellner, C., Bruenke, J., Stieglmaier, J., Schwemmlein, M., Schwenkert, M., Singer, H., Mentz, K., Peipp, M., Lang, P., Oduncu, F. et al. (2008) A novel CD19-directed recombinant bispecific antibody derivative with enhanced immune effector functions for human leukemic cells. *J. Immunother.*, **31**, 871–884.

109. Singer, H., Kellner, C., Lanig, H., Aigner, M., Stockmeyer, B., Oduncu, F., Schwemmlein, M., Stein, C., Mentz, K., Mackensen, A. et al. (2010) Effective elimination of acute myeloid leukemic cells by recombinant bispecific antibody derivatives directed against CD33 and CD16. *J. Immunother.*, **33**, 599–608.
110. Kügler, M., Stein, C., Kellner, C., Mentz, K., Saul, D., Schwenkert, M., Schubert, I., Singer, H., Oduncu, F., Stockmeyer, B. et al. (2010) A recombinant trispecific single-chain Fv derivative directed against CD123 and CD33 mediates effective elimination of acute myeloid leukaemia cells by dual targeting. *Br. J. Haematol.*, **150**, 574–586.
111. Roopenian, D.C. and Akilesh, S. (2007) FcRn: the neonatal Fc receptor comes of age. *Nat. Rev. Immunol.*, **7**, 715–725.
112. Merchant, A.M., Zhu, Z., Yuan, J.Q., Goddard, A., Adams, C.W., Presta, L.G., and Carter, P. (1998) An efficient route to human bispecific IgG. *Nat. Biotechnol.*, **16**, 677–681.
113. Xie, Z., Guo, N., Yu, M., Hu, M., and Shen, B. (2005) A new format of bispecific antibody: highly efficient heterodimerization, expression and tumor cell lysis. *J. Immunol. Methods*, **296**, 95–101.
114. Jendreyko, N., Popkov, M., Beerli, R.R., Chung, J., McGavern, D.B., Rader, C., and Barbas, C.F. III (2003) Intradiabodies, bispecific, tetravalent antibodies for the simultaneous functional knockout of two cell surface receptors. *J. Biol. Chem.*, **278**, 47812–47819.
115. Michaelson, J.S., Demarest, S.J., Miller, B., Amatucci, A., Snyder, W.B., Wu, X., Huang, F., Phan, S., Gao, S., Doern, A. et al. (2009) Anti-tumor activity of stability-engineered IgG-like bispecific antibodies targeting TRAIL-R2 and LTβR. *mAbs*, **1**, 128–141.
116. Orcutt, K.D., Ackerman, M.E., Cieslewicz, M., Quiroz, E., Slusarczyk, A.L., Frangioni, J.V., and Wittrup, K.D. (2010) A modular IgG-scFv bispecific antibody topology. *Protein Eng. Des. Sel.*, **23**, 221–228.
117. Lu, D., Zhang, H., Ludwig, D., Persaud, A., Jimenez, X., Burtrum, D., Balderes, P., Liu, M., Bohlen, P., Witte, L. et al. (2004) Simultaneous blockade of both the epidermal growth factor receptor and the insulin-like growth factor receptor signaling pathways in cancer cells with a fully human recombinant bispecific antibody. *J. Biol. Chem.*, **279**, 2856–2865.
118. Wu, C., Ying, H., Grinnell, C., Bryant, S., Miller, R., Clabbers, A., Bose, S., McCarthy, D., Zhu, R.R., Santora, L. et al. (2007) Simultaneous targeting of multiple disease mediators by a dual-variable-domain immunoglobulin. *Nat. Biotechnol.*, **25**, 1290–1297.
119. Wu, C., Ying, H., Bose, S., Miller, R., Medina, L., Santora, L., and Ghayur, T. (2009) Molecular construction and optimization of anti-human IL-1alpha/beta dual variable domain immunoglobulin (DVD-Ig) molecules. *mAbs*, **1**, 339–347.
120. Lu, D., Zhang, H., Koo, H., Tonra, J., Balderes, P., Prewett, M., Corcoran, E., Mangalampalli, V., Bassi, R., Anselma, D. et al. (2005) A fully human recombinant IgG-like bispecific antibody to both the epidermal growth factor receptor and the insulin-like growth factor receptor for enhanced antitumor activity. *J. Biol. Chem.*, **280**, 19665–19672.
121. Park, S.S., Ryu, C.J., Kang, Y.J., Kashmiri, S.V., and Hong, H.J. (2000) Generation and characterization of a novel tetravalent bispecific antibody that binds to hepatitis B virus surface antigens. *Mol. Immunol.*, **37**, 1123–1130.
122. Marvin, J.S. and Zhu, Z. (2005) Recombinant approaches to IgG-like bispecific antibodies. *Acta Pharmacol. Sin.*, **26**, 649–658.
123. Asano, R., Kawaguchi, H., Watanabe, Y., Nakanishi, T., Umetsu, M., Hayashi, H., Katayose, Y., Unno, M., Kudo, T., and Kumagai, I. (2008) Diabody-based recombinant formats of humanized IgG-like bispecific antibody with effective retargeting of lymphocytes to tumor cells. *J. Immunother.*, **31**, 752–761.

124. Dimasi, N., Gao, C., Fleming, R., Woods, R.M., Yao, X.T., Shirinian, L., Kiener, P.A., and Wu, H. (2009) The design and characterization of oligospecific antibodies for simultaneous targeting of multiple disease mediators. *J. Mol. Biol.*, **393**, 672–692.
125. Shen, J., Vil, M.D., Jimenez, X., Iacolina, M., Zhang, H., and Zhu, Z. (2006) Single variable domain–IgG fusion. A novel recombinant approach to Fc domain-containing bispecific antibodies. *J. Biol. Chem.*, **281**, 10706–10714.
126. Shen, J., Vil, M.D., Jimenez, X., Zhang, H., Iacolina, M., Mangalampalli, V., Balderes, P., Ludwig, D.L., and Zhu, Z. (2007) Single variable domain antibody as a versatile building block for the construction of IgG-like bispecific antibodies. *J. Immunol. Methods*, **318**, 65–74.
127. Cao, Y. and Lam, L. (2003) Bispecific antibody conjugates in therapeutics. *Adv. Drug Deliv. Rev.*, **55**, 171–197.
128. Fischer, N. and Leger, O. (2007) Bispecific antibodies: molecules that enable novel therapeutic strategies. *Pathobiology*, **74**, 3–14.
129. Repp, R., van Ojik, H.H., Valerius, T., Groenewegen, G., Wieland, G., Oetzel, C., Stockmeyer, B., Becker, W., Eisenhut, M., Steininger, H. et al. (2003) Phase I clinical trial of the bispecific antibody MDX-H210 (anti-FcgammaRI × anti-HER-2/neu) in combination with filgrastim (G-CSF) for treatment of advanced breast cancer. *Br. J. Cancer*, **89**, 2234–2243.
130. Fury, M.G., Lipton, A., Smith, K.M., Winston, C.B., and Pfister, D.G. (2008) A phase-I trial of the epidermal growth factor receptor directed bispecific antibody MDX-447 without and with recombinant human granulocyte-colony stimulating factor in patients with advanced solid tumors. *Cancer Immunol. Immunother.*, **57**, 155–163.
131. Bokemeyer, C. (2010) Catumaxomab – trifunctional anti-EpCAM antibody used to treat malignant ascites. *Expert Opin. Biol. Ther.*, **10**, 1259–1269.
132. Kiewe, P. and Thiel, E. (2008) Ertumaxomab: a trifunctional antibody for breast cancer treatment. *Expert Opin. Investig. Drugs*, **17**, 1553–1558.
133. Wolf, E., Hofmeister, R., Kufer, P., Schlereth, B., and Baeuerle, P.A. (2005) BiTEs: bispecific antibody constructs with unique anti-tumor activity. *Drug Discov. Today*, **10**, 1237–1244.
134. Baeuerle, P.A. and Reinhardt, C. (2009) Bispecific T-cell engaging antibodies for cancer therapy. *Cancer Res.*, **69**, 4941–4944.
135. Dreier, T., Baeuerle, P.A., Fichtner, I., Grun, M., Schlereth, B., Lorenczewski, G., Kufer, P., Lutterbuse, R., Riethmuller, G., Gjorstrup, P. et al. (2003) T cell costimulus-independent and very efficacious inhibition of tumor growth in mice bearing subcutaneous or leukemic human B cell lymphoma xenografts by a CD19-/CD3-bispecific single-chain antibody construct. *J. Immunol.*, **170**, 4397–4402.
136. Nagorsen, D., Bargou, R., Ruttinger, D., Kufer, P., Baeuerle, P.A., and Zugmaier, G. (2009) Immunotherapy of lymphoma and leukemia with T-cell engaging BiTE antibody blinatumomab. *Leuk. Lymphoma*, **50**, 886–891.
137. Bargou, R., Leo, E., Zugmaier, G., Klinger, M., Goebeler, M., Knop, S., Noppeney, R., Viardot, A., Hess, G., Schuler, M. et al. (2008) Tumor regression in cancer patients by very low doses of a T cell-engaging antibody. *Science*, **321**, 974–977.
138. Topp, M.S., Zugmaier, G., Goekbuget, N., Kufer, P., Goebeler, M., Klinger, M., Degenhard, E., Baeuerle, P.A., Schmidt, M., Nagorsen, D. et al. (2009) Report of a phase II trial of single-agent BiTE™ antibody blinatumomab in patients with minimal residual disease (MRD) positive B-precursor acute lymphoblastic leukemia (ALL). *Blood*, **114**, 840.
139. Brischwein, K., Schlereth, B., Guller, B., Steiger, C., Wolf, A., Lutterbuese, R., Offner, S., Locher, M., Urbig, T., Raum, T. et al. (2006) MT110: a novel bispecific single-chain antibody construct with high efficacy in eradicating established tumors. *Mol. Immunol.*, **43**, 1129–1143.

140. Friedrich, M., Drache, D., Amann, M., Filusch, S., Voelkel, M., Thomas, O., Baeuerle, P.A., Rattel, B. (2010) Eradication of established pancreatic tumors in mice by engagement of extra-tumoral human T cells with BiTE antibody MT110, AACR 101st Annual Meeting, Washington, DC, poster.

141. Osada, T., Hsu, D., Hammond, S., Hobeika, A., Devi, G., Clay, T.M., Lyerly, H.K., and Morse, M.A. (2010) Metastatic colorectal cancer cells from patients previously treated with chemotherapy are sensitive to T-cell killing mediated by CEA/CD3-bispecific T-cell-engaging BiTE antibody. *Br. J. Cancer*, **102**, 124–133.

142. Lutterbuese, R., Raum, T., Kischel, R., Lutterbuese, P., Schlereth, B., Schaller, E., Mangold, S., Rau, D., Meier, P., Kiener, P.A. *et al.* (2009) Potent control of tumor growth by CEA/CD3-bispecific single-chain antibody constructs that are not competitively inhibited by soluble CEA. *J. Immunother.*, **32**, 341–352.

143. Huhalov, A., Adams, S., Paragas, V., Oyama, S., Overland, R., Luus, L., Gibbons, F., Zhang, B., Nguyen, S., Nielsen, U.B. *et al.* (2010) MM-111, an ErbB2/ErbB3 bispecific antibody with potent activity in ErbB2-overexpressing cells, positively combines with trastuzumab to inhibit growth of breast cancer cells driven by the ErbB2/ErbB3 oncogenic unit, AACR 101st Annual Meeting, Washington, DC, poster.

144. Vallera, D.A., Chen, H., Sicheneder, A.R., Panoskaltsis-Mortari, A., and Taras, E.P. (2009) Genetic alteration of a bispecific ligand-directed toxin targeting human CD19 and CD22 receptors resulting in improved efficacy against systemic B cell malignancy. *Leuk. Res.*, **33**, 1233–1242.

145. Hartmann, F., Renner, C., Jung, W., da Costa, L., Tembrink, S., Held, G., Sek, A., Konig, J., Bauer, S., Kloft, M. *et al.* (2001) Anti-CD16/CD30 bispecific antibody treatment for Hodgkin's disease: role of infusion schedule and costimulation with cytokines. *Clin. Cancer Res.*, **7**, 1873–1881.

146. Hartmann, F., Renner, C., Jung, W., Deisting, C., Juwana, M., Eichentopf, B., Kloft, M., and Pfreundschuh, M. (1997) Treatment of refractory Hodgkin's disease with an anti-CD16/CD30 bispecific antibody. *Blood*, **89**, 2042–2047.

147. Hartmann, F., Renner, C., Jung, W., and Pfreundschuh, M. (1998) Anti-CD16/CD30 bispecific antibodies as possible treatment for refractory Hodgkin's disease. *Leuk. Lymphoma*, **31**, 385–392.

148. Arndt, M.A., Krauss, J., Kipriyanov, S.M., Pfreundschuh, M., and Little, M. (1999) A bispecific diabody that mediates natural killer cell cytotoxicity against xenotransplantated human Hodgkin's tumors. *Blood*, **94**, 2562–2568.

149. Hecht, J.R., Mitchell, E., Chidiac, T., Scroggin, C., Hagenstad, C., Spigel, D., Marshall, J., Cohn, A., McCollum, D., Stella, P. *et al.* (2009) A randomized phase IIIB trial of chemotherapy, bevacizumab, and panitumumab compared with chemotherapy and bevacizumab alone for metastatic colorectal cancer. *J. Clin. Oncol.*, **27**, 672–680.

150. Tol, J., Koopman, M., Cats, A., Rodenburg, C.J., Creemers, G.J., Schrama, J.G., Erdkamp, F.L., Vos, A.H., van Groeningen, C.J., Sinnige, H.A. *et al.* (2009) Chemotherapy, bevacizumab, and cetuximab in metastatic colorectal cancer. *N. Engl. J. Med.*, **360**, 563–572.

Polymer-Based Systems

17
Design of Polymer–Drug Conjugates

Jindřich Kopeček and Pavla Kopečková

17.1
Introduction

The idea of using macromolecules as carriers of (anticancer) drugs has developed continuously over the last 100 years. In 1906, Ehrlich coined the phrase "magic bullet," recognizing the importance of biorecognition [1]. The conjugation of drugs to synthetic and natural macromolecules was initiated nearly 50 years ago. Jatzkewitz used a dipeptide (GL) spacer to attach a drug (mescaline) to polyvinylpyrrolidone in the early 1950s [2], and Ushakov's group synthesized numerous water-soluble polymer–drug conjugates in the 1960s and 1970s, focusing on conjugates of polyvinylpyrrolidone and various antibiotics [3–5]. Mathé et al. pioneered conjugation of drugs to immunoglobulins, setting the stage for targeted delivery [6]. DeDuve discovered that many enzymes are localized in the lysosomal compartment and the lysosomotropism of macromolecules [7] – an important phenomenon for the design of polymer–drug conjugates. Finally, Ringsdorf presented the first clear concept of the use of polymers as targetable drug carriers [8].

The major rationale for the use of water-soluble polymers as carriers of anticancer drugs is based on the mechanism of cell entry [9, 10]. Whereas the majority of low-molecular-weight drugs enter the cell by diffusion across the plasma membrane, the entry of macromolecules is restricted to endocytosis [11, 12]. Macromolecules captured by this mechanism are usually channeled to the lysosomal compartment of the cell.

Moieties incorporated into the macromolecular structure that complement cell surface receptors or antigens of a subset of cells render the macromolecule biorecognizable [4, 5]. For efficiency, targetable polymer–drug conjugates should be biorecognizable at two levels [6–8]: at the plasma membrane, eliciting selective recognition and internalization by a subset of target cells, and intracellularly, where lysosomal enzymes induce the release of drug from the carrier. The latter is a prerequisite for transport of the drug across the lysosomal membrane into the cytoplasm and translocation into the organelle decisive for biological activity.

There are numerous reviews that summarize the rationale, design, synthesis, and evaluation of macromolecular therapeutics [9, 10, 13–18]. This chapter will focus on structural factors important in the *design* of water-soluble polymer conjugates, present novel designs, and briefly discuss possible future developments. Polymeric carriers based on copolymers of N-(2-hydroxypropyl)methacrylamide (HPMA) [19] will be used as a frequent example. However, the conclusions can be considered generally applicable to water-soluble carriers with other chemical structures.

17.2
Polymer Carriers

Polymers chosen as drug carriers must meet certain requirements in order to maximize their potential. The polymers must be well characterized and easily synthesized; the structure should provide drug attachment/release sites for the incorporation of drugs. The carrier and all metabolic products should be nontoxic and nonantigenic. Likewise, the carriers should display the ability to be directed to predetermined cell types and, ideally, they should be biodegradable or eliminated from the organism after fulfilling their function [20].

Macromolecules as drug carriers may be divided into degradable and non-degradable types based on their fate within the organism. Biodegradable polymeric drug carriers are traditionally derived from natural products (polysaccharides, poly(amino acids), proteins) in the hope that the body's natural catabolic mechanisms will act to break down the macromolecular structure into small, easily eliminated fragments. However, the substitution of natural macromolecules with covalently linked drug molecules generally hampers the host's ability to effectively enzymatically degrade the polymeric carrier, because enzymes that cleave peptide or saccharide bonds have considerably large active sites that accommodate several amino acid or saccharide "monomer" units. Substitution along the macromolecular backbone renders the formation of the enzyme–substrate complex energetically less favorable. Therefore, drug substitution of a polymeric carrier, such as poly(amino acids) [21] or polysaccharides [22], may result in the inability of a naturally occurring, normally biodegradable macromolecule, to be degraded into small fragments able to cross the lysosomal membrane [23]. The larger fragments may accumulate in the lysosomes and increase the osmotic pressure with a potentially negative impact on biocompatibility.

Synthetic macromolecules can be tailormade to have properties matching the biological situation. However, to enhance elimination via glomerular filtration, the entire molecular weight distribution must be under the renal threshold – about 45 kDa for neutral hydrophilic random coils. Further, to prevent the nonspecific reuptake of the macromolecule after being released into the bloodstream following cell death, its structure must be designed in such a way that internalization occurs by fluid-phase pinocytosis. The absence of nonspecific interactions with plasma membranes will minimize the accumulation of the carrier in nontargeted cells and thus increase the biocompatibility of the carrier. Examples of polymer–drug conjugates are shown in Figure 17.1.

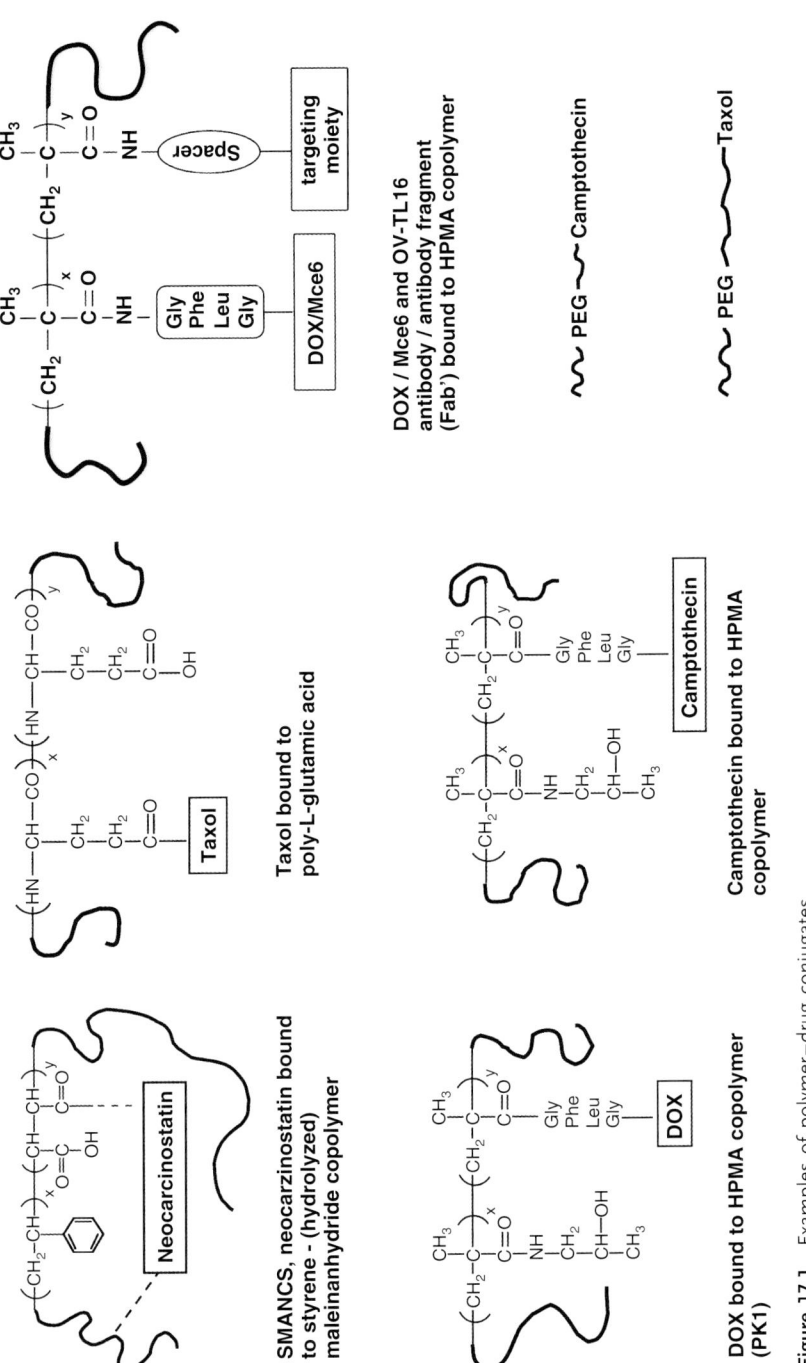

Figure 17.1 Examples of polymer–drug conjugates.

17.2.1
Impact of the Molecular Weight of the Polymer Carrier on its Fate and Efficiency

Molecular weight has an important impact on the fate of soluble polymers. The higher the molecular weight, the longer the intravascular half-life and slower the elimination of polymers from the organism, as shown in early papers on the fate of polyHPMA [24, 25], polyvinylpyrrolidone [26], dextran and pullulan [27], and other structures (reviewed in [28, 29]). Recently, Lammers et al. [30] evaluated the effect of physicochemical modification on the biodistribution and tumor accumulation of HPMA copolymers. Similar to other authors [24–28], they observed that increasing the molecular weight of HPMA copolymers resulted in prolonged circulation times and enhanced tumor concentration. Interestingly, they found that modification of the structure with carboxyl and hydrazide groups or attachment of oligopeptide spacers terminated in drug decreased the intravascular half-life; consequently, lower levels of polymer were found in tumor and all organs except kidney. Importantly, the tumor/tissue ratio did not change, indicating that functionalization did not affect the targetability of the conjugates [30].

Kopeček et al. demonstrated the impact of the molecular weight of HPMA copolymer–doxorubicin (DOX) conjugates on solid tumor treatment. To verify the hypothesis that therapeutic efficacy of conjugates will be molecular weight dependent, they designed and synthesized branched, water-soluble HPMA copolymer–DOX conjugates containing lysosomally degradable oligopeptide sequences as cross-links and side-chains terminated in DOX [31]. Four conjugates with M_w of 22, 160, 895, and 1230 kDa were prepared. Their biodistribution and treatment efficacy were evaluated in *nu/nu* mice bearing subcutaneous human ovarian OVCAR-3 carcinoma xenografts [32]. The half-life of HPMA copolymer–DOX conjugate ($M_w = 1230$ kDa) in blood was up to 28 times longer and the elimination rate from the tumor was 25 times slower than that of free DOX. The results clearly demonstrated that M_w of conjugates has a significant effect on solid tumor treatment. The higher the molecular weight of the HPMA copolymer–DOX conjugates, the higher the tumor accumulation with a concomitant increase in therapeutic efficacy (Figure 17.2) [32].

Figure 17.2 Long-circulating HPMA copolymer–DOX conjugates of different molecular weight (M_w). (a) The copolymers were synthesized by copolymerization of HPMA, N-methacryloylglycylphenylalanylleucylglycyl–DOX, and a cross-linker, N^2,N^5-bis(N-methacryloylglycylphenylalanylleucylglycyl) ornithine. The copolymerization was stopped short of the gel point and narrow-molecular-weight fractions prepared by SEC [31]. (b) Accumulation of DOX in subcutaneous OVCAR-3 human ovarian tumor xenografts in *nu/nu* mice after administration of free DOX and DOX bound to HPMA copolymer carriers of different molecular weight [32]. (c) Growth inhibition of subcutaneous OVCAR-3 human ovarian tumor xenografts in *nu/nu* mice by long-circulating HPMA copolymer–DOX conjugates. The mice received intravenous injection of 2.2 mg/kg DOX equivalent dose as HPMA copolymer conjugates of different M_w [32].

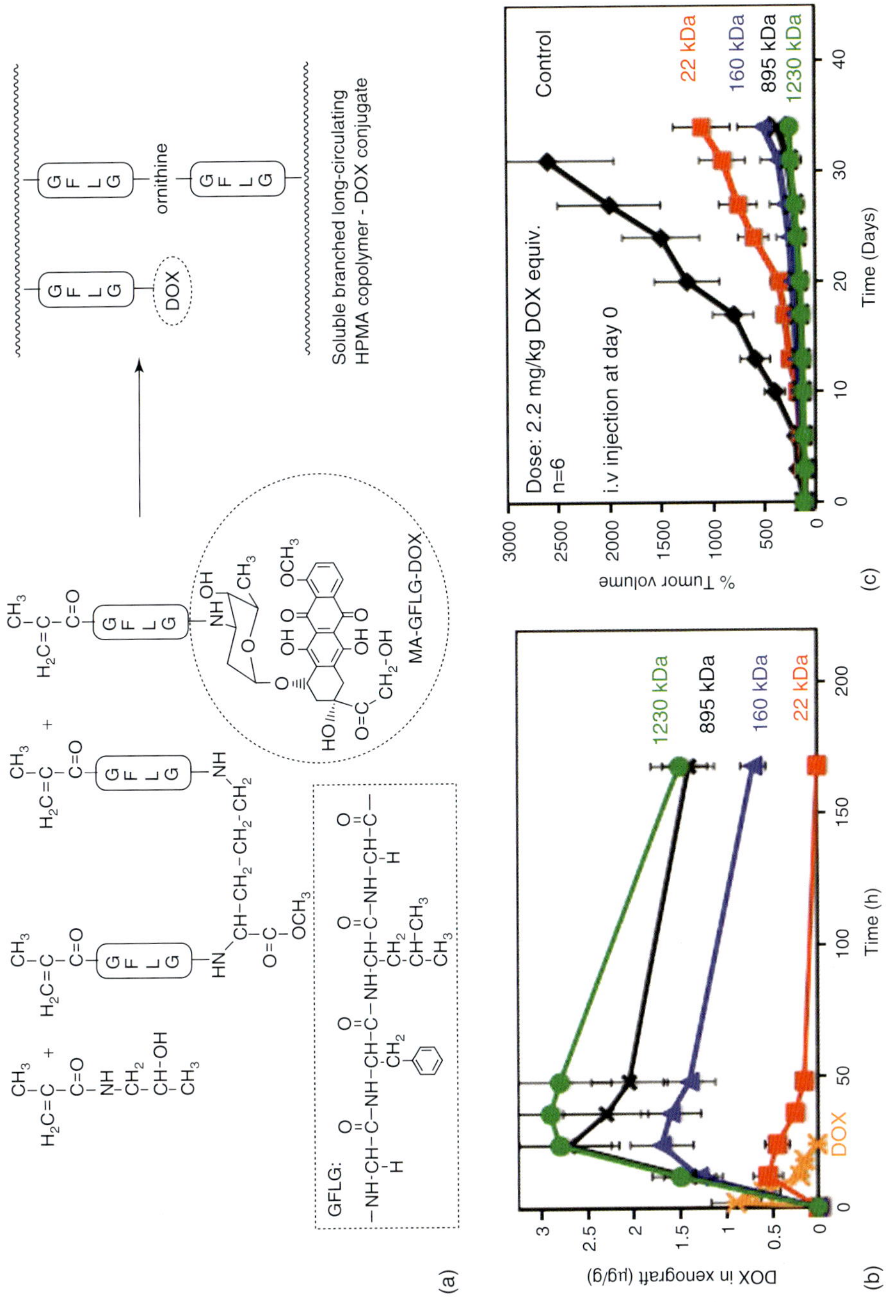

(a)
GFLG:
ornithine
DOX
MA-GFLG-DOX
Soluble branched long-circulating HPMA copolymer - DOX conjugate
(b)
DOX in xenograft (μg/g)
Time (h)
1230 kDa
895 kDa
160 kDa
22 kDa
DOX
(c)
% Tumor volume
Time (Days)
Dose: 2.2 mg/kg DOX equiv.
n=6
i.v injection at day 0
Control
22 kDa
160 kDa
895 kDa
1230 kDa

17.2.2
Structural Factors Influencing the Cellular Uptake and Subcellular Fate of Macromolecules

A suitable macromolecular drug carrier should possess highly efficient cellular uptake and preferential subcellular trafficking. These biological properties are determined to a large extent by physicochemical characteristics of the macromolecular drug carriers. For instance, positively charged macromolecular drug carriers are internalized by cells more efficiently than negatively charged carriers; however, due to the positive charge, their uptake occurs in the majority of cells [33]. Understanding the uptake and subcellular trafficking of macromolecular drug carriers by cells relies on knowledge of the complexity and diversity of endocytic pathways ([12]; see also [38]). Several endocytic pathways have been identified and a variety of classification schemes have been proposed. Based on the cargo, endocytosis is classified as phagocytosis or pinocytosis (fluid-phase endocytosis) [34]. Based on receptors, endocytosis can be designated as receptor-mediated endocytosis specified by involvement of specific high-affinity receptors, adsorptive endocytosis denoted by nonspecific binding of solutes to the cell membrane, and regular endocytosis taking up surrounding fluid nonspecifically [11]. Most common classification schemes of endocytosis are based on protein machinery that facilitate the process, such as clathrin-mediated endocytosis and clathrin-independent endocytosis [11, 35, 36]. Clathrin-independent endocytosis is further categorized as caveolae-mediated endocytosis, and clathrin- and caveolin-independent endocytosis [11, 35] or dynamin-dependent and dynamin-independent endocytosis [35, 36]. Dynamin is a GTPase protein that surrounds the neck of vesicle pits and facilitates the scission of many, but not all vesicles, such as clathrin-coated, caveolae-mediated, and clathrin- and caveolin-independent vesicles [37]. Macropinocytosis is a distinct pathway of pinocytosis [11, 38, 39]; traditionally, macropinocytosis was designated as bulk nonselective and constitutive uptake of extracellular fluid through plasma membrane protrusion or ruffling. It has been recently recognized as an elaborately coordinated process including actin-mediated membrane reorganization and regulation of signaling, such as phosphoinositide 3-kinases [38, 39].

General conclusions on the relationship between structure (charge, molecular weight, hydrophobicity) and internalization are known [40–42]. However, depending on the type of cell and detailed structure of conjugate, the subcellular trafficking may vary. The understanding of the endocytic pathways is important in the design of effective conjugates and should be individually evaluated for each design and target.

Recently, using fluorescently labeled HPMA copolymers, the basic physicochemical properties that determine the distribution and fate of synthetic macromolecules in living cells have been characterized [12, 43]. Twelve different classes of water-soluble copolymers were created by incorporating eight different functionalized comonomers. These comonomers possessed functional groups with positive or negative charges, or contained short hydrophobic peptides. The copolymers were fractionated to create parallel "ladders" consisting of 10 fractions of narrow polydispersity with molecular weights ranging from 10 to 200 kDa (Figure 17.3) [43].

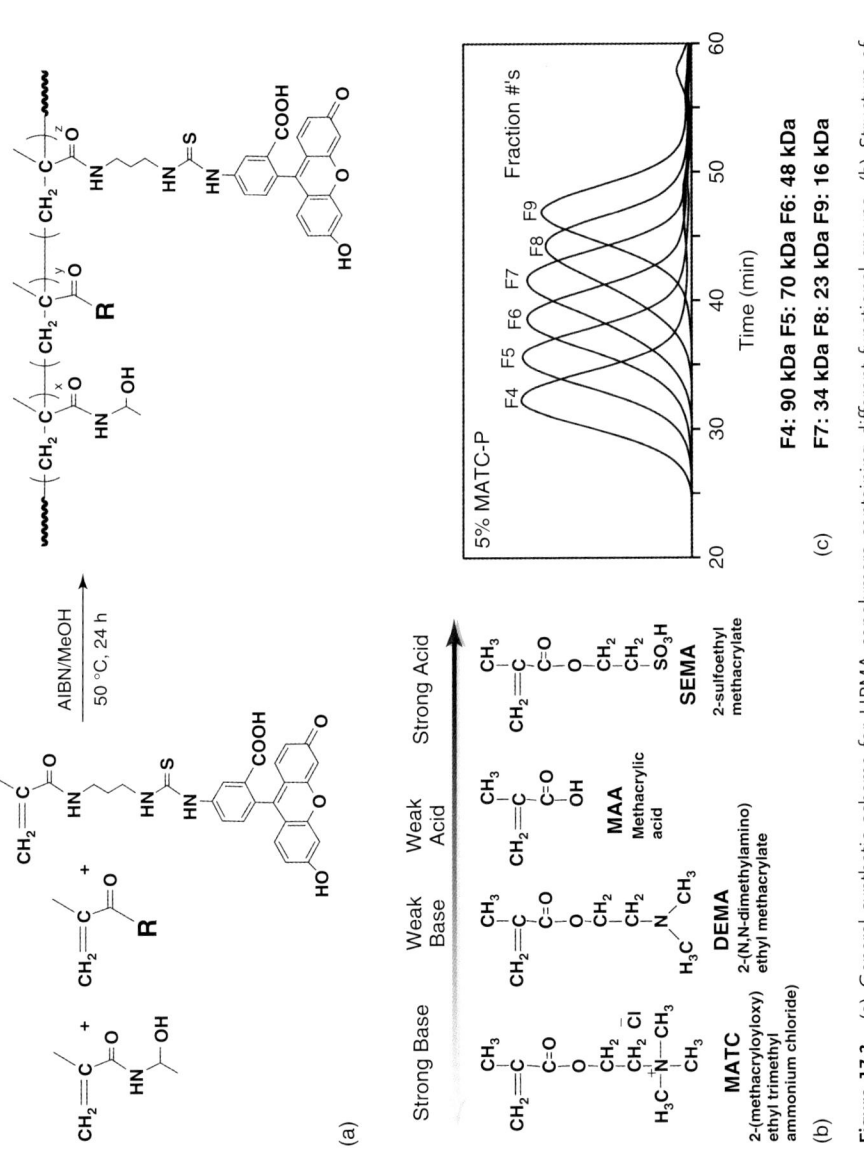

Figure 17.3 (a) General synthetic scheme for HPMA copolymers containing different functional groups. (b) Structure of comonomers used to produce the copolymer array. (c) Molecular weight profiles of P-MATC5 (copolymer of HPMA with 5 mol% MATC) fractions obtained by SEC [43].

Liu et al. [12] studied the endocytic uptake and subcellular trafficking of this large array of HPMA-based copolymers (Figure 17.3) by flow cytometry and living cell confocal microscopy in cultured prostate cancer cells. The degrees of cellular uptake of various copolymer fractions with narrow polydispersities were quantified. The copolymer charge was the predominant physicochemical feature in terms of cellular uptake. Fast and efficient uptake occurred in positively charged copolymers due to nonspecific adsorptive endocytosis, whereas slow uptake of negatively charged copolymers was observed. The uptake of positively and negatively charged copolymers correlated distinctly with molecular weight. The positively charged copolymers with higher molecular weight contain more positively charged groups and generate a stronger attractive electrostatic force, leading to elevated uptake. On the contrary, the negatively charged copolymers with higher molecular weight have more negatively charged groups and produce a stronger repulsive electrostatic force, resulting in diminished uptake. The copolymers were internalized into the cells through multiple endocytic pathways: positively charged copolymers robustly engaged clathrin-mediated endocytosis, macropinocytosis, and dynamin-dependent endocytosis, while weakly negatively charged copolymers weakly employed these pathways; strongly negatively charged copolymers only mobilized macropinocytosis. All copolymers ultimately localized in late endosomes/lysosomes via early endosomes, with varying kinetics among the copolymers [12].

Callahan et al. studied the nuclear entry of this large array of HPMA-based copolymers (Figure 17.3). Once macromolecules are delivered to the cytosol (e.g., by endosomal escape in the "real world"; by microinjection in the experiments), a number of methods may be employed to traffic them to specific subcellular compartments, such as the nucleus, in order to enhance their therapeutic efficacy [43]. Nuclear localization of macromolecules has been mediated by targeting peptides [44, 45]. However, macromolecules (without subcellular targeting moieties) are typically excluded from entering membrane-limited organelles, with the exception of any nucleus whose membrane possesses channels that allow the passive uptake of intermediate-sized macromolecules. The nuclear pore complex (NPC) of the nuclear envelope is composed of about 30 different nucleoporin proteins, and is the conduit for both nuclear import and export of macromolecules, such as proteins and nucleic acids. In active transport, cargo as large as 40 nm possessing nuclear localization sequence or nuclear export sequence signaling peptides are guided through the channel after binding to nuclear transport receptor proteins [46]. For smaller macromolecules below 10 nm, however, NPCs have been shown to act as nonspecific pores that allow exchange between the nucleus and cytoplasm by diffusion [47]. As a conduit for nonbiological macromolecules, the NPCs have been shown to transport poly(ethylene glycol)-coated gold colloid particles 4–7 nm in diameter [48].

The intracellular distributions were characterized for copolymer solutions microinjected into the cytoplasm of cultured ovarian carcinoma cells. Even the highest molecular weight HPMA copolymers were shown to quickly and evenly diffuse throughout the cytoplasm, and remain excluded from membrane-bound organelles, regardless of composition. The exceptions were the strongly cationic copolymers of

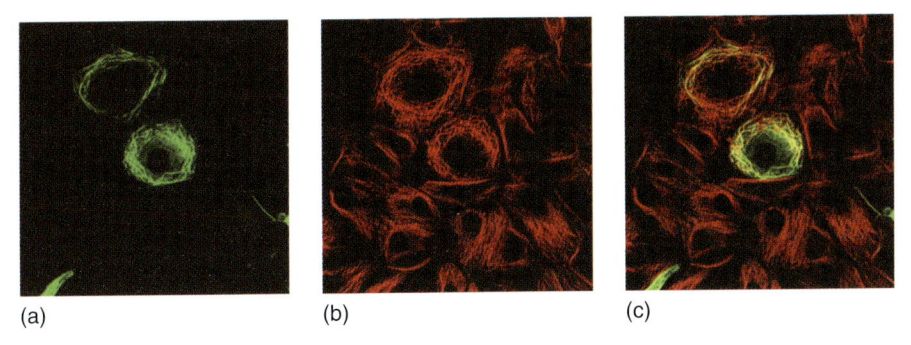

Figure 17.4 Typical images of fixed human ovarian carcinoma MDAH2774 cells after microinjection with strongly cationic copolymer 20% MATC-P-F4 (copolymer of HPMA with 20 mol% MATC; fraction F4 of $M_w = 103$ kDa), thereby demonstrating its localization on microtubules [43]. Cells were microinjected with copolymer 24 h before fixation with 3% paraformaldehyde. Microtubules were labeled using E7 antitubulin primary antibody, which was visualized using a goat antimouse AlexaFluor® 555 secondary antibody. The green channel (a) is from the fluorescein isocyanate-labeled copolymer and the red channel (b) shows microtubule staining. Overlay fluorescent image (c) demonstrated microtubule colocalization with the copolymer although some inhibition of the antitubulin antibody was evident when injected cell were compared with noninjected cells. Note: for these experiments large cells were selected to provide better images of subcellular structures.

HPMA with 2-methacryloyloxyethyl trimethylammonium chloride (MATC), which demonstrated a pronounced localization to microtubules (Figure 17.4). For all copolymers, nuclear entry was consistent with passive transport through the NPC. Nuclear uptake was shown to be largely dictated by the molecular weight of the copolymers; however, detailed kinetic analyses showed that nuclear import rates were moderately, but significantly, affected by differences in comonomer composition. HPMA copolymers containing amide-terminated phenylalanine–glycine (FG) sequences, analogous to those found in the NPC channel protein, demonstrated a potential to regulate import to the nuclear compartment. Kinetic analyses showed that 15-kDa copolymers containing **GGFG**, but not those containing **GGLFG**, peptide pendant groups altered the size-exclusion characteristics of NPC-mediated nuclear import [43]. One possible explanation is that the GGFG moieties were able to weakly bind to FG-domain cross-links in a way that altered the dynamics of a putative nucleoporin hydrogel structure, whereas GGLFG peptides would be expected to bind more strongly and prevent a rapid transfer of cross-links in the hydrogel-like structure of the nucleopore proteins [49].

17.2.3
Other Design Factors

The conformation and behavior of macromolecules usually change when a drug and/or a targeting moiety is attached to the polymer backbone. In aqueous solutions, polyHPMA assumes a random coil conformation [50]. Incorporation of hydrophobic side-chains into HPMA copolymers may result in intra- and/or intermolecular association between the hydrophobic moieties. The critical role of side-chain terminal moieties on the association of macromolecules was demonstrated in experiments with HPMA copolymers containing azobenzene side-chains. The association of the copolymer was reversibly controlled by photoirradiation. Photoinduced change of the azobenzene configuration from *trans* (apolar) to *cis* (high dipole moment) resulted in decreased polymer interactions with concomitant decrease of the aggregation degree [51, 52].

The distinction between the inter- and intramolecular association of side-chains (Figure 17.5) can be made using a combination of physicochemical methods. For example, HPMA copolymers containing side-chains terminated in chlorin e_6 (a photosensitizer) were evaluated by determination of the quantum yield of singlet oxygen formation and by light scattering. The decrease of the quantum yield indicated polymer association, while minimal changes in the hydrodynamic volumes of the conjugates (as observed by dynamic light scattering) indicated that the association was intramolecular [53, 54].

Various techniques have been used to study conformational changes in polymer nanomedicines, such as: size-exclusion chromatography (SEC) [55], quasi-elastic light scattering [56], nuclear magnetic resonance [57], and fluorescence resonance energy transfer (FRET) [58]. The energy transfer efficiency in FRET is a direct function of the distance between the fluorescent donor and acceptor. Polymer association usually occurs along with alterations in chain conformation, resulting in changes in FRET efficiency. Enhancement of FRET efficiency is indicative of decreased distance between fluorophore pair, which is then an indication of a more compact polymer chain conformation. FRET is particularly useful for conformation analyses of macromolecules in complicated conditions. Kataoka's group used FRET to detect conformational changes of plasmid DNA in a nonviral delivery system, using DNA modified with fluorescein (donor) and X-rhodamine (acceptor) [59].

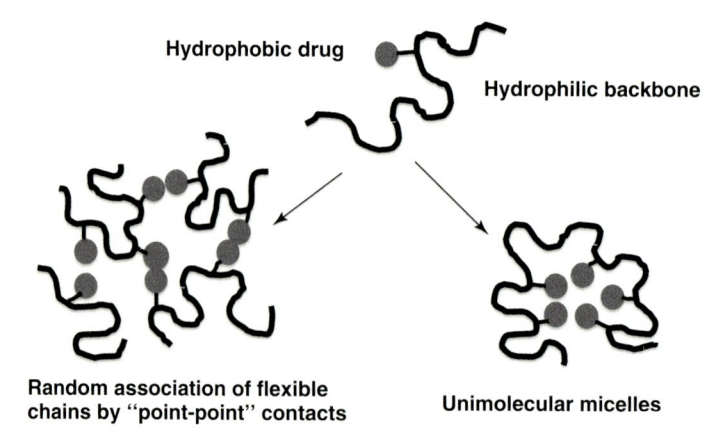

Figure 17.5 Schematics of intramolecular and intermolecular association of hydrophobic side-chains in a water-soluble polymer–drug conjugate.

This system was used to track the internalization and subcellular fate of DNA complexes [60].

Multifunctional polymeric drug carriers containing several components, such as targeting modules, drug-releasing modules, and endosome-disruptive modules, have showed the potential to perform multiple functions within a single structure [61]. Ideally, each component within the delivery system should function independently, without affecting the functionality of the other components. However, the physical and biological properties of multifunctional conjugates can be expected to exert some influence on the other components [55, 62]. Therefore, awareness of the complexities caused by the introduction of each component is needed to design multicomponent drug carriers [63]. For example, higher amounts of the hydrophobic drug prostaglandin E_1 bound to polyHPMA macromolecules resulted in a lower rate of drug release [62]. Ding et al. studied the self-association of HPMA copolymers containing an amphipathic CD21-binding heptapeptide (YILIHRN) using FRET, light scattering, and SEC [64]. The process of association, largely the result of intrapolymer hydrophobic interactions, resulted in a unimolecular micelle structure. The degree of self-association increased with increased heptapeptide content. The self-association of HPMA copolymer–peptide conjugate was disrupted by the incorporation of acrylic acid comonomers into the HPMA copolymer backbone; the ionization of COOH groups along the polymer chains induced a conformational change into an extended conformation. On the other hand, the formation of unimolecular micelles (in the absence of ionizable comonomer) resulted in decreased enzyme biorecognizability and accessibility of oligopeptide side-chains (GFLG) by papain (Figure 17.6). A better understanding of the relationship between the

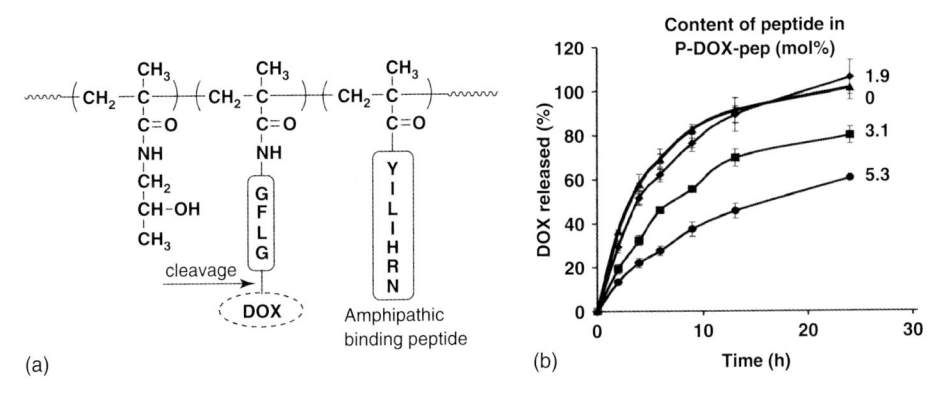

Figure 17.6 Multifunctional HPMA copolymer conjugate containing DOX and varying amounts of hydrophobic targeting heptapeptide (YILIHRN). Enhanced heptapeptide content may improve targetability of the conjugate. However, the association induced conformational changes of the conjugate have an impact on the rate of DOX release. (a) Structure of the copolymer and (b) in vitro enzymatic release of doxorubicin from HPMA copolymer–DOX conjugates containing various amounts of peptide heptapeptide (the numbers indicate the mol% of peptide in the copolymer). Papain 10 µM, glutathione 250 mM, DOX equivalent 100 µM, 0.1 M phosphate buffer containing 1 mM EDTA, 37 °C [64].

self-association of polymer conjugates and biological significance is a prerequisite for the rational design of polymeric drug delivery systems.

Polymer architecture has an important impact on the activity of the conjugates. Ulbrich's group studied in detail the relationship between the architecture of HPMA copolymers – linear conjugates, branched conjugates, grafted conjugates, self-assembled micellar conjugates, and grafted dendritic star conjugates – and their activity (reviewed in [65]). Szóka and Fréchet performed careful studies on the impact of molecular architecture (hydrodynamic volume, conformation, flexibility, and branching) on the fate of polymers in the organism. They concluded that molecular architecture has a serious impact on the elimination of the carrier via glomerular filtration, but a much smaller impact on the extravasation of the polymer into the tumor (reviewed in [66]).

17.3
Binding Drugs to Polymer Carriers

Two major routes can be used for the synthesis of polymer–drug conjugates: copolymerization, and polymer-analogous attachment (Figure 17.7). Copolymerization of HPMA with a polymerizable derivative of a drug (e.g., N-(4-aminobenzenesulfonyl)-N'-butylurea) is one example of the first route [67]. Attachment of insulin [68] and ampicillin [69] to HPMA copolymers by aminolysis of reactive polymeric precursors are examples of the latter.

The lysosomal membrane is not permeable to macromolecules [23]. Consequently, drug–polymer linkages have to be designed to be stable in the bloodstream and interstitial space, but susceptible to hydrolysis in the lysosomal compartment. One option is to use the change of pH inside subcellular vesicles during internalization, by binding drugs via acid-labile bonds [70, 71]. However, one problem is that the difference of two pH units between the bloodstream and the lysosomal compartment is not high enough to ensure both excellent stability in the bloodstream and fast hydrolysis in prelysosomal and lysosomal compartments. Nevertheless, this is an acceptable and functional design.

Alternately, the design of the bond between the HPMA copolymer carrier and the (anticancer) drug can be based on the activity of lysosomal enzymes. From the several options available (oligonucleotide, oligosaccharide, and oligopeptide sequences), oligopeptide sequences have been used most frequently as drug attachment/release points [19]. The choice of the optimal sequence was based on the detailed study of the relationship between oligopeptide sequences attached to HPMA copolymers and their degradability by proteolytic enzymes. Early studies with model enzymes, chymotrypsin [72], trypsin [73], and papain [74], resulted in recognition of the main factors responsible for the release of drugs bound at oligopeptide side-chain termini: length and detailed structure of the oligopeptide sequence, drug loading and related solution properties of the conjugate, structure of the drug, and steric hindrance [75]. The observation of *in vivo* degradability of oligopeptide sequences [76] and their stability in blood plasma and serum

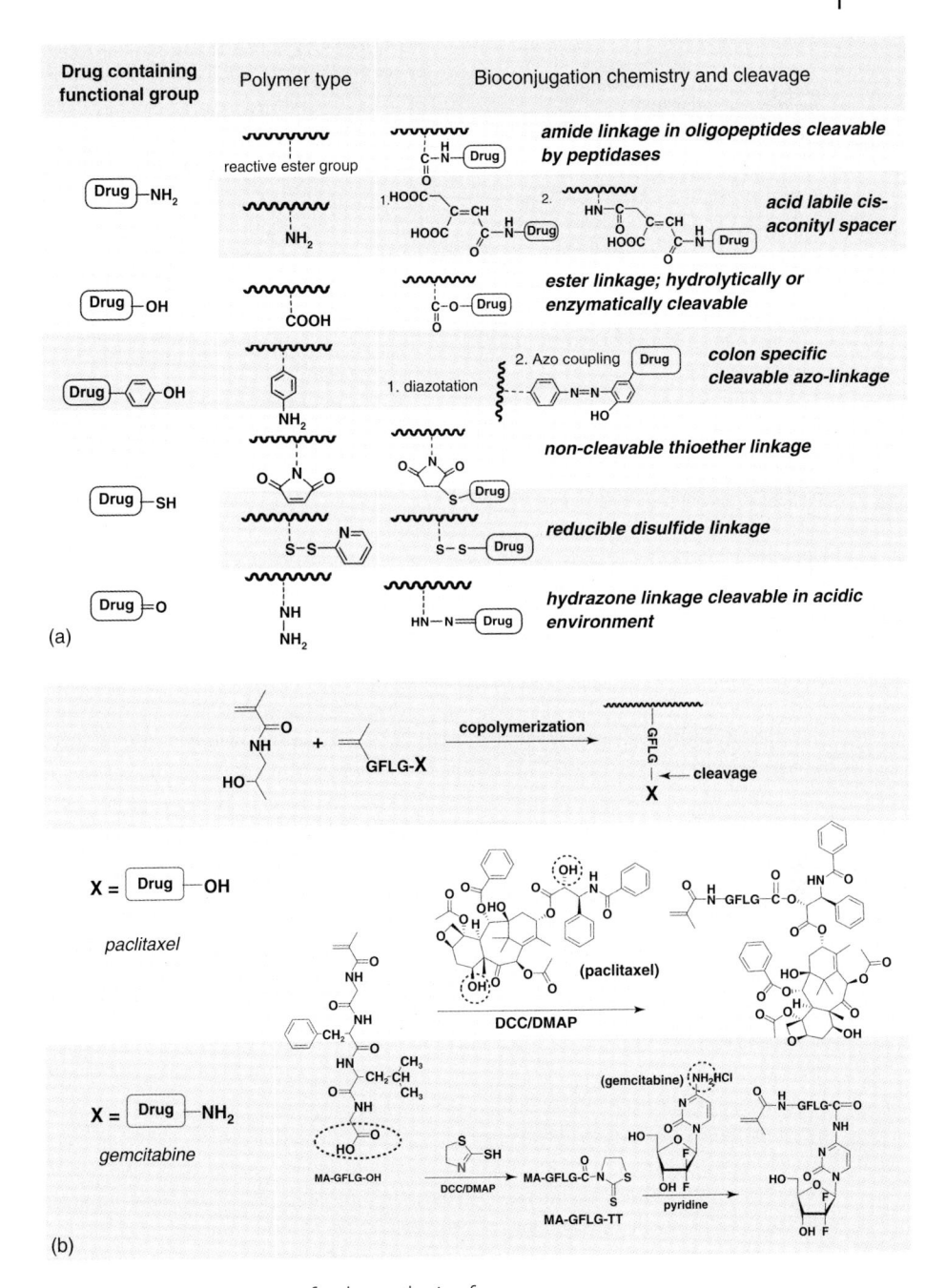

Figure 17.7 Two main routes for the synthesis of water-soluble polymer–drug conjugates: (a) attachment by polymer-analogous reaction and (b) copolymerization with a polymerizable drug derivative (monomeric form of drug).

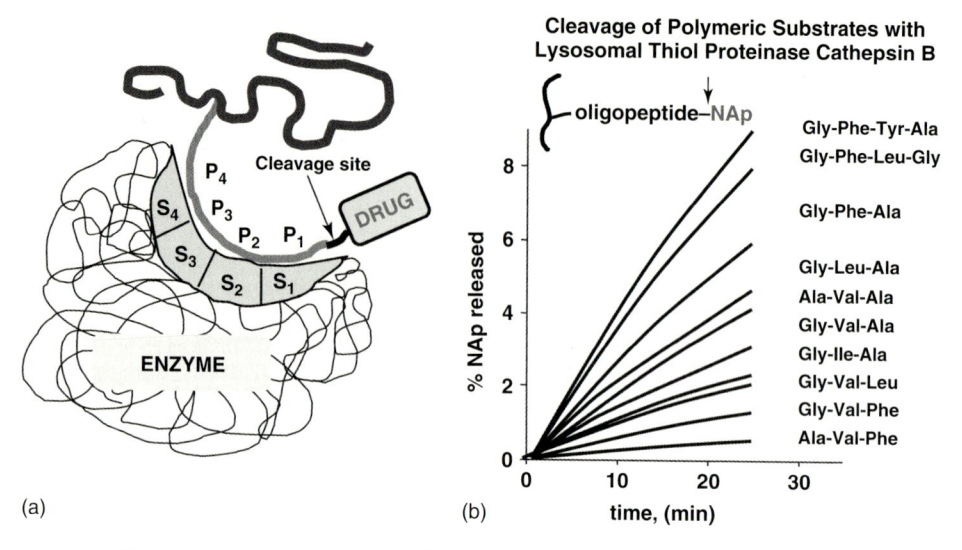

Figure 17.8 Design of enzymatically cleavable oligopeptide spacers. (a) Arrangement of a polymer–drug conjugate in the active site of an enzyme ($S_1 - S_4$ are enzyme subsites; $P_1 - P_4$ are amino acid residues that interact with the corresponding subsite). (b) Relationship between the structure of oligopeptide spacers and the release of a drug model (NAp = p-nitroaniline) from HPMA copolymer conjugates by cathepsin B, an important lysosomal thiol proteinase [79].

[44] clearly indicated lysosomal degradation. Degradation studies with isolated lysosomal enzyme mixtures [77] and individual lysosomal enzymes [78] followed. The study with cathepsin B, the most important lysosomal cysteine proteinase, resulted in the recognition of the GFLG sequence [79], which is incorporated in all conjugates used in clinical trials (Figure 17.8).

Elongated spacers, where the enzymatically cleavable bond is separated from the drug by a self-eliminating group, have been designed by several groups [62, 80]. Alternatively, the self-eliminating groups can be activated by the reduction of aromatic azo bonds [81, 82] – a suitable design for colon-specific oral drug delivery (Figure 17.9).

17.4
Attachment of Targeting Moieties

Active targeting of polymer–drug conjugates can be achieved by the incorporation of cancer cell-specific ligands, such as carbohydrates, lectins, antibodies, antibody fragments, and peptides, resulting in enhanced uptake of conjugates by cancer cells through receptor-mediated endocytosis with concomitant improvement in therapeutic efficacy [19]. The advantage of polymeric carriers is the fact that several targeting moieties can be attached to one macromolecule. This results in a multivalency effect with enhanced avidity of the conjugate. Examples include

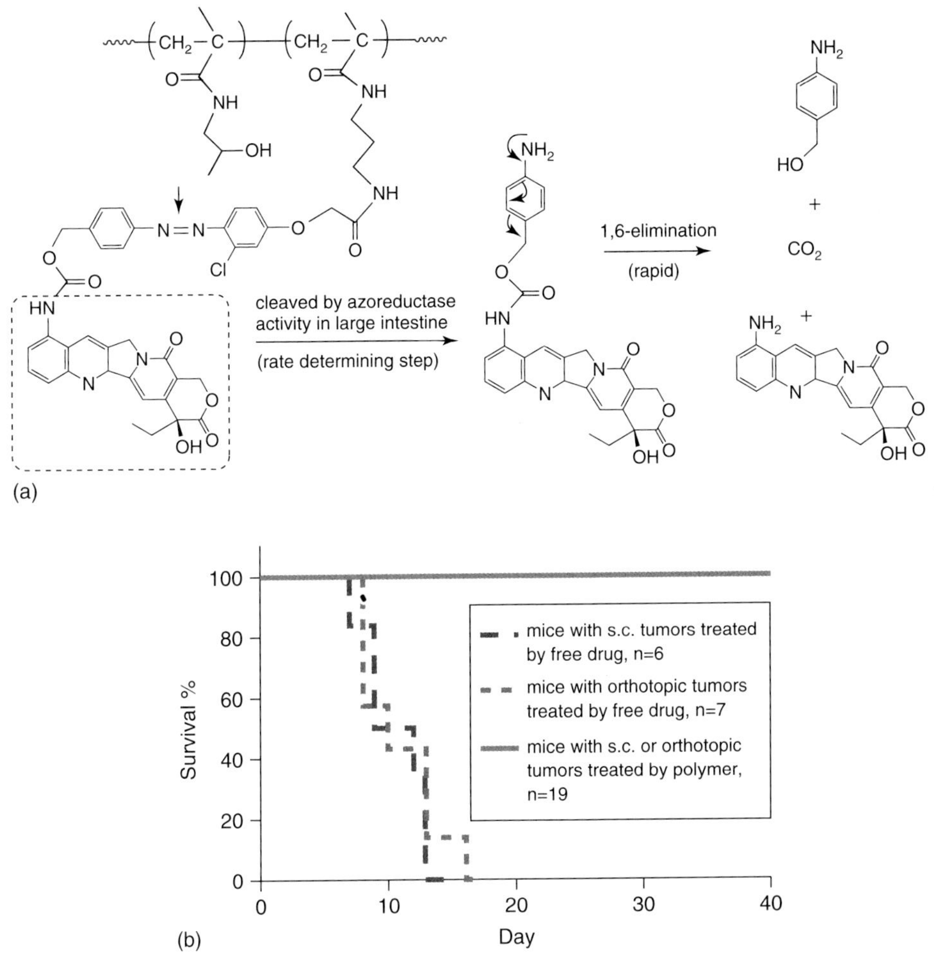

Figure 17.9 HPMA copolymer–9-aminocamptothecin (9-AC) conjugate (P-9-AC) containing an elongated spacer composed from a reducible aromatic azo bond and a 1,6-elimination unit. (a) Structure and scheme of release of unmodified 9-AC from HPMA copolymer–9-AC conjugates by a two-step process: rate-controlling aromatic azo bond cleavage, followed by fast 1,6-elimination [81]. (b) Survival curves of mice bearing human colon carcinoma xenografts treated by 9-AC and P-9-AC at a dose of 3 mg/kg of 9-AC or 9-AC equivalent [82].

binding several Fab′ antibody fragments per HPMA macromolecule [83] or binding a number of peptides [84]. The multivalency effect resulted in enhanced biological activity of the conjugates.

Chemistry of binding of the targeting moiety can have an impact on the activity of the conjugate. The influence of different methods of coupling the OV-TL16 antibody and its Fab′ fragment to HPMA copolymer–drug (DOX or mesochlorin e_6 mono(N-2-aminoethylamide) (Mce$_6$)) carriers on the binding affinity of the

Polymer-drug conjugates containing targeting moieties — Ab/Fab'				
Binding approach	Random amide linkage	Site-specific binding via *hydrazone* linkage with sugar chains near hinge region	Site-specific binding via *thiol-maleimide* reaction	Native Ab
K_a (M^{-1}×10^{-8})	1.0	3.2	3.0	8.0

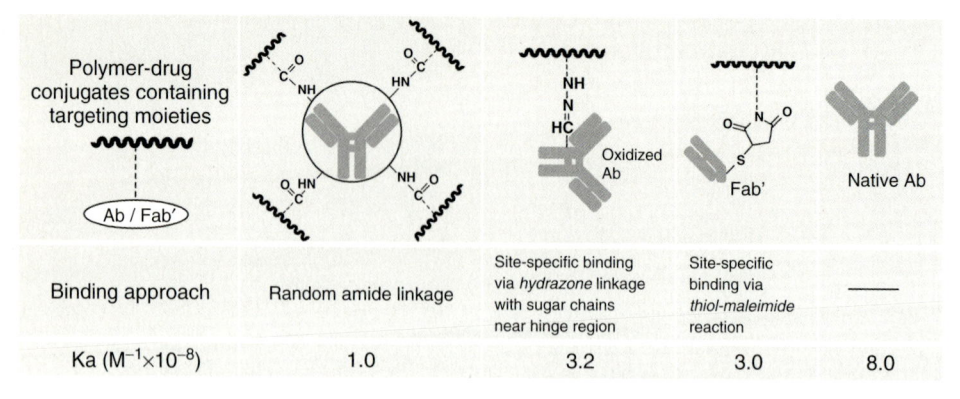

Figure 17.10 Influence of different methods of binding the OV-TL16 antibody and its Fab' fragment to HPMA copolymer–drug (DOX or Mce$_6$) conjugates on the affinity of conjugates to the ovarian carcinoma OVCAR-3 cell-associated CD47 antigen. Affinity constants K_a (M^{-1} × 10^{-8}) are shown for free antibody; antibody bound via amino groups, antibody bound via oxidized saccharide units in the hinge region, and Fab' fragment bound via thioether bonds [85].

conjugates to the CD47 antigen associated with ovarian carcinoma (OVCAR-3) cells was studied. Three different methods of covalently binding the antibody or Fab' to polymers were used [85]:

Method A: binding via amide bonds formed by aminolysis of active ester groups on the HPMA copolymer–drug (DOX or Mce$_6$) conjugates by amino groups on the antibody.

Method B: binding via hydrazone bonds formed by the reaction of aldehyde groups on the oxidized antibody with hydrazo groups on the HPMA copolymer–Mce$_6$ conjugates.

Method C: binding via thioether bonds formed by the reaction of sulfhydryl groups of Fab' fragments with maleimido groups on the side-chain termini of the HPMA copolymer–Mce$_6$ conjugates.

Differences in K_a were observed as shown in Figure 17.10.

17.4.1
Subcellular Targeting

Recently, research has been focusing on the identification of different routes of cell entry with the aim to deliver drugs into subcellular compartments different from lysosomes [86, 87]. This direction was mainly driven by attempts to deliver genes or oligonucleotides (i.e., compounds) that may degrade in the lysosomes; however, other rationales may be important: (i) the activity of many drugs depends on their subcellular location and (ii) the mechanism of action of polymer-bound drugs may be different than that of the free drug. Consequently, manipulation of

17.4.1.1 Mitochondrial Targeting

A wide variety of therapeutic agents may benefit by specifically directing them to the mitochondria in tumor cells. To design delivery systems that would enable a combination of tumor and mitochondrial targeting, novel HPMA copolymer-based delivery systems that employ triphenylphosphonium (TPP) ions as mitochondriotropic agents [88] were developed [86]. Constructs were initially synthesized with fluorescent labels substituted for drug, which were used for validation experiments. Microinjection and incubation experiments performed using these fluorescently labeled constructs confirmed the mitochondrial targeting ability [89]. Subsequently, HPMA copolymer–drug conjugates were synthesized using a photosensitizer Mce_6. Mitochondrial targeting of HPMA copolymer-bound Mce_6 enhanced cytotoxicity as compared to nontargeted HPMA copolymer–Mce_6 conjugates (Figure 17.11) [86].

17.4.1.2 Hormone-Mediated Nuclear Delivery

Steroid hormone receptors (SHRs) are known to shuttle between the cytoplasm and nucleus of cells. The rationale for using SHRs as vehicles for transporting drugs from the cytoplasm into the nucleus is based upon the binding of the steroid ligand to receptors such as glucocorticoid receptor (GR); the ligand–receptor complex actively migrates to the nucleus [90]. Analysis of the structure of SHRs [91] indicated that hormone structure might be modified without impairing binding to the receptor. Indeed, Rebuffat *et al.* used steroid receptors as shuttles to facilitate the uptake of transfected DNA into the nucleus of GR-positive cells [92]. Using a similar strategy, we synthesized a hormone-modified photosensitizer (cortisol-modified Mce_6 (Cort-Mce_6) capable of binding to GR in the cytoplasm and then localizing to the nucleus [93].

Novel HPMA copolymer-based delivery systems of this derivative were also synthesized. After internalization of a HPMA copolymer–Cort-Mce_6 conjugate (via lysosomally degradable GFLG spacer) by endocytosis, Cort-Mce_6 was cleaved, translocated to the cytoplasm, bound to the GR, and translocated to the nucleus [93]. To verify that coupling of cortisol to Mce_6 maintains the capacity to form a complex with the cytosolic GR resulting in nuclear localization, we investigated the subcellular fate of the modified drug. Cort-Mce_6 was monitored in 1471.1 cells transfected with plasmid that expresses Green Fluorescent Protein (GFP)-labeled GR (GFP-GR). Cortisol and Mce_6 served as positive and negative controls, respectively. GR translocated to the nucleus after attachment of a glucocorticoid analog (e.g., cortisol). The fluorescent GFP label permits the movement of the GR to be monitored in real-time. The data clearly indicated the time- and concentration-dependent nuclear localization of Cort-Lys-Mce_6 and cortisol. In contrast, cells incubated with Mce_6 did not show any alteration in receptor localization following treatment [93].

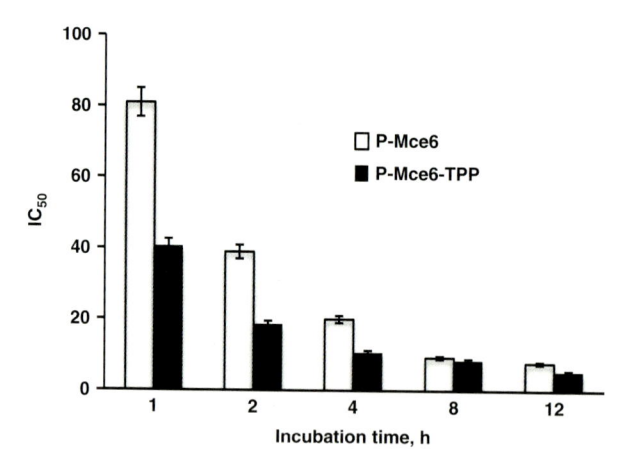

Figure 17.11 Mitochondrial targeting of HPMA copolymer–Mce$_6$ conjugates containing drug bound via a disulfide linker. Cytotoxicity of TPP targeted P-SS-TPP-lysine-Mce$_6$ conjugate (P is the HPMA copolymer backbone) and the nontargeted conjugate P-SS-Mce$_6$ in human ovarian cancer SKOV-3 cells for different times of incubation [86]. IC$_{50}$ doses determined by incubating serial dilutions (Mce$_6$ concentration) of HPMA copolymer–drug conjugates with SKOV-3 cells for specified periods of time. Illumination was achieved using a lamp assembly for 30 min. Viability determined by CCK-8 bioassay, and used to construct dose–response curves and determine IC$_{50}$. Values expressed as mean IC$_{50}$ values with standard deviations calculated from three to four replicates in each case.

17.5
Novel Designs of Polymer Therapeutics

17.5.1
Design of Backbone Degradable, Long-Circulating Polymer Carriers

As discussed above, high-molecular-weight (long-circulating) polymer conjugates accumulate efficiently in tumor tissue due to the enhanced permeability and retention (EPR) effect. However, the intravascular half-life of the HPMA copolymer conjugates evaluated in clinical trials has been suboptimal [30]. To achieve substantial accumulation of the polymer–drug conjugate in solid tumor (due to the EPR effect) a sustained concentration gradient is needed. The concentration depends on the administered dose and the circulation time of the molecular weight of the carrier. Higher-molecular-weight drug carriers with a nondegradable backbone deposit and accumulate in various organs, impairing biocompatibility. Previous attempts to design and synthesize long-circulating conjugates produced branched, partially cross-linked copolymers with enzymatically degradable sequences [31]. The synthetic process and the polymer structure were difficult to control; consequently, the reproducibility was poor. Nevertheless, the results proved that higher molecular weight of carrier transfers into higher efficacy [32].

To this end we designed new, second-generation anticancer nanomedicines based on high-molecular-weight HPMA copolymer–drug carriers containing enzymatically degradable bonds in the main chain (polymer backbone) [94–96]. The proposed new design permits tailormade synthesis of well-defined backbone degradable HPMA copolymers. The synthetic process consists of two main steps: first, the synthesis of a telechelic HPMA copolymer by RAFT polymerization, followed in the second step by chain extension using alkyne-azide [94, 95, 97] or thiol-ene [96] click reactions. A series of experiments were conducted as feasibility studies. We have designed and synthesized new chain transfer agents (CTAs) with different functionalities [94–96]. One of CTAs is a trithiocarbonate flanked with alkyne groups at both ends. Telechelic polyHPMA was synthesized via RAFT polymerization using this new CTA and the polymer chain was further extended using azido-modified GFLG tetrapeptide by Cu(I)-catalyzed click reaction [94, 95, 98] as shown in Figure 17.12.

Multiblock polyHPMAs with M_w as high as 350 kDa and containing degradable GFLG sequences were obtained by chain extension followed by isolation using SEC. The exposure of the multiblock HPMA copolymer to model enzyme papain (pH 6, 37 °C; similar activity as lysosomal cathepsin B) resulted in complete degradation of GFLG segments and decrease of the molecular weight of the carrier to the initial one [94–96]. These data support our hypothesis and bode well for the success of the proposed design of backbone degradable HPMA copolymers composed of alternating segments of HPMA copolymer with molecular weight below the renal threshold and lysosomally degradable tetrapeptide GFLG.

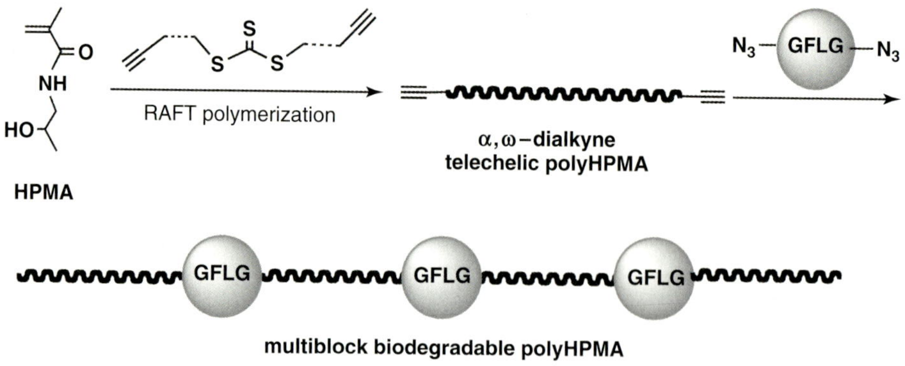

Figure 17.12 Design of backbone degradable HPMA copolymer carriers [95].

17.5.2
Drug-Free Macromolecular Therapeutics

Molecular biorecognition is at the center of all biological processes and it forms the basis for the design of precisely defined smart systems, including targeted therapeutics, imaging agents, biosensors, and stimuli-sensitive and self-assembled biomaterials. In parallel to the cancer program, we study the self-assembly of hybrid materials, composed of synthetic and biological macromolecules, mediated by the biorecognition of biological motifs [99]. Recently, we designed a pair of oppositely charged pentaheptad peptides (CCE and CCK) that formed antiparallel coiled-coil heterodimers and served as physical cross-linkers for HPMA graft copolymers [99]. HPMA graft copolymers, CCE-P and CCK-P (P is the HPMA copolymer backbone), self-assembled into hybrid hydrogels with a high degree of biorecognition [100, 101].

We hypothesized that this unique biorecognition of CCK and CCE peptide motifs could be expanded past biomaterials design, and be applied to a living system and mediate a biological process. This would provide a bridge between the designs of biomaterials and macromolecular therapeutics. To verify this hypothesis we chose to study the induction of apoptosis in CD20$^+$ cells [102]. CD20 is one of the most reliable biomarkers for B cell non-Hodgkin's lymphoma (NHL) [103], which functions as a cell cycle regulatory protein [104] that either controls or functions as a store-operated calcium channel. CD20 is expressed on most NHL malignant cells as well as on normal B cells. However, it is not expressed on stem cells and mature plasma cells. Consequently, normal numbers of B cells can be restored after treatment [105]. It is a noninternalizing antigen that remains on the cell surface when bound to a complementary antibody [105]. Although, cross-linking of CD20-bound antibodies with a secondary antibody results in apoptosis [106]. To exploit this phenomenon, we designed a system composed of CCE and CCK peptides, Fab' fragment of the 1F5 anti-CD20 antibody, and HPMA copolymer (Figure 17.13). The exposure of CD20$^+$ Raji B cells to Fab'–CCE resulted in the decoration of the cell surface with multiple copies of

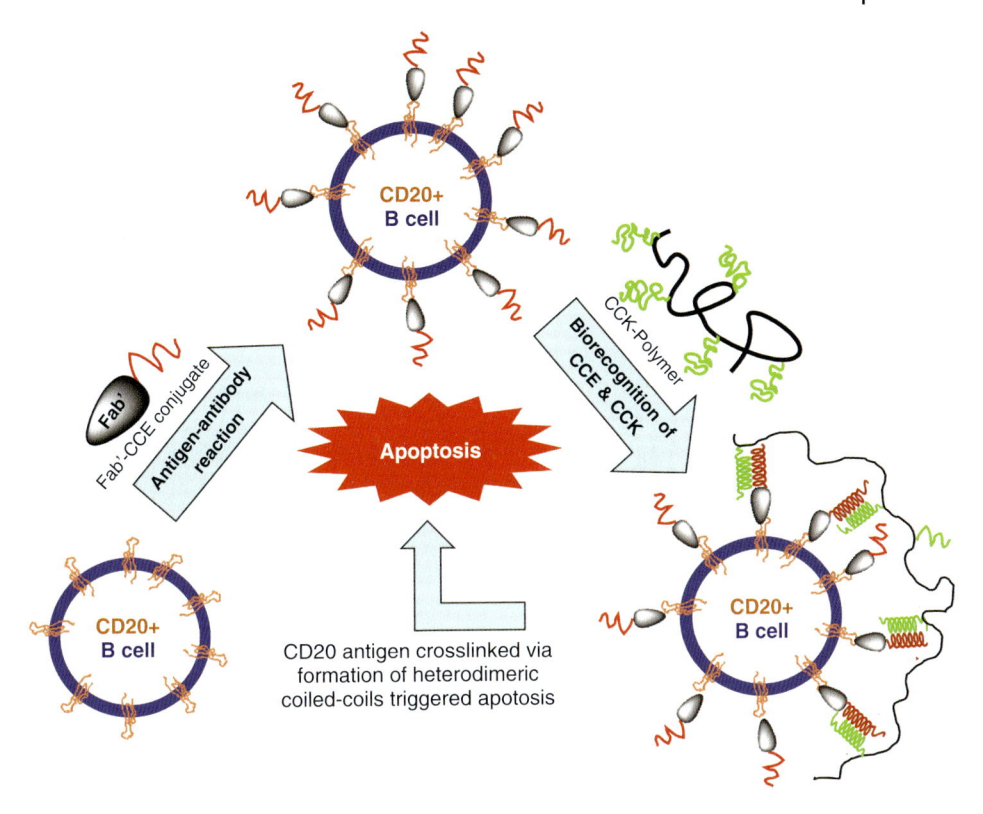

Figure 17.13 Design of drug-free macromolecular therapeutics [102]. Induction of apoptosis in human Burkitt's NHL Raji B cells by cross-linking of its CD20 antigens mediated by antiparallel coiled-coil heterodimer formation at the cell surface. Fab′–CCE is a conjugate of the Fab′ fragment of the 1F5 antibody and the CCE peptide (YGGEVSALEKEVSALEKKN-SALEKEVSALEKEVSALEK); CCK-Polymer is a HPMA copolymer containing nine grafts of the CCK peptide (CYGGKVSALKEKVSAL-KEEVSANKEKVSALKEKVSALKE).

the CCE peptide via antigen–antibody fragment biorecognition. Further exposure of the decorated cells to HPMA copolymer grafted with multiple copies of CCK resulted in the formation of CCE–CCK coiled-coil heterodimers on the cell surface. This second biorecognition event induced cross-linking of CD20 receptors and triggered apoptosis of Raji B cells as detected by three apoptosis assays: caspase-3 activity assay, Annexin-V/propidium iodide assay, and terminal deoxynucleotidyl transferase dUTP nick end-labeling (TUNEL) assay [102].

This is a new paradigm in apoptosis induction mediated by biorecognition of coiled-coil-forming peptide segments at the cell surface. The important feature of this design is the absence of low-molecular-weight cytotoxic compounds. The fact that biorecognition of coiled-coils at the cell surface occurred in media containing 10% bovine serum indicates the specificity of the CCE–CCK interaction and bodes well for the development of efficient drug-free macromolecular therapeutics. This conclusion is supported by our recent data that demonstrate the effectiveness of this approach in a mouse model of NHL (Wu et al., in preparation).

17.6
Conclusions and Perspectives

The advantages of polymer-bound drugs (when compared to low-molecular-weight drugs) are [19]: (i) active uptake by fluid-phase pinocytosis (nontargeted polymer-bound drug) or receptor-mediated endocytosis (targeted polymer-bound drug), (ii) increased *passive* accumulation of the drug at the tumor site by the EPR effect, (iii) increased *active* accumulation of the drug at the tumor site by targeting, (iv) long-lasting circulation in the bloodstream, (v) decreased nonspecific toxicity of the conjugated drugs, (vi) potential to overcome multidrug resistance, (vii) decreased immunogenicity of the targeting moiety, (viii) immunoprotecting and immunomobilizing activities, and (ix) modulation of the cell signaling and apoptotic pathways. In addition to preclinical evaluation on animal cancer models, these advantages were also recognized in numerous clinical trials of water-soluble polymer–drug conjugates (reviewed in [17]). However, the translation of laboratory research into the clinics has been slow. To enhance the development and translation, new approaches are needed. Research areas to be pursued are [107]:

- Design of conjugates for the treatment of noncancerous diseases.
- Further studies on combination therapy.
- New targeting strategies.
- Relationship between detailed structure of the conjugates and their properties.
- Mechanism of action.
- Mechanism of internalization and subcellular trafficking.
- Subcellular targeting.
- Design of backbone degradable, long-circulating polymer carriers.

We certainly hope that a concerted effort of pharmaceutical chemists, molecular biologists, biomedical engineers, and physicians along these lines will achieve translation of water-soluble polymer–drug conjugates into the clinic within the current decade.

Acknowledgments

The research in the authors' laboratory was supported in part by the National Institutes of Health (recently grants CA51578, CA132831, GM69847, and EB5288), Department of Defense grant W81XWH-04-1-0900, and the University of Utah Research Foundation. Thanks to Dr. Jiyuan Yang and Michael Jacobsen for editing the artwork and the text. We thank our past and present coworkers and numerous collaborators. We are truly indebted to all of them; their scientific contributions are reflected in the references.

References

1. Ehrlich, P. (1906) *Studies in Immunity*, Plenum Press, New York.
2. Jatzkewitz, H. (1955) Peptamin (glycyl-L-leucyl-mescaline) bound to blood plasma expander (polyvinylpyrrolidone) as a new depot form of a biologically active primary amine (mescaline). *Z. Naturforsch.*, **10b**, 27–31.
3. Givetal, N.I., Ushakov, S.N., Panarin, E.F., and Popova, G.O. (1965) [Experimental studies on penicillin polymer derivatives]. *Antibiotiki*, **10**, 701–706.
4. Shumikina, K.I., Panarin, E.F., and Ushakov, S.N. (1966) [Experimental study of polymer salts of penicillins]. *Antibiotiki*, **11**, 767–770.
5. Panarin, E.F. and Ushakov, S.N. (1968) [Synthesis of polymer salts and amidopenicillines]. *Khim. Pharm. Zhur.*, **2**, 28–31.
6. Mathé, G., Loc, T.B., and Bernard, J. (1958) Effect sur la leucémie L1210 de la Souris d'une combinaison par diazotation d'a méthoptérine et de γ-globulines de hamsters porteurs de cette leucémie par hétérogreffe. *C.R. Acad. Sci.*, **3**, 1626–1628.
7. De Duve, C., De Barsy, T., Poole, B., Trouet, A., Tulkens, P., and van Hoof, F. (1974) Lysosomotropic agents. *Biochem. Pharmacol.*, **23**, 2495–2531.
8. Ringsdorf, H. (1975) Structure and properties of pharmacologically active polymers. *J. Polym. Sci. Polym. Symp.*, **51**, 135–153.
9. Kopeček, J. (1977) Soluble biomedical polymers. *Polim. Med.*, **7**, 191–221.
10. Putnam, D. and Kopeček, J. (1995) Polymers with anticancer activity. *Adv. Polym. Sci.*, **122**, 55–123.
11. Conner, S.D. and Schmid, S.L. (2003) Regulated portals of entry into the cell. *Nature*, **422**, 37–44.
12. Liu, J., Bauer, H., Callahan, J., Kopečková, P., Pan, H., and Kopeček, J. (2010) Endocytic uptake of a large array of HPMA copolymers: elucidation into the dependence on the physicochemical characteristics. *J. Control. Release*, **143**, 71–79.
13. Duncan, R. (2003) The dawning era of polymer therapeutics. *Nat. Rev. Drug Discov.*, **2**, 347–360.
14. Ulbrich, K. and Šubr, V. (2004) Polymeric anticancer drugs with pH-controlled activation. *Adv. Drug Deliv. Rev.*, **56**, 1023–1050.
15. Haag, R. and Kratz, F. (2006) Polymer therapeutics: concepts and applications. *Angew. Chem. Int. Ed.*, **45**, 1198–1215.
16. Khandare, J. and Minko, T. (2006) Polymer–drug conjugates: progress in polymer prodrugs. *Prog. Polym. Sci.*, **31**, 359–397.
17. Li, C. and Wallace, S. (2008) Polymer–drug conjugates: recent development in clinical oncology. *Adv. Drug Deliv. Rev.*, **60**, 886–898.
18. Pan, H. and Kopeček, J. (2008) Multifunctional water-soluble polymers for drug delivery in *Multifunctional Pharmaceutical Nanocarriers*, Fundamental Biomedical Technologies, vol. 4 (ed. V.P. Torchilin), Springer, New York, pp. 81–142.
19. Kopeček, J. and Kopečková, P. (2010) HPMA copolymers: origins, early developments, present, and future. *Adv. Drug Deliv. Rev.*, **62**, 122–149.
20. Krinick, N.L. and Kopeček, J. (1991) Soluble polymers as targetable drug carriers in *Targeted Drug Delivery*, Handbook of Experimental Pharmacology, vol. 100 (ed. R.L. Juliano), Springer, Berlin, pp. 105–179.
21. Chiu, H.-C., Kopečková, P., Deshmane, S.S., and Kopeček, J. (1997) Lysosomal degradation of poly(α-amino acids). *J. Biomed. Mater. Res.*, **34**, 381–392.
22. Chiu, H.-C., Koňák, Č., Kopečková, P., and Kopeček, J. (1994) Enzymatic degradation of poly(ethylene glycol) modified dextrans. *J. Bioact. Comp. Polym.*, **9**, 388–410.
23. Lloyd, J.B. (2000) Lysosomal membrane permeability: implications for drug delivery. *Adv. Drug Deliv. Rev.*, **41**, 189–200.
24. Šprincl, L., Exner, J., Štěrba, O., and Kopeček, J. (1976) New types of synthetic infusion solutions. III Elimination and retention of poly

[N-(2-hydroxypropyl)methacrylamide] in a test organism. *J. Biomed. Mater. Res.*, **10**, 953–963.

25. Seymour, L.W., Duncan, R., Strohalm, J., and Kopeček, J. (1987) Effect of molecular weight of N-(2-hydroxypropyl)methacrylamide copolymers on body distribution and rate of excretion after subcutaneous, intraperitoneal and intravenous administration to rats. *J. Biomed. Mater. Res.*, **21**, 1341–1358.

26. Hespe, W., Meier, A.M., and Blankwater, Y.J. (1977) Excretion and distribution studies in rats with two forms of 14 carbon-labeled polyvinylpyrrolidone with a relatively low mean molecular weight after intravenous administration. *Drug Res.*, **27**, 1158–1162.

27. Yamaoka, T., Tabata, Y., and Ikada, Y. (1993) Body distribution profile of polysaccharides after intravenous administration. *Drug Deliv.*, **1**, 75–82.

28. Kopeček, J. (1981) Soluble polymers in medicine, in *Systemic Aspects of Biocompatibility*, vol. II (ed. D.F. Williams), CRC Press, Boca Raton, FL, pp. 159–180.

29. Yamaoka, T., Tabata, Y., and Ikada, Y. (1995) Fate of water-soluble polymers administered via different routes. *J. Pharm. Sci.*, **84**, 349–354.

30. Lammers, T., Kühnlein, R., Kissel, M., Šubr, V., Etrych, T., Pola, R., Pechar, M., Ulbrich, K., Storm, G., Huber, P., and Peschke, P. (2005) Effect of physicochemical modification on the biodistribution and tumor accumulation of HPMA copolymers. *J. Control. Release*, **110**, 103–118.

31. Dvořák, M., Kopečková, P., and Kopeček, J. (1999) High-molecular weight HPMA copolymer–adriamycin conjugates. *J. Control. Release*, **60**, 321–332.

32. Shiah, J.-G., Dvořák, M., Kopečková, P., Sun, Y., Peterson, C.M., and Kopeček, J. (2001) Biodistribution and antitumor efficacy of long-circulating N-(2-hydroxypropyl)methacrylamide copolymer–doxorubicin conjugates in nude mice. *Eur.J. Cancer*, **37**, 131–139.

33. McCormick, L.A., Seymour, L.C.W., Duncan, R., and Kopeček, J. (1986) Interaction of a cationic N-(2-hydroxypropyl)methacrylamide copolymer with rat visceral yolk sac cultured *in vitro* and rat liver *in vivo*. *J. Bioact. Compat. Polym.*, **1**, 901–905.

34. Mukherjee, S., Ghosh, R.N., and Maxfield, F.R. (1997) Endocytosis. *Physiol. Rev.*, **77**, 759–803.

35. Mayor, S. and Pagano, R.E. (2007) Pathways of clathrin-independent endocytosis. *Nat. Rev. Mol. Cell Biol.*, **8**, 603–612.

36. Gong, Q., Huntsman, C., and Ma, D. (2008) Clathrin-independent internalization and recycling. *J. Cell Mol. Med.*, **12**, 126–144.

37. Praefcke, G.J. and McMahon, H.T. (2004) The dynamin superfamily: universal membrane tubulation and fission molecules? *Nat. Rev. Mol. Cell Biol.*, **5**, 133–147.

38. Jones, A.T. (2007) Macropinocytosis: searching for an endocytic identity and role in the uptake of cell penetrating peptides. *J. Cell Mol. Med.*, **11**, 670–684.

39. Kerr, M.C. and Teasdale, R.D. (2009) Defining macropinocytosis. *Traffic*, **10**, 364–371.

40. Duncan, R., Rejmanová, P., Kopeček, J., and Lloyd, J.B. (1981) Pinocytic uptake and intracellular degradation of N-(2-hydroxypropyl)methacrylamide copolymers. A potential drug delivery system. *Biochim. Biophys. Acta*, **678**, 143–150.

41. Duncan, R., Cable, H.C., Rejmanová, P., Kopeček, J., and Lloyd, J.B. (1984) Tyrosinamide residues enhance pinocytic capture of N-(2-hydroxypropyl)methacrylamide copolymers. *Biochim. Biophys. Acta*, **799**, 1–8.

42. Liu, J., Kopečková, P., Bühler, P., Wolf, P., Pan, H., Bauer, H., Elsässer-Beile, U., and Kopeček, J. (2009) Biorecognition and subcellular trafficking of HPMA copolymer–anti-PMSA antibody conjugates by prostate cancer cells. *Mol. Pharm.*, **6**, 959–970.

43. Callahan, J., Kopečková, P., and Kopeček, J. (2009) The intracellular

trafficking and subcellular distribution of a large array of HPMA copolymer conjugates. *Biomacromolecules*, **10**, 1704–1714.
44. Tijerina, M., Kopečková, P., and Kopeček, J. (2003) Correlation of subcellular compartmentalization of HPMA copolymer–Mce$_6$ conjugates with chemotherapeutic activity in human ovarian carcinoma cells. *Pharm. Res.*, **20**, 728–737.
45. Tijerina, M., Kopečková, P., and Kopeček, J. (2003) Mechanism of cytotoxicity in human ovarian carcinoma cells exposed to free Mce$_6$ or HPMA copolymer–Mce$_6$ conjugates. *Photochem. Photobiol.*, **77**, 645–652.
46. Panté, N. and Kann, M. (2002) Nuclear pore complex is able to transport macromolecules with diameters of about 39 nm. *Mol. Biol. Cell*, **13**, 425–434.
47. Paine, P.L., Moore, L.C., and Horowitz, S.B. (1975) Nuclear envelope permeability. *Nature*, **254**, 109–114.
48. Feldherr, C.M. and Akin, D. (1997) The location of the transport gate in the nuclear pore complex. *J. Cell Sci.*, **110**, 3065–3070.
49. Frey, S., Richter, R.P., and Görlich, D. (2006) FG-rich repeats of nuclear pore proteins form a three-dimensional meshwork with hydrogel-like properties. *Science*, **314**, 815–817.
50. Bohdanecký, M., Bažilová, H., and Kopeček, J. (1974) Poly[N-(2-hydroxypropyl)methacrylamide]. II. Hydrodynamic properties of dilute solutions. *Eur. Polym. J.*, **10**, 405–410.
51. Koňák, Č., Kopečková, P., and Kopeček, J. (1992) Photoregulated association of N-(2-hydroxypropyl)methacrylamide copolymers with azobenzene containing side-chains. *Macromolecules*, **25**, 5451–5456.
52. Kopeček, J., Kopečková, P., and Koňák, Č. (1997) Biorecognizable polymers: design, structure, and bioactivity. *J. Macromol. Sci. Pure Appl. Chem.*, **A34**, 2103–2117.
53. Shiah, J.G., Koňák, Č., Spikes, J.D., and Kopeček, J. (1997) Solution and photoproperties of N-(2-hydroxypropyl)methacrylamide copolymer–meso-chlorin e$_6$ conjugates. *J. Phys. Chem.*, **B101**, 6803–6809.
54. Shiah, J.G., Koňák, Č., Spikes, J.D., and Kopeček, J. (1998) Influence of pH on aggregation and photoproperties of N-(2-hydroxypropyl)methacrylamide copolymer–meso-chlorin e$_6$ conjugates. *Drug Deliv.*, **5**, 119–126.
55. Ulbrich, K., Koňák, Č., Tuzar, Z., and Kopeček, J. (1987) Solution properties of drug carriers based on poly[N-(2-hydroxypropyl)methacrylamide] containing biodegradable bonds. *Makromol. Chem.*, **188**, 1261–1272.
56. Noda, T. and Morishima, Y. (1999) Hydrophobic association of random copolymers of sodium 2-(acrylamido)-2-methylpropanesulfonate and dodecyl methacrylate in water as studied by fluorescence and dynamic light scattering. *Macromolecules*, **32**, 4631–4640.
57. Nagayama, T., Hashidzume, A., and Morishima, Y. (2002) Characterization of self-association in water of polycations hydrophobically modified with hydrocarbon and siloxane chains. *Langmuir*, **18**, 6775–6782.
58. Sparr, E., Ash, W.L., Nazarov, P.V., Rijkers, D.T., Hemminga, M.A., Tieleman, D.P., and Killian, J.A. (2005) Self-association of transmembrane alpha-helices in model membranes: importance of helix orientation and role of hydrophobic mismatch. *J. Biol. Chem.*, **280**, 39324–39331.
59. Itaka, K., Harada, A., Nakamura, K., Kawaguchi, H., and Kataoka, K. (2002) Evaluation of fluorescence resonance energy transfer of the stability of nonviral gene delivery vectors under physiological conditions. *Biomacromolecules*, **3**, 841–845.
60. Itaka, K., Harada, A., Yamasaki, Y., Nakamura, K., Kawaguchi, H., and Kataoka, K. (2004) In situ single cell observation of fluorescence resonance energy transfer reveals fast intra-cytoplasmic delivery and easy release of plasmid DNA complexed with linear polyethyleneimine. *J. Gene Med.*, **6**, 76–84.
61. Ding, H., Prodinger, W.M., and Kopeček, J. (2006) Two-step fluorescence screening of

CD21-binding peptides with one-bead one-compound library and investigation of binding properties of N-(2-hydroxypropyl)methacrylamide copolymer-peptide conjugates. *Biomacromolecules*, **7**, 3037–3046.

62. Pan, H., Kopečková, P., Wang, D., Yang, J., Miller, S., and Kopeček, J. (2006) Water-soluble HPMA copolymer–prostaglandin E1 conjugates containing a cathepsin K sensitive spacer. *J. Drug Target.*, **14**, 425–435.

63. Lee, B.S., Fujita, M., Khazenzon, N.M., Wawrowsky, K.A., Wachsmann-Hogiu, S., Farkas, D.L., Black, K.L., Ljubimova, J.Y., and Holler, E. (2006) Polycefin, a new prototype of a multifunctional nanoconjugate based on poly(beta-L-malic acid) for drug delivery. *Bioconjug. Chem.*, **17**, 317–326.

64. Ding, H., Kopečková, P., and Kopeček, J. (2007) Self-association properties of HPMA copolymers containing an amphipathic heptapeptide. *J. Drug Target.*, **15**, 465–474.

65. Ulbrich, K. and Šubr, V. (2010) Structural and chemical aspects of HPMA copolymers as drug carriers. *Adv. Drug Deliv. Rev.*, **62**, 150–166.

66. Fox, M.E., Szóka, F.C., and Fréchet, J.M. (2009) Soluble polymer carriers for the treatment of cancer: the importance of molecular architecture. *Acc. Chem. Res.*, **42**, 1141–1151.

67. Obereigner, B., Burečová, B., Vrána, A., and Kopeček, J. (1979) Preparation of polymerizable derivatives of N-(4-aminobenzenesulfonyl)-N'-butylurea. *J. Polym. Sci. Polym. Symp.*, **66**, 41–52.

68. Chytrý, V., Vrána, A., and Kopeček, J. (1978) Synthesis and activity of a polymer which contains insulin covalently bound on a copolymer of N-(2-hydroxypropyl)methacrylamide and N-methacryloylglycylglycine 4-nitrophenyl ester. *Makromol. Chem.*, **179**, 329–336.

69. Solovskij, M.V., Ulbrich, K., and Kopeček, J. (1983) Synthesis of N-(2-hydroxypropyl)methacrylamide copolymers with antimicrobial activity. *Biomaterials*, **4**, 44–48.

70. Shen, W.-C. and Ryser, H.J.-P. (1981) Cis-aconityl spacer between daunomycin and macromolecular carriers: a model of pH-sensitive linkage releasing drug from a lysosomotropic conjugate. *Biochem. Biophys. Res. Commun.*, **102**, 1048–1054.

71. Chytil, P., Etrych, T., Koňák, Č., Šírová, M., Mrkvan, T., Říhová, B., and Ulbrich, K. (2006) Properties of HPMA copolymer–doxorubicin conjugates with pH-controlled activation: effect of polymer chain modification. *J. Control. Release*, **115**, 26–36.

72. Kopeček, J., Rejmanová, P., and Chytrý, V. (1981) Polymers containing enzymatically degradable bonds 1. Chymotrypsin catalyzed hydrolysis of p-nitroanilides of phenylalanine and tyrosine attached to side-chains of copolymers of N-(2-hydroxypropyl)methacrylamide. *Makromol. Chem.*, **182**, 799–809.

73. Ulbrich, K., Strohalm, J., and Kopeček, J. (1981) Polymers containing enzymatically degradable bonds. 3. Poly[N-(2-hydroxypropyl)methacrylamide] chains connected by oligopeptide sequences cleavable by trypsin. *Makromol. Chem.*, **182**, 1917–1928.

74. Ulbrich, K., Zacharieva, E.I., Obereigner, B., and Kopeček, J. (1980) Polymers containing enzymatically degradable bonds. 5. Hydrophilic polymers degradable by papain. *Biomaterials*, **1**, 199–204.

75. Kopeček, J. (1984) Controlled degradability of polymers – a key to drug delivery systems. *Biomaterials*, **5**, 19–25.

76. Kopeček, J., Cífková, I., Rejmanová, P., Strohalm, J., Obereigner, B., and Ulbrich, K. (1981) Polymers containing enzymatically degradable bonds. 4. Preliminary experiments in vivo. *Makromol. Chem.*, **182**, 2941–2949.

77. Duncan, R., Cable, H.C., Lloyd, J.B., Rejmanová, P., and Kopeček, J. (1983) Polymers containing enzymatically degradable bonds. 7. Design of oligopeptide side-chains in poly[N-(2-hydroxypropyl)methacrylamide] copolymers to promote efficient

degradation by lysosomal enzymes. *Makromol. Chem.*, **184**, 1997–2008.
78. Šubr, V., Kopeček, J., Pohl, J., Baudyš, M., and Kostka, V. (1988) Cleavage of oligopeptide side-chains in *N*-(2-hydroxypropyl)methacrylamide copolymers by mixtures of lysosomal enzymes. *J. Control. Release*, **8**, 133–140.
79. Rejmanová, P., Pohl, J., Baudyš, M., Kostka, V., and Kopeček, J. (1983) Polymers containing enzymatically degradable bonds. 8. Degradation of oligopeptide sequences in *N*-(2-hydroxypropyl)methacrylamide copolymers by bovine spleen cathepsin B. *Makromol. Chem.*, **184**, 2009–2020.
80. Toki, B.E., Cerveny, C.G., Wahl, A.F., and Senter, P.D. (2002) Protease-mediated fragmentation of *p*-amidobenzyl ethers: a new strategy for the activation of anticancer prodrugs. *J. Org. Chem.*, **67**, 1866–1872.
81. Gao, S.-Q., Lu, Z.-R., Petri, B., Kopečková, P., and Kopeček, J. (2006) Colon-specific 9-aminocamptothecin–HPMA copolymer conjugates containing a 1,6-elimination spacer. *J. Control. Release*, **110**, 323–331.
82. Gao, S.-Q., Sun, Y., Kopečková, P., Peterson, C.M., and Kopeček, J. (2009) Antitumor efficacy of colon-specific HPMA copolymer–9-aminocamptothecin conjugates in mice bearing human colon carcinoma xenografts. *Macromol. Biosci.*, **9**, 1135–1142.
83. Johnson, R.N., Kopečková, P., and Kopeček, J. (2009) Synthesis and evaluation of multivalent branched HPMA copolymer-Fab′ conjugates targeted to the B-cell antigen. *Bioconjug. Chem.*, **20**, 129–137.
84. Tang, A., Kopečková, P., and Kopeček, J. (2003) Binding and cytotoxicity of HPMA copolymers to lymphocytes mediated by receptor-binding epitopes. *Pharm. Res.*, **20**, 360–367.
85. Omelyanenko, V., Kopečková, P., Gentry, C., Shiah, J.-G., and Kopeček, J. (1996) HPMA copolymer–anticancer drug–OVTL16 antibody conjugates. 1. Influence of the method of synthesis on the binding affinity to OVCAR-3 ovarian carcinoma cells *in vitro*. *J. Drug Target.*, **3**, 357–373.
86. Cuchelkar, V., Kopečková, P., and Kopeček, J. (2008) Novel HPMA copolymer-bound constructs for combined tumor and mitochondrial targeting. *Mol. Pharm.*, **5**, 696–709.
87. Nori, A. and Kopeček, J. (2005) Intracellular targeting of polymer-bound drugs for cancer chemotherapy. *Adv. Drug Deliv. Rev.*, **57**, 609–636.
88. Muratovska, A., Lightowlers, R.N., Taylor, R.W., Turnbull, D.M., Smith, R.A., Wilce, J.A., Martin, S.W., and Murphy, M.P. (2001) Targeting peptide nucleic acid (PNA) oligomers to mitochondria within cells by conjugation to lipophilic cations: implications for mitochondrial DNA replication, expression and disease. *Nucleic Acids Res.*, **29**, 1852–1863.
89. Callahan, J. and Kopeček, J. (2006) Semitelechelic HPMA copolymers functionalized with triphenylphosphonium as drug carriers for membrane transduction and mitochondrial localization. *Biomacromolecules*, **7**, 2347–2356.
90. Mangelsdorf, D.J., Thummel, C., Beato, M., Herrlich, P., Schutz, G., Umesono, K., Blumberg, B., Kastner, P., Mark, M., Chambon, P., and Evans, R.M. (1995) The nuclear receptor superfamily: the second decade. *Cell*, **83**, 835–839.
91. Williams, S.P. and Sigler, P.B. (1998) Atomic structure of progesterone complexed with its receptor. *Nature*, **393**, 392–396.
92. Rebuffat, A., Bernasconi, A., Ceppi, M., Wehrli, H., Brenz Verca, S., Ibrahim, M., Frey, B.M., Frey, F.J., and Rusconi, S. (2001) Selective enhancement of gene transfer by steroid-mediated gene delivery. *Nat. Biotechnol.*, **19**, 1155–1161.
93. Cuchelkar, V. (2008) Strategies for enhancing the photodynamic effect of *N*-(2-hydroxypropyl)methacrylamide copolymer bound mesochlorin e_6 PhD Dissertation, Department of Bioengineering, University of Utah.

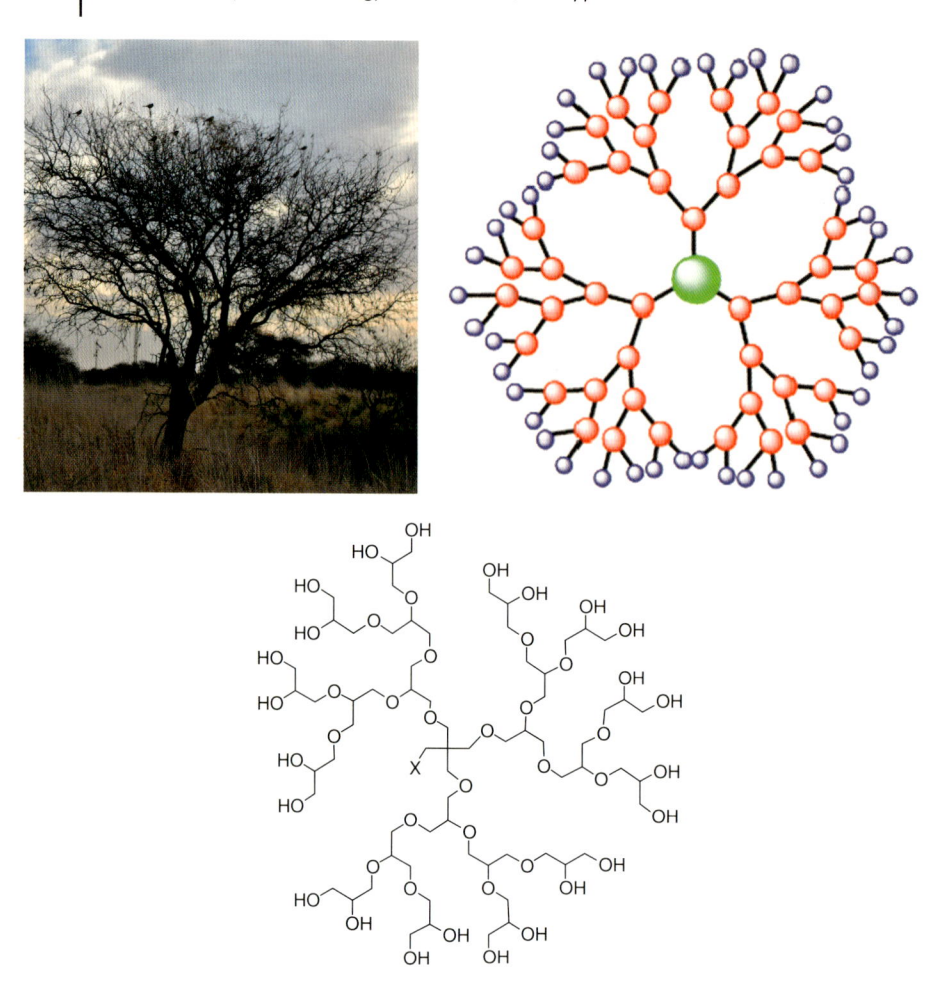

Figure 18.1 Branching as a structural motif: from nature to the molecule of a dendrimer. Reproduced with kind permission from Valeria Albornoz, Merlo (San Luis, Argentina).

and technologies. Such a huge surge in engaging dendrimers in biomedicine stems from several unparalleled biological properties of dendrimers not offered by conventional polymers or self-assembled nanostructures like liposome or micelles. These advantages include rapid cellular passage, higher cell membrane permeability, reduced macrophage activation, and controllable toxicity, along with targetability and adjustable cell-trafficking profile.

The use of dendrimers in medicine mainly follows two major streams, the first one being the utilization of supramolecular voids within dendritic structure to encapsulate guest molecules. Pioneered by the work of Maciejewski [9], this concept led the way toward dendritic nanocarriers, where a wide range of drug molecules are noncovalently attached within the dendritic core [10]. The so-called "unimolecular micelle" or "dendritic box" type architecture has been demonstrated with PAMAM dendrimers, and is often referred to as an "unimolecular micelle" [11, 12]. Following this approach of noncovalent interaction, a wide range of dendritic structures have been used for the delivery of therapeutic agents to intracellular target sites for disease management via oral, topical, ocular, and transdermal routes [13]. A similar concept was adopted for loading the dendrimer molecule with magnetic resonance imaging (MRI) contrast agents and fluorescent dyes for diagnostic purposes.

The other application stream of dendrimers in medicine involves the utilization of Ringsdorf's concept of drug–polymer conjugates utilized upon the dendritic scaffold [14]. The idea involves the attachment of bioactive molecule(s) directly or via spacer molecules to dendrimer terminal groups. The attachments are cellularly hydrolyzable and in most cases ester or amide bonds are employed. To improve therapeutic efficiency, targeting fragments/marker proteins can also be attached to the dendritic scaffold. Thanks to multiple functional group features of dendrimers, it is possible to attach several copies of the same drug, or different drug(s), and targeting fragment upon one carrier molecule.

Owing to the special chemical, physical, and biological features of dendrimers, and their application mechanism as described above, an extensive effort has been made to utilize these special molecules in therapeutic and diagnostic purposes for the treatment of cancer. Frequent challenges confronted by current cancer therapies include nonspecific systemic distribution of antitumor agents, inadequate drug concentrations in tumor tissues, an inadequate ability to monitor therapeutic response, and finally the issue of multidrug resistance due to insufficient concentration of the active agents at the target sites [15].

The application of dendrimers in cancer therapeutics mainly embraces three major fields:

1) Delivery of antineoplastic and contrast agents.
2) Boron neutron capture therapy (BNCT).
3) Photodynamic therapy (PDT).

This chapter deals with the application of dendrimers toward the treatment of cancer. The basic chemical concepts in designing such therapeutic agents, their distinct biological effects, and their mechanism of action will be discussed. The specialized effects displayed by dendritic architectures toward the biological milieu, including cellular uptake, membrane interaction, organelle targeting, and biodistribution, will be emphasized and their applicability in cancer biology will be elaborated.

18.2
Chemistry and Architecture

Synthetically, dendrimers can be prepared by either a divergent or convergent approach, each of which has its own synthetic advantages and limitations. In the divergent method, as pioneered by Tomalia *et al.* [16], dendrimers are synthesized radially from a central core molecule (Figure 18.2, top panel). In this approach, the

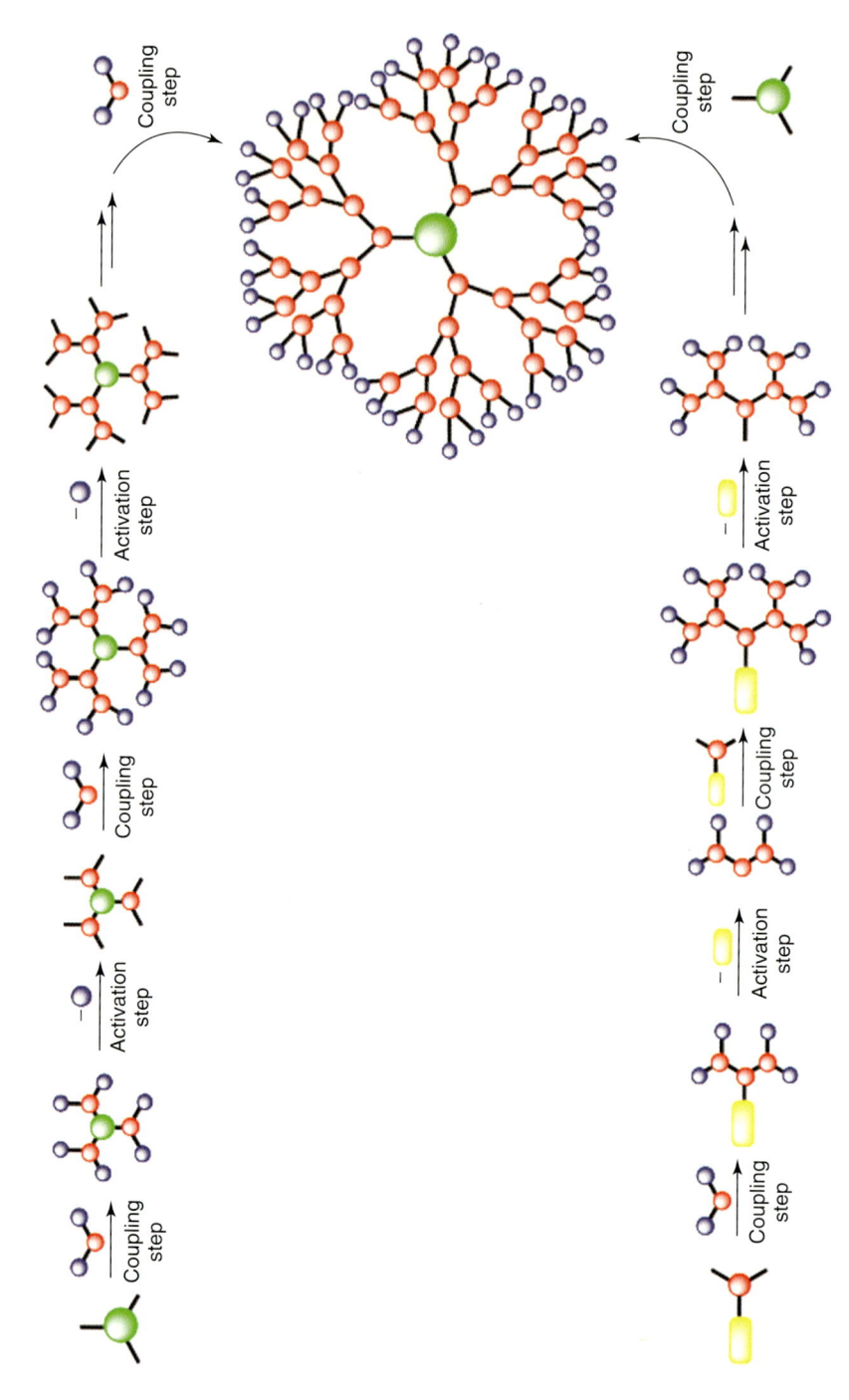

Figure 18.2 Divergent (top) and convergent (bottom) synthesis of dendrimers [17].

dendrimer synthesis takes place through a stepwise layer-by-layer modification that starts from the focal core and builds up the molecule toward the periphery using two basic chemical maneuvers: (i) the building blocks are coupled to the core and (ii) the end-group functionalities of the attached building block are modified for further growth. The divergent approach is strategically straightforward and controllable. Nevertheless, synthesis of high-generation dendrimers is often problematic due to steric effects and purification of the final product is usually difficult.

On the other hand, the convergent method reported by Fréchet and Hawker involves the preferential construction of branched subunits (dendrons), which are then attached to a multifunctional core (Figure 18.2, bottom panel) [4]. The convergent approach overcomes some of the problems associated with the divergent approach, mainly those associated with purification due to a difference of molecular weight between the preformed branches and the core molecule. The major disadvantage of dendrimer synthesis by this method is again the steric crowding. As the dendrimer generation increases, the reactive groups are buried at the focal point of the dendrons and the attachment of the preformed units to the core fragment becomes increasingly difficult.

The branching units of a dendrimer are described by generation. The centrally branched core molecule is designated as generation 0 (G0) and the generation number increases with each successive addition of branching points (Gn). The number of end-groups increases exponentially with each successive generation, resulting in a more globular molecule and linear increment of molecular diameter. Tomalia-type PAMAM dendrimers, which are commercially available, have been investigated heavily for their biomedical applicability. However, various dendrimers of diversified chemical architectures have been synthesized and their biological activity has been explored as presented in Figure 18.3 [8].

The core feature of the application of dendrimers in anticancer therapeutics lies in the fact that each of the structural parameters (i.e., size, molecular shape, end-group functionality, charge density, and basicity of a dendritic molecule) can be controlled to modulate their:

- Nanoscopic size and size-dependent targetability.
- Bioconjugation properties with drugs, signaling fragments, and markers.
- Interaction with cellular membrane, biodistribution, and biocompatibility.

Such structure-dependent activity control can be used as a useful strategy to design and devise efficient dendrimer-based therapeutic agents for cancer management.

18.3
Dendritic Architectures and Oncology: Background and Application

Tissue targeting, selectivity, and effective delivery of antineoplastic agents to the cancer tissues are the primary objectives that define clinical success in cancer treatment [15]. In an ideal scenario, a drug will accumulate in the tumor cells at a

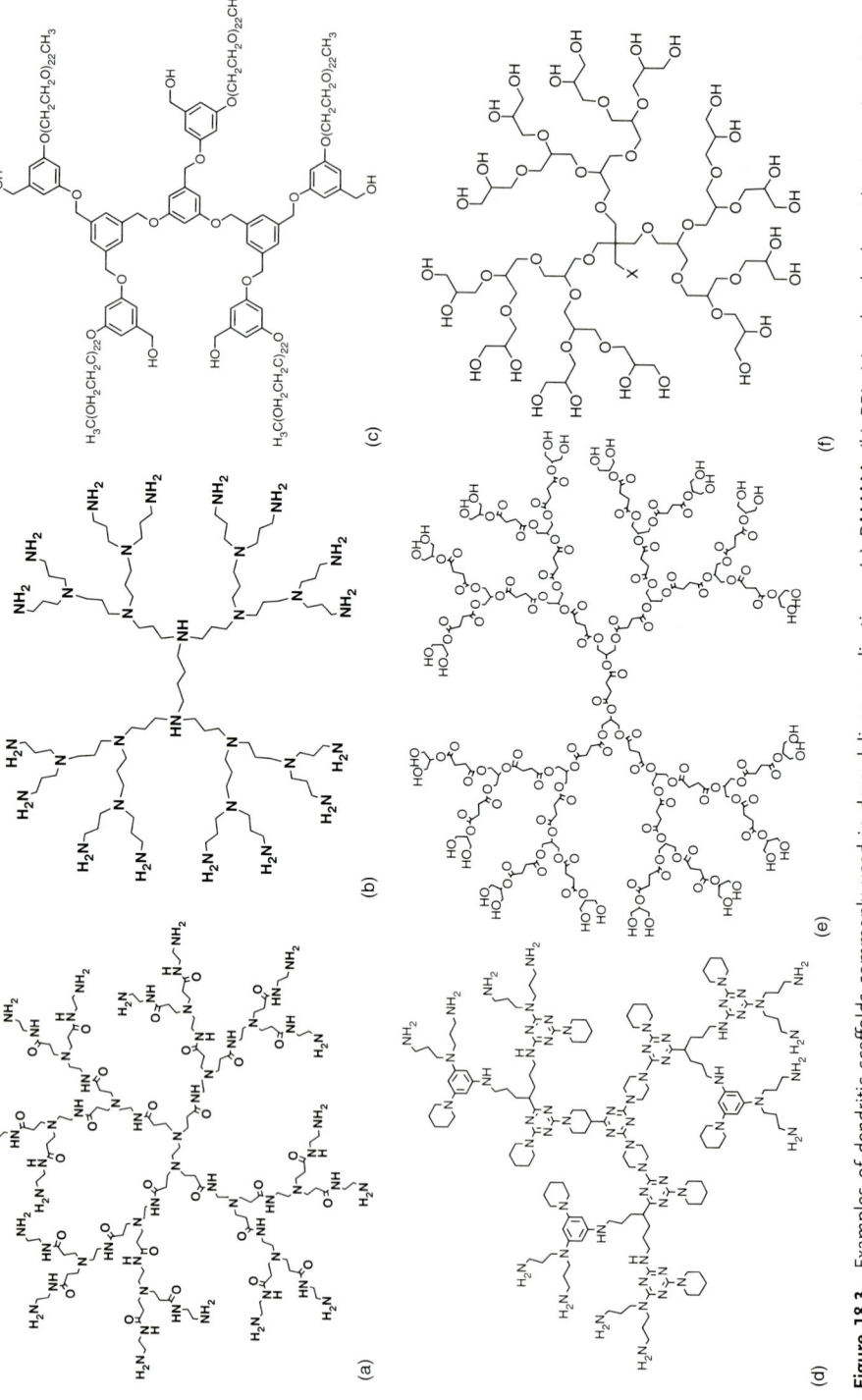

Figure 18.3 Examples of dendritic scaffolds commonly used in drug delivery applications. (a) PAMAM, (b) PPI, (c) polyaryl ether, (d) triazine-based dendrimer, (e) poly(glycerol succinic acid) dendrimer, and (f) polyglycerol dendrimer. (Adapted with permission from [8]. © 2010 Elsevier.)

desired therapeutic concentration with almost no collateral damage to the normal tissues. Most of the anticancer drugs are small molecules with a molecular weight typically within the size range of 200–500 g/mol. One of the major disadvantages of such small-molecular-weight drugs lies in the fact that they rapidly reach their maximum plasma concentration after systemic administration, with apparently no specific selectivity over their volume of distribution. This results in acute to chronic toxicity and nonspecific side-effects, with relatively small therapeutic indices and a high risk/benefit ratio of the treatment. Secondly, rapid biotransformation of small-molecule drugs by drug-metabolizing enzymes in the liver and subsequent removal by excretory systems requires repeated dosing for maintaining steady-state plasma concentration of the antineoplastic. Such frequent drug administration causes further worsening of side-effects and the toxicity-related situation. In the case of cancer diagnostic agents, the problem is associated mainly with selectivity, where a sharp tumor/background ratio is necessary along with a longer residence time of the diagnostic agent in the diseased tissues. Furthermore, systemic circulation of the free drug/contrast agent results in enzymatic deactivation and nonspecific binding to plasma proteins, which substantially affects their pharmacokinetic and bioavailability profile. Another problem associated with conventional anticancer therapy is related to the molecular size of the drug and vasculature properties of tumor blood vessels. While the exact size of molecules that can easily transverse vascular pores from the bloodstream and reach tumor tissue is unclear, it is probably limited to the size of proteins (less than 20 nm). Studies have documented that molecules 100 nm in diameter do not effectively diffuse across the vascular endothelium and even molecules 40 nm in diameter are problematic unless the vasculature is traumatized by radiation or heating [18]. Therefore, it needs a complex interplay between the size and multifunctionality of a drug carrier system, which can load multiple therapeutic agents, and the same time be small enough to exit the vasculature in order to intimately interact with and specifically eliminate the cancer cells.

Dendrimers can offer solutions to these problems by the following mechanisms:

- Anticancer agents can be noncovalently loaded onto dendrimers.
- Anticancer agents can be covalently conjugated to the functional end-groups of a dendritic molecule.
- Dendritic scaffolds can be tailored to respond to the tumor microenvironment.
- Dendrimers can extravasate into the interstitial spaces to promote delivery of the active agent to the vicinity of the tumor site.
- Interaction with cell membrane, intracellular trafficking, and the toxicity profile of a dendrimer entirely depend on its end-group functionality.
- Modifying dendritic end-groups largely affects the pharmacokinetics of the dendrimer and the anticancer cargo loaded onto it.

These highlighted factors will now be discussed with relevant citations to illustrate the techniques and strategies involved in using dendrimers in cancer treatment. Special application of dendrimers in other broad fields of anticancer therapeutics (i.e., BNCT, PDT, and gene therapy) will be discussed separately along with the delivery of diagnostic agents. This chapter will focus on the key concepts prevailing in this area. A number of reviews have already been published in this field where particular and detailed references are available [13, 19–23].

18.3.1
Complexation of Anticancer Agents by Dendritic Architectures

The supramolecular voids formed within the dendritic molecule units can non-covalently harbor anticancer agents (Figure 18.4) [24]. The drug molecules can stabilize themselves within these spaces assembly within the branching fragments through secondary interactions (hydrogen bonding, electrostatic interactions, and dipole–dipole interactions). Such a spontaneous supramolecular self-assembly enables the utilization of dendrimers as a drug delivery vehicle and offers several distinct advantages, such as hydrotropic solubilization of nonpolar drugs in aqueous media and minimization of nonspecific interaction of the complexed drug with plasma components.

Initial work following this principle involved the preparation of fourth-generation poly(glycerol sodium succinate) dendrimer that noncovalently stabilizes 10-hydroxycampothecins, a group of naturally derived anticancer agents. With MCF-7 human breast cancer cell lines, drug-encapsulated dendrimers elicited substantial cytotoxic activity compared to unloaded dendrimers at a comparable concentration [25]. The anticancer drug doxorubicin (DOX) or etoposide has similarly been encapsulated within the dendritic cavities of the star-shaped amphiphilic PAMAM block copolymers containing poly(ε-caprolactone) spacer and poly(ethylene glycol) (PEG) arms [26]. Although the encapsulation efficiency showed polarity dependence, etoposide-loaded dendrimer showed comparable cytotoxic activity in porcine kidney epithelial cell lines relative to unloaded dendrimer.

New dendritic structures have continually been prepared and their noncovalent encapsulation properties toward anticancer agents have been extensively

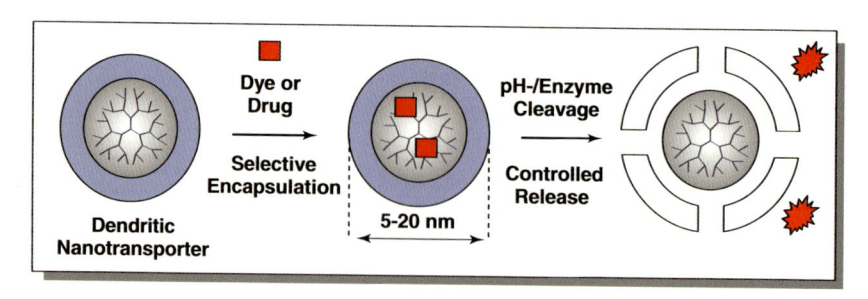

Figure 18.4 Principle of supramolecular drug entrapment within a dendritic structure and further released after an *in vivo* trigger.

investigated. Melamine-based dendrimers were used to encapsulate the anticancer drugs methotrexate (MTX) and 6-mercaptopurene to improve water solubility and decrease toxicity of the active guest. It was found that dendrimer-encapsulated drugs were less hepatotoxic in terms of alanine transaminase levels compared to control to a substantial extent during subchronic dosing in C3H mice [27]. Recently, dextran conjugated poly(propylene imine) (PPI) dendrimers were synthesized and further loaded with DOX. The formulation was tested for *in vitro* drug release, cell uptake, and cytotoxicity studies in A549 cell lines, and for hemolytic activity. The dextran-conjugated dendrimer construct was found to be less hemolytic and more cytotoxic than the free drug. Although the complex showed initial rapid release, the cell uptake studies showed that the drug-loaded dendrimers were preferably uptaken by the tumor cells when compared to free drug [28]. Such dendrimer-stabilized drug delivery systems are straightforward to construct, but suffer from a nonuniform drug release profile that mostly occurs within a short span of time.

Based on this concept, a simple and general method for the generation of core–shell-type architectures from readily accessible dendritic polymers was extensively explored by Haag et al. [29–32]. Several pH-sensitive nanocarriers have been prepared by attaching pH-sensitive shells through acetal or imine bonds to commercially available dendritic core structures, such as polyglycerol and poly(ethylene imine) (PEI). In some cases, the pH-responsive nanocarriers showed a very high transport capacity, which is an important criterion for efficient drug delivery. Various guest molecules, such as polar dyes, oligonucleotides, and anticancer drugs, have been encapsulated inside these dendritic core–shell architectures. Furthermore, an optimal release behavior was observed: fast release at pH 5–6 and slow release at pH 7.4. Among them were several water-soluble systems that localize in tumors *in vivo* as demonstrated by fluorescence imaging in tumor-bearing mice with an indotricarbocyanine–nanocarrier complex.

An effective and easy method for the synthesis of unimolecular micelles was developed by Brooks *et al.* [33]. The obtained structures carried alkyl chains at a polyglycerol core and PEG moieties grafted on the shell. Due to their low intrinsic viscosity, these scaffolds were an extremely promising candidate for human serum albumin substitutes [34]. The encapsulation efficiency was evaluated using paclitaxel and pyrene as model compounds. Fluorescence studies revealed that the hydrophobic molecules are most likely to be located in the hydrophobic pockets of the unimolecular structures. The solubility of paclitaxel in water was increased from 0.3–1 up to 2 mg/ml after encapsulation in the nanocarriers, without any considerable effect on the size of the unimolecular micelles. The release profile was characterized by a rapid-release phase followed by a slower sustained-release phase, reaching 80% of paclitaxel released. Since these structures presented mucoadhesive properties, their complex with paclitaxel was evaluated as an intravesical agent against non-muscle-invasive bladder cancer [35]. Although the encapsulated paclitaxel was slightly less potent than the free drug *in vitro*, the *in vivo* studies in a orthotopic mouse model showed

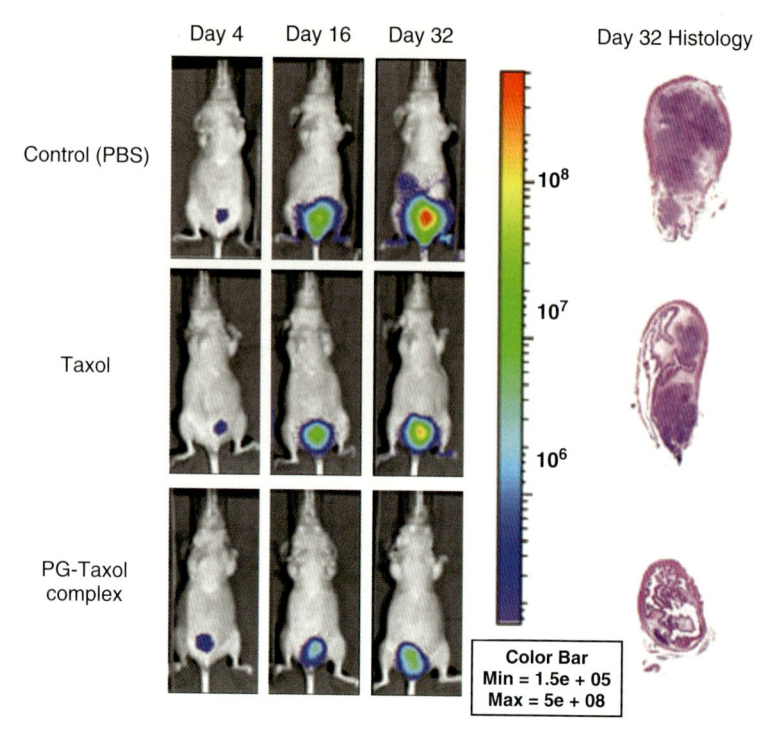

Figure 18.5 *In vivo* evaluation of hydrophobic polyglycerol–paclitaxel complex against orthotopic bladder tumor. (Adapted with permission from [35]. © 2009 Wiley-VCH Verlag GmbH & Co. KGaA.)

that the mucoadhesive formulation of paclitaxel was significantly more effective in reducing orthotopic bladder tumor growth than the standard Cremophor-EL® formulation of paclitaxel (Figure 18.5). Relative tumor growth with the paclitaxel complex was reduced to 15% of the control compared to 66% for the free paclitaxel group. The complex was well tolerated in mice, and the resulting stabilized level of hematuria and body weight with zero mortality indicated no sign of systemic toxicity.

The principle of secondary interaction between the dendritic structure and the guest molecules also operates for delivering genes, oligonucleotides, or metal-complexed therapeutic/contrast agents, the detailed mechanism of which will be discussed separately. For example, organic-coated superparamagnetic iron oxide nanoparticles were transferred from organic media to water using PAMAM dendrimers modified with 6-TAMRA fluorescent dye and folic acid (FA) molecules to form dendrimer-coated superparamagnetic iron oxide nanoparticles (DC-SPIONs). Selective targeting and internalization of the DC-SPIONs to KB cancer cells *in vitro* was observed [36]. Table 18.1 summarizes examples of dendritic systems used in the supramolecular loading and transport of anticancer agents.

Table 18.1 Dendritic polymers used in drug encapsulation.

Dendrimer	Drug, diagnostic probes, or targeting moiety	Cell line	Main finding	References
G4 poly(glycerol sodium succinate)	camptothecins	MCF-7 human breast cancer	cell toxicity	[25]
Star-shaped PAMAM–poly(ε-caprolactone)–PEG	DOX or etoposide	porcine kidney epithelial	improved solubility of lipophilic drugs	[26]
Melamine-based	MTX and 6-mercaptopurene	male C3H mice	improved solubility and decreased hepatotoxicity	[27]
Dextran-conjugated PPI	DOX	A549 cell lines	less hemolytic and more cytotoxic; increased cellular uptake	[28]
Dendritic polyglycerol and PEI	DOX and fluorescence probes	F9 teratocarcinoma	fast release at pH 5–6 and slow release at pH 7.4, which localize in tumors *in vivo*	[29–32]
Dendritic polyglycerol–alkyl chains–PEG	paclitaxel	orthotopic bladder tumor	4.5-fold reduction in relative tumor growth as compared with the free drug	[35]
PAMAM-coated SPIONs	6-TAMRA fluorescent dye and FA	KB cancer cells	selective targeting and internalization	[36]

18.3.2
Anticancer Agents can be Chemically Conjugated with Dendrimer Functional Groups

Peripheral end-groups of a dendrimer can be used as points of attachment to couple anticancer drugs to a dendritic scaffold. Following Ringsdorf's idea of polymer–drug conjugates, not only the active, but also the targeting fragment and/or solubilizing moiety can be linked to the carrier molecule to confer a multifunctional drug delivery platform of dendritic origin. The key principle in designing this conjugate lies in the fact that multiple copies of the same or different drug molecules can be attached to each dendrimer molecule by classical coupling reactions between the orthogonal and complementary functional groups of the two species. Release kinetics of the active agents from the dendrimer is largely governed by the chemical linkage by which the drug is coupled. In most of the cases, the linkage is of ester or amide type [37, 38]. However, a wide range of linking chemistry is used that is responsive to the tumor microenvironment. In addition to ester or amide types, drugs are also linked to the dendritic scaffold through hydrazone, imine, carbamate, disulfide, carbazate bonds, and enzymatically cleavable peptide sequences.

Substantial research has been directed to forming anticancer drug conjugates with dendrimers (Table 18.2), the driving force of which is to make a more stable and synthesis of linking segments and utilizing novel dendritic architecture. The work involves the synthesis of triazine-based dendrimers where the anticancer drug paclitaxel was linked by acylation of 2-hydroxyl group and also contains disulfide linkages. Installation of the paclitaxel group relies on reacting 12 primary amines of a G2 triazine dendrimer with a dichlorothiazine bearing the drug. The dichlorothiazine group was again generated by (i) reacting paclitaxel with glutaric anhydride, (ii) activating with N-hydroxysuccinimide (NHS), (iii) treating the resulting ester with either 1,3-diaminopropane or cystamine, and (iv) finally reacting with cyanuric chloride. The conjugate was finally PEGylated and the constructs were tested for their cytotoxicity in PC-3 prostate cancer cells. The IC_{50} values were found to be in the low nanomolar range with dithiothreitol and glutathione enhancing the toxicity of the disulfide-containing constructs [46].

A novel polymer conjugate of camptothecin using a core-functionalized, symmetrically PEGylated poly(L-lysine) (PLL) dendrimer was synthesized. This PEGylated scaffold consisted of a lysine dendrimer functionalized with aspartic acid, which was used as an attachment site for PEG and camptothecin. The molecular weight of the conjugate was in the range of 40 kDa, containing 4–6 wt% camptothecin. The dendrimer-bound camptothecin showed substantially prolonged blood circulation time and high tumor uptake. Compared to control, the PEGylated lysine-based dendrimer also manifested superior efficacy in murine (C26) and human colon carcinoma (HT-29) as evident with higher survival rates of the tumor-inflicted mice in both cases [47].

18.3.3
Tumor Microenvironment and Attachment of Targeting Moiety to the Dendrimer

The tumor microenvironment can be intelligently used to improve selective drug accumulation within cancer tissues by modification of either the active drug or its carrier. Hyperproliferative cancer cells have marked and observable effects on their surrounding microenvironment. Tumors are evolved to perform hypoxic metabolism to obtain extra energy, resulting in an acidic microenvironment. In addition, cancer cells overexpress and release some enzymes and/or marker proteins that are crucial for tumor migration, invasion, and metastasis. These enzymes or proteins comprise a broad range of signature compounds, including FA, biotin, and matrix metalloproteinases (MMPs) specific for a particular cancer type [50].

Secondly, angiogenesis is crucial to tumor progression and angiogenic blood vessels in tumor tissues, unlike those in normal tissues, have gaps as large as 600–800 nm between adjacent endothelial cells [51, 52]. This defective vascular architecture coupled with poor lymphatic drainage is a well-established factor for attaining passive targeting of antineoplastic drugs in the cancer tissues when they are coupled with a macromolecular carrier – the phenomena widely known as the enhanced permeation and retention (EPR) effect [51, 53]. Intelligent utilization of the tumor microenvironment along with engineering of the dendritic nanostructure can be of importance in increasing specific accumulation of drugs within the tumor tissues (Figure 18.8) [14, 54].

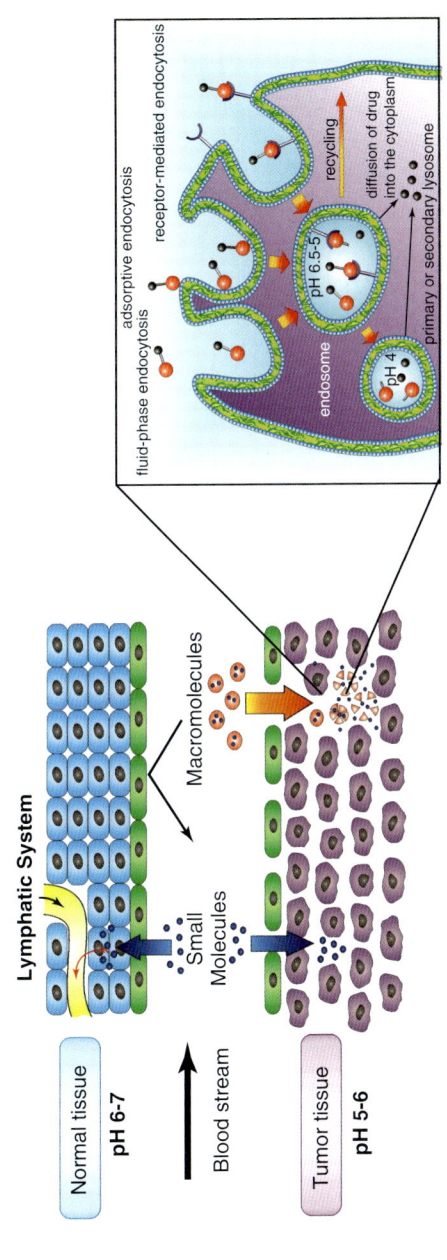

Figure 18.8 Schematic representation of the loose vasculature of tumor tissue – the "EPR" effect.

Table 18.3 Dendritic polymers used in combination with targeting modalities.

Dendrimer	Drug, diagnostic probes, or targeting moiety	Cell line	Main finding	References
PEGylated PAMAM	^{99m}Tc, FA	KB cancer cells	higher uptake and substantial accumulation in tumor area	[59]
G5 PAMAM	FA, fluorescein, and MTX or paclitaxel	KB cancer cells	general proof of FA targeting in vitro and in vivo	[60–62]
G5 PAMAM	FGFR	cell lines expressing FGFR	used in cancer, wound healing, or angiogenesis	[72]
G4 PAMAM	biotin	ovarian cancer (OVCAR-3)	Cellular uptake was substantially higher	[64, 65]
G5 PAMAM	LHRH	–	–	[68]
G5 PAMAM	mAb cetuximab, MTX	EGFR-expressing rat glioma cell line F98(EGFR)	potential benefit from using EGFR in vitro	[73]
G5 PAMAM	anti-prostate-specific membrane antigen (PSMA)	PMSA-positive (LNCaP.FGC) cells	unconjugated dendrimer was not taken up by cells	[75]
G6 lysine	humanized mAb, trastuzumab	HER2-positive (SKBR3)	specifically bound to SKBR3 cells in a dose-dependent manner	[77]
G5 PAMAM	PhiPhiLux G1D2, FA	Jurkat	5-fold increase in intracellular fluorescence	[63]
DOTA-conjugated mono-, di-, and tetravalent dendrimeric alkynes	cRGDs	human umbilical vein endothelial cells	$\alpha_v\beta_3$ integrin targeting	[69, 70]
PEPE	D-glucosamine, MTX	U87 MG and U343 MGa	enhanced endocytosis and increased BBB permeability	[80]

Active targeting of an anticancer agent to the site of tumor is realized by attaching different targeting moieties/cancer signature molecules to the multiple functional groups present within the dendritic carrier (examples described in Table 18.3). In most of the cases, these targeting moieties include the endogenous molecules that are highly demanded or analogs for receptors that are overexpressed in the tumor tissues, such as FA, biotin, proteins like transferrin, or specific markers like monoclonal antibodies (mAbs), MMPs or peptides. A general schematic illustration of the concept of ligand targeted application of dendrimers is shown in Figure 18.9.

On the other hand, nonspecific or passive targeting of tumors is usually achieved by increasing the hydrodynamic radius of the dendrimer through PEGylation or cross-linking, or by simply creating larger carrier molecules, leading to the accumulation of dendrimers in tumor tissue by the EPR effect. EPR has been widely used to achieve passive tumor localization of macromolecular anticancer agents to angiogenic solid tumors. The intravenous injection of platinate conjugate with G3.5 PAMAM dendrimer resulted in an approximately 50-fold increase in selectively targeting platinum reagents to subcutaneous B16F10 tumors compared to intravenous administration of cisplatin at its maximum tolerated dose in C57 [48].

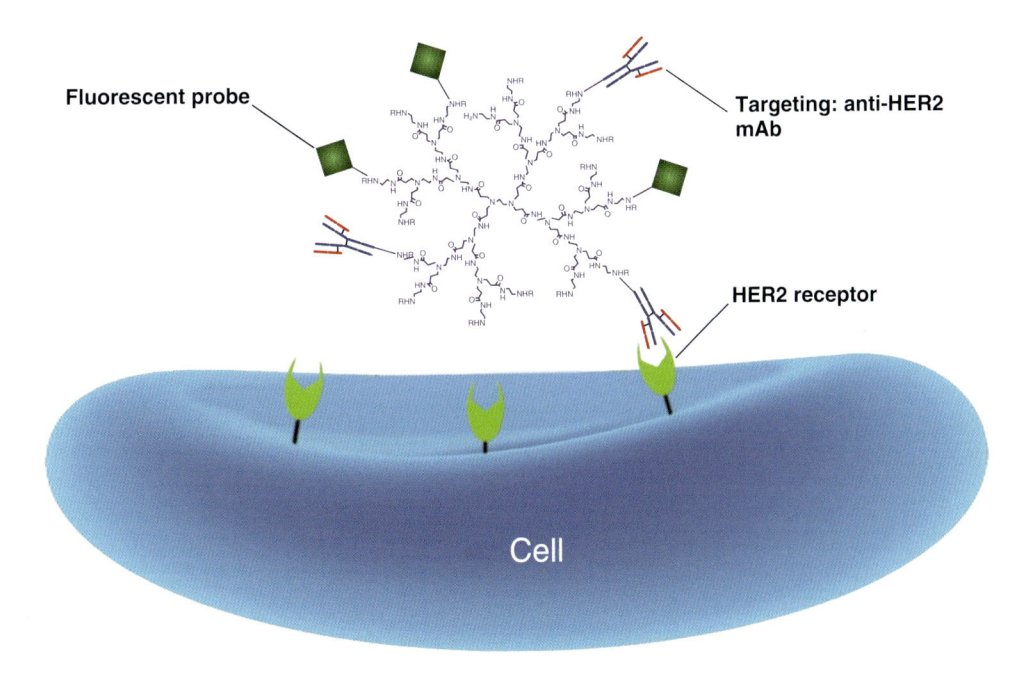

Figure 18.9 Ligand-targeted approach for targeted delivery. The ligand used is anti-HER2 mAb. A fluorescent probe is used for visualization of target binding. (Adapted with permission from [20]. © 2008 Elsevier. The lengh scale of the elements in the figure is schematic and does not represents the reality.)

One of the mostly studied targeting fragments is FA. Reports show that FA-conjugated dendrimers preferentially target tumor cells that overexpress FA receptors (FARs) [55–58]. Hong et al. reported 5-fold augmentation of binding avidity of FAR-overexpressing cells toward multivalent targeted G5 PAMAM containing different numbers of FA molecules. It was suggested that aggregates of five to six FARs are preassembled on the membrane and the enhanced residence time of the FA-containing PAMAM on the cell surface has been considered as the key feature of such observation. Very recently, ^{99m}Tc-labeled PEGylated PAMAM dendrimer conjugated to FA has been subjected to cell-uptake and micro-single photon emission computed tomography (micro-SPECT) imaging studies. The cell-uptake experiment showed a much higher uptake of the radiolabeled conjugate in FAR-positive KB cells and substantial accumulation in the tumor area [59].

The Baker group thoroughly and systematically investigated the effect of FA conjugation on active targeting. In one of their primary studies, PAMAM dendrimers were conjugated to FA, fluorescein, and MTX, and investigated *in vitro* against KB cells [60]. Antiproliferative activity was observed that was slightly lower for the dendrimer–drug conjugates compared to free MTX. Binding to KB cells was found to be dose-dependent. Targeting was diminished yet still significant against KB cells underexpressing FARs and surprisingly the drug dendrimer complex became ineffective when the cells were pretreated with FA. The cytotoxicity and specificity of dendrimer–FA and –MTX were characterized by a novel "coculture assay" in which FAR-positive and -negative cells were cultured together, and preferential killing of the former was observed. The coculture experiment showed cytotoxicity and specific killing of FAR-positive cells by dendritic conjugate [61]. A similar principle seems to be operating with FA, fluorescein, and paclitaxel conjugated to partially acetylated PAMAM dendrimer [62]. Again, FA targeting occurred, preferentially delivering paclitaxel-conjugated dendrimers to KB cells. Internalization was not detected when dendrimers were exposed to KB cells in which the expression of the FAR was downregulated.

The apoptotic sensor PhiPhiLux G1D2 was conjugated to multifunctional FA-targeted PAMAM delivery vehicles in order to detect the extent of apoptosis or cell killing caused by a delivered antiproliferative agent [63]. PhiPhiLux G1D2 is a caspase-specific fluorescence resonance energy transfer (FRET)-based agent that responds to the release of the apoptosis-inducing agent, staurosporine. The internalization of the conjugated dendrimers occurred within the first 30 min of incubation with Jurkat cells and upon apoptosis, and a 5-fold increase in intracellular fluorescence was detected, demonstrating the potential of chemotherapeutic delivery as well as monitoring cell-killing efficacy *in vivo*.

Biotin is another essential micronutrient for cell survival and its level is high in rapidly proliferating cancer cells, which implies that if conjugated with a dendritic scaffold, the biotin molecule can contribute to enhanced cancer cell-specific uptake. To this end, PAMAM dendrimers were coupled to biotin using sulfo-NHS-LC-biotin. The effect of generation and the mechanism of cellular uptake of biotin–G4 PAMAM conjugate in OVCAR-3 and human embryonic kidney HEK-293T) cells was determined by fluorescent microscopy and flow cytometry. The cellular uptake of biotin–PAMAM was found to be substantially higher in the OVCAR-3 cells compared to the HEK-293T cells, and biotinylated PAMAM was found to be internalized by biotin receptor-mediated endocytosis and charge-mediated adsorptive endocytosis [64]. Wen *et al.* also observed higher cellular uptake of fluorescein isothiocyanate (FITC) and biotin-conjugated G5 PAMAM into HeLa cells than the conjugate without biotin. The uptake pattern they found was energy- and dose-dependent [65].

Peptides like luteinizing hormone-releasing hormone (LHRH) and cyclic peptides with the RGD (arginine–glycine–aspartate) motif can be used as a targeting fragment to receptors that are overexpressed in the plasma membrane of many types of cancer cells [66, 67]. A dendrimer–peptide conjugate has been synthesized based on G5 PAMAM as a platform and LHRH peptide as a targeting moiety. The conjugate was characterized from a structural and stability point of view [68]. Cyclic (c) RGDs have recently been used quite extensively as another active targeting ligand. cRGDs have been attached to DOTA (1,4,7,10-tetraazacyclododecane-1,4,7,10-tetraacetic acid)-conjugated mono-, di-, and tetravalent dendrimeric alkynes for $\alpha_v\beta_3$ integrin targeting [63]. Binding characteristics were evaluated *in vitro* and *in vivo* in mice with human SK-RC-52 tumors. Biodistribution studies revealed that the tetrameric RGD–dendrimer showed the highest level of tumor targeting [69, 70]. A similar approach has also been reported by Khan *et al.*, who coupled cRGD to G5 PAMAM [71]. The nanodevice specifically binds to the $\alpha_v\beta_3$ integrins, apparently much stronger than the cyclic cRGD peptide itself.

The Baker group also reported for the first time the utilization of fibroblast growth factor (FGF), whose receptor is overexpressed in a wide variety of tumors as an active targeting fragment to be used in cancer, wound-healing, or angiogenesis. Purified recombinant FGF-1 was coupled to a G5 PAMAM dendrimer. The specific binding and internalization of this conjugate labeled with FITC was investigated by flow cytometry and confocal microscopic analysis in cell lines expressing FGF receptor (FGFR). While the binding and uptake of FGF-conjugated dendrimers was completely blocked by excess nonconjugated FGF-1, confocal microscopic analysis showed cytosolic as well as nuclear localization [72].

Green-Church *et al.* constructed a drug delivery vehicle that targeted the epidermal growth factor receptor (EGFR) and its mutant isoform EGFRvIII. The mAb, cetuximab, previously known as C225, which binds to both EGFR and EGFRvIII, was covalently linked via its Fc region to a G5 PAMAM dendrimer containing the cytotoxic drug MTX. Specific binding and cytotoxicity of the bioconjugate were evaluated against the EGFR-expressing rat glioma cell line F98(EGFR). Using a competitive binding assay, it was shown that the bioconjugate retained its affinity for F98(EGFR) cells. Only cetuximab completely inhibited binding of the bioconjugate, which was unaffected by MTX or dendrimer. Cetuximab alone was not cytotoxic to F98(EGFR) cells at the concentration tested, whereas the conjugate shows a decrease in toxicity over that of free MTX.

However, the *in vivo* test did not show the substantial selectivity offered by the dendritic conjugate. Nevertheless, the experiment revealed the potential utilization benefit of using EGFR, at least so far as cell-study-based experiments are concerned [73].

The G5 PAMAM dendrimer was labeled with AlexaFluor® 488 and conjugated to anti-HER2 mAb (Figure 18.9). The binding and internalization of the antibody-conjugated dendrimer to HER2-expressing cells were evaluated by flow cytometry and confocal microscopy. Uniquely, the conjugate demonstrated better cellular uptake and internalization in HER2-expressing cells than with free antibody. The time course of internalization and blocking experiments with free antibody suggests that the rapid and efficient cellular internalization of the dendrimer–antibody conjugate was achieved without alterations in specificity of targeting. Animal studies demonstrated that the conjugate targets HER2-expressing tumors. Similarly, mAb conjugation to PAMAM has evolved as a robust technique for specific targeting of tumor cells that overexpress certain antigens [74–77]. Similarly many other peptides such as the neuropeptide neurotensin and transferrin have also been reported as targeting fragments for peptide-mediated tumor-selective therapy [78, 79].

Targeting fragments of cell-penetrating small molecules have been attached to dendritic molecules to permeate more complicated physiological barriers like blood–brain barriers (BBBs). Therapeutic benefit in glial tumors is often limited due to low permeability of delivery systems across the BBB, drug resistance, and poor penetration into the tumor tissue. In an attempt to overcome these hurdles, polyether-*co*-polyester (PEPE) dendrimers were evaluated as drug carriers for the treatment of gliomas [80]. Dendrimers were conjugated to D-glucosamine as the ligand for enhancing BBB permeability and tumor targeting. The efficacy of MTX-loaded dendrimers was established against U87 MG and U343 MGa cells. Permeability of rhodamine-labeled dendrimers and MTX-loaded dendrimers across the *in vitro* BBB model and their distribution into avascular human glioma tumor spheroids has also been reported. Glucosylated dendrimers were found to be endocytosed in significantly higher amounts than nonglucosylated dendrimers by both cell lines. The IC_{50} of MTX after loading in dendrimers was lower than that of the free MTX, which suggests that loading MTX in PEPE dendrimers increased its potency. A similar higher activity of MTX-loaded glucosylated and nonglucosylated dendrimers was found in the reduction of tumor spheroid size. These MTX-loaded dendrimers were able to kill even MTX-resistant cells, highlighting their ability to overcome MTX resistance. In addition, the amount of MTX transported across the BBB was 3–5 times more after loading in the dendrimers. Glucosylation further increased the cumulative permeation of dendrimers across the BBB and hence increased the amount of MTX available across it. Glucosylated dendrimers distributed throughout the avascular tumor spheroids within 6 h, while nonglucosylated dendrimers could do so in 12 h. The results show that glucosamine can be used as an effective ligand not only for targeting glial tumors, but also for enhanced permeability across BBB.

18.4
Intracellular Trafficking, Cytotoxicity, and Pharmacokinetics of a Dendritic Architecture are Tunable

Translocation of anticancer molecules from the blood vessel to interstitial places through the endothelial cells lining the blood vessels is critically important for enrichment of the tumor site with therapeutic concentrations of the active agent. The phenomenon, otherwise known as "tissue extravasation," is an important structural feature in dendritic architecture, and is essential for high clinical benefit and reduction of the risk of drug resistance. Kitchens et al. systemically studied the influence of size and molecular weight as functions of tissue extravasation for a PAMAM dendrimer series [81]. Extravasation time was found to increase exponentially with an increase in molecular weight and size of the PAMAM dendrimers. The order of extravasation time for PAMAM dendrimers was sequential from G0 to G4 (G0 < G1 < G2 < G3 < G4), G0 having the lowest extravasation time of 143.9 s, while G4 manifested the longest time required for extravasation (422.7 s). The size of the endothelial pores (4–5 nm), molecular size of PAMAM-NH_2 series (1.5–4.5 nm), surface positive charges of the dendrimers, and their interaction with negatively charged cellular glycocalyx may be the originating factors for such an observation [1].

The mechanistic reports from Tomalia et al. and Baker et al., as well as from Kitchen's work group, have revealed several important mechanisms regarding how dendrimers traffic intracellularly, and can be used as guidelines to describe their transport across cell membranes:

- Dendrimers are more effectively translocated across epithelial barriers than their linear water-soluble counterparts [82].
- Charged dendrimers exhibit higher permeability than their neutral analogs, such as those that are hydroxyl-terminated.
- In addition to molecular size, weight, and generation, the translocation is largely affected by the specific cell type and translocation pathway involved [83–85].

By modifying the structure of the dendrimers, it is fairly easy to exercise control over their cellular interaction. For instance, additional branching on the dendritic core can be performed to manipulate tissue extravasation, PEGylation can be executed over the scaffold to increase solubility and hydrodynamic radii, and organic transformation of terminal functional groups can be done to change the charge distribution of dendritic species [86].

In terms of cytotoxicity, large doses of cationic dendrimer-based drug delivery systems are problematic. Since the dendrimers follow transcellular and/or paracellular pathways, the cytotoxicity profile of a dendrimer is closely associated with its bioefficiency. In PAMAM dendrimers, as a corollary to the permeability issue, both anionic and neutral species were found to be substantially less cytotoxic as well as the lower-generation dendrimers (G0–G1) [23, 26, 87]. There are fortunately several intelligent tactics to minimize dendrimer-related cytotoxicity issues. These strategies encompass surface modifications that restrict the size of the conjugates at the nanoscale (particularly below 10 nm), enhancement of rapid renal clearance, and imparting biodegradability of the parent scaffold. Changing these parameters affects bioavailability, biodistribution pattern, and the associated pharmacokinetic profile of the therapeutics as well as the carrier molecule.

Selecting the precise size within the nano range can facilitate passive targeting efficiency by enhancing EPR effects or cancer tissue-specific localization. Baker *et al.* has shown that surface amidation of amine functional groups in PAMAM dendrimers can markedly reduce cytotoxicity of the conjugate [88]. In the case of the Caco-2 cell line, amidation of dendrimer amine surface groups led to a 10-fold reduction in cytotoxicity while retaining desirable transepithelial permeability across the cell layer [82]. A linear relationship between the number of bare amine surface groups and cytotoxicity was observed. Capping the dendrimer end-groups with four chains of PEG 2000 and six chains of lauroyl functionality also led to reduced toxicity of cationic PAMAM (G2–G4) dendrimers toward Caco-2 cells compared to unmodified dendrimers. To improve the charge-dependent toxicity-related issues, positively charged groups are often capped with neutral molecules such as acetyl and glycidol groups or poly(ethylene oxide) chains. It is a well-documented fact that cloaking or masking the dendritic end-groups with suitable functionality can be used as an effective strategy to modulate dendrimer-related cytotoxicity [89].

PEGylation of PAMAM dendrimers has now become a very realistic technique to improve bioavailability and modify dendritic pharmacokinetics. The fabrication of so-called "stealth-type" dendrimers is one of the robust approaches to avoid the macrophage deactivation of the dendritic scaffold bearing anticancer drug. PAMAM dendrimers with a PEG shell attached onto them showed 40% increase in endothelial cell viability after 24 h incubation compared to free PAMAM [90]. PEGylated PAMAM dendrimers with acetylated amines showed 2–9 times less cytotoxicity than non-PEGylated actylated PAMAM [91].

The Simanek group also reported the effect of surface groups on cytotoxicity, hemolysis, and acute *in vivo* toxicity with melamine polymers as drug delivery vehicles [92]. To improve the cytotoxicity profile of unmodified melamine dendrimers, amine, Boc-protected amine, guanidine, carboxylate, sulfonate, phosphonate, and PEGylated G3 melamine dendrimers were synthesized, and investigated for acute toxicity and hemolysis. It was found that positively charged amine and guanidine groups demonstrated dose- and time-dependent hemolytic activity, whereas negatively charged sulfonate, phosphonate, and carboxylate dendrimers resulted in decreased hemolysis only at high concentrations. PEGylated melamine showed minimal activity. In rat liver cells, the PEGylated dendrimers were noncytotoxic, as evidenced by insignificant increases in urea nitrogen or liver enzyme levels.

In an attempt to explore the potential of dendritic polyglycerol systems for the development of effective anticancer drug delivery systems, Haag et al. explored a simple modular approach of preparing polyglycerol–DOX prodrugs, with flexibility for drug loading using an acid-sensitive hydrazone linker and further postmodification with a PEG shell. The resulting drug–polymer conjugates showed optimal properties for *in vitro* and *in vivo* applications because of their high water solubility, appropriate size for passive tumor toxicity, high stability at physiological conditions, pronounced acid-sensitive properties, cellular internalization, and favorable toxicity profile. DOX–polyglycerol conjugates with a high drug-loading ratio clearly showed improved antitumor efficacy over DOX in an ovarian xenograft tumor model (A2780), inducing transient complete remissions and thus demonstrating the potential of developing efficient multifunctional dendritic drug delivery using this modular approach [93].

Finally, Okuda *et al.* reported the biodistribution characteristics of G4, G5, and G6 amino acid dendrimers based on PLL or poly(L-ornithine) and their PEGylated derivatives, and their report illustrates how PEGylation modulated the pharmacokinetics of the dendrimer conjugates [94]. G4, G5, and G6 amino acid dendrimers containing no PEG were all eliminated from circulation within minutes of injection, with accumulation primarily in the liver and kidneys. Larger-generation polymers were accumulated in the liver with subsequent reduction of renal accumulation. PEGylation of the G6 PLL increased blood retention time from minutes to over 24 h with substantially reduced liver accumulation. The two PEGylated G6–lysine dendrimers possessing low (10) or high (around 76) numbers of PEG 5000-Da chains attached to the periphery groups (66 000 versus 396 000 Da) were investigated for EPR-mediated tumor selectivity in normal and tumor-bearing mice [95]. The remaining unmodified end-groups consisted of primary amines. It was observed that the PEGylated derivatives did not accumulate in the kidney. The dendrimer with the highest PEG content accumulated effectively in tumor tissue with enhanced retention in the plasma, while the nonPEGylated lysine dendrimer showed negligible tumor accumulation and rapid clearance, illustrating the proof-of-concept of changing the biodistribution and pharmacokinetic pattern by PEGylation of the dendritic carrier.

18.5
Other Medical Applications of Dendritic Polymers

18.5.1
Photodynamic Therapy

PDT is defined as the activation of a photosensitizing agent with visible or near-IR electromagnetic radiation resulting in the formation of a highly energetic state of the photoactive agent, which upon reaction with oxygen affords a reactive singlet oxygen capable of inducing necrosis and apoptosis in tumor cells [96]. For the last few decades, PDT has been used to reduce tumors, direct cell killing, disrupt tumor blood vessels, and trigger acute inflammatory response, these being the key features of PDT's antitumor mechanism. Dendrimers have been used to deliver PDT agents, and its potential has been investigated utilizing the native properties of target specificity and structural modifiability of dendrimers [97–100].

In one of their recent works, Kataoka *et al.* developed the dendrimer phthalocyanine (DPc)-encapsulated polymeric micelle (DPc/m). The DPc/m induced efficient and unprecedentedly rapid cell death accompanied by characteristic morphological changes such as blebbing of cell membranes when the cells were photoirradiated using a low-power halogen lamp or a high-power diode laser. The DPc/m was found to accumulate in the endo/lysosomes; however, upon photoirradiation, DPc/m might be promptly released into the cytoplasm and photodamage the mitochondria, which was speculated for the enhanced photocytotoxicity of DPc/m. This study also demonstrated that DPc/m showed significantly higher *in vivo* PDT efficacy than clinically used Photofrin (polyhematoporphyrin esters (PHEs)) in mice bearing human lung adenocarcinoma A549 cells. Furthermore, the DPc/m-treated mice did not show skin phototoxicity, which was apparently observed for the PHE-treated mice, under the tested conditions [101].

Nanocapsules of photosensitizers using PEG-attached dendrimers for application to PDT were prepared [99]. Two PEG-attached dendrimers derived from PAMAM and PPI dendrimers (PEG–PAMAM and PEG–PPI) were synthesized, and Rose Bengal and protoporphyrin IX (PpIX) were used as photosensitizers. Results showed that fewer PpIX molecules were encapsulated by both PEG-attached dendrimers than Rose Bengal, but the complexes were more stable under physiological conditions. Furthermore, PEG–PPI held photosensitizers in a more stable manner than PEG–PAMAM because of their inner hydrophobicity. The complex of PpIX with PEG–PPI exhibited efficient cytotoxicity, compared with free PpIX. It was suggested that the cytotoxicity was caused by the high level of singlet oxygen production and the efficient delivery to mitochondria.

18.5.2
Boron Neutron Capture Therapy

The principle of BNCT focuses upon the lethal $^{10}B(n, \alpha)^{7}Li$ capture reaction that occurs when ^{10}B is irradiated with low-energy thermal neutrons to produce high-energy α-particles and ^{7}Li nuclei. The limitation of BNCT lies in the fact that the therapy critically requires sufficient tumor targeting or therapeutic ^{10}B accumulation (around 10^9 atoms/cell) in malignant tissues. To this end, dendritic delivery vehicles have been utilized [102, 103]. The basic architectural design includes the attachment of boron-complexing agent to the dendritic scaffold reinforced for targeting to cancer tissues by attachment of marker molecule/targeting moieties. PAMAM has long been used as the dendritic system of choice for BNCT [104].

Fenstermaker and Wikstrand proposed to evaluate a boronated EGFRvIII-specific mAb, L8A4, for BNCT of the receptor-positive rat glioma, F98(npEGFRvIII) [105]. A heavily boronated PAMAM dendrimer (BD) was conjugated to L8A4 by two heterobifunctional reagents, *N*-succinimidyl 3-(2-pyridyldithio)propionate and *N*-(κ-maleimidoundecanoic acid)hydrazide. For *in vivo* studies, F98 wild-type receptor-negative or EGFRvIII human gene-transfected receptor-positive F98(npEGFRvIII) glioma cells were implanted intracerebrally into the brains of Fischer rats. Animals received ^{125}I-BD–L8A4 by either convection enhanced delivery (CED) or direct intratumoral injection and were euthanized at specific time intervals. At 6 h, equivalent amounts of the bioconjugate were detected in receptor-positive and receptor-negative tumors, but by 24 h the amounts retained by receptor-positive gliomas were 60.1% following CED and 43.7% following intratumoral injection compared with 14.6% ID/g by receptor-negative tumors. Boron concentrations in normal brain, blood, liver, kidneys, and spleen were all at nondetectable levels (below 0.5 µg/g) at the corresponding times. Based on these favorable biodistribution data, BNCT studies were initiated and rats received BD–L8A4 (around 40 µg ^{10}B/750 µg protein) by CED either alone or in combination with intravenous boronophenylalanine (BPA; 500 mg/kg). BNCT was carried out 24 h after administration of the bioconjugate and 2.5 h after intravenous injection of BPA for those animals that received both agents. Rats that received BD–L8A4 by CED in combination with intravenous BPA had a mean survival time of 85.5 days with 20% long-term survivors (greater than six months) and those that received BD–L8A4 alone had a mean survival time of 70.4 days with 10% long-term survivors compared with 40.1 days for intravenous BPA and 30.3 and 26.3 days for irradiated and untreated controls, respectively. These data convincingly show the therapeutic efficacy of molecular targeting of EGFRvIII using either boronated mAb L8A4 alone or in combination with BPA.

Neutron capture therapy (NCT) has also been used for tumor vasculature and micrometastatic lymphatics. Backer *et al.* synthesized boronated G5 PAMAM (BD) with vascular endothelial growth factor (VEGF) and near-IR Cy5 dye (VEGF–BD/Cy5) for targeting upregulated VEGF receptors overexpressed in tumor neovasculature [106]. Accumulation of VEGF–BD/Cy5 was evident in 4T1 mouse breast carcinoma with increased concentrations at the tumor periphery by near-IR imaging compared to BD/Cy5 conjugate. Kobayashi *et al.* investigated gadolinium-labeled PAMAM dendrimers for the delivery of MRI contrast agents that can be also used in NCT to the sentinel lymph node, which is often indicated for breast cancer management [107]. It was found that G6 PAMAM with a particle size of 9 nm produced the earliest and most intense opacification of the sentinel lymph nodes with sufficient gadolinium concentrations for NCT. Conversely, G2 and G4 PAMAM drained out of the lymphatic vessels, while G8 PAMAM is large enough for rapid uptake. Based on these results, it was determined that gadolinium-labeled G6 PAMAM could be a suitable alternative for treatment and diagnostic of primary tumors or micrometastasis in the sentinel lymph nodes.

18.5.3
Diagnostic Application of Dendrimers

Dendrimers have found applications in the field of cancer diagnostics, particularly in MRI techniques. Dendritic molecules are used to encapsulate/complex gadolinium paramagnetic contrast agents for MRI for contrast enhancement, tissue retention, and improved clearance characteristics [55, 108]. Initial work with gadolinium-labeled PAMAM systems has still been used as an attractive system for visualizing tumor location, vasculature, and lymphatic involvement. It was possible to observe changes in tumor vasculature by using gadolinium-labeled G8 PAMAM contrast agents after a single large dose of radiation treatment

18.5.4
Gene Delivery with Dendrimers

With the advent of molecular biology, a large number of diseases are addressed by interfering with the nucleic material of the diseased cells. Such treatment procedure calls for transferring oligonucleotides in the form of small interfering RNA (siRNA) or DNA. The associated treatment limitation is the destruction of therapeutic nucleotides by the systemic environment before they reach the target tissues. Dendrimers have been used to complex these therapeutic oligonucleotides either by electrostatic bonding or supramolecular interaction of noncovalent origin (Figure 18.11). Again, the dendritic carrier can provide 2-fold advantages where it can act as a carrier and, additionally, targeting fragments can be attached to the functional group of the dendrimer to enhance tissue selectivity.

Of the recent works on this topic, ornithine-conjugated G4 PAMAM dendrimers have been prepared, and their gene transfection efficiency and cytotoxicity have been assessed. Ornithine-conjugated G4 PAMAM dendrimers were prepared by Fmoc synthesis. A comparative gene transfection study between G4 PAMAM dendrimers and the surface-modified dendrimers was conducted in HEK-293T, GM7373, and NCI H157G cell lines. Cytotoxicity of the dendriplexes was tested in HEK-293T cells by 3-(4,5-dimethylthiazol-2-yl)-2,5-diphenyltetrazolium bromide (MTT) assay. Structurally, about 60 molecules of ornithine were conjugated to a G4 PAMAM

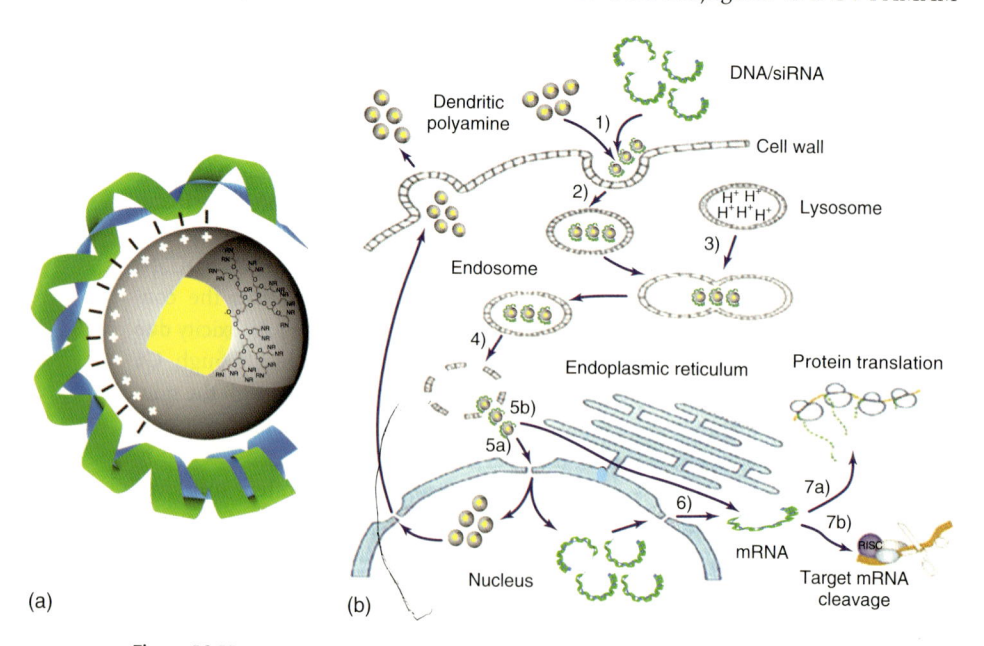

Figure 18.11 (a) Principle of nucleotide binding over a dendritic scaffold and (b) mechanism of DNA/siRNA delivery in the form of a dendriplex.

dendrimer. Preliminary studies indicated that serum does not affect the transfection efficiency of the dendriplexes. Transfection efficiency of PAMAM–ORN60 dendriplexes was slightly higher in cancer cells (NCI H157G) than in HEK-293T cells. Transfection efficiency of the PAMAM–ORN60 dendrimers decreased in the presence of excess of ornithine while there was no effect on the parent G4 PAMAM dendrimers. Cytotoxicity assay has shown that G4 PAMAM–ORN60 dendriplexes at N/P 10 were safe at concentrations equal or less than 50 μg/ml [114].

Haag et al. recently synthesized dendritic polyglycerolamine (polyglycerol-NH_2) with average molecular weight of 10 kDa in an attempt to explore the effects of postmodification of dendritic polyglycerol with primary amines in the favorable 1,2-orientation [115–117]. In a previous study, the polyglycerol-NH_2 architecture, which consists of primary amine groups spread all around the polyglycerol structure, showed promising properties as a prospective system for gene delivery (i.e., high charge with a relative low cytotoxicity and an optimal charge/pH behavior so far as the buffering capacity is concerned) [118]. Of all the polyglycerol systems analyzed for gene transfection [119], dendritic polyglycerol-NH_2 showed the highest affinity toward DNA fragments, according to the ethidium bromide displacement assay. The polymer was able to complex siRNA yielding slightly positive charged globular polyplexes. The knockdown efficiency of the siRNA polyplex was comparable to HiPerFect for the proteins lamin, CDC2, and mitogen-activated protein kinase 2 in HeLAS3 cells. In a comparison of silencing efficiency and cytotoxicity with PEI derivates, the polyglycerol-NH_2 architecture showed a better toxicity profile at concentrations relevant for its activity. It was found that the siRNA polyplex was internalized into glioblastoma cells within 24 h by the endo/lysosome/mediated system. More interestingly, siRNA-polyglycerol-NH_2 polyplex was administered intratumorally or intravenously to tumor-bearing mice, resulting in a major silencing effect and no apparent toxicity (Figure 18.12). High levels of fluorescently labeled siRNA were detected in the tumor and not in other healthy organs examined.

In the case of targeted delivery of antisense oligonucleotides, FA–PAMAM conjugates were prepared. These therapeutic antisense oligonucleotides are designed to inhibit the growth of C6 glioma cells. FA was coupled to the surface amino groups of G5 PAMAM dendrimer through a 1-[3-(dimethylamino) propyl]-3-ethylcarbodiimide bond and the nucleotides corresponding to rat EGFR were then complexed with FA–PAMAM conjugate. At a nucleotide/PAMAM ratio of 16 : 1, agarose electrophoresis indicated that antisense oligonucleotides were completely complexed with PAMAM or FA–PAMAM. The nucleotide transfection rates mediated by FA–PAMAM and PAMAM were superior to oligofectamine, resulting in greater suppression of EGFR expression and glioma cell growth. Stereotactic injection of EGFR antisense oligonucleotide:FA–PAMAM complexes into established rat C6 intracranial gliomas resulted in greater suppression of tumor growth and longer survival time of tumor-bearing rats compared with PAMAM and oligofectamine-mediated EGFR antisense oligonucleotide therapy. The study demonstrated the suitability of FA–PAMAM dendrimer conjugates for efficient EGFR antisense oligonucleotide delivery into glioma cells, wherein they release the

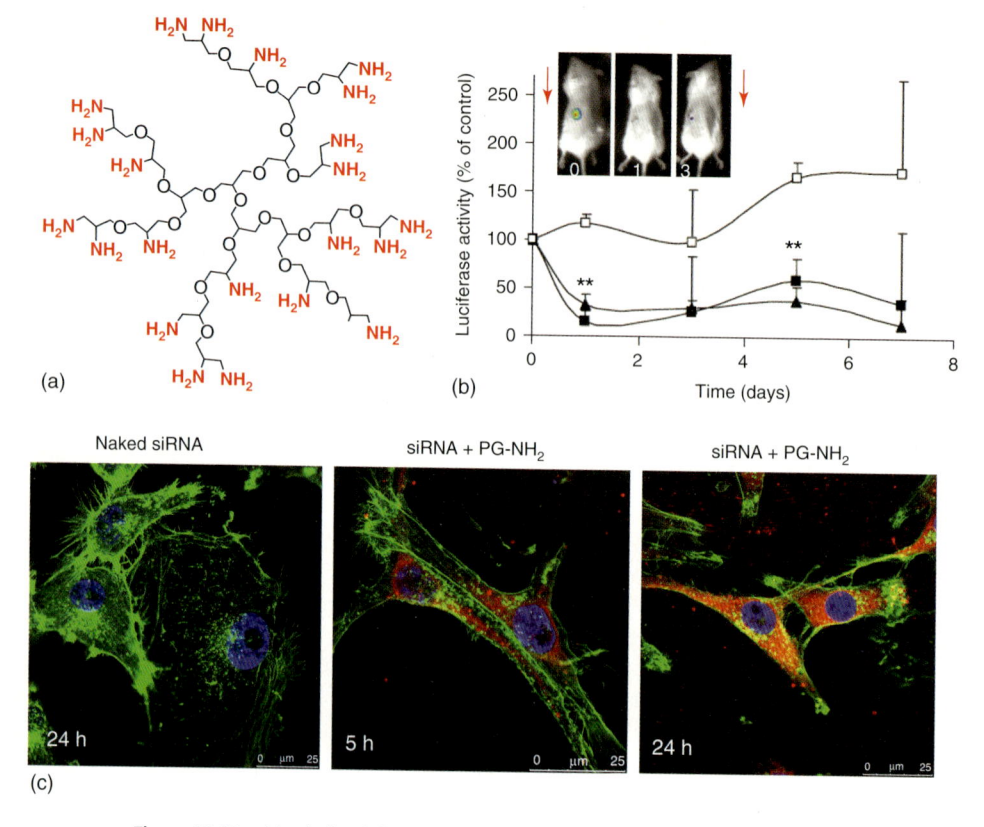

Figure 18.12 (a) Idealized fragment of polyglycerolamine and (b) SCID mice bearing U87-Luc tumors treated with 10 mg/kg polyglycerol-NH$_2$, complexed with 2.5 mg/kg luciferase siRNA (■), 20 mg/kg polyglycerol-NH$_2$, complexed with 5 mg/kg luciferase siRNA (▲), or saline as control (□). (c) siRNA-polyglycerol-NH$_2$ polyplex intracellular uptake. U87-Luc cells were incubated with TRITC-labeled siRNA (red) either alone ("Naked siRNA") or complexed with polyglycerol-NH$_2$ ("siRNA + PG − NH$_2$"). Actin filaments were stained with phalloidin (green). Scale bar = 25 mm. (Adapted with permission from [120]. © 2010 Wiley-VCH Verlag GmbH & Co. KGaA.)

nucleotide from the FA–PAMAM to knockdown EGFR expression in C6 glioma cells, both *in vitro* and *in vivo* [121].

The low penetration ability of siRNA through the cellular plasma membrane combined with its limited stability in blood limits the effectiveness of the systemic delivery of siRNA. In order to overcome such difficulties, a nanocarrier-based delivery system was constructed with PPI dendrimers. To provide lateral and steric stability to withstand the aggressive environment in the bloodstream, the formed siRNA nanoparticles were caged with a dithiol containing cross-linker molecules followed by coating them with PEG. A synthetic analog of LHRH peptide was conjugated to the distal end of the PEG polymer to direct the siRNA nanoparticles specifically to the cancer cells. It was found that this layer-by-layer modification and targeting approach conferred the siRNA nanoparticles stability in plasma and intracellular bioavailability, and provided for their specific uptake by tumor cells, accumulation of siRNA in the cytoplasm of cancer cells, and efficient gene silencing [122].

Structurally flexible triethanolamine core PAMAM dendrimers have been prepared which are able to deliver an Hsp27 siRNA effectively into PC-3 cells by forming stable nanoparticles with siRNA, protecting the siRNA nanoparticles from enzymatic degradation, and enhancing cellular uptake of siRNA. The Hsp27 siRNA resulted in potent and specific gene silencing of heat-shock protein 27, an attractive therapeutic target in castrate-resistant prostate cancer. Silencing of the Hsp27 gene led to induction of caspase-3/7-dependent apoptosis and inhibition of PC-3 cell growth *in vitro*. In addition, the siRNA–dendrimer complexes are noncytotoxic under the conditions used for siRNA delivery and proved to be a promising approach for combating castrate-resistant prostate cancer [123].

18.6
Novel Therapeutic Approaches with Dendrimers

This section deals with novel approaches where the dendritic scaffold itself can be utilized as a therapeutic agent or innovative approaches that are adopted to utilize dendrimers in treatment. Of course, the first kinds that have already entered into phase II human clinical trials are the anionic functionalized PLL dendrimers, commercialized as VivaGel®, developed by Starpharma (Melbourne, Australia). VivaGel is the first dendrimer-based product to receive Fast Track Status from the US Food and Drug Administration under an Investigational New Drug Application for the prevention of genital herpes. A G4 PLL-based dendrimer with naphthalene disulfonic acid surface groups (i.e., SPL7013) is the active ingredient in VivaGel. Another innovative approach is based on the so-called "self-immolative dendrimers" designed by Shabat *et al*. This innovative prodrug concept can open the way to stimuli-responsive dendrimers that release the drug upon activation by specific molecular markers overexpressed in cancer tissues [124].

Activated $\alpha_v\beta_3$ integrin occurs specifically on tumor cells and on endothelial cells of the tumor-associated vasculature and plays a key role in invasion and metastasis. The PHSCN peptide (Ac-PHSCN-NH$_2$) preferentially binds activated $\alpha_v\beta_3$, to block invasion *in vitro* and inhibits growth, metastasis, and tumor recurrence in preclinical models of prostate cancer. In a phase I clinical trial, systemic Ac-PHSCN-NH$_2$ monotherapy was well tolerated and metastatic disease progression was prevented for 4–14 months in one-third of the treated patients. A significantly more potent derivative, the PHSCN-PLL dendrimer, has been prepared [125]. Using *in vitro* invasion assays with naturally serum-free basement membranes, PHSCN dendrimer was found to be 130- to 1900-fold more potent than the PHSCN peptide at blocking $\alpha_v\beta_3$-mediated invasion by DU-145 and PC-3 human prostate cancer cells. The PHSCN dendrimer was also approximately 800 times more effective than PHSCN peptide at preventing DU-145 and PC-3 extravasation in the lungs of athymic mice. A single pretreatment with the PHSCN dendrimer was 100-fold more affective than the PHSCN peptide at reducing lung colony formation. Since many patients newly diagnosed with prostate cancer already have locally advanced or metastatic disease, the availability of a well-tolerated, nontoxic systemic therapy, like the PHSCN dendrimer, which prevents metastatic progression by inhibiting invasion, could be very beneficial. The PHSCN dendrimer is also found to be useful in the treatment of breast cancer [126].

Tumors frequently contain hypoxic regions that result from a shortage of oxygen due to poorly organized tumor vasculature. Cancer cells in these areas are resistant to radiation and chemotherapy, limiting the treatment efficacy. Macrophages have inherent hypoxia-targeting ability and are therefore very advantageous for targeted delivery of anticancer therapeutics to cancer cells in hypoxic areas. However, most anticancer drugs cannot be directly loaded into macrophages because of their toxicity. A novel drug delivery vehicle hybridizing macrophages with nanoparticles through cell surface modification has been reported with PAMAM dendrimer scaffolded nanoparticles. Nanoparticles immobilized on the cell surface provide numerous new sites for anticancer drug loading, hence potentially minimizing the toxic effect of anticancer drugs on the viability and hypoxia-targeting ability of the macrophage vehicles. 5-(Aminoacetamido) fluorescein-labeled G4.5 PAMAM dendrimer, both of which were coated with amine-derivatized PEG, were immobilized to the sodium periodate-treated surface of macrophages through a transient Schiff base linkage. Furthermore, a reducing agent, sodium cyanoborohydride, was applied to reduce Schiff bases to stable secondary amine linkages. The distribution of nanoparticles on the cell surface was confirmed by fluorescence imaging and it was found to be dependent on the stability of the linkages coupling nanoparticles to the cell surface [127].

The Baker group has studied the utilization of dendrimers on carbon nanotubes (CNTs), which hold great promise for their use as a platform in nanomedicine, especially in drug delivery, medical imaging, and cancer targeting and therapeutics. The group reported a facile approach for modifying CNTs with multifunctional G5 PAMAM dendrimers for cancer cell targeting and imaging. In this approach, FITC and FA-modified amine-terminated G5 PAMAM dendrimers were covalently linked to acid-treated multiwalled CNTs (MWNTs), followed by acetylation of the remaining primary amine groups of the dendrimers. The resulting MWNT/dendrimer composites are water-dispersible, stable, and biocompatible. *In vitro* flow cytometry and confocal microscopy data show that the formed composites can specifically target to cancer cells overexpressing high-affinity FARs. The results of this study suggest that, through modification with multifunctional dendrimers, complex CNT-based materials can be fabricated, thereby providing many possibilities for various applications in biomedical sensing, diagnosis, and therapeutics [128]. These newer architectures have not only paved the way toward designing novel molecular structures, but also demonstrate the potential of congregating different areas of biological and chemical sciences for designing therapeutic scaffolds for anticancer therapy.

18.7
Conclusions

This chapter covers the basic features of dendritic architectures that make them a specifically applicable new platform for cancer diagnosis and therapy. A complex array of biochemical and pathological parameters and resultant innovative therapeutic tools and techniques are needed to devise new cancer therapeutics. The new molecular scaffolds of dendritic macromolecules can be used to provide novel approaches for cancer treatment. For commercialization of dendritic architectures for anticancer drug delivery, a prime requirement is the standardization of the synthesis and conjugation techniques. Up to now, the major limitation in utilizing dendrimers in the clinical setup has been due to their synthetic and characterization protocol. Although low-molecular-weight dendrimers are easy to prepare and characterize, dendrimers with increasingly high generation numbers and molecular weights are more complex. In addition, drug-loaded dendrimers suffer from issues associated with a precise release of the active molecule. In spite of accelerated efforts to add targeting efficiency to dendrimer based drug-delivery systems, it is still difficult to specifically target such delivery systems to affected tissues. Dendrimer biopharmacokinetics, toxicity, and immunogenicity have not yet been fully explored, not to mention their impact on the environment and ecology. Despite these technical limitations, several dendrimer-based scaffolds have already made their way to clinical trials. Novel coupling methodologies and orthogonal synthetic procedures to design dendritic scaffolds of diversified architectures have been developed and investigated. Converging with new findings in cancer biology, newer markers and targets are being discovered and attached onto dendrimers to attain tissue specificity. Nonetheless, extensive biomedical evaluation still remains one of the most critically important parameters for the translation of dendritic scaffolds from the laboratory to the clinic.

Acknowledgments

We thank Dr. Pamela Winchester for proofreading and Mr. Diego Galliari for graphical support.

References

1. Menjoge, A.R., Kannan, R.M., and Tomalia, D.A. (2010) *Drug Discov. Today*, **15**, 171.
2. Buhleier, E., Wehner, W., and Vogtle, F. (1978) *Synthesis*, 155.
3. Newkome, G.R., Yao, Z.-Q., Baker, G.R., and Gupta, V.K. (1985) *J. Org. Chem.*, **50**, 2003.
4. Hawker, C.J. and Frechet, J.M.J. (1990) *J. Am. Chem. Soc.*, **112**, 7638.
5. Worner, C. and Muhlhaupt, R. (1993) *Angew. Chem. Int. Ed. Engl.*, **105**, 1367.
6. De Brabander-van den Berg, E.M.M. and Meijer, E.W. (1993) *Angew. Chem. Int. Ed. Engl.*, **105**, 1370.

75. Patri, A.K., Myc, A., Beals, J., Thomas, T.P., Bander, N.H., and Baker, J.R. Jr. (2004) *Bioconjug. Chem.*, **15**, 1174.
76. Chang, S.S., O'Keefe, D.S., Bacich, D.J., Reuter, V.E., Heston, W.D., and Gaudin, P.B. (1999) *Clin. Cancer Res.*, **5**, 2674.
77. Miyano, T., Wijagkanalan, W., Kawakami, S., Yamashita, F., and Hashida, M. (2010) *Mol. Pharm.*, **7**, 1318.
78. Koppu, S., Oh, Y.J., Edrada-Ebel, R., Blatchford, D.R., Tetley, L., Tate, R.J., and Dufès, C. (2010) *J. Control. Release*, **143**, 215.
79. Falciani, C., Fabbrini, M., Pini, A., Lozzi, L., Lelli, B., Pileri, S., Brunetti, J., Bindi, S., Scali, S., and Bracci, L. (2007) *Mol. Cancer Ther.*, **6**, 2441.
80. Dhanikula, R.S., Argaw, A., Bouchard, J.F., and Hildgen, P. (2008) *Mol. Pharm.*, **5**, 105.
81. Kitchens, K.M. (2005) *Adv. Drug Deliv. Rev.*, **57**, 2163.
82. Kolhatkar, R.B. (2007) *Bioconjug. Chem.*, **18**, 2054.
83. Kitchens, K.M. (2008) *Mol. Pharm.*, **5**, 364.
84. Perumal, O.P. (2008) *Biomaterials*, **29**, 3469.
85. Saovapakhiran, A. (2009) *Bioconjug. Chem.*, **20**, 693.
86. Fox, M.E., Szoka, F.C., and Frechet, J.M. (2009) *Acc. Chem. Res.*, **42**, 1141.
87. Hong, S., Leroueil, P.R., Janus, E.K., Peters, J.L., Kober, M.M., Islam, M.T., Orr, B.G., Baker, J.R. Jr., Banaszak Holl, M.M. (2006) *Bioconjug. Chem.*, **17**, 728.
88. Kukowska-Latallo, J.F. (2005) *Cancer Res.*, **65**, 5317.
89. Jevprasesphant, R. (2003) *Int. J. Pharm.*, **252**, 263.
90. Yang, H. (2008) *J. Mater. Sci. Mater. Med.*, **19**, 1991.
91. Kim, Y. (2008) *Bioconjug. Chem.*, **19**, 1660.
92. Chen, H.T., Neerman, M.F., Parrish, A.R., and Simanek, E.E. (2004) *J. Am. Chem. Soc.*, **126**, 10044.
93. Calderon, M., Welker, P., Licha, K., Graeser, R., Fichtner, I., Haag, R., Kratz, F. (2011) *J. Control. Release*, **151**, 295, [Epub ahead of print].
94. Okuda, T., Kawakami, S., Maeie, T., Niidome, T., Yamashita, F., and Hashida, M. (2006) *J. Control. Release*, **114**, 69.
95. Okuda, T., Kawakami, S., Akimoto, N., Niidome, T., Yamashita, F., and Hashida, M. (2006) *J. Control. Release*, **116**, 330.
96. Triesscheijn, M., Baas, P., Schellens, J.H., and Stewart, F.A. (2006) *Oncologist*, **11**, 1034.
97. Nishiyama, N., Stapert, H.R., Zhang, G.D., Takasu, D., Jiang, D.L., Nagano, T., Aida, T., and Kataoka, K. (2003) *Bioconjug. Chem.*, **14**, 58.
98. Battah, S.H., Chee, C.E., Nakanishi, H., Gerscher, S., MacRobert, A.J., and Edwards, C. (2001) *Bioconjug. Chem.*, **12**, 980.
99. Kojima, C., Toi, Y., Harada, A., and Kono, K. (2007) *Bioconjug. Chem.*, **18**, 663.
100. Battah, S., Balaratnam, S., Casas, A., O'Neill, S., Edwards, C., Batlle, A., Dobbin, P., and MacRobert, A.J. (2007) *Mol. Cancer Ther.*, **6**, 876.
101. Nishiyama, N., Nakagishi, Y., Morimoto, Y., Lai, P.S., Miyazaki, K., Urano, K., Horie, S., Kumagai, M., Fukushima, S., Cheng, Y., Jang, W.D., Kikuchi, M., and Kataoka, K. (2009) *J. Control. Release*, **133**, 245.
102. Wu, G., Barth, R.F., Yang, W., Lee, R.J., Tjarks, W., Backer, M.V., and Backer, J.M. (2006) *Anticancer Agents Med. Chem.*, **6**, 167.
103. Yang, W., Barth, R.F., Adams, D.M., and Soloway, A.H. (1997) *Cancer Res.*, **57**, 4333.
104. Barth, R.F., Adams, D.M., Soloway, A.H., Alam, F., and Darby, M.V. (1994) *Bioconjug. Chem.*, **5**, 58.
105. Yang, W., Barth, R.F., Wu, G., Kawabata, S., Sferra, T.J., Bandyopadhyaya, A.K., Tjarks, W., Ferketich, A.K., Moeschberger, M.L., Binns, P.J., Riley, K.J., Coderre, J.A., Ciesielski, M.J., Fenstermaker, R.A., and Wikstrand, C.J. (2006) *Clin. Cancer Res.*, **12**, 3792.
106. Backer, M.V., Gaynutdinov, T.I., Patel, V., Bandyopadhyaya, A.K., Thirumamagal, B.T., Tjarks, W., Barth,

R.F., Claffey, K., and Backer, J.M. (2005) *Mol. Cancer Ther.*, **4**, 1423.

107. Kobayashi, H., Kawamoto, S., Bernardo, M., Brechbiel, M.W., Knopp, M.V., and Choyke, P.L. (2006) *J. Control. Release*, **111**, 343.

108. Wiener, E.C., Brechbiel, M.W., Brothers, H., Magin, R.L., Gansow, O.A., Tomalia, and D.A., Lauterbur, P.C. (1994) *Magn. Reson. Med.*, **31**, 1.

109. Kobayashi, H., Reijnders, K., English, S., Yordanov, A.T., Milenic, D.E., Sowers, A.L., Citrin, D., Krishna, M.C., Waldmann, T.A., Mitchell, J.B., and Brechbiel, M.W. (2004) *Clin. Cancer Res.*, **10**, 7712.

110. Langereis, S., de Lussanet, Q.G., van Genderen, M.H., Meijer, E.W., Beets-Tan, R.G., Griffioen, A.W., van Engelshoven, J.M., and Backes, W.H. (2006) *NMR Biomed.*, **19**, 133.

111. Fu, Y., Nitecki, D.E., Maltby, D., Simon, G.H., Berejnoi, K., Raatschen, H.J., Yeh, B.M., Shames, D.M., and Brasch, R.C. (2006) *Bioconjug. Chem.*, **17**, 1043.

112. Xu, R., Wang, Y., Wang, X., Jeong, E.K., Parker, D.L., and Lu, Z.R. (2007) *Exp. Biol. Med.*, **232**, 1081.

113. Thomas, T.P., Myaing, M.T., Ye, J.Y., Candido, K., Kotlyar, A., Beals, J., Cao, P., Keszler, B., Patri, A.K., Norris, T.B., and Baker, J.R. Jr. (2004) *Biophys. J.*, **86**, 3959.

114. Gupta, U., Dwivedi, S.K., Bid, H.K., Konwar, R., and Jain, N.K. (2010) *Int. J. Pharm.*, **393**, 185.

115. Fischer, W., Calderon, M., Ofek, P., Satchi-Fainaro, R., and Haag, R. (2009) International Dendrimer Symposium, Stockholm.

116. Ofek, P., Fischer, W., Calderon, M., Haag, R., and Satchi-Fainaro, R. (2010) *FASEB J.*, **24**, 3122.

117. Fischer, W., Calderon, M., Schulz, A., Andreou, I., Weber, M., and Haag, R. (2010) *Bioconjug. Chem.*, **21**, 1744.

118. Khandare, J., Mohr, A., Calderon, M., Welker, P., Licha, K., and Haag, R. (2010) *Biomaterials*, **31**, 4268.

119. Fischer, W., Calderon, M., and Haag, R. (2010) *Top. Curr. Chem.*, **296**, 95.

120. Ofek, P., Miller, K., Eldar-Boock, A., Polyak, D., Segal, E., and Satchi-Fainaro, R. (2010) *Israel J. Chem.*, **50**, 185.

121. Kang, C., Yuan, X., Li, F., Pu, P., Yu, S., Shen, C., Zhang, Z., and Zhang, Y. (2010) *J. Biomed. Mater. Res. A*, **93**, 585.

122. Taratula, O., Garbuzenko, O.B., Kirkpatrick, P., Pandya, I., Savla, R., Pozharov, V.P., He, H., and Minko, T. (2009) *J. Control. Release*, **140**, 284.

123. Liu, X.X., Rocchi, P., Qu, F.Q., Zheng, S.Q., Liang, Z.C., Gleave, M., Iovanna, J., and Peng, L. (2009) *ChemMedChem*, **4**, 1302.

124. Amir, R.J., Pessah, N., Shamis, M., and Shabat, D. (2003) *Angew. Chem. Int. Ed.*, **42**, 4494.

125. Yao, H., Veine, D.M., Zeng, Z.Z., Fay, K.S., Staszewski, E.D., and Livant, D.L. (2010) *Clin. Exp. Metastasis*, **27**, 173.

126. Yao, H., Veine, D.M., Fay, K.S., Staszewski, E.D., Zeng, Z.Z., and Livant, D.L. (2010) *Breast Cancer Res. Treat.*, **125**, 363.

127. Holden, C.A., Yuan, Q., Yeudall, W.A., Lebman, D.A., and Yang, H. (2010) *Int. J. Nanomed.*, **5**, 25.

128. Shi, X., Wang, S.H., Shen, M., Antwerp, M.E., Chen, X., Li, C., Petersen, E.J., Huang, Q., Weber, W.J., and Baker, J.R. Jr. (2009) *Biomacromolecules*, **10**, 1744.

19
Site-Specific Prodrug Activation and the Concept of Self-Immolation
André Warnecke

19.1
Introduction

Research in drug delivery is currently one of the major sources of innovation in many therapeutic areas such as cancer, rheumatic diseases, and immunosuppression. In order to improve the potential of the respective drug, several carrier technologies are currently available or under development, such as drug conjugates using monoclonal antibodies or synthetic polymers as carriers, or drugs encapsulated in liposomes or other micro- or nanoparticles.

Attaching anticancer drugs to suitable carriers is normally performed with the goal of significantly altering the pharmacokinetic properties of the drug. The carrier is intended to act as a vehicle by ensuring a direct transport to the site of action without being excreted or trapped by other organs. During this migration process the drug plays the passive role of a sleeping payload. Sleeping means that the drug should not exert any activity or toxicity before reaching its target and moreover should not negatively influence the transport properties of the carrier. As soon as the site of action is reached, the ideal carrier-bound drug should awake, thus gaining full activity to start its designated work – the killing of cancer cells.

A prerequisite for the activation of the drug is obviously the detachment from its carrier. In the case of covalently bound drugs at least one chemical bond has to be broken during the process of drug release. In most cases this bond should be fully stable in the bloodstream and in healthy tissue in order to prevent the conjugate from prematurely releasing the drug. At the target site, however, the drug should be efficiently liberated in an active form.

In this chapter, the significance of the concept of self-immolation for the design of carrier-bound anticancer drugs and related drug delivery systems will be elucidated. Sections 19.2.1 and 19.2.2 will focus on the chemical aspects of these reaction types. By comparing self-immolative with analogous classic systems, the scope of applying self-immolative linkers (SILs) will be evaluated in Section 19.2.3. Section 19.3 deals with the development of tumor-specific activated trigger groups based on benzyl elimination reactions. The concept of self-immolation can be extended to dendritic

Drug Delivery in Oncology: From Basic Research to Cancer Therapy, First Edition.
Edited by Felix Kratz, Peter Senter, and Henning Steinhagen.
© 2012 Wiley-VCH Verlag GmbH & Co. KGaA. Published 2012 by Wiley-VCH Verlag GmbH & Co. KGaA.

or polymeric carriers that consist of branched SILs. In these materials, activation of a single trigger leads to a chemical breakdown of the whole structure and concomitant drug release by a cascade of elimination reactions. These and other carrier systems that are based on multiple elimination linkers will be introduced in Section 19.4. Finally, the clinical impact and the future prospects of this technology will be discussed in Sections 19.5 and 19.6.

19.2
Rationale and Chemical Aspects of the Concept of Self-Immolation

Solid tumors are characterized by biochemical and pathophysiological features, such as the upregulation of certain proteases (e.g., cathepsins or matrix metalloproteases), a decreased pH in tumor tissue or – more pronounced – intracellularly in endosomes and/or lysosomes as well as a reductive milieu due to hypoxia. These site-specific features can be exploited for the cleavage reaction by incorporating a predetermined breaking point or trigger that is labile under tumortropic conditions. Meanwhile, a number of more or less elegant ways of how to construct cleavable drug–carrier conjugates have been developed. The different features of the general design of carrier-linked drugs are depicted in Figure 19.1.

In simply constructed drug–carrier conjugates (Figure 19.1a) an accessible moiety of the drug is directly bound to a suitable functional group of the carrier. These types of conjugates often suffer from either being too labile and prone to hydrolysis (e.g., ester bonds) or being too stable and thus cannot be cleaved effectively (e.g., amide or ether bonds). However, there are a few examples of directly conjugated cytotoxic drugs that have proven sufficiently stable while showing a tumor-specific release. One of them, poly(glutamic acid)-bound paclitaxel (Xyotax®), was shown to release the drug after proteolytic degradation of the carrier by cathepsin B [1].

All other types of conjugate architecture utilize a special bridging molecule, the so-called (cross)linker or spacer. With the aid of this building block, it is possible to link carriers and drugs with orthogonal functionalities. When no specific predetermined breaking point is defined (Figure 19.1b), the conjugates suffer from the same drawbacks as those resulting from direct coupling. Therefore, the chemical potential of introducing an additional defined structural unit should be exploited: the incorporation of tumor-specific cleavable moieties such as proteolytically cleavable peptides, disulfides for a reductive cleavage or acid-sensitive acetal or hydrazone groups [2]. Regardless of the type of the scissile bond, its position determines whether the drug itself is released (Figure 19.1d) or a drug derivative with a persistent fragment of the former linker attached (Figure 19.1c). It is obvious that releasing the native drug is the preferred strategy (although there may be examples of released drug derivatives that "accidently" show a higher activity than the parent compound) so that the focus is normally set on the development of carrier–drug conjugates having a breaking point adjacent to the drug (Figure 19.1d). This favorable strategy, however, is often associated with

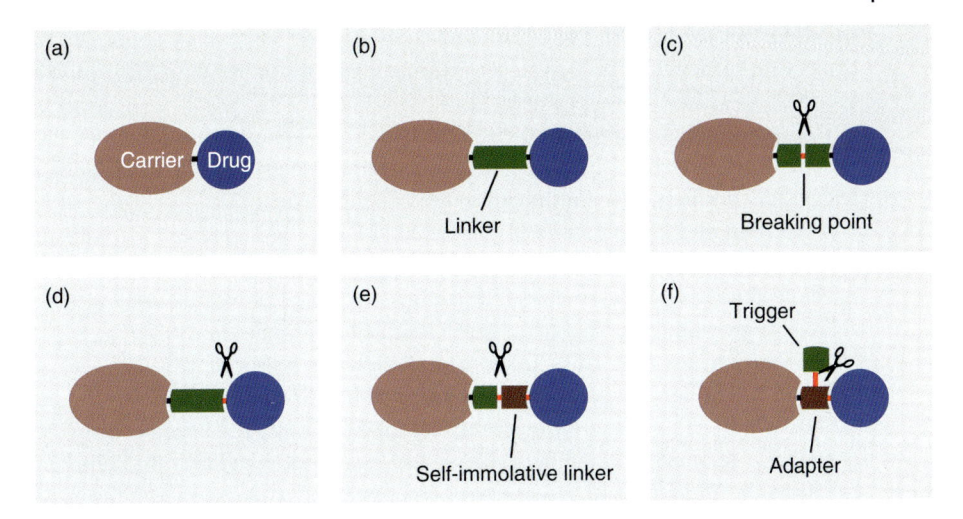

Figure 19.1 Main architectures of 1 : 1 carrier–drug conjugates: (a) direct coupling, (b) with a noncleavable linker, (c) with a predetermined breaking point incorporated in the linker, (d) with a predetermined breaking point adjacent to the drug, (e) with a SIL, and (f) with an adapter (SIL with an additional attachment point) and a trigger unit. Cleavable bonds are highlighted red.

various problems. In many cases, drugs do not offer a suitable functional group for the design of a labile bond. Another disadvantage affects enzymatically cleavable conjugates. Due to steric hindrance produced by bulky drugs, the conjugate might turn out to be a poor substrate for the respective enzyme and the rate of cleavage is not sufficient.

To overcome these drawbacks, an elegant way of controlled drug release was developed by introducing a SIL as an additional transient spacer group between the breaking point and the drug (Figure 19.1e). The SIL is designed to be stable under normal physiological conditions. As soon as the scissile bond is cleaved, an intermediate SIL–drug derivative is released from the carrier that decomposes spontaneously, liberating the free drug and a derivative of the SIL (Figure 19.2).

By placing the cleavable bond more or less at the center of the overall linker construct, enzymes generally have an improved access to their substrates. Furthermore, an SIL fills the gap between incompatible functional groups of

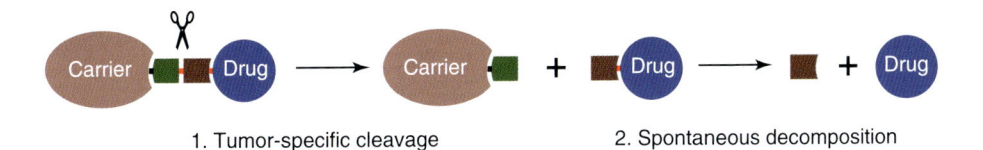

Figure 19.2 Two-step mechanism of drug release using a SIL.

the drug and the breaking point, thus making this release strategy applicable to drugs with nucleophilic groups such as amino, mercapto, or the abundant hydroxy groups.

This approach is equivalent to the double-prodrug concept that describes the design of pro-prodrugs (sometimes also called tripartate prodrugs) consisting of a trigger (or specifier), a (self-immolative) linker, and the drug [3].

A variation of the above strategy is depicted in Figure 19.1f. Here, a SIL with an additional attachment point, the so-called adaptor, is used as a trifunctional linker to connect the drug, the carrier, and the labile moiety responsible for tumor-specific release (trigger unit) [4]. This concept will be elucidated in Section 19.5.

The prerequisites for a cross-linker to be classified as self-immolative are easy to describe. (i) The bond between the effector group (drug or dye) and the linker should be sufficiently stable under various chemical conditions. (ii) The bond between the trigger and the linker should be stable as well except for conditions prevailing in the tumor or tumor cells where cleavage takes place. (iii) After cleavage of the bond between the trigger and the linker, a chemical reaction takes place that results in a rapid and irreversible breakage of the linker–effector bond. Thus, SILs can be regarded as effective transmitters of chemical signals. Due to the irreversibility of this process, however, applications are limited to those that do not require a recovery of the system.

Principally, the spontaneous fragmentation of the SIL–drug intermediate can be chemically achieved by two different reaction types: cyclization and elimination reactions. Selected examples for each type will now be discussed (a comprehensive overview can be found in [5, 6]).

19.2.1
Cyclization Strategies

Cyclization linkers designed to undergo self-immolation rely on three key features. (i) The drug is bound via an amino, hydroxyl, or thiol group (Z) to the carbonyl function of the linker forming a carboxylic or carbonic acid derivative. (ii) At the other end of the linker a nucleophilic group X (amino, hydroxyl, or thiol) is chemically masked. (iii) After demasking (activation of the trigger), the liberated nucleophilic group X is capable of attacking the carbonyl group of the -C(O)-Z-drug function resulting in a release of the drug and the formation of a cyclic byproduct (see Figure 19.3).

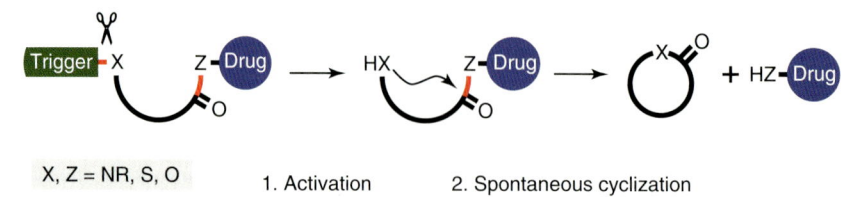

X, Z = NR, S, O   1. Activation   2. Spontaneous cyclization

Figure 19.3 General principle of drug release from a cyclization-based SIL.

19.2 Rationale and Chemical Aspects of the Concept of Self-Immolation

Normally, cyclization strategies exploit the energetically favored formation of five- and six-membered rings. Hence, the formed cyclic byproduct is a γ- or δ-lactone or lactam, a cyclic urea, or carbamate. The trimethyl lock (TML) lactonization is an example of a cyclization strategy that exploits the facile formation of benzo δ-lactones. It describes the spontaneous ring-closure of esters or amides based on 2-hydroxyphenyl propionic acid:

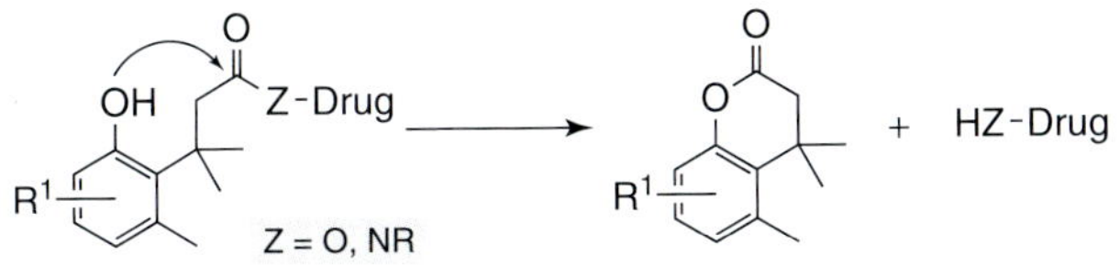

In initial studies it was found that the presence of three methyl groups is crucial for a rapid cyclization [7]. The TML reaction is one of only a few examples for a hydroxyl group acting as the nucleophile that is capable of attacking an amide bond under physiological conditions. This linker has been used for the design of poly(ethylene glycol) (PEG) conjugates of daunorubicin (DNR) by Greenwald et al. [8].

The cyclization strategy with the largest spectrum of applications is undoubtedly the formation of imidazolidinones from acylated ethylene diamines:

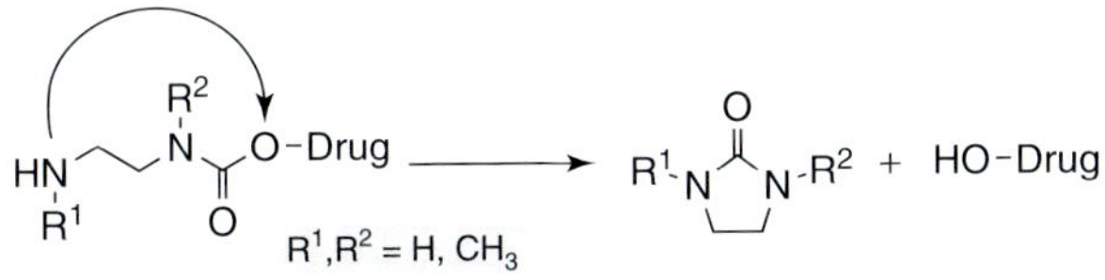

This reaction offers a useful release strategy for hydroxyl-functionalized drugs and proceeds fastest when both amino groups are methylated. For N,N'-dimethylethylene diamine derivatives the half-life was reported to be 36 min under physiological conditions [9]. Moreover, by linking two alcohols as carbamates via an ethylene bridge the above strategy provides a reasonable synthetic alternative for using carbonates:

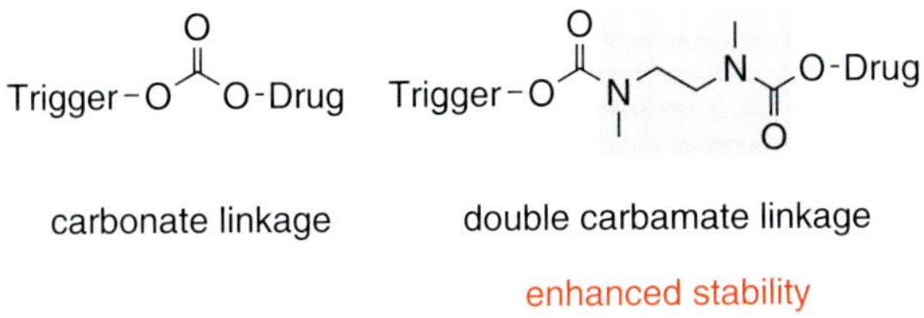

carbonate linkage   double carbamate linkage
                           enhanced stability

Compared to carbonates, carbamate bonds generally display a higher stability under physiologic conditions. Examples for this strategy are found in a N-(2-hydroxypropyl)methacrylamide (HPMA) copolymer conjugate of etoposide

[10] and prodrugs of camptothecin in which the drug is released from a PEGylated self-immolative dendrimer scaffold (see also Section 19.4) [11].

19.2.2
Elimination Strategies

Compared to cyclization reactions, elimination-based release strategies have gained more importance in the design of prodrugs due to their versatility and the possibility of creating multiple elimination linkers (see Section 19.4). Therefore, the underlying reaction types will be discussed in more detail. Principally, the release of drugs from elimination linkers occurs similarly to that of cyclization linkers depicted in Figure 19.3 with the difference that the spontaneous step is an elimination reaction and the formed byproduct has at least one double bond (although there are examples of elimination-based linkers that are able to react in a competing cyclization reaction [12] so that in some cases the actual mechanism of self-immolation is not apparent). As in most elimination reactions, the quality of the leaving group is crucial for achieving high reaction rates.

One of the shortest elimination linkers is the -O-C(O)- (oxycarbonyl) group that readily eliminates carbon dioxide from the intermediary formed carbonic or carbamic acids:

$$HO-C(O)-Z\text{-Drug} \longrightarrow CO_2 + HZ\text{-Drug}$$
$$Z = O, NR, S$$

This reaction is often used in combination with other elimination linkers. Alcohols (not phenols [13]) and amines are usually poor leaving groups so that the incorporation of an oxycarbonyl group strongly enhances the rate of elimination.

Another type of one-atom elimination linker is the methylene group that is also used in combination with other linkers. Formacetals, aminals, and N,O-acetals are markedly stable at physiological pH. In contrast, the respective hemiacetals or hemiaminals undergo hydrolysis to release the amino or hydroxyl drug, formaldehyde, and – for the hemiaminals – ammonia:

$$HX\text{-}CH_2\text{-}Z\text{-Drug} \xrightarrow{H_2O} H_2X + HCHO + HZ\text{-Drug}$$
$$X = O, NH$$
$$Z = O, NR$$

This method has proven useful for tethering the antimetabolite 5-fluorouracil (5-FU) since direct coupling produces a carbamate bond that lacks stability in human plasma [14]. The incorporation of an aminal group significantly enhances the stability [15]:

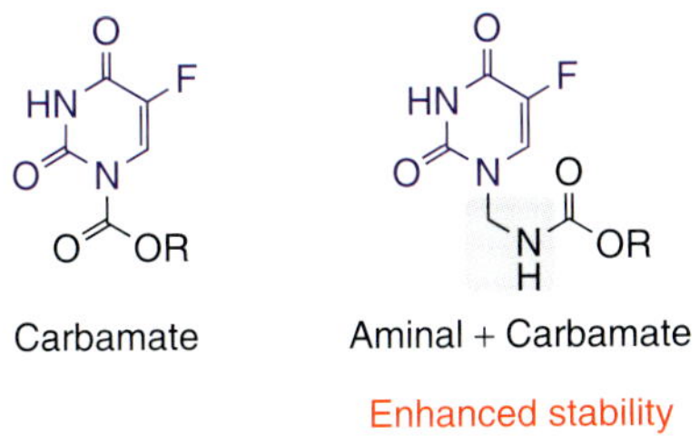

19.2 Rationale and Chemical Aspects of the Concept of Self-Immolation

Carbamate **Aminal + Carbamate**

Enhanced stability

The above examples of one-atom linkers are special cases. Although commonly not regarded as self-eliminating linkers, they play an important role when combined with SIL. Classic self-elimination linkers exploit benzyl eliminations (also denoted as quinone methide elimination) or related reactions for the release of drugs. The term benzyl elimination describes the spontaneous 1,4- or 1,6-eliminations of vinylogous hemiacetals, N,O-hemiacetals, or S,O-hemiacetals:

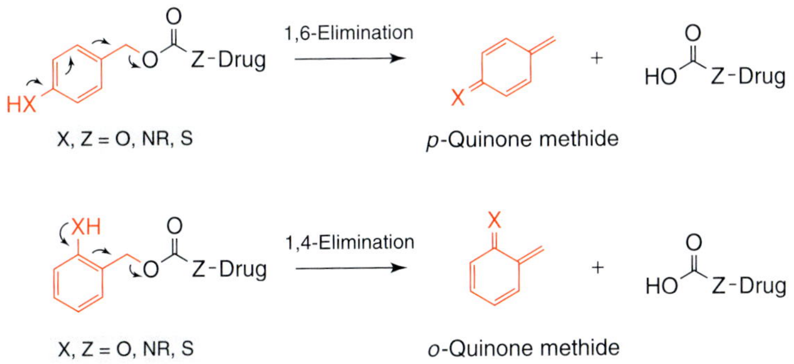

1,6-Elimination → p-Quinone methide

X, Z = O, NR, S

1,4-Elimination → o-Quinone methide

X, Z = O, NR, S

As a result, a quinone methide and the instable carbamic or carbonic esters are formed, which decompose to carbon dioxide and the respective drug (see above). Quinone methides and iminoquinone methides are strong electrophiles that readily react with nucleophiles, primarily with the abundant water:

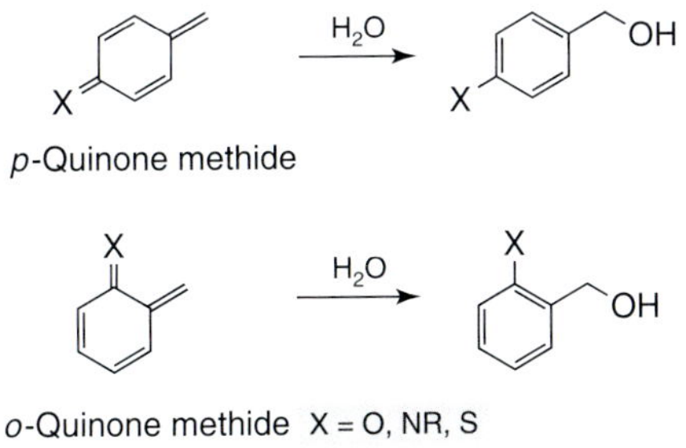

p-Quinone methide

o-Quinone methide X = O, NR, S

Through a Michael-type addition of water, the aromatic system is regenerated. However, there are some concerns about potential alkylating activity *in vivo* that may produce DNA damage or an inhibition of enzymes since quinone methides are known to form adducts with nucleic bases and to label enzymes [16, 17]. For prodrugs with single SILs, however, these possible side-reactions do not seem to hamper clinical development since the first drug candidates employing this type of elimination linker have been tested in clinical trials and were well-tolerated (see Section 19.6).

Generally, 1,6-eliminations proceed faster than respective 1,4-eliminations [18, 19]. The reaction rate further depends on the electron-donating qualities of the group X [20]. Since acylated X are weak electron donors, acylation is an effective way to mask the group X in order to prevent the system from a premature elimination. In the past years, many other methods for masking X have been developed that allow a specific triggering (see Section 19.3).

The most efficient and most widespread type of linker is the aniline-based *p*-aminobenzyloxycarbonyl (PABC) system first introduced by Katzenellenbogen et al. [21]. At neutral pH, the 1,6-elimination proceeds very rapidly with a half-life of 16 s [22] so that the demasking of the amino group (i.e., the cleavage of the trigger) normally becomes the rate-determining step of drug release.

An attractive alternative for the 1,4- and 1,6-benzyl elimination linkers was recently published by Shabat et al. who have shown that elimination also takes place when one carbon atom of the phenyl ring is replaced by nitrogen [23]. Although the mechanism for the so-called pyridinone-methide elimination as well as the reaction rate do not differ substantially from those of their phenyl analogs, the use of pyridine derivatives significantly enhances the water solubility of the linker. Besides pyridines, elimination reactions from five-ring heterocyclic compounds have been reported as well. Substituted furans and thiophenes can also undergo 1,6-elimination as has been shown for bioreductively activated phosporamidate prodrugs [24]:

Similar 1,6-elimination linkers were also derived from imidazole [25]:

De Groot et al. focused on systems that eliminate over a longer distance. For this purpose styrene, naphthalene, and biphenyl derivatives were developed [26, 27] that were supposed to react in 1,8- and 1,10-eliminations, respectively:

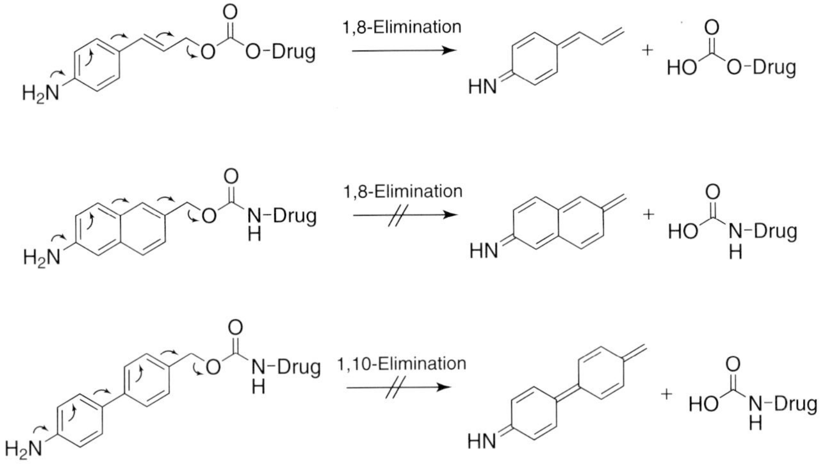

Interestingly, the styrene derivative displayed a complete release of the drug, whereas neither the related 1,8-elimination from the naphthalene derivative nor the postulated 1,10-elimination from the biphenyl derivative could be observed even under harsh conditions. The authors suggested that the energetically unfavorable loss of aromaticity of two ring systems hinders these elimination reactions [27]. A noteworthy application of a 1,8-elimination linker was recently presented by Shabat et al. who developed a self-eliminating derivative of the fluorophore umbelliferone [28]:

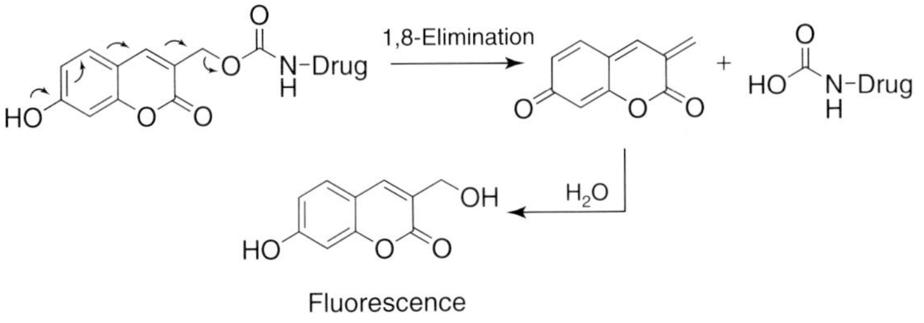

After 1,8-elimination and regeneration of the aromatic system by addition of a water molecule, a fluorescence signal indicates the release of the drug so that this system is suitable for a real-time monitoring of drug release as shown in *in vitro* experiments.

Table 19.1 Half-lives of enzymatically cleavable prodrugs of DOX (PABC-containing prodrugs are highlighted in italics).

Substrate	$t_{1/2}$	Cleavage conditions	References
Z-Phe–Lys–DOX	ND	cathepsin B (40 nM)	[29]
Z-Phe–Lys–PABC–DOX	8 min	cathepsin B (40 nM)	[29]
Z-Val–Cit–DOX	ND	cathepsin B (40 nM)	[29]
Z-Val–Cit–PABC–DOX	4 h	cathepsin B (40 nM)	[29]
H-Ser–Leu–DOX	>20 h	LNCaP tumor tissue homogenate	[30]
H-Ser–Leu–PABC–DOX	<1 h	LNCaP tumor tissue homogenate	[30]
H-Ser–Leu–DOX	>24 h	LNCaP cell lysate	[30]
H-Ser–Leu–PABC–DOX	~10 h	LNCaP cell lysate	[30]
H-D-Ala–Phe–Lys–PABC–DOX	1.66 h	plasmin (0.025 U/ml)	[27]
H-D-Ala–Phe–Lys–(PABC)$_2$–DOX	0.82 h	plasmin (0.025 U/ml)	[27]
H-D-Ala–Phe–Lys–(PABC)$_3$–DOX	0.57 h	plasmin (0.025 U/ml)	[27]

ND, not detectable.

19.2.3
Self-Immolative versus Classic Strategies – A Comparison

One important goal of incorporating SILs into prodrugs that are activated enzymatically is to reduce the influence of sterically demanding drugs on the cleavage reaction. In the literature some impressive examples with the bulky drug doxorubicin (DOX) can be found that strongly support the strategy of using an additional SIL. Dubowchik *et al.* have shown that the cathepsin B substrates Z-Phe–Lys and Z-Val–Cit are not cleaved by the enzyme when directly coupled to the drug's amino group [29]. In both cases, the incorporation of the PABC linker resulted in an effective cleavage which proceeded very rapidly for the Z-Phe–Lys substrate (see Table 19.1).

Another example was recently given by Kratz *et al.* who designed an albumin-binding prodrug of DOX with a heptapeptide linker as a substrate for the enzymatically active prostate-specific antigen (PSA). The activation follows a two-step mechanism [30]:

19.2 Rationale and Chemical Aspects of the Concept of Self-Immolation

First, the prodrug is cleaved by the target enzyme PSA releasing a Ser–Leu dipeptide–drug derivative. This intermediate is further degraded by unspecified proteases to liberate the active drug. It was found that the second step was only successful when a PABC linker was incorporated, whereas the H-Ser–Leu–DOX derivative was either not hydrolyzed or formed stable H-Leu–DOX when incubated with tumor cell lysates or homogenates, respectively (see Table 19.1). The *in vitro* cytotoxicity of H-Ser–Leu-PABC–DOX and H-Ser–Leu–DOX also reflected the cleavage properties with the latter being 20 times less toxic than the one incorporating PABC.

The effect of facilitating enzymatic cleavage by means of a PABC linker can be further enhanced by introducing multiple PABC groups as shown by de Groot *et al.* who developed prodrugs of DOX with the plasmin-cleavable D-Ala–Phe–Lys linker [27]. Compared to the prodrug with one PABC linker, the elongation using a triple linker [(PABC)$_3$] resulted in a significant acceleration of the cleavage rate (see Table 19.1). Similar results were also obtained for analogous paclitaxel prodrugs.

SILs cannot only enhance the cleavage efficiency of proteolytically activated prodrugs by reducing steric hindrance, they can also act as versatile trigger groups for tumor-specific prodrug activation or as building blocks for rather complex release systems as illustrated in the following two sections.

19.3
Elimination-Based Trigger Groups for Tumor-Specific Activation

Since benzyl elimination reactions can be easily triggered by deblocking or generating a suitable nucleophilic group in an *ortho* or a *para* position from the oxymethyl group, there are many possibilities to design tumor-specific trigger groups based on these SILs. This section will give a comprehensive overview including also examples that do not actually deal with prodrug activation, but may provide some fruitful inspirations.

19.3.1
Enzymatic and Related Biocatalytic Activation

For a proteolytic activation (e.g., by the tumor-associated proteases cathepsins, PSA, plasmin), the simplest way is to acylate the aniline group of a PABC linker with a peptide that is cleaved at the C-terminus. While this type of trigger group has already been introduced in Section 19.2.3, the focus will be set on other enzymatic methods of activating SIL. A method similar to proteolytic activation is the frequently employed cleavage by penicillin-G amidase (PGA) that was used for the activation of cascade release systems such as self-immolative dendrimers or polymers (see Section 19.4). Acylation of the PABC system with phenylacetic acid produces trigger groups that are readily deblocked by PGA [31]:

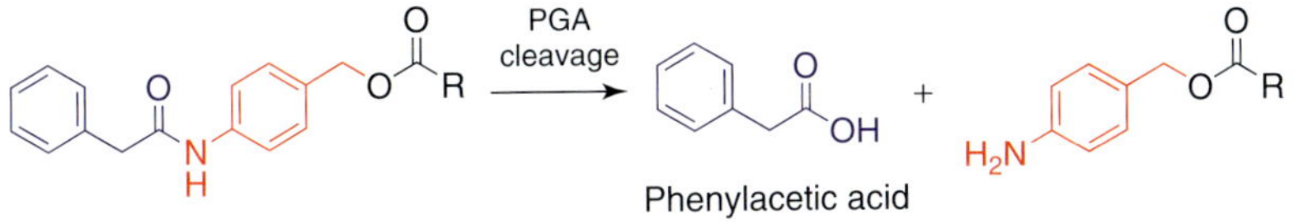

19.3 Elimination-Based Trigger Groups for Tumor-Specific Activation | 565

Although most frequently applied in model compounds, the use of this enzyme and the related penicillin-V amidase was also suggested for various antibody-directed enzyme prodrug therapy (ADEPT) approaches (see 6) [32–34]. ADEPT was also studied in a number of glycoside prodrugs that are cleaved by exogenous enzymes such as α-galactosidase from coffee beans or β-glucuronidase from *Escherichia coli*, and many methods have been developed that utilize these enzymes for a specific triggering of glycosylated *p*-hydroxybenzyl or *p*-aminobenzyl groups [6, 35]:

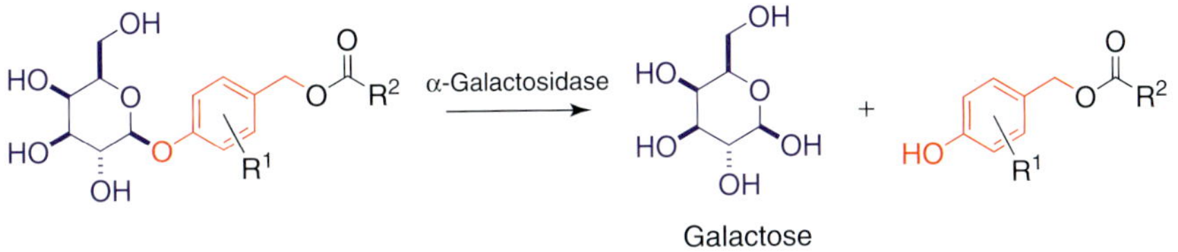

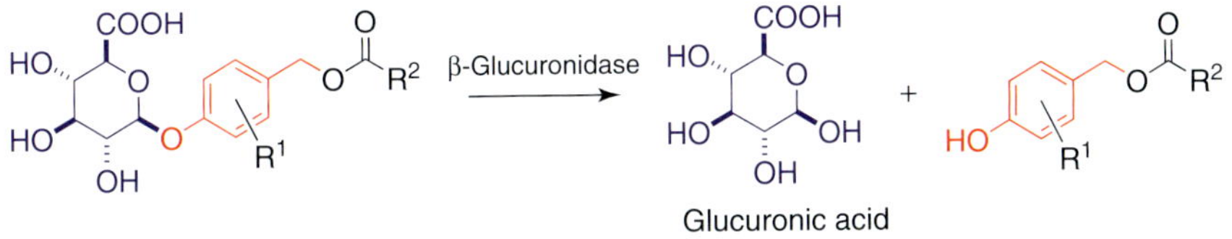

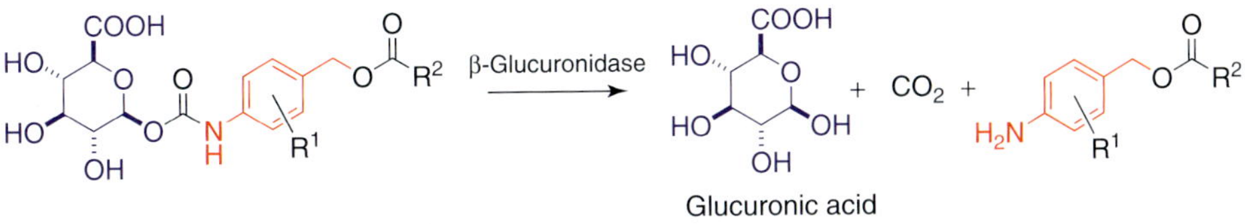

Other enzymatic reactions that were reported to initiate benzyl elimination are the hydrolysis of sulfates [36] and phosphates [37] by human steroid sulfatase and tyrosine phosphatases, respectively:

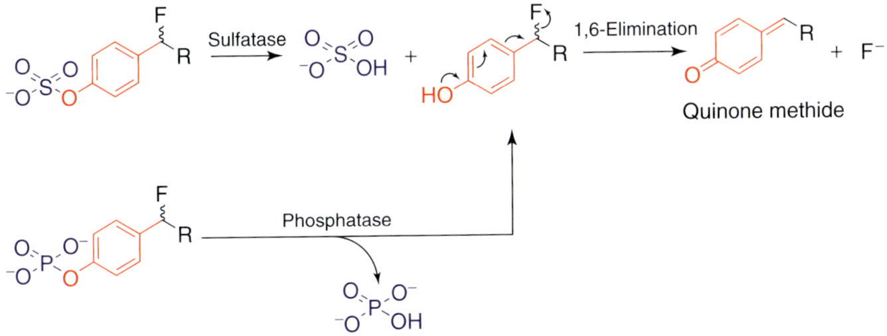

Although these substrates were designed as activity probes for enzyme labeling by the reactive quinone methide (so-called suicide substrates), it is likely that related techniques can also find application in the field of prodrug activation.

Apart from enzymes, there are other biocatalysts that can be exploited for selective activation of trigger groups. Shabat et al. used the substrate specificity of catalytic antibody 38C2 for the design of prodrugs. 38C2 catalyzes a retro-aldol–retro-Michael tandem reaction [31, 38, 39]:

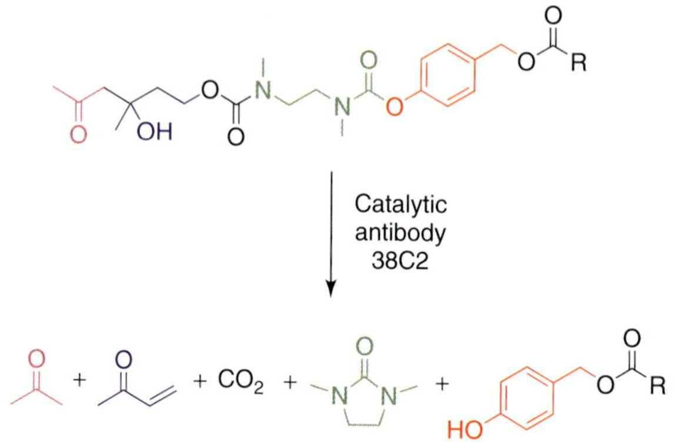

The substrate is combined with an ethylene diamine-based cyclization linker and the self-eliminating p-hydroxybenzyloxycarbonyl group that undergoes 1,6-elimination. The trigger group was used for the design of a combination prodrug that simultaneously releases the drugs DOX, etoposide, and camptothecin [40]. Due to the specificity of this activation mechanism, Shabat et al. suggested its use in analogy to a polymer-directed enzyme prodrug therapy [41] approach in which a polymer conjugate of the antibody should warrant passive tumor targeting and thus a site-specific activation of low-molecular-weight prodrugs [42].

A simple retro-Michael reaction could also be exploited for trigger activation utilizing the catalytic activity of bovine serum albumin (BSA) [43]:

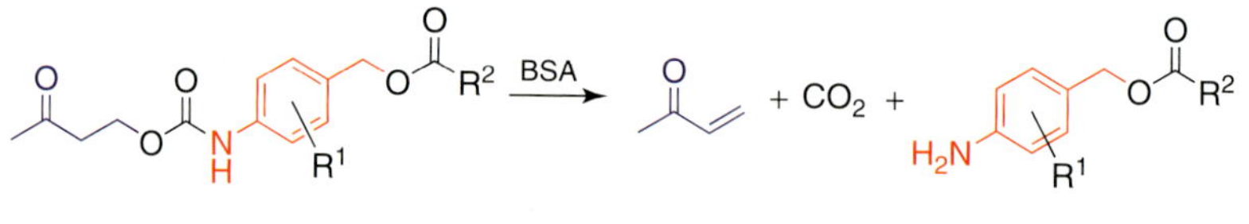

Although BSA is a transport protein and no enzyme, it catalyzes the retro-Michael reaction of the 3-oxobutyl group and enables cascade elimination reactions [44, 45].

19.3.2
Reductive Activation

Many solid tumors are deprived of oxygen due to insufficient blood supply, a situation described as hypoxia. The lack of oxygen gives rise to a reductive milieu

19.3 Elimination-Based Trigger Groups for Tumor-Specific Activation | 567

in tumor tissue that can be exploited for the site-specific activation of prodrugs by bioreduction processes. One of the most popular strategies is to mask the aromatic amino group of a PABC linker as a nitro group (see also Section 19.2.2) [26]:

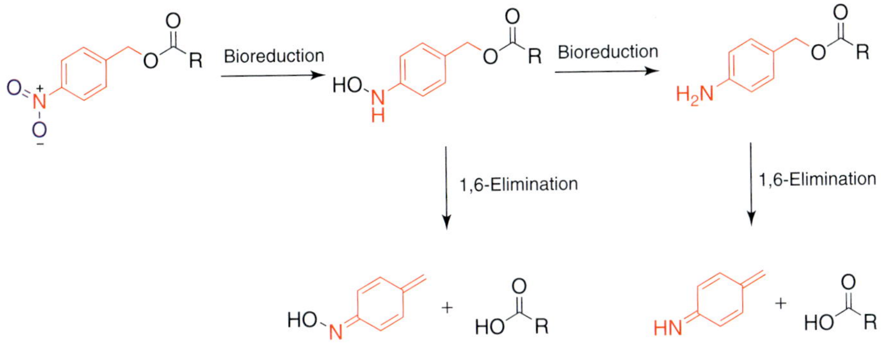

Interestingly, it does not matter whether the nitro group is fully reduced to the amine or the reduction stops at the stage of the hydroxylamine since both undergo 1,6-elimination. Due to its ease of chemical activation (e.g., by reduction with Zn/AcOH), the nitro group was also used to trigger elimination in model compounds [19, 46].

Apart from aromatic nitro compounds, phenylazides were also evaluated for their use as bioreductive trigger groups, albeit with less success [26]. Azides, however, undergo some very chemoselective reactions that can be exploited for prodrug activation. One of them is the Staudinger reaction that describes the reduction of azides by phosphines. The group of Robillard presented an azido prodrug of DOX that can be activated with a water-soluble phosphine [47]:

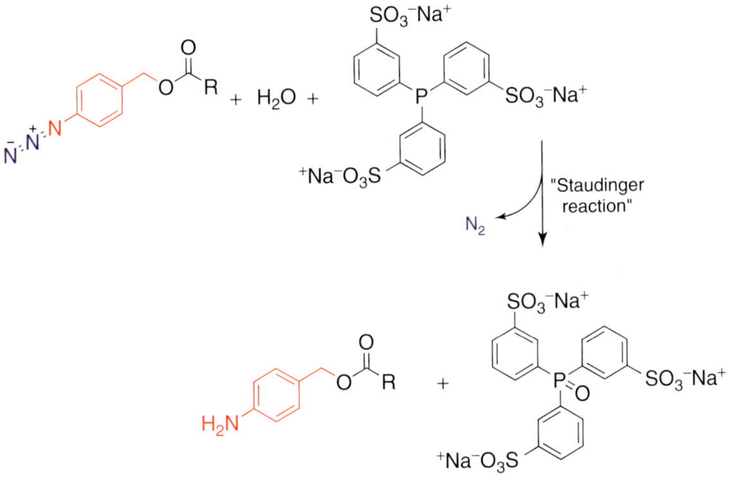

Benzyl eliminations from thiophenol derivatives, although fairly uncommon, can also be used for tumor-specific triggering as Senter *et al.* have shown by studying the release behavior of a number of mitomycin prodrugs [48]. The compounds proved to be stable in aqueous solution indicating an efficient masking of the thiol group. After reductive cleavage of the disulfide, however, a fast release of mitomycin was observed for the *para*- and *ortho*-substituted compounds whereas the *meta* derivative was found to be stable as expected:

Mitomycin

Another example for a thiol-sensitive trigger group was recently reported by Zhu et al. who found that a PABC derivative with an additional amino group can be masked by reaction with selenium dioxide [49]. The resulting benzoselenadiazol derivative reacts with organic dithiols such as 1,4-dithiothreitol (DTT) and 1,2-dimercaptoethane but not or to a much lesser extent with monothiols or other reductive agents such as ascorbic acid:

With a fluorescent probe using 4-aminonaphthalimide as the reporter, Zhu et al. showed that activation takes place in the cytosol of HeLa cells leading to an imaging of thiol reactivity. In contrast, prior incubation with the thiol-blocking agent N-ethylmaleimide resulted in a distinct decrease in fluorescence.

19.3.3
Oxidative Activation

For tumor-specific activation, oxidative strategies do not play an important role. However, it should be mentioned that there is a very sensitive method for using hydrogen peroxide as the triggering agent. Lo and Chu have reported that boronic acids are readily oxidized by hydrogen peroxide. The resulting boric acid ester is hydrolyzed in aqueous solutions, thus demasking the benzyl elimination linker [50]:

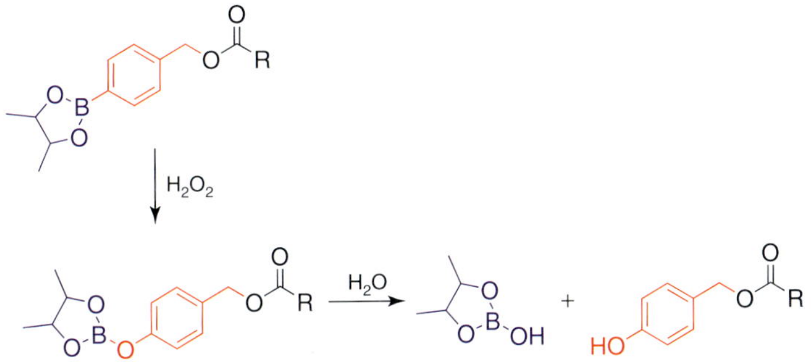

Apart from fluorescence probes, Shabat et al. presented an interesting application of the above reaction – the so-called dendritic chain reaction (see Figure 19.4) [51–53]. In a first step, a boronic acid trigger group is activated with hydrogen peroxide as described above. As a result of a cascade of elimination reactions, one molecule of the reporter 4-nitroaniline as well as two molecules of choline are liberated. Choline acts as a cosubstrate for the enzyme choline oxidase that produces hydrogen peroxide, which further reacts in the same way.

This is an example for an exponential autocatalysis and signal amplification since the triggering agent is multiplied by a factor of 4 after each cycle of the chain reaction. Recently, Shabat et al. also published a thiol-triggered variation of this reaction type [54].

19.3.4
pH-Dependent Activation

It is not surprising that the popular amine protective groups *tert*-butoxycarbonyl (Boc) and fluorenylmethyloxycarbonyl (Fmoc) can also be employed for effectively masking the PABC's amino group. These types of model triggers have been applied to complex release systems such as self-immolative dendrimers [55] or

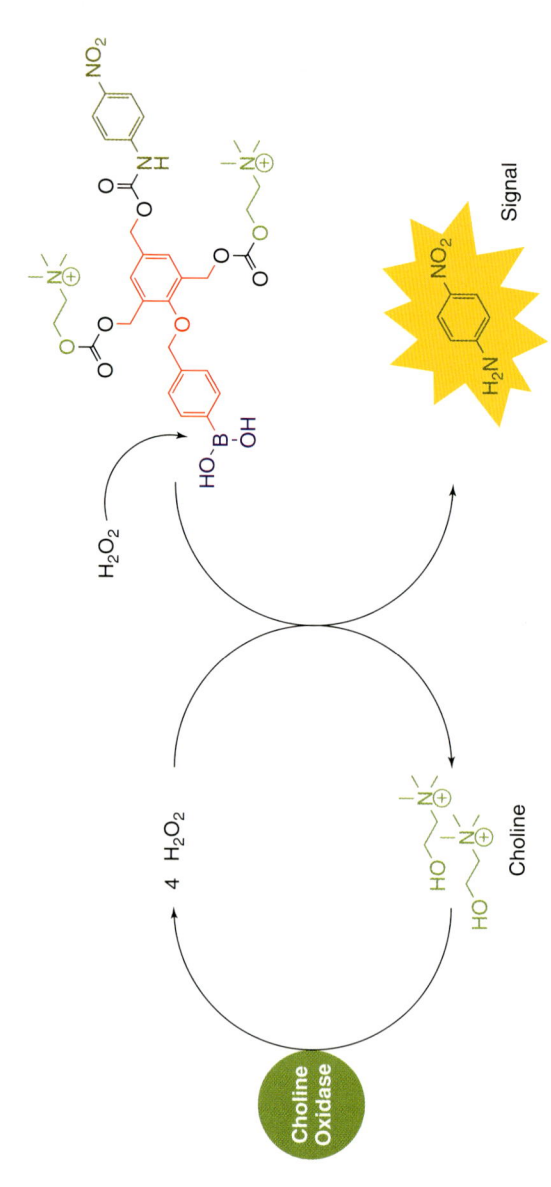

Figure 19.4 Dendritic chain reaction triggered by hydrogen peroxide. The triple elimination linker releases one molecule of the dye 4-nitroaniline as the reporter. Furthermore, two molecules of choline are liberated that act as a cosubstrate for the enzyme choline oxidase, which produces four molecules of hydrogen peroxide. Each of them will initiate another cycle of the chain reaction.

self-immolative microcapsules [56]. Whereas Boc is cleaved in strongly acidic media (typically trifluoroacetic acid), the Fmoc group requires alkaline conditions to be removed (secondary amines such as piperidine or diethylamine). However, for tumor-specific release of carrier-bound drugs, an activation under mild acidic conditions proved to be a very promising approach since tumor tissue is characterized by a slightly decreased pH that is often 0.5–1.0 units lower than in normal tissue [57]. A more pronounced shift in pH from 7.2 to 7.4 in the blood or extracellular spaces to 4.0–6.5 in the various intracellular compartments takes place during cellular uptake of the carrier-linked prodrugs [58]. Warnecke et al. could recently show that Schiff bases derived from benzaldehydes and p-aminobenzyl alcohol act as efficient trigger groups for an acid-catalyzed activation of fluorogenic model compounds [22]:

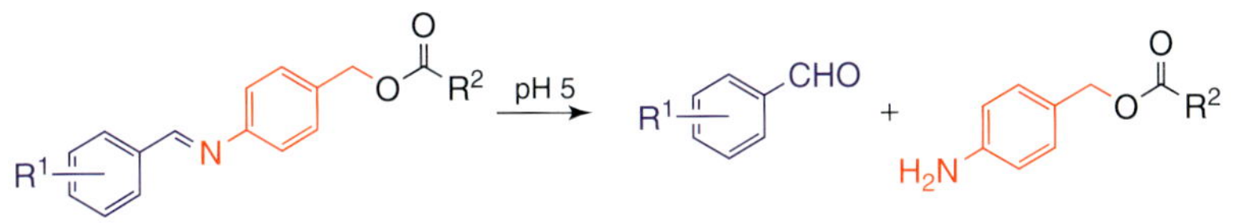

By varying the substituent R^1 it was possible to adjust the stability at neutral pH as well as the rate of hydrolysis at pH 5 with the tetra- and pentafluoro derivatives showing promising release kinetics. This approach should be applicable for the development of pH-responsive anticancer prodrugs.

19.3.5
Other Methods of Activation

Unspecific hydrolysis of various esters, amides, carbonates, and carbamates was studied in PEG conjugates of DNR by Greenwald et al. [59]. While all of the tested compounds displayed a long-term stability in buffer, the esters and carbonates experienced a fast cleavage in rat plasma, whereas the amides proved to be stable. Interestingly, the orientation of the -NH-C(O)-O- group played a crucial role for plasma stability of the carbamates, with the PABC derivative being significantly more stable:

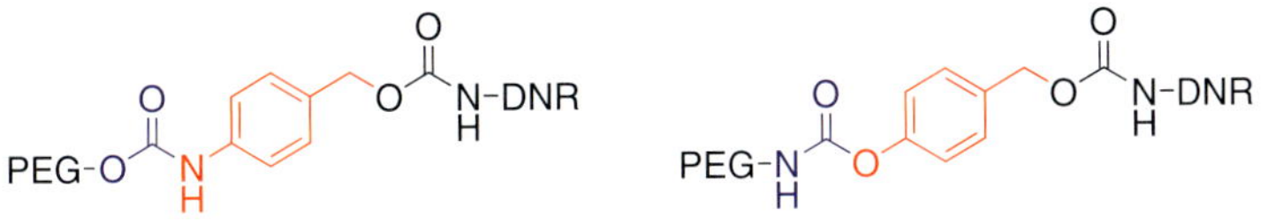

stable in rat plasma   half-live in rat plasma: 4 h

A rather exotic method of prodrug activation was reported by Azoulay et al. [60]. The release strategy relies on the Staudinger ligation, which is an extension of the Staudinger reaction (see Section 19.3.2). An azide serves as the triggering agent which reacts in a first step with the phosphino group of the prodrug to form a reactive aza-ylide intermediate:

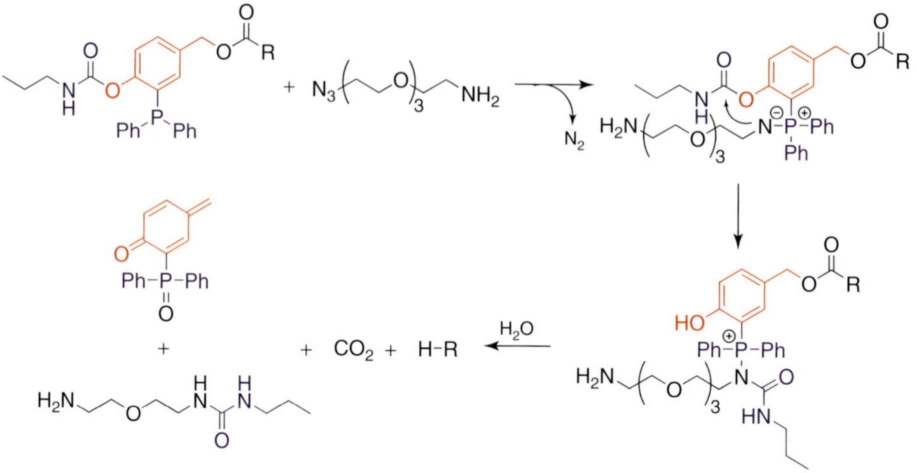

In a second step, an intramolecular shift of the carbamate demasks the phenolic OH group so that the system undergoes 1,6-elimination. This reaction is very chemoselective and it could be shown that prodrugs of DOX were fully stable in the absence of azides.

Photochemical activation is a method frequently used to trigger model compounds [55, 61], but photoactivated prodrugs of 5-FU have also been reported [62]. Generally, 2-nitrobenzyl compounds such as the nitroveratryloxycarbonyl (Nvoc) [63] protective group are suitable photolabile trigger groups. The mechanism of activation is a rather complex multistep reaction involving an intramolecular cyclization and the hydrolysis of an hemiacetal:

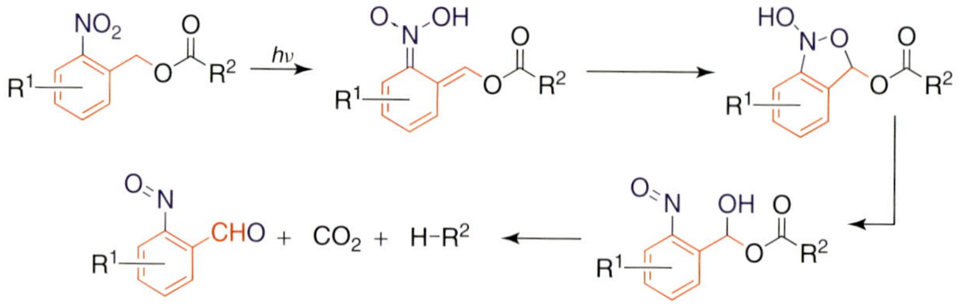

Although not actually a benzyl elimination linker, this reaction broadens the spectrum of activation methods.

All the trigger groups that were introduced in this section are characterized by their ability to initiate a cascade of elimination reactions upon a specific triggering signal. From a chemical point of view, the trigger groups are essentially equivalent and can be exchanged with minimal synthetic effort. In the future, these and other groups may thus be valuable building blocks for the rational design of prodrugs.

19.4
Branched Elimination Linkers–Chemical Adaptors or Building Blocks for More Complex Self-Immolative Architectures

SILs can be modified by the introduction of additional functional groups. For those having merely an extra attachment point that is not involved in the elimination cascade, the term "chemical adaptor system" was coined [4]. With the aid of this type of trifunctional linker it is possible to realize the general prodrug architecture depicted in Figure 19.1f. The feasibility of this approach was first demonstrated in polymer conjugates of the drug etoposide (see Figure 19.5) [10]. In this example, 4-hydroxymandelic acid was used as an adapter to form the link between a HPMA copolymer carrier, the drug, and a trigger group that is activated by the catalytic antibody 38C2 (see Section 19.3.1).

One advantage over the "linear" architecture (Figure 19.1e) is that the trigger group is placed in a more exposed position that may enhance the activation reaction. The second, more important, benefit results from the modular character of the prodrug. With this architecture it is possible to vary the components with less synthetic effort, which facilitates the optimization of each of them individually. This may form the basis for a combinatorial development of carrier-bound drugs in the future.

Apart from adaptor units, other modified SILs have been developed that display a more sophisticated release behavior. The underlying concept is rather simple: introducing additional hydroxymethyl groups (or their vinylogs) to elimination linkers leads to so-called AB_n linkers that are capable of undergoing multiple eliminations to release n tail groups as illustrated in the following example of an AB_2-type SIL:

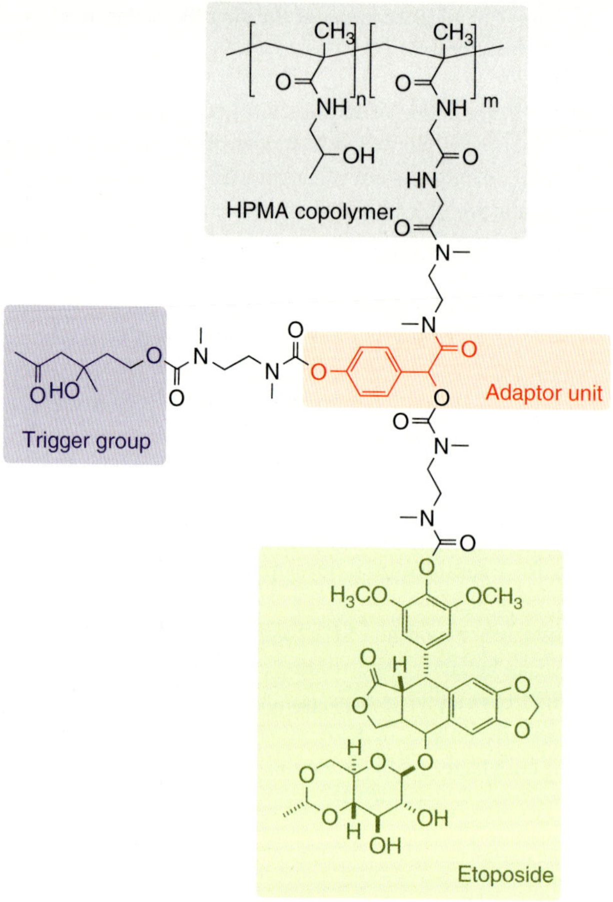

Figure 19.5 HPMA copolymer conjugate of etoposide comprising an adaptor unit (red) and a trigger group (blue) that is activated by the catalytic antibody 38C2 [10].

After activation of the trigger group, the faster 1,6-elimination takes place releasing the first residue R^1. Regeneration of the quinone methide intermediate by addition of one water molecule allows the second elimination step to proceed, resulting in the liberation of the residue R^2 [18, 19]. There are many possibilities to construct multiple elimination linkers and various examples can be found in the literature [39, 64–67]. The most spectacular instance of this class of compounds was presented by Shabat et al., who designed an AB_6 elimination linker that was shown to react in subsequent 1,6- and 1,8-elimination steps [68]:

19.4 Branched Elimination Linkers--Chemical Adaptors or Building Blocks

$\xrightarrow{\text{1,6- and 1,8-Eliminations}}$

$+ 6\ CO_2 + 6\ H\text{-}R$

Replacing single by multiple elimination linkers can be used to improve the drug loading of drug–carrier conjugates [69]. Furthermore, it offers the opportunity to create innovative multicomponent drugs with a defined ratio of the components. An example of such a combination prodrug was also given by the group of Shabat who combined a triple (AB_3) elimination linker with the drugs DOX, camptothecin, and etoposide plus a trigger group that is activated by the catalytic antibody 38C2 (see Figure 19.6) [40].

However, there is no pharmacological rationale for the used 1 : 1 : 1 drug combination and thus the prodrug merely serves as an example for the viability of the underlying technology. In addition to prodrug design, AB_2 linkers have also been employed to construct nanoparticles from photolabile polymers that were shown to encapsulate dyes and release them upon radiation [70]. Moreover, double elimination linkers have been used to develop even more complex self-immolative architectures. In 2003, the groups of Shabat, de Groot, and McGrath independently reported on the development of perfectly branched molecular scaffolds composed of double-elimination linkers [46, 55, 71, 72]. These dendrimers, either classified as self-immolative (Shabat), cascade-release (de Groot), or geometrically disassembling (McGrath), are characterized by an efficient disassembly of the whole dendritic scaffold upon a single triggering event. The trigger is placed at the focal point so that the elimination cascade reaction can spread from there to the tail units to release the effector payload (see Figure 19.7).

Shabat and McGrath presented chemically [71] or photochemically [61] triggered G1 and G2 [55, 73] dendrons, each of which releasing eight molecules of the dyes 4-nitroaniline and 4-nitrophenol, respectively, whereas de Groot developed a reductively triggered G1 dendron [46] capable of releasing four molecules of the anticancer drug paclitaxel (see Figure 19.8).

Although different types of double elimination linkers have been employed (de Groot: double 1,8-elimination; Shabat: double 1,4-elimination combined with ethylene diamine-based cyclization linkers; McGrath: 1,6- and 1,4- elimination), the dendrons reacted according to the same overall mechanism. Due to their ability to act as molecular amplifiers ensuring a simultaneous multiple release of drugs, self-immolative dendrimers have been proposed as ideal drug delivery vehicles, but there are a number of reasons explaining why this class of compounds still lacks application. The use of hydrophobic linker groups results in a poor water

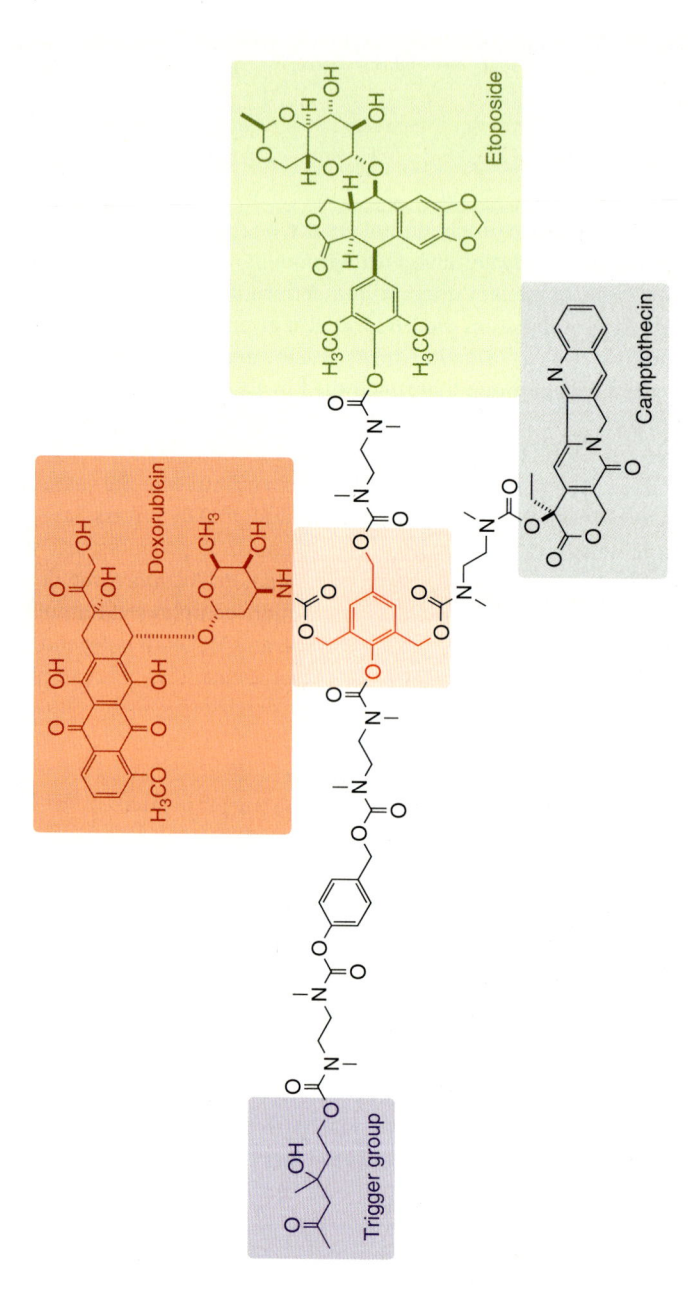

Figure 19.6 Prodrug based on a triple elimination linker (red) to ensure a nearly simultaneous release of a 1 : 1 : 1 combination of the anticancer drugs etoposide, DOX, and camptothecin. The prodrug is activated by the catalytic antibody 38C2 [40].

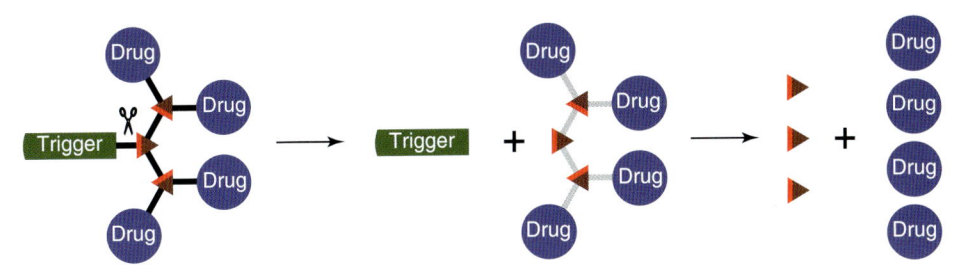

Figure 19.7 General principle of drug release from self-immolative dendrimers as exemplified by a G1 dendrimer based on AB$_2$ linkers. After activation and cleavage of the trigger group, a cascade of elimination reaction takes place that results in a complete fragmentation of the carrier with a concomitant release of n drug molecules and $n - 1$ linker groups.

solubility of the dendrimers. Moreover, their molecular masses have been too low for a use as drug delivery systems that make use of the EPR effect. To circumvent these drawbacks, the group of Shabat developed an enzymatically triggered G1 self-immolative dendrimer loaded with four molecules of the anticancer drug camptothecin (see Figure 19.9) [11]. For improving the water solubility, the system was grafted with two PEG chains using click chemistry. *In vitro* data show that the cytotoxicity of the prodrug is increased 100-fold in the presence of the enzyme PGA, but no *in vivo* data have been published so far.

Another limitation of self-immolative dendrimers results from the dendritic structure itself. Due to the exponentially growing steric demands of the outer shell from generation to generation, it seems that a G2 dendron with a loading capacity of eight drugs marks the limit for the perfect dendritic structure. To overcome this drawback, linear self-immolative structures have been developed that – at least in theory – should be capable of releasing an unlimited number of side-chain-bound drugs. The simplest self-immolative polymer uses the PABC linker as the monomer unit and was presented by the group of Shabat [44]. Since poly(PABC) is not water soluble, Shabat *et al.* also developed a slightly modified polymer with solubilizing side-chains and a terminal 4-nitroaniline group as a reporter (see Figure 19.10).

Depolymerization is triggered by BSA (see Section 19.3.1). The complete degradation of the chain was proven both by the increase in fluorescence of the liberated monomer units and the appearance of a yellow color resulting from the release of the terminal reporter group. A polymer with the potential for a controlled release of drugs was also published by Shabat *et al.* who employed double 1,6-elimination linkers as monomer units [45]. However, the resulting self-immolative system,

Figure 19.8 Self-immolative G1 dendron of de Groot [46] (a), and G2 dendrons of McGrath [73] (b) and Shabat [55] (c). The double elimination linkers are highlighted red. (In contrast to the nomenclature used by Shabat who specified the above dendrimer G3 and a branched SIL as a G1 dendrimer [74], this chapter follows the official nomenclature classifying the first branching unit as G0.)

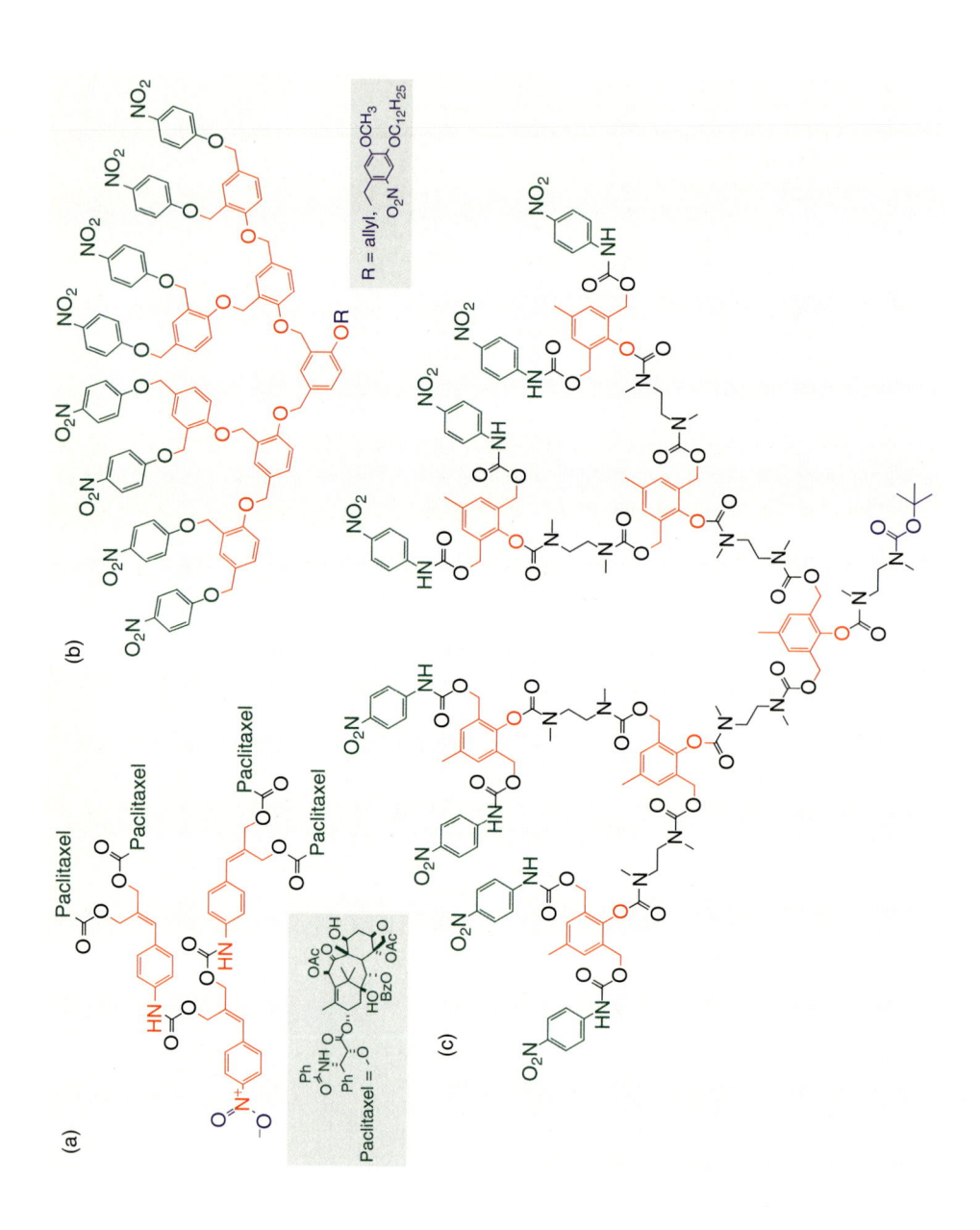

578 | *19 Site-Specific Prodrug Activation and the Concept of Self-Immolation*

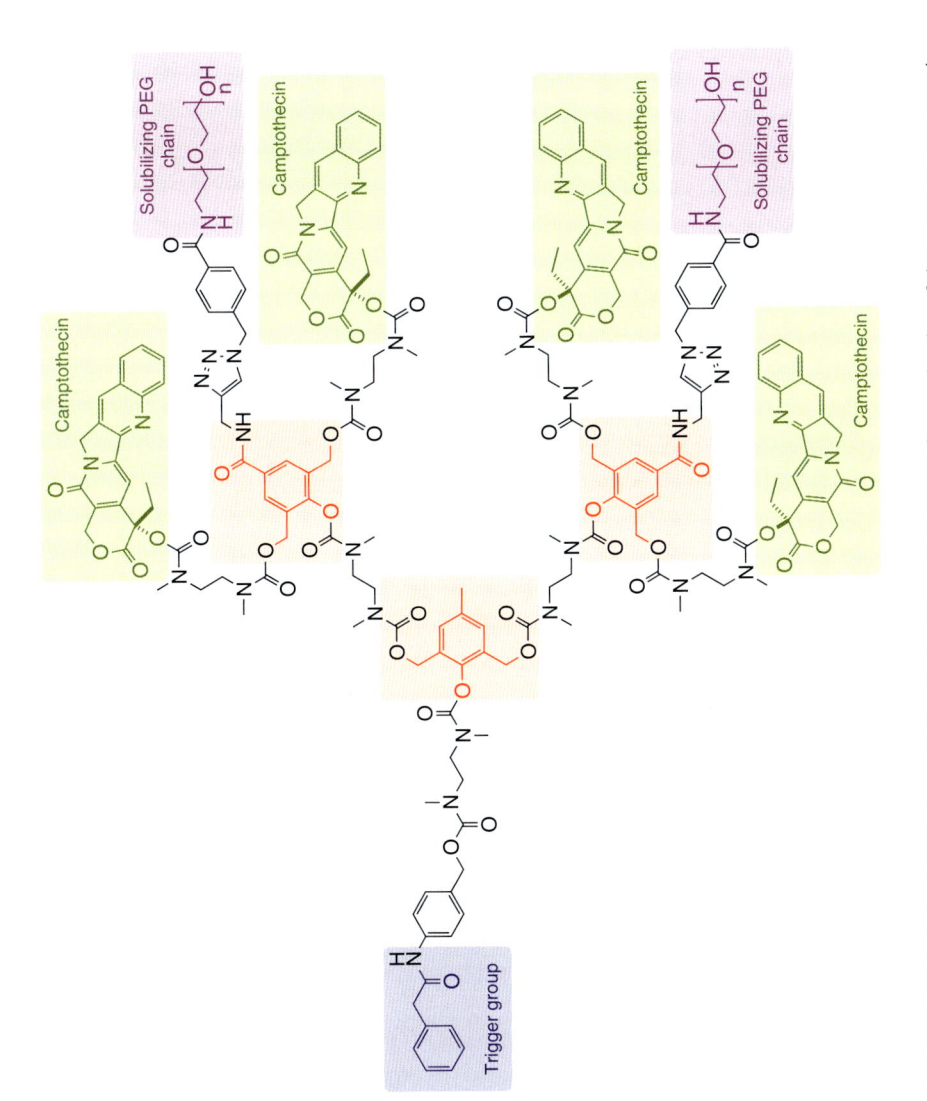

Figure 19.9 PEG chain-grafted water-soluble G1 dendrimer loaded with four molecules of the cytotoxic compound camptothecin [11].

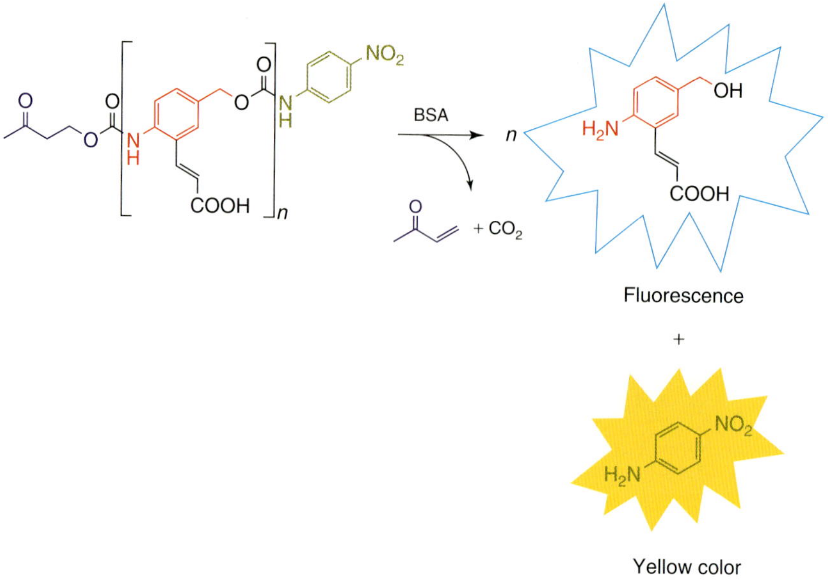

Figure 19.10 Self-immolative polymer releasing fluorogenic monomer units and the reporter 4-nitroaniline [44].

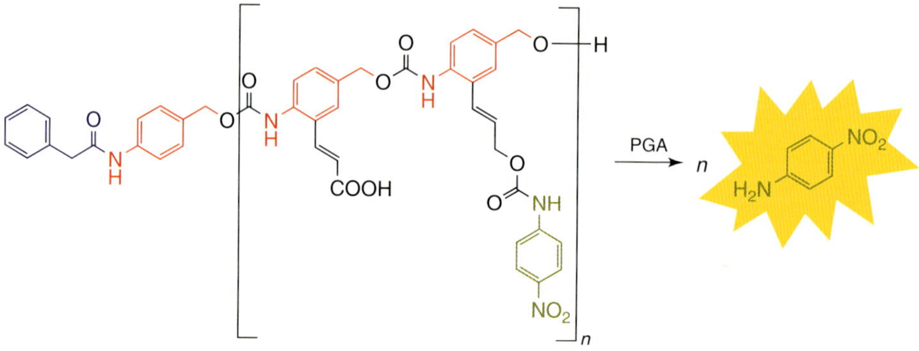

Figure 19.11 Self-immolative comb polymer releasing n molecules of the reporter 4-nitroaniline [45].

a comb polymer with 4-nitroaniline as the side chain-bound reporter, was too hydrophobic to be investigated in aqueous solution. Therefore, Shabat et al. developed a water-soluble polymer with alternating solubilizing and double release monomers (see Figure 19.11).

This polymer releases n molecules of the reporter after enzymatic activation by PGA (see Section 19.3.1). Shabat determined that the polymer consists of approximately 13 repeating units, which corresponds to a molecular weight of

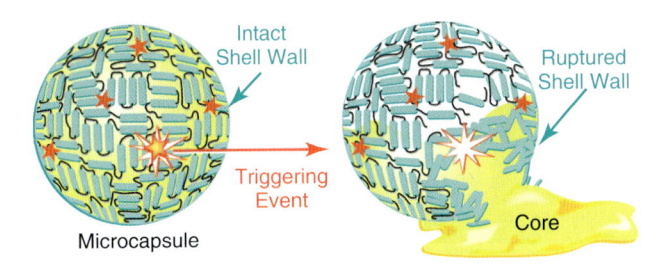

Figure 19.12 General principle of the release of encapsulated content from microcapsules based on self-immolative polymers [56]. (Reproduced with permission from [56], © 2010 American Chemical Society.)

around 8 kDa. Although the loading with effector molecules is significantly higher when compared to self-immolative dendrimers, the molecular weight has to be further increased to obtain a carrier suitable for passive tumor targeting that is worth being loaded with anticancer drugs instead of dyes. While this has been the only approach of comb polymers as linear congeners of self-immolative dendrimers so far, there are some other recent developments making use of self-immolative polymers that are worth mentioning.

The group of Gillies developed an amphiphilic block copolymer comprising a hydrophilic PEG and a hydrophobic polyurethane block, with the latter being a self-immolative polymer that consists of alternate cyclization and elimination linkers similar to the self-immolative dendrimer of Shabat et al. [75]:

The system forms aggregates in aqueous solutions that were shown to effectively encapsulate the dye Nile Red. The ester bond serves as the trigger group that slowly hydrolyzes at neutral pH so that a sustained release of the encapsulated dye from the nanoparticles was observed.

Recently, another application of self-immolative polymers has been published – the construction of cleavable microcapsules (see Figure 19.12) [56]. In this example, a slight modification of the self-immolative poly(PABC) polymer of Shabat (as described above) was used to form the shell wall of the microcapsules. The synthesis was performed by cross-linking the linear polymer chains to obtain a spherically shaped polymer network sized 5–40 µm. Either Boc or Fmoc protective groups were used as trigger units.

Using scanning electron microscopy it could be impressively demonstrated that only the exposure of the microcapsules to the designated cleavage conditions

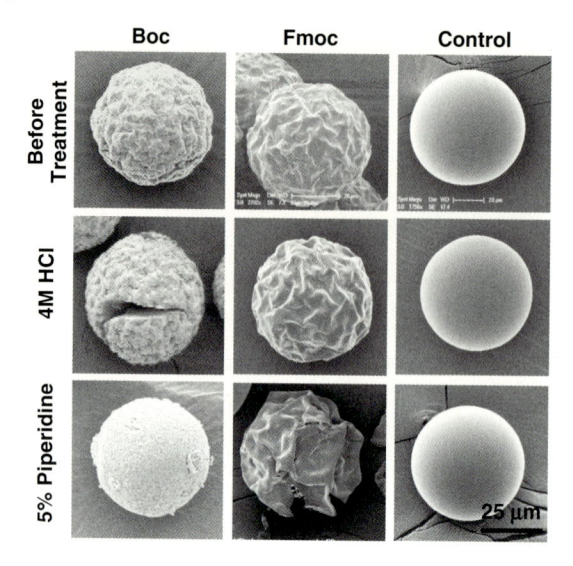

Figure 19.13 Scanning electron microscopy images of Boc- and Fmoc-triggered capsules before and after 48 h exposure to the respective triggering conditions. Triggered capsules bear a distinct cracking pattern on the outsides of their shell walls. (Reproduced with permission from [56], © 2010 American Chemical Society.)

(4 M HCl for Boc- and 10% piperidine for Fmoc-triggered capsules) resulted in a rupture of the shell wall and a release of the content (see Figure 19.13). This technology might have a great potential for future applications as universal drug delivery systems.

The technology of self-immolative polymeric architectures introduced in this section is still relatively new and the majority of the presented examples do not exceed the status of model compounds in which dyes were used as effectors to study the release behavior. For an application in the field of drug delivery, the systems have to be optimized with respect to basic pharmacological properties such as water solubility and pharmacokinetics. The dyes used as effectors must be replaced by pharmaceutically active compounds (or suitable dyes for imaging agents) and, last but not least, the trigger groups have to be adapted to the field of application.

19.5
Clinical Impact

Apart from the large number of more or less complex model compounds that have been synthesized for studying the release behavior of self-immolative systems, several prodrugs comprising a PABC or related SIL have been preclinically developed. Recent examples for SIL-incorporating prodrugs for which *in vivo* data has been presented are albumin-binding prodrugs of DOX or paclitaxel that are

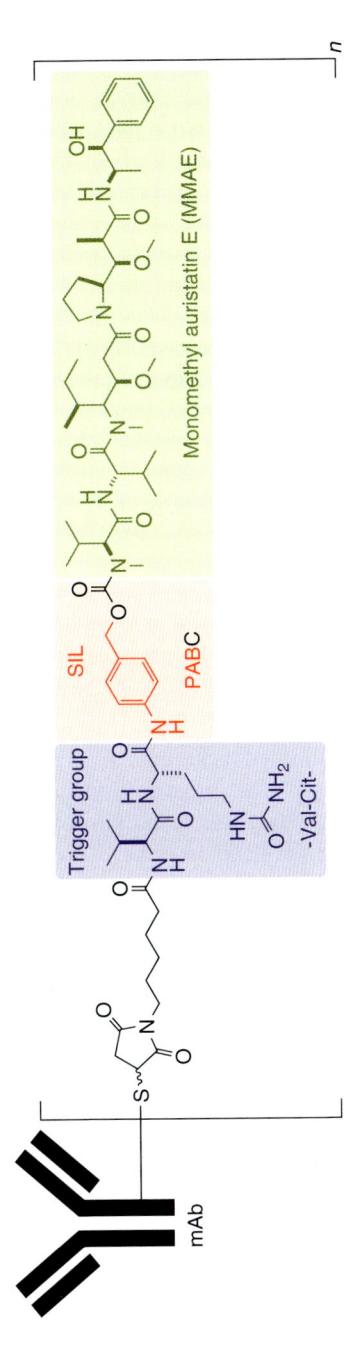

Figure 19.14 General design of clinically assessed conjugates of MMAE with different antibodies and variable drug loading. The prodrugs consist of the carrier mAb, a lysosomally cleavable Val–Cit trigger group, a self-immolative PABC linker, and the drug.

cleaved by cathepsin B [76] or PSA [77, 78], or antibody conjugates of highly potent camptothecin analogs [79]. However, the number of compounds comprising a SIL that have reached a clinical stage of development is limited to a few examples given by various antibody conjugates of the highly potent drug monomethyl auristatin E (MMAE) that is too toxic to be administered as a single agent (see also Chapter 10). The overall prodrug design follows the one depicted in Figure 19.1e with one to several drugs bound to the carrier through cleavable peptides in combination with the self-immolative PABC linker (see Figure 19.14). The choice of the Val–Cit sequence is a result of a longer optimization process and was mainly due to the excellent stability in the circulation.

This technology seems to be applicable to a number of antibodies. Meanwhile, six different antibody conjugates of auristatin are undergoing clinical trials [80]. The most advanced candidate, brentuximab vedotin (SGN-35), which is based on the chimeric anti-CD30 mAb cAC10 has proven very efficacious against relapsed $CD30^+$ Hodgkin's lymphoma. In a phase I study, the maximum tolerated dose of brentuximab vedotin was merely 1.8 mg/kg administered every 3 weeks due to the potency of MMAE with grades 1–2 toxic effects being observed. Seventeen of the 45 treated patients showed objective response (38%) including 11 complete remissions [81]. This drug is currently being assessed in phase III studies (*www.seagen.com*).

19.6
Conclusion and Perspectives

Thirty years after Katzenellenbogen *et al.* introduced the PABC linker for the design of prodrugs, the incorporation of SILs in drug–carrier conjugates has meanwhile become a well-established technique of modern prodrug design and the first antibody–drug conjugates comprising PABC linkers have reached the clinical setting. Especially in the last few years, the concept of self-immolation has received growing attention due to the work of Shabat and some other groups who have impressively demonstrated how to broaden the scope of this research area. Employing SIL as building blocks for polymeric architectures is a promising approach to novel smart materials. Compared to other fully degradable polymers, dendritic as well as linear self-immolative systems have the intriguing advantage of signal amplification, which means that a single stimulus is sufficient to initiate a complete depolymerization of the macromolecule. For drug delivery, polymeric self-immolative compounds can be either designed as water-soluble carriers or as insoluble degradable materials. In particular, the most recent developments such as the construction of microcapsules from self-immolative polymers or the formation of nanoparticles from block copolymers with a self-immolative block pave the way from classic drug–carrier conjugates to modern nanomedical drug delivery. These technologies, however, are still at their beginning and the full potential of self-immolative structures for prodrug design needs to be evaluated preclinically as the next important step in the development of clinically relevant drug delivery systems in the field of oncology.

References

1. Singer, J.W., Baker, B., De Vries, P., Kumar, A., Shaffer, S., Vawter, E., Bolton, M., and Garzone, P. (2003) Poly-(L)-glutamic acid–paclitaxel (CT-2103) [XYOTAX], a biodegradable polymeric drug conjugate: characterization, preclinical pharmacology, and preliminary clinical data. *Adv. Exp. Med. Biol.*, **519**, 81–99.
2. Kratz, F., Müller, I.A., Ryppa, C., and Warnecke, A. (2008) Prodrug strategies in anticancer chemotherapy. *ChemMedChem*, **3**, 20–53.
3. Bundgaard, H. (1989) The double prodrug concept and its applications. *Adv. Drug Deliv. Rev.*, **3**, 39–65.
4. Shabat, D., Amir, R.J., Gopin, A., Pessah, N., and Shamis, M. (2004) Chemical adaptor systems. *Chem. Eur. J.*, **10**, 2626–2634.
5. Papot, S., Tranoy, I., Tillequin, F., Florent, J.-C., and Gesson, J.-P. (2002) Design of selectively activated anticancer prodrugs: elimination and cyclization strategies. *Curr. Med. Chem. Anticancer Agents*, **2**, 155–185.
6. Tranoy-Opalinski, I., Fernandes, A., Thomas, M., Gesson, J.P., and Papot, S. (2008) Design of self-immolative linkers for tumour-activated prodrug therapy. *Anticancer Agents Med. Chem.*, **8**, 618–637.
7. Milstien, S. and Cohen, L.A. (1972) Stereopopulation control. I. Rate enhancement in the lactonizations of o-hydroxyhydrocinnamic acids. *J. Am. Chem. Soc.*, **94**, 9158–9165.
8. Greenwald, R.B., Choe, Y.H., Conover, C., Shum, K., Wu, D., and Royzen, M. (2000) Drug delivery systems based on trimethyl lock lactonization: poly(ethylene glycol) prodrugs of amino-containing compounds. *J. Med. Chem.*, **43**, 475–487.
9. Saari, W.S., Schwering, J.E., Lyle, P.A., Smith, S.J., and Engelhardt, E.L. (1990) Cyclization-activated prodrugs. Basic carbamates of 4-hydroxyanisole. *J. Med. Chem.*, **33**, 97–101.
10. Gopin, A., Pessah, N., Shamis, M., Rader, C., and Shabat, D. (2003) A chemical adaptor system designed to link a tumor-targeting device with a prodrug and an enzymatic trigger. *Angew. Chem. Int. Ed.*, **42**, 327–332.
11. Gopin, A., Ebner, S., Attali, B., and Shabat, D. (2006) Enzymatic activation of second-generation dendritic prodrugs: conjugation of self-immolative dendrimers with poly(ethylene glycol) via click chemistry. *Bioconjug. Chem.*, **17**, 1432–1440.
12. Lee, H.Y., Jiang, X., and Lee, D. (2009) Kinetics of self-immolation: faster signal relay over a longer linear distance? *Org. Lett.*, **11**, 2065–2068.
13. Toki, B.E., Cerveny, C.G., Wahl, A.F., and Senter, P.D. (2002) Protease-mediated fragmentation of p-amidobenzyl ethers: a new strategy for the activation of anticancer prodrugs. *J. Org. Chem.*, **67**, 1866–1872.
14. Buur, A. and Bundgaard, H. (1986) Prodrugs of 5-fluorouracil. V. 1-Alkoxycarbonyl derivatives as potential prodrug forms for improved rectal or oral delivery of 5-fluorouracil. *J. Pharm. Sci.*, **75**, 522–527.
15. Madec-Lougerstay, R., Florent, J.-C., and Monneret, C. (1999) Synthesis of self-immolative glucuronide spacers based on aminomethylcarbamate. Application to 5-fluorouracil prodrugs for antibody-directed enzyme prodrug therapy. *J. Chem. Soc. Perkin Trans. 1*, 1369–1375.
16. Weinert, E.E., Dondi, R., Colloredo-Melz, S., Frankenfield, K.N., Mitchell, C.H., Freccero, M., and Rokita, S.E. (2006) Substituents on quinone methides strongly modulate formation and stability of their nucleophilic adducts. *J. Am. Chem. Soc.*, **128**, 11940–11947.
17. Weinstain, R., Baran, P.S., and Shabat, D. (2009) Activity-linked labeling of enzymes by self-immolative polymers. *Bioconjug. Chem.*, **20**, 1783–1791.
18. Erez, R. and Shabat, D. (2008) The azaquinone-methide elimination: comparison study of 1,6- and 1,4-eliminations under physiological conditions. *Org. Biomol. Chem.*, **6**, 2669–2672.

19. Warnecke, A. and Kratz, F. (2008) 2,4-Bis(hydroxymethyl)aniline as a building block for oligomers with self-eliminating and multiple release properties. *J. Org. Chem.*, **73**, 1546–1552.
20. Wakselman, M. (1983) 1,4-Eliminations and 1,6-eliminations from hydroxy-substituted and amino-substituted benzyl systems – chemical and biochemical applications. *Nouv. J. Chem.*, **7**, 439–447.
21. Carl, P.L., Chakravarty, P.K., and Katzenellenbogen, J.A. (1981) A novel connector linkage applicable in prodrug design. *J. Med. Chem.*, **24**, 479–480.
22. Müller, I.A., Kratz, F., Jung, M., and Warnecke, A. (2010) Schiff bases derived from p-aminobenzyl alcohol as trigger groups for pH-dependent prodrug activation. *Tetrahedron Lett.*, **51**, 4371–4374.
23. Perry-Feigenbaum, R., Baran, P.S., and Shabat, D. (2009) The pyridinone-methide elimination. *Org. Biomol. Chem.*, **7**, 4825–4828.
24. Borch, R.F., Liu, J., Schmidt, J.P., Marakovits, J.T., Joswig, C., Gipp, J.J., and Mulcahy, R.T. (2000) Synthesis and evaluation of nitroheterocyclic phosphoramidates as hypoxia-selective alkylating agents. *J. Med. Chem.*, **43**, 2258–2265.
25. Hay, M.P., Sykes, B.M., Denny, W.A., and Wilson, W.R. (1999) A 2-nitroimidazole carbamate prodrug of 5-amimo-1-(chloromethyl)-3-[(5,6,7-trimethoxyindol-2-yl)carbonyl]-1,2-dihydro-3H-benz[e]indole (amino-seco-CBI-TMI) for use with ADEPT and GDEPT. *Bioorg. Med. Chem. Lett.*, **9**, 2237–2242.
26. Damen, E.W., Nevalainen, T.J., van den Bergh, T.J., de Groot, F.M., and Scheeren, H.W. (2002) Synthesis of novel paclitaxel prodrugs designed for bioreductive activation in hypoxic tumour tissue. *Bioorg. Med. Chem.*, **10**, 71–77.
27. de Groot, F.M., Loos, W.J., Koekkoek, R., van Berkom, L.W., Busscher, G.F., Seelen, A.E., Albrecht, C., de Bruijn, P., and Scheeren, H.W. (2001) Elongated multiple electronic cascade and cyclization spacer systems in activatible anticancer prodrugs for enhanced drug release. *J. Org. Chem.*, **66**, 8815–8830.
28. Weinstain, R., Segal, E., Satchi-Fainaro, R., and Shabat, D. (2010) Real-time monitoring of drug release. *Chem. Commun.*, **46**, 553–535.
29. Dubowchik, G.M. and Firestone, R.A. (1998) Cathepsin B-sensitive dipeptide prodrugs. 1. A model study of structural requirements for efficient release of doxorubicin. *Bioorg. Med. Chem. Lett.*, **8**, 3341–3346.
30. Elsadek, B., Graeser, R., Warnecke, A., Unger, C., Saleem, T., El-Melegy, N., Madkor, H., and Kratz, F. (2010) Optimization of an albumin-binding prodrug of doxorubicin that is cleaved by prostate-specific antigen. *ACS Med. Chem. Lett.*, **1**, 234–238.
31. Pessah, N., Reznik, M., Shamis, M., Yantiri, F., Xin, H., Bowdish, K., Shomron, N., Ast, G., and Shabat, D. (2004) Bioactivation of carbamate-based 20 (S)-camptothecin prodrugs. *Bioorg. Med. Chem.*, **12**, 1859–1866.
32. Zhang, Q., Xiang, G., Zhang, Y., Yang, K., Fan, W., Lin, J., Zeng, F., and Wu, J. (2006) Increase of doxorubicin sensitivity for folate receptor positive cells when given as the prodrug N-(phenylacetyl) doxorubicin in combination with folate-conjugated PGA. *J. Pharm. Sci.*, **95**, 2266–2275.
33. Vrudhula, V.M., Senter, P.D., Fischer, K.J., and Wallace, P.M. (1993) Prodrugs of doxorubicin and melphalan and their activation by a monoclonal antibody–penicillin-G amidase conjugate. *J. Med. Chem.*, **36**, 919–923.
34. Bignami, G.S., Senter, P.D., Grothaus, P.G., Fischer, K.J., Humphreys, T., and Wallace, P.M. (1992) N-(4′-hydroxyphenylacetyl)palytoxin: a palytoxin prodrug that can be activated by a monoclonal antibody–penicillin G amidase conjugate. *Cancer Res.*, **52**, 5759–5564.
35. Gesson, J.P., Jacquesy, J.C., Mondon, M., Petit, P., Renoux, B., Andrianomenjanahary, S., Dufat-Trinh Van, H., Koch, M., Michel, S., Tillequin, F. et al. (1994) Prodrugs of anthracyclines for chemotherapy via

enzyme–monoclonal antibody conjugates. *Anticancer Drug Des.*, **9**, 409–423.
36. Lu, C.P., Ren, C.T., Wu, S.H., Chu, C.Y., and Lo, L.C. (2007) Development of an activity-based probe for steroid sulfatases. *ChemBioChem*, **8**, 2187–2190.
37. Lo, L.C., Pang, T.L., Kuo, C.H., Chiang, Y.L., Wang, H.Y., and Lin, J.J. (2002) Design and synthesis of class-selective activity probes for protein tyrosine phosphatases. *J. Proteome Res.*, **1**, 35–40.
38. Shabat, D., Rader, C., List, B., Lerner, R.A., and Barbas, C.F. III (1999) Multiple event activation of a generic prodrug trigger by antibody catalysis. *Proc. Natl. Acad. Sci. USA*, **96**, 6925–6930.
39. Shamis, M., Lode, H.N., and Shabat, D. (2004) Bioactivation of self-immolative dendritic prodrugs by catalytic antibody 38C2. *J. Am. Chem. Soc.*, **126**, 1726–1731.
40. Haba, K., Popkov, M., Shamis, M., Lerner, R.A., Barbas, C.F., and Shabat, D. III (2005) Single-triggered trimeric prodrugs. *Angew. Chem. Int. Ed.*, **44**, 716–720
41. Duncan, R., Gac-Breton, S., Keane, R., Musila, R., Sat, Y.N., Satchi, R., and Searle, F. (2001) Polymer–drug conjugates, PDEPT and PELT: basic principles for design and transfer from the laboratory to clinic. *J. Control. Release*, **74**, 135–146.
42. Satchi-Fainaro, R., Wrasidlo, W., Lode, H.N., and Shabat, D. (2002) Synthesis and characterization of a catalytic antibody–HPMA copolymer conjugate as a tool for tumor selective prodrug activation. *Bioorg. Med. Chem.*, **10**, 3023–3029.
43. Jourdain, N., Carlón, R.P., and Reymond, J.-L. (1998) A stereoselective fluorogenic assay for aldolase: detection of an anti-selective aldolase catalytic antibody. *Tetrahedron Lett.*, **39**, 9415–9418.
44. Sagi, A., Weinstain, R., Karton, N., and Shabat, D. (2008) Self-immolative polymers. *J. Am. Chem. Soc.*, **130**, 5434–5435.
45. Weinstain, R., Sagi, A., Karton, N., and Shabat, D. (2008) Self-Immolative comb-polymers: multiple-release of side-reporters by a single stimulus event. *Chem. Eur. J.*, **14**, 6857–6861.
46. de Groot, F.M., Albrecht, C., Koekkoek, R., Beusker, P.H., and Scheeren, H.W. (2003) "Cascade-release dendrimers" liberate all end groups upon a single triggering event in the dendritic core. *Angew. Chem. Int. Ed.*, **42**, 4490–4494.
47. van Brakel, R., Vulders, R.C., Bokdam, R.J., Grull, H., and Robillard, M.S. (2008) A doxorubicin prodrug activated by the Staudinger reaction. *Bioconjug. Chem.*, **19**, 714–718.
48. Senter, P.D., Pearce, W.E., and Greenfield, R.S. (1990) Development of a drug-release strategy based on the reductive fragmentation of benzyl carbamate disulfides. *J. Org. Chem.*, **55**, 2975–2978.
49. Zhu, B., Zhang, X., Jia, H., Li, Y., Liu, H., and Tan, W. (2010) A highly selective ratiometric fluorescent probe for 1,4-dithiothreitol (DTT) detection. *Org. Biomol. Chem.*, **8**, 1650–1654.
50. Lo, L.C. and Chu, C.Y. (2003) Development of highly selective and sensitive probes for hydrogen peroxide. *Chem. Commun.*, 2728–2729.
51. Sella, E. and Shabat, D. (2009) Dendritic chain reaction. *J. Am. Chem. Soc.*, **131**, 9934–9936.
52. Sella, E., Lubelski, A., Klafter, J., and Shabat, D. (2010) Two-component dendritic chain reactions: experiment and theory. *J. Am. Chem. Soc.*, **132**, 3945–3952.
53. Avital-Shmilovici, M. and Shabat, D. (2010) Dendritic chain reaction: responsive release of hydrogen peroxide upon generation and enzymatic oxidation of methanol. *Bioorg. Med. Chem.*, **18**, 3643–3647.
54. Sella, E., Weinstain, R., Erez, R., Burns, N.Z., Baran, P.S., and Shabat, D. (2010) Sulfhydryl-based dendritic chain reaction. *Chem. Commun.*, **46**, 6575–6577.
55. Amir, R.J., Pessah, N., Shamis, M., and Shabat, D. (2003) Self-immolative dendrimers. *Angew. Chem. Int. Ed.*, **42**, 4494–4499.
56. Esser-Kahn, A.P., Sottos, N.R., White, S.R., and Moore, J.S. (2010) Programmable microcapsules from

self-immolative polymers. *J. Am. Chem. Soc.*, **132**, 10266–10268.
57. Tannock, I.F. and Rotin, D. (1989) Acid pH in tumors and its potential for therapeutic exploitation. *Cancer Res.*, **49**, 4373–4384.
58. Kratz, F., Beyer, U., and Schütte, M.T. (1999) Drug–polymer conjugates containing acid-cleavable bonds. *Crit. Rev. Ther. Drug Carrier Sys.*, **16**, 245–288.
59. Greenwald, R.B., Pendri, A., Conover, C., Zhao, H., Choe, Y.H., Martinez, A., Shum, K., and Guan, S. (1999) Drug delivery systems employing 1,4- or 1,6-elimination: poly(ethylene glycol) prodrugs of amine-containing compounds. *J. Med. Chem.*, **42**, 3657–3667.
60. Azoulay, M., Tuffin, G., Sallem, W., and Florent, J.C. (2006) A new drug-release method using the Staudinger ligation. *Bioorg. Med. Chem. Lett.*, **16**, 3147–3149.
61. Szalai, M.L. and McGrath, D.V. (2004) Phototriggering of geometric dendrimer disassembly: an improved synthesis of 2,4-bis(hydroxymethyl)phenol based dendrimers. *Tetrahedron*, **60**, 7261–7266.
62. Zhang, Z., Hatta, H., Ito, T., and Nishimoto, S. (2005) Synthesis and photochemical properties of photoactivated antitumor prodrugs releasing 5-fluorouracil. *Org. Biomol. Chem.*, **3**, 592–596.
63. Amit, B., Sehavi, V., and Patchornik, A. (1974) Photosensitive protecting groups of amino sugars and their use in glycoside synthesis. 2-Nitrobenzyloxycarbonylamino and 6-nitroveratryloxycarbonylamino derivatives. *J. Org. Chem.*, **39**, 192–196.
64. Adler-Abramovich, L., Perry, R., Sagi, A., Gazit, E., and Shabat, D. (2007) Controlled assembly of peptide nanotubes triggered by enzymatic activation of self-immolative dendrimers. *ChemBioChem*, **8**, 859–862.
65. Danieli, E. and Shabat, D. (2007) Molecular probe for enzymatic activity with dual output. *Bioorg. Med. Chem.*, **13**, 7318–7324.
66. Perry, R., Amir, R.J., and Shabat, D. (2007) Substituent-dependent disassembly of self-immolative dendrimers. *New J. Chem.*, **31**, 1307–1312.
67. Sagi, A., Segal, E., Satchi-Fainaro, R., and Shabat, D. (2007) Remarkable drug-release enhancement with an elimination-based AB3 self-immolative dendritic amplifier. *Bioorg. Med. Chem.*, **15**, 3720–3727.
68. Shamis, M. and Shabat, D. (2007) Single-triggered AB6 self-immolative dendritic amplifiers. *Chem. Eur. J.*, **13**, 4523–4528.
69. Erez, R., Segal, E., Miller, K., Satchi-Fainaro, R., and Shabat, D. (2009) Enhanced cytotoxicity of a polymer–drug conjugate with triple payload of paclitaxel. *Bioorg. Med. Chem.*, **17**, 4327–4335.
70. Fomina, N., McFearin, C., Sermsakdi, M., Edigin, O., and Almutairi, A. (2010) UV and near-IR triggered release from polymeric nanoparticles. *J. Am. Chem. Soc.*, **132**, 9540–9542.
71. Szalai, M.L., Kevwitch, R.M., and McGrath, D.V. (2003) Geometric disassembly of dendrimers: dendritic amplification. *J. Am. Chem. Soc.*, **125**, 15688–15689.
72. Meijer, E.W. and Van Genderen, M.H. (2003) Chemistry: dendrimers set to self-destruct. *Nature*, **426**, 128–129.
73. McGrath, D.V. (2005) Dendrimer disassembly as a new paradigm for the application of dendritic structures. *Mol. Pharm.*, **2**, 253–263.
74. Amir, R.J. and Shabat, D. (2006) Domino dendrimers. *Adv. Polym. Sci.*, **192**, 59–93.
75. DeWit, M.A. and Gillies, E.R. (2009) A cascade biodegradable polymer based on alternating cyclization and elimination reactions. *J. Am. Chem. Soc.*, **131**, 18327–18334.
76. Abu Ajaj, K., Graeser, R., Fichtner, I., and Kratz, F. (2009) *In vitro* and *in vivo* study of an albumin-binding prodrug of doxorubicin that is cleaved by cathepsin B. *Cancer Chemother. Pharmacol.*, **64**, 413–418.
77. Elsadek, B., Graeser, R., Esser, N., Schafer-Obodozie, C., Tsurumi, C., Abu Ajaj, K., Warnecke, A., Unger, C., Saleem, T., and Kratz, F. (2011) *In vivo* evaluation of a novel albumin-binding prodrug of doxorubicin in an orthotopic mouse model of prostate cancer

(LNCaP). *Prostate Cancer Prostatic Dis.*, **14**, 14–21.

78. Elsadek, B., Graeser, R., Esser, N., Schafer-Obodozie, C., Ajaj, K.A., Unger, C., Warnecke, A., Saleem, T., El-Melegy, N., Madkor, H., and Kratz, F. (2010) Development of a novel prodrug of paclitaxel that is cleaved by prostate-specific antigen: an *in vitro* and *in vivo* evaluation study. *Eur. J. Cancer*, **46**, 3434–3444.

79. Burke, P.J., Senter, P.D., Meyer, D.W., Miyamoto, J.B., Anderson, M., Toki, B.E., Manikumar, G., Wani, M.C., Kroll, D.J., and Jeffrey, S.C. (2009) Design, synthesis, and biological evaluation of antibody–drug conjugates comprised of potent camptothecin analogues. *Bioconjug. Chem.*, **20**, 1242–1250.

80. Alley, S.C., Okeley, N.M., and Senter, P.D. (2010) Antibody–drug conjugates: targeted drug delivery for cancer. *Curr. Opin. Chem. Biol.*, **14**, 529–537.

81. Younes, A., Bartlett, N.L., Leonard, J.P., Kennedy, D.A., Lynch, C.M., Sievers, E.L., and Forero-Torres, A. (2010) Brentuximab vedotin (SGN-35) for relapsed CD30-positive lymphomas. *N. Engl. J. Med.*, **363**, 1812–1821.

20
Ligand-Assisted Vascular Targeting of Polymer Therapeutics

Anat Eldar-Boock, Dina Polyak, and Ronit Satchi-Fainaro

20.1
Overview of Tumor Angiogenesis

Angiogenesis – the generation of new blood vessels from pre-existing vasculature [1] – may be considered as an organizing principle in biomedicine [2], and measured as an healthy essential process in embryogenesis, body growth, and wound healing. The expansion of the vasculature provides nutrients and oxygen to growing tissues, and allows cell movement. Normal blood vessels are lined by a thin monolayer of smooth, tightly joined endothelial cells that forms a barrier between the circulation and the tissue, controlling the transport of different components from one side to the other. Healthy vessels are organized stable structures lined with mural cells to form functional basement membranes [3].

Angiogenesis is regulated by a number of different growth factors [4], and is dependent on the balance between pro- and antiangiogenic factors. The vascular endothelial growth factor (VEGF) family of proteins is one of the noticeable proangiogenic factors [5]. Judah Folkman was the first to propose that tumor growth is angiogenesis dependent, and that antiangiogenic drugs may serve as a potent and successful anticancer therapy [6]. Angiogenesis is a crucial process in tumor growth and progression. This multistep process involves (i) activation of earlier quiescent endothelial cells, (ii) dissolution of the basement membrane followed by stromal invasion, (iii) increase in the proliferation and migration of endothelial cells accompanied by tube formation and vessel anastomosis, and finally (iv) coalescence of the sprouts to newly formed vasculature stabilized with smooth muscle cells and pericytes. Tumor growth is angiogenesis dependent, yet blood vessels in tumors are abnormal at many levels. Defects in the endothelial monolayer makes the tumor vessels leaky and, together with the poor lymphatic drainage, allows for the selective accumulation of macromolecules – a phenomenon defined as the enhanced permeability and retention (EPR) effect [7] (Figure 20.1).

Ever since angiogenesis inhibitors were recognized as a promising strategy to fight cancer, many potential compounds have been identified and isolated; several are currently undergoing clinical trials, 14 have been clinically approved (Table 20.1),

Drug Delivery in Oncology: From Basic Research to Cancer Therapy, First Edition.
Edited by Felix Kratz, Peter Senter, and Henning Steinhagen.
© 2012 Wiley-VCH Verlag GmbH & Co. KGaA. Published 2012 by Wiley-VCH Verlag GmbH & Co. KGaA.

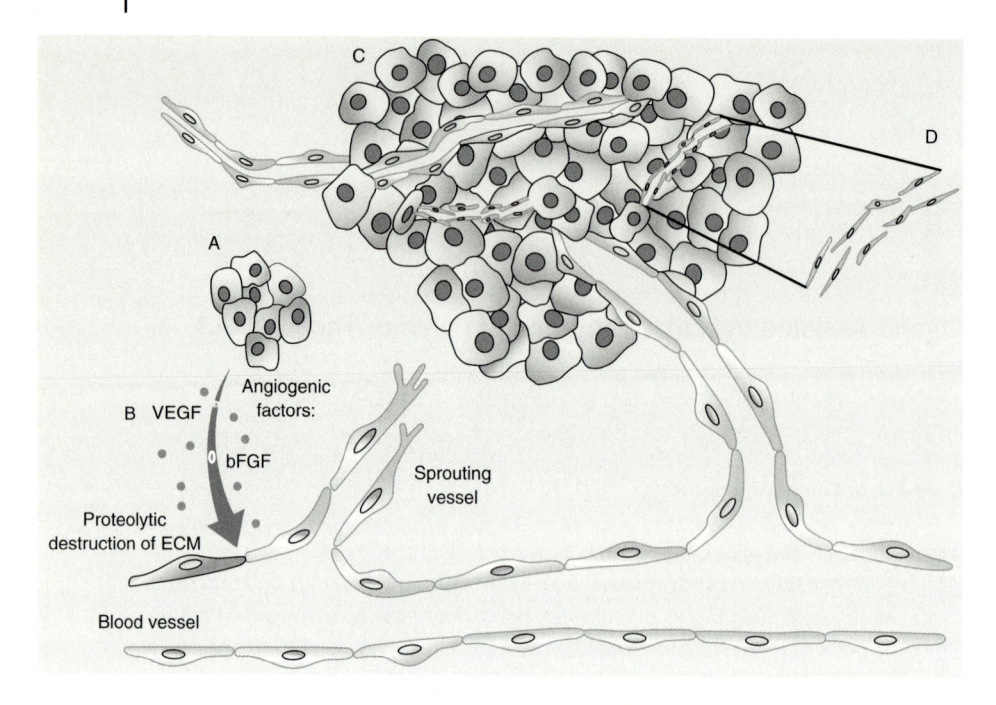

Figure 20.1 Angiogenic steps. Schematic representation of the angiogenesis process in tumors. (A) A dormant avascular tumor prior to the "angiogenic switch" followed by (B) tumor secretion of angiogenic factors, leading to endothelial cells proliferation and migration, resulting in new capillaries sprouting followed by tubular formation and vascular stabilization. (C) Large, vascularized tumor mass nurtured by blood vessels which are disorganized, bearing blunt-ends, characterized by irregular sluggish blood flow, poor lymphatic drainage, and (D) hyperpermeable, allowing polymer therapeutics to extravasate by the EPR effect.

and other clinically approved drugs were found to induce antiangiogenic activity in addition to their known activity [2, 8].

The objective of targeting toxic agents to proliferating endothelial cells in the tumor neovasculature rather than tumor cells presents three main advantages:

1) Aiming the drugs to proliferating endothelial cells in the tumor microenvironment can be effective against a variety of malignancies, since the therapeutic target is not subject to tumor type.
2) Acquired drug resistance resulting from genetic and epigenetic mechanisms often reduces the effectiveness of available drugs [9–11]. Antiangiogenic therapy targets the endothelial cells of the tumor vasculature, which are considered genetically stable relatively to tumor cells. Therefore, antiangiogenic therapy possesses the potential to overcome chemotherapy-associated resistance [12] and reduce the incidence of drug resistance [13, 14], especially when direct inhibitors are used.
3) Since cancer cells depend upon endothelial cells for survival and growth, damaging the proliferating tumor endothelial cells may amplify the antiangiogenic

Table 20.1 Approved antiangiogenicaly therapies for cancer.

Drug	Trade name/ code name	Manufacturer/ sponsor	Mechanism	Approved indications	Route of administration	Year of approval
mAbs						
Bevacizumab	Avastin®	Genentech	mAb to VEGF	combined with conventional chemotherapy for mCRC, NSCLC, and advanced breast cancer	intravenous	2004
Cetuximab	Erbitux®	ImClone; Bristol-Myers Squibb; Merck	mAb to EGFR	combined with conventional chemotherapy and radiation therapy for mCRC and head and neck cancer	intravenous	2004
Panitumumab	Vectibix™	Amgen	mAb to EGFR	EGFR-expressing mCRC in patients who have failed prior chemotherapy	intravenous	2006
Trastuzumab	Herceptin®	Genentech	mAb to extracellular domain of HER2	combined with conventional chemotherapy or as second-line monotherapy for breast cancer	intravenous	1998
Small-molecule TKIs						
Erlotinib	Tarceva®	Genentech; OSI Pharmaceuticals; Roche	small-molecule TKI of EGFR	monotherapy for NSCLC or in as combined with conventional chemotherapy for pancreatic cancer	oral	2004
Gefitinib	Iressa®	AstraZeneca; Teva	small-molecule TKI of EGFR	second-line therapy for NSCLC	oral	2003
Lapatinib	Tykerb®	GlaxoSmithKline	small-molecule TKI of EGFR and HER2/neu	first-line therapy in triple-positive breast cancer and for Herceptin-progressed breast cancer	oral	2007
Sorafenib	Nexavar®	Bayer; Onyx	small-molecule TKI of VEGFR (1, 2, and 3), PDGFR-β, and Raf-1	renal cell carcinoma and hepatocellular carcinoma	oral	2005
Sunitinib	Sutent®	Pfizer	small-molecule TK of VEGFR (1, 2, and 3) and PDGFR-β and RET	renal cell carcinoma, second-line treatment of GIST	oral	2006

(continued overleaf)

Table 20.1 (continued)

Drug	Trade name/ code name	Manufacturer/ sponsor	Mechanism	Approved indications	Route of administration	Year of approval
Imatinib	Gleevec®/ Glivec®	Novartis	inhibition of Bcr–Abl tyrosine kinase, PDGFR, and c-Kit kinase	CML	oral	2001
Vatalanib[a]	PTK787	Novartis	inhibition of VEGFR(1, 2, and 3), PDGFR and c-Kit kinase	combined with conventional chemotherapy for mCRC	oral	–
Inhibitors of mTOR						
Temsirolimus	Torisel™	Wyeth	–	advanced renal cell carcinoma	intravenous	2007
Other antiangiogenic agents						
Bortezomib	Velcade®	Millennium Pharmaceuticals	proteasome inhibitor	second-line treatment in multiple myeloma and MCL	intravenous	2003
Thalidomide	Thalomid®	Celgene	unknown	combined with dexamethasone for multiple myeloma	oral	2003
Neovastat[a]	AE-941	AEterna Zentaris	natural MMP inhibitor, and VEGF–VEGFR binding inhibitor	combined with conventional chemotherapy and radiation therapy for NSCLC, treatment of metastatic kidney cancer, refractory multiple myeloma, advanced breast cancer, and colorectal cancer	intravenous	–
Rebimastat[a]	BMS275291	Bristol-Myers Squibb	second-generation MMP inhibitor	combined with conventional chemotherapy for prostate cancer, HIV-related Kaposi's sarcoma, and metastatic NSCLC	intravenous	–
Endostatin	Endostar	EntreMed	inhibits endothelial proliferation	lung cancer	intravenous	2005 (in China)

mAb, monoclonal antibody; mCRC, metastatic colorectal cancer; NSCLC, non-small-cell lung cancer; EGFR, epidermal growth factor receptor; TKI, tyrosine kinase inhibitor; PDGFR, platelet-derived growth factor receptor; GIST, gastrointestinal stromal tumor; CML, chronic multiple myeloma; mTOR, mammalian target of rapamycin; MCL, mantle cell lymphoma.
[a]Phase III clinical study.

therapeutic effect. This is particularly promising since the elimination of a single endothelial cell may act as an initiator to a series of actions, causing hundreds of tumor cells to undergo apoptosis [15].

Tumor angiogenic blood vessels carry unique molecular markers such as integrin $\alpha_v\beta_3$ and $\alpha_v\beta_5$, aminopeptidase N (APN/CD13), VEGF receptors (VEGFRs), basic fibroblast growth factor receptor (bFGFR), matrix metalloproteases (MMPs), P- and E-selectin, some of which are targeted by certain peptides, antibody fragments, or some small molecules [16–20] (Figure 20.2). Based on the Ringsdorf model [21], polymeric carriers that can actively target the tumor vasculature by ligand-mediated interactions can be utilized to improve the therapeutic index of chemotherapeutic agents by increasing the time of drug exposure to the tumor vasculature and can thus enhance treatment potency [15].

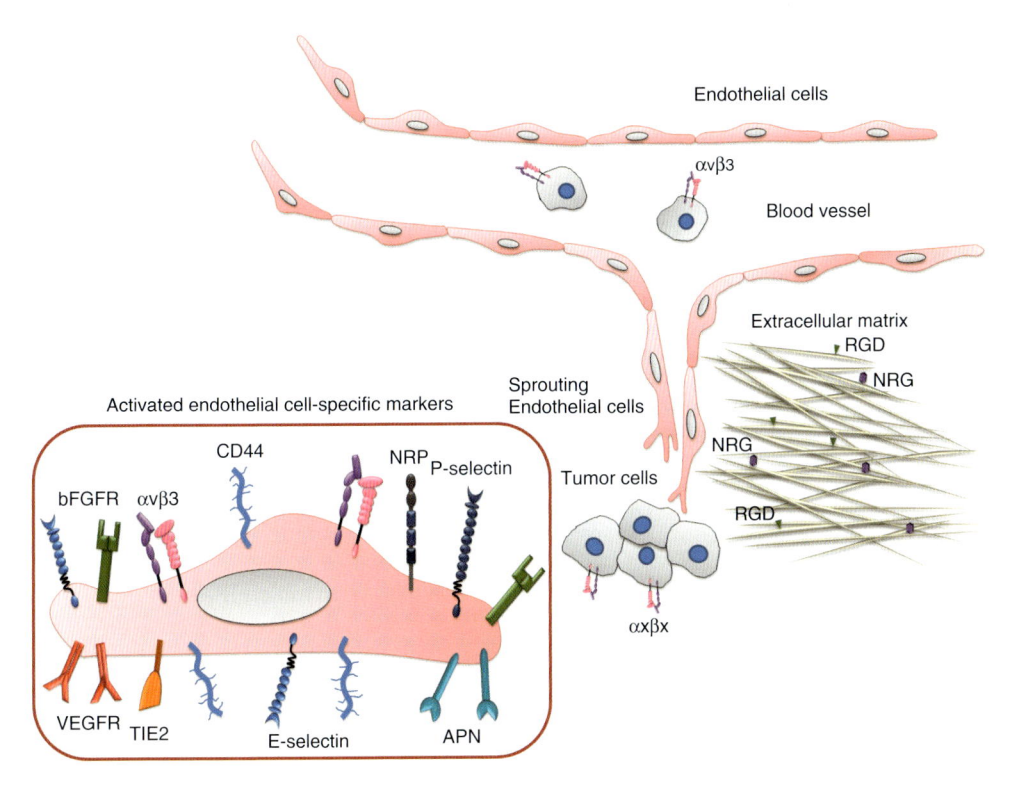

Figure 20.2 Neovasculature endothelial cell markers: sprouting microvessels emerging from normal blood vessels toward the tumor tissue upon secretion of proangiogenic factors (such as VEGF). The proliferating endothelial cells intrude the ECM by adhering to ECM motifs (such as RGD- or NGR-containing molecules). Endothelial cell adherence molecules and other overexpressed receptors are specified.

20.2
Potential Angiogenic Markers

20.2.1
Integrins

Integrins are heterodimeric cell surface receptors that mediate cell attachment to the extracellular matrix (ECM), but can also interact with cell surface and soluble ligands. There are 18 different α subunits and eight different β subunits, which form 24 different α/β known integrin combinations [22, 23]. Each individual transmembrane subunit includes a large extracellular domain and a short cytoplasmic tail [24, 25]. Dimerization of the α and β subunits forms the functional receptor, allowing integrins the ability of bidirectional signal transmission. Extracellular ligand binding is modulated from inside the cell (inside-out signaling), whereas the binding of the ECM proteins activates intracellular signal transduction (outside-in signaling). The promiscuity of integrins enables them to bind a large number of different ECM proteins (Table 20.2), while ECM components can also be recognized by more than one integrin. Cells can display a variable repertoire of integrins on their surface, which predispose to ECM–cell interaction. These unique features, as well as their anchorage ability, allow integrins to coordinate cell–ECM, cell–cell, and cell–soluble ligand cross-talk, and to modulate tissue architecture.

Integrins are tightly linked to cancer due to their dual involvement. On the one hand, these adhesion molecules communicate tumor cell proliferation, migration, invasion, and survival. On the other hand, they play a key role by activating different cellular pathways in the formation of new capillary blood vessels [37, 38]. Integrin $\alpha_v\beta_3$ is probably the most-studied and best-characterized adhesion receptor in the context of cancer and angiogenesis. This integrin is highly expressed on proliferating vascular endothelial cells during pathological angiogenesis, but not on the quiescent endothelial cells lining adult vasculature, which makes it an attractive target for antiangiogenic therapies.

20.2.2
Selectins

Selectins are a family of C-type lectins – cell adhesion molecules known mainly as mediators of the earliest stages of leukocyte trafficking. The selectins are a family of carbohydrate-binding proteins, expressed on cytokine-activated endothelial cells (E-selectin/CD62E and P-selectin/CD62P), platelets (P-selectin), and leukocytes (L-selectin/CD62L) [39, 40].

E-selectin is a molecular marker associated with the tumor vasculature and represents another excellent target for therapeutic agents intended to destroy tumor endothelial cells. It is expressed exclusively by vascular endothelial cells during inflammation and cancer [41–43], and its expression has been associated with tumor angiogenesis and metastasis in a variety of cancers [44, 45]. E-selectin is a 97-kDa protein that binds the tetrasaccharide sialyl Lewis X (sLe^x) structure. Several

Table 20.2 Endothelial cell-targeted polymer therapeutics.

Compound	Polymeric carrier	Effector moiety	Targeting moiety	Target	Cell types expressing the target	References
HPMA–AM-GDM–cRGDfK	HPMA copolymer	aminohexylamino geldanamycin	cyclic RGDfK	$\alpha_v\beta_3$ integrin	vasculature endothelial cells and PC-3 (prostate cancer cells)	[26, 27]
PGA–PTX–E-[c(RGDfK)$_2$]	PGA	PTX	bis-cyclic RGDfK	$\alpha_v\beta_3$ integrin	vasculature endothelial cells	[28]
PEG–DOX–E-[c(RGDfK)$_2$]	PEG	DOX	bis-cyclic RGDfK	$\alpha_v\beta_3$ integrin	vasculature endothelial cells and U87 glioblastoma cells	[29]
G3–[PEG–cRGDfK]–[DOX]	G3 poly(L-lysine) dendrimers	DOX siRNA (luciferase gene)	cyclic RGDfK	$\alpha_v\beta_3$ integrin	U87 glioblastoma cells	[30]
c(RGDfK)–PEG–PLys/pDNA polyplex micelle	PEG-P(Lys) micelles	plasmid DNA	cyclic RGDfK	$\alpha_v\beta_3$ integrin	HeLa human epithelial cervical cancer cells	[31]
RGD-4C–PEG-b-P(CL-Hyd-DOX) RGD-4C–PEG-b-P(CL-Ami-DOX)	(PEO-b-PCL) micelles	DOX	double cyclic RGD-4C	$\alpha_v\beta_3/\alpha_v\beta_5$ integrin	human MDA-435 breast cancer cells[a] (sensitive and resistant to DOX)	[32]
HPMA–Esbp–DOX	HPMA	DOX	Esbp	E-selectins	immortalized vascular endothelial cells	[33]
HPMA-D-(KLAKLAK)$_2$–NGR	HPMA	D-(KLAKLAK)$_2$ peptide	NRG	APN (CD13)	human fibrosarcoma HT-1080 cells	[34]
siRNA/(PEI-SS)-b-HA complex	PEI	siRNA (VEGF gene)	HA	HA receptor (CD44)	B16/F1 melanoma	[35]

[a]MDA-MB-435 cells are derived from the M14 melanoma cell line and cannot be considered a model of breast cancer [36].

E-selectin-mediated targeting strategies were previously exploited for the delivery of macromolecules into inflamed and tumor tissues, such as immunoliposomes and nanoparticles, using the natural ligand sLe^x, or its derivatives, as the targeting agent [46].

20.2.3
APN (CD13)

APN is a type 2 transmembrane zinc-dependent metallopeptidase of the superfamily of gluzincins (molecular weight 150 kDa) [47, 48], which forms a noncovalently bound homodimer on the cellular membrane. It has a conserved pentapeptide consensus sequence His–Glu–X–X–His representing a zinc-binding motif in its extracellular metalloprotease domain and therefore belongs to the M1 family of aminopeptidase [49].

APN is expressed in many cells and tissues, including myeloids, fibroblasts, brain cells, hepatocytes, osteoclasts, endometrial cells, epithelial cells of the liver, kidney, and intestine, and in synaptic membranes of the central nervous system [50, 51]. Due to wide expression of APN, its function strongly depends on its location [49].

APN has been identified as one of the important tumor markers overexpressed on the surface of tumor vascular endothelial cells, and involved in cancer angiogenesis, invasion, and metastasis [52, 53]. APN participates in tumor angiogenesis through regulating filopodia formation and endothelial invasion [54]; furthermore, it is present on tumor neovasculature, thus differentiating it from existing blood vessels [55]. The proteolytic degradation of the ECM, through the activity of APN and other proteases such as MMPs, contributes to the growth and metastasis of tumors [49].

The NGR motif (Asn–Gly–Arg) has been confirmed to bind exclusively to APN expressed in tumors, and not to the other types of APN isoforms expressed in normal epithelia and myeloid cells [55, 56].

20.2.4
Hyaluronic Acid Binding Receptor (CD44)

CD44 is a cell surface carbohydrate receptor and a component of the ECM [57]. CD44 is a 90-kDa transmembrane receptor expressed by many cell types, including leukocytes, fibroblasts, epithelial cells, keratinocytes, and some endothelial cells. Changes in CD44 expression are associated with a wide variety of tumors and metastasis. The physical and functional properties that are common to CD44 receptors include the high binding affinity to hyaluronic acid (HA, also referred to as hyaluronan or hyaluronate). HA is a linear, negatively charged polysaccharide that is composed of two alternating and repeating units of D-glucuronic acid (GlcUA) and N-acetyl-D-glucosamine (GlcNAc) linked together [58]. In contrast to other HA-binding proteins, CD44 binds HA at the cell surface, where multiple, closely arrayed CD44 receptor molecules interact with the highly multivalent repeating disaccharide chain of HA [59].

HA – a prevalent component of the ECM and pericellular matrixes – is a nonsulfated glycosaminoglycan ubiquitously expressed by various cell types in almost all animal tissues [60]. HA has been demonstrated to play a key role in several biological processes, including embryonic development, wound healing, tumor growth, and angiogenesis, mainly by providing a provisional matrix for supporting cellular migration and adherence [60–64].

HA–CD44 interactions are often crucial in tumor malignancy; hence, they are a target for new liposomal, stabilized nanoparticles, and polymer therapeutics [59, 65–67].

20.3
Drug Delivery Strategy: Targeted Polymer Therapeutics

Most of the antiangiogenic or chemotherapeutic agents are low-molecular-weight compounds that are administered systemically, and exhibit nonspecific biodistribution profile, low tumor site accumulation, short plasma circulation time, and rapid systemic elimination. Consequently, relatively small amounts of the drug reach the target site, and therapy is associated with side-effects and low efficacy [68, 69].

The poor pharmacokinetics and limited therapeutic effect of the compounds can be improved by incorporation of these agents with polymeric delivery systems. The attachment of low-molecular-weight anticancer drugs to water-soluble polymers facilitates improvement of tumor tissue specificity due to the EPR effect [7]. The EPR phenomenon, which enables passive accumulation of macromolecules and other nanoparticles in solid tumors, is attributed to the leaky and fenestrated tumor vasculature and to poor lymphatic drainage (see Figure 20.1).

N-(2-Hydroxypropyl)methacrylamide (HPMA) copolymer–TNP-470 conjugate (caplostatin) is the first example of passive antiangiogenic targeting to the tumor site using the EPR effect. The antiangiogenic properties of TNP-470 – a low-molecular-weight analog of fumagillin – were established in 1990 by Ingber et al. [70]. Treatment with TNP-470 showed promising antitumor activity in clinical trials, either as monotherapy or in combination with conventional chemotherapy [71, 72]. Nevertheless, neurotoxicity occurred at the optimal anticancer dose, significantly limiting the efficacy of the drug [73, 74]. Satchi-Fainaro et al. synthesized and characterized HPMA copolymer–Gly–Phe–Leu–Gly–TNP-470 conjugate, sized 30 kDa [75], which they named caplostatin (Figure 20.3a). HPMA copolymer is a nondegradable, water-soluble, and biocompatible polymer that has been studied intensively for therapeutic applications for almost three decades. The tetrapeptide linker (Gly–Phe–Leu–Gly) conjugating TNP-470 with the HPMA copolymer is stable in circulation [76] and is cleavable by lysosomal thiol-dependent proteases, particularly cathepsin B, which is overexpressed in many tumor cells and tumor endothelial cells [77]. Caplostatin is selectively accumulated in the tumor microvasculature by passive targeting phenomenon due to the EPR effect [7, 78]. Furthermore, this conjugate does not cross the blood–brain barrier and does not induce the neurotoxicity associated with treatment with unconjugated TNP-470 (Figure 20.3b).

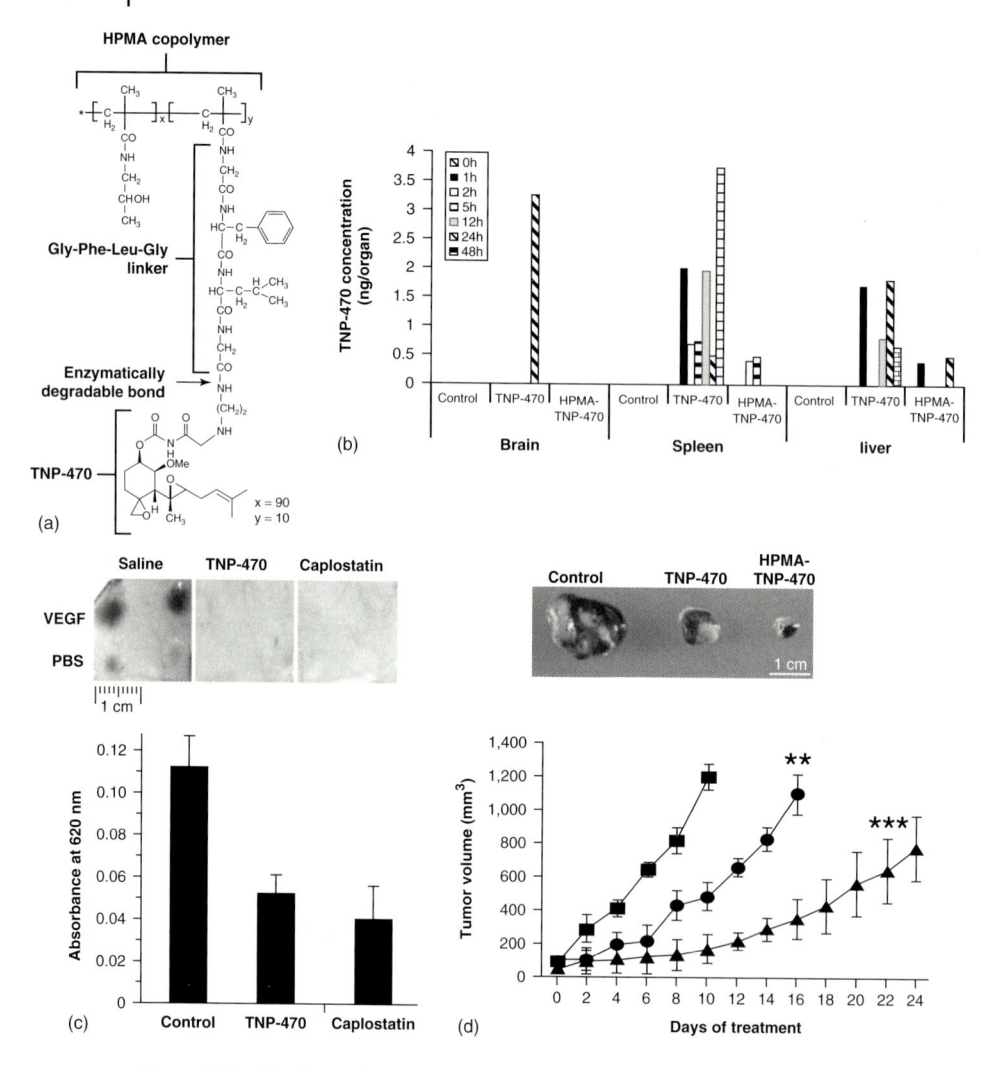

Figure 20.3 (a) Chemical structure HPMA copolymer–TNP-470 conjugate (caplostatin). (b) HPMA copolymer–TNP-470 conjugate does not accumulate in the brain compared with free TNP-470 that does TNP-470 extracted from brain, spleen, and liver. Values represent mean ± standard error ($n = 3$ mice per group). (c) Inhibition of vessel hyperpermeability by TNP-470 and caplostatin. (d) Effects of TNP-470 (closed circles), HPMA copolymer–TNP-470 conjugate (closed triangles), and saline (closed squares) on mice bearing A2058 human melanoma ($n = 5$ mice per group). Excised tumors on day 8 of treatment. Taken from [75] and [79].

Caplostatin is significantly effective on a large variety of cancer types and can be administered over a dose range more than 10-fold that of the original TNP-470 without any toxicity [75, 79, 80]. In addition to its antiangiogenic activity, caplostatin is the most potent known inhibitor of vascular hyperpermeability [2]. Caplostatin prevented vascular leakage induced by VEGF, bradykinin, histamine, and platelet-activating factor, and prevented pulmonary edema induced by interleukin-2 (Figure 20.3c and d). The vascular hyperpermeability inhibition mechanism can be partly explained by the ability of TNP-470 to hinder VEGF-induced phosphorylation of its receptor (VEGFR2), calcium influx, and RhoA activation in endothelial cells.

Caplostatin represents the most broad-spectrum anticancer agent known, while it is not restricted to any specific targeting to endothelial cell receptors [79].

The lack of tumor specificity displayed by low-molecular-weight drugs for cancer treatments often results in significant toxicity to noncancerous tissues. A well-designed polymeric carrier that can actively target tumor vasculature by ligand-mediated interactions may improve the therapeutic index of chemotherapeutic agents by increasing the time of drug exposure to the tumor vasculature and can thus enhance treatment potency.

20.4
Novel Targeted Polymeric Drug Delivery Systems Directed to Tumor Endothelial Cells

In general, an ideal delivery system is one that can enable the conjugation of any targeting moiety and the active entity in a simple chemical platform fashion.

A diversity of ongoing research in various fields of drug delivery is being combined to target angiogenesis and cancer. Polymers, polymerized liposomes, encapsulated nano- and microparticles, dendrimers, and microspheres are being loaded with or conjugated to a variety of entities. One such entity will be a specific targeting moiety to proliferating endothelial cells, such as an antibody (to VEGF, endosialin, endothelial cell caveolae proteins, or others), a peptide (i.e., Arg–Gly–Asp (RGD), NRG, or HA), or any ligand to the upregulated molecules present on the surface of proliferating endothelial cells. Other entities will include an active moiety, which may be an angiogenesis inhibitor, a low-molecular-weight drug, a viral vector/gene expressing an angiogenesis-inhibiting protein or toxin, coagulation factors, vasoactive molecules, or cytotoxic drugs [78].

This chapter's focus is on macromolecules bearing a toxic effector moiety conjugated with a targeting motif directed mainly to the tumor vasculature. In situations where a tumor is well-vascularized, but vasculature permeability is poor, this strategy might be essential since the tumor endothelial cells are directly exposed to the conjugate in the blood circulation without the need to extravasate from the tumor vasculature into the tumor tissue (Figure 20.4).

20.4.1
RGD-Based Polymer–Drug Conjugates

The tripeptide sequence RGD is all that is required as a fundamental recognition site for cells and proteins. This short but highly conserved sequence was found by Erkki Ruoslahti's group some 25 years ago [82]. In order to explore the structure–activity relationship between fibronectin and its receptor (later recognized as $\alpha_v\beta_3$ integrin), this group substituted every amino acid in the RGDS

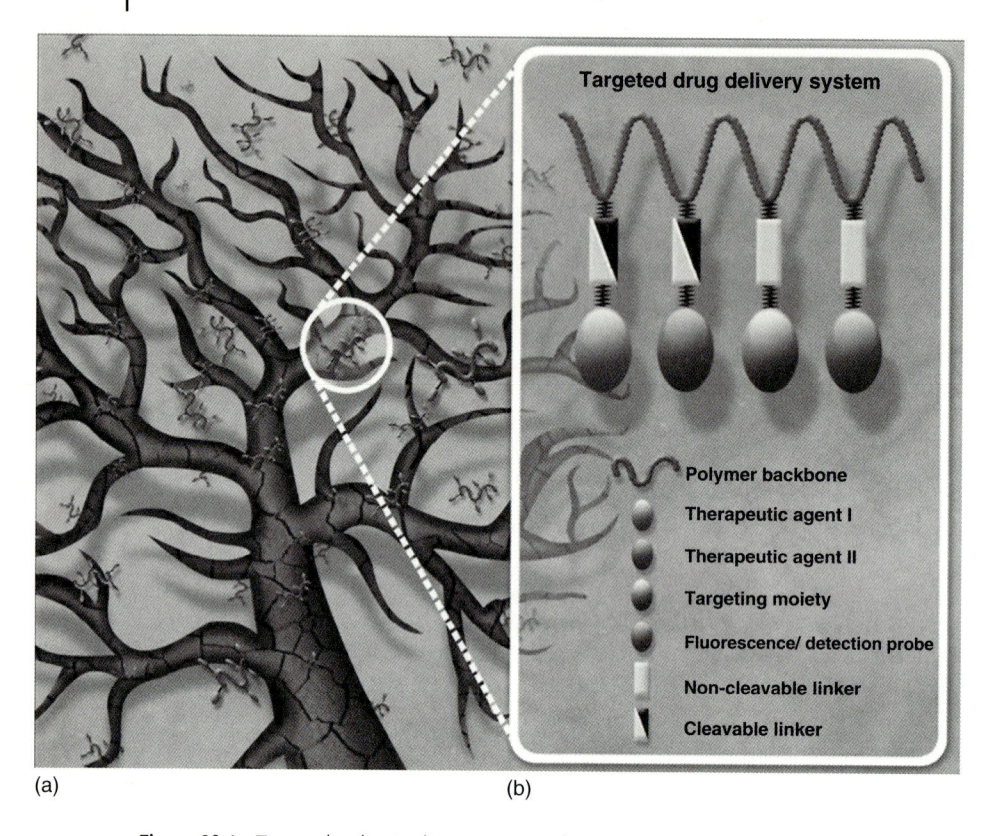

Figure 20.4 Targeted polymer therapeutics to the tumor endothelium and cancer cells at the tumor site. (a) Permeable neovasculature in the tumor site allows passive extravasation of polymer therapeutics by the EPR effect and their accumulation in the tumor. (b) Schematic illustration of a targeted polymer–drug delivery system comprised of (i) polymer backbone, (ii) one or more chemotherapeutic and antiangiogenic drugs conjugated via degradable linkers, (iii) targeting moiety bound through nondegradable linker, and (iv) optional detection moiety. The targeting moiety leads the polymer directly to the tumor endothelial cells exposed to the bloodstream and to marker-expressing tumor cells, allowing cellular internalization of the polymer–drug conjugate, degradation of the linker, and release of the toxic effectors only within the target cells. (From [81].)

tetrapeptide with a different one. Using this simple approach they were able to discover that even the most conservative substitution in the first three amino acids (RGD) renders cell attachment activity, while the fourth position can undergo changes without altering attachment ability.

As years have passed, it was realized that this essential recognition epitope is present not only in fibronectin, but in other ECM proteins [83] (Table 20.3), and involved in cell–ECM, cell–cell, and cell–virus/bacteria interaction [84, 85]. The promiscuity of the tripeptide motif, and its biological and pharmaceutical importance, has led to utilization approaches by mimicking and blocking this adherence system (Figure 20.5a).

Table 20.3 Common integrins and their ECM ligands as potential targets for polymer therapeutics.

Integrin	Natural ligands (ECM proteins)	Tumor types	Associated phenotypes
$\alpha_4\beta_1$	vascular cellular adhesion molecule	ovarian	increased peritoneal metastasis
$\alpha_5\beta_1$	fibronectin, fibrin	non-small-cell lung cancer	decreased survival in patients with lymph node-negative tumors
		melanoma	vertical growth phase and lymph node metastasis
$\alpha_6\beta_1$	laminins	prostate	perineural invasion and bone metastasis
$\alpha_6\beta_4$	laminins	breast	increased tumor size and grade and decreased survival
$\alpha_v\beta_3$	vitronectin, fibronectin, laminin, thrombospondin, tenascin, osteopontin, bone sialoprotein, nonfibrillar collagen, denatured collagen, MMP2, basic fibroblast growth factor, von Willebrand factor, thrombin	melanoma	vertical growth phase and lymph node metastasis
		breast	increased bone metastasis
		prostate	increased bone metastasis
		pancreatic	lymph node metastasis
		ovarian	tumor proliferation
		cervical	associated with decreased patient survival
		glioblastoma	tumor cell expression, a possible role in invasion
$\alpha_v\beta_5$	vitronectin	glioblastoma	tumor cell expression, a possible role in invasion
$\alpha_v\beta_6$	fibronectin	colon	reduced patient survival

Given that the RGD sequence is conserved so that any change in it will abrogate its functionality, modification of flanking amino acids, particularly the two subsequent to the aspartic acid, achieves higher affinity and specificity [86], different conformational features, and better stability. Chemical instability of the linear RGD peptides and its high susceptibility to degradation due to the reaction of the terminal aspartic acid with the peptide backbone is often overcome with cyclization. Cyclization is used to improve the binding properties of RGD peptides for a specific subtype of integrin and to improve its stability [87, 88].

The finding that structural restriction within the cyclic RGD backbone can lead to selective integrin-subtype antagonists took the immense research by the group of Kessler a step forward to the discovery of the potent $\alpha_v\beta_3/\alpha_v\beta_5$ inhibitor c(RGDf[NMe]V), known as cilengitide (Figure 20.5b) [89, 90].

The clinical potential of cilengitide (EMD121974) was promptly recognized and eagerly translated to the clinical setting, which was the beginning of an era for the integrin inhibitor class as investigational agents for antiangiogenic and anticancer therapies [91]. Presently, cilengitide is being tested in several clinical trials as monotherapy or in combination with conventional chemotherapy ([91, 92] and *http://clinicaltrials.gov/search/intervention=Cilengitide*). Despite the reported clinical

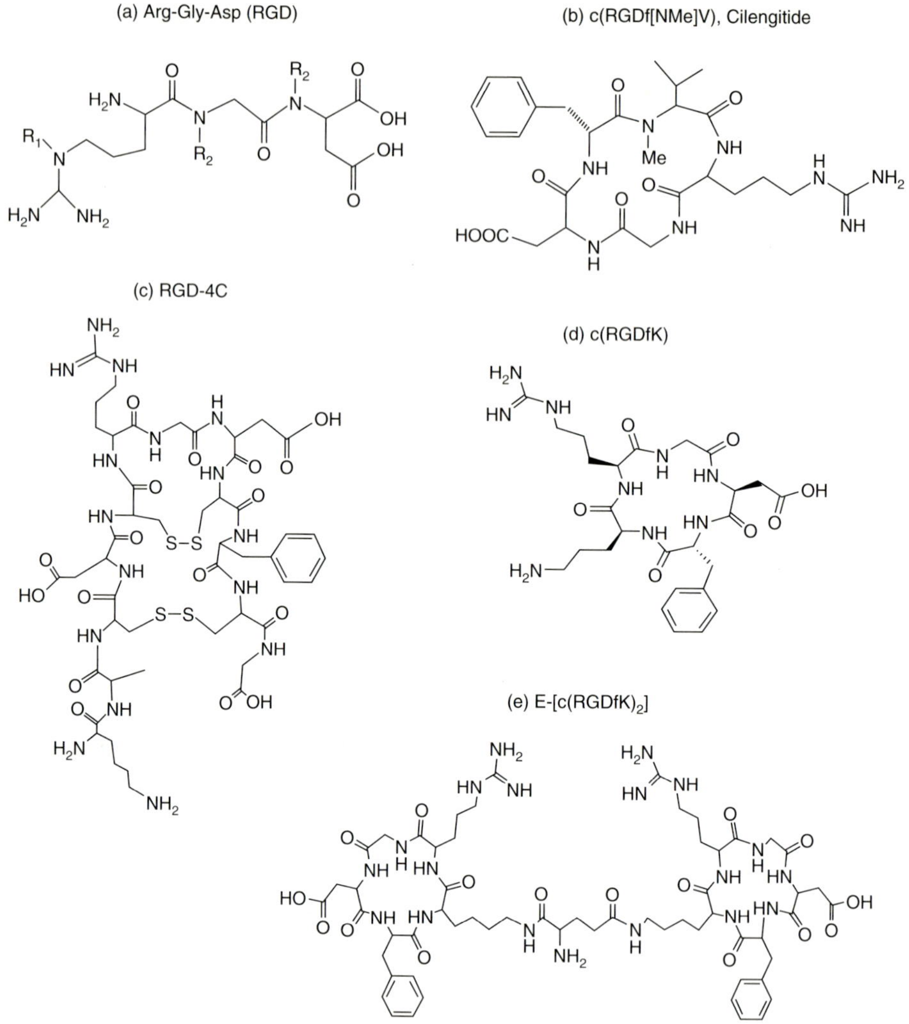

Figure 20.5 (a)–(e) Chemical structures of various RGD-containing peptide derivatives.

advances of cilengitide, it was reported in two distressing publications in 2009 that RGD-mimetic agents, at well-defined experimental settings, may promote, rather than inhibit, angiogenesis. Undoubtedly, the complex effects of integrin antagonists should be further explored experimentally and evaluated in properly designed clinical trials [24, 93].

To set aside the potential use of integrin antagonists as therapeutic agents *per se*, these compounds can be successfully applied in RGD ligand-guided drug delivery polymeric systems. After the discovery of the selective $\alpha_v\beta_3$ integrin inhibitor and the growing understanding of its importance, it was only natural that new RGD-containing peptides would be designed and evaluated. In a pioneering work

20.4 Novel Targeted Polymeric Drug Delivery Systems Directed to Tumor Endothelial Cells

by Arap et al. [94], in vivo selection of phage-display libraries led to the identification of RGD-4C (Figure 20.5c). CDCRGDCFC, a small RGD-containing cyclic peptide, was conjugated to the chemotherapeutic agent doxorubicin (DOX), giving rise to the covalent construct RGD-4C–DOX. This conjugate showed improved activity and toxicity profile over free DOX in several models; in some the tumor cells did not express integrin $\alpha_v\beta_3$, suggesting a direct endothelial effect [95]. Despite these encouraging results, the interest in the RGD-4C targeting platform for drug delivery has decreased. This may be attributed to the presence of a reversible disulfide bridge connecting the cysteine components, which may lead to structural heterogeneity and is associated with the chemical instability of the RGD-4C construct. Quite the opposite, a number of stable peptide derivatives based on cilengitide had been developed, which demonstrate specific tumor-targeting properties [96–98].

The objective of enhancing the affinity of RGD ligands to their binding site has been further pursued by designing multimeric RGD-containing systems, according to the general concepts of multivalency. By embedding multiple copies of the RGD recognition motif on a central scaffold, multimeric RGD systems have served to increase integrin affinity and avidity, facilitate their clustering, and induce an active integrin-mediated internalization [99, 100].

One of the derivatives is the stable cyclic RGD-based pentapeptide c(RGDfK) (Figure 20.5d) – an $\alpha_v\beta_3$-specific and potent RGD motif – that was conjugated by Borgman et al. through the lysine (K) residue to a HPMA copolymer system for tumor delivery of 17-(6-aminohexylamino)-17-demethoxygeldanamycin (AH-GDM) derivatives [26]. Geldanamycin (GDM) – a benzoquinone ansamycin antibiotic – had demonstrated anticancer activity through the inhibition of heat-shock protein 90 (HSP90) chaperone function [101]. This antitumor antibiotic was found to be effective against neoplastic cells at concentrations greater than 0.1 µg/ml in in vitro studies. However, in vivo studies showed short systemic duration of the drug and high hepatotoxicity [102]. GDM conjugation to HPMA copolymer was first introduced by Kasuya et al. in order to extend the plasma half-life of GDM and to reduce its toxicity [103]. Conjugation of GDM with the polymeric carrier required substitution of the methoxy group on the 17-position of the antibiotic. Among the synthesized polymer-bound GDM derivatives, AH-GDM conjugated with HPMA copolymer showed superior stability and favorable in vitro activity. Borgman et al. further modified the HPMA copolymer–AH-GDM by equipping it with c(RGDfK) peptide (Figure 20.6) to extend GDM's known antiangiogenic activity and to enhance its accumulation in the tumor vascular bed [26, 104]. In vitro endothelial cell binding assays showed that the HPMA copolymer–c(RGDfK)–AH-GDM conjugate had similar binding ability to that of free c(RGDfK). The IC_{50} of the targetable conjugated AH-GDM was similar to the IC_{50} of free AH-GDM, whereas unmodified free GDM was much more potent. c(RGDfK)-containing polymer–drug conjugate exhibited higher maximum tolerated dose than the free modified drug and significant tumor localization of the targeted copolymer conjugate was seen in a biodistribution assay (Figure 20.7). Finally, accumulation in other organs was decreased with the exception of the kidneys, where large accumulation took place [26].

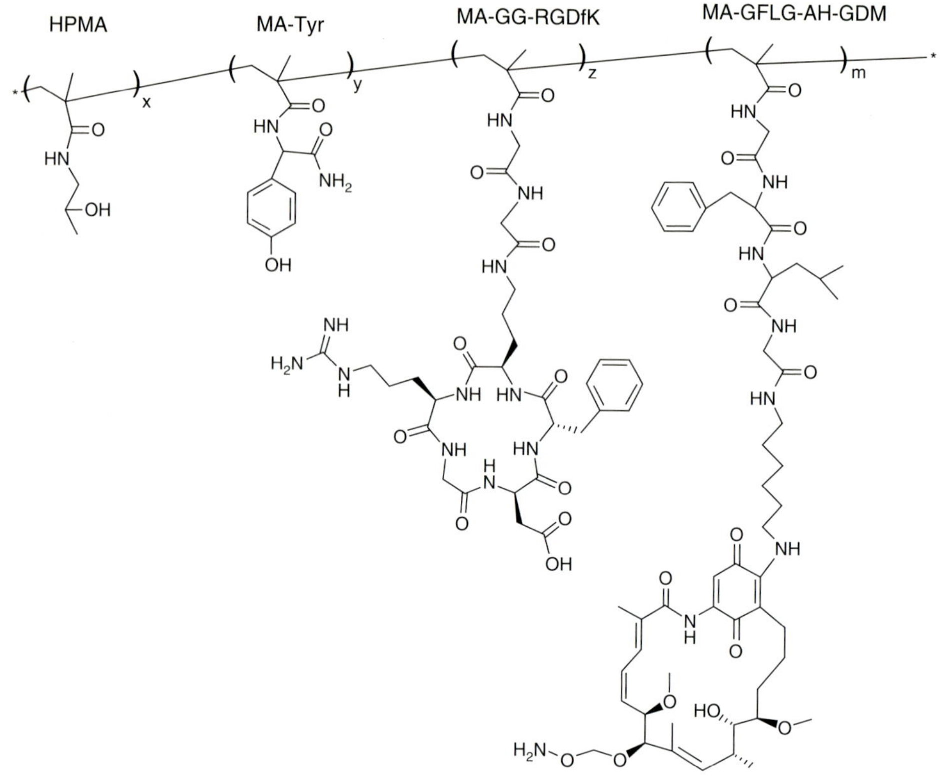

Figure 20.6 Structure of HPMA copolymer–RGDfK–AH-GDM conjugate.

Further diagnostic studies by Janssen et al. [97] demonstrated that a dimeric form of c(RGDfK), E-[c(RGDfK)$_2$], has improved tumor-targeting properties over the monomeric form (Figure 20.5e). Encouraged by these results, Ryppa et al. [105] coupled the antimicrotubule and antiangiogenic drug paclitaxel (PTX) with the E-[c(RGDfK)$_2$]. PTX is a potent, cytotoxic, and hydrophobic drug, that causes side-effects such as neutropenia and neuropathies. When solubilized in Cremophor EL®, PTX causes hypersensitivity reactions. While the *in vitro* evaluation in this study showed somewhat favorable results toward E-[c(RGDfK)$_2$]–PTX, no antitumor efficacy was demonstrated in the *in vivo* studies in an OVCAR-3 xenograft model for E-[c(RGDfK)$_2$]–PTX as compared to the moderate efficacy of PTX.

The objective of improving PTX's delivery and accumulation to the tumor site have been further pursued by designing a polyglutamic acid (PGA)–PTX–E-[c(RGDfK)$_2$] conjugate (Figure 20.8). Opaxio™, a PGA–PTX conjugate, is currently undergoing phase III clinical trials, showing promising results [106–108]. PGA is a water-soluble, biocompatible, nontoxic, and biodegradable polymer that accumulates in the tumor bed by the EPR effect when it is used at a nanoscaled size of 10–150 nm. Eldar-Boock et al. [28] conjugated PGA with PTX and E-[c(RGDfK)$_2$] as a targeting moiety, resulting in a roughly 30-nm diameter nanoconjugate.

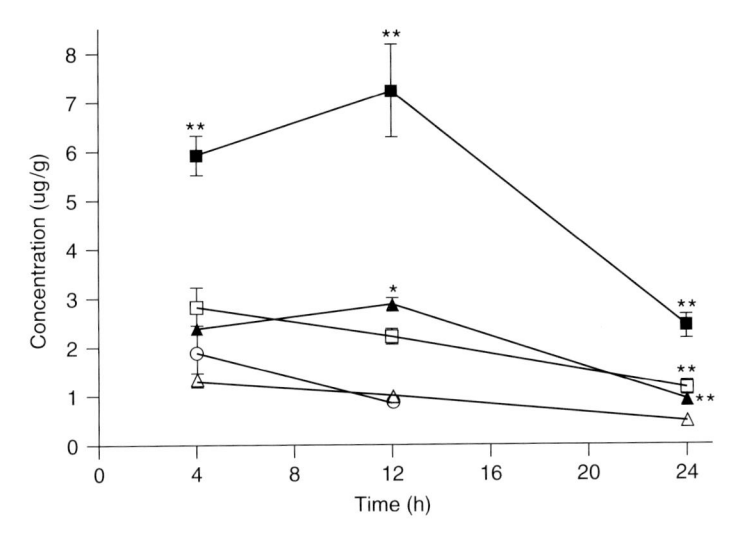

Figure 20.7 Tumor accumulation of free AH-GDM at 4, 12, and 24 h post-intravenous administration of HPMA copolymer–AH-GDM–RGDfK conjugate (P1) and HPMA copolymer–AH-GDM conjugate (P2) copolymer conjugates at 30 and 60 mg/kg drug-equivalent and 30 mg/kg AH-GDM hydrochloride. Data shows increasing tumor concentrations of drug for copolymer P1 treatments compared with nontargeted copolymer P2. Tumor concentrations following treatment with AH-GDM 30 mg/kg fall rapidly and are not detectable at 24 h. Closed triangles: P1 30 mg/kg. Closed squares: P1 60 mg/kg. Open triangles: P2 30 mg/kg. Open squares: P2 60 mg/kg. Open circle: AH-GDM 30 mg/kg. Data expressed as mean ± standard deviation. Significant differences for polymer treatment groups compared with drug alone at each time point indicated as *$P < 0.05$, **$P < 0.001$. Taken from [26].

Figure 20.8 Chemical structure of PGA–PTX–E-[c(RGDfK)$_2$] conjugate.

The ester linker between the polymer and the drug is hydrolytically labile, and PTX release occurs under lysosomal acidic pH, while the PGA itself is degradable by lysosomal enzymes such as cysteine proteases, particularly cathepsin B. PGA–PTX–E-[c(RGDfK)$_2$] nanoconjugate inhibited endothelial cell proliferation *in vitro*; their migration toward VEGF, their formation as capillary-like tubular structures, and their adhesion to fibrinogen-coated wells. These results warrant PGA–PTX–E-[c(RGDfK)$_2$] as a novel targeted antiangiogenic anticancer therapy, yet further *in vivo* investigation is required to determine its tumor accumulation ability and, more importantly, its anticancer effect *in vivo*.

In addition to PTX, several reports exist where cyclic RGD-based vehicles were exploited to carry other consignments to tumor vasculature and cells. One such example is DOX that was PEGylated and conjugated with E-[c(RGDfK)$_2$]. Poly(ethylene glycol) (PEG) is a water-soluble, biocompatible, nontoxic, and nonimmunogenic polymer used for various applications. The fact that PEG is commercially available and approved by the US Food and Drug Administration makes it an attractive polymeric carrier for drug delivery [68, 109–111].

DOX is an effective anthracycline antibiotic that is widely used in the clinic to treat several types of cancer. Nevertheless, its use is constricted due to acquired tumor drug resistance and cumulative dose-related cardiotoxicity. The coupling of DOX to PEG via the (6-maleimidocaproyl)-hydrazone derivative of the drug (DOX–EMCH) and to the bis-cyclic RGD resulted in a 13-kDa PEG–DOX–E-[c(RGDfK)$_2$] conjugate (Figure 20.9). The hydrazone linker is relatively stable under neutral pH, yet it is hydrolyzed at the acidic environment of the cellular lysosomes, allowing a rapid intracellular release of DOX [112]. Fluorescent properties of DOX were utilized to follow PEG–DOX–E-[c(RGDfK)$_2$] internalization into U87-MG cells overexpressing $\alpha_v\beta_3$ integrin. Both DOX and PEG–DOX–E-[c(RGDfK)$_2$] conjugate entered the cells rapidly; however, the route of internalization was probably different. The low-molecular-weight DOX entered the cells by diffusion, whereas PEG–DOX–E-[c(RGDfK)$_2$] conjugate was designed to internalize into the cells through $\alpha_v\beta_3$ integrin-mediated endocytosis. PEG–DOX–E-[c(RGDfK)$_2$] conjugate exhibited a similar cytotoxicity effect on human umbilical vein endothelial cells (HUVECs) and U87-MG glioblastoma cells as free DOX, thus demonstrating that the conjugation of E-[c(RGDfK)$_2$] to PEG–DOX did not alter its cytotoxicity. Furthermore, the adhesion of endothelial cells to fibrinogen-coated wells was inhibited by PEG–DOX–E-[c(RGDfK)$_2$] conjugate, whereas the nontargeted control PEG–DOX–c(RADfK) conjugate had no effect. In order to study the tumor-specific accumulation and preferential biodistribution profile of PEG–E-[c(RGDfK)$_2$] *in vivo*, the conjugate was coupled to a near-IR cyanine dye tetrasulfoindotricarbocyanine-aryl (TSCA). Accumulation of PEG–TSCA–E-[c(RGDfK)$_2$] in a DA3 mammary tumor inoculated in BALB/c mice was 15- and 7-fold higher than PEG–TSCA–c(RADfK) and PEG–TSCA, respectively. Additionally, the biodistribution profile of PEG–TSCA–E-[c(RGDfK)$_2$] was tumor specific, bypassing other selected organs. Although DA3 cells expressed low levels of $\alpha_v\beta_3$ integrin, the presence of this integrin on tumor endothelial cells was sufficient for active delivery of PEG–TSCA–E-[c(RGDfK)$_2$] to the tumor

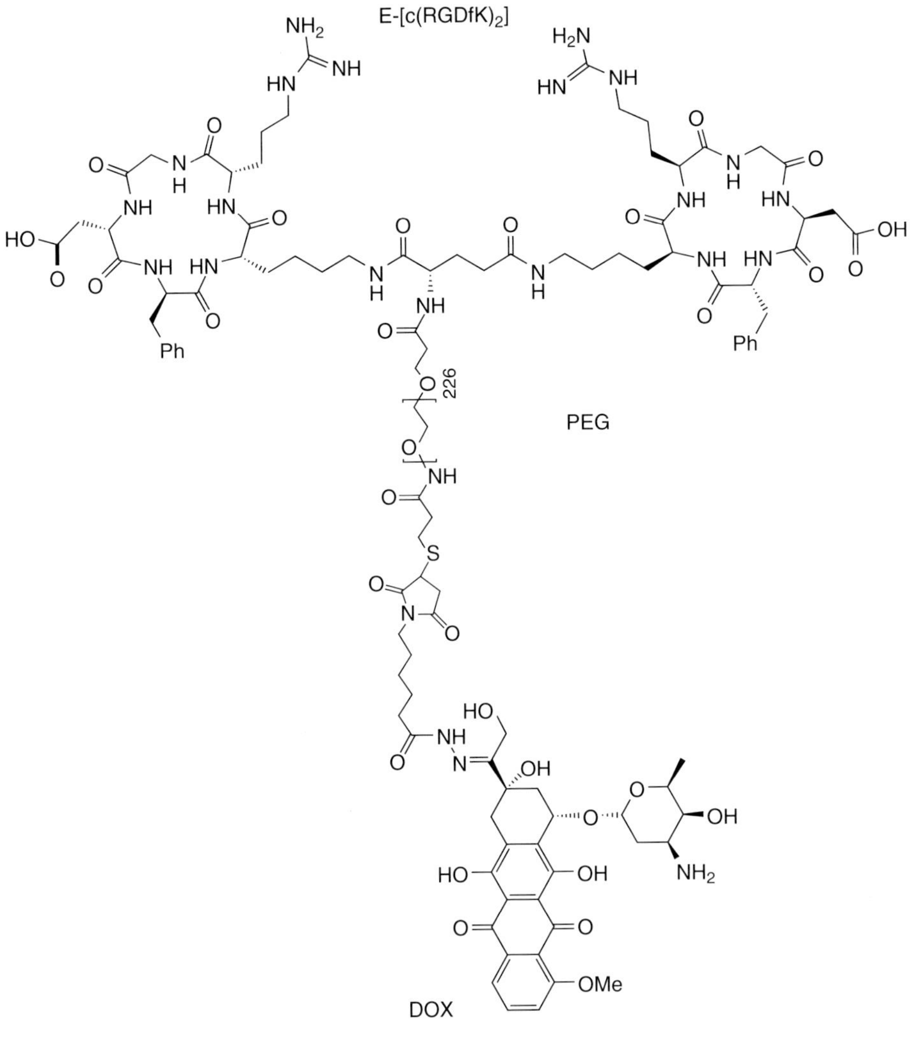

Figure 20.9 Chemical structure of PEG–DOX–E-[c(RGDfK)₂] conjugate.

vasculature. While the conjugation of DOX with PEG facilitates passive tumor tissue accumulation, the addition of the specific targeting moiety, bis-cyclic RGD, to the macromolecule enables direct delivery of PEG–DOX–E-[c(RGDfK)₂] to endothelial cells and tumor cells overexpressing the $\alpha_v\beta_3$ integrin (Figure 20.10) [29].

Another example is a generation-3 (G3) poly(L-lysine) dendrimer with a three-dimensional compact globular morphology. The nanoglobular c(RGDfK)-targeted dendrimeric platform is a codelivery system for DOX and small interfering RNA (siRNA). A siRNA is a short double-stranded RNA, which is regarded as a novel potential therapeutic for the treatment of various diseases by specific gene silencing of the complementary mRNA. However, the efficiency of gene silencing

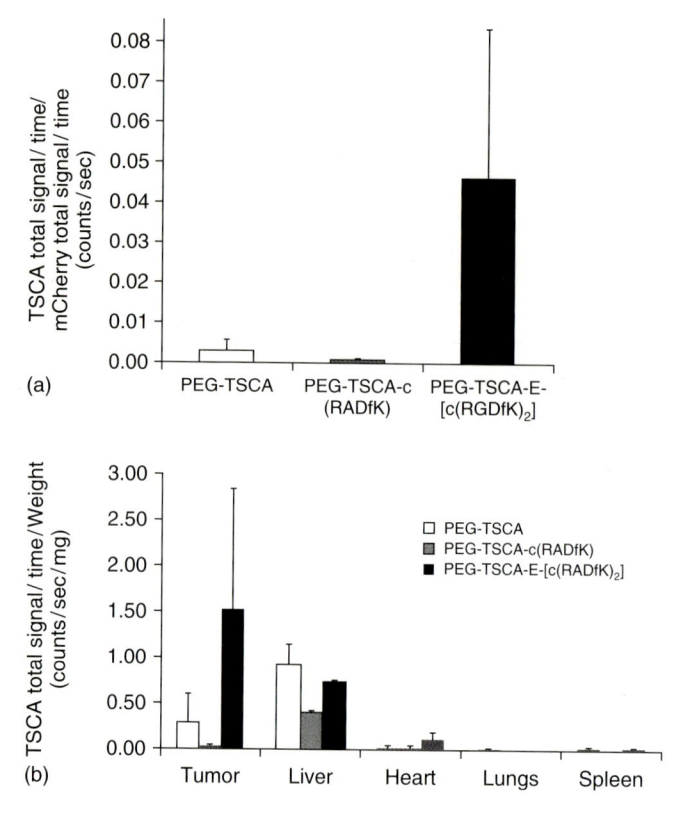

Figure 20.10 Biodistribution and tumor accumulation of PEG–TSCA conjugates in DA3-mCherry tumor-bearing BALB/c mice. (a) Accumulation of PEG–TSCA–E-[c(RGDfK)$_2$] (black) in a DA3 mammary tumor was 15- and 7-fold higher than PEG–TSCA–c(RADfK) (gray) and PEG–TSCA (white), respectively. (b) Accumulation of PEG–TSCA–E-[c(RGDfK)$_2$] in a mammary tumor was much higher than in other selected organs. The fluorescent signal was followed using the CRI Maestro™ noninvasive fluorescence imaging system. Taken from [29].

by siRNA is very low because of its extensive degradation by nucleases in the plasma and rapid renal clearance [113]. Accordingly, siRNA delivery has emerged as a key issue for the development of siRNA therapeutics [114] (Figure 20.11). The siRNA complexes of the targeted conjugate G3–[PEG-RGD]–[DOX] were readily internalized in U87-MG cells via receptor-mediated endocytosis, followed by intracellular accumulation. Codelivery of DOX and siRNA resulted in significantly high gene silencing in U87-Luc cells due to the combination effects of cytotoxicity and RNA interference activity. It was shown that the compact and three-dimensional nanoglobules are promising carriers for the combined delivery of nucleic acids and chemotherapeutic agents [30].

The RGD peptide-mediated delivery of therapeutic nucleic acids, siRNAs, and nonviral and viral gene macromolecules represents a prosperous area of research. Herein, a representative model is discussed to give a glance into this

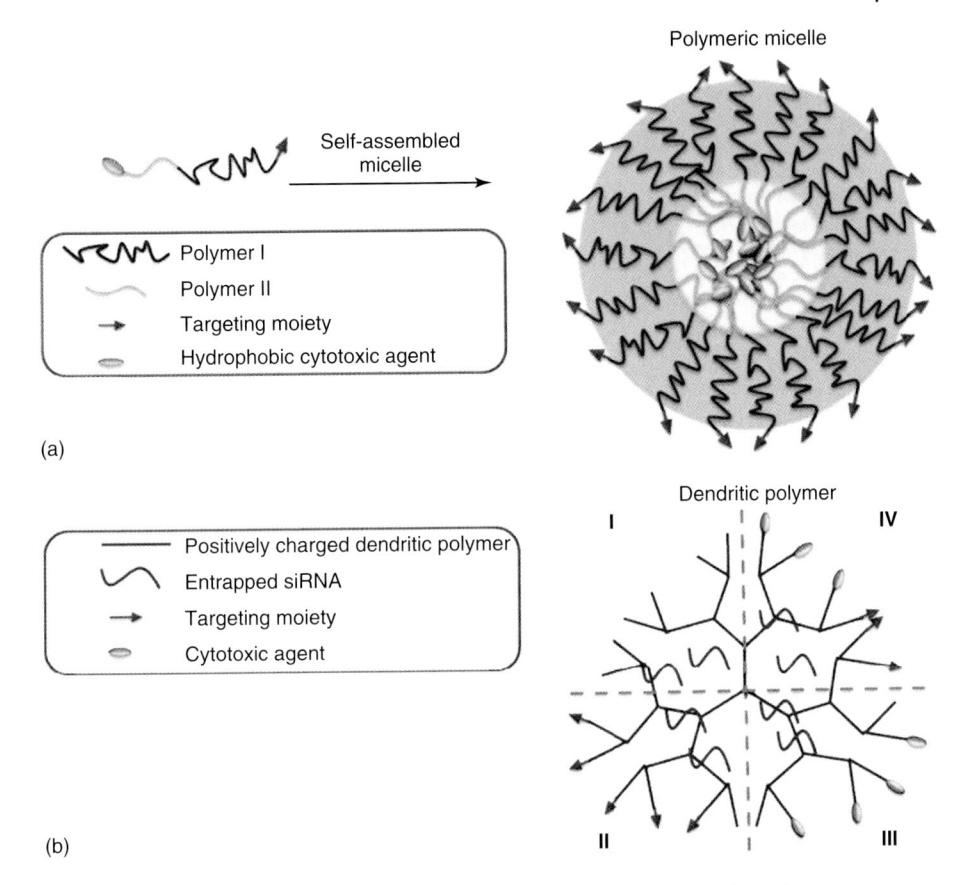

20.4 Novel Targeted Polymeric Drug Delivery Systems Directed to Tumor Endothelial Cells

Figure 20.11 Schematic structures of (a) self-assembled micellar structure of a polymer bound to hydrophobic and hydrophilic molecules. (b) (I) siRNA entrapped within a polymeric dendrimer by electrostatic interaction, (II) targeted dendritic delivery system of siRNA, (III) nontargeted combined drug and siRNA dendritic system, and (IV) combined system using siRNA, drug, and targeting moiety.

promising research area. Kataoka et al. [31] constructed a cyclic RGD peptide conjugated to a block copolymer, c(RGDfK)–PEG–poly(L-lysine), by connecting a PEG–poly(L-lysine) carboxyaldehyde to cysteine-terminated cyclic RGD peptide via a thiazolidine ligation procedure. Next, the polyplex micelle associated with plasmid DNA showed outstanding transfection efficiency in $\alpha_v\beta_3/\alpha_v\beta_5$ integrin-overexpressing HeLa cells. These results were established by flow cytometric analysis, which confirmed a superior uptake of the RGD micelles as compared to a non-RGD counterpart. Using confocal microscopy it was observed that the plasmid DNA in RGD-targeted micelles preferentially accumulated in the perinuclear region of the HeLa cells, whilst RGD-free micelles did not. Taken together, these results imply that the superior transfection efficiency induced by the RGD ligand within the micelle can be attributed to an increase in cellular uptake and to accelerated intracellular trafficking to the perinuclear region, and paves the way for a promising use of such micellar formulations in site-specific targeted gene delivery intervention.

Multidrug resistance (MDR) is a mechanism by which cancer cells protect themselves from chemotherapy; it is also one of the major obstacles of currently available cancer chemotherapy. The ATP-dependent transmembrane transporter P-glycoprotein (P-gp) is responsible for the dominant mechanism that reduces intracellular levels of cytotoxic drugs below lethal thresholds by active pumping of the drug out from the tumor cell.

The bypass of P-gp and/or controlled delivery of cytotoxic agents (e.g., DOX) to alternative subcellular sites in cancer cells may enhance the efficacy of the drugs in resistant tumors.

Xiong et al. [32] developed two polymeric nanocarriers; (i) RGD-4C–PEO-b-P(CL-Hyd-DOX), linked by pH-sensitive hydrazone (Hyd) bond, and (ii) RGD-4C–PEO-b-P(CL-Ami-DOX), linked by a more stable amide (Ami) bond, with the objective to increase the therapeutic efficacy of DOX for sensitive and resistant cancers. The delivery systems are based on biodegradable poly(ethylene oxide)-block-poly(3-caprolactone) (PEO-b-PCL) micelles functionalized on the micellar shell (PEO) as well as the micellar core (PCL). Both micellar conjugates were stable in physiological pH 7.2, but at pH 5.0, DOX was released from P(CL-Hyd-DOX) due to degradation of the acid-labile linker and from P(CL-Ami-DOX) due to micellar core degradation. In both formulations, RGD-4C-containing micelles significantly increased the cellular uptake of DOX in a DOX-sensitive cancer cell line (MDA-435/LCC6^{WT}) and a DOX-resistant cancer cell line (a clone expressing a high level of P-gp, MDA-435/LCC6^{MDR}). In MDA-435/LCC6^{WT}, the best cytotoxic response was achieved using RGD-4C–PEO-b-P(CL-Hyd-DOX), that correlated with the highest cellular uptake and preferential nuclear accumulation of DOX. In MDA-435/LCC6^{MDR}, RGD-4C–PEO-b-P(CL-Ami-DOX) was the most cytotoxic and this effect correlated with the accumulation of DOX in the mitochondria. Consistent with those in vitro results, RGD-4C–PEO-b-P(CL-Hyd-DOX) and RGD-4C–PEO-b-P(CL-Ami-DOX) nanoformulations were found to be more effective than free DOX in inhibiting the in vivo growth of DOX-sensitive and DOX-resistant tumors, respectively.

20.4.2
Selectin-Targeted Polymer–Drug Conjugates

E-selectin was targeted with a high-affinity peptide named E-selectin-binding peptide (Esbp) for the selective delivery of drugs to tumor vascular endothelium. The Esbp moiety contains the DITWDQLWDLMK sequence – exclusively binding E-selectin, but not its family members, P-selectin and L-selectin. Polymers carrying drugs and/or diagnostic agents would benefit from E-selectin-mediated targeting using Esbp since it can be easily attached to a polymeric scaffold. In addition, Esbp binds E-selectin at a low nanomolar range concentrations [115] and in a noncompetitive manner, compared with sLe^x (another well-characterized binding peptide).

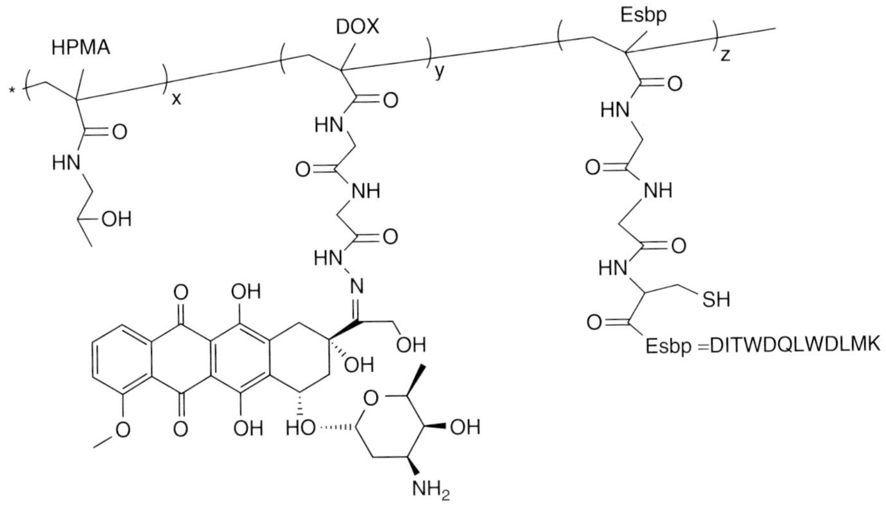

Figure 20.12 Chemical structure of HPMA copolymer–Esbp containing a terminal hydrazone-bound DOX moiety.

Shamay et al. [33] demonstrated that copolymers carrying Esbp and anticancer drug possess strong cytotoxicity against E-selectin-expressing vascular endothelium, by using the water-soluble HPMA copolymer as the polymeric drug carrier. The passive localization associated with the EPR effect was shown to be significantly improved by active mechanism involving receptor–ligand interactions [116].

In this study, Esbp-targeted HPMA copolymer was conjugated with DOX via a spacer containing a hydrazide group. Esbp peptide significantly increased the HPMA–DOX conjugate's endocytosis efficiency into immortalized vascular endothelial cells (IVECs) expressing E-selectin upon tumor necrosis factor-α activation [117]. This was attributed to multivalent interactions between the HPMA–Esbp copolymers and the cell surface-associated E-selectin (Figure 20.12). The cellular binding and uptake of the conjugate, as observed by confocal fluorescence images, were consistent with the increased cytotoxicity of P–(Esbp)–DOX. This cytotoxicity of P–(Esbp)–DOX requires cellular uptake of the copolymer followed by the release of the active DOX moieties in endosomal and lysosomal compartments. Esbp peptide was found, for the first time, to be capable of delivering elevated amounts of DOX to E-selectin-expressing vascular endothelium. This is the first successful attempt to implement Esbp-directed chemotherapy to activated endothelial cells using a peptide–polymer–drug conjugate for specific binding to E-selectin [33].

20.4.3
APN-Targeted Polymer Therapeutics

APN/CD13 acts as an endothelial (and cancer) cell target, as described by Adar et al. [34]. They recently reported the design and synthesis of CD13-targeted

HPMA copolymers for the selective delivery of proapoptotic drug into cancer and endothelial cells [34]. The use of the NGR motif facilitates active targeting to the CD13 receptor. A significant benefit of using polymers carrying multivalent display of NGR motifs is that they can act simultaneously on more than one CD13 receptor, to markedly improve the binding affinity [118, 119].

Peptides capable of invading mitochondria of mammalian cells and triggering apoptosis are a new therapeutic method for cancer treatment [120–122]. The mitochondria-disrupting peptide D-(KLAKLAK)$_2$, a 14-amino-acid cationic and α-helical-forming peptide, had been shown to induce apoptosis in cancer cells [123]. This D-(KLAKLAK)$_2$ peptide does not penetrate the zwitterionic plasma membranes of eukaryotic cells, but when internalized, it can disrupt the negatively charged mitochondrial membrane [124], resulting in cell death by mitochondrial-dependent apoptosis [120]. The use of this peptide for enhancing the apoptotic activity is therefore promising, but must involve targeting and internalization strategies. The peptide was attached to the polymer, as described before, through an acid-sensitive hydrazone linkage that is stable in the blood circulation at pH 7.4, but hydrolytically degradable in mildly acidic environment [125] and can be used for controlled release of the D-(KLAKLAK)$_2$ moieties.

The novel water-soluble HPMA copolymer bearing a multivalent display of NGR motifs targets the proapoptotic drug to CD13-overexpressing cells (Figure 20.13). Several NGR sequences of various structural conformations were examined, but the dimeric and cyclic NGR sequences demonstrated superior binding affinity to

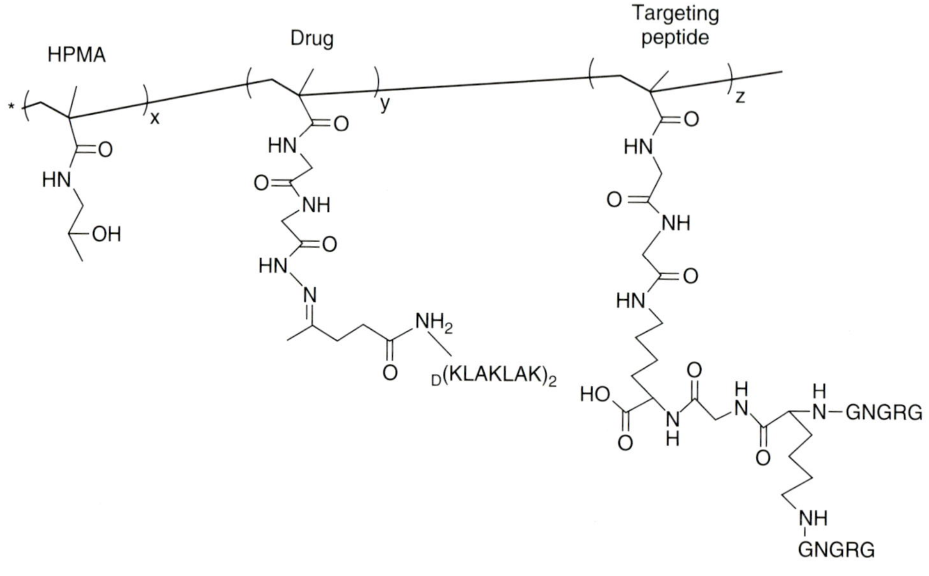

Figure 20.13 Chemical structure of targeted HPMA copolymer bearing (GNGRG)$_2$ as targeting ligand and D-(KLAKLAK)$_2$ as cytotoxic moiety.

CD13-overexpressing cells over the linear peptide. The attachment of the drug to a polymeric carrier markedly increased the cytotoxicity and the proapoptotic activity of the active peptide relative to free D-(KLAKLAK)$_2$ in CD13$^+$ cells. Apoptosis was the major mechanism for induction of cell death following exposure to the polymeric drug. Altogether, this conjugate showed an improved intracellular delivery and cytotoxicity of polymer–D-(KLAKLAK)$_2$ conjugate in endothelial cells and various cancer cells [34].

20.4.4
HA-Based Polymer Therapeutics

HA is a natural anionic polysaccharide that is efficiently taken up by cells via HA receptor (CD44)-mediated endocytosis. Jere et al. reported the conjugation of HA to polyethyleneimine (PEI); PEI-g-HA conjugate reduced the cytotoxicity of PEI and enabled target specific delivery to tissues with various HA receptors. Among several candidates, branched PEI (bPEI, molecular weight 25 kDa) has been regarded as one of the most effective nonviral vehicles for *in vitro* gene silencing. It is highly positively charged; hence, forming tight electrostatic interaction with the negatively charged siRNA [126].

Park et al. synthesized reducible bPEI by the cross-linking of low-molecular-weight PEI with cystamine bisacrylamide (CBA). PEI with a molecular weight of 2000 Da has relatively negligible cytotoxicity, but also low siRNA delivery efficiency. The cross-linked PEI containing disulfide bonds (PEI-SS) showed comparable siRNA delivery capability to high-molecular-weight bPEI with remarkably reduced cytotoxicity. The amine groups of PEI-SS were further conjugated to the carboxyl groups of HA in the form of block copolymer by reductive amidation, resulting in (PEI-SS)-*b*-HA conjugate complexed with siRNA.

Among other methods, various synthetic polymers such as PEI [127] were investigated for intracellular delivery of siRNA. Tumor angiogenesis was reported to be suppressed efficiently by downregulating the gene expression of VEGF. Moreover, there were many reports on therapeutic application of VEGF siRNA (siVEGF) for the treatment of cancer [128].

The cytotoxicity of (PEI-SS)-*b*-HA appeared to be negligible; the effective cellular uptake of siRNA/(PEI-SS)-*b*-HA complex by HA receptor-mediated endocytosis was confirmed by flow cytometric and confocal microscopic analyses. In addition, siRNA/(PEI-SS)-*b*-HA complex showed an *in vitro* gene silencing with 50–80% efficiency. HA on the outer surface of siRNA/(PEI-SS)-*b*-HA complex contributed to not only effective cellular uptake by HA receptor-mediated endocytosis, but also enhanced serum stability, alleviating the non-specific binding with serum proteins.

(PEI-SS)-*b*-HA conjugate was developed as a target specific and nontoxic delivery system of siRNA therapeutics and was proved successful when siVEGF/(PEI-SS)-*b*-HA complex was applied to the treatment of cancer, dramatically retarding the tumor growth (Figure 20.14) [35].

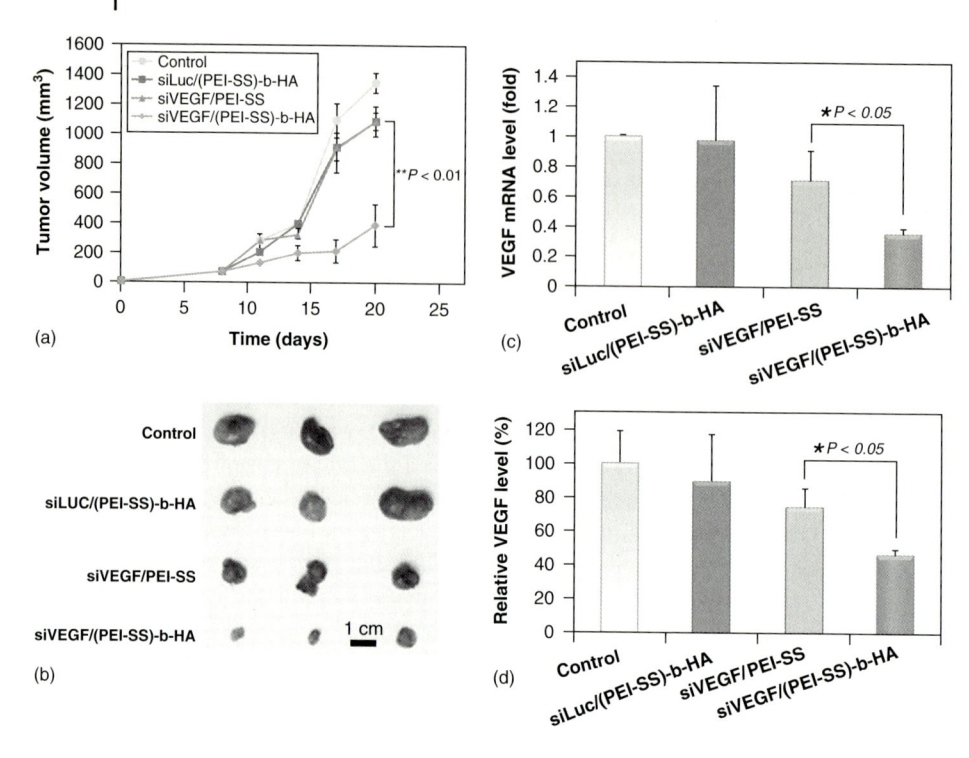

Figure 20.14 Antitumoral therapeutic effect of siVEGF/(PEI-SS)-b-HA complex in female BALB/c mice where CT-26 colon cancer cells were injected for tumor inoculation and growth. (a) Tumor volume change with increasing time after intratumoral injection of a control of 5% glucose solution, siVEGF/PEI-SS, nonspecific Luc siRNA (siLuc)/(PEI-SS)-b-HA, and siVEGF/(PEI-SS)-b-HA complexes. The treatments were performed 3 times after 8, 11, and 14 days. The results represent mean ± standard deviation ($n = 3$). *$P < 0.05$ versus the control. (b) Photo-images of dissected tumor tissues after 20 days. (c) VEGF mRNA levels in tumor tissues 1 day after last treatment with the samples (after 15 days). The data were normalized with mouse GAPDH mRNA level. *$P < 0.05$ versus siVEGF/PEI-SS. (d) Comparison of VEGF levels in tumor tissues after 20 days. *$P < 0.05$ versus siVEGF/PEI-SS. Taken from [35].

20.5
Opportunity for Dual Targeting of Angiogenesis-Related Markers

Cancer is a complex and dynamic disease that involves genetic alterations in tumor cells, accelerated cell proliferation followed by unrestrained tumor mass growth. Limitations in clinical therapy may develop during cancer treatment due to emerging tumor cell resistance mechanisms or life-threatening healthy organ toxicities. One approach to overcome this drawback is to use combination therapy. Combination and simultaneous delivery of different therapies to the tumor tissue holds great therapeutic potential. One example is a specific targeted delivery system for treatment of bone metastasis, which is composed of HPMA copolymer conjugated via an enzymatically cleavable linker with the chemotherapeutic agent PTX or the antiangiogenic agent TNP-470 in combination with the bone-targeted aminobisphosphonate alendronate [129, 130].

All the conjugates described above share two main characteristics. (i) Their structure – a polymer–toxic agent–targeting moiety. (ii) They are all directed to molecules presented on endothelial cells forming new capillaries within the tumor tissue, where they can attack and destroy the endothelial cells, and hence cause tumor starvation. But, is that all? Cancer is a "smart" disease, constantly changing, presenting different forms from its original specific tissue-characterized cell origin. Some of those very common changes are expression of different receptors that enable and increase the cancer cell's ability to grow, migrate, attach to the ECM, extravasate through the blood vessels to new locations, and allow homing of metastasis. Those receptors are frequently the same molecules used by other proliferating/migrating/attaching cells, such as angiogenesis-related endothelial cells. Different tumor types were characterized and their cells are known to express the homing molecules presented herein. The activity of the targeted polymer–toxic agent conjugates was evaluated either on endothelial cells, cancer cells, or both. The expression of integrins, selectins, and HA by different tumor cells (summarized in Table 20.4) offers a huge advantage to the conjugates presented above, conferring them a dual-targeting capability, both to the endothelial cells nurturing the tumor and the tumor cells themselves.

20.6 Tumor Angiogenesis-Targeted Polymeric Drug Delivery Systems: Summary and Lessons Learnt

We have presented the formation of a new combined tactic for the treatment of cancer. This team of newly formed and characterized molecules is yet to be completed and further recruitment is needed. The leading tactics forming all these nanoscaled smart drug delivery systems were based on an approach combining various well-known strategies – the combination of antiangiogenesis, together with antitumor activity, polymer therapeutics, and targeted drug delivery. However, these combined nanomedicines are still in their formative stage. Three critical stages are required for cytotoxic activity of targeted polymer–drug conjugates: (i) cellular recognition site for the polymer, (ii) release of free drug from the polymer (kinetics, intracellular site of release, and intracellular trafficking), and (iii) sensitivity of the cell toward the drug [26]. All the conjugates presented were designed to follow this strategy, and to follow it in *in vitro* studies on both endothelial and various cancer cell lines. There are two crucial barriers yet to be conquered: showing preferred accumulation of the drug in the tumor site and an enhancement in *in vivo* efficacy.

Targeted polymer therapeutics gradually focus on the neovasculature of tumors and growing metastases. There is no barrier between the systemic circulation, which transports the nanoscaled polymer therapeutics, and the targeted cells. Each target cell (i.e., the tumor endothelial cell) is exposed directly to the systemic

Table 20.4 Endothelial cell marker expression on different tumor cell types.

Marker	Ligand	Endothelial expression	Expressing human cancer cells	References
$\alpha_v\beta_3$ integrin	RGD-containing sequence	HUVECs	glioblastoma (U87-MG), melanoma (M21), breast (MDA-MB-231, T47D, MDA-MB-435[a], pancreatic (Panc-1), ovarian carcinoma (MLS), prostate (PC-3), cervical (HeLa)	[29, 31, 83, 92, 118, 131]
APN/CD13	NGR sequence	HUVECs	prostate (PC3-MM2), non-small-cell lung carcinoma (H1299)	[34, 49, 132, 133]
		IVECs	fibrosarcoma (HT-1080)	
		HBMECs	promyelocytic leukemia (HL-60), ovarian (ES-2), lung (A549), hepatic (PLC/PRF/5, HepG2, H7402, A172, HuH-7), glioblastoma (U87)	
CD44/HA receptor	HA	HUVECs	lung (HTB58)	[35, 64, 134, 135]
			breast (MDA-MB-231), melanoma (M21, B16/F1)	[131, 136]
E-selectin	Esbp synthetic analog of sLe^x	IVECs	promyelocytic leukemia (HL-60)	[33, 137]
		HUVECs	–	

HBMECs, human brain microvascular endothelial cells.
[a]MDA-MB-435 cells are derived from the M14 melanoma cell line and can no longer be considered a model of breast cancer.

supply route and hence the therapeutics. Extravasation of the macromolecules to the tumor site due to the EPR effect renders the conjugate activity. Moreover, better penetration is presented by an additional targeting moiety, which allows for receptor-mediated endocytosis of the conjugate and release of the drug specifically within the tumor endothelial cells or cancer cells. Antiangiogenic therapy, tumor targeting, and polymer therapeutics are all being investigated separately. However, the idea that gathering the knowledge collected from different fields might hold the key to conquering cancer has long been suggested. Although the multidisciplinary approach is well established, this chapter presents a revolutionary and exciting therapeutic approach – a unique combination of several different strategies in the war against cancer. Further investigation of the different cytotoxic agent-targeted polymer therapeutics presented here is required, and many different combinations are yet to be explored in order to complete this team and render it as an active force in this ongoing war.

References

1. Folkman, J. and Kalluri, R. Tumor angiogenesis (2003) in *Cancer Medicine* (ed. D.W. Kufe), Decker, Hamilton, pp. 161–194.
2. Folkman, J. (2007) Angiogenesis: an organizing principle for drug discovery. *Nat. Rev. Drug Discov.*, **6**, 273–286.
3. McDonald, D.M. Angiogenesis and vascular remodeling in inflammation and cancer: biology and architecture of the vasculature (2008) in *Angiogenesis: An Integrative Approach from Science to Medicine* (eds W.D. Figg and J. Folkman), Springer, New York, pp. 17–35.
4. Matsumoto, T. and Claesson-Welsh, L. (2001) VEGF receptor signal transduction. *Sci. STKE*, **2001**, RE21.
5. Neufeld, G., Cohen, T., Gengrinovitch, S., and Poltorak, Z. (1999) Vascular endothelial growth factor (VEGF) and its receptors. *FASEB J.*, **13**, 9–22.
6. Folkman, J. (1971) Tumor angiogenesis therapeutic implications. *N. Engl. J. Med.*, **285**, 1182–1186.
7. Matsumura, Y. and Maeda, H. (1986) A new concept for macromolecular therapeutics in cancer chemotherapy: mechanism of tumoritropic accumulation of proteins and the antitumor agent smancs. *Cancer Res.*, **46**, 6387–6392.
8. Ferrara, N. and Kerbel, R.S. (2005) Angiogenesis as a therapeutic target. *Nature*, **438**, 967–974.
9. Germano, S. and O'Driscoll, L. (2009) Breast cancer understanding sensitivity and resistance to chemotherapy and targeted therapies to aid in personalised medicine. *Curr. Cancer Drug Targets*, **9**, 398–418.
10. Pastorino, F. et al. (2003) Vascular damage and anti-angiogenic effects of tumor vessel-targeted liposomal chemotherapy. *Cancer Res.*, **63**, 7400–7409.
11. Stordal, B., Pavlakis, N., and Davey, R. (2007) A systematic review of platinum and taxane resistance from bench to clinic: an inverse relationship. *Cancer Treat. Rev.*, **33**, 688–703.
12. Browder, T. et al. (2000) Antiangiogenic scheduling of chemotherapy improves efficacy against experimental drug-resistant cancer. *Cancer Res.*, **60**, 1878–1886.
13. Klement, G. et al. (2000) Continuous low-dose therapy with vinblastine and VEGF receptor-2 antibody induces sustained tumor regression without overt toxicity. *J. Clin. Invest.*, **105**, R15–R24.
14. Man, S. et al. (2002) Antitumor effects in mice of low-dose (metronomic)

cyclophosphamide administered continuously through the drinking water. *Cancer Res.*, **62**, 2731–2735.
15. Hlatky, L., Hahnfeldt, P., and Folkman, J. (2002) Clinical application of antiangiogenic therapy: microvessel density, what it does and doesn't tell us. *J. Natl. Cancer Inst.*, **94**, 883–893.
16. Funovics, M., Montet, X., Reynolds, F., Weissleder, R., and Josephson, L. (2005) Nanoparticles for the optical imaging of tumor E-selectin. *Neoplasia*, **7**, 904–911.
17. Landon, L.A. and Deutscher, S.L. (2003) Combinatorial discovery of tumor targeting peptides using phage display. *J. Cell. Biochem.*, **90**, 509–517.
18. Ruoslahti, E. (2002) Specialization of tumour vasculature. *Nat. Rev. Cancer*, **2**, 83–90.
19. Ruoslahti, E. (2002) Drug targeting to specific vascular sites. *Drug Discov. Today*, **7**, 1138–1143.
20. Ruoslahti, E. and Rajotte, D. (2000) An address system in the vasculature of normal tissues and tumors. *Annu. Rev. Immunol.*, **18**, 813–827.
21. Ringsdorf, H. (1975) Structure and properties of pharmacologically active polymers. *J. Polym. Sci. Symp.*, **51**, 135–153.
22. Hynes, R.O. (2002) Integrins: bidirectional, allosteric signaling machines. *Cell*, **110**, 673–687.
23. Cai, W. and Chen, X. (2006) Anti-angiogenic cancer therapy based on integrin alphavbeta3 antagonism. *Anticancer Agents Med. Chem.*, **6**, 407–428.
24. Alghisi, G.C., Ponsonnet, L., and Ruegg, C. (2009) The integrin antagonist cilengitide activates alphaVbeta3, disrupts VE-cadherin localization at cell junctions and enhances permeability in endothelial cells. *PLoS ONE*, **4**, e4449.
25. Hood, J.D. et al. (2002) Tumor regression by targeted gene delivery to the neovasculature. *Science*, **296**, 2404–2407.
26. Borgman, M.P. et al. (2009) Targetable HPMA copolymer–aminohexylgeldanamycin conjugates for prostate cancer therapy. *Pharm. Res.*, **26**, 1407–1418.
27. Pike, D.B. and Ghandehari, H. (2010) HPMA copolymer–cyclic RGD conjugates for tumor targeting. *Adv. Drug Deliv. Rev.*, **62**, 167–183.
28. Eldar-Boock, A., Miller, K., Sanchis, J., Lupu, R., Vicent, M.J. and Satchi-Fainaro, R. (2010) Integrin assisted drug delivery of nano-scaled polymer therapeutics bearing paclitaxel. *Biomaterials*, **32**, 3862–3874.
29. Polyak, D. et al. (2011) Development of PEGylated doxorubicin–E-[c(RGDfK)$_2$] conjugate for integrin-targeted cancer therapy. *Polym. Adv. Technol.*, **22**, 103–113.
30. Kaneshiro, T.L. and Lu, Z.R. (2009) Targeted intracellular codelivery of chemotherapeutics and nucleic acid with a well-defined dendrimer-based nanoglobular carrier. *Biomaterials*, **30**, 5660–5666.
31. Oba, M. et al. (2007) Cyclic RGD peptide-conjugated polyplex micelles as a targetable gene delivery system directed to cells possessing alphavbeta3 and alphavbeta5 integrins. *Bioconjug. Chem.*, **18**, 1415–1423.
32. Xiong, X.B., Ma, Z., Lai, R., and Lavasanifar, A. (2010) The therapeutic response to multifunctional polymeric nano-conjugates in the targeted cellular and subcellular delivery of doxorubicin. *Biomaterials*, **31**, 757–768.
33. Shamay, Y., Paulin, D., Ashkenasy, G., and David, A. (2009) E-selectin binding peptide-polymer-drug conjugates and their selective cytotoxicity against vascular endothelial cells. *Biomaterials*, **30**, 6460–6468.
34. Adar, L., Shamay, Y., Journo, G., and David, A. (2011) Pro-apoptotic peptide–polymer conjugates to induce mitochondrial-dependent cell death. *Polym. Adv. Technol.*, **22**, 199–208.
35. Park, K., Lee, M.-Y., Kim, K.S., and Hahn, S.K. (2010) Target specific tumor treatment by VEGF siRNA complexed with reducible polyethyleneimine–hyaluronic acid conjugate. *Biomaterials*, **31**, 5258–5265.
36. Rae, J.M., Creighton, C.J., Meck, J.M., Haddad, B.R., and Johnson, M.D. (2007) MDA-MB-435 cells are derived from M14 melanoma cells – a

loss for breast cancer, but a boon for melanoma research. *Breast Cancer Res. Treat.*, **104**, 13–19.
37. Mitra, S.K. and Schlaepfer, D.D. (2006) Integrin-regulated FAK–Src signaling in normal and cancer cells. *Curr. Opin. Cell Biol.*, **18**, 516–523.
38. Guo, W. and Giancotti, F.G. (2004) Integrin signalling during tumour progression. *Nat. Rev. Mol. Cell Biol.*, **5**, 816–826.
39. Bertozzi, C.R. (1995) Cracking the carbohydrate code for selectin recognition. *Chem. Biol.*, **2**, 703–708.
40. Rosen, S.D. and Bertozzi, C.R. (1994) The selectins and their ligands. *Curr. Opin. Cell Biol.*, **6**, 663–673.
41. Barthel, S.R., Gavino, J.D., Descheny, L., and Dimitroff, C.J. (2007) Targeting selectins and selectin ligands in inflammation and cancer. *Expert Opin. Ther. Targets*, **11**, 1473–1491.
42. McEver, R.P. (1997) Selectin–carbohydrate interactions during inflammation and metastasis. *Glycoconj. J.*, **14**, 585–591.
43. Kobayashi, H., Boelte, K.C., and Lin, P.C. (2007) Endothelial cell adhesion molecules and cancer progression. *Curr. Med. Chem.*, **14**, 377–386.
44. Kannagi, R., Izawa, M., Koike, T., Miyazaki, K., and Kimura, N. (2004) Carbohydrate-mediated cell adhesion in cancer metastasis and angiogenesis. *Cancer Sci.*, **95**, 377–384.
45. Laferriere, J., Houle, F., and Huot, J. (2002) Regulation of the metastatic process by E-selectin and stress-activated protein kinase-2/p38. *Ann. NY Acad. Sci.*, **973**, 562–572.
46. Ehrhardt, C., Kneuer, C., and Bakowsky, U. (2004) Selectins – an emerging target for drug delivery. *Adv. Drug Deliv. Rev.*, **56**, 527–549.
47. Hooper, N.M. (1994) Families of zinc metalloproteases. *FEBS Lett.*, **354**, 1–6.
48. Look, A.T., Ashmun, R.A., Shapiro, L.H., and Peiper, S.C. (1989) Human myeloid plasma membrane glycoprotein CD13 (gp150) is identical to aminopeptidase N. *J. Clin. Invest.*, **83**, 1299–1307.
49. Wang, X. et al. (2010) Activity screening and structure-activity relationship of the hit compounds targeting APN/CD13. *Fundam. Clin. Pharmacol.*, **25**, 217–228.
50. Lendeckel, U. et al. (2000) Review: the role of membrane peptidases in immune functions. *Adv. Exp. Med. Biol.*, **477**, 1–24.
51. Shipp, M.A. and Look, A.T. (1993) Hematopoietic differentiation antigens that are membrane-associated enzymes: cutting is the key! *Blood*, **82**, 1052–1070.
52. Luan, Y. and Xu, W. (2007) The structure and main functions of aminopeptidase N. *Curr. Med. Chem.*, **14**, 639–647.
53. Bhagwat, S.V. et al. (2001) CD13/APN is activated by angiogenic signals and is essential for capillary tube formation. *Blood*, **97**, 652–659.
54. Petrovic, N. et al. (2007) CD13/APN regulates endothelial invasion and filopodia formation. *Blood*, **110**, 142–150.
55. Pasqualini, R. et al. (2000) Aminopeptidase N is a receptor for tumor-homing peptides and a target for inhibiting angiogenesis. *Cancer Res.*, **60**, 722–727.
56. Curnis, F. et al. (2002) Differential binding of drugs containing the NGR motif to CD13 isoforms in tumor vessels, epithelia, and myeloid cells. *Cancer Res.*, **62**, 867–874.
57. Isacke, C.M. and Yarwood, H. (2002) The hyaluronan receptor, CD44. *Int. J. Biochem. Cell Biol.*, **34**, 718–721.
58. Bajorath, J., Greenfield, B., Munro, S.B., Day, A.J., and Aruffo, A. (1998) Identification of CD44 residues important for hyaluronan binding and delineation of the binding site. *J. Biol. Chem.*, **273**, 338–343.
59. David, A. (2010) Carbohydrate-based biomedical copolymers for targeted delivery of anticancer drugs. *Isr. J. Chem.*, **50**, 204–219.
60. Laurent, T.C. and Fraser, J.R. (1992) Hyaluronan. *FASEB J.*, **6**, 2397–2404.
61. Knudson, W. (1996) Tumor-associated hyaluronan. Providing an extracellular matrix that facilitates invasion. *Am. J. Pathol.*, **148**, 1721–1726.

62. Camenisch, T.D. and McDonald, J.A. (2000) Hyaluronan: is bigger better. *Am. J. Respir. Cell Mol. Biol.*, **23**, 431–433.
63. Lee, J.Y. and Spicer, A.P. (2000) Hyaluronan: a multifunctional, megaDalton, stealth molecule. *Curr. Opin. Cell Biol.*, **12**, 581–586.
64. Szczepanek, K., Kieda, C., and Cichy, J. (2008) Differential binding of hyaluronan on the surface of tissue-specific endothelial cell lines. *Acta Biochim. Pol.*, **55**, 35–42.
65. Eliaz, R.E. and Szoka, F.C. Jr. (2001) Liposome-encapsulated doxorubicin targeted to CD44: a strategy to kill CD44-overexpressing tumor cells. *Cancer Res.*, **61**, 2592–2601.
66. Peer, D. and Margalit, R. (2004) Tumor-targeted hyaluronan nanoliposomes increase the antitumor activity of liposomal doxorubicin in syngeneic and human xenograft mouse tumor models. *Neoplasia*, **6**, 343–353.
67. Peer, D., Park, E.J., Morishita, Y., Carman, C.V., and Shimaoka, M. (2008) Systemic leukocyte-directed siRNA delivery revealing cyclin D1 as an anti-inflammatory target. *Science*, **319**, 627–630.
68. Haag, R. and Kratz, F. (2006) Polymer therapeutics concepts and applications. *Angew. Chem. Int. Ed. Engl.*, **45**, 1198–1215.
69. Eichhorn, M.E., Strieth, S., and Dellian, M. (2004) Anti-vascular tumor therapy: recent advances, pitfalls and clinical perspectives. *Drug Resist. Updat.*, **7**, 125–138.
70. Ingber, D. et al. (1990) Synthetic analogues of fumagillin that inhibit angiogenesis and suppress tumour growth. *Nature*, **348**, 555–557.
71. Kudelka, A.P. et al. (1997) A phase I study of TNP-470 administered to patients with advanced squamous cell cancer of the cervix. *Clin. Cancer Res.*, **3**, 1501–1505.
72. Kudelka, A.P., Verschraegen, C.F., and Loyer, E. (1998) Complete remission of metastatic cervical cancer with the angiogenesis inhibitor TNP-470. *N. Engl. J. Med.*, **338**, 991–992.
73. Bhargava, P. et al. (1999) A phase I and pharmacokinetic study of TNP-470 administered weekly to patients with advanced cancer. *Clin. Cancer Res.*, **5**, 1989–1995.
74. Dezube, B.J. et al. (1998) Fumagillin analog in the treatment of Kaposi's sarcoma: a phase I AIDS Clinical Trial Group study. AIDS Clinical Trial Group No. 215 Team. *J. Clin. Oncol.*, **16**, 1444–1449.
75. Satchi-Fainaro, R. et al. (2004) Targeting angiogenesis with a conjugate of HPMA copolymer and TNP-470. *Nat. Med.*, **10**, 255–261.
76. Mendichi, R., Rizzo, V., Gigli, M., and Schieroni, A.G. (2002) Fractionation and characterization of a conjugate between a polymeric drug-carrier and the antitumor drug camptothecin. *Bioconjug. Chem.*, **13**, 1253–1258.
77. Duncan, R., Cable, H.C., Rejmanova, P., Kopecek, J., and Lloyd, J.B. (1984) Tyrosinamide residues enhance pinocytic capture of N-(2-hydroxypropyl)methacrylamide copolymers. *Biochim. Biophys. Acta*, **799**, 1–8.
78. Satchi-Fainaro, R. (2002) Targeting tumor vasculature: reality or a dream. *J. Drug Target.*, **10**, 529–533.
79. Satchi-Fainaro, R. et al. (2005) Inhibition of vessel permeability by TNP-470 and its polymer conjugate, caplostatin. *Cancer Cell*, **7**, 251–261.
80. Chesler, L. (2007) Malignant progression and blockade of angiogenesis in a murine transgenic model of neuroblastoma. *Cancer Res.*, **67**, 9435–9442.
81. Ofek, P., Miller, K., Eldar-Boock, A., Polyak, D., Segal, E., and Satchi-Fainaro, R. (2010). Special theme issue: polymer therapeutics as novel nanomedicines. *Isr. J. Chem.*, **50**, 185–203.
82. Pierschbacher, M.D. and Ruoslahti, E. (1984) Cell attachment activity of fibronectin can be duplicated by small synthetic fragments of the molecule. *Nature*, **309**, 30–33.
83. Liu, S. (2009) Radiolabeled cyclic RGD peptides as integrin

alpha$_v$beta$_3$-targeted radiotracers: maximizing binding affinity via bivalency. *Bioconjug. Chem.*, **20**, 2199–2213.
84. Bergelson, J.M., Shepley, M.P., Chan, B.M., Hemler, M.E., and Finberg, R.W. (1992) Identification of the integrin VLA-2 as a receptor for echovirus 1. *Science*, **255**, 1718–1720.
85. Leininger, E. et al. (1991) Pertactin, an Arg–Gly–Asp-containing *Bordetella pertussis* surface protein that promotes adherence of mammalian cells. *Proc. Natl. Acad. Sci. USA*, **88**, 345–349.
86. Pierschbacher, M.D. and Ruoslahti, E. (1987) Influence of stereochemistry of the sequence Arg–Gly–Asp–Xaa on binding specificity in cell adhesion. *J. Biol. Chem.*, **262**, 17294–17298.
87. Goodman, S.L., Holzemann, G., Sulyok, G.A., and Kessler, H. (2002) Nanomolar small molecule inhibitors for alphav(beta)6, alphav(beta)5, and alphav(beta)3 integrins. *J. Med. Chem.*, **45**, 1045–1051.
88. Bogdanowich-Knipp, S.J., Chakrabarti, S., Williams, T.D., Dillman, R.K., and Siahaan, T.J. (1999) Solution stability of linear vs. cyclic RGD peptides. *J. Pept. Res.*, **53**, 530–541.
89. Dechantsreiter, M.A. et al. (1999) N-Methylated cyclic RGD peptides as highly active and selective alpha$_v$beta$_3$ integrin antagonists. *J. Med. Chem.*, **42**, 3033–3040.
90. Aumailley, M. et al. (1991) Arg–Gly–Asp constrained within cyclic pentapeptides. Strong and selective inhibitors of cell adhesion to vitronectin and laminin fragment P1. *FEBS Lett.*, **291**, 50–54.
91. Paolillo, M., Russo, M.A., Serra, M., Colombo, L., and Schinelli, S. (2009) Small molecule integrin antagonists in cancer therapy. *Mini. Rev. Med. Chem.*, **9**, 1439–1446.
92. Desgrosellier, J.S. and Cheresh, D.A. (2010) Integrins in cancer: biological implications and therapeutic opportunities. *Nat. Rev. Cancer*, **10**, 9–22.
93. Reynolds, A.R. et al. (2009) Stimulation of tumor growth and angiogenesis by low concentrations of RGD-mimetic integrin inhibitors. *Nat. Med.*, **15**, 392–400.
94. Arap, W., Pasqualini, R., and Ruoslahti, E. (1998) Cancer treatment by targeted drug delivery to tumor vasculature in a mouse model. *Science*, **279**, 377–380.
95. Kim, J.W. and Lee, H.S. (2004) Tumor targeting by doxorubicin–RGD-4C peptide conjugate in an orthotopic mouse hepatoma model. *Int. J. Mol. Med.*, **14**, 529–535.
96. Janssen, M. et al. (2002) Comparison of a monomeric and dimeric radiolabeled RGD-peptide for tumor targeting. *Cancer Biother. Radiopharm.*, **17**, 641–646.
97. Janssen, M.L. et al. (2002) Tumor targeting with radiolabeled alpha$_v$beta$_3$ integrin binding peptides in a nude mouse model. *Cancer Res.*, **62**, 6146–6151.
98. Janssen, M. et al. (2004) Improved tumor targeting of radiolabeled RGD peptides using rapid dose fractionation. *Cancer Biother. Radiopharm.*, **19**, 399–404.
99. Wester, H.J. and Kessler, H. (2005) Molecular targeting with peptides or peptide–polymer conjugates: just a question of size. *J. Nucl. Med.*, **46**, 1940–1945.
100. Sancey, L. et al. (2009) Clustering and internalization of integrin alphavbeta3 with a tetrameric RGD-synthetic peptide. *Mol. Ther.*, **17**, 837–843.
101. Holzbeierlein, J.M., Windsperger, A., and Vielhauer, G. (2010) Hsp90: a drug target. *Curr. Oncol. Rep.*, **12**, 95–101.
102. Lattouf, J.B., Srinivasan, R., Pinto, P.A., Linehan, W.M., and Neckers, L. (2006) Mechanisms of disease: the role of heat-shock protein 90 in genitourinary malignancy. *Nat. Clin. Pract. Urol.*, **3**, 590–601.
103. Kasuya, Y., Lu, Z.R., Kopeckova, P., Tabibi, S.E., and Kopecek, J. (2002) Influence of the structure of drug moieties on the *in vitro* efficacy of HPMA copolymer–geldanamycin derivative conjugates. *Pharm. Res.*, **19**, 115–123.
104. Kaur, G. et al. (2004) Antiangiogenic properties of 17-(dimethylaminoethylamino)-17-demethoxygeldanamycin: an orally bioavailable heat shock protein 90

modulator. *Clin. Cancer Res.*, **10**, 4813–4821.

105. Ryppa, C., Mann-Steinberg, H., Biniossek, M.L., Satchi-Fainaro, R., and Kratz, F. (2009) In vitro and in vivo evaluation of a paclitaxel conjugate with the divalent peptide E-[c(RGDfK)$_2$] that targets integrin alpha v beta 3. *Int. J. Pharm.*, **368**, 89–97.

106. Paz-Ares, L. et al. (2008) Phase III trial comparing paclitaxel poliglumex vs docetaxel in the second-line treatment of non-small-cell lung cancer. *Br. J. Cancer*, **98**, 1608–1613.

107. O'Brien, M.E. et al. (2008) Randomized phase III trial comparing single-agent paclitaxel Poliglumex (CT-2103, PPX) with single-agent gemcitabine or vinorelbine for the treatment of PS 2 patients with chemotherapy-naive advanced non-small cell lung cancer. *J. Thorac. Oncol.*, **3**, 728–734.

108. Langer, C.J. et al. (2008) Phase III trial comparing paclitaxel poliglumex (CT-2103, PPX) in combination with carboplatin versus standard paclitaxel and carboplatin in the treatment of PS 2 patients with chemotherapy-naive advanced non-small cell lung cancer. *J. Thorac. Oncol.*, **3**, 623–630.

109. Satchi-Fainaro, R., Duncan, R., and Barnes, C.M. (eds) (2006) *Polymer Therapeutics for Cancer: Current Status and Future Challenges*, Springer, Heidelberg, pp. 1–65.

110. Qu, G., Yao, Z., Zhang, C., Wu, X., and Ping, Q. (2009) PEG conjugated N-octyl-O-sulfate chitosan micelles for delivery of paclitaxel: in vitro characterization and in vivo evaluation. *Eur. J. Pharm. Sci.*, **37**, 98–105.

111. Tekade, R.K., Kumar, P.V., and Jain, N.K. (2009) Dendrimers in oncology: an expanding horizon. *Chem. Rev.*, **109**, 49–87.

112. Willner, D. et al. (1993) (6-Maleimidocaproyl)hydrazone of doxorubicin – a new derivative for the preparation of immunoconjugates of doxorubicin. *Bioconjug. Chem.*, **4**, 521–527.

113. Aagaard, L. and Rossi, J.J. (2007) RNAi therapeutics: principles, prospects and challenges. *Adv. Drug Deliv. Rev.*, **59**, 75–86.

114. Ofek, P., Fischer, W., Calderon, M., Haag, R., and Satchi-Fainaro, R. (2010) In vivo delivery of small interfering RNA to tumors and their vasculature by novel dendritic nanocarriers. *FASEB J.*, **24**, 3122–3134.

115. Martens, C.L. et al. (1995) Peptides which bind to E-selectin and block neutrophil adhesion. *J. Biol. Chem.*, **270**, 21129–21136.

116. Rihova, B. (1998) Receptor-mediated targeted drug or toxin delivery. *Adv. Drug Deliv. Rev.*, **29**, 273–289.

117. Shamay, Y., Paulin, D., Ashkenasy, G., and David, A. (2009) Multivalent display of quinic acid based ligands for targeting E-selectin expressing cells. *J. Med. Chem.*, **52**, 5906–5915.

118. Kiessling, L.L. and Pohl, N.L. (1996) Strength in numbers: non-natural polyvalent carbohydrate derivatives. *Chem. Biol.*, **3**, 71–77.

119. Roy, R. (1996) Syntheses and some applications of chemically defined multivalent glycoconjugates. *Curr. Opin. Struct. Biol.*, **6**, 692–702.

120. Ellerby, H.M. et al. (1999) Anti-cancer activity of targeted pro-apoptotic peptides. *Nat. Med.*, **5**, 1032–1038.

121. Law, B., Quinti, L., Choi, Y., Weissleder, R., and Tung, C.H. (2006) A mitochondrial targeted fusion peptide exhibits remarkable cytotoxicity. *Mol. Cancer Ther.*, **5**, 1944–1949.

122. Mai, J.C., Mi, Z., Kim, S.H., Ng, B., and Robbins, P.D. (2001) A proapoptotic peptide for the treatment of solid tumors. *Cancer Res.*, **61**, 7709–7712.

123. Javadpour, M.M. et al. (1996) De novo antimicrobial peptides with low mammalian cell toxicity. *J. Med. Chem.*, **39**, 3107–3113.

124. Wallace, D.C. (2005) Mitochondria and cancer: Warburg addressed. *Cold Spring Harb. Symp. Quant. Biol.*, **70**, 363–374.

125. Etrych, T., Jelinkova, M., Rihova, B., and Ulbrich, K. (2001) New HPMA copolymers containing doxorubicin bound via pH-sensitive linkage: synthesis and preliminary in vitro and in vivo biological properties. *J. Control. Release*, **73**, 89–102.

126. Jere, D. et al. (2009) Degradable polyethylenimines as DNA and small interfering RNA carriers. *Expert Opin. Drug Deliv.*, **6**, 827–834.
127. Urban-Klein, B., Werth, S., Abuharbeid, S., Czubayko, F., and Aigner, A. (2005) RNAi-mediated gene-targeting through systemic application of polyethylenimine (PEI)-complexed siRNA *in vivo*. *Gene Ther.*, **12**, 461–466.
128. Choi, Y.S. et al. (2010) The systemic delivery of siRNAs by a cell penetrating peptide, low molecular weight protamine. *Biomaterials*, **31**, 1429–1443.
129. Segal, E. et al. (2009) Targeting angiogenesis-dependent calcified neoplasms using combined polymer therapeutics. *PLoS ONE*, **4**, e5233.
130. Miller, K., Erez, R., Segal, E., Shabat, D., and Satchi-Fainaro, R. (2009) Targeting bone metastases with a bispecific anticancer and antiangiogenic polymer–alendronate–taxane conjugate. *Angew. Chem. Int. Ed. Engl.*, **48**, 2949–2954.
131. Samanna, V., Wei, H., Ego-Osuala, D., and Chellaiah, M.A. (2006) Alpha-V-dependent outside-in signaling is required for the regulation of CD44 surface expression, MMP-2 secretion, and cell migration by osteopontin in human melanoma cells. *Exp. Cell Res.*, **312**, 2214–2230.
132. Moffatt, S., Wiehle, S., and Cristiano, R.J. (2005) Tumor-specific gene delivery mediated by a novel peptide–polyethylenimine–DNA polyplex targeting aminopeptidase N/CD13. *Hum. Gene Ther.*, **16**, 57–67.
133. Inagaki, Y. et al. (2010) Novel aminopeptidase N (APN/CD13) inhibitor 24F can suppress invasion of hepatocellular carcinoma cells as well as angiogenesis. *Biosci. Trends*, **4**, 56–60.
134. Blaheta, R.A. et al. (2009) Tumor–endothelium cross talk blocks recruitment of neutrophils to endothelial cells: a novel mechanism of endothelial cell anergy. *Neoplasia*, **11**, 1054–1063.
135. Jiang, G. et al. (2008) Hyaluronic acid–polyethyleneimine conjugate for target specific intracellular delivery of siRNA. *Biopolymers*, **89**, 635–642.
136. Mun, G.I. and Boo, Y.C. (2010) Identification of CD44 as a senescence-induced cell adhesion gene responsible for the enhanced monocyte recruitment to senescent endothelial cells. *Am. J. Physiol.*, **298**, H2102–H2111.
137. Banquy, X. et al. (2008) Selectins ligand decorated drug carriers for activated endothelial cell targeting. *Bioconjug. Chem.*, **19**, 2030–2039.

21
Drug Conjugates with Poly(Ethylene Glycol)
Hong Zhao, Lee M. Greenberger, and Ivan D. Horak

21.1
Introduction

Many drug candidates, as well as marketed drug products, suffer from deficiencies in pharmaceutical properties including poor solubility, toxic side-effects, poor pharmacokinetics profile, immunogenicity, and antigenicity. In an attempt to overcome these problems, a variety of drug delivery methodologies have been explored and developed. Particularly notable among these delivery approaches is PEGylation, the chemical conjugation of a poly(ethylene glycol) (PEG) to the drug molecule [1–7]. More than 30 years ago, in the laboratories of Professor Frank Davis at Rutgers University, PEGylation was found to increase circulation half-life ($t_{1/2}$) and reduce immunogenicity of various enzymes while still preserving activity [8]. These effects are mediated by protection of the PEG–enzyme species from proteolytic degradation, reduction of renal elimination, and interaction with antibody that can further reduce $t_{1/2}$ and activity. Consequently, PEGylation has become a validated approach to improve enzyme performance. The technology has been applied to market products that improve the pharmaceutical properties of ligands, antibodies, and aptamers. New releasable PEGylation technology can also improve the solubility and efficacy of small molecules (i.e., molecular weight under 1000 Da). In addition, PEG can help prolong the circulation half-life of nanoparticles including liposomes and other particles by shielding the surface of these formulations.

21.2
Rationale for PEGylation and PEG-Drug Conjugates

There are many reasons why PEG has become one of the chosen methodologies for drug conjugates.

- PEG is an amphiphilic polymer that has been used both as a formulation excipient and as a drug conjugate. As an amphiphilic compound, PEG has the

Drug Delivery in Oncology: From Basic Research to Cancer Therapy, First Edition.
Edited by Felix Kratz, Peter Senter, and Henning Steinhagen.
© 2012 Wiley-VCH Verlag GmbH & Co. KGaA. Published 2012 by Wiley-VCH Verlag GmbH & Co. KGaA.

ability to solubilize compounds that have inherently poor aqueous solubility and, at the same time, be amenable to various chemistries that require dissolution in organic solvents.
- PEG has a very favorable toxicity profile that has allowed it to be safely used even long term (years) in humans. It is well tolerated at high doses after chronic or acute administration. The metabolism of PEG itself is simple and primarily involves the oxidation of alcohol groups on the PEG to carboxylic groups [9–11]. Renal and bile excretion are the two major elimination routes for PEG, with the size of the PEG largely determining the elimination route.
- The PEG polymer can be modified synthetically and therefore easily adapted to optimize biological features. Important variables for PEG conjugates are morphology, linker stability, site of PEGylation, loading, and size of PEG. PEG itself is a linear polymer comprised of ethylene glycol repeating units with hydroxyl functional groups at the distal ends. Variations and modifications of the linear polymer can be made. The linear polymer commonly includes capping one end with a methyl group forming methoxy PEG (methoxy poly(ethylene glycol or mPEG-OH), which allows chemical derivatization of the free hydroxyl group. Further synthetic chemistry can be applied to produce different geometries including U-shaped (branched) PEG [11] and multiarm PEG that can alter PEG loading onto the drug product [12].
- Chemical modification of functional groups linking the drug to PEG allows greater flexibility. PEG conjugates can have either very stable bonds ("permanent" linkages) or relatively labile bonds ("releasable" linkages) depending on the requirements for the drug. This feature is often coupled with altered PEG morphology. For example, a branched PEG often is used for conjugation to proteins via a permanent linkage to prolong circulation time while preserving activity of the conjugated drug. In this case, care must be taken to avoid masking the active region of the protein so that adequate drug activity remains in the PEGylated compound and hence site-specific PEGylation techniques may be necessary. In contrast, a multiarm PEG is common in small-molecule delivery systems, where multiple cytotoxic compounds might be linked to a single PEG molecule through various linking chemistries, providing different release characteristics [3, 7]. In the case of such small molecules, a permanent linkage would likely obliterate drug activity; therefore, releasable linkers are necessary and the release rate can be altered by changing linker chemistry to optimize pharmacokinetic properties.

The PEG backbone is extensively hydrogenated in aqueous solution. The radius of the hydrogenated PEG molecule could be as large as 5–10 times the actual size of the polymer. This effect may potentially provide a layer of shield when conjugated with drug molecules and minimize renal permeability (Figure 21.1) [13, 14].

The size of the PEG conjugate is of critical importance in determining $t_{1/2}$ of drugs (see Figure 21.2) [14]. This is most easily demonstrated by altering the length of PEG since the effective size of a PEGylated compound is much larger than that of a highly folded protein for any given molecular weight. The circulation $t_{1/2}$ of PEG

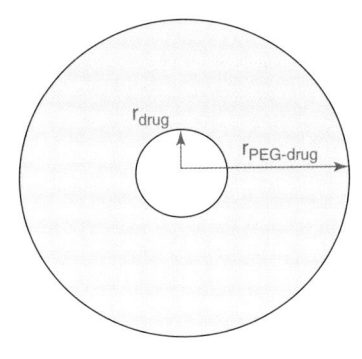

Figure 21.1 Hydrodynamic radius (r) of a PEGylated drug is dependent on PEG mass and will markedly exceed that of the unmodified drug molecule such as protein.

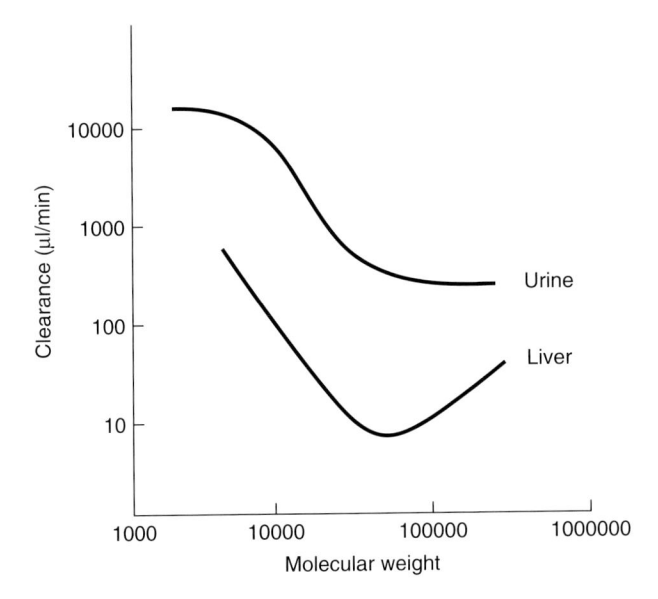

Figure 21.2 Effect of molecular weight of PEG on renal and hepatic clearance.

polymers in mice has been shown to increase as the size of the PEG increases, up to a point at which any further size increase has no effect (Figure 21.3) [15]. The effect demonstrated in this curve is largely due to exclusion of high-molecular-weight (high molecular weightHMW) compounds from sieving through the glomerulus and the subsequent urinary excretion. However, the $t_{1/2}$ can be enhanced by a very long single PEG or by adding a large number of short PEGs.

The current chapter will demonstrate how these principles of PEG have been applied principally in the oncology field.

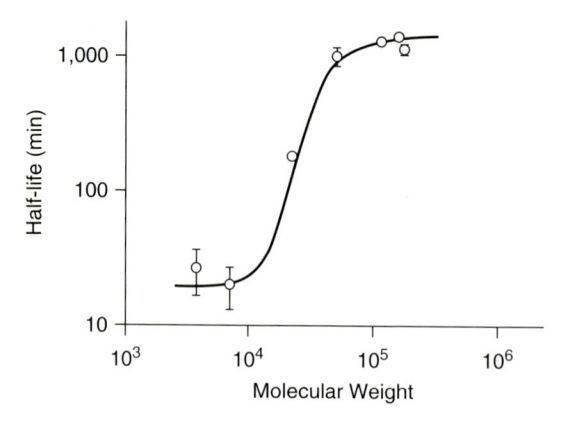

Figure 21.3 Relationship between molecular weight of PEG polymer and half-life of circulation in mice.

21.3
Permanent PEGylation

Permanent PEGylated conjugates have been used in many US Food and Drug Administration (FDA)-approved PEG drugs. The method is well suited to use with enzymes or ligands, where activity of the parent molecule is sufficiently retained in the conjugated form.

21.3.1
First-Generation PEG Linker: SS-PEG

A first-generation PEG linker is mPEG-OH succinimidyl succinate (SS-PEG) and is reviewed elsewhere [8, 16]. During drug conjugation, SS-PEG reacts with the nucleophilic groups (e.g., amino groups) of the drug molecules to form stable amide bonds (Scheme 21.1). Since protein molecules generally have multiple free amino groups, many of which located on the surface of the protein and hence readily available for conjugation, multiple SS-PEG strands can be conjugated to one protein molecule. This type of PEGylation approach is referred to as global PEGylation or random PEGylation.

Scheme 21.1 Conjugation of SS-PEG with protein.

PEGylation of adenosine deaminase (ADA) and L-asparaginase (L-ASNase) with 5-kDa SS-PEG has led to two FDA-approved products: Adagen® (pegadamase bovine) and Oncaspar® (pegaspargase), respectively. Adagen is used as an enzyme-replacement therapy for ADA deficiency in patients with severe combined immunodeficiency [17]. Oncaspar is used as a component of a multiagent chemotherapeutic regimen for the treatment of patients with acute lymphoblastic leukemia (ALL) [18, 19]. Approximately 22 of the 33 free amino groups (N-terminus and lysine side-chains) are PEGylated in Oncaspar to give the final PEGylated protein with a molecular weight of approximately 245 kDa. The PEG conjugate has reserved a little bit over 50% of the original enzyme activity. As described below, the PEGylation of L-ASNase offers many advantages compared with unPEGylated L-ASNase formulations.

Asparagine (ASN) is critical to the survival of leukemic cells, which, due to their low level of ASN synthetase, are unable to perform sufficient *de novo* ASN synthesis [20–22]. L-ASNase depletes plasma ASN by converting it to L-aspartate. Thus, leukemic cells cannot derive sufficient extracellular L-ASNase and ultimately die due to the inhibition of protein synthesis. Some of the advantages of Oncaspar compared to the unPEGylated ASNase are that clinical hypersensitivity (up to 75%), acute allergic reactions, and high rates of immunogenicity compared with native ASNase are minimized [23–29]. In addition, anti-ASNase antibodies can neutralize its enzymatic activity and because of the short $t_{1/2}$ and rapid clearance of unPEGylated ASNase, there is a need for frequent administration [24, 30, 31]. In particular, pharmacokinetics studies have shown that pegaspargase has a serum $t_{1/2}$ of 5.73 ± 3.24 days ($n = 10$) in humans, which is considerably longer than that of unPEGylated L-ASNase (1.28 ± 0.35 days ($n = 9$)) [20]. The significantly longer $t_{1/2}$ of pegaspargase allows for 26–34 days of ASN depletion for pegaspargase versus 14–23 days for unPEGylated L-ASNase [20].

Consistent with the enhanced pharmacokinetics with Oncaspar, a single administration of pegaspargase during the induction period has been shown to be as efficacious as nine doses of the unPEGylated enzyme [32]. Beyond this, Oncaspar has induced a more rapid lymphoblast clearance from bone marrow by pegaspargase at days 7 and 14 versus L-ASNase, and 3-year event-free survival after Oncaspar was 85 versus 78% with L-ASNase. SS-PEG has also been widely used in the research and development of many other protein–drug conjugates [33, 34].

21.3.2
Second-Generation PEG Linkers

21.3.2.1 SC-PEG
While SS-PEG conjugates continue to be useful in the clinic, the ester bond in the succinimidyl spacer can be hydrolyzed when the conjugate is stored under standard drug storage conditions, thereby reducing the pegylation of the parent molecule and increasing the free enzyme in the product overtime.

To overcome this problem, another stable PEG linker, mPEG-OH succinimidyl carbonate (SC-PEG) [35], was developed. Similar to SS-PEG, SC-PEG will react

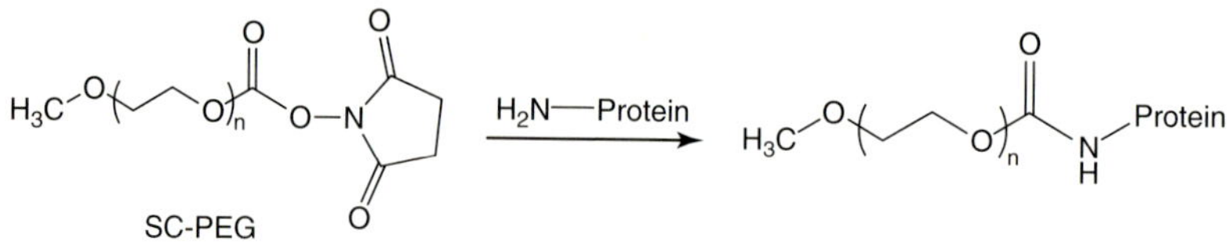

Scheme 21.2 Conjugation of SC-PEG with protein.

preferentially with the amino groups of drug molecules (Scheme 21.2) provided the pH is high enough (in the range of 8–9) so that lysines are adequately deprotonated and consequently become nucleophilic. This is a very simple and straightforward chemistry; only a stable carbamate bond is formed between the PEG polymer and the drug molecule (Scheme 21.2). At a lower pH, reactivity at other amino acids containing nucleophilic groups can become significant sites of reactivity. The utility of Oncaspar versus SC-PEG–ASNase is currently being evaluated in clinical trials.

One successful application of the SC-PEG linker is the development of the marketed drug PegIntron® (peginterferon-α2b), a 12-kDa mono-PEGylated interferon (IFN-α2b) conjugate with a molecular weight about 31.3 kDa [36]. IFN proteins are naturally occurring cytokines that have a broad spectrum of antiviral, antitumor, and immunomodulatory properties [37–39]. In 1986, the FDA approved Intron A® (IFN-α2b) – the first approved recombinant IFN-α, for the treatment of hairy cell leukemia [40].

Although there are numerous reactive groups within IFN-α2b that could be conjugated with SC-PEG, the pH of the conjugation reaction was sufficiently low (pH 6.5) such that approximately 95% of peginterferon-α2b was present as the mono-PEGylated form, with PEG-derivatized His34 and Cys1 comprising 48 and 13%, respectively, and lower amounts of positional isomers PEGylated predominantly on various lysine residues [41]. Although peginterferon-α2b retained about 28% of the original activity of IFN-α2b, the *in vivo* activity of the molecule is equivalent to that of the unPEGylated IFN-α2b [42].

Beyond this, the serum $t_{1/2}$ of peginterferon-α2b was approximately 40 h, or 10-fold longer than that of IFN-α-2b [43], and clinically significant levels persisted for the entire week after a single administration. Peginterferon-α2b has also been evaluated in several clinical studies of patients with glioblastoma multiforme (GBM) and other solid tumors. Some clinical benefit of peginterferon-α2b has been observed in GBM when given with temozolomide [44].

21.3.2.2 PEG-Aldehyde

The PEG-aldehyde linker is a widely used site-specific PEG linker. When PEG-aldehyde reacts with a protein or a polypeptide under acidic pH conditions, it selectively reacts with the N-terminal amino group to form the imine bond, which is reduced *in situ* by sodium cyanoborohydride to a stable amine bond (Scheme 21.3). The ability for PEG-aldehyde to specifically react with the N-terminal amino group is based on the pK_a value difference of the α-amino group of the N-terminal amino acid (7.6–8.0) [45] and the ε-amino groups of

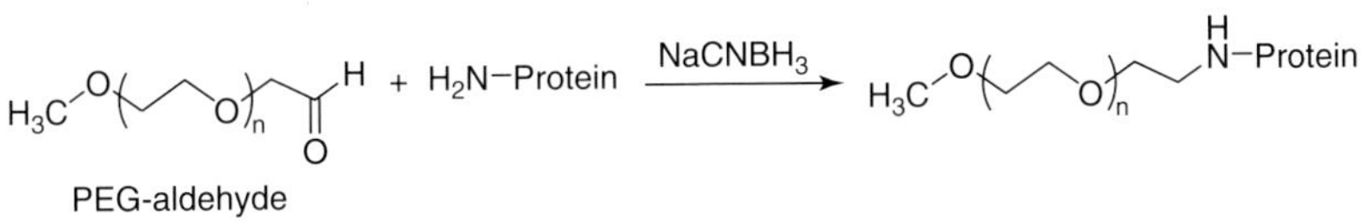

$H_3C-O-(-CH_2-CH_2-O-)_n-CH_2-CHO$ + H_2N-Protein $\xrightarrow{\text{NaCNBH}_3}$ $H_3C-O-(-CH_2-CH_2-O-)_n-CH_2-CH_2-NH$-Protein

PEG-aldehyde

Scheme 21.3 Reductive alkylation of protein by PEG-aldehyde.

the lysine residues (10.0–10.2) [46] in the polypeptide backbone. The advantage of this site-selective PEGylation is that conjugation at the protein N-terminus will minimize undesirable PEG interference with other, potentially biologically important, amino acid residues in the protein.

PEG-aldehyde has been successfully used to conjugate with the N-terminal amino group of granulocyte colony-stimulating factor (G-CSF) – a protein used to treat neutropenia in patients with cancer [46]. G-CSF is a naturally occurring myeloid growth factor that stimulates the growth and differentiation of neutrophils. Filgrastim (Neupogen®) is a human recombinant form of G-CSF [46–49]. Filgrastim was shown to be effective in reducing the incidence of infections as a result of febrile neutropenia in patients with neomyeloid malignancies receiving myeosuppressive chemotherapy. It also improved adherence to the dose and schedule of chemotherapy [47–51]. However, the rapid renal elimination of filgrastim and short $t_{1/2}$ (approximately 3.5 h) necessitated daily injections until neutrophil recovery, which is undesirable in patients with cancer [50].

Pegfilgrastim (Neulasta®) is prepared by reductive alkylation of the G-CSF protein and consists of a 20-kDa linear PEG molecule covalently linked to the N-terminal methionine residue of filgrastim to give a final conjugate with a molecular weight of approximately 39 kDa [52]. Since the functional molecular size of pegfilgrastim is more than twice the molecular weight of the parental molecule (18.8 kDa), renal elimination is minimized and serum $t_{1/2}$ (approximately 15–80 h) of pegfilgrastim is 4- to 23-fold greater than that of filgrastim. Clinically, the improved pharmacokinetic and pharmacodynamic properties of pegfilgrastim relative to the non-PEGylated molecule allow for its administration once per chemotherapy cycle without compromising its biological effect [53, 54].

Pegfilgrastim has also demonstrated a favorable safety profile in clinical trials involving patients with breast cancer, lung cancer, and lymphoma (including non-Hodgkin's) [55–61]. It has been demonstrated that a single injection of pegfilgrastim given once per chemotherapy cycle had similar efficacy and safety to that provided by an average of 11 daily injections of filgrastim [56, 58, 59, 62, 63].

21.3.2.3 U-PEG

PEGylation of proteins with linear-strand PEG linkers has greatly improved the pharmaceutical properties of different drugs. However, PEGylation generally will reduce protein activities, even though the lost activity can be compensated for by prolonged presence of the protein conjugate in the circulation. To minimize the potential loss of protein activity, new PEG linkers with a different geometry have been invented. The U-shaped PEG linkers (U-PEG) [13] can provide more surface

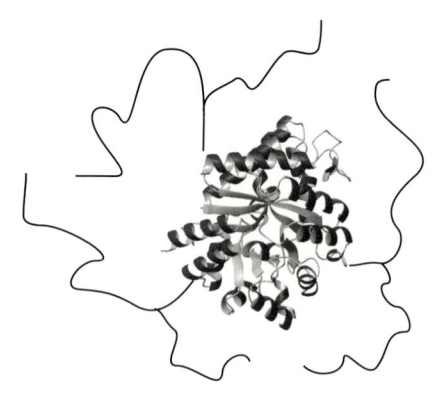

Figure 21.4 PEGylation with U-PEG linker.

coverage of parental drug per PEG attachment (Figure 21.4). As such, U-PEG can provide equivalent shielding effects with a lesser extent of modification of the parental drug molecule.

U-PEG can be prepared by first reacting mPEG-OH with a properly protected trifunctional linker such as lysine ethyl ester, followed by deprotection and activation of the acid group (Scheme 21.4a). U-PEGs will react with the amino groups of protein molecules to form a stable amide bond (Scheme 21.4b). U-PEGs have successfully improved the pharmaceutical properties of various types of drug molecules including cytokines (e.g., IFN-α) [64], oligonucleotides (e.g., anti-vascular endothelial growth factor (VEGF)) [65], and antibody fragments (e.g., anti-tumor necrosis factor (TNF)) [66].

21.3.2.3.1 Peginterferon-α2a Peginterferon-α2a (Pegasys®) is indicated for the treatment of adults with chronic hepatitis C who have compensated liver disease and have not been previously treated with IFN-α [64]. To prepare peginterferon-α2a, 40-kDa U-PEG-Lys-NHS is reacted with IFN-α2a under slightly basic pH. After purification, peginterferon-α2a is composed mainly of the mono-PEGylated species with a molecular weight of about 60 kDa. Like peginterferon-α2b, peginterferon-α2a has significantly improved the pharmacokinetic and PD properties of the cytokine protein, and, when given together with antiviral drug ribivarin, has achieved clinical benefits for patients with hepatitis C. The combination of peginterferon-α2a and ribivarin is currently considered the standard therapy for patients with hepatitis C and this combination is the backbone for the development of novel targeted therapies for hepatitis C [67, 68]. Peginterferon-α2a has been evaluated and continues evaluation in multiple clinical trials to treat various types of cancers including intermediate- and high-risk melanoma and chronic-phase chronic myeloid leukemia (CML) (http://clinicaltrials.gov/ct2/show/NCT00573378).

21.3.2.3.2 PEGylated Antibody Fragments Antibodies and antibody fragments have become successful therapeutic modalities in recent years, as evidenced by

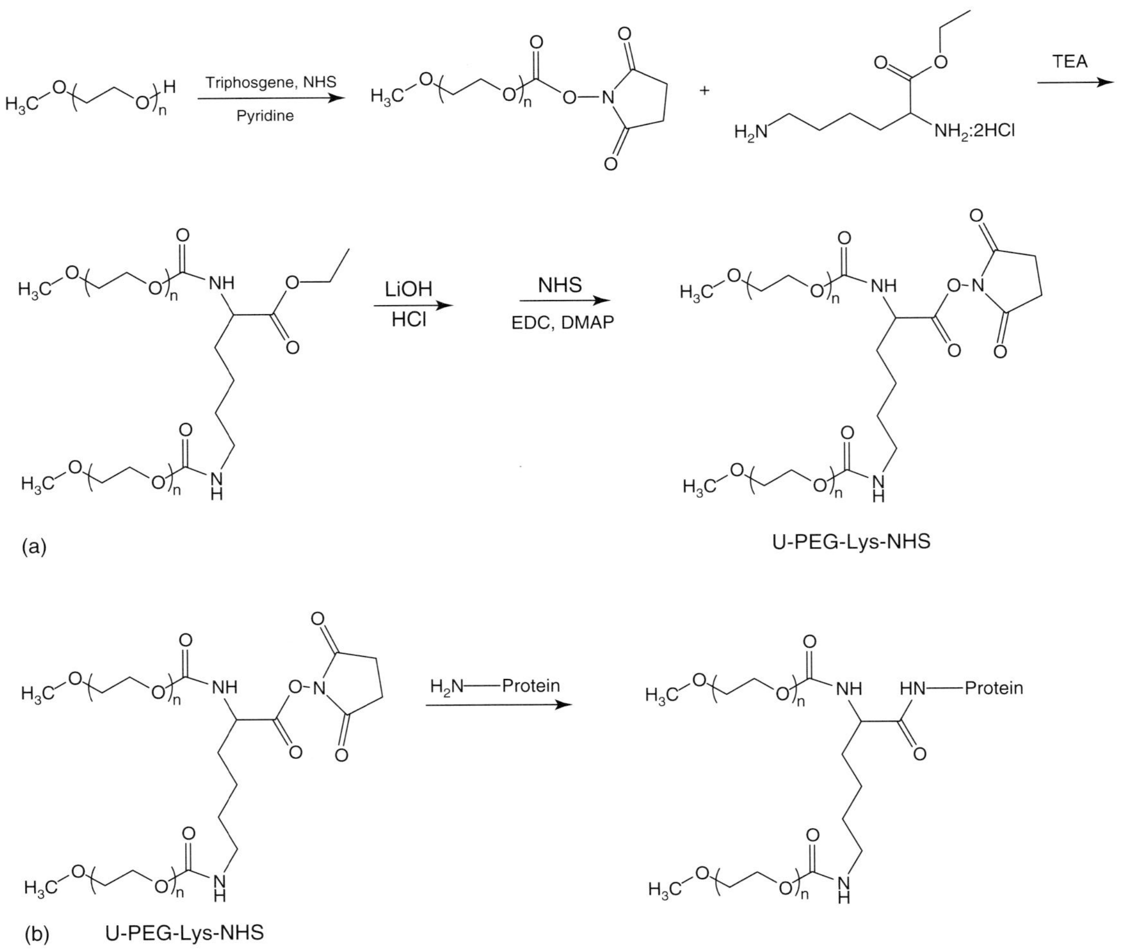

Scheme 21.4 (a) Preparation of activated U-PEG; (b) Conjugation of U-PEG with protein

multiple FDA-approved antibody-based drugs [69]. Antibody fragments including Fab', single-chain antibody, and so on have binding affinity and therapeutic potential comparable to that of a full-length antibody, yet the reduced size enables them to more rapidly penetrate in body tissues such as tumors [70]. However, due to the much smaller size of the antibody fragments, they tend to have relatively shorter circulation half-lives *in vivo*, which may hamper their therapeutic efficacies [70]. PEGylation provides an ideal solution to overcome this challenge and improve the pharmacokinetics of antibody fragments. The effect of the number of PEG strands and size of the PEG polymer on the circulation $t_{1/2}$ of antibody fragments in rats and monkeys has been systemically studied [70]. It was found that both Fab' and chemically cross-linked diFab' were cleared very rapidly from the circulation, whereas a 40-kDa PEG-conjugated Fab' persisted to an extent similar to the IgG control (Figure 21.5) [70]. It is worthwhile to point out that despite its molecular weight of approximately 95 kDa, which exceeds the glomerular filtration limit, the chemically cross-linked diFab' used in the study still had a relatively short $t_{1/2}$. Apparently, elimination via nonrenal mechanisms is substantial.

The utility of PEGylation for antibody fragments is demonstrated by the FDA approvals of certolizumab (Cimzia®) for Crohn's disease (2008) and rheumatoid arthritis (2009) [66, 71, 72]. TNF-α is a proinflammatory cytokine. Certolizumab is a PEGylated humanized anti-TNF-α Fab' fragment using the 40-kDa U-PEG-Lys-maleimide linker that site-specifically conjugates through the cysteine residue engineered at a nonbinding site of the antibody fragment with a molecular

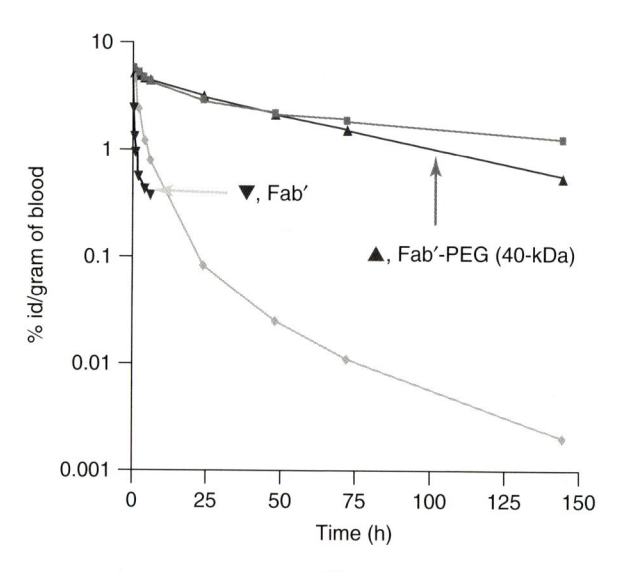

Figure 21.5 Pharmacokinetics of ^{125}I-labeled conjugates in rats: comparison of IgG (■), Fab' (▼), diFab' (♦), and site-specifically attached PEG–Fab' (▲).

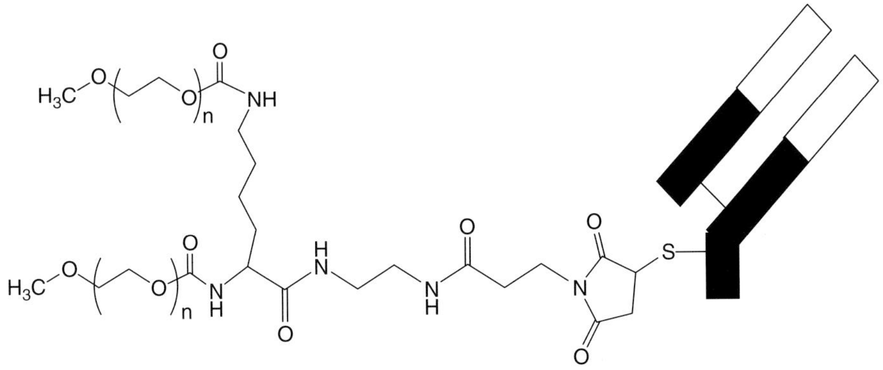

Figure 21.6 U-PEG-Lys-maleimide-Fab'.

weight of about 91 kDa [72]. PEGylation has successfully prolonged the circulating $t_{1/2}$ of Fab' to approximately 14 days in humans from hours [72, 73]. As a result, certolizumab can be administered every 2–4 weeks subcutaneously to patients in whom good efficacy and favorable toxicity profiles have been demonstrated [67].

The U-PEG technology has been used to PEGylate an antibody fragment VEGF that binds to VEGF receptor 2 (vascular endothelial growth factor receptorVEGFR2) that is involved in the formation of new blood vessels in tumors (angiogenesis), allowing cancer cells to receive nutrients for growth. To improve the pharmacokinetics of this antibody fragment, a 40-kDa U-PEG-maleimide linker also was used to site-selectively conjugate with the cysteine presented at the cross-linker, which covalently connects the two Fab' molecules (CDP791) to render a PEG conjugate with a molecular weight of approximately 140 kDa (Figure 21.6) [74].

PEGylation significantly improved the pharmacokinetic profile of VEGFR2 Fab' fragments alone [74]. When CDP791 was administered at doses of 10 mg/kg or higher, the plasma level of the conjugate remained biologically relevant for at least 3 weeks. No dose-limiting toxicity (DLT) was observed, and the conjugate was well tolerated. Initial phase II trials suggest that CDP791 in combination with chemotherapy increased response rate of overall survival (but not progression-free survival (PFS)) in patients with small-cell lung cancer compared to chemotherapy alone.

21.3.2.4 Other Permanent Linkers

Other permanent PEG linker chemistries have been used for site-specific conjugation to minimize the negative impact on the efficacy of drug molecules. Three distinct chemistries bind to thiol [75, 76] or disulfides [77]. Site-specific, permanent PEGylation to the side-chain of arginine of proteins has been achieved [78]. In addition, site-specific conjugation to glutamines by enzymatic PEGylation using a microbial transglutaminase has recently been described [79].

21.4
Releasable PEGylation

While permanent PEGylation has achieved great success in the delivery of antibodies, enzymes, and cytokines, this approach has certain limitations. In many cases, drug molecules will lose most or all of their biological activities after permanent PEGylation because PEG may hinder the drug from binding to its receptor. If the binding affinity is not totally lost, the PEG–drug conjugate may still have superior *in vivo* biological activity because of the prolonged presence of the drug in the circulation compared to the native drug. In the cases where the drug lost all its biological activity after PEGylation, releasable (or reversible) PEGylation may provide a practical solution. The releasable linker may allow the drug to reach full activity after being released from the PEG polymer. This technology is versatile since several types of releasable PEG have been described [3, 7]. Consequently, the benefit of PEGylation may now be extended to small molecules, peptides, and other drug molecules that were not previously considered candidates for polymeric delivery.

For a releasable PEG conjugate, the stability of the drug conjugate linkage and its potential for predetermined degradation is an important consideration in determining the effectiveness of the prodrug. For example, rapid breakdown of the prodrug can lead to spiking of the parent drug and possible toxicity, while a slow release rate will compromise the drug's efficacy. In addition, consideration of the site of release may be important, since release in the plasma or other site (i.e., tumor) may achieve optimal efficacy. At the target site, the active principal should preferably be released by a specific, enzymatic mechanism. The rate and site of release for a particular PEG conjugate cannot be fully predicted at this time and therefore an empirical approach using preclinical models is needed to optimize the conjugate.

21.4.1
Releasable PEG Linkers Based on Ester Linkage

The most-often employed prodrugs generally are based on hydrolyzable or enzymatically cleavable bonds such as esters, carbonates, aryl carbamates, and hydrazones, among which esters are the most ubiquitous in the literature, no doubt since they are often the easiest to synthesize. Prodrugs of this sort can be designed from either an alcohol with an acid parent drug or an alcohol parent drug with an acid. The rate of breakdown of the ester typically is more easily controlled for an alcohol drug by modification of the associated acid structure.

21.4.1.1 PEG–Paclitaxel

Paclitaxel (Taxol®) is a small molecule that is used to treat a variety of cancers. It binds to and inhibits the function of tubulin, leading to inhibition of cell division. Although the molecule has very poor water solubility, this is overcome by systemic administration of paclitaxel in Cremophor® along with steroids to reduce hypersensitivity reactions to the formulation [80]. Esterification of paclitaxel (containing a secondary alcohol that is required for activity) with a PEG acid directly or through the amino acid glycine yielded highly water-soluble 2′-PEG esters of paclitaxel [7, 81, 82]. The polymer conjugates were shown to function as prodrugs (i.e., breakdown occurred in a predictable fashion *in vitro*). Cell tissue culture employing P338/0 and L1210 murine leukemia cells gave IC_{50} values that were comparable to those of paclitaxel (Table 21.1) [7].

The *in vivo* efficacy of the conjugate was superior to paclitaxel in the P388 mouse leukemia model (Table 21.1) and was active in a variety of solid tumor models (Table 21.2). The molecular weight of the PEG dramatically influences the efficacy. For example, while 40 000-Da PEG–Gly–paclitaxel increased the ILS to 82%, no efficacy was seen when the paclitaxel was conjugated to a 5000-Da PEG. This was presumably due to the rapidly elimination of the conjugate by the kidneys and not due to the lack of release of the conjugate since this conjugate had equivalent activity compared to paclitaxel *in vitro* where no such elimination is possible. This example clearly illustrates the necessity for *in vivo* testing to verify *in vitro* cytotoxicity results.

The basis for the improved efficacy of the HMW PEG–paclitaxel prodrug conjugates is likely to be due to two mechanisms. (i) The HMW of the polymer and the relatively slower rate of cleavage of the ester bond provides an *in vitro* $t_{1/2}$ of the released paclitaxel of 0.5–1 h in rat plasma. This probably allows several circulatory passages to be completed *in vivo*, thereby altering the biodistribution of paclitaxel. (ii) The HMW polymer–drug conjugate is expected to selectively accumulate in the tumor. This accumulation, known as the enhanced permeability and retention (EPR) effect, or passive tumor targeting [83–85], may occur for HMW polymer conjugate therapeutics. The EPR effect is achieved because blood vessels are leaky and lymphatic drainage is slow in tumor, which allows HMW molecules to accumulate within the tumor. In addition, the reduced toxicity exhibited by these conjugates probably results from a more controlled ester bond hydrolysis, possibly from an altered biodistribution, compared with the nonattenuated release of unconjugated paclitaxel. The two properties, passive targeting and continuous release from a depot of the polymeric prodrug, provide what has been termed double targeting [86] and is thought to produce enhanced efficacy.

PEG–Gly–paclitaxel entered phase I clinical trials to determine the safety, tolerability, and pharmacology in patients with advanced solid tumors and lymphomas [87]. As with paclitaxel, neutropenia was the predominant hematological toxicity observed following administration of PEG–Gly–paclitaxel. Other side-effects of PEG–Gly–paclitaxel administration consisted of peripheral neuropathy, vomiting, and diarrhea. Preliminary pharmacokinetic monitoring following administration of PEG–Gly–paclitaxel demonstrated detectable levels (above 5 ng/ml) of free paclitaxel still present after 48 h.

Recently, another PEG–taxane conjugate, NKTR-105, was reported using releasable chemistry that would allow slow release of docetaxel. NKTR-105 is a PEGylated docetaxel conjugate with a glycine linker that has shown good preclinical activity in colon and lung cancer xenograft models [88]. This conjugate has

Table 21.1 In vitro[a] and in vivo results of PEG–paclitaxel derivatives.

Compound	IC$_{50}$ (nM) P388/0	$t_{1/2}$ (h)[b]		P388 in vivo[c]			% ILS[e]	P values versus control	P values versus paclitaxel
		Phosphate-buffered saline, pH 7.4	Rat plasma	Total dose (mg/kg)	Mean time to death (days)[d] (cures/group)				
Control	–	–	–	–	13.2 ± 1.2 (0/10)		–	–	–
Paclitaxel	6	–	–	75	17.5 ± 1.7 (0/10)		33	0.0151	–
	–	–	–	100	13.7 ± 1.3 (0/10)		4	0.7714	–
PEG⏞O⏞O-2'-PCT PEG MW 40000	10	5.5	0.4	75	19.0 ± 1.1 (0/10)		44	0.0013	0.3850[f]
mPEG⏞O⏞O-2'-PCT mPEG MW 5000	15	5.5	0.5	75	14.1 ± 2.3 (0/10)		13	0.06	<0.0001
PEG⏞O⏞N(H)⏞O-2'-PCT PEG MW 40000	14	7.0	0.4	75	21.8 ± 1.0 (0/10)		65	0.0001	0.0151[f]
	–	–	–	100	24.0 ± 8.9 (1/10)		82	<0.0001	<0.0001[g]

[a] All experiments were performed in duplicate: standard deviation of measurements = ±10%.
[b] These results more appropriately represent the half-lives of disappearance of the transport form.
[c] In vivo efficacy study of the water-soluble paclitaxel derivatives using the P388/0 murine leukemia model. Paclitaxel or prodrug derivatives were given, in equivalent doses of paclitaxel, daily (intraperitoneal × 5), 24 h following an injection of P388/0 cells into the abdominal cavity with survival monitored for 40 days.
[d] Kaplan–Meier estimates with survivors censored.
[e] Increased lifespan (% ILS) is (T/C − 1) × 100.
[f] Paclitaxel at 75 mg/kg.
[g] Paclitaxel at 100 mg/kg.

Table 21.2 Antitumor activity of PEG–Gly–paclitaxel against subcutaneous human tumor xenografts in nude mice.

Tumor type	Treatment schedule[a]	Total dose (mg/kg)[b]	% T/C[c]
HT-29 (colon)	3 cycles of daily × 5 at intervals of 14 days, intraperitoneal	225	11.3[d]
A549 (lung)	daily × 5 for 2 weeks, intraperitoneal	150	9.5[d]
SKOV-3 (ovarian)	weekly × 2 for 4 weeks, intravenous	200	8.1[d]

[a]Treatments initiated when tumor volumes reached around 100 mm^3.
[b]Based on paclitaxel content.
[c]Treatment and control groups were measured when the control group's median tumor volume reached around 800–1100 mm^3.
[d]$p < 0.01$.

entered phase I clinical studies enrolling approximately 30 patients with refractory solid tumors who failed all prior available therapies.

21.4.1.2 PEG–Camptothecin Analogs

Camptothecins (CPTs) are natural products that potently inhibit topoisomerase I [89]. Due to the poor solubility of the parent compound, two water-soluble analogs were developed. Topotecan is approved for second-line chemotherapy for ovarian and small cell lung cancers, while CPT-11 (irinotecan) is used to treat colon cancers [90]. Upon release of the water-solubilizing group from CPT-11, SN-38 is formed. SN-38 is approximately 100-fold more potent than CPT-11 and is believed to be the active ingredient in CPT-11. However, the amount of SN-38 released from CPT-11 is 3–4% [91, 92] and therefore this may blunt the antitumor activity of CPT-11.

PEGylation of CPT, CPT-11, or SN-38 has been used to overcome solubility and potency issues of this class of chemotherapeutic agents. PEGylation with a 40-kDa PEG linker improved the solubility of CPT and SN-38 by 80- and 1000-fold, respectively. PEG–CPT conjugates have been shown to hydrolyze *in vivo* and gradually release unPEGylated CPT [93]. Fortuitously, it was found that modifying CPT and SN-38 at the 20-OH position as a PEG ester additionally stabilizes the active lactone ring (essential for activity) under physiological conditions [94]. Stabilization by acylation of the 20-OH group of CPT has been shown to be due to a low degree of intramolecular hydrogen bonding [94, 95]. The introduction of various spacer groups between the PEG-solubilizing portion of the molecule and the CPT alcohol again led to significant differences in biological activity [96], as observed for paclitaxel.

Both PEG–Ala–camptothecin (Pegamotecan®) and PEG–SN-38 (EZN-2208) had excellent antitumor activity in preclinical models. In particular, PEG–SN-38 had superior antitumor activity compared to CPT-11 in all tested human solid and hematological xenograft tumor models investigated to date [97–99]. Pegamotecan was examined in phase I and II studies [100–102]. The drug was given as a 1-h infusion once every 3 weeks. Maximal concentrations of free CPT in plasma were observed about 24 h after infusion, reflecting the interplay between the release of CPT from the PEG conjugate, clearance of the conjugate, and clearance of the released CPT. A phase II study with 7000 mg/m^2 PEG–CPT (equivalent to 120 mg/m^2 of CPT) in 37 patients with advanced and metastatic adenocarcinomas of the stomach and gastroesophageal junction demonstrated that five patients (14%) had a partial response. An additional 14 patients (40%) had stable disease [102].

Although this data was interesting, a more active conjugate, EZN-2208, has been pursued further. To do so, a new PEGylation technology has been used to link the multiarm PEG to four SN-38 molecules through different amino acid linkers [12]. The lead compound (EZN-2208) was obtained by coupling a four-arm PEG (40 kDa) with SN-38, through a glycine spacer. The coupling strategy was developed to selectively link the 20-OH group of SN-38, thus preserving the E-ring of SN-38 in the active lactone form (similar to Pegamotecan), while leaving the drug 10-OH group free (Scheme 21.5).

EZN-2208 showed an increase in drug loading, reaching a value of 3.7 wt% or higher compared with 1.7 wt% for Pegamotecan [12]. The conjugate acts as a prodrug with a half-life of SN-38 release in human plasma of 12.3 min [12]. It was found that irinotecan had a very rapid clearance from circulation compared with EZN-2208 (Figure 21.7a). Accordingly, SN-38 released from irinotecan was cleared from the circulation much faster compared with EZN-2208. The longer circulation half-life of EZN-2208 resulted in high exposure of both EZN-2208 and released SN-38. In tumors, exposure of EZN-2208 was 468-fold higher than that of irinotecan (Figure 21.7). This resulted in 207-fold higher exposure to free SN-38 when injected as EZN-2208 compared with irinotecan [97]. This passive accumulation of HMW EZN-2208 conjugate in solid tumors was attributed to the EPR effect [83–85].

EZN-2208 has demonstrated promising antitumor activity *in vivo* with activity superior to that observed with CPT-11 and frequently associated with cures in animal models [97–99]. Curative activity has been found in models of breast cancer, hematological malignancies, and neuroblastoma. Beyond this, mice harboring CPT-11-resistant human colorectal tumors that progressed through multiple doses of CPT-11 showed tumor regression when treated with EZN-2208 (Figure 21.8) [97–99]. Although the basis for superior activity with EZN-2208 is incompletely understood, sustained delivery of SN-38 within the tumor was associated with suppression of hypoxia inducible factor (HIF)-1α as well as inhibition of angiogenesis [99, 103], known to be controlled by HIF-1α [104]. Thus, prolonged exposure to SN-38 by administration of PEG-SN-38 accentuates the antiangiogenic effects that have been previously observed with other topoisomerase I inhibitors [105].

EZN-2208 was evaluated in two phase I studies with different administration schedules. In the first study [106], EZN-2208 was administered as a 1-h intravenous infusion once every 3 weeks, with or without G-CSF. In the second study, EZN-2208 was administered for 3 weeks of every 4-week treatment

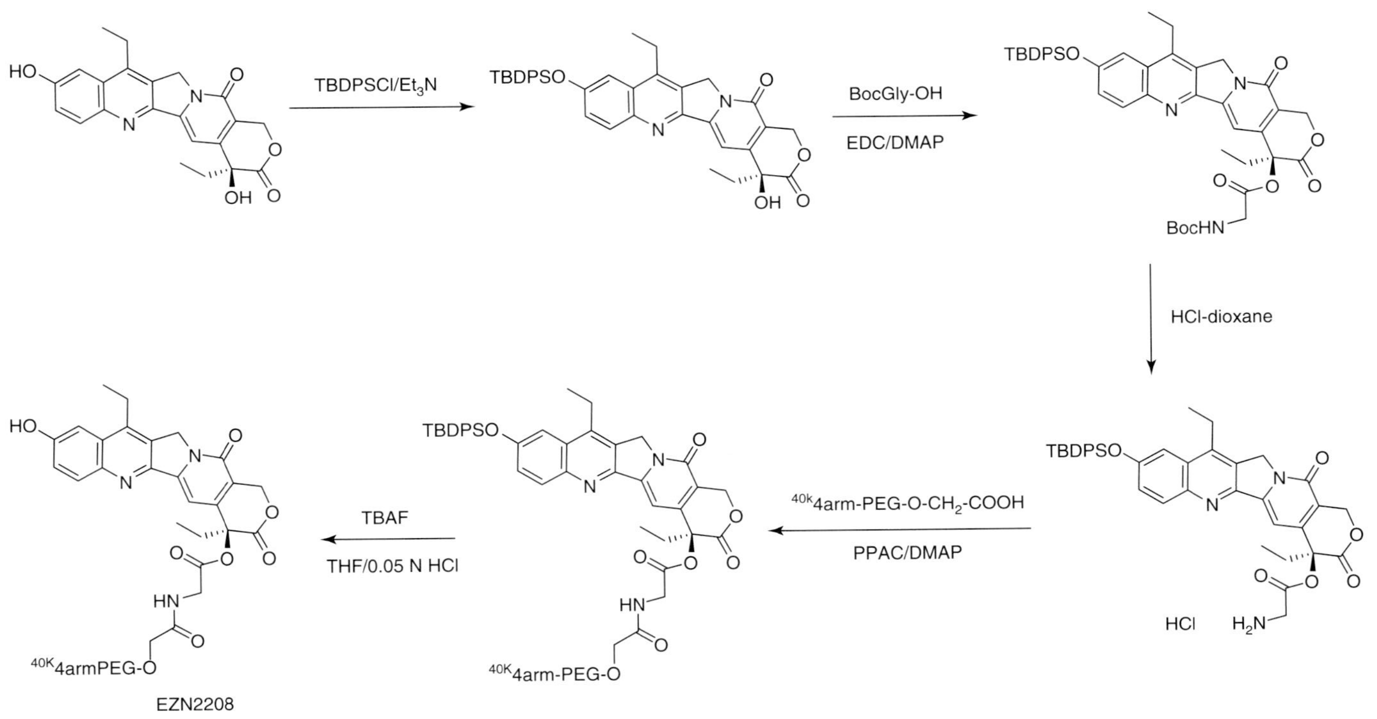

Scheme 21.5 Preparation of EZN-2208 (PEG–SN-38).

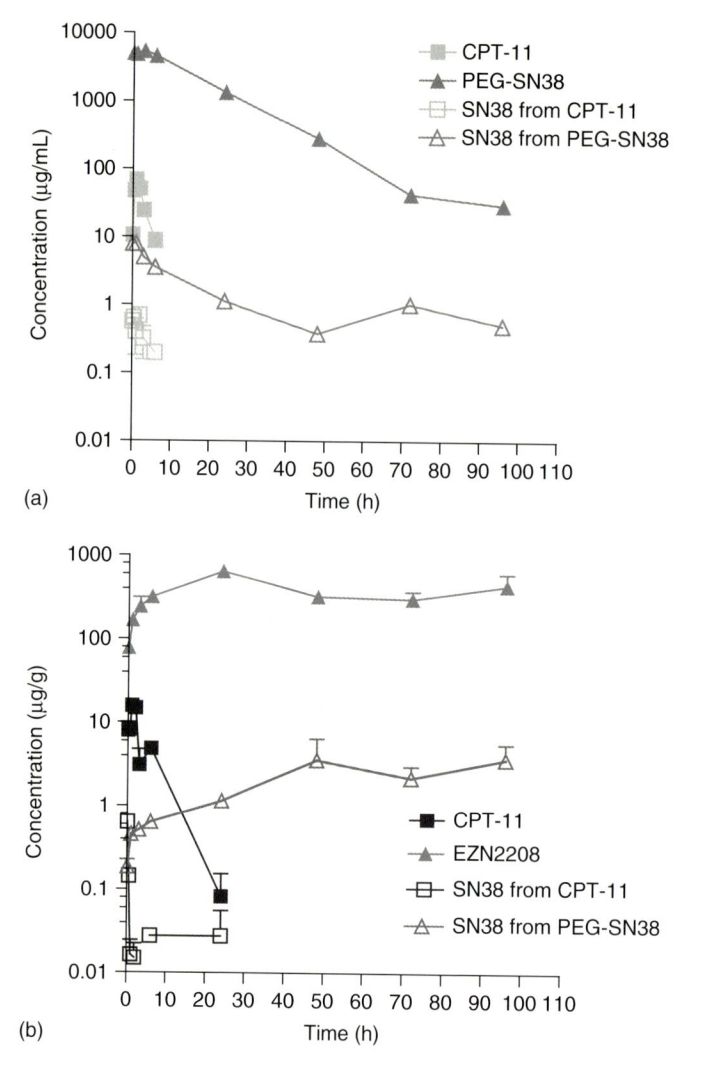

Figure 21.7 Plasma (a) and tumor (b) concentration–time curves of drugs after an intravenous bolus MTD treatment of EZN-2208 and CPT-11 to MX-1 xenografts ($n = 3$). Mice were sacrificed at various timepoints, and blood and tumor samples were obtained. The concentrations of PEG-SN-38 (▲), CPT-11 (■), and released SN-38 (from EZN-2208 (△) or from CPT-11 (□)) were determined using high-performance liquid chromatography analysis.

cycle [107]. In both studies, PEG-SN-38 was found to be well tolerated in previously treated patients with advanced malignancies. For both studies, the DLT was neutropenia with or without fever, in distinction to the DLT of CPT-11, which is diarrhea. In both studies, stable disease or sometimes prolonged PFS associated with tumor shrinkage was observed. For some patients, the duration of EZN-2208 was longer than the duration of their prior therapies. EZN-2208

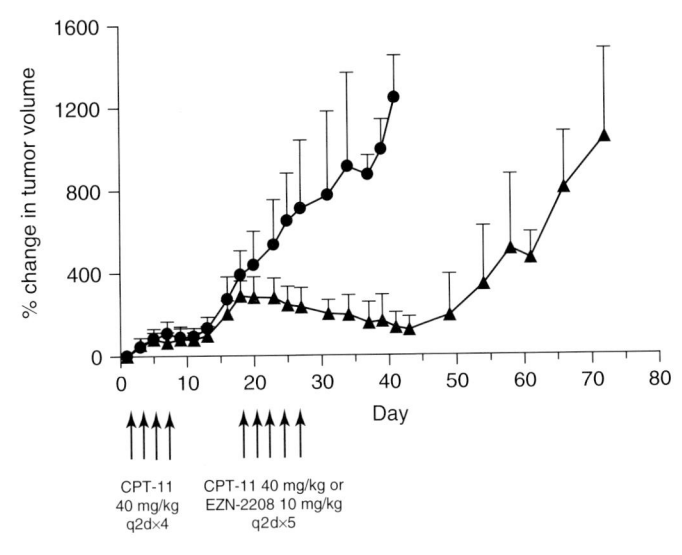

Figure 21.8 Activity of EZN-2208 in CPT-11-resistant colorectal tumor xenografts. Nude mice bearing human colorectal (HT-29) xenografts with resistance to CPT-11 were randomized and treated with either PEG-SN-38 (●) or CPT-11 (▲) ($n = 7$). Arrow denotes time of administration of the indicated drugs.

currently is being evaluated in phase II studies in patients with metastatic colorectal cancer (http://clinicaltrials.gov/ct2/show/NCT00931840) and metastatic breast cancer (http://clinicaltrials.gov/ct2/show/NCT01036113). EZN-2208 is also being evaluated in a phase I study of pediatric cancers. The maximum tolerated dose (MTD) and recommended phase II dose for EZN-2208 administered for 3 weeks per 4-week cycle is 9 mg/m^2 (SN-38 equivalent) [107]. In contrast, the recommended dosage for irinotecan in patients with recurrent colorectal cancer is 125 mg/m^2 given every week for 4 weeks or 350 mg/m^2 given once every 3 weeks. The higher doses of irinotecan reflect the reduce potency of the parent compound, as the low amount of SN-38 released from irinotecan [91, 92].

21.4.1.2.1 NKTR-102 NKTR-102 is a PEGylated CPT-11 using 40-kDa star-like four-arm PEG and a glycine spacer, similar to EZN-2208. In preclinical human ovarian and colorectal tumor xenograft models grown in mice, NKTR-102 had superior efficacy when compared to CPT-11 (Figure 21.9) [108, 109]. The lowest dose of NKTR-102 had superior activity when compared to the highest dose of CPT-11. NKTR-102 has also improved the pharmacokinetics and tumor distribution of CPT-11 and its active metabolite SN-38 [110]. When administered to rats through intravenous administration, NKTR-102 resulted in an 80-fold increase in SN-38 plasma area under the curve (AUC) versus CPT-11 and an extended SN-38 plasma half-life of 40 h compared to 3.5 h for CPT-11 at equivalent doses. In phase I trials where NKTR-102 was given as monotherapy, SN-38 levels were sustained, which

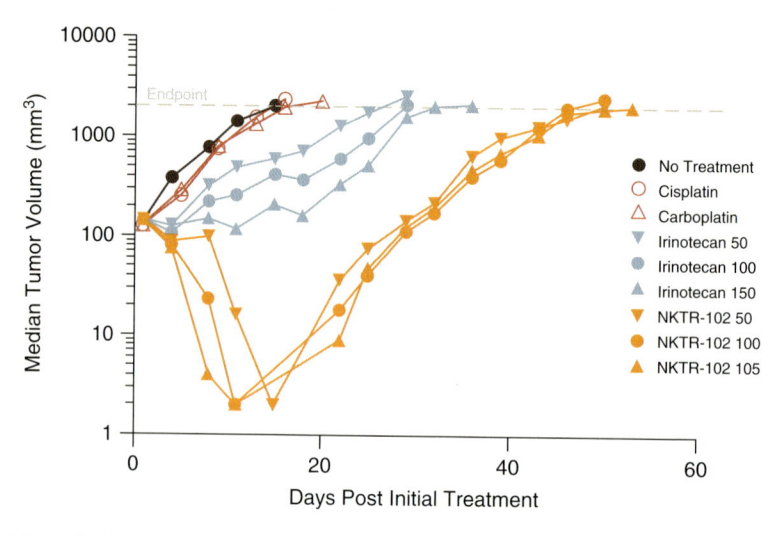

Figure 21.9 NKTR-102 showed superior activity over CPT-11 in platinium-resistant 2780 ovarian cancer models.

is similar to what was observed in animals. The response rate was 13% in heavily pretreated patients including 11% with a confirmed partial response. Antitumor activity was seen in patients with a variety of tumors.

In the phase II clinical studies in women with platinum-resistant ovarian cancer, NKTR-102 resulted in a response rate of 27 and 22% in the every 2-week and every 2-week schedule, respectively. A favorable toxicity profile [111] was observed. The study showed that women who received NKTR-102 once every 21 days had a median PFS of 21.0 weeks. Current agents approved by FDA to treat women with platinum-resistant ovarian cancer have a median PFS of between 9.1 and 13.6 weeks. NKTR-102 currently is in phase II clinical development for patients with solid tumor malignancies, including colorectal, breast, ovarian, and cervical cancers.

21.4.2
Releasable PEG Linkers Based on Amide or Other Amino-Derived Linkages

PEG conjugates linked by an amide bond are generally stable linkages that are susceptible to cleavage by proteases. Four types of amide linkages have been used to achieve efficient linkage with desired release properties. They include benzyl elimination (BE), trimethyl lock (TML), bis-N-2-hydroxyethylglycinamide (BCN), and aromatic linkers.

21.4.2.1 Releasable PEG Linkers Based on Aromatic Systems
The BE system employs a double prodrug strategy whereby hydrolysis initially results in release of the PEG polymer, followed by the classical and rapid 1,4- or 1,6-BE reaction and molecular decomposition [112, 113]. Further refinement of

Figure 21.10 PEG-BE prodrug.

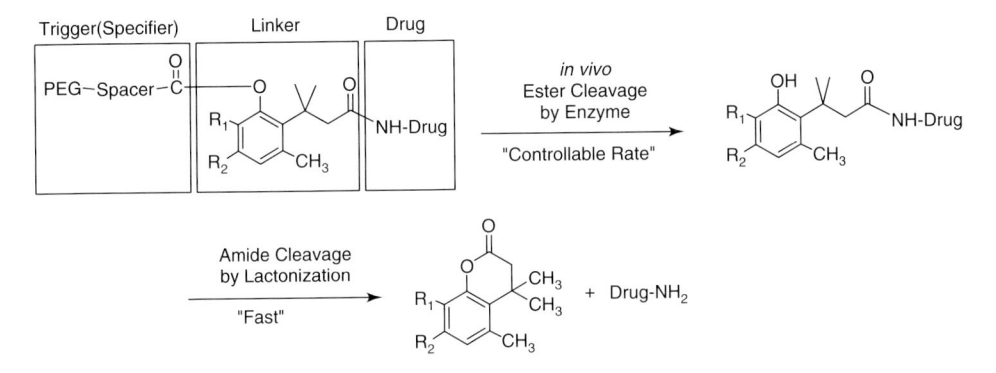

Figure 21.11 PEG-TML prodrug.

release kinetics is accomplished by the introduction of steric hindrance as *ortho* side-chains on the benzyl ring. The rate of release is relatively slow and therefore may be useful when the desired blood residency time of the active compound is hours to days, similar to what is achieved with permanently PEGylated proteins (Figure 21.10) [112].

The TML system is a similar releasing system based on an intramolecular cyclization reaction (lactonization) of a hindered amide [77, 78]. The TML was developed with various methodologies that allowed the efficient synthesis of different acyl functionalities (triggers) such as esters, carbonates, and carbamates on the phenolic hydroxyl group (Figure 21.11) [84]. The acylating agents were bifunctional by necessity and offered a site for easy PEGylation. Thus, introduction of PEG into the TML system as part of the specifier or trigger resulted in a neutral and highly water-soluble tripartate polymeric prodrug [84].

The BE and TML systems were first applied to the delivery of amino-containing anthracyclines such as doxorubicin (DOX) and daunorubicin [84, 112, 113]. A series of PEG conjugates were prepared and different releasing profiles in plasma were achieved. In addition, quite a few conjugates demonstrated enhanced anticancer efficacy compared to unPEGylated drugs. A comparable study between TML and BE also was reported [114].

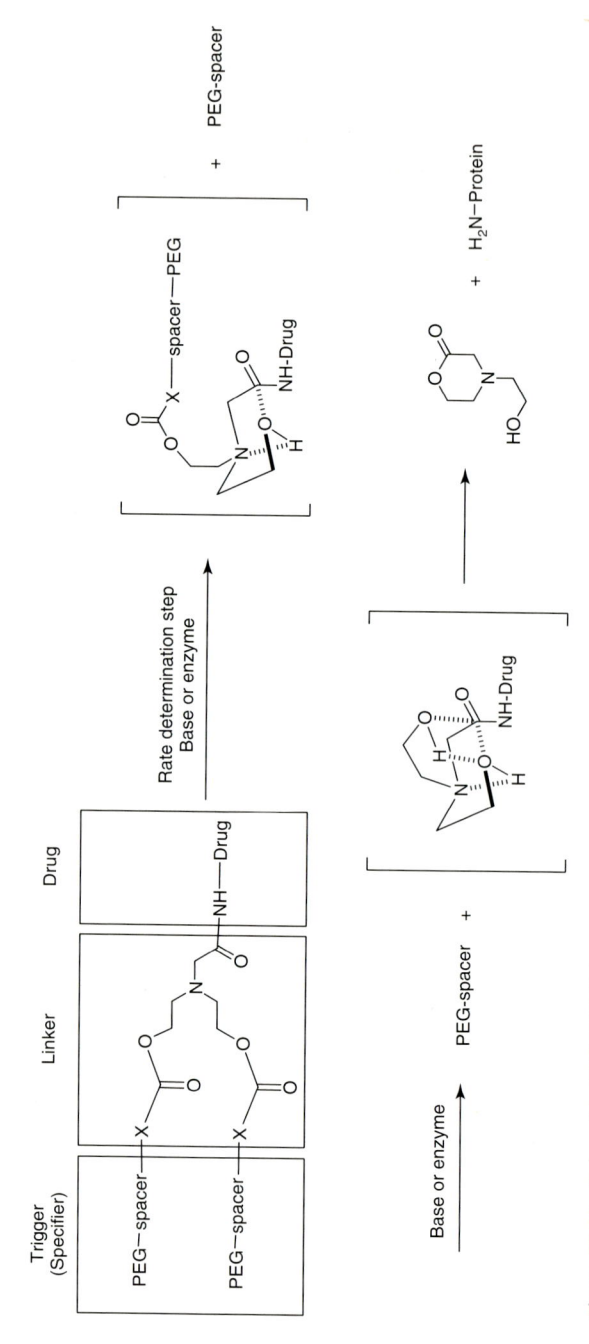

648 *21 Drug Conjugates with Poly(Ethylene Glycol)*

Figure 21.12 Releasable PEG-BCN linkers.

Another potential application of PEG-BE linkers is the delivery of oligonucleotides. In general, oligonucleotides are susceptible to enzymatic degradation and short plasma half-life, which can limit the utility of oligonucleotides as potential therapeutics. To overcome these hurdles, various releasable PEG-BE linkers with a molecular weight of 20 000 Da were used to conjugate with a model anti-Bcl-2 oligonucleotide (5′-aminoalkyl-oligonucleotide which has the same base sequence as G3139) [115, 116].

21.4.2.2 Releasable PEG Linkers Based on an Aliphatic System

In some cases, development of a versatile format for releasable PEGylation utilizing only aliphatic structures is desirable. The chemical foundation for this approach is the observed deamidation mechanism of bis-BCN [90]. This basic design (Figure 21.12) was further engineered to tailor the release rates of the prodrug by introduction of an α-heteroatom on the acid portion of the ester or by provision of anchimeric assistance by inclusion of additional side-chains [117, 118]. Diminishing the release rates was accomplished by introducing steric hindrance and by adding α-substituents. This overall approach also provided a facile strategy for designing branched linkers as well as linear linkers whereby either one [117] or multiple [118] PEGs could be attached per linker. The branched PEG linkers (U-PEG or umbrella PEG) are preferred in many applications of protein PEGylation [13, 119, 120]. PEG-BCN linkers have been used to deliver various types of drug molecules, including small molecules, enzymes, and immunotoxins.

In the case of immunotoxins, a BCN releasable linker was designed to discharge the biologically active molecule after it was internalized into the cell. This was done since the antibody-conjugated toxin (designated SS1P and composed of the Fv portion of an antibody to mesothelin genetically engineered to also express truncated *Pseudomonas* exotoxin A) exhibits toxicities and suboptimal pharmacology that limit the dose and frequency of administration when used to control the growth of mesothelin-expressing tumors in animal models. In addition, permanent PEGylation of SS1P where a single large PEG was attached to N-terminus of the SS1P heterodimer (and therefore near the antigen-binding site) blocked antigen binding and eliminated cytotoxic activity in cell culture [121]. Using the releasable PEG-BCN3 linker, SS1P was conjugated with three strands of branched 24-kDa PEG as random attachments. If the release of this PEG conjugate was prevented, it was inactive in cell-based cytotoxicity assays. In contrast, PEG-BCN3–SS1P conjugates showed superior bioactivity *in vivo* when compared to either unmodified SS1P or permanently PEGylated counterparts [121]. For example, complete regression was achieved in 25 and 75% of mice receiving 2.0 and 3.0 mg/kg, respectively. In mice receiving two doses of 2.0 mg/kg, 50% of mice showed complete regression of the tumors (Figure 21.13a). Doses at these levels exceed the median lethal dose (LD_{50}) for the unmodified SS1P and are therefore not feasible for the parent drug. PEGylation of SS1P with releasable linkers thus provided both reduced toxicity and improved efficacy.

The enhanced efficacy of the PEG-SS1P releasable may be explained partially by three beneficial features. First, the PEGylated conjugate (Figure 21.13b) had a

21 Drug Conjugates with Poly(Ethylene Glycol)

Table 21.3 Summary of in vitro and in vivo results of PEG–Ara-C.

Compound	$t_{1/2} >$ (h)[a], phosphate = buffered saline, pH 7.4	$t_{1/2}$(h)[a], human plasma	Solubility (mg/ml)[b]	Dose (mg/kg)	%TGI[c] (LX-1) solid tumor
Ara-C	–	–	–	100	26.2
(PEG–Ara-C structure 1)	32	2.9	~300	20	50.5
(PEG–Ara-C structure 2)	32	4.4	~400	40	66.3
(PEG–Ara-C structure 3)	30	4.1	>500	60	78.2

[a] All experiments were performed at 37°C in duplicate and $t_{1/2}$ was measured by the disappearance of PEG derivatives. Standard deviation of measurements ±10%.
[b] Solubility in acidic formulated buffer.
[c] Percentage tumor growth inhibition (% TGI) was calculated from the quotient of the median tumor volume of the treatment group divided by the median tumor volume of the control group ((1 − T/C) × 100) when the latter reached 1000.

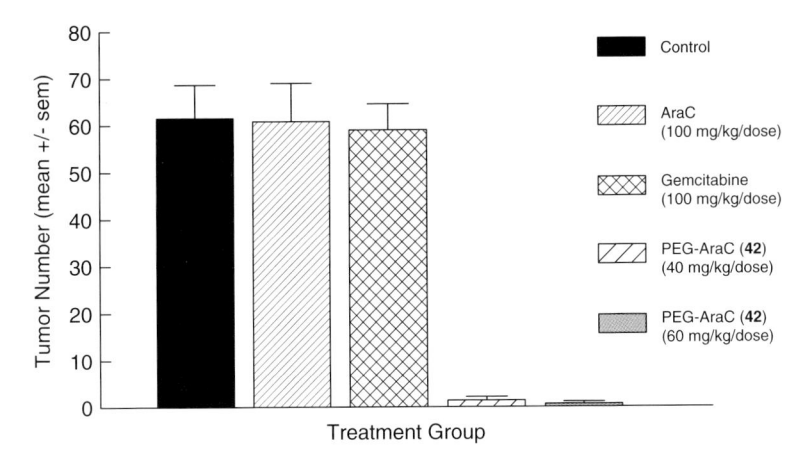

Figure 21.14 Response of orthotopic human pancreatic ductal adenocarcinoma (PANC-1) xenografts to intravenous treatment with PEG–Ara-C (**42**). Seven days post-tumor implantation, mice were dosed q3d × 5 and their abdominal cavities were then examined on day 40 for tumor proliferation. PEG–Ara-C doses were based on –ara-C content.

21.4.2.5 Other Releasable Linkers

Many other prodrug strategies for releasable PEGylation have been described in the literature; however, most of them were not used directly in the oncology field. These releasable strategies include utilizing oligo-lactic acid linkages [130] or succinic esters [131]. A format for reversible PEGylation based on maleimide-9-hydroxymethyl-7-sulfofluorene-N-hydroxysuccinimide ester heterobifunctional linkers, a derivative of the familiar amino reversible protecting reagent Fmoc [132–134], was also developed. A disulfide-substituted benzyl carbamate [135] system was used in which the linker design provides amide modification of molecular amines that are cleavable by thiolysis to regenerate the original molecule. Several disulfide-based reversible designs may be possible [136]. This approach was explored with thiol-PEG modifications of papain using a 4-pyridyl disulfide linker [134]. Releasable linkers based on succinimidyl esters also have been evaluated [137–139]. Some pioneering research also was performed on releasable PEGylation using a maleic anhydride-designed linker [140]. All of these linkers ultimately will need further testing to confirm the extent to which complete linker release and parental drug regeneration can be achieved.

21.5
Summary of Clinical Status

Many PEG–drug conjugates have been developed to treat human malignancies over the years. The parental drug molecules that can potentially benefit from

Table 21.4 Status of PEG–drug conjugates as anticancer therapeutics that have entered clinical trials or been approved by the FDA.

Name	Parental drug	PEG and molecular weight	PEGylation rationale	Status
Oncaspar (pegaspargase)	L-ASNase	5-kDa SS-PEG	prolong circulation time, reduce immunogenicity	approved in 1994 for ALL
Pegintron (peginterferon-α2b)	IFN-α2b	12-kDa SC-PEG	prolong circulation time, enhance *in vivo* activity	approved in 2001 for hepatitis C virus; in phase II clinical studies for melanoma and plexiform neurofibromas in children and young adults
Pegasys (peginterferon-α2a)	IFN-α2a	40-kDa U-PEG-NHS	prolong circulation time, enhance *in vivo* activity	approved in 2002 for hepatitis C virus; In phase II study for CML
Neulasta (pegfilgrastim)	G-CSF	5-kDa mPEG-aldehyde	prolong circulation time	approved in 2002 for chemotherapy-induced neutropenia
CDP791 (pegylated anti-VEGFR2 antibody fragment)	anti-VEGFR2 antibody fragment	40-kDa U-PEG-maleimide	prolong circulation	completed phase I study for lung cancer
PEG–paclitaxel	paclitaxel	40-kDa PEG-diol	increase solubility, improve pharmacokinetic profile	completed phase I studies for advanced solid tumors
NKTR-105 (pegylated DOX)	DOX	40-kDa four-arm star PEG	increase solubility, improve pharmacokinetic profile	in phase I studies for advanced solid tumors
Pegamotecan (PEG–CPT)	CPT	40-kDa PEG-diol	increase solubility, improve pharmacokinetic profile	finished phase II studies for stomach and gastroesophageal junction cancers
EZN-2208 (PEG–SN-38)	SN-38	40-kDa four-arm PEG	increase solubility, improve pharmacokinetic profile	in phase II studies for colorectal cancer, metastatic breast cancer, and pediatric malignancies
NKTR-102 (pegylated irinotecan)	irinotecan	40-kDa four-arm star PEG	increase solubility, improve pharmacokinetic profile	in phase II studies for colorectal cancer, metastatic breast, ovarian, and gastrointestinal cancers

PEGylation vary from enzymes, cytokines, antibody fragments, and other proteins to small-molecule cytotoxic agents. Both permanent and releasable linkers have been applied to address the specific delivery needs of the parental drugs. A couple of PEG–drug conjugates have already been approved to treat human cancer and cancer-related diseases. Many other compounds are now at different stages in clinical trials for various kinds of human malignancies. Table 21.4 summarizes the status of these PEG conjugates.

Oncaspar was the first approved PEG conjugate for cancer treatment. Currently a much more stable version of PEG–ASNase using SC-PEG instead of SS-PEG is in clinical trials to establish the desired pharmacokinetic profile and identify the optimal dose to achieve equivalent biological efficacy. Both PegIntron and Pegasys were originally approved for hepatitis C virus indication, but later on found anticancer activities in human. They are both in phase II clinical trials in combination with other chemotherapeutics to treat metastatic cancers. It appears that the choices of chemo-agents, combined dose regimens, and type of cancers to treat are the focus of on-going studies. While CDP791 is the first PEG conjugate of an antibody fragment that entered clinical trials to treat cancer, PEG–paclitaxel, NKTR-105, Pegamotecan, NKTR-102, and EZN-2208 are all PEGylated small-molecule cytotoxics. PEG–paclitaxel and Pegamotecan both used a 40-kDa molecular weight linear PEG diol, and there were two drug molecules conjugated to each PEG polymer. Due to the loading limitations, relatively high amounts of dosing were needed in clinical trials based on PEG mass. Both agents have met their endpoints in phase I and phase II studies, respectively, and demonstrated favorable toxicity profiles compared to native drugs and anticancer activities. NKTR-105, NKTR-102, and EZN-2208 have used different types of HMW four-arm PEG polymers in order to increase drug loading. As a result, the doses used in clinics based on PEG mass are much less for these conjugates. This improvement may potentially reduce any injection-related adverse events, and add convenience to both clinicians and patients. Recently, it has been reported that both NKTR-102 and EZN-2208 have shown excellent anticancer activities in several phase II studies in different solid tumors besides improved toxicity profiles.

21.6
Conclusions and Perspectives

PEGylation was introduced as a drug delivery technology more than 30 years ago. Multiple PEGylated drugs, several in the oncology field, have been marketed. The clinical success of PEGylation has encouraged improvements in this technology that provide new or better applications for the delivery of small molecules, proteins, peptides, and other molecules through customized linkers. Initially, permanent PEG linkers and nonselective conjugation were the major approaches. However, the demand for extending the benefit of this technology from enzymes to other types of therapeutics has led to the development of new ways to conduct PEGylation.

These include new linker chemistries for PEG attachments that have been designed to degrade at a controlled rate *in vivo* and dispatch the active drug cargo, which was biologically inert in its starting prodrug bioconjugate.

In contrast to the PEGylation of proteins and antibody fragments, other roles of PEGylation in the enhancement of pharmaceutical properties of small molecules or oligonucleotides remain unproven in humans even though significant therapeutic benefits have been achieved in preclinical models. The recent advancement of several PEGylated small-molecule conjugates into clinical trials certainly provides the opportunities to demonstrate the utility of this technology for small-molecule agents. Owing to the HMW of PEG required to prevent rapid clearance of the drug conjugate, the unPEGylated small-molecule drug employed in the conjugate needs to possess initial high activity (nanomolar or greater) to minimize the amount of PEG conjugate required for administration. The utility of multiarm PEG and the development of terminal branching permit a payload of eight drug molecules or more without difficulty and appear sufficient for most applications. The utility of the PEG prodrug approach to drug delivery provides a way to solubilize insoluble drugs in a nonionic matrix and to reduce drug clearance while extending the plasma concentration, thereby providing a greater apparent AUC. Applications of this concept to water-soluble drugs also may serve to prevent rapid clearance from the body and lead to a greater apparent AUC. PEG prodrugs can be used for agents with amino, hydroxyl, or carboxyl functions, thus giving them great versatility for drug delivery. The chemistry of the PEG linker seems adequately designed at this point leaving only the choice of the small-molecule candidate to be determined. Releasable PEGylation allows the regeneration of physically and functionally equivalent unPEGylated drugs from their PEG conjugates in a therapeutically relevant period of minutes to days. The benefits of a prodrug designed to avoid early systemic clearance mechanisms and the incremental deposition of released active therapeutics offer a new scope for the application of PEGylation science.

HMW PEG conjugation has passive targeting potential, which allows for accumulation of drug molecules in solid tumors and therefore reduces off-target damage to healthy tissues. Ultimately, combining PEGylation properties with molecules that are actively targeting the tumor (i.e., antibodies) will further enhance the therapeutic index of anticancer drugs. Inevitably, PEGylation technology will continue to advance and more examples will be generated to demonstrate its versatility to meet the need of modern drug delivery.

Acknowledgments

We would like to thank Dr. Zheng Wang and Ms. Arlene Reiss for their assistance in editing this chapter.

References

1. Pasut, G. and Veronese, F.M. (2009) PEGylation for improving the effectiveness of therapeutic biomolecules. *Drugs Today*, **45**, 687–695.
2. Kang, J.S., DeLuca, P.P., and Lee, K.C. (2009) Emerging PEGylated drugs. *Expert Opin. Emerg. Drugs*, **14**, 363–380.
3. Filpula, D. and Zhao, H. (2008) Releasable PEGylation of proteins with customized linkers. *Adv. Drug Deliv. Rev.*, **60**, 29–49.
4. Bailon, P. and Won, C.Y. (2009) PEG-modified biopharmaceuticals. *Expert Opin. Drug Deliv.*, **6**, 1–16.
5. Pasut, G. and Veronese, F.M. (2009) PEG conjugates in clinical development or use as anticancer agents: an overview. *Adv. Drug Deliv. Rev.*, **61**, 1177–1188.
6. Jevsevar, S., Kunstelj, M., and Porekar, V.G. (2010) PEGylation of therapeutic proteins. *Biotechnol. J.*, **5**, 113–128.
7. Greenwald, R.B. and Zhao, H. (2007) Poly (ethylene glycol) prodrugs: altered pharmacokinetics and pharmacodynamics in, *Prodrugs: Challenges and Rewards*, Part 1 (eds V.J. Stella, R.T. Borchardt, M.J. Hageman, R. Oliyai, H. Maag, and J.W. Tilley), Springer, New York, pp. 283–338.
8. Abuchowski, A., van Es, T., Palczuk, N.C., and Davis, F.F. (1977) Alteration of immunological properties of bovine serum albumin by covalent attachment of polyethylene glycol. *J. Biol. Chem.*, **252**, 3578–3581.
9. Hunt, D.F., Giordiani, A.B., Rhodes, G., and Herold, D.A. (1982) Mixture analysis by triple-quadrupole mass spectrometry: metabolic profiling of urinary carboxylic acids. *Clin. Chem.*, **28**, 2387–2392.
10. Friman, S., Leandersson, P., Tagesson, C., and Svanvik, J. (1990) Biliary excretion of different sized polyethylene glycols in the cat. *J. Hepatol.*, **11**, 215–220.
11. Friman, S., Egestad, B., Sjövall, J., and Svanvik, J. (1993) Hepatic excretion and metabolism of polyethylene glycols and mannitol in the cat. *J. Hepatol.*, **17**, 48–55.
12. Zhao, H., Rubio, B., Sapra, P., Wu, D., Reddy, P., Sai, P., Martinez, A., Gao, Y., Lozanguiez, Y., Longley, C., Greenberger, L.M., and Horak, I.D. (2008) Novel prodrugs of SN-38 using multiarm poly(ethylene glycol) linkers. *Bioconjug. Chem.*, **19**, 849–859.
13. Martinez, A., Pendri, A., and Greenwald, R.B. (1997) Branched poly(ethylene glycol) linkers. *Macromol. Chem. Phys.*, **198**, 2489–2498.
14. Yamaoka, T., Tabata, Y., and Ikada, Y. (1994) Distribution and tissue uptake of poly(ethylene glycol) with different molecular weights after intravenous administration to mice. *J. Pharm. Sci.*, **83**, 601–606.
15. Harris, J.M., Martin, N.E., and Modi, M. (2001) Pegylation: a novel process for modifying pharmacokinetics. *Clin. Pharmacokinet.*, **40**, 539–551.
16. Abuchowski, A., Kazo, G.M., Verhoest, C.R. Jr., Van Es, T., Kafkewitz, D., Nucci, M.L., Viau, A.T., and Davis, F.F. (1984) Cancer therapy with chemically modified enzymes. I. Antitumor properties of polyethylene glycol–asparaginase conjugates. *Cancer Biochem. Biophys.*, **7**, 175–186.
17. Enzon Pharmaceuticals (2008) Adagen® (pegademase bovine) [package insert]. Enzon Pharmaceuticals, Bridgewater, NJ.
18. Dinndorf, P.A., Gootenberg, J., Cohen, M.H., Keegan, P., and Pazdur, R. (2007) FDA drug approval summary: pegaspargase (Oncaspar®) for the first-line treatment of children with acute lymphoblastic leukemia (ALL). *Oncologist*, **12**, 991–998.
19. Enzon Pharmaceuticals (2006) Oncaspar® (pegaspargase) [package insert]. Enzon Pharmaceuticals Bridgewater, NJ.
20. Asselin, B.L., Whitin, J.C., Coppola, D.J., Rupp, I.P., Sallan, S.E., and Cohen, H.J. (1993) Comparative pharmacokinetic studies of three asparaginase preparations. *J. Clin. Oncol.*, **11**, 1780–1786.
21. Kafkewitz, D. and Bendich, A. (1983) Enzyme-induced asparagine and

glutamine depletion and immune system function. *Am. J. Clin. Nutr.*, **37**, 1025–1030.

22. Rizzari, C., Zucchetti, M., Conter, V., Diomede, L., Bruno, A., Gavazzi, L., Paganini, M., Sparano, P., Lo Nigro, L., Arico, M., Milani, M., and D'Incalci, M. (2000) L-Asparagine depletion and L-asparaginase activity in children with acute lympoblastic leukemia receiving i.m. or i.v. *Erwinia C.* or *E. coli* L-asparaginase as first exposure. *Ann. Oncol.*, **11**, 189–193.

23. Amgen (2010) Neulasta® (pegfilgrastim) [package insert]. Amgen, Thousand Oaks, CA.

24. Douer, D., Yampolsky, H., Cohen, L.J., Watkins, K., Levine, A.M., Periclou, A.P., and Avramis, V.I. (2007) Pharmacodynamics and safety of intravenous pegaspargase during remission induction in adults aged 55 years or younger with newly diagnosed acute lymphoblastic leukemia. *Blood*, **109**, 2744–2750.

25. Silverman, L.B., Gelber, R.D., Dalton, V.K., Asselin, B.L., Barr, R.D., Clavell, L.A., Hurwitz, C.A., Moghrabi, A., Samson, Y., Schorin, M.A., Arkin, S., Declerck, L., Cohen, H.J., and Sallan, S.E. (2001) Improved outcome for children with acute lymphoblastic leukemia: results of Dana-Farber Consortium Protocol 91-01. *Blood*, **97**, 1211–1218.

26. Seibel, N.L., Steinherz, P.G., Sather, H.N., Nachman, J.B., Delaat, C., Ettinger, L.J., Freyer, D.R., Mattano, L.A. Jr., Hastings, C.A., Rubin, C.M., Bertolone, K., Franklin, J.L., Heerema, N.A., Mitchell, T.L., Pyesmany, A.F., La, M.K., Edens, C., and Gaynon, P.S. (2008) Early postinduction intensification therapy improves survival for children and adolescents with high-risk acute lymphoblastic leukemia: a report from the Children's Oncology Group. *Blood*, **111**, 2548–2555.

27. Wang, B., Relling, M.V., Storm, M.C., Woo, M.H., Ribeiro, R., Pui, C.H., and Hak, L.J. (2003) Evaluation of immunologic crossreaction of antiasparaginase antibodies in acute lymphoblastic leukemia (ALL) and lymphoma patients. *Leukemia*, **17**, 1583–1588.

28. Wacker, P., Land, V.J., Camitta, B.M., Kurtzberg, J., Pullen, J., Harris, M.B., and Shuster, J.J. (2007) Allergic reactions to *E. coli* L-asparaginase do not affect outcome in childhood B-precursor acute lymphoblastic leukemia: a Children's Oncology Group study. *J. Pediatr. Hematol. Oncol.*, **29**, 627–632.

29. Ovation Pharmaceuticals (2007) Elspar® (asparaginase) [package insert]. Ovation Pharmaceuticals, Deerfield, IL.

30. Graham, M.L. (2003) Pegaspargase: a review of clinical studies. *Adv. Drug Deliv. Rev.*, **55**, 1293–1302.

31. Avramis, V.I., Sencer, S., Periclou, A.P., Sather, H., Bostrom, B.C., Cohen, L.J., Ettinger, A.G., Ettinger, L.J., Franklin, J., Gaynon, P.S., Hilden, J.M., Lange, B., Majlessipour, F., Mathew, P., Needle, M., Neglia, J., Reaman, G., Holcenberg, J.S., and Stork, L. (2002) A randomized comparison of native *Escherichia coli* asparaginase and polyethylene glycol conjugated asparaginase for treatment of children with newly diagnosed standard-risk acute lymphoblastic leukemia: a Children's Cancer Group study. *Blood*, **99**, 1986–1994.

32. Ettinger, L.J., Kurtzberg, J., Voûte, P.A., Jürgens, H., and Halpern, S.L. (1995) An open-label, multicenter study of polyethylene glycol–L-asparaginase for the treatment of acute lymphoblastic leukemia. *Cancer*, **75**, 1176–1181.

33. Wang, M., Basu, A., Palm, T., Hua, J., Youngster, S., Hwang, L., Liu, H., Li, X., Peng, P., Zhang, Y., Zhao, H., Zhang, Z., Longley, C., Mehlig, M., Borowski, V., Sai, P., Viswanathan, M., Jang, E., Petti, G., Liu, S., Yang, K., and Filpula, D. (2006) Engineering an arginine catabolizing bioconjugate: biochemical and pharmacological characterization of PEGylated derivatives of arginine deiminase from mycoplasma arthritidis. *Bioconjug. Chem.*, **17**, 1447–1459.

34. Sherman, M.R., Saifer, M.G.P., and Perez-Ruiz, F. (2008) PEG–uricase in

the management of treatment-resistant gout and hyperuricemia. *Adv. Drug Deliv. Rev.*, **60**, 59–68.
35. Zalipsky, S., Seltzer, R., and Menon-Rudolph, S. (1992) Evaluation of a new reagent for covalent attachment of polyethylene glycol to proteins. *Biotechnol. Appl. Biochem.*, **15**, 100–114.
36. Schering-Plough (2009) PegIntron® (peginterferon-α2b) [package insert]. Schering-Plough, Kenilworth, NJ.
37. Spiegel, R.J. (1989) Alpha interferons: a clinical overview. *Urology*, **34** (Suppl. 4), 75–79; discussion 87–96.
38. Pestka, S., Langer, J.A., Zoon, K.C., and Samuel, C.E. (1987) Interferons and their actions. *Annu. Rev. Biochem.*, **56**, 727–777.
39. Baron, S., Tyring, S.K., Fleischmann, W.R. Jr., Coppenhaver, D.H., Niesel, D.W., Klimpel, G.R., Stanton, G.J., and Hughes, T.K. (1991) The interferons. Mechanisms of action and clinical applications. *J. Am. Med. Assoc.*, **266**, 1375–1383.
40. Schering-Plough (2009) Intron® (interferon-α2b) [package insert] Schering-Plough, Kenilworth, NJ.
41. Wang, Y.S., Youngster, S., Grace, M., Bausch, J., Bordens, R., and Wyss, D.F. (2002) Structural and biological characterization of pegylated recombinant interferon α2b and its therapeutic implications. *Adv. Drug Deliv. Rev.*, **54**, 547–570.
42. Grace, M., Youngster, S., Gitlin, G., Sydor, W., Xie, L., Westreich, L., Jacobs, S., Brassard, D., Bausch, J., and Bordens, R. (2001) Structural and biologic characterization of pegylated recombinant IFN-α2b. *J. Interferon Cytokine Res.*, **21**, 1103–1115.
43. Glue, P., Fang, J.W.S., Rouzier-Panis, R., Raffanel, C., Sabo, R., Gupta, S.K., Salfi, M., and Jacobs, S. (2000) Pegylated interferon-α2b: pharmacokinetics, pharmacodynamics, safety, and preliminary efficacy data. *Clin. Pharmacol. Ther.*, **68**, 556–567.
44. Groves, M.D., Puduvalli, V.K., Gilbert, M.R., Levin, V.A., Conrad, C.A., Liu, V.H., Hunter, K., Meyers, C., Hess, K.R., and Yung, W.K.A. (2009) Two phase II trials of temozolomide with interferon-α2b (pegylated and non-pegylated) in patients with recurrent glioblastoma multiforme. *Br. J. Cancer*, **101**, 615–620.
45. Yamamoto, Y., Tsutsumi, Y., Yoshioka, Y., Nishibata, T., Kobayashi, K., Okamoto, T., Mukai, Y., Shimizu, T., Nakagawa, S., Nagata, S., and Mayumi, T. (2003) Site-specific PEGylation of a lysine-deficient TNF-α with full bioactivity. *Nat. Biotechnol.*, **21**, 546–552.
46. Amgen (2010) Neupogen® (filgrastim) [package insert]. Amgen, Thousand Oaks, CA.
47. Heil, G., Hoelzer, D., Sanz, M.A., Lechner, K., Liu Yin, J.A., Papa, G., Noens, L., Szer, J., Ganser, A., O'Brien, C., Matcham, J., and Barge, A., The International Acute Myeloid Leukemia Study Group (1997) A randomized, double-blind, placebo-controlled, phase III study of filgrastim in remission induction and consolidation therapy for adults with de novo acute myeloid leukemia. *Blood*, **90**, 4710–4718.
48. Dale, D.C., Bonilla, M.A., Davis, M.W., Nakanishi, A.M., Hammond, W.P., Kurtzberg, J., Wang, W., Jakubowski, A., Winton, E., Lalezari, P., Robinson, W., Glaspy, J.A., Emerson, S., Gabrilove, J., Vincent, M., and Boxer, L.A. (1993) A randomized controlled phase III trial of recombinant human granulocyte colony-stimulating factor (filgrastim) for treatment of severe chronic neutropenia. *Blood*, **81**, 2496–2502.
49. Blackwell, S. and Crawford, J. (1994) Filgrastim (r-metHuC-CSF) in the chemotherapy setting in *Filgrastim (r-metHuG-CSF) in Clinical Practice* (eds G. Morstyn and T.M. Dexter), Dekker, New York, pp. 103–116.
50. Crawford, J., Ozer, H., Stoller, R., Johnson, D., Lyman, G., Tabbara, I., Kris, M., Grous, J., Picozzi, V., Rausch, G., Smith, R., Gradishar, W., Yahanda, A., Vincent, M., Stewart, M., and Glaspy, J. (1991) Reduction by granulocyte colony-stimulating factor of fever and neutropenia induced by chemotherapy in patients with

small-cell lung cancer. *N. Engl. J. Med.*, **325**, 164–170.

51. Pettengell, R., Gurney, H., Radford, J.A., Deakin, D.P., James, R., Wilkinson, P.M., Kane, K., Bentley, J., and Crowther, D. (1992) Granulocyte colony-stimulating factor to prevent dose-limiting neutropenia in non-Hodgkin's lymphoma: a randomized controlled trial. *Blood*, **80**, 1430–1436.

52. Kinstler, O., Molineux, G., Treuheit, M., Ladd, D., and Gegg, C. (2002) Mono-N-terminal poly(ethylene glycol)–protein conjugates. *Adv. Drug Deliv. Rev.*, **54**, 477–485.

53. Molineux, G., Kinstler, O., Briddell, B., Hartley, C., McElroy, P., Kerzic, P., Sutherland, W., Stoney, G., Kern, B., Fletcher, F.A., Cohen, A., Korach, E., Ulich, T., McNiece, I., Lockbaum, P., Miller-Messana, M.A., Gardner, S., Hunt, T., and Schwab, G. (1999) A new form of filgrastim with sustained duration *in vivo* and enhanced ability to mobilize PBPC in both mice and humans. *Exp. Hematol.*, **27**, 1724–1734.

54. Molineux, G. (2004) The design and development of pegfilgrastim (PEG-rmetHuG-CSF, Neulasta®). *Curr. Pharm. Des.*, **10**, 1235–1244.

55. George, S., Yunus, F., Case, D., Yang, B.B., Hackett, J., Shogan, J.E., Meza, L.A., Neumann, T.A., and Liang, B.C. (2003) Fixed-dose pegfilgrastim is safe and allows neutrophil recovery in patients with non-Hodgkin's lymphoma. *Leuk. Lymphoma*, **44**, 1691–1696.

56. Green, M.D., Koelbl, H., Baselga J., Galid, A., Guillem, V., Gascon, P., Siena, S., Lalisang, R.I., Samonigg, H., Clemens, M.R., Zani, V., Liang, B.C., Renwick, J., and Piccart, M.J., The International Pegfilgrastim 749 Study Group (2003) A randomized double-blind multicenter phase III study of fixed-dose single-administration pegfilgrastim versus daily filgrastim in patients receiving myelosuppressive chemotherapy. *Ann. Oncol.*, **14**, 29–35.

57. Grigg, A., Solal-Celigny, P., Hoskin, P., Taylor, K., McMillan, A., Forstpointner, R., Bacon, P., Renwick, J., and Hiddemann, W., The International Study Group (2003) Open-label, randomized study of pegfilgrastim vs. daily filgrastim as an adjunct to chemotherapy in elderly patients with non-Hodgkin's lymphoma. *Leuk. Lymphoma*, **44**, 1503–1508.

58. Holmes, F.A., Jones, S.E., O'Shaughnessy, J., Vukelja, S., George, T., Savin, M., Richards, D., Glaspy, J., Meza, L., Cohen, G., Dhami, M., Budman, D.R., Hackett, J., Brassard, M., Yang, B.B., and Liang, B.C. (2002) Comparable efficacy and safety profiles of once-per-cycle pegfilgrastim and daily injection filgrastim in chemotherapy-induced neutropenia: a multicenter dose-finding study in women with breast cancer. *Ann. Oncol.*, **13**, 903–909.

59. Holmes, F.A., O'Shaughnessy, J.A., Vukelja, S., Jones, S.E., Shogan, J., Savin, M., Glaspy, J., Moore, M., Meza, L., Wiznitzer, I., Neumann, T.A., Hill, L.R., and Liang, B.C. (2002) Blinded, randomized, multicenter study to evaluate single administration pegfilgrastim once per cycle versus daily filgrastim as an adjunct to chemotherapy in patients with high-risk stage II or stage III/IV breast cancer. *J. Clin. Oncol.*, **20**, 727–731.

60. Johnston, E., Crawford, J., Blackwell, S., Bjurstrom, T., Lockbaum, P., Roskos, L., Yang, B.B., Gardner, S., Miller-Messana, M.A., Shoemaker, D., Garst, J., and Scyhwab, G. (2000) Randomized, dose-escalation study of SD/01 compared with daily filgrastim in patients receiving chemotherapy. *J. Clin. Oncol.*, **18**, 2522–2528.

61. Vose, J.M., Crump, M., Lazarus, H., Emmanouilides, C., Schenkein, D., Moore, J., Frankel, S., Flinn, I., Lovelace, W., Hackett, J., and Liang, B.C. (2003) Randomized, multicenter, open-label study of pegfilgrastim compared with daily filgrastim after chemotherapy for lymphoma. *J. Clin. Oncol.*, **21**, 514–519.

62. Danova, M., Chiroli, S., Rosti, G., and Doan, Q.V. (2009) Cost-effectiveness of pegfilgrastim versus six days of filgrastim for preventing febrile neutropenia

63. Lyman, G.H., Lalla, A., Barron, R.L., and Dubois, R.W. (2009) Cost-effectiveness of pegfilgrastim versus filgrastim primary prophylaxis in women with early-stage breast cancer receiving chemotherapy in the United States. *Clin. Ther.*, **31**, 1092–1104.
64. Genentech (2010) Pegasys® (peginterferon-α2a) [package insert]. Genentech, South San Francisco, CA.
65. Eyetech (2006) Macugen® (pegaptanib sodium injection) [package insert]. Eyetech, Cedar Knolls, NJ.
66. UCB (2010) Cimzia® (certolizumab pegol) [package insert]. Eyetech, Smyrna, GA.
67. Vogel, W. (2003) Peginterferon-alpha 2a (40 kDa)/ribavirin combination for the treatment of chronic hepatitis C infection. *Expert Rev. Anti Infect. Ther.*, **1**, 423–431.
68. McHutchison, J.G., Manns, M.P., Muir, A.J., Terrault, N.A., Jacobson, I.M., Afdhal, N.H., Heathcote, E.J., Zeuzem, S., Reesink, H.W., Garg, J., Bsharat, M., George, S., Kauffman, R.S., Adda, N., and Di Bisceglie, A.M. (2010) Telaprevir for previously treated chronic HCV infection. *N. Engl. J. Med.*, **362**, 1292–1303.
69. Oldham, R.K. and Dillman, R.O. (2008) Monoclonal antibodies in cancer therapy. *J. Clin. Oncol.*, **26**, 1774–1777.
70. Chapman, A.P. (2002) PEGylated antibodies and antibody fragments for improved therapy: a review. *Adv. Drug Deliv. Rev.*, **54**, 531–545.
71. Sandborn, W.J., Feagan, B.G., Stoinov, S., Honiball, P.J., Rutgeerts, P., Mason, D., Bloomfield, R., and Schreiber, S., PRECISE 1 Study Investigators (2007) Certolizumab pegol for the treatment of Crohn's disease. *N. Engl. J. Med.*, **357**, 228–238.
72. Choy, E.H.S., Hazleman, B., Smith, M., Moss, K., Lisi, L., Scott, D.G.I., Patel, J., Sopwith, M., and Isenberg, D.A. (2002) Efficacy of a novel PEGylated humanized anti-TNF fragment (CDP870) in patients with rheumatoid arthritis: a phase II double-blinded, randomized, dose-escalating trial. *Rheumatology*, **41**, 1133–1137.
73. Nesbitt, A., Fossati, G., Bergin, M., Stephens, P., Stephens, S., Foulkes, R., Brown, D., Robinson, M., and Bourne, T. (2007) Mechanism of action of certolizumab pegol (CDP870): in vitro comparison with other anti-tumor necrosis factor α agents. *Inflamm. Bowel Dis.*, **13**, 1323–1332.
74. Ton, N.C., Parker, G.J.M., Jackson, A., Mullamitha, S., Buonaccorsi, G.A., Roberts, C., Watson, Y., Davies, K., Cheung, S., Hope, L., Power, F., Lawrance, J., Valle, J., Saunders, M., Felix, R., Soranson, J.A., Rolfe, L., Zinkewich-Peotti, K., and Jayson, G.C. (2007) Phase I evaluation of CDP791, a PEGylated di-Fab' conjugate that binds vascular endothelial growth factor receptor 2. *Clin. Cancer Res.*, **13**, 7113–7118.
75. Wang, W., Jiang, J., Ballard, C.E., and Wang, B. (1999) Prodrug approaches to the improved delivery of peptide prodrugs. *Curr. Pharm. Des.*, **5**, 265–287.
76. Shan, D., Nicolaou, M.G., Borchardt, R.T., and Wang, B. (1997) Prodrug strategies based on intramolecular cyclization reactions. *J. Pharm. Sci.*, **86**, 765–767.
77. Shaunak, S., Godwin, A., Choi, J.W., Balan, S., Pedone, E., Vijayarangam, D., Heidelberger, S., Teo, I., Zloh, M., and Brocchini, S. (2006) Site-specific PEGylation of native disulfide bonds in therapeutic proteins. *Nat. Chem. Biol.*, **2**, 312–313.
78. Oya, T., Hattori, N., Mizuno, Y., Miyata, S., Maeda, S., Osawa, T., and Uchida, K. (1999) Methylglyoxal modification of protein. Chemical and immunochemical characterization of methylglyoxal-arginine adducts. *J. Biol. Chem.*, **274**, 18492–18502.
79. Maullu, C., Raimondo, D., Caboi, F., Giorgetti, A., Sergi, M., Valentini, M., Tonon, G., and Tramontano, A. (2009) Site-directed enzymatic PEGylation of the human granulocyte colony-stimulating factor. *FEBS J.*, **276**, 6741–6750.

demonstrates improved pharmacokinetics with sustained exposure of irinotecan and its active metabolite. 14th European Cancer Conference, Barcelona.
112. Lee, S., Greenwald, R.B., McGuire, J., Yang, K., and Shi, C. (2001) Drug delivery systems employing 1,6-elimination: releasable poly(ethylene glycol) conjugates of proteins. *Bioconjug. Chem.*, **12**, 163–169.
113. Greenwald, R.B., Yang, K., Zhao, H., Conover, C.D., Lee, S., and Filpula, D. (2003) Controlled release of proteins from their poly(ethylene glycol) conjugates: drug delivery systems employing 1,6-elimination. *Bioconjug. Chem.*, **14**, 395–403.
114. Greenwald, R.B., Choe, Y.H., Conover, C.D., Shum, K., Wu, D., and Royzen, M. (2000) Drug delivery systems based on trimethyl lock lactonization: poly(ethylene glycol) prodrugs of amino-containing compounds. *J. Med. Chem.*, **43**, 475–487.
115. Zhao, H., Greenwald, R.B., Reddy, P., Xia, J., and Peng, P. (2005) A new platform for oligonucleotide delivery utilizing the PEG prodrug approach. *Bioconjug. Chem.*, **16**, 758–766.
116. Zhao, H., Peng, P., Longley, C., Zhang, Y., Borowski, V., Mehlig, M., Reddy, P., Xia, J., Borchard, G., Lipman, J., Benimetskaya, L., and Stein, C.A. (2007) Delivery of G3139 using releasable PEG-linkers: impact on pharmacokinetic profile and anti-tumor efficacy. *J. Control. Release*, **119**, 143–152.
117. Zhao, H., Yang, K., Martinez, A., Basu, A., Chintala, R., Liu, H.C., Janjua, A., Wang, M., and Filpula, D. (2006) Linear and branched bicin linkers for releasable PEGylation of macromolecules: controlled release in vivo and in vitro from mono- and multi-PEGylated proteins. *Bioconjug. Chem.*, **17**, 341–351.
118. Greenwald, R.B., Zhao, H., Yang, K., Reddy, P., and Martinez, A. (2004) A new aliphatic amino prodrug system for the delivery of small molecules and proteins utilizing novel PEG derivatives. *J. Med. Chem.*, **47**, 726–734.
119. Yang, K., Basu, A., Wang, M., Chintala, R., Hsieh, M.C., Liu, S., Hua, J., Zhang, Z., Zhou, J., Li, M., Phyu, H., Petti, G., Mendez, M., Janjua, H., Peng, P., Longley, C., Borowski, V., Mehlig, M., and Filpula, D. (2003) Tailoring structure–function and pharmacokinetic properties of single-chain Fv proteins by site-specific PEGylation. *Protein Eng.*, **16**, 761–770.
120. Bailon, P., Palleroni, A., Schaffer, C.A., Spence, C.L., Fung, W.J., Porter, J.E., Ehrlich, G.K., Pan, W., Xu, Z.X., Modi, M.W., Farid, A., Berthold, W., and Graves, M. (2001) Rational design of a potent, long-lasting form of interferon: a 40 kDa branched polyethylene glycol-conjugated interferon α-2a for the treatment of hepatitis C. *Bioconjug. Chem.*, **12**, 195–202.
121. Filpula, D., Yang, K., Basu, A., Hassan, R., Xiang, L., Zhang, Z., Wang, M., Wang, Q., Ho, M., Beers, R., Zhao, H., Peng, P., Zhou, J., Li, X., Petti, G., Janjua, A., Liu, J., Wu, D., Yu, D., Zhang, Z., Longley, C., FitzGerald, D., Kreitman, R.J., and Pastan, I. (2007) Releasable PEGylation of mesothelin targeted immunotoxin SS1P achieves single dosage complete regression of a human carcinoma in mice. *Bioconjug. Chem.*, **18**, 773–784.
122. Duncan, R. (2006) Polymer conjugates as anticancer nanomedicines. *Nat. Rev. Cancer*, **6**, 688–701.
123. Hadfield, A.F. and Sartorelli, A.C. (1984) The pharmacology of prodrugs of 5-fluorouracil and 1-beta-D-arabinofuranosylcytosine. *Adv. Pharmacol. Chemother.*, **20**, 21–67.
124. Fadl, T.A., Hasegawa, T., Youssef, A., Farag, H., Omar, F., and Kawaguchi, T. (1995) Synthesis and investigation of N^4-substituted cytarabine derivatives as prodrugs. *Pharmazie*, **50**, 382–387.
125. Wipf, P., Wenjie, L., and Vasu, S. (1991) Synthesis of chemoreversible prodrugs of ARA-C. *Bioorg. Med. Chem. Lett.*, **1**, 745–750.
126. Wipf, P., Li, W., Adeyeye, C.M., Rusnak, J.M., and Lazo, J.S. (1996) Synthesis of chemoreversible prodrugs of ara-C with variable time-release profiles. Biological evaluation of their

apoptotic activity. *Bioorg. Med. Chem.*, **4**, 1585–1596.

127. Choe, Y.H., Conover, C.D., Wu, D., Royzen, M., and Greenwald, R.B. (2002) Anticancer drug delivery systems: N^4-acyl poly(ethyleneglycol) prodrugs of ara-C I. Efficacy in solid tumors. *J. Control. Release*, **79**, 41–53.

128. Choe, Y.H., Conover, C.D., Wu, D., Royzen, M., Gervacio, Y., Borowski, V., Mehlig, M., and Greenwald, R.B. (2002) Anticancer drug delivery systems: multi-loaded N^4-acyl poly(ethylene glycol) prodrugs of ara-C. II. Efficacy in ascites and solid tumors. *J. Control. Release*, **79**, 55–70.

129. Rodrigues, P.C., Beyer, U., Schumacher, P., Roth, T., Fiebig, H.H., Unger, C., Messori, L., Orioli, P., Paper, D.H., Mülhaupt, R., and Kratz, F. (1999) Acid-sensitive polyethylene glycol conjugates of doxorubicin: preparation, *in vitro* efficacy and intracellular distribution. *Bioorg. Med. Chem.*, **7**, 2517–2524.

130. Choi, S.H., Lee, H., and Park, T.G. (2003) PEGylation of G-CSF using cleavable oligo-lactic acid linkage. *J. Control. Release*, **89**, 271–284.

131. Ferruti, P., Tanzi, M.C., Rusconi, L., and Cecchi, R. (1981) Succinic half-esters of poly(ethylene glycol)s and their benzotriazole and imidazole derivatives as oligomeric drug-binding matrixes. *Makromol. Chem.*, **182**, 2183–2192.

132. Tsubery, H., Mironchik, M., Fridkin, M., and Shechter, Y. (2004) Prolonging the action of protein and peptide drugs by a novel approach of reversible polyethylene glycol modification. *J. Biol. Chem.*, **279**, 38118–38124.

133. Shechter, Y., Tsubery, H., Mironchik, M., Rubinstein, M., and Fridkin, M. (2005) Reversible PEGylation of peptide YY3-36 prolongs its inhibition of food intake in mice. *FEBS Lett.*, **579**, 2439–2444.

134. Peleg-Shulman, T., Tsubery, H., Mironchik, M., Fridkin, M., Schreiber, G., and Shechter, Y. (2004) Reversible PEGylation: a novel technology to release native interferon $\alpha 2$ over a prolonged time period. *J. Med. Chem.*, **47**, 4897–4904.

135. Zalipsky, S., Qazen, M., Walker, J.A. II, Mullah, N., Quinn, Y.P., and Huang, S.K. (1999) New detachable poly(ethylene glycol) conjugates: cysteine-cleavable lipopolymers regenerating natural phospholipid, diacyl phosphatidylethanolamine. *Bioconjug. Chem.*, **10**, 703–707.

136. Pomroy, N.C. and Deber, C.M. (1998) Solubilization of hydrophobic peptides by reversible cysteine PEGylation. *Biochem. Biophys. Res. Commun.*, **245**, 618–621.

137. Woghiren, C., Sharma, B., and Stein, S. (1993) Protected thiol-polyethylene glycol: a new activated polymer for reversible protein modification. *Bioconjug. Chem.*, **4**, 314–318.

138. Zhao, X. and Harris, J.M. (1997) Novel degradable poly(ethylene glycol) esters for drug delivery in *Poly(ethylene Glycol) Chemistry and Biological Applications*, ACS Symposium Series 680 (eds J.M. Harris and S. Zalipsky), American Chemical Society, Washington, DC, pp. 458–472.

139. Roberts, M.J. and Harris, J.M. (1998) Attachment of degradable poly(ethylene glycol) to proteins has the potential to increase therapeutic efficacy. *J. Pharm. Sci.*, **87**, 1440–1445.

140. Garman, A.J. and Kalindjian, S.B. (1987) The preparation and properties of novel reversible polymer–protein conjugates. 2-ω-Methoxypolyethylene (5000) glycoxymethylene-3-methylmaleyl conjugates of plasminogen activators. *FEBS Lett.*, **223**, 361–365.

22
Thermo-Responsive Polymers

Drazen Raucher and Shama Moktan

22.1
Introduction

Cancer is a complex disease, and in addition to forming locally aggressive tumor as it progresses, cancer cells from primary tumors may invade the lungs, liver, brain, and other organs. The failure to achieve control of localized cancers is associated not only with the potential morbidity of local recurrence, but also a higher propensity to develop metastatic disease. Tumor cell metastasis is a major cause of death amongst cancer patients. Therefore, it is necessary to contain locally and to treat effectively primary solid tumors. Current treatment for solid tumors is limited by the fact that only a small percentage of the administered drug dose reaches the tumor site, while the rest of the drug is distributed throughout the body, thereby leading to increased toxicity in normal tissues. Since traditional therapies (such as radical surgery or radiation therapy) applied either alone or in combination often fail to eradicate local tumors, it is necessary to consider alternative, novel therapies.

Solid tumors have unique pathophysiological characteristics. Unlike normal tissue, tumors haphazardly undergo angiogenesis that is characterized by aberrant branching and twisted, leaky blood vessels. Additionally, this irregular vasculature leads to impaired lymphatic drainage. Tumors also inappropriately produce a number of permeability mediators and growth factors. All these factors will lead to uneven and slow blood flow, and abnormal fluid dynamics, especially for macromolecules and drug–polymer conjugates, which will tend to preferentially accumulate in tumor tissues. This property is defined as the enhanced permeability and retention (EPR) effect [1–3], and it is the key to the clinical success of passive targeting of anticancer macromolecular drug carriers to solid tumors. Passive targeting exploits the specific tumor architecture that preferentially traps and retains macromolecular drug carriers, thus diminishing systemic toxicity associated with carrier-free drug delivery. Many different systems, such as liposomes, micro- and nanoparticles, and macromolecular prodrugs, have been developed to utilize this passive targeting principle (reviewed in [4–6]) in the treatment of solid tumors. Several natural and synthetic water-soluble polymers, such as poly(ethylene

Drug Delivery in Oncology: From Basic Research to Cancer Therapy, First Edition.
Edited by Felix Kratz, Peter Senter, and Henning Steinhagen.
© 2012 Wiley-VCH Verlag GmbH & Co. KGaA. Published 2012 by Wiley-VCH Verlag GmbH & Co. KGaA.

glycol) (PEG), dextrans, and N-(2-hydroxypropyl)methacrylamide copolymers, are in clinical trials (reviewed in [3, 7, 8]).

The application of polymer carriers not only increases specificity in drug delivery by these passively targeting drugs to solid tumors, but may also enhance tissue selectivity by actively directing the release or accumulation of the drug at the tumor site. Polymers that respond to external stimuli in order to actively target drugs are called stimuli-responsive polymers. These polymers respond to small or modest environmental changes. Changes in light, salt concentration, pH, or temperature may contribute to the solubility and/or conformation, due to alteration of the hydrophobic/hydrophilic equilibrium of the polymer carrier. These solubility and conformational effects may lead to local accumulation of polymeric drug carrier and/or drug release in tissues or organs where external stimulus is applied. This chapter will focus on temperature as an external stimulus, and it will cover the basic principles and selected thermo-responsive polymers.

In addition to longer circulation time, improved pharmacokinetics, and potential for passive tumor targeting, thermo-responsive polymers that undergo a lower critical solution temperature (LCST) phase transition are also capable of thermal targeting to externally heated tumors. These polymers are soluble in aqueous solution below their LCST, but at temperatures above their LCST there polymers undergo an inverse phase transition and hydrophobic collapse, and form insoluble aggregates. Therefore, the main hypothesis of thermo-responsive drug–polymer systems is that intravenously delivered thermo-responsive polypeptides are likely to be cleared under physiological conditions (37 °C). However, they will accumulate in solid tumors where externally induced local heat (40–42 °C) is applied (Figure 22.1). Thermo-responsive polymers are designed to have a LCST between 40 and 42 °C, because this temperature is higher than physiological body temperature (37 °C), but lower than the temperature that is commonly used for hyperthermia treatment in cancer patients.

22.2
Hyperthermia in Cancer Treatment

Hyperthermia is a noninvasive method of increasing tumor temperature to enhance oxygenation, stimulate blood flow, and sensitize cancer cells to chemotherapy and radiation. Hyperthermia has been introduced in the treatment of glioblastoma, head and neck cancer, breast cancer, cancer of the gastrointestinal or urogenital tract, and sarcomas (reviewed in [9–11]). At present, hyperthermia is used in multimodal tumor therapy approaches, combined with chemotherapy or radiochemotherapy. Randomized clinical trials have shown that hyperthermia is a very potent radio- as well as chemo-sensitizer and results in improved disease-free survival and local tumor control. Due to the significant technical improvements that have allowed selective heating of superficial and deep-seated tumors, and thermal mapping of tumors with magnetic resonance imaging (MRI), hyperthermia is becoming more accepted clinically. Hyperthermia is accomplished using microwave,

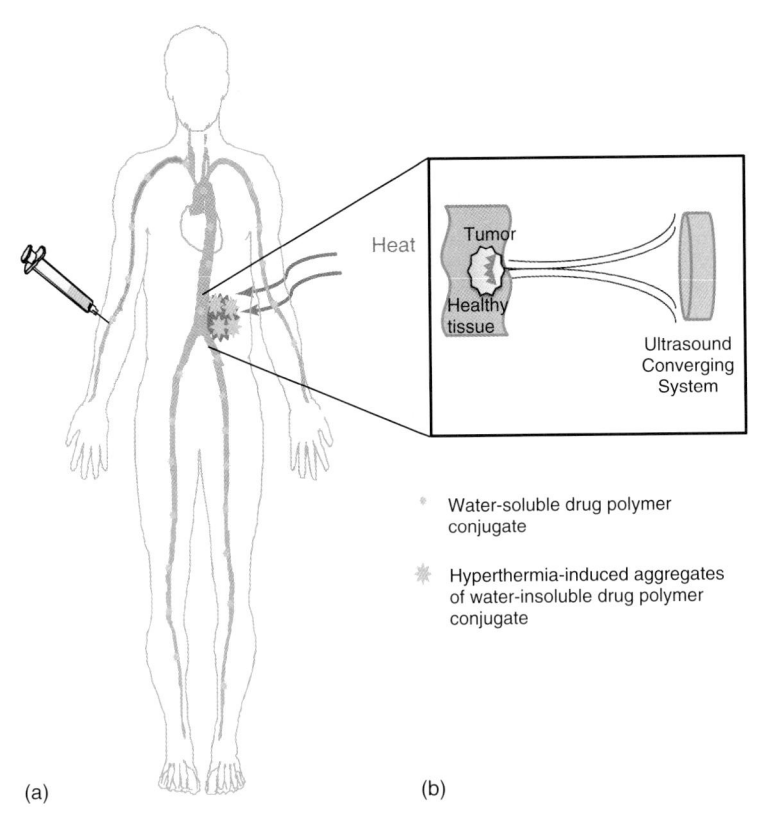

Figure 22.1 Thermo-responsive polymers as anticancer delivery vehicles. (a) Intravenously delivered thermo-responsive polymers carrying anticancer therapeutics (green) are likely to have low blood concentration and they will be rapidly cleared under physiological conditions ($T < T_t$). However, they will aggregate at heated sites (red colored area) where $T > T_t$, allowing preferential accumulation of anticancer drugs at the heated area. (b) Schematic diagram of an ultrasound-based heating system that can be used to precisely focus heat in the tumor area.

radiofrequency, and high-intensity focused ultrasound (HIFU). Of these, HIFU technology has garnered much attention because it is emerging as a potentially noninvasive modality for the treatment of many solid tumors. In HIFU-mediated thermal ablation, a high-intensity convergent ultrasound beam is generated by high-power transducers to produce heat. As an acoustic wave propagates through the tissue, part of it is absorbed and converted to heat [12]. With focused beams, a small area of interest can be precisely heated deep in tissues (Figure 22.2a). As the target tumor tissue accumulates heat, it overtime leads to lesion formation and subsequently coagulative necrosis [13]. What makes HIFU even more attractive is that it can be coupled with ultrasound or MRI to monitor the change in tumor volume to precisely guide HIFU treatment (Figure 22.2b). These imaging systems can also be useful in monitoring the progression of tissue damage due to treatment

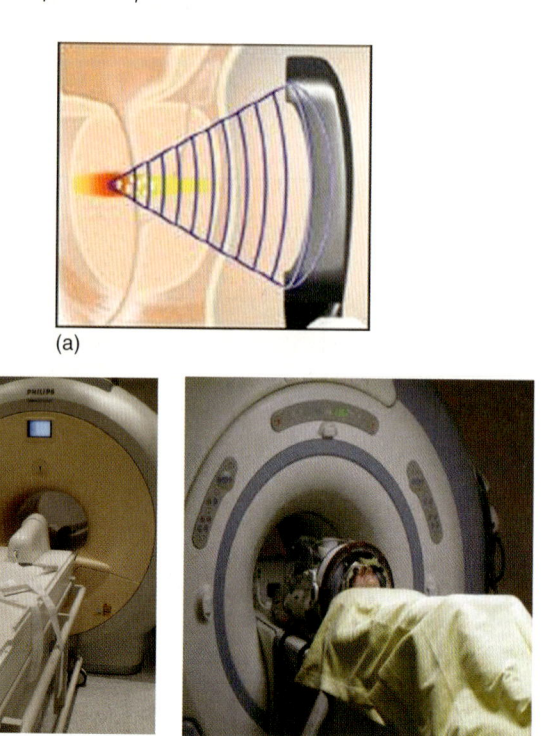

Figure 22.2 HIFU. (a) Schematic of HIFU transducers that focus a high-intensity ultrasound beam to a specific point in tissue to generate localized heat. (b) MRI-guided HIFU can progressively scan HIFU treatment in real-time, allowing for precise control of hyperthermia temperatures.

in real-time. HIFU exposure settings can be optimized to produce mild hyperthermia temperatures (around 42 °C) for thermal targeting of thermo-responsive drug polymers [14].

Consequently the methods and techniques necessary to employ thermal targeting of thermo-responsive polymers are already available in the clinical setting.

22.3
Synergistic Advantages of Combining Thermo-Responsive Polymers and Hyperthermia

There are several advantages to using thermo-responsive polymers in combination with hyperthermia. One advantage is that hyperthermia increases the permeability of the tumor vasculature more than the normal vasculature and therefore will enhance the preferential delivery of drugs by thermo-responsive carriers to tumors [15–17]. A second advantage is that with appropriate sources of hyperthermia and selective local heating, thermo-responsive polymers can target solid tumors in any organ or tissue. Furthermore, due to abnormal tumor vasculature, aberrant vascular architecture, and insufficient lymphatic drainage, tumors cannot perfuse heat adequately. Consequently heat dissipation is slower in tumors than that in normal tissues, and as the temperature of the tumor continues to rise, tumor targeting and retention of thermo-responsive polymer drug carriers are enhanced. Finally, the significant advantage of these polypeptides over other thermally sensitive carriers, such as temperature-sensitive liposomes [18], is that accumulation of the drug in the target tissue occurs through the LCST transition of the carrier rather than through heat-triggered release of the drug. Unlike other delivery systems, a concentration gradient is therefore not required to drive thermo-responsive polymers into the heated tumor. Even when the blood concentration is less than the total concentration in the tumor, thermo-responsive polypeptides continue to accumulate because of aggregation in the heated tumor and alteration of its parent form. Therefore, the polypeptide–drug conjugate may be injected at a low concentration systemically, while still achieving a higher concentration in the tumor. The strategy of using thermo-responsive polymers in conjunction with hyperthermia is therefore very promising for the delivery of anticancer drugs to solid tumors

22.4
Selected Thermo-Responsive Polymer Classes

22.4.1
Synthetic Polymers

Synthetic polymers are of increasing interest in targeted drug delivery systems as their therapeutic values are being vigorously investigated. Like their biological counterparts, thermo-responsive synthetic polymers also display LCSTs in aqueous solution. Therefore, a thermo-responsive polymer undergoes a phase transition from being water soluble at temperatures below its LCST to being water insoluble at temperatures above its LCST. This unique physiochemical behavior is attributed primarily to gains in entropy following increases in temperature. Thermally sensitive synthetic polymers can be employed as drug delivery systems because increases in temperature beyond the polymer's LCST will trigger a phase transition, make the polymer water insoluble, and thereby expel any drug that may be entrapped within the structure (Figure 22.3). A few prominent examples of thermo-responsive synthetic polymers are highlighted here.

22.4.2
N-Isopropylacrylamide-Based Polymers

N-Isopropylacrylamide (NIPAAm) (Figure 22.4a) is the building block of one of the most studied temperature-sensitive synthetic polymeric carrier systems, poly(NIPAAm) (PNIPAAm). With a phase transition temperature between 30 and

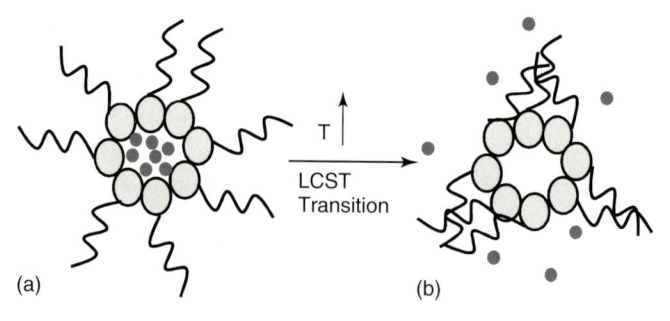

Figure 22.3 Schematics of a thermo-responsive PNIPAAm-based drug delivery micelle. (a) Below its LCST, the micelle exists in a soluble form entrapping the drug. (b) Above its LCST, the micelle structure collapses, releasing the entrapped drug.

Figure 22.4 Chemical structures of selected thermo-responsive synthetic polymers. (a) PNIPAAm, (b) PEO, and (c) PPZ.

34 °C [19, 20], PNIPAAm is an excellent candidate for therapeutic drug delivery. It is hydrated and displays an extended coil conformation below the LCST, whereas it becomes dehydrated and displays a globular conformation above the LCST. Cross-linked PNIPAAm chains known as "hydrogels" provide an excellent meshwork to entrap small-molecule chemotherapeutics. PNIPAAm hydrogels display water-soluble swelling behavior below the LCST and water-insoluble deswelling behavior above the LCST; therefore, drugs remain entrapped below the LCST and are expelled above the LCST. The LCST of PNIPAAm hydrogels can be modified by the addition of a hydrophobic or hydrophilic group. The former decreases the LCST, whereas the latter increases the LCST. When the LCST of a PNIPAAm drug delivery system is close to body temperature, it will remain aqueous at room temperature; however, it will deswell at body temperature upon injection in response to a temperature-triggered phase transition. The advantage of such a system is the "smart" release of the drug cargo at the injection site where a subcutaneous tumor is located. However, a potential problem with an injectable hydrogel system is premature gel formation, inhibiting the drug from reaching deep tissue [21]. Furthermore homomers or copolymers of PNIPAAm are not amenable for physiological use because they are toxic and not biodegradable [22]. Therefore, temperature-responsive

PNIPAAm polymer chains are often complexed with biodegradable polymers to form microspheres or micellar drug delivery systems.

PNIPAAm, which is a weak poly-acid, can be copolymerized with other proton-accepting polymer segments to form amphiphilic block copolymers that self-assemble into a biodegradable micellar system. The advantage of such a system is the encapsulation of chemotherapeutic agents that are stable and water soluble. This is especially important when delivering drugs that have no or limited aqueous solubility. PNIPAAm-based drug carriers are synthesized by first dissolving the participating block copolymers of PNIPAAm and a second polymer in a suitable solvent along with the drug of choice. Stable micelles are then prepared by dialyzing the sample against water and forcing the hydrophobic segments of the block copolymers to self-interact, as well as to interact with the drugs. This essentially leads to micelle formation with the hydrophobic groups forming the inner core (encapsulating the drug) and the PNIPAAm chain forming the outer hydrophilic shell. An alternative to this method of synthesizing drug-loaded micelles is to heat the mixture of drug and block copolymers close to the LCST, and then to slowly cool down the solution to room temperature in the presence of the drug, allowing the drug to be entrapped within the micelle core. Below its LCST, such a micelle would remain structurally stable, entrapping the drug (Figure 22.3a); however, above its LCST, a hyperthermia-triggered change in PNIPAAm structure would collapse the micelle, facilitating the controlled release of the drug at the target site (Figure 22.3b). The composition of the hydrophobic block, the chain length, and the molar ratio of the hydrophobic and the thermo-responsive blocks are essential for the design of a physiologically relevant drug delivery system.

Typically, the LCST of a polymeric drug delivery system is modified to clinically relevant temperatures so that the phase transition can occur slightly above body temperature. In this way the system remains aqueous at room temperature; however, when injected into the body, its structure collapses in response to focused localized hyperthermia at the tumor site, effectively releasing the drug cargo. Therefore, a thermo-responsive PNIPAAm-based polymer system cannot only be targeted to the tumor by passive targeting due to the EPR effect, it can also be targeted to the tumor by active targeting through the application of mild hyperthermia at the tumor site. Since the hydrophobic core is constructed of biodegradable polymers, the eventual decrease in the overall polymer molecular weight will result in easier elimination from the body. PNIPAAm-based hydrogels, microspheres, and micelles have been developed as temperature-sensitive drug delivery systems. A summary of examples of these systems specific to the delivery of chemotherapeutic agents in diverse cell culture and/or preclinical studies is shown in Table 22.1.

There are other polymers, like PNIPAAm, that also exhibit temperature sensitive behavior through the LCST phenomenon. Most notable are poly(N-vinylcaprolactam) (PVCL), PEG, poly(ethylene oxide) (PEO), and poly(propylene oxide) (PPO).

Table 22.1 Illustrative examples of PNIPAAm-based temperature-sensitive carriers of chemotherapeutics.

Nanocarrier type	Polymer	Drug	LCST (°C)	Therapeutic outcome	References
Hydrogel	PEG and PNIPAAm-co-n-butyl methacrylate	DOX	20	subcutaneous injection of a single dose of 5 mg/kg of DOX-hydrogel inhibited the tumor growth of a U87MG xenograft and decreased the tumor weight by about 6-fold compared to the untreated controls and about 5-fold compared to the free DOX treatment	[23]
Micelle	(PNIPAAm-co-acrylamide)-b-poly(DL-lactide)	docetaxel	41	in combination with hyperthermia, intravenous injection resulted in a superior antitumor activity against subcutaneous Lewis lung carcinoma tumor xenograft in C57BL/6 mice with reduced weight loss compared to equivalent free docetaxel dose (Figure 22.5)	[24]
Micelle	(PNIPAAm-co-acrylamide)-b-poly(DL-lactide)	docetaxel and paclitaxel	39.8 39.7	inhibition of more than 80% of the tumor volume in a human gastric BGC mouse xenograft model	[25]
Micelle	PLLA-sb-PNIPAAm	methotrexate	31	90% sustained release of the drug was observed at 37°C in vitro	[26]

22.4.3
PEO-Based Polymers

Temperature-sensitive diblock and triblock copolymers of PEO and poly(L-lactic acid) (PLLA) are soluble at 45 °C so drug loading is done at this higher temperature. For the chemical structure of PEO, see Figure 22.4b. When this soluble system is injected into the body (37 °C), it gels, and facilitates the sustained and controlled release of the entrapped drug [22]. PLLA is a hydrophobic block and forms the hydrophobic core of the resulting micelle structure. At the same time it is also biodegradable so that its biodegradation leads to a decrease in the molecular weight of the overall system, facilitating elimination from the body. The sol–gel transition temperature is dependent on both the concentration and composition

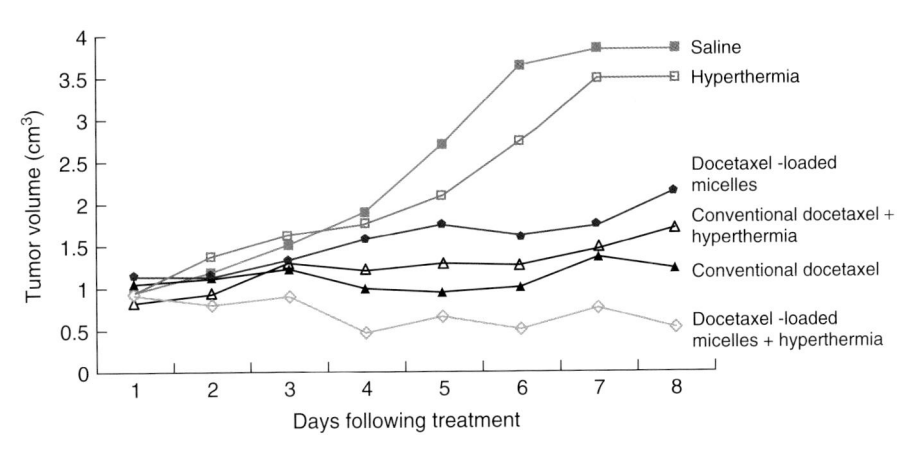

Figure 22.5 Antitumor effect of PNIPAAm-based thermo-sensitive docetaxel. Mice bearing Lewis lung carcinoma xenografts were treated intravenously through the tail vein with 20 mg/kg/day of conventional docetaxel, or 74 mg/kg/day of docetaxel-loaded micelles on days 0, 4, and 8 with or without hyperthermia. Control groups were given saline with or without hyperthermia. After injection, hyperthermia was achieved by totally immersing the tumor-bearing limb of the animal in a water bath at 43 °C for 30 min [24]. Needs permission to print the figure.

of the block copolymers. The copolymers along with the chemotherapeutic agent of interest can be dissolved at higher temperatures to form polymeric micelles owing to the hydrophobic interaction of the PLLA blocks. Upon cooling to lower temperatures, the micelles aggregate and form gels. In the case of the PEO–PLLA triblock copolymers, the polymeric micelles of a model drug (fluorescein isocyanate (FITC)–dextran, M_r 20 kDa) were formulated above the body temperature (45 °C). When the system was injected into rats (37 °C), the micelles aggregated and formed gels, which precipitated a sustained release of the incorporated dextran. The more hydrophobic the entrapped drug is, the longer it is anticipated to get released in an aqueous environment. A major drawback of this system is that it can only be applied to treat subcutaneous tumors as gel formation occurs *in situ* upon injection. Furthermore, mixing of the drug delivery system at higher temperatures could denature biological therapeutics, such as proteins and peptides and unstable chemotherapeutic drugs.

A large variety of PEO and PPO block copolymers commercially known as poloxamers (or under the tradename Pluronics) exhibit phase transitions as well [27]. The $PEO_x - PPO_y - PEO_x$ triblock copolymers with various molecular weights and PEG/PEO ratios were originally developed as surfactants to be used in the pharmaceutical industry. The LCST of Pluronic copolymers vary with the PEO content and the overall polymer concentration. The LCST increases with increase in the PEO content. For drug delivery purposes, copolymers that have LCSTs ranging from about 20 to 40 °C are mostly used [28]. For the most part, the LCST behavior is mainly applied to synthesize polymeric drug micelles and not necessarily to thermally target the drug to the tumor. Micelle formation of the copolymers occurs at concentrations above the critical micelle concentration (CMC). In aqueous solutions above the CMC, the copolymers self-assemble into a micelle composed of a core of PPO and a shell of PEO. Solute molecules that are incorporated within the micelle core are transferred to the surrounding aqueous environment until equilibrium is reached due to the dynamic partitioning of the incorporated molecule within the micelle and in the surrounding environment [29]. Injectable Pluronic drugs can in effect be released over a longer time period, with reports of 17% of initial dose of the polymer still being found in circulation 19 h postadministration. Drug micelle complex are prepared by (i) injecting the drug solution (solvent has to be water miscible) into the micelle solution of Pluronic, (ii) dissolving the drug and the block copolymer first in a common organic solvent, then adding the aqueous component, followed by removal of the organic solvent by dialysis or evaporation, or (iii) evaporating the organic solvent from a solution mix of the drug and the block copolymer to generate a dry film of the mixture, which can then be micellized in an aqueous media [29].

For application in cancer therapy, Pluronic® F127 or poloxamer 407 has been extensively investigated for the thermo-sensitive *in situ* delivery of various chemotherapeutics. Pluronic F127 (M_r 12.6 kDa) consists of 200.45 average number of PEO units and 65.17 average number of PPO units. A 20 wt% (0.5–1.0 mg/ml) Pluronic F127 gels at 25 °C so that it exists as a mobile viscous liquid at room temperature and transforms into a semisolid transparent gel at body temperature. Therefore, this formulation of Pluronic F127 is widely used for the topical delivery of chemotherapeutics. Intratumoral delivery of docetaxel-loaded mixed micelles of Pluronic F127 and Tween 80 increased the pharmacokinetics of the drug in SKOV-3 ovarian tumor xenograft mice (more than 6 days postinjection) as shown in Figure 22.6 [30]. Likewise the intratumoral administration of Pluronic F127 formulation of paclitaxel delayed the growth rate of B16F1 melanoma tumors in mice and was associated with better survival (91%) compared to the control group (58%) [31]. Pluronic F127 was also applied in mice bearing colon CT-26 subcutaneous tumors. The study showed that Pluronic F127 could be thermally targeted to the tumor region by the application of mild hyperthermia. The heated tumor had 2.5-fold greater release of the cargo than the nonheated tumors [32]. Intrapertioneal injection of Pluronic F127 also resulted in sustained release of mitomycin that resulted in the enhancement of the therapeutic effects of mitomycin against a sarcoma-180 ascites tumor in mice [33].

Pluronic systems enhance drug stability and drug solubility, and facilitate a sustained drug release. Furthermore, depending on the composition, the hydrodynamic radii of Pluronic micelles range from 20 to 100 nm, which is within the optimum range of passive targeting due to the EPR effect. Therefore, drug-loaded Pluronic systems are attractive chemotherapeutics. Although not used as a thermo-responsive formulation, the most prominent Pluronic-based drug delivery system is SP1049C (Supratek Pharma, Montreal, CA), which is doxorubicin (DOX) formulated with the mixed micelle of Pluronics L61 and F127. This micelle formulation of DOX has recently completed phase II clinical trials in patients with

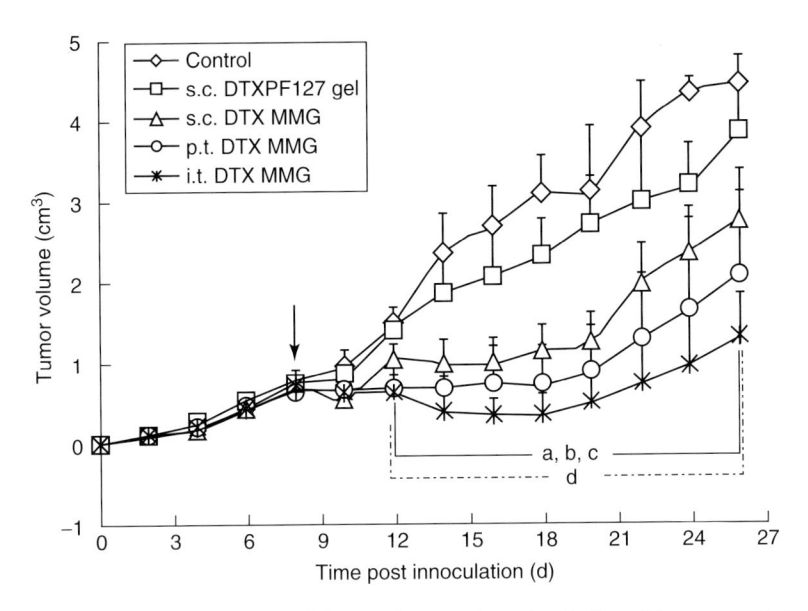

Figure 22.6 Antitumor effect of docetaxel-loaded mixed micelles of Pluronic F127 (PF127) and Tween 80. Mice bearing SKOV-3 ovarian carcinoma xenografts were treated with a single dose of docetaxel (DTX) in mixed micelle gel (MMG) formulation via intratumoral, peritumoral, or subcutaneous injections or docetaxel in PF127 formulation via subcutaneous injections. A dose of 10 mg docetaxel equivalent per kilogram of body weight was given on day 8 after tumor implantation (indicated by an arrow). Animals were sacrificed 18 days after treatment. $^aP < 0.05$, subcutaneous docetaxel MMG versus control at the same timepoint, $^bP < 0.05$, peritumoral docetaxel MMG versus control at the same timepoint, $^cP < 0.05$, intratumoral docetaxel MMG versus control at the same time-point; $^dP < 0.05$, intratumoral docetaxel MMG versus subcutaneous DTX PF127 gel at the same time-point [30].

advanced adenocarcinoma of the esophagus and gastroesophageal junction. The outcome suggests that the drug has significant anticancer activity with minimum safety risk [34]. The completed studies thus far all strongly support that polymer drugs are a strong contender in the next generation of chemotherapeutics.

22.4.4
Poly(Organophosphazene)-Based Polymers

Poly(organophosphazene) (PPZ) (Figure 22.4c) hydrogels that are amphiphilic in nature also exhibit sol–gel phase transition as a function of temperature. For this reason they have also been examined as a thermosensitive drug delivery system. They are biodegradable and nontoxic, making them an attractive for delivery of chemotherapeutics. A PPZ bearing α-amino-ω-methoxy-PEO and hydrophobic L-isoleucine ethyl ester as side-groups was carboxylic acid terminated and conjugated to the 3′-amino position of DOX. This formulation of DOX remained at sol state at room temperature. Upon intratumoral injection, gelation occurred due to the hydrophobic interaction between the side-chain fragments of L-isoleucine ethyl ester. The resulting polymer DOX–conjugate gel localized to the tumor in which DOX was released over a prolonged period of time effectively inhibiting the tumor growth of SNU-601 human gastric cancer in mice [35].

22.4.5
Miscellaneous

There are several other synthetic polymers that undergo phase transitions with transition temperatures ranging from 33 °C for PVCL to 37 °C for poly(methyl vinyl ether) (PMVE) to 62 °C for poly(N-ethyl oxazoline) (PEtOx). A dual-stimuli-responsive diblock copolymer of PEtOx and PLLA was shown to form a micelle [36]. A DOX-loaded PetOx–PLLA micelle was stable at 37 °C and pH 7.4. However, at 37 °C and pH 5.0, DOX was continuously released (about 65% in 24 h) and inhibited cell viability of non-small-cell lung carcinoma CL3 cells.

22.5
Elastin-Like Biopolymers

Derived from the hydrophobic domain of tropoelastin, an elastin-like polypeptide (ELP) is composed of pentapeptide repeats of Val-Pro-Gly-Xaa-Gly (VPGXaaG), where Xaa is any amino acid except proline. ELPs undergo an inverse phase transition at a specified temperature, known as the inverse transition temperature (T_t) [37]. ELPs are structurally disordered and soluble in aqueous solution below their T_t (Figure 22.7a); however, they are desolvated and aggregated above their T_t (Figure 22.7a and b) [38, 39]. This process is fully reversible when the temperature of the media is lowered below T_t. The T_t of ELP is inversely related to the hydrophobicity of the ELP molecule. It is also dependent on chain length of the pentapeptide repeat. Since ELP is genetically encoded, the T_t of ELP can be tuned to any desired temperature by varying the composition and mole fraction of Xaa, which influences the hydrophobicity of the molecule, and the chain length of the pentapeptide repeat [40, 41]. Furthermore, because ELPs are expressed in a bacterial system they can be purified in large quantities by simple inverse transition cycling [42].

22.5.1
ELP Synthesis

ELP constructs with varying molecular weight and hydrophobicity profile are made by recursive directional ligation of oligomers encoding a short (10–16) pentapeptide repeat of the desired ELP in pUC19 [43]. The resulting gene is then cloned in between a translation initiation codon and two termination codons in a pET25b+ expression vector. In addition, a pentapeptide spacer of Ser-Lys-Gly-Pro-Gly is

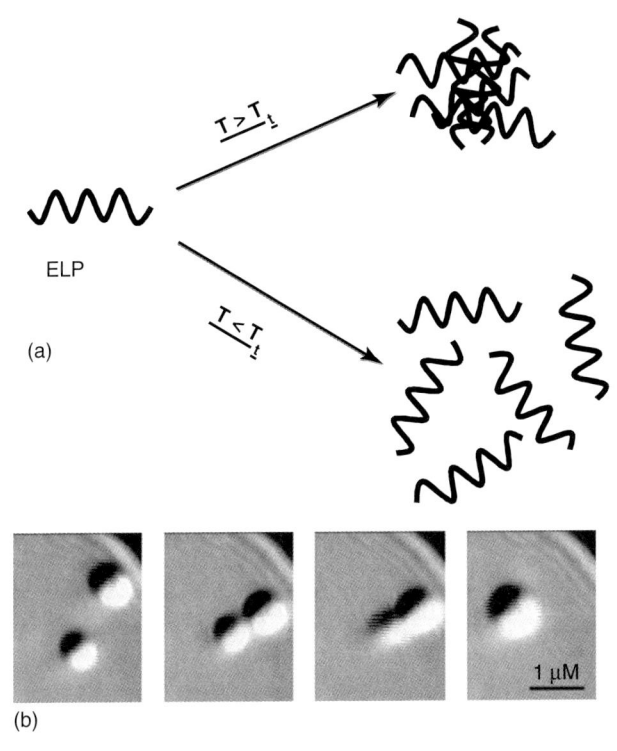

Figure 22.7 Thermo-responsive ELP biopolymer. (a) Schematic representation of the ELP shows that below its T_t it is water soluble; however, above its T_t ELP aggregates. (b) Panel of differential interference microscopy images shows the progression of formation of an aggregate of two ELP molecules in response to rise in temperature beyond the T_t.

encoded at the N-terminus of the ELP sequence and a dipeptide spacer of Trp–Pro is encoded at the C-terminus of the ELP sequence. The polypeptides are eventually expressed in the BLR(DE3) *Escherichia coli* strain. The ELP protein is first separated in the soluble fraction of the cell lysate [44]. It is further purified by repeated inverse thermal cycling procedure [42]. At room temperature the ELP molecules are soluble in an aqueous solution of phosphate-buffered saline (PBS) (Figure 22.8a). When ELP molecules are exposed to a temperature slightly higher than the LCST in a water bath, the solution turns turbid, reflective of ELP aggregation (Figure 22.8b). Centrifugation of this solution will result in the separation of the ELP proteins in the pellet fraction and impurities in the supernatant fraction (Figure 22.8c). The ELP protein pellet can be redissolved in PBS and centrifuged again to remove impurities that are now going to be in the pellet fraction as the room temperature soluble ELP proteins separate in the supernatant fraction. This cycling procedure can be repeated to generate ELP proteins with high purity.

(a) At room temperature; $T < T_t$

(c) After centrifugation

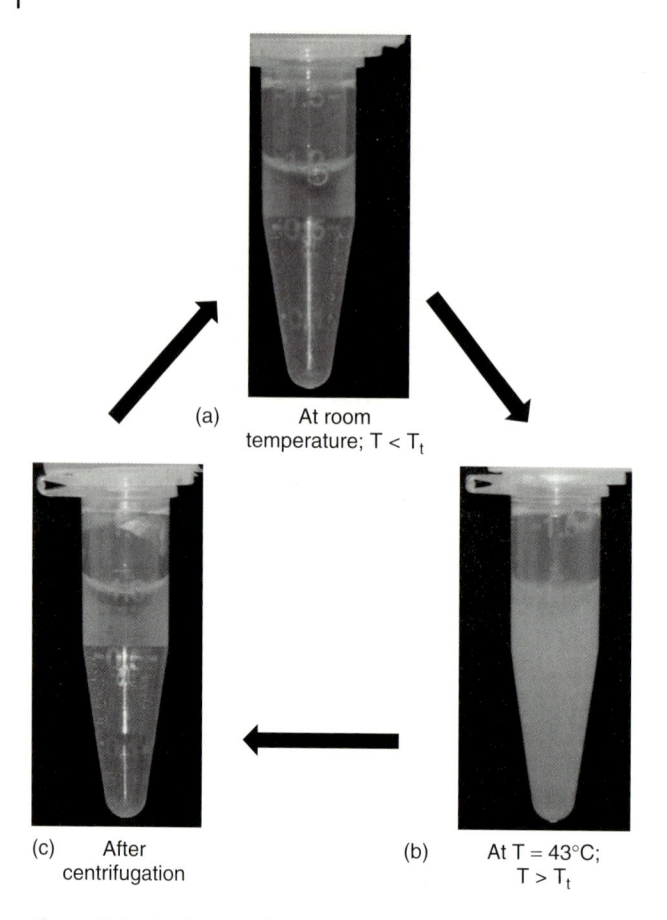

(b) At $T = 43°C$; $T > T_t$

Figure 22.8 Purification of ELPs by inverse thermal cycling. (a) ELPs are soluble at room temperature and exist as a clear solution in PBS. (b) Upon exposure to mild hyperthermia, ELPs aggregate and the solution becomes cloudy. (c) When the turbid ELP solution is centrifuged, ELP aggregates are fractionated in the pellet. Supernatant fraction containing impurities can be decanted. The ELP pellet can be dissolved in PBS, and the cycle can be repeated to obtain ELP proteins of high purity.

22.5.2
Cell-Penetrating Peptides for Intracellular Delivery of ELPs

In order to exhibit therapeutic efficacy and reach intracellular molecular targets in tumor cells, macromolecular drug carriers must successfully overcome the transport barriers, such as tumor microvessel walls and the plasma membrane of the tumor cells. The plasma membrane is impermeable to large hydrophilic compounds, thus making drug carriers such as polypeptides or macromolecules of limited therapeutic value. One approach for delivering polypeptides or macromolecules into target cells is to couple them to cell-penetrating peptides (CPPs). The ELP drug carrier used for thermal targeting (ELP1) has a molecular weight of

22.5 Elastin-Like Biopolymers

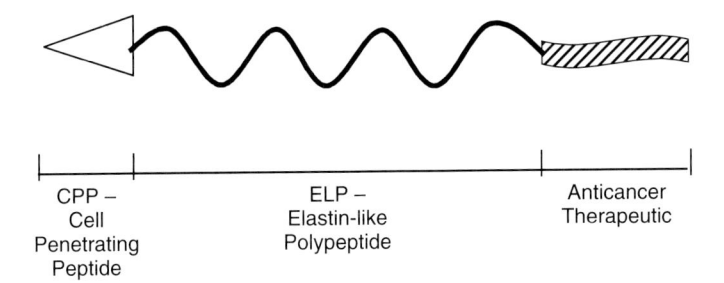

Figure 22.9 Graphical representation of CPP-ELP. The thermo-responsive ELP polypeptide is modified at its N-terminus to contain a CPP to mediate uptake of the macromolecule across the plasma membrane and dictate intracellular localization. A therapeutic peptide is added at the C-terminus.

Table 22.2 CPPs used for intracellular delivery of ELPs.

CPP	Amino acid sequence	References
Pen	RQIKIWFQNRRMKWKK	[46]
Tat	YGRKKRRQRRR	[47]
hMTS	AAVALLPAVLLALLAP	[48]
Bac	RRIRPRPPRLPRPRPRPLPFPRPG	[49]

59.1 kDa [43] and it enters eukaryotic cells at low levels by an endocytic mechanism. To improve the efficiency of tumor penetration and cellular internalization of ELP, ELP was modified at its N-terminus with several CPPs (Figure 22.9) [45]. The sequences of CPPs conjugated to ELP, which are used to deliver various therapeutic peptides, are shown in Table 22.2. Four CPPs were used in previous studies, including penetratin (Pen) peptide from the *Drosophila* transcription factor Antennapedia [46], Tat peptide from the HIV-1 Tat protein [47], membrane translocating sequence (MTS) derived from Kaposi fibroblast growth factor [48], and Bac peptide derived from the bactenecin antimicrobial peptide [49].

22.5.3
Efficiency and Mechanism of CPP-ELP Cellular Uptake

Although CPPs are progressively drawing more interest as a noninvasive delivery technology for peptides, small molecules, macromolecules, proteins, oligonucleotides, liposomes, and nanoparticles, the mechanism of CPP internalization remains elusive. Several mechanisms, such as direct penetration, inverted micelles [50], or simple endocytosis [51, 52], have been proposed. CPPs have been shown to cross cell membranes through an energy-independent, temperature-insensitive mechanism that is not receptor mediated. From previous studies it is clear that the mechanism is dependent on the cargo attached to the CPP (reviewed in [53, 54]). Therefore, improving the efficiency of cellular uptake by fusing ELPs to CPPs and understanding the mechanism of their cellular internalization could contribute to development of new therapeutic approaches. To compare different CPPs, Pen, Tat, and MTS were fused to ELPs, and their efficiency and mechanism of cellular uptake were evaluated [45]. The internalization of all CPP-ELPs was impaired dramatically at 4 °C, under ATP-depletion conditions, indicating that CPP-ELP uptake was temperature and energy dependent. Significant inhibition of polypeptide internalization was also observed when clathrin-coated pits were blocked with hyperosmolar sucrose [55]. However, depletion of the membrane cholesterol and blocking of the clathrin-independent endocytosis via caveolae by using methyl-β-cyclodextrin [56] had very little effect on CPP-ELP internalization, indicating that CPP-ELP internalization occurs via a caveolae-independent endocytic mechanism.

To further investigate the mechanism of internalization, cellular localization of CPP-ELPs was examined by confocal microscopy. Figure 22.10 shows confocal fluorescence images of cells incubated with CPP-ELPs labeled with rhodamine immediately after a 1-h incubation (left panel) and 24 h later (right panel). After 1 h of incubation, little or no fluorescent polypeptides were observed in the cytoplasm and all CPP-ELPs were localized at the plasma membrane as concluded from intense plasma membrane fluorescence. Twenty-four hours later, punctate cytoplasmic aggregates of polypeptides and some uniform diffuse staining of the cytoplasm was observed (right panel). CPP-ELP aggregates were mainly concentrated in the perinuclear region of cells, suggesting that the localization of CPP-ELP polypeptides mainly occurs in endocytotic vesicles.

In light of the findings that only a fraction of CPP-ELPs are internalized at 4 °C or in conditions of depleted intracellular ATP, the internalization of CPP-ELPs cannot be fully explained by an endocytotic mechanism. Therefore, more than one uptake route for CPP-ELPs may be possible and their relative contributions may be CPP dependent.

Further studies including cell growth experiments have shown that the CPP-ELP carrier was able to deliver therapeutics and reach its intracellular target without becoming confined to endosomes. These results were independent of the internalization mechanism and CPP identity.

22.5.4
ELPs for Delivery of Peptides

Peptide therapy is an emerging anticancer approach that exploits bioactive therapeutic peptides to specifically target deregulated proteins in cancer cells. These peptides are designed to block interactions of specific oncogenic proteins with their partners that would otherwise cause uncontrolled cell proliferation. The development of therapeutic peptides has advanced rapidly because these molecules have such diverse activity and show great promise as targeted drugs. They are easily

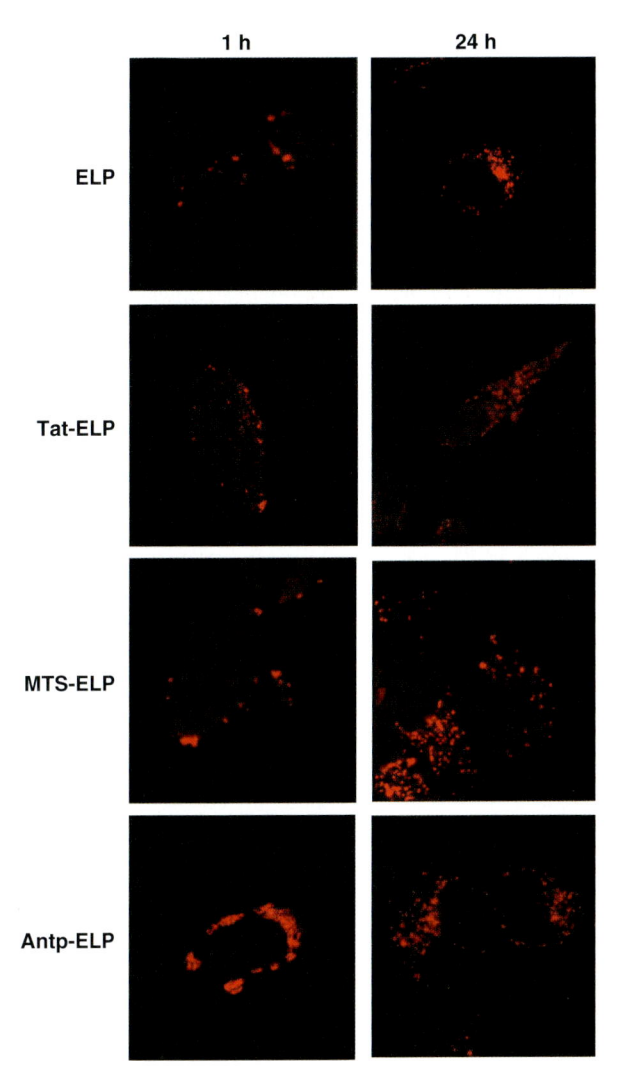

Figure 22.10 Subcellular localization of CPP-ELPs. HeLa cells were treated with rhodamine-labeled CPP-ELP (20 μM) for 1 h at 37°C. Confocal images were taken 1 and 24 h later. Owing to the considerable difference in fluorescence uptake between CPP-ELPs, the gain was adjusted individually during each image acquisition. Image intensities were adjusted for clarity and do not represent the actual level of polypeptide in the cells.

produced, using chemical synthesis or molecular biology techniques, and their sequence is easily modified. When applied *in vivo*, peptides are rapidly degraded in circulation and their charged nature makes them impermeable to cancer cell membranes. Therefore, the utility of therapeutic peptides for cancer therapy is currently limited by poor tumor penetration [57, 58] and pharmacokinetic parameters. As the field of peptide therapy grows, much attention is being focused on improving delivery systems. CPPs can be used to overcome poor tumor and cell membrane penetration, and permit noninvasive delivery of drugs to their appropriate intracellular molecular target. Pharmacokinetics of therapeutic peptides may be improved by using polymers or macromolecules as carriers.

Since it is genetically encoded, an ELP may be easily applied as a targeted macromolecular carrier for therapeutic peptides. Therapeutic peptides can be attached to the ELP by simply modifying the coding sequence, using molecular biology techniques. This approach eliminates the need for expensive peptide synthesis and chemical conjugation of the peptide and the carrier. The genetically encoded nature also allows for expression of the ELP in *E. coli* and large quantities of the molecule can be purified by simple thermal cycling (42). In this chapter we describe the application of CPP-ELP for delivery of a peptide that inhibits the transcriptional activity of the c-Myc oncogene and a peptide that arrests the cell cycle by mimicking the cyclin-dependent kinase (CDK) inhibitor p21.

22.5.5
Delivery of c-Myc Inhibitory Peptides by ELPs

Cell proliferation, differentiation, and survival are regulated by a number of cellular hormones, growth factors, and cytokines in complex organisms. These molecules, such as proto-oncogenes, serve as ligands for cellular receptors and communicate with the nucleus of the cell through a network of intracellular pathways. Although proto-oncogenes have a normal function in growth and differentiation of cells, these genes, when overexpressed or mutated, cause deregulated cell signaling and proliferation, and ultimately cancer. Studies of aberrant oncogene signaling have greatly contributed to our understanding of the molecular mechanisms of tumor maintenance and survival.

One of the oncogenes, c-Myc, is associated with numerous types of human cancer. c-Myc is a transcriptional regulator, and deregulated expression of c-Myc causes uncontrolled cell growth and cancer cell proliferation, confirming its strong oncogenic potential. Therefore, the inhibition of c-Myc transcriptional activity represents an attractive target for tumor therapy. For its oncogenic activity, c-Myc has to dimerize with its partner protein Max. By inhibiting c-Myc and Max interaction, c-Myc transcriptional activity and cancer cell may be inhibited. Peptides that bind only to a specific oncogene, such as c-Myc, would be expected to provide targeted therapy for specific cancer cells that are overexpressing that particular oncogene. To target c-Myc, a peptide that was derived from helix 1 (H1) of the helix–loop–helix region of c-Myc (H1-S6A, F8A) to disrupt the c-Myc signaling pathway was fused to the C-terminus of the ELP carrier. To increase the efficiency of ELP delivery to tumor cells, Pen CPP was added to the N-terminus (Pen-ELP-H1). The addition of a CPP increased cellular uptake of Pen-ELP-H1 3-fold when compared to ELP alone. Furthermore cellular uptake in MCF-7 cells was increased 13-fold when aggregation of the polypeptide was induced by hyperthermia treatment [59]. A single 1-h exposure to the Pen-ELP-H1 polypeptide resulted in a 30% inhibition of the cell proliferation rate. In addition, when the Pen-ELP-H1 treatment was combined with hyperthermia treatment, the antiproliferative effect was enhanced 2-fold (Figure 22.11a).

To investigate the mechanism of inhibition of cell proliferation by Pen-ELP1-H1, the cellular localization of c-Myc and its dimerization partner Max was examined by confocal immunofluorescence microscopy in Pen-ELP1-H1 untreated and treated cells. In untreated cells, Max and c-Myc display primarily a nuclear distribution, and the overlay of images of Max and c-Myc (Figure 22.11b) shows nuclear colocalization of these two proteins, as shown by the yellow color. The localization of c-Myc and Max is unchanged when cells are treated with Pen-ELP1. Treatment of cells with Pen-ELP1-H1 caused redistribution of c-Myc from mostly nuclear to cytoplasmic localization, thus preventing colocalization of c-Myc and Max. Since Pen-ELP1-H1 inhibits c-Myc–Max heterodimerization, it is also expected that it will inhibit c-Myc transcriptional activity. The ability of Pen-ELP1-H1 to inhibit the transcriptional activity of c-Myc was evaluated by assaying expression levels of c-Myc-responsive genes, ornithine decarboxylase (ODC) [60] and lactate dehydrogenase-A (LDH-A) [61]. As shown in Figure 22.11c, treatment with Pen-ELP1-H1 led to a strong decrease in mRNA expression of ODC and LDH-A, whereas glyceraldehyde 3-phosphate dehydrogenase (GAPDH; a gene that is not regulated by c-Myc) mRNA levels were unaffected by the polypeptide treatments. The redistribution of c-Myc from mostly nuclear to cytoplasmic localization and the decreased expression of c-Myc controlled genes suggest the following model shown in Figure 22.12. The binding of ligand to mitogen receptor stimulates production of c-Myc mRNA and c-Myc is translated in the cytoplasm. However, before it enters the nucleus and interacts with Max, newly synthesized c-Myc protein is sequestered by Pen-ELP-H1, which localizes it in the cytoplasm. As a result, expression of c-Myc controlled genes is decreased, which inhibits cancer cell proliferation.

22.5.6
ELP-Based Delivery of a Cell Cycle Inhibitory p21 Mimetic Peptide

Inhibitors of the cell cycle are important anticancer drug candidates because of their potential to restore control of the cell cycle in deregulated cancer cells. $p21^{CIP1/WAF1}$ is a p53-inducible CDK inhibitor protein that plays an important role in the regulation of the cell cycle and cell growth [62]. In an attempt to restore or mimic the inhibitory actions of p21, a peptide derived from the $p21^{CIP1/WAF1}$ [63] was fused to the C-terminus of a thermo-responsive ELP (ELP-p21). Since p21 is a nuclear protein, CPP Bac, which has been shown to deliver ELP to nucleus, was added at the N-terminus of the ELP to form a thermo-responsive therapeutic polypeptide, Bac-ELP-p21. The addition of Bac not only improves tumor and cancer cell membrane translocation, but it also enhances the polypeptide's nuclear delivery and potency. The ability of Bac-ELP1-p21 to inhibit cancer cell proliferation was evaluated in three cancer cells lines: SKOV-3 (ovarian), MCF-7 (breast), and Panc-1 (pancreatic) [64]. As shown in Figure 22.13a, Bac-ELP1-p21 at 37 °C inhibited only 20% of SKOV-3 cells proliferation even at the highest concentration of 40 µM.

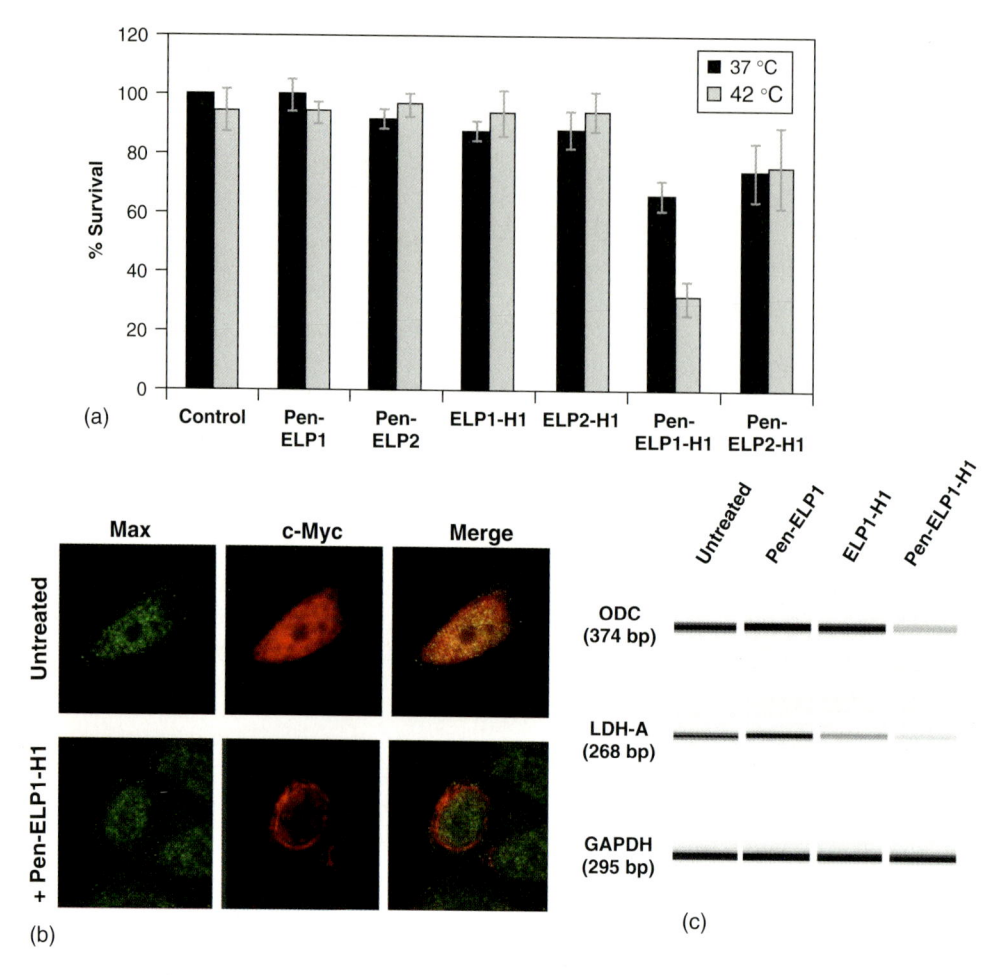

Figure 22.11 Antiproliferative effect of Pen-ELP-H1. (a) Proliferation of MCF-7 cells was determined 11 days after a single 1-h treatment with the indicated polypeptide (18 µM) at 37 or 42 °C. Cells were counted using the Trypan Blue dye-exclusion assay. Results represent the mean ± SE of three to five experiments performed in duplicate. (b) Subcellular localization of c-Myc and Max was determined by confocal immunofluorescence microscopy in untreated cells (top row) and in cells treated with 18 µM Pen-ELP1-H1 (bottom row) for 1 h. Images were taken 24 h after polypeptide treatment with a × 100 oil immersion objective. (c) mRNA levels for the c-Myc-responsive genes ODC (top panel) and LDH-A (middle panel), and a control gene GAPDH (bottom panel) were assayed by reverse transcription-polymerase chain reaction. MCF-7 cells were untreated (lane 1) or treated with 18 µM Pen-ELP1 (lane 2), ELP1-H1 (lane 3), or Pen-ELP1-H1 (lane 4) for 1 h. RNA was purified 48 h after treatment. Polymerase chain reaction products were analyzed by capillary electrophoresis using a Bioanalyzer Labchip with fluorescence detection. The fluorescence data was converted to a simulated gel using Agilent software. The experiment was repeated twice.

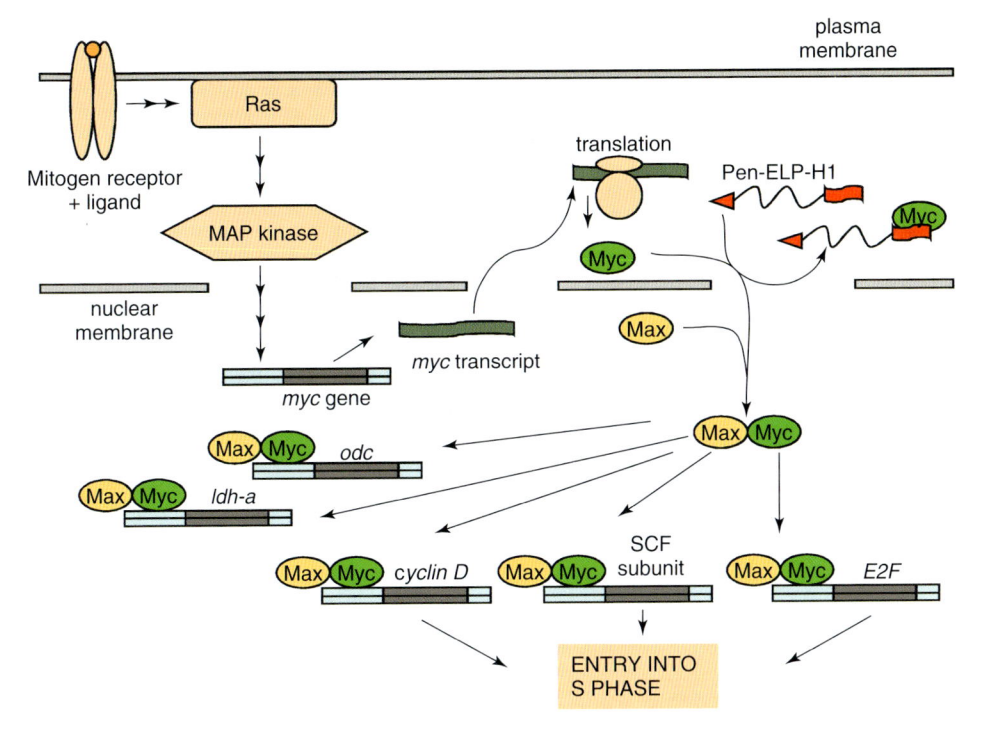

Figure 22.12 Proposed model for c-Myc inhibition by Pen-ELP-H1. Mitogen stimulation induces transcription of mRNA from the c-Myc gene. When cells are treated with Pen-ELP-H1, newly translated c-Myc is bound by the polypeptide in the cytoplasm. Once bound, c-Myc cannot be imported into the nucleus and interact with Max. This results in the downregulation of c-Myc–Max-responsive genes and leads to inhibition of cell proliferation.

However, treatment of the cells with the polypeptide at 42 °C completely inhibited cell proliferation. Bac-ELP1-p21 treatment combined with hyperthermia was also very effective in the inhibition of MCF-7 breast cancer (Figure 22.13a, middle panel) and Panc-1 pancreatic cancer cell proliferation (Figure 22.13a, lower panel). Inhibition of cell proliferation was enhanced primarily by the nuclear localization of the Bac-ELP-p21 construct (Figure 22.13b).

One of the possible targets of p21 cell cycle inhibition is the tumor suppressor protein Rb. In the hypophosphorylated state, Rb inhibits cell cycle progression. When Rb is phosphorylated, it releases transcription factor E2F and cell cycle progression occurs. Therefore, to investigate whether Bac-ELP-p21 causes cell cycle inhibition through inhibition of Rb phosphorylation, pRb levels were determined in cells that were treated with Bac-ELP-p21 (Figure 22.13c). Treatment of the SKOV-3 cells with Bac-ELP1-p21 for 1 h at 42 °C resulted in a decrease in pRb levels as compared to untreated or Bac-ELP1 treated cells. Twenty-four hours after treatment with Bac-ELP1-p21 for 1 h at 42 °C, SKOV-3 cells showed a considerable

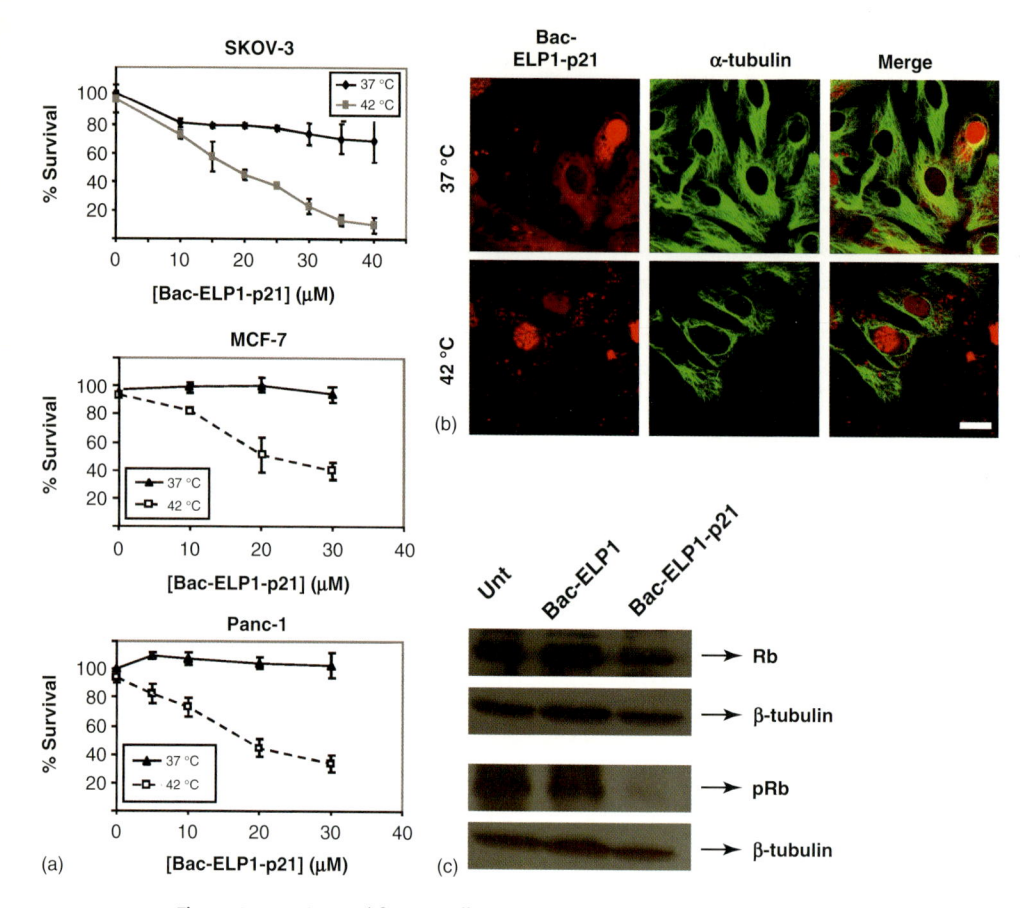

Figure 22.13 Antiproliferative effect Bac-ELP-p21 polypeptides. (a) Inhibition of proliferation by Bac-ELP-p21 was examined in SKOV-3, MCF-7, and Panc-1 cells. Cells were exposed to the indicated concentration of Bac-ELP2-p21 at 37 or 42°C for 1 h and cell proliferation was determined 6 days later (SKOV-3) or 3 days later (MCF-7 and Panc-1) using the 3-(4,5-dimethylthiazol-2-yl)-5-(3-carboxymethoxyphenyl)-2-(4-sulfophenyl)-2H-tetrazolium assay. Data represent the mean ± SE of three independent experiments. (b) Subcellular localization of rhodamine-labeled Bac-ELP1-p21 in SKOV-3 cells was visualized by confocal microscopy. Cells were treated with 20 μM Bac-ELP1-p21 at 37 or 42°C for 1 h. Confocal images were taken 24 h later. Tubulin was stained as a reference for cellular structure. Scale bar = 20 μm. The subcellular distribution of Bac-ELP1-p21 was also confirmed in live cells 24 h after a 1 h exposure at 37 or 42°C (not shown). (c) For sodium dodecyl sulfate–polyacrylamide gel electrophoresis analysis of Rb protein in SKOV-3 cells following treatment with Bac-ELP1-p21, cells were treated with the indicated polypeptide (30 μM) at 42°C for 1 h, harvested 24 h later, and lyzed. Equal amounts of samples were loaded onto a 12% sodium dodecyl sulfate gel and transferred to a blot that was probed with the indicated antibodies.

decrease in the pRb levels as compared to untreated or Bac-ELP1 treated cells. The total Rb level was unchanged and β-tubulin blotting was used to confirm accurate gel loading. These results suggest that Bac-ELP1-p21 most likely inhibits cell proliferation by inhibiting the phosphorylation of the Rb protein and thus blocking the cell cycle.

This cell cycle arrest may also be due to the interaction of various cell cycle regulators, like cyclins and CDKs, with Bac-ELP1-p21 that inhibits complex formation, as modeled in Figure 22.14. Bac-ELP1-p21, which mimics p21 protein, may inhibit interaction of CDK2 with cyclin A and cyclin E, and disrupt cell cycle progression into the S phase. Similarly, the cell cycle can also be arrested in the M phase, by inhibition of the CDC2 and CDK4/6 interaction with cyclin B and cyclin E, respectively. Delivery and therapeutic efficacy of Bac-ELP-p21 is currently being tested in mouse and rat breast cancer models, a mouse ovarian cancer model, and a mouse pancreatic cancer model.

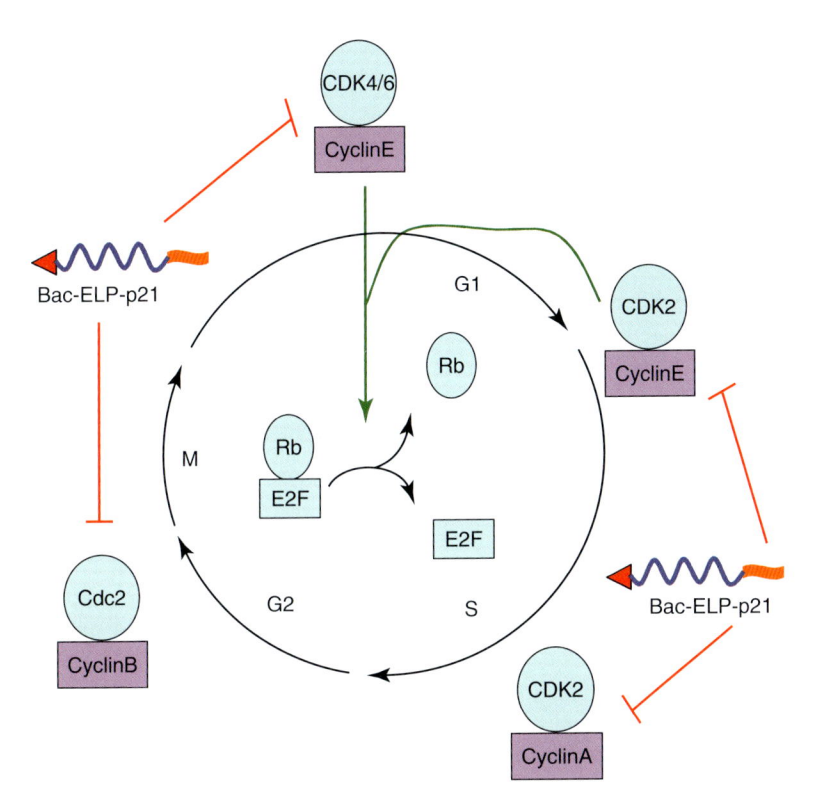

Figure 22.14 Model for cell cycle inhibition by Bac-ELP-fused p21 peptide. Inhibitors of CDKs are important drug candidates because of their potential to restore the inhibitory control of the cell cycle that is frequently lost in cancer cells. The kinase activity of the activated cyclin D1–cdk4 is required to commit cells to the S phase. Bac-ELP-p21 inhibits the kinase activity of cyclin D1–cdk4 and cyclin E–cdk2 by binding to these complexes.

22.5.7
ELP Delivery of Conventional Drugs

The thermo-responsive ELP has also been applied to enhance the delivery of conventional chemotherapeutics in the presence of mild hyperthermia in various cell culture studies, with animal studies underway. Various strategies have been implemented to both conjugate a drug to the ELP and then to release the drug from the ELP once the ELP is inside the cancer cells. A built-in cysteine residue(s) in the C-terminus of the ELP provides an efficient means to conjugate thiol-reactive derivatives of conventional chemotherapeutics. It is crucial that once in the tumor the drug be released from the attached ELP to act on the appropriate cellular target. Two approaches can be taken to facilitate the release of the drug:

1) Derivatize an acid-labile drug that self-cleaves in the acidic environment of the tumor microenvironment and/or in the lysosomes.
2) Incorporate an enzyme-degradable substrate either in the ELP sequence or in the drug structure that gets cleaved by extracellular and/or lysosomal proteases.

Ideally, a cleavage strategy that releases the drug in its native state is most desirable. However, even when a slightly modified DOX was released from a cathepsin cleavable Tat-ELP-GFLG-DOX complex (Figure 22.15), the drug was still potent against cancer cells, especially in the presence of hyperthermia [65]. Furthermore, DOX distribution was mostly seen at the nuclear periphery as opposed to the conventional drug that had mostly nuclear distribution [65]. This clearly indicates that the DOX cleaved from Tat-ELP-GFLG-DOX could have a different mechanism of cytotoxicity compared to the conventional DOX. DOX was coupled to Tat-ELP through a maleimide group on DOX by S-alkylation of the reduced thiol on the ELP to generate a stable thioether Tat-ELP-GFLG-DOX conjugate. The lysosomal protease cathepsin cleavable tetrapeptide linker of Gly-Phe-Leu-Gly was designed upstream of the reactive cysteine residue at the ELP C-terminus (Figure 22.15). Although the free drug was relatively more toxic than the conjugated drug, the latter was highly potent against DOX-resistant uterine sarcoma and breast cancer cells because the DOX conjugate is able circumvent the P-glycoprotein pump [66]. A pH-sensitive hydrazone derivative of a thiol-reactive DOX also displayed similar subcellular localization when delivered by ELP [67]. A maleimide linker composed of succinimidyl-4-(N-maleimidomethyl)cyclohexane-1-carboxylate was used for conjugation with ELP. The cytotoxicity of this formulation of ELP–DOX was comparable to the free drug in a squamous carcinoma cell line. Acid-sensitive ELP–DOX showed 80% drug release over a 72-h period in the presence of low pH (pH 4.0) [68]. These findings demonstrate that ELPs can be used as carriers of chemotherapeutics for selective delivery to tumors.

Characterization of 6-maleimidocaproyl hydrazone derivatives of DOX and paclitaxel conjugated to CPP-ELP in cell culture and in animal models is currently ongoing.

22.5 Elastin-Like Biopolymers | 691

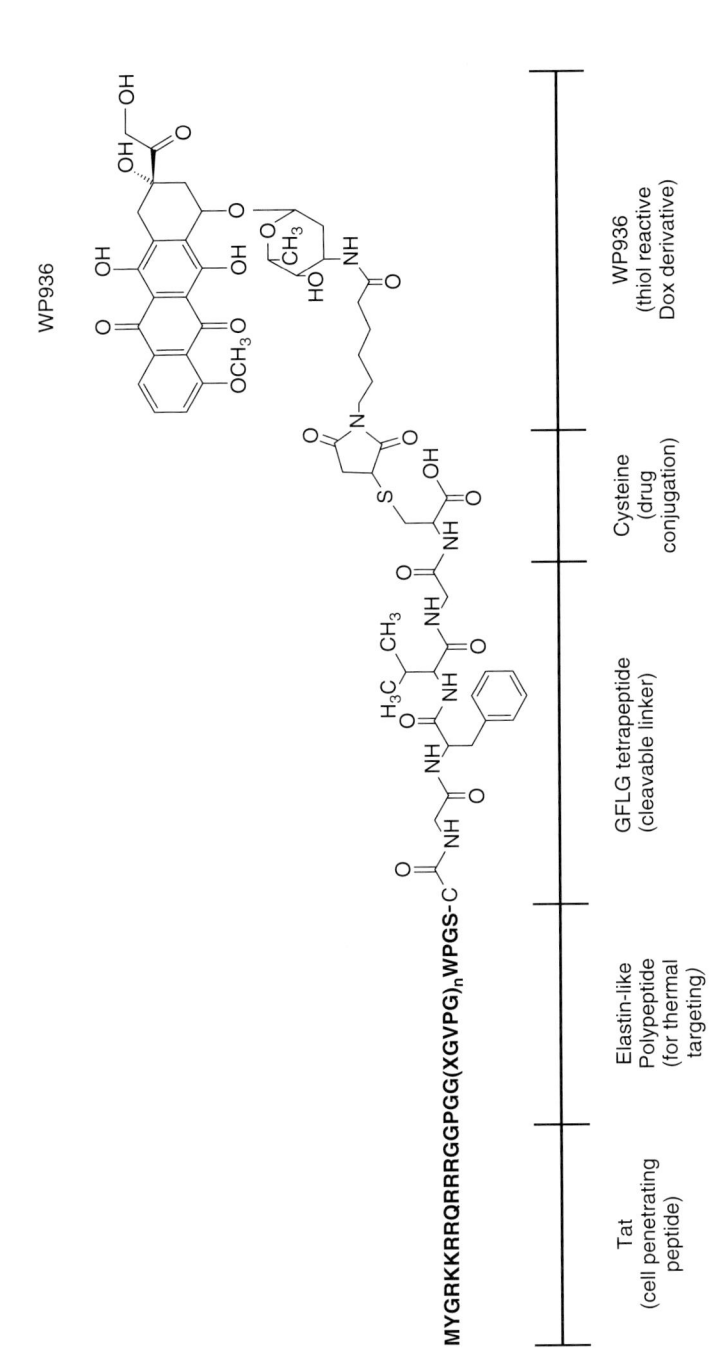

MYGRKKRRQRRRGGPGG(XGVPG)ₙWPGS-C

| Tat (cell penetrating peptide) | Elastin-like Polypeptide (for thermal targeting) | GFLG tetrapeptide (cleavable linker) | Cysteine (drug conjugation) | WP936 (thiol reactive Dox derivative) |

Figure 22.15 Schematic of the Tat-ELP carrier of DOX. The N-terminus of ELP was modified with the addition of the Tat peptide. A tetrapeptide cleavable linker (Gly-Phe-Leu-Gly) was coded in the C-terminus of ELP. A single terminal cysteine residue at the ELP C-terminus was used for the conjugation of a thiol-reactive DOX derivative.

22.5.8
In Vivo Studies with Thermo-Responsive ELP Carriers

ELPs can be thermally targeted to solid tumors by the application of local mild hyperthermia. *In vivo* studies of ELP delivery to human tumors implanted in nude mice demonstrated that focused hyperthermia at the tumor site resulted in a 2-fold increase in tumor localization of ELPs compared to localization without hyperthermia [69]. Over half of the increased accumulation was attributed to the thermally triggered aggregation of the ELP that was caused by the phase transition of the ELP in response to hyperthermia. In our own lab, we have conducted preliminary studies with Tat-ELP-GFLG-DOX in a uterine sarcoma rat xenograft model to evaluate the level of drug–polymer accumulation in locally heated tumors. In this study, the protein component of the drug–polymer conjugate was labeled with ^{125}I. Four hours after injection, tumors that were heated showed approximately 3-fold higher accumulation of Tat-ELP-GFLG-DOX compared to tumors that were left unheated (Figure 22.16). These findings demonstrate that conjugation of anticancer agents to ELPs can result in an enhanced delivery of such agents, due to the combined action of the EPR effect (passive targeting) and hyperthermia (active targeting).

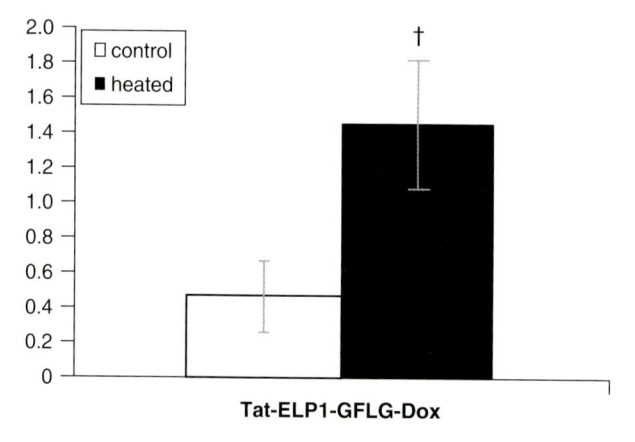

Figure 22.16 Accumulation of Tat-ELP1-GFLG-DOX in MES-SA tumors. ^{125}I-Tat-ELP1-GFLG-DOX was injected intravenously into athymic RNU nude rats bearing MES-SA tumors in each hind leg. One tumor was heated to a core temperature of 42 °C for 1 h after injection, while the second was left at normal body temperature. The animal was sacrificed and the tumors frozen 4 h after injection. The tumors were serially sliced and exposed to film, and images were digitized and quantitated using NIH Image. Between 25 and 30 tumor slices from each animal were averaged, and data from five animals was pooled (bars = SEM). †Difference between heated and unheated tumors is statistically significant as assessed by Student's t-test, $P < 0.05$.

22.5.9
Optimizing *In Vivo* Delivery of ELP Carriers with CPPs

Although hyperthermia application devices such as microwaves, radiofrequency, and HIFU are clinically available, a heating device feasible for laboratory use is the IR light-emitting diode (LED) laser (Figure 22.17a). A pilot study was conducted with Laser Sys*Stim 540® (Mettler Electronics, Anaheim, CA) to determine the optimum settings to generate the required hyperthermia temperature of 42 °C at the tumor. Sprague-Dawley rats bearing two bilateral tumors were use: one tumor was heated, while the other was unheated as a control. The LED probe was positioned approximately 1 mm from the skin over the tumor site with the area surrounding the tumor shielded from illumination. An IR light output at 805 nm was sufficient to reach hyperthermia temperature within 20 min at a 10-kHz pulse frequency (Figure 22.17b). Then a 5-kHz pulse frequency maintained the temperature at 42 °C for the next 40 min. As shown in Figure 22.17b, heating of the tumor at 42 °C did not alter the body temperature of the animal. The control unheated tumor remained near 35 °C during the heating period. Furthermore, the skin surface was not significantly heated by IR illumination. Therefore, this IR LED device is effective in producing the desired hyperthermia temperatures for preclinical *in vivo* studies.

The goal of targeted delivery of cancer therapeutics is to deliver drugs both at the tumoral level and at the cellular level. Drug delivery systems should be specifically targeted to the tumor site to minimize drug exposure in healthy tissues and they should reach their molecular target in the cancer cells to effectively inhibit their growth. Therefore, after administration, drug carriers must overcome transport barriers to drug delivery that are posed by unique structural properties of tumors, extravasate from the tumor blood vessels, and transport the drug cargo through the plasma membrane of cancer cells. The major impediments to drug delivery in solid tumors are: (i) heterogeneous distribution of blood vessels, combined with aberrant branching and tortuosity, all of which result in uneven and slowed blood flow and (ii) the high permeability of tumor vessels combined with the absence of a functional lymphatic system resulting in an elevated interstitial pressure, which retards convective transport of high-molecular-weight (above 2000 Da) drugs. An efficient means to address these challenges is to use CPPs. These short peptides are able to translocate cargo peptides or drugs as described above. Our previous studies with ELPs designed with CPPs at the N-terminus have shown that CPPs fused with ELP carriers enhance uptake into the tumor cells *in vitro* [42, 45, 64, 65, 70]. Furthermore, preliminary *in vivo* studies show that CPPs can also mediate escape of the polypeptide from the tumor vasculature and entry into the tumor cells (Figure 22.18). The thermo-responsive c-Myc inhibitory polypeptide, Bac-ELP1-H1, was intravenously administered to an animal bearing two bilateral tumors. As shown in Figure 22.18, Bac-ELP1-H1 was present not only in the tumor blood vessels, but it also escaped circulation and entered the tumor cells. This marks the first direct observation that ELPs aided by a CPP can escape the tumor vasculature and enter the tumor cells.

(a)

(b)

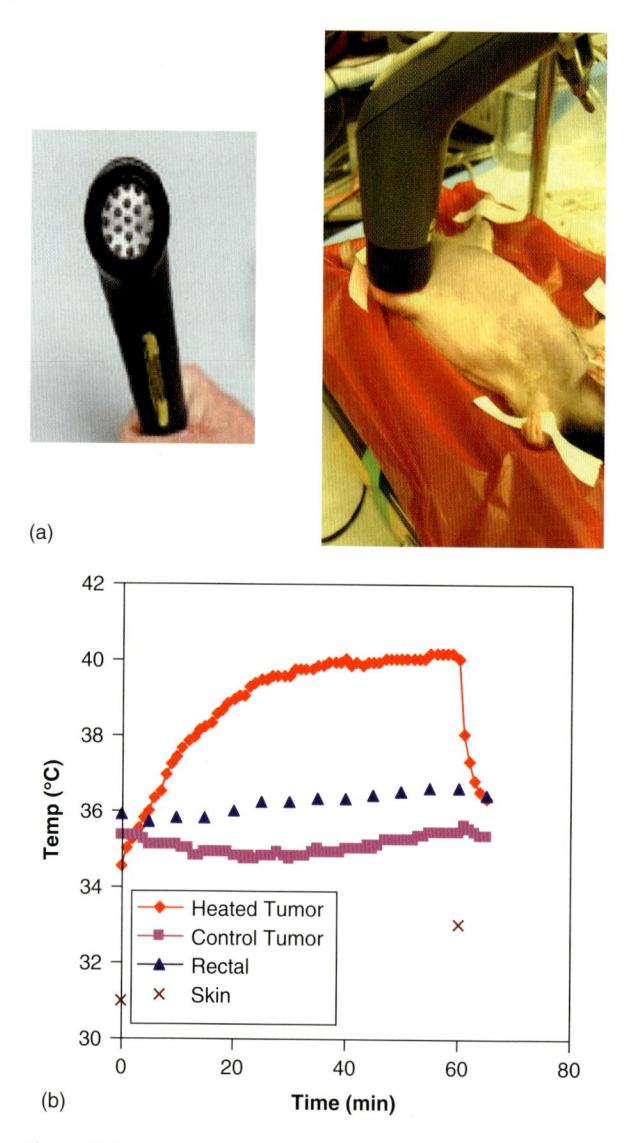

Figure 22.17 Heating tumors using IR light. (a) An IR LED applicator (Laser Sys*Stim 540) can be used to heat subcutaneous tumors in small animals in the laboratory. (b) Subcutaneous tumors of rat glioma C6 cells were established in Sprague-Dawley rats by injecting 3×10^6 cells into each flank. Heating trial was commenced when the tumors reached 8×10 mm. One tumor was used for hyperthermia treatment, while the second was left at normal body temperature as a control. A needle thermocouple was placed in the core of both the heated and control tumors. The body temperature was monitored by a rectal probe. Tumors were heated with the LED set to a 10-kHz pulse frequency for 20 min. The hyperthermia temperature was maintained at or near 40°C for the remainder of the hour.

	Hoescht	FITC-Dextran	Bac-ELP1-H1	Merge
T<T_t				
T>T_t				

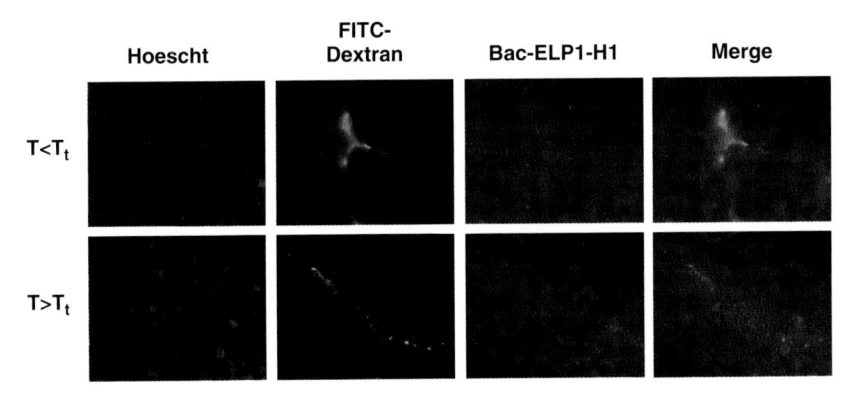

Figure 22.18 Imaging intratumor distribution of the ELP therapeutic peptide carrier. Rhodamine-labeled Bac-ELP1-H1 was intravenously injected in rats bearing C6 tumors. One tumor was heated for 60 min using IR illumination as described in the text. One minute prior to euthanasia, high-molecular-weight (500-kDa) FITC–dextran was injected intravenously in order to mark the perfused vessels. The tumors were removed, rapidly frozen, and sectioned using a cryomicrotome. Tumor sections were fixed and stained with Hoechst 33342, and imaged using a Nikon fluorescence microscope with a CoolSnap CCD camera. A representative section from multiple tumor sections from duplicate animals is shown.

These results along with the *in vivo* data demonstrate that rationally designed ELPs have not only targeting capability, but that they can also overcome transport barriers to delivery, reach the molecular site of action within the cancer cells, and inhibit their growth. Animal experiments to evaluate the therapeutic efficacy of ELP carrier systems are currently underway in our lab.

22.6
Conclusions and Perspectives

Advancement in polymer science and molecular bioengineering and recombinant DNA techniques has led to the development of new polymers for targeted and controlled delivery of therapeutic drugs. Polymers carriers are macromolecules that can improve the pharmacokinetics of small-molecule drugs. They also accumulate preferentially in tumors relative to normal tissues due to the EPR effect. This passive targeting capability and extended pharmacological effect of polymers can be further improved and optimized by designing polymers, termed stimuli-responsive polymers, which change their physicochemical properties in response to environmental signals.

One class of stimuli-responsive polymer, thermo-responsive polymers, have been of increasing interest in recent years for anticancer drug delivery. These polymers are designed to have a LCST above 40–42 °C and therefore they will be cleared under physiological conditions (37 °C). However, they will hydrophobically collapse and undergo an inverse phase transition, leading to drug release of the polymer–drug conjugate in tumors where externally induced local hyperthermia is applied. There are two main classes of thermo-responsive polymers: (i) synthetic polymers, such as NIPAAm and acrylamide coploymers, and (ii) genetically engineered polypeptides, such as ELPs. PNIPAAm and its copolymers have been used for drug delivery, mainly as a polymeric micelles and cross-linked hydrogels, which are designed to release anticancer drugs when the tumor site is heated above their LCST. Thermo-responsive genetically engineered ELPs have been also tested in preclinical animal models to deliver therapeutic peptides and conventional chemotherapeutics. Although both polymers are designed to have an LCST in the same range (39–42 °C), each polymer system has different advantages and disadvantages in the application of targeted drug delivery. PNIPAAm-based polymers are synthetic polymers that can be produced in large quantities and whose properties can be modified by the incorporation of monomers. However, their polydispersity, sequence, chain length, and conjugation stoichiometry with therapeutics cannot be controlled to the extent possible with genetically engineered biopolymers. Genetically engineered biopolymers are genetically encodable, which provides complete control of their sequence.

Preclinical studies in xenograft tumor animal models with synthetically and genetically engineered thermo-responsive polymers have shown that these carriers in combination with hyperthermia accumulate in solid tumors significantly more than the same polymers without hyperthermia. Although these studies confirm that the thermal targeting approach is very promising, further optimization is necessary to increase the efficiency of targeted delivery and to apply this approach in clinical trials. Optimizing the injected dose and polymer concentration, mode of administration, and polymer macromolecular weight may further enhance the accumulation of thermo-responsive polymers in solid tumors. Also, the addition of a fusion peptide sequence or a specific ligand that recognizes specific cancers cells to these genetically engineered biopolymers may improve the specificity and targeted delivery of drug cargo.

The clinical and translational potential of thermal targeting approaches and the application of thermo-responsive polymers as anticancer drug carriers have been furthered by recent advances not only in biopolymer science and biotechnology, but also in the development of new hyperthermia applicators based on ultrasound transducers and microwave arrays.

Acknowledgements

This research was partially supported by research grants from National Institutes of Health grants R21 CA113813-01A2 and R43 CA135799-01A2, and National Science Foundation award CBET-0931041. We would also like to thank Emily H. Thomas for critical reading of the manuscript.

References

1. Greish, K. (2007) Enhanced permeability and retention of macromolecular drugs in solid tumors: a royal gate for targeted anticancer nanomedicines. *J. Drug Target.*, **15**, 457–464.
2. Iyer, A.K. et al. (2006) Exploiting the enhanced permeability and retention effect for tumor targeting. *Drug Discov. Today*, **11**, 812–818.
3. Maeda, H., Bharate, G.Y., and Daruwalla, J. (2009) Polymeric drugs for efficient tumor-targeted drug delivery based on EPR-effect. *Eur. J. Pharm. Biopharm.*, **71**, 409–419.
4. Talelli, M. et al. (2010) Micelles based on HPMA copolymers. *Adv. Drug Deliv. Rev.*, **62**, 231–239.
5. Matsumura, Y. (2008) Poly(amino acid) micelle nanocarriers in preclinical and clinical studies. *Adv. Drug Deliv. Rev.*, **60**, 899–914.
6. Vicent, M.J. and Duncan, R. (2006) Polymer conjugates: nanosized medicines for treating cancer. *Trends Biotechnol.*, **24**, 39–47.
7. Hu, X. and Jing, X. (2009) Biodegradable amphiphilic polymer-drug conjugate micelles. *Expert Opin. Drug Deliv.*, **6**, 1079–1090.
8. Khare, P. et al. (2009) Bioconjugates: harnessing potential for effective therapeutics. *Crit. Rev. Ther. Drug Carrier Syst.*, **26**, 119–155.
9. Falk, M.H. and Issels, R.D. (2001) Hyperthermia in oncology. *Int. J. Hyperthermia*, **17**, 1–18.
10. Dewhirst, M.W. et al. (1997) Hyperthermic treatment of malignant diseases: current status and a view toward the future. *Semin. Oncol.*, **24**, 616–625.
11. Takahashi, I. et al. (2002) Clinical application of hyperthermia combined with anticancer drugs for the treatment of solid tumors. *Surgery*, **131**, S78–S84.
12. ter Haar, G.R. (2001) High intensity focused ultrasound for the treatment of tumors. *Echocardiography*, **18**, 317–322.
13. Hu, Z. et al. (2007) Investigation of HIFU-induced anti-tumor immunity in a murine tumor model. *J. Transl. Med.*, **5**, 34.
14. Wang, S., Frenkel, V., and Zderic, V. (2009) Preliminary optimization of non-destructive high intensity focused ultrasound exposures for hyperthermia applications. *Conf. Proc. IEEE Eng. Med. Biol. Soc.*, 3055–3059.
15. Issels, R.D. (1995) Regional hyperthermia combined with systemic chemotherapy of locally advanced sarcomas: preclinical aspects and clinical results. *Recent Results Cancer Res.*, **138**, 81–90.
16. Feyerabend, T. et al. (1997) Rationale and clinical status of local hyperthermia, radiation, and chemotherapy in locally advanced malignancies. *Anticancer Res.*, **17**, 2895–2897.
17. van Vulpen, M. et al. (2002) Prostate perfusion in patients with locally advanced prostate carcinoma treated with different hyperthermia techniques. *J. Urol.*, **168**, 1597–1602.
18. Kong, G. and Dewhirst, M.W. (1999) Hyperthermia and liposomes. *Int. J. Hyperthermia*, **15**, 345–370.
19. Schild, H.G. (1992) Poly (N-isopropylacrylamide): experiment, theory and application. *Prog. Polym. Sci.*, **17**, 163.
20. Shibayama, M.N., Norisuye, T., and Nomura, S. (1996) Cross-link density dependence of spatial inhomogeneities and dynamic fluctuations of poly (N-isopropylacrylamide) gels. *Macromolecules*, **29**, 8746–8750.
21. Bajpai, A.K., Shukla, S.K., Bhanu, S., and Kankane, S. (2008) Responsive polymers in controlled drug delivery. *Prog. Polym. Sci.*, **33**, 1088–1118.
22. Jeong, B. et al. (1997) Biodegradable block copolymers as injectable drug-delivery systems. *Nature*, **388**, 860–862.
23. Arai, T. et al. (2006) Novel drug delivery system using thermoreversible gelation polymer for malignant glioma. *J. Neurooncol.*, **77**, 9–15.
24. Liu, B. et al. (2008) The antitumor effect of novel docetaxel-loaded thermosensitive micelles. *Eur. J. Pharm. Biopharm.*, **69**, 527–534.

25. Liu, B. et al. (2008) Enhanced efficiency of thermally targeted taxanes delivery in a human xenograft model of gastric cancer. *J. Pharm. Sci.*, **97**, 3170–3181.
26. Wei, H. et al. (2007) Self-assembled thermosensitive micelles based on poly (L-lactide-star block-N-isopropylacrylamide) for drug delivery. *J. Biomed. Mater. Res. A*, **83**, 980–989.
27. Alexandridis, P.H. and Hatton, T.A. (1995) Poly(ethylene oxide)–poly(propylene oxide)–poly(ethylene oxide) block-copolymer surfactants in aqueous-solutions and at interfaces – thermodynamics, structure, dynamics, and modeling. *Colloid Surf.*, **96**, 1–46.
28. Ron, E.S. and Bromberg, L.E. (1998) Temperature-responsive gels and thermogelling polymer matrices for protein and peptide delivery. *Adv. Drug Deliv. Rev.*, **31**, 197–221.
29. Kabanov, A.V., Batrakova, E.V., and Alakhov, V.Y. (2002) Pluronic block copolymers as novel polymer therapeutics for drug and gene delivery. *J. Control. Release*, **82**, 189–212.
30. Yang, Y. et al. (2009) A novel mixed micelle gel with thermo-sensitive property for the local delivery of docetaxel. *J. Control. Release*, **135**, 175–182.
31. Amiji, M.M. et al. (2002) Intratumoral administration of paclitaxel in an *in situ* gelling poloxamer 407 formulation. *Pharm. Dev. Technol.*, **7**, 195–202.
32. Wells, J., Sen, A., and Hui, S.W. (2003) Localized delivery to CT-26 tumors in mice using thermosensitive liposomes. *Int. J. Pharm.*, **261**, 105–114.
33. Miyazaki, S. et al. (1992) Antitumor effect of Pluronic F-127 gel containing mitomycin C on sarcoma-180 ascites tumor in mice. *Chem. Pharm. Bull. (Tokyo)*, **40**, 2224–2226.
34. Valle, J.W. et al. (2010) A phase 2 study of SP1049C, doxorubicin in P-glycoprotein-targeting pluronics, in patients with advanced adenocarcinoma of the esophagus and gastroesophageal junction. *Invest. New Drugs*, Epub ahead of print.
35. Chun, C. et al. (2009) Doxorubicin–polyphosphazene conjugate hydrogels for locally controlled delivery of cancer therapeutics. *Biomaterials*, **30**, 4752–4762.
36. Hsiue, G.H. et al. (2006) Environmental-sensitive micelles based on poly(2-ethyl-2-oxazoline)-b-poly (L-lactide) diblock copolymer for application in drug delivery. *Int. J. Pharm.*, **317**, 69–75.
37. Urry, D.W. (1988) Entropic elastic processes in protein mechanisms. I. Elastic structure due to an inverse temperature transition and elasticity due to internal chain dynamics. *J. Protein Chem.*, **7**, 1–34.
38. Urry, D.W. (1992) Free energy transduction in polypeptides and proteins based on inverse temperature transitions. *Prog. Biophys. Mol. Biol.*, **57**, 23–57.
39. Li, B. et al. (2001) Hydrophobic hydration is an important source of elasticity in elastin-based biopolymers. *J. Am. Chem. Soc.*, **123**, 11991–11998.
40. Urry, D.W. et al. (1991) Temperature of polypeptide inverse temperature transition depends on mean residue hydrophobicity. *J. Am. Chem. Soc.*, **113**, 4346–4348.
41. Meyer, D.E. and Chilkoti, A. (2004) Quantification of the effects of chain length and concentration on the thermal behavior of elastin-like polypeptides. *Biomacromolecules*, **5**, 846–851.
42. Bidwell, G.L. and Raucher, D. III (2005) Application of thermally responsive polypeptides directed against c-Myc transcriptional function for cancer therapy. *Mol. Cancer Ther.*, **4**, 1076–1085.
43. Meyer, D.E. and Chilkoti, A. (2002) Genetically encoded synthesis of protein-based polymers with precisely specified molecular weight and sequence by recursive directional ligation: examples from the elastin-like polypeptide system. *Biomacromolecules*, **3**, 357–367.
44. Meyer, D.E. and Chilkoti, A. (1999) Purification of recombinant proteins by fusion with thermally responsive polypeptides. *Nat. Biotechnol.*, **17**, 1112–1115.
45. Massodi, I., Bidwell, G.L., and Raucher, D. III (2005) Evaluation of cell penetrating peptides fused to elastin-like

polypeptide for drug delivery. *J. Control. Release*, **108**, 396–408.

46. Derossi, D. et al. (1994) The third helix of the Antennapedia homeodomain translocates through biological membranes. *J. Biol. Chem.*, **269**, 10444–10450.

47. Vives, E., Brodin, P., and Lebleu, B. (1997) A truncated HIV-1 Tat protein basic domain rapidly translocates through the plasma membrane and accumulates in the cell nucleus. *J. Biol. Chem.*, **272**, 16010–16017.

48. Lin, Y.Z. et al. (1995) Inhibition of nuclear translocation of transcription factor NF-kappa B by a synthetic peptide containing a cell membrane-permeable motif and nuclear localization sequence. *J. Biol. Chem.*, **270**, 14255–14258.

49. Sadler, K. et al. (2002) Translocating proline-rich peptides from the antimicrobial peptide bactenecin 7. *Biochemistry*, **41**, 14150–14157.

50. Derossi, D., Chassaing, G., and Prochiantz, A. (1998) Trojan peptides: the penetratin system for intracellular delivery. *Trends Cell Biol.*, **8**, 84–87.

51. Richard, J.P. et al. (2003) Cell-penetrating peptides. A reevaluation of the mechanism of cellular uptake. *J. Biol. Chem.*, **278**, 585–590.

52. Vives, E. et al. (2003) TAT peptide internalization: seeking the mechanism of entry. *Curr. Protein Pept. Sci.*, **4**, 125–132.

53. Edenhofer, F. (2008) Protein transduction revisited: novel insights into the mechanism underlying intracellular delivery of proteins. *Curr. Pharm. Des.*, **14**, 3628–3636.

54. Heitz, F., Morris, M.C., and Divita, G. (2009) Twenty years of cell-penetrating peptides: from molecular mechanisms to therapeutics. *Br. J. Pharmacol.*, **157**, 195–206.

55. Heuser, J.E. and Anderson, R.G. (1989) Hypertonic media inhibit receptor-mediated endocytosis by blocking clathrin-coated pit formation. *J. Cell Biol.*, **108**, 389–400.

56. Thyberg, J. (2002) Caveolae and cholesterol distribution in vascular smooth muscle cells of different phenotypes. *J. Histochem. Cytochem.*, **50**, 185–195.

57. Talmadge, J.E. (1998) Pharmacodynamic aspects of peptide administration biological response modifiers. *Adv. Drug Deliv. Rev.*, **33**, 241–252.

58. Lipka, E., Crison, J., and Amidon, G.L. (1996) Transmembrane transport of peptide type compounds: prospects for oral delivery. *J. Control. Release*, **39**, 121–129.

59. Bidwell, G.L., Davis, A.N., and Raucher, D. III (2009) Targeting a c-Myc inhibitory polypeptide to specific intracellular compartments using cell penetrating peptides. *J. Control. Release*, **135**, 2–10.

60. Walhout, A.J.M. et al. (1997) c-Myc/Max heterodimers bind cooperatively to the E-box sequences located in the first intron of the rat ornithine decarboxylase (ODC) gene. *Nucleic Acids Res.*, **25**, 1516–1525.

61. Shim, H. et al. (1997) c-Myc transactivation of LDH-A: implications for tumor metabolism and growth. *Proc. Natl. Acad. Sci. USA*, **94**, 6658–6663.

62. Mutoh, M. et al. (1999) A p21$^{Waf1/Cip}$ carboxyl-terminal peptide exhibited cyclin-dependent kinase-inhibitory activity and cytotoxicity when introduced into human cells. *Cancer Res.*, **59**, 3480–3488.

63. Ball, K.L. et al. (1997) Cell-cycle arrest and inhibition of Cdk4 activity by small peptides based on the carboxy-terminal domain of p21^{WAF1}. *Curr. Biol.*, **7**, 71–80.

64. Massodi, I. et al. (2010) Inhibition of ovarian cancer cell proliferation by a cell cycle inhibitory peptide fused to a thermally responsive polypeptide carrier. *Int. J. Cancer*, **126**, 533–544.

65. Bidwell, G.L. III et al. (2007) Development of elastin-like polypeptide for thermally targeted delivery of doxorubicin. *Biochem. Pharmacol.*, **73**, 620–631.

66. Bidwell, G.L. III et al. (2007) A thermally targeted elastin-like polypeptide–doxorubicin conjugate overcomes drug resistance. *Invest. New Drugs*, **25**, 313–326.

67. Dreher, M.R. et al. (2003) Evaluation of an elastin-like polypeptide–doxorubicin

conjugate for cancer therapy. *J. Control. Release*, **91**, 31–43.

68. Furgeson, D.Y., Dreher, M.R., and Chilkoti, A. (2006) Structural optimization of a "smart" doxorubicin–polypeptide conjugate for thermally targeted delivery to solid tumors. *J. Control. Release*, **110**, 362–369.

69. Meyer, D.E. *et al.* (2001) Drug targeting using thermally responsive polymers and local hyperthermia. *J. Control. Release*, **74**, 213–224.

70. Bidwell, G.L. III *et al.* (2010) A thermally targeted peptide inhibitor of symmetrical dimethylation inhibits cancer-cell proliferation. *Peptides*, **31**, 834–841.

23
Polysaccharide-Based Drug Conjugates for Tumor Targeting

Gurusamy Saravanakumar, Jae Hyung Park, Kwangmeyung Kim, and Ick Chan Kwon

23.1
Introduction

Conventional cancer chemotherapy is limited by the indiscriminate distribution of drugs in the body and multidrug resistance in cancer. Therefore, there has been a tremendous effort focused on the design of carriers that can effectively deliver drugs to the tumor tissue, thereby reducing side-effects and maximizing their therapeutic efficacy [1, 2]. Over the past few decades, polymer therapeutics have received increasing attention for tumor-targeted therapy because they are often accumulated to the solid tumor in high concentrations, which is due to anatomical and pathophysiological abnormalities of the tumor tissue, such as large vascular permeability, high diffusivity, and lack of lymphatic drainage [3–6]. The polymer–drug conjugate is a representative example of polymer therapeutics and its concept was first proposed by Ringsdorf in 1975 [7]. In general, the conjugates consist of a water-soluble polymeric carrier, the drug attached via a cleavable spacer, and a targeting moiety complementary to an antigen or receptor on the surface of the target cell. Conjugation of drugs to polymers offers several distinct advantages over traditional low-molecular-weight drugs, including enhancement of the aqueous solubility of anticancer drugs, prolonged circulation of the drugs in the bloodstream, protection of the drugs from undesired *in vivo* enzymatic degradation, decrease in nonspecific toxicity, and increase in the accumulation of the drugs at the tumor site by either active targeting (receptor-mediated endocytosis) and/or passive targeting [8]. In addition, polymer–drug conjugates allow delivering two or more drugs with different properties to induce synergistic effects *in vivo*.

Various macromolecules, such as polysaccharides, proteins, antibodies, lectins, and synthetic polymers, have been used for the conjugation of anticancer drugs [9–12]. Among them, natural polysaccharides have often been used for the conjugates as they are biocompatible and abundant in nature. Polysaccharides are a class of macromolecules consisting of repeating mono- or disaccharides linked via glycosidic bonds. The chemical structures of the polysaccharides extensively used for conjugates are shown in Table 23.1, and their sources and some special characteristics are summarized in Table 23.2. Polysaccharides are available in

Drug Delivery in Oncology: From Basic Research to Cancer Therapy, First Edition.
Edited by Felix Kratz, Peter Senter, and Henning Steinhagen.
© 2012 Wiley-VCH Verlag GmbH & Co. KGaA. Published 2012 by Wiley-VCH Verlag GmbH & Co. KGaA.

Table 23.1 Chemical structure of polysaccharides used for polymer–drug conjugates.

Polysaccharide	Chemical structure
Dextran	
Chitosan	
Hyaluronic acid	

Chondroitin sulfate

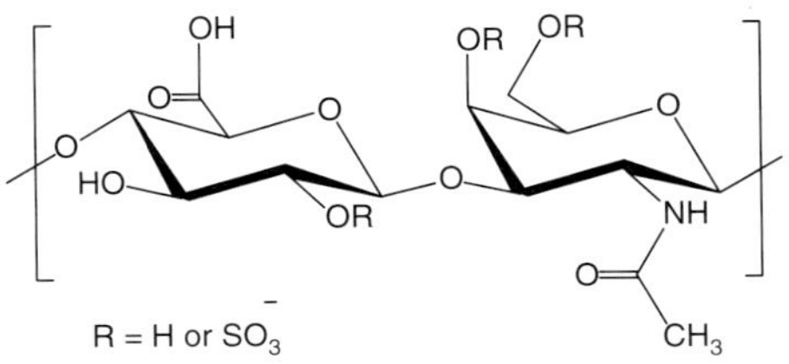

R = H or SO$_3^-$

Heparin

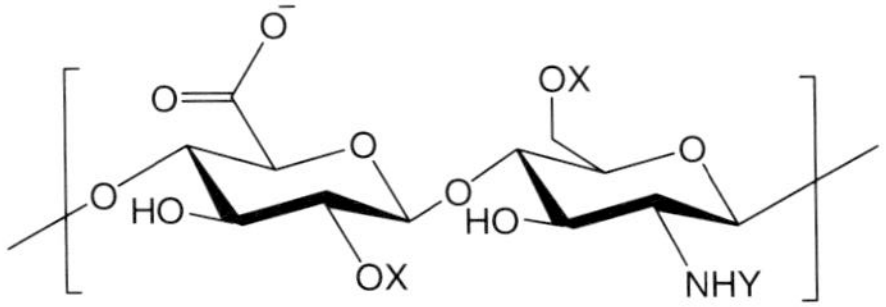

X = H or SO$_3^-$
Y = Ac, SO$_3^-$ or H

Alginate

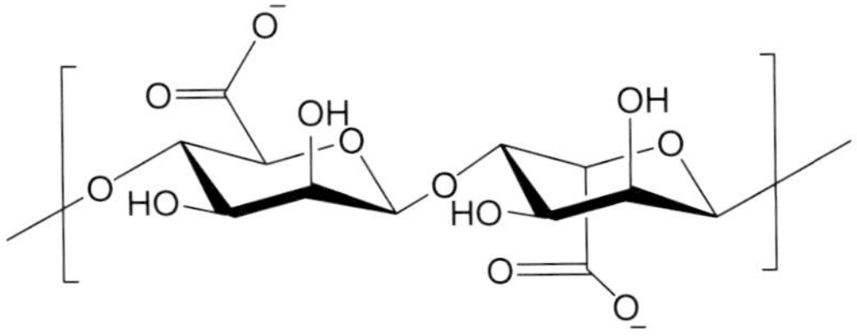

(continued overleaf)

Table 23.1 (continued).

Polysaccharide	Chemical structure
Pullulan	

Table 23.2 Characteristics of polysaccharides used for polymer–drug conjugates.

Polysaccharides	Source	Comments
Dextran	bacterial (*Streptococcus mutans* and *Leuconostoc mesenteroides*)	degree of branching, length of branch chains, and molecular weight distribution could influence the physicochemical properties of Dex; low-molecular-weight Dex eliminated from circulation via kidney, while high-molecular-weight Dex exhibits longer half-life and degraded by the reticuloendothelial system; Dex of molecular weight between 40 and 70 kDa preferable as carrier for drug conjugates; plausible mechanism of uptake for Dex conjugates is most likely via fluid-phase endocytosis; Dex metabolized by different exo- and endodextranases present in various parts of the body, including liver, spleen, and colon
Chitosan	exoskeleton of crustaceans (such as crabs and shrimp)	physicochemical characteristics are greatly influenced by its degree of deacetylation and molecular weight; mucoadhesive and absorption enhancer in its protonated form, and this increases *in vivo* residence time of dosage forms; capable of opening tight junctions between epithelial cells; degraded by lysozyme and bacterial enzymes in the colon
Hyaluronic acid	human and animal (found in ECM, especially of soft connective tissues)	nonsulfated glycosaminoglycan, with a wide range of molecular weights (1000–10 000 000 Da), plays a crucial role in cell adhesion, growth, and migration; HA has been implicated in metastatic disease process; various tumors overexpress HA receptors such as CD44 and RHAMM; CD44 could interact with a minimum HA length of six to eight saccharides; HA is degraded by hyaluronidase; the major concern of HA-based carriers is their rapid clearance from the blood circulation by means of recognition by HA receptors of the reticuloendothelial systems of the liver and spleen

(continued overleaf)

Table 23.2 (continued)

Polysaccharides	Source	Comments
Chondroitin sulfate	human, other mammals, and invertebrates (commercially derived from such as shark cartilage and chicken keel)	involved in intracellular signaling, cell orientation, and connection between ECM and cells; could be used as a carrier for colon-targeted delivery
Heparin	mammalian (mucosa tissue)	highly sulfated glycosaminoglycan with a molecular weight range of 15–40 kDa, average molecular weight of 15 kDa, and average negative charge of approximately −75 mV; widely used as an anticoagulant drug in the clinic and also involved in other physiological process, including cell proliferation, differentiation, and inflammation; also influences cancer progression and metastasis; strongly interferes with the activity of growth factors (basic FGF), thereby inhibiting angiogenesis essential for tumor progression; potential is limited by its strong anticoagulant activity and undesirable side-effects, such as bleeding complications and heparin-induced thrombocytopenia
Alginate	extracted from marine brown algae or soil bacteria	possesses broad molecular weight (10–1000 kDa) depending on the source and processing; with divalent cations such as Ca^{2+}, alginates could form a gel network (egg-box structure); stimulates the production of the cytokines tumor necrosis factor-α, interleukin-1, and interleukin-6 from human monocytes; exhibits inherent antitumor activity against murine tumor models; lack of clear evidence for enzymatic degradation and *in vivo* clearance of high-molecular-weight alginate
Pullulan	produced from starch by a certain polymorphic fungus, *Aureobasidium pullulans*	nonionic polysaccharide, with a molecular weight range of thousands to more than 2 000 000 Da depending upon the growth conditions of organisms; can selectively bind to ASGP receptors, which are expressed exclusively on the surface of liver parenchymal cells

various molecular weights, chemical composition, and architectures. They also possess abundant functional groups on their backbone for chemical conjugation of diverse drug molecules. Some of the polysaccharides have inherent properties of recognizing specific receptors on the tumor cells, rendering them attractive as targeting moieties. For example, hyaluronic acid (HA) can specifically bind to CD44, which is a specific cell surface receptor overexpressed on many tumor cells [13].

In this chapter, we focus our attention primarily on polysaccharide-based drug conjugates for tumor targeting. Other macromolecular prodrugs such as antibody–drug conjugates and protein–drug conjugates are presented in detail in other chapters in this volume. This chapter is divided into three major parts. In Section 23.2, we discuss various synthetic methodologies available for the conjugation of drugs to polysaccharides. Although numerous synthetic methods are available for the modification of polysaccharides depending upon functionality both at the polysaccharide backbone and the drugs to be conjugated, we highlight the most widely used methods with representative examples. Section 23.3 is subdivided into several sections, where we discuss individual polysaccharide-based drug conjugates for cancer therapy. Although a number of studies have used polysaccharides in protein/small interfering RNA conjugation to enhance the biopharmaceutical properties, this chapter deals only with traditional low-molecular-weight drugs. In Section 23.4, we briefly describe cyclodextrin-containing polymer–drug conjugates.

23.2
Chemistry of Polysaccharide–Drug Conjugation

In addition to other favorable physicochemical and biological characteristics, an essential prerequisite of the polymer as the constituent of the conjugate is the availability of adequate reactive functional groups for chemical fixation of therapeutic drugs. As described above, many polysaccharides possess a large number of reactive functional groups (e.g., hydroxyl, amino, and carboxyl) on their backbone, which can be exploited as active sites for the conjugation of drugs either directly or through spacers. The spacer group between the polysaccharide backbone and drug is critical for the therapeutic efficacy of the conjugate. The spacer can be appropriately chosen to control the release rate of the drug. In general, spacers should be stable in the bloodstream, but susceptible to cleavage at the target site (e.g., lysosomal compartment of the cells). Various spacers that are sensitive to pH, enzyme, or reduction have been used for the preparation of polymer–drug conjugates, exhibiting release of the drug in its active form at the site of interest [14, 15].

Depending on the functional groups, a variety of methods have been employed to prepare polysaccharide–drug conjugates [16]. However, it is of importance to select a facile conjugation method, being performed under mild reaction conditions without altering the chemical structure and biological activity of the parent drugs. In most cases, the drugs have been conjugated to amine-

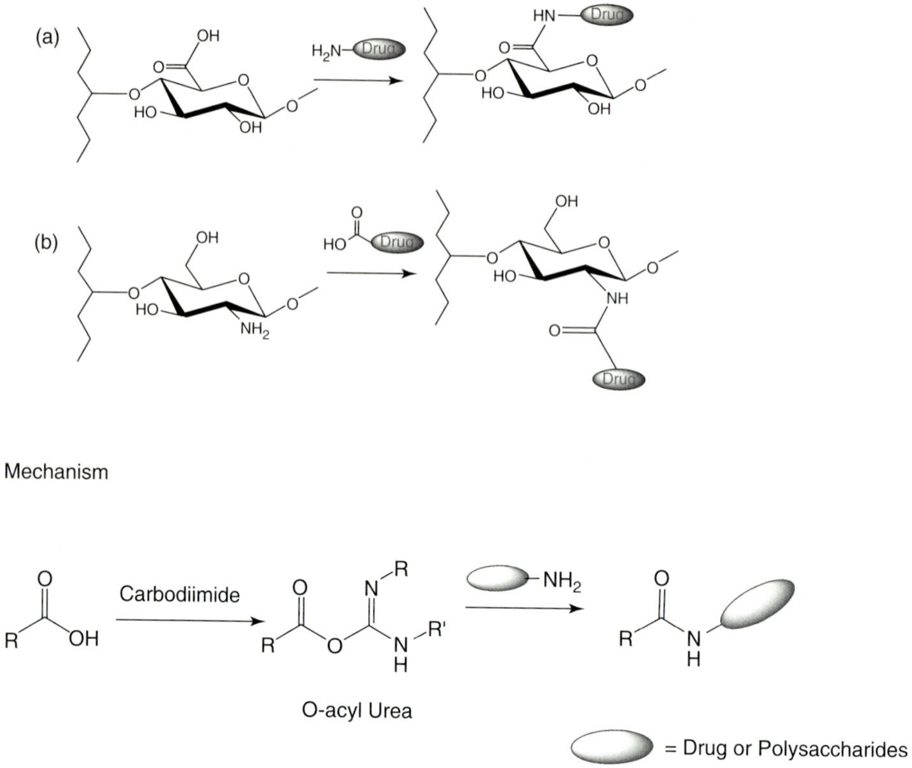

Figure 23.1 Synthesis of polysaccharide–drug conjugates. (a) and (b) Drugs can be conjugated to polysaccharides bearing carboxylic acid or amine groups through the carbodiimide-mediated coupling reaction. Polysaccharides bearing hydroxyl groups can often be converted to other reactive groups for chemical conjugation with the drugs.

or carboxyl-containing polysaccharides, either directly or through a spacer, via formation of an amide bond by the carbodiimide-mediated coupling reaction (Figure 23.1a). This method involves activation of the carboxylic groups using cross-linking agents, called zero-length cross-linkers, to form an O-acylisourea intermediate that is capable of acylating amines. Representative agents for conjugation reactions are carbodiimides, including 1-ethyl-3-(3-dimethylaminopropyl) carbodiimide hydrochloride (EDC; a water-soluble carbodiimide), N,N'-dicyclohexyl carbodiimde, or N,N'-diisopropyl carbodiimide.

For polysaccharides that contain only a hydroxyl group, drugs containing a carboxylic group can directly react with the polysaccharides to produce esters. Otherwise, the hydroxyl groups of the polysaccharide have often been converted to other functional groups for facile conjugation of drugs (Figure 23.1b). For example, an aldehyde group is introduced into the polysaccharide in the presence of periodates and reacted with the amino group of the drug to yield the Schiff base

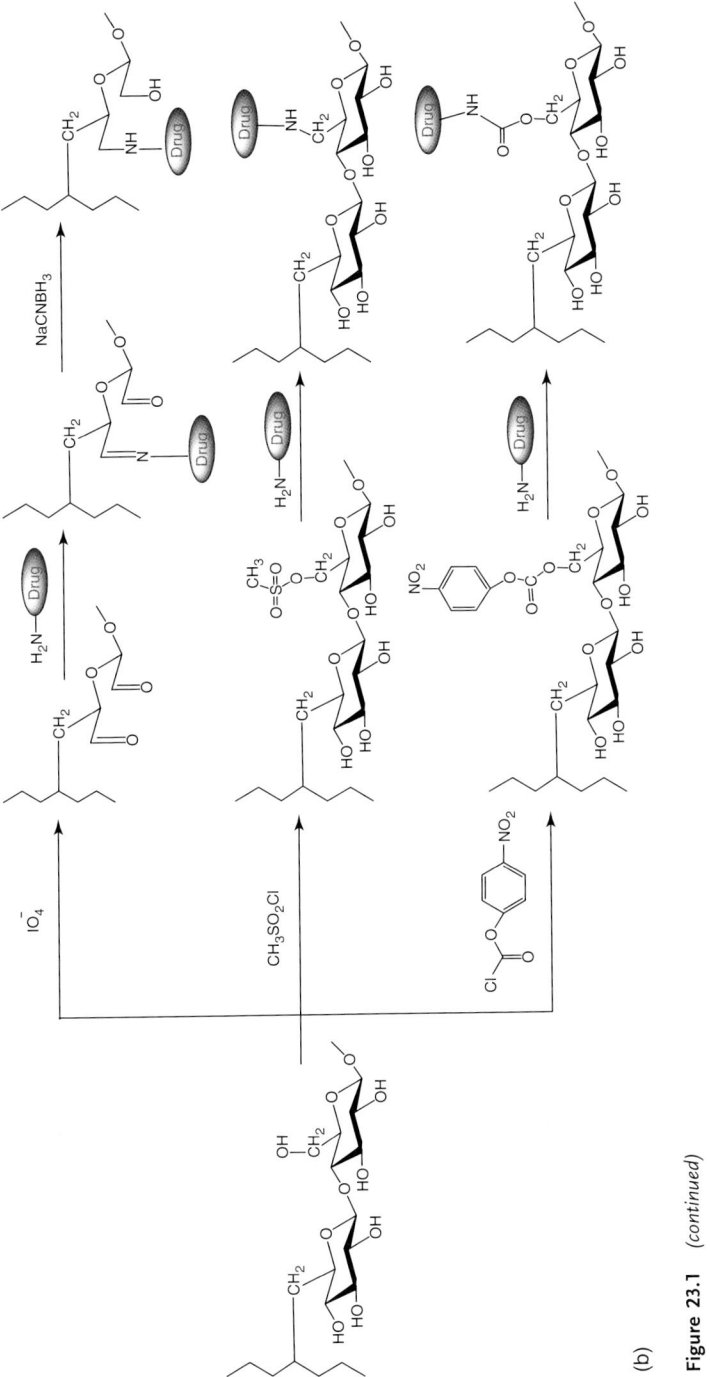

Figure 23.1 *(continued)*

(c)

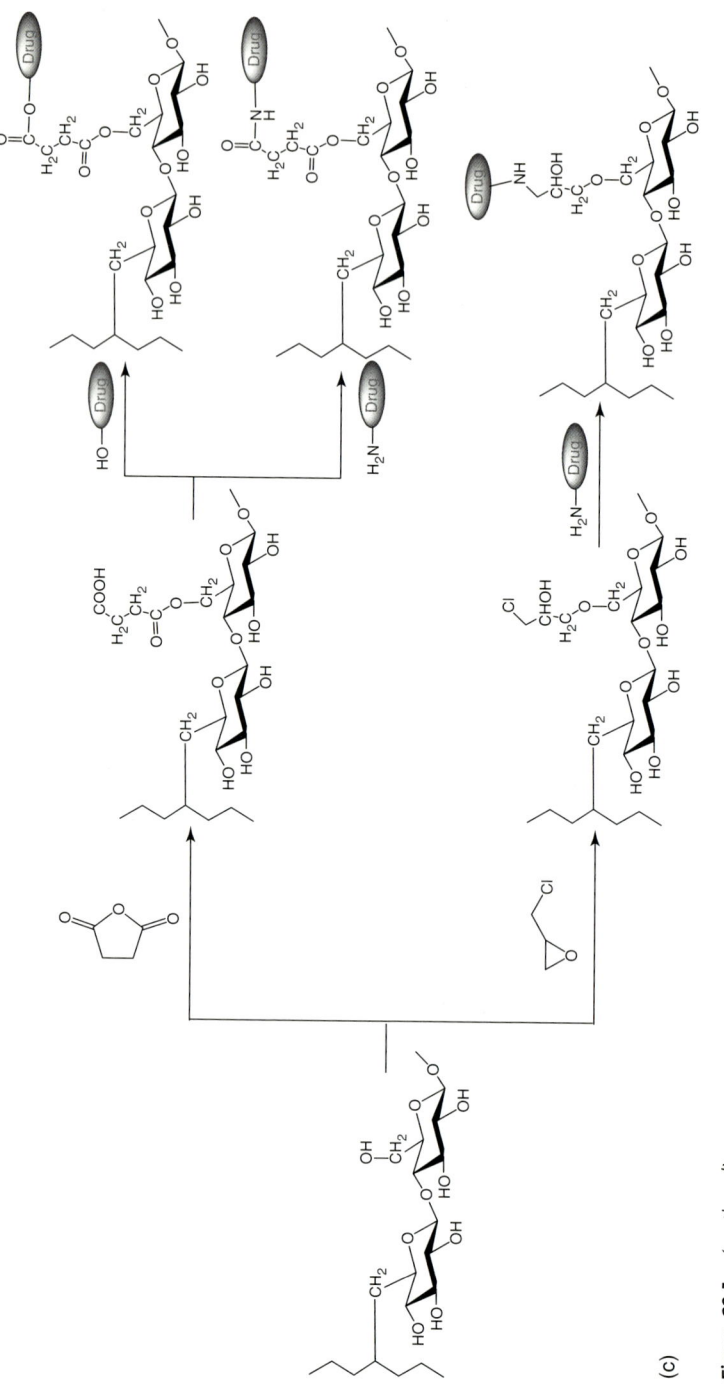

Figure 23.1 (continued)

(imino-conjugates), which is relatively unstable and can release the drug rapidly. The subsequent reduction of the Schiff base with sodium cyanoborohydride results in the production of hydrolytically stable conjugates. Based on this method, polysaccharides have been conjugated with various anticancer drugs, such as doxorubicin (DOX), daunomycin (DNM), and methotrexate (MTX) [17]. Also, this method is preferred for the conjugation of proteins to polysaccharides without significant loss of their biological activities [18].

The hydroxyl groups of polysaccharides have been modified with tosylate or mesylate as the functional leaving group on the polymer chains to form sulfonyl esters, which can further react with amine-containing drugs (Figure 23.1b and c). The reaction conditions for the activation are important for this process, since they influence the resulting activation products, sulfonyl esters. For example, the reaction of pullulan with mesyl chloride produces O-mesyl pullulan in pyridine, whereas chlorodeoxy pullulan is obtained as the main product in N,N-dimethylformamide [19]. To obtain the reactive carbonate ester, the hydroxyl group of the polysaccharide can be activated using chloroformate, which is useful to attach amine-containing drugs via a stable carbamate linkage. The hydroxyl group of the polysaccharide is often converted to a carboxylic group using succinic anhydride. The carboxylated polysaccharides can be then coupled with amine- or hydroxyl group-containing drugs. A wide range of polysaccharides, such as dextran (Dex), pullulan, and chitosan, have been activated using succinic anhydride to introduce more active carboxylic groups for the preparation of drug conjugates. The reaction of polysaccharide with epichlorohydrin under strong alkaline conditions or with $Zn(BF_4)_2$ as catalyst is known to yield 3-chloro-2-hydropropyl derivatives, available for the coupling of amine-containing drugs. Using this method, drugs like 6-purinethiol and 5-fluorouracil (5-FU) have been conjugated to Dex [20].

23.3
Polysaccharide-Drug Conjugates

23.3.1
Dex-Based Drug Conjugates

Dex is a water-soluble microbial polysaccharide composed of linear α1–6-linked glucopyranose units with some degree of 1–3-linked branches [21]. The degree of branching depends on the source of dextran and varies from 0.5 to 60%. Dex is one of the promising candidates for the preparation of drug conjugates because it has many advantages, such as a well-defined chemical structure, availability in different molecular weights, good aqueous solubility, high stability, lack of intrinsic toxicity, and presence of numerous hydroxyl groups for derivatization.

Dex–MMC conjugates have been extensively studied for cancer therapy. They were prepared by reacting an ε-aminocaproic acid spacer to the dextran activated using cyanogen bromide, followed by conjugation of MMC to the carboxylic acid via the carbodiimide-catalyzed reaction [22]. These conjugates (Figure 23.2a) released

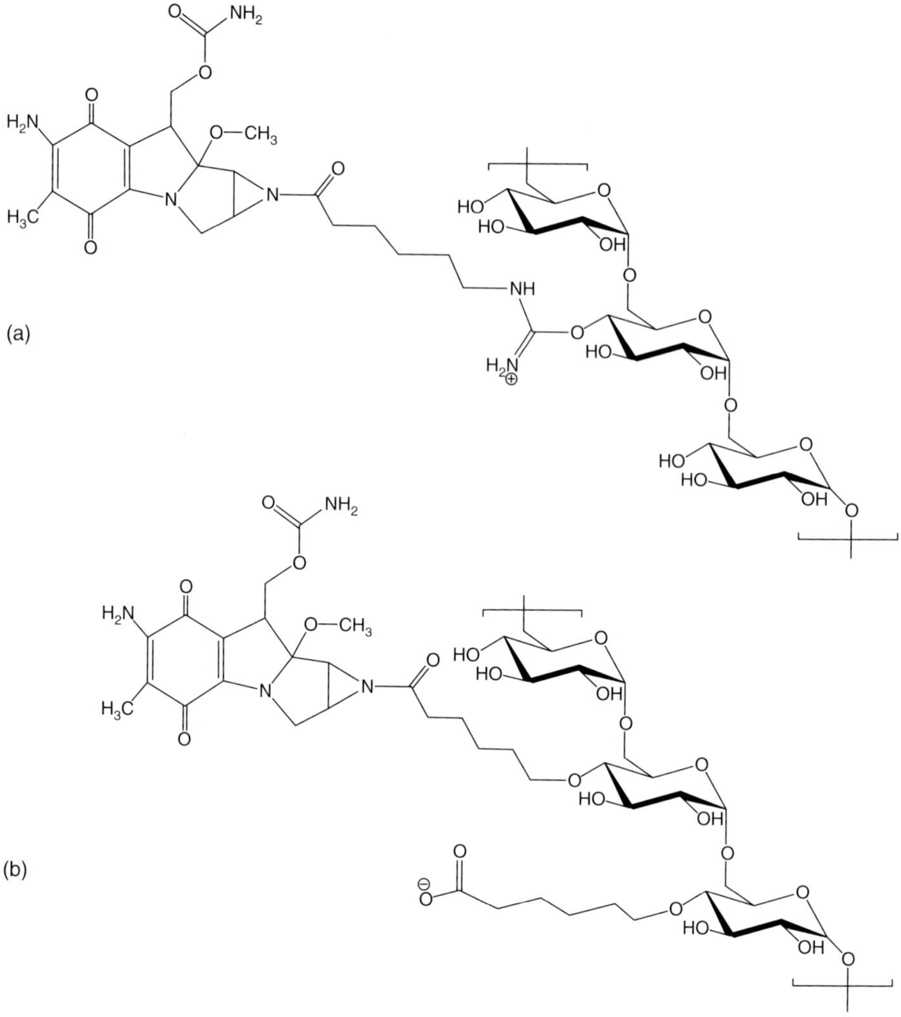

Figure 23.2 Chemical structure of Dex-based drug conjugates: (a) cationic Dex–MMC and (b) anionic Dex–MMC.

MMC in a sustained manner and the release rate was controlled by changing the length of the spacer [23, 24]. The conjugates showed significant antitumor activity to mice bearing P388 leukemia or B16 melanoma [22, 23]. Anionic Dex–MMC (Figure 23.2b) was prepared by reacting Dex with 6-bromohexanoic acid under strong alkaline conditions, followed by conjugation of MMC [25]. When administrated systemically into mice, anionic Dex–MMC showed a higher concentration in both plasma and tumor than free drug. A recent study demonstrated that when the conjugates were administered intratumorally, cationic Dex–MMC is retained in the tumor more than anionic Dex–MMC and free drug [26]. When cationic Dex–MMC was administered to rats through intramuscular injection, the conjugates were retained at the injection site for 48 h and then transferred to the lymphatic system [27]. The results indicated that conjugation of MMC to high-molecular-weight cationic Dex has promising potential for the treatment of lymph node metastasis.

DOX was conjugated to oxidized Dex via Schiff base formation without further reduction of the conjugate [28]. As the Schiff base moiety is acid labile, DOX could be released from the conjugates in the acidic endo/lysosomal compartments of the cell. The Dex–DOX conjugate exhibited higher antitumor activity and less toxicity than free DOX. The area under the plasma concentration curve for Dex–DOX, injected intravenously into the mice, was about 160-fold higher than that for free DOX. Effective inhibition of tumor growth was observed in various tumor models, including Lewis lung carcinoma and Walker 256 carcinosacrcoma [28, 29]. Lam *et al.* also showed that Dex–DOX conjugates exerted superior activity to free DOX in multidrug-resistant cell lines, due to a decrease in the removal rate of DOX by P-glycoprotein [30]. Similar results were obtained for Dex–DOX conjugates against a multidrug-resistant subline of human epidermal carcinoma (KB-3-1) [31]. Preclinical toxicological studies carried out in mice, rats, and dogs demonstrated that the LD_{50} value was 5 times higher for the conjugates, compared with free DOX. In mice and rats, plasma and tumor levels of the conjugate were higher than those of free DOX [28, 29, 32]. However, a clinical phase I trial conducted by intravenous administration of the conjugates showed significant clinical toxicities, such as thrombocytopenia and hepatotoxicity, presumably due to uptake of the conjugate by the reticuloendothelial cells [33].

Paclitaxel (PTX) was conjugated to carboxymethyl-Dex (CM-Dex) through a tetrapeptide Gly–Gly–Phe–Gly (GGFG) linker (Figure 23.3) [34]. *In vitro* drug release experiments showed that more than 80% of PTX was released from the conjugate after 24–48 h in plasma or serum. PTX showed broad cytotoxicity against a range of human tumor cell lines, whereas CM-Dex-GGFG-PTX was inactive *in vitro*. However, the antitumor efficacy of CM-Dex-GGFG-PTX was superior to that of free PTX against colon26 carcinoma-bearing mice, which might be due to release of the active drug at the target site (Figure 23.4). In addition, the maximum tolerated dose of CM-Dex-GGFG-PTX was more than twice that of free PTX.

In an attempt to improve the pharmaceutical properties and pharmacokinetics of camptothecin (CPT), a macromolecular prodrug (T-0128) (Figure 23.5) was synthesized by conjugating a CPT analog (T-2513: 7-ethyl-10-aminopropyloxy-CPT) to CM-Dex through a peptide linker Gly–Gly–Gly (GGG) [35]. T-0128 was resistant to various kinds of enzymes, whereas it was effectively cleaved by cysteine proteinases (cathepsin B). The *in vivo* antitumor study against Walker-256 carcinoma demonstrated that T-0128 was 10 times as active as the CPT analog, T-2513. Also, comparative efficacy studies performed using a panel of human tumor xenografts in nude mice showed that T-0128 was effective in the suppression of tumors refractory to CPT analogs, including irinotecan, topotecan, and T-2513 (Figure 23.6a and b) [36]. However, T-0128 was found to be a very weak inhibitor

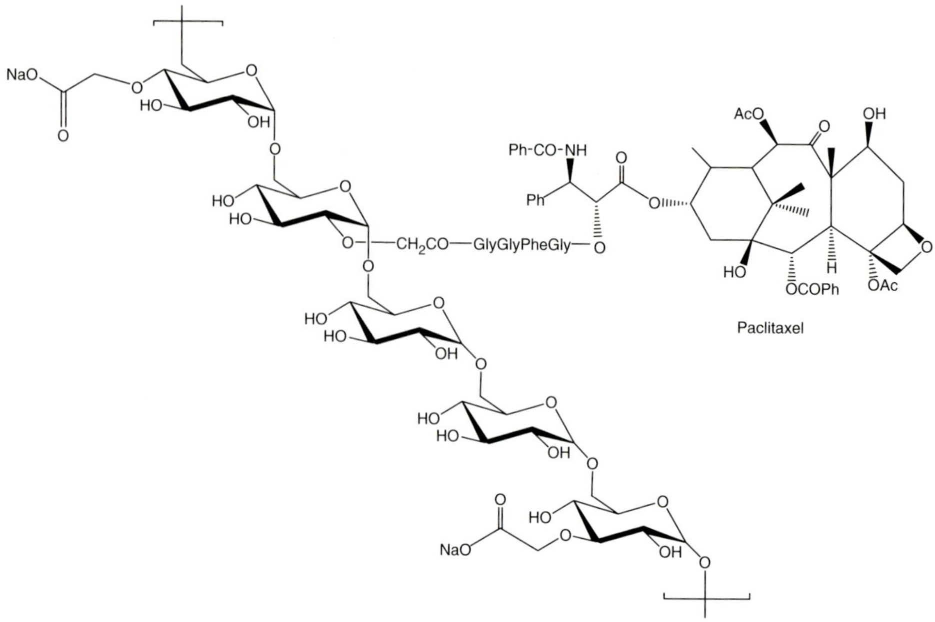

Figure 23.3 Chemical structure of CM-Dex-GGFG-PTX conjugate.

of cell proliferation *in vitro*, indicating that the cellular uptake and release of the linked drug is critical for its activity. Comparative efficacy studies showed that the conjugate was more effective against B16 melanoma cells cocultured with J774.1 macrophages than those without macrophages (Figure 23.6c and d). This indicates that macrophages play a crucial role in the antitumor activity of the conjugate, and its efficiency lies in the internalization and release of drugs into the tumor cells [37].

Cisplatin (CDDP; *cis*-diaminedichloroplatinum(II)), one of the most potent antitumor platinum complexes, was complexed to CM-Dex by Schechter et al. [38]. The complexes were less toxic than free drug *in vivo*. When tested *in vivo* against a CDDP-sensitive tumor, the complexes were more effective than free drug. CDDP was also conjugated to oxidized Dex (OX-Dex–CDDP) and dicarboxymethylated Dex (DCM-Dex–CDDP) by Nakashima et al. [39]. They found that DCM-Dex–CDDP shows longer *in vitro* antitumor activity in serum compared with OX-Dex–CDDP. *In vivo* studies also revealed that retention of DCM-Dex–CDDP in blood circulation was much higher than that of OX-Dex–CDDP.

In order to target hepatoma cells, CDDP was immobilized to DCM-Dex having branched galactose units (Gal4A) to obtain a macromolecular prodrug (DCM-Dex-Gal4A-CDDP) (Figure 23.7) [40]. The *in vitro* cytotoxicity of DCM-Dex-Gal4A-CDDP against HepG2 human hepatoma cells was higher than free CDDP and the conjugate without the galactose residue. The addition of free galactose or Gal4A into the media decreased the cytotoxic activity of the conjugate,

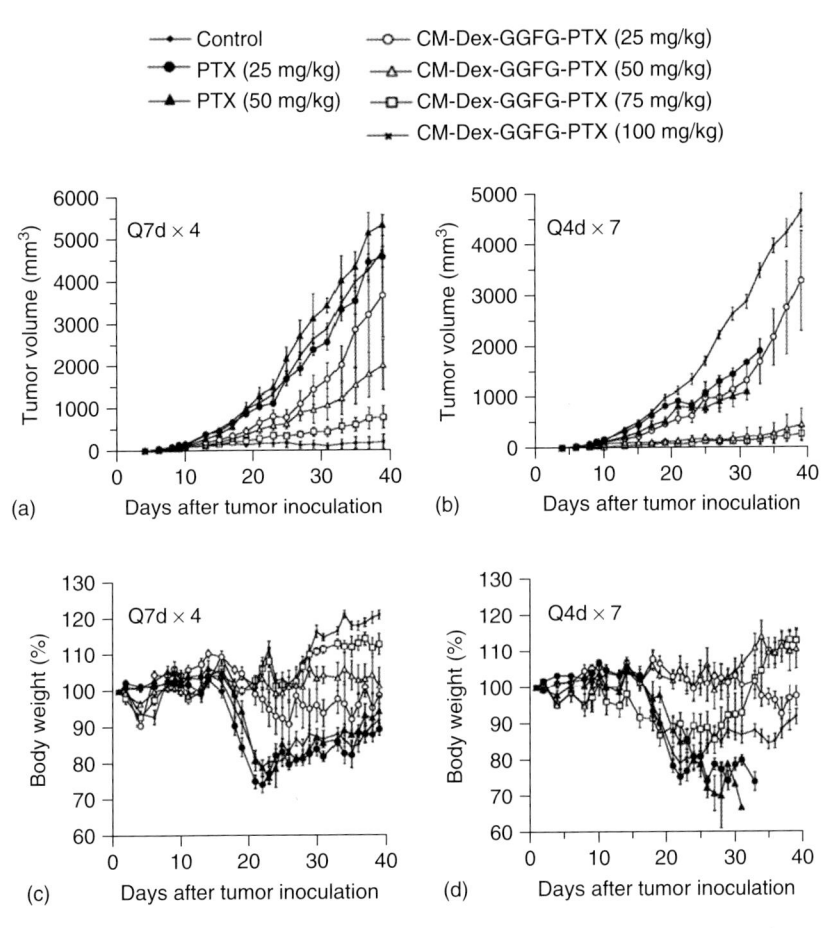

Figure 23.4 In vivo efficacy of CM-Dex-GGFG-PTX conjugates and free PTX in mice bearing colon26 carcinoma cells: (a) and (c) tumor growth and (b) and (d) body weight changes of mice (Q7d × 4 represents four injections administered with a 7-day interval and Q4d × 7 indicates seven injections administered with a 4-day interval). (Adapted from [34].)

while no effect was observed for free CDDP. Overall, it could be concluded that the conjugate with branched galactose units has high affinity to hepatoma cells, which may enhance the therapeutic effect of the conjugate.

Another Dex-based macromolecular prodrug has been synthesized using MTX [41]. A Dex-peptide-MTX conjugate was prepared via the multistep solid-phase synthetic procedure, where the peptide linker (Pro–Val–Gly–Leu–Ile–Gly) was specifically cleavable by the enzymes matrix metalloproteinase-2 and -9 (Figure 23.8). The conjugates exhibited satisfactory stability in the serum condition, while the peptide linker was cleaved to allow the release of MTX in the presence of the enzymes, suggesting that the conjugate could remain intact in systemic circulation.

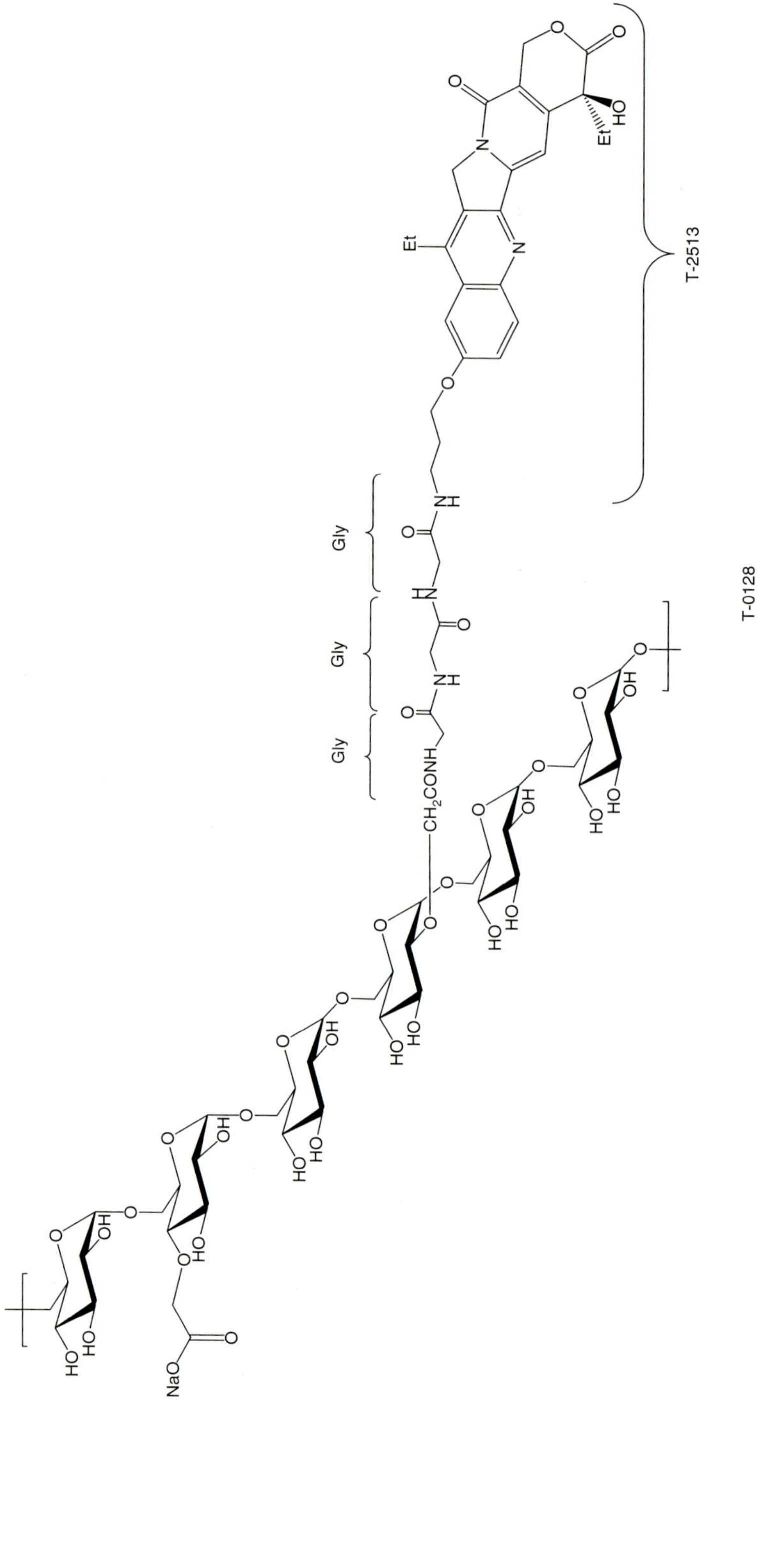

Figure 23.5 Chemical structure of Dex–CPT conjugate.

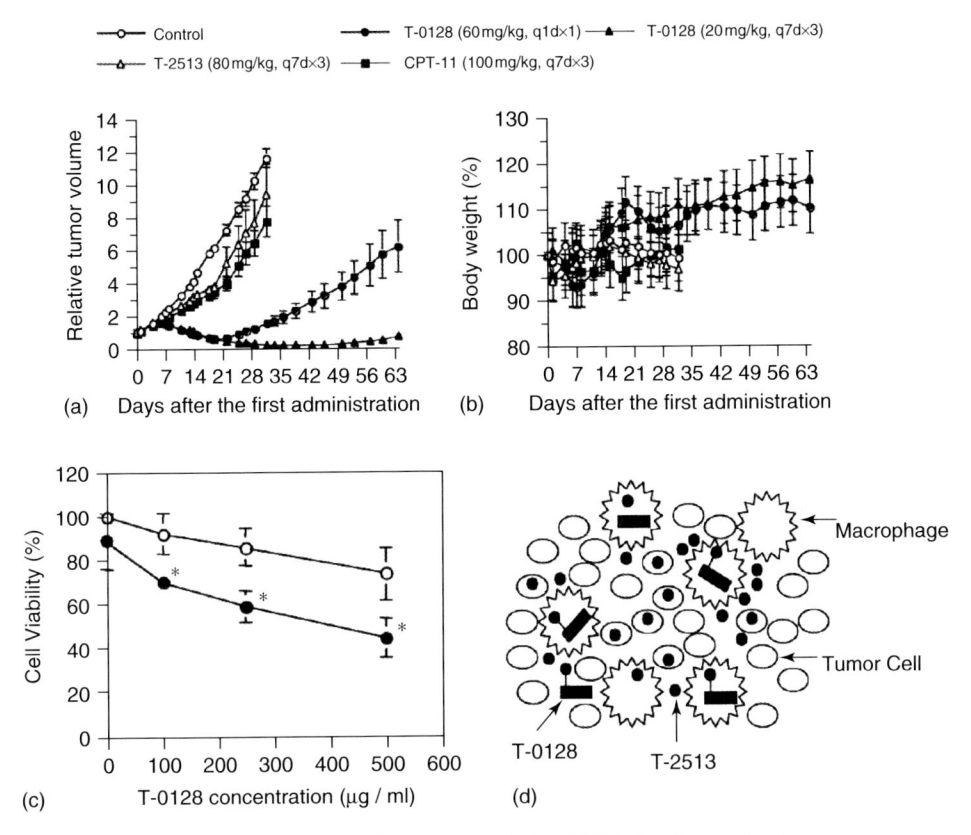

Figure 23.6 In vivo efficacy of CPT analogs in HT-29 human colorectal tumor xenograft model: (a) tumor growth and (b) body weight change. (c) Inhibitor effect of T-0218 on B16 melanoma cell growth in the presence (●) and absence (○) of J774.1 macrophage-like cells. (d) Proposed mechanism for the action of T-0218. After tumor accumulation, T-0218 is taken up by phagocytes, like macrophages, in the tumor tissue. The peptidyl linker is then cleaved intracellularly and the entry of released T-2513 into tumor cells through passive diffusion is responsible for the antitumor activity of T-0218. (Adapted from [36] and [37].)

23.3.2
Chitin– and Chitosan–Drug Conjugates

Chitosan, composed of D-glucosamine and N-acetyl glucosamine, is a linear aminopolysaccharide obtained by deacetylation of chitin – a natural polysaccharide found in the exoskeleton of crustaceans such as crab and shrimp [42, 43]. The physicochemical characteristics of chitosan are greatly influenced by its degree of deacetylation and molecular weight. The mucoadhesive property of chitosan increases the *in vivo* residence time of the dosage forms in the gastrointestinal tract and improves the bioavailability of various drugs. In the physiological environment, chitosan can be readily digested by enzymes such as lysozymes or chitinases,

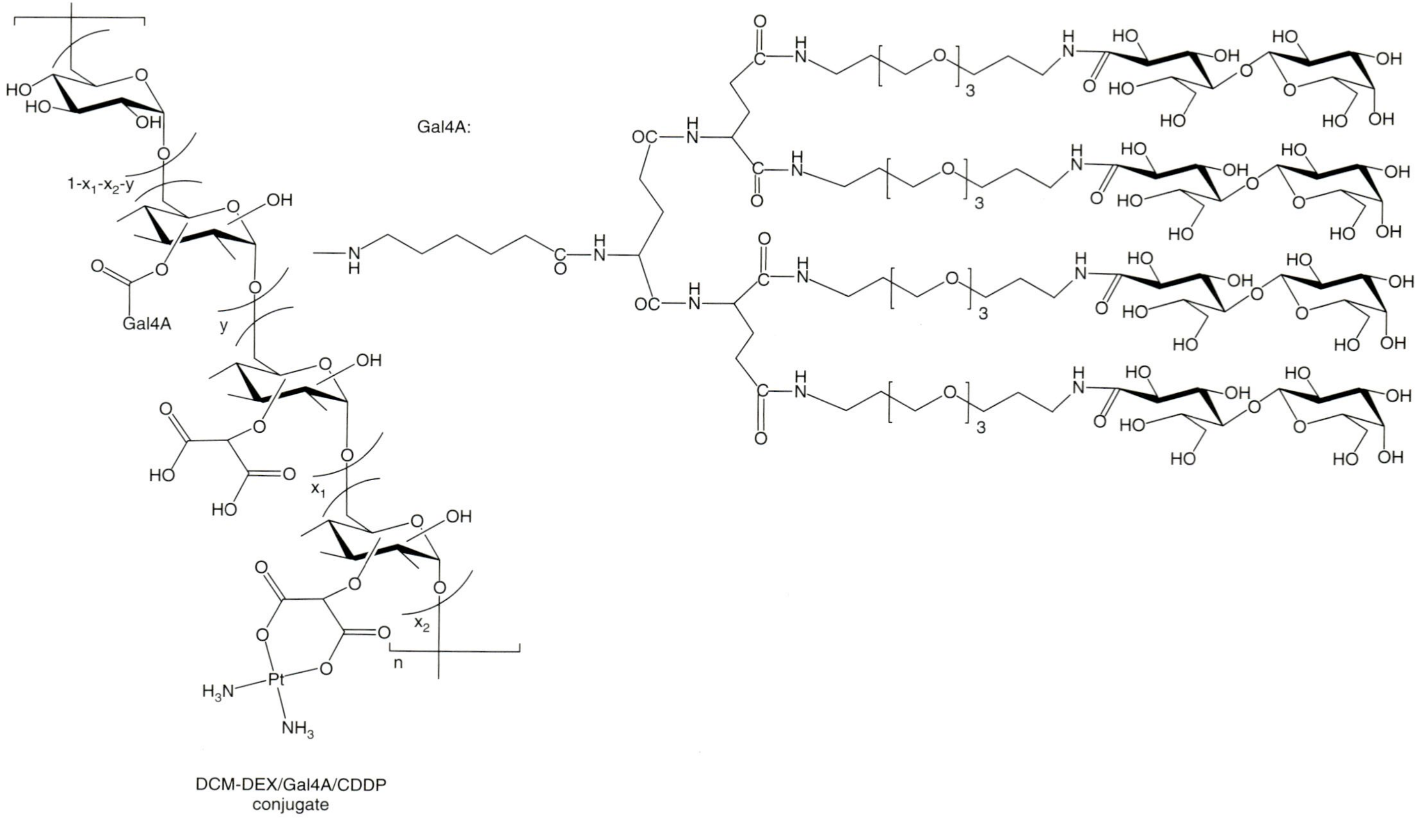

718 *23 Polysaccharide-Based Drug Conjugates for Tumor Targeting*

Figure 23.7 Chemical structure of DCM-Dex-Gal4A-CDDP conjugate.

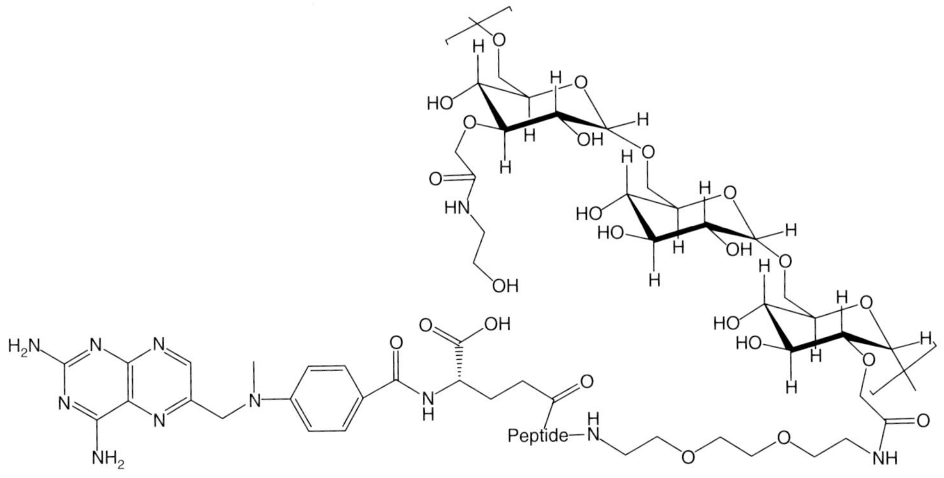

Figure 23.8 Chemical structure of Dex-peptide-MTX conjugate.

which can be produced by the normal flora in the human intestine [44]. Therefore, chitosan has been investigated as a carrier for colon-specific drug delivery. The reactive functional groups on the backbone of chitosan offer great opportunity to synthesize various chitosan derivatives such as thiolated chitosan, carboxyalkyl chitosan, N-trimethyl chitosan, N-succinimidyl chitosan, and bile acid-modified chitosan [42, 45]. These chitosan derivatives have unique properties for specific applications. For example, thiolation of chitosan improves the mucoadhesive properties, whereas its succinylation prolongs *in vivo* half-life of the polymers after intravenous administration [46, 47]. These special physicochemical and biological properties of chitosan have paved the way for its use in the delivery of various therapeutic agents [48, 49].

Chitin conjugates were prepared by chemical attachment of DOX to 6-O-carboxymethyl-chitin (CM-Chit) through a lysosomally digestible tetrapeptide spacer Gly–Phe–Leu–Gly (CM-Chit-GFLG-DOX) and an alkyl penthamethylene spacer (CM-Chit-C$_5$-DOX) using carbodiimide chemistry (Figure 23.9) [50]. The release rate of DOX from CM-Chit-GFLG-DOX increased in the presence of cathepsin B, whereas no significant change in the release behavior was observed for CM-Chit-C$_5$-DOX. The conjugates showed lower cytotoxicity compared to free DOX, in which bioactivity of the CM-Chit-GFLG-DOX conjugate was higher than CM-Chit-C$_5$-DOX, attributed to release of the drug after internalization by enzyme-mediated hydrolysis. The survival effects of these conjugates were investigated against mice bearing P388 lymphocytic leukemia cells. The results demonstrated that CM-Chit-GFLG-DOX conjugates exhibited higher survival rate, compared to the untreated mice [51].

Since conjugation of hydrophobic drugs to the hydrophilic polymers induces amphiphilic characteristics to the resulting prodrugs, some of the conjugates self-assemble into nanoparticles [52]. Kwon *et al.* prepared glycol chitosan–DOX

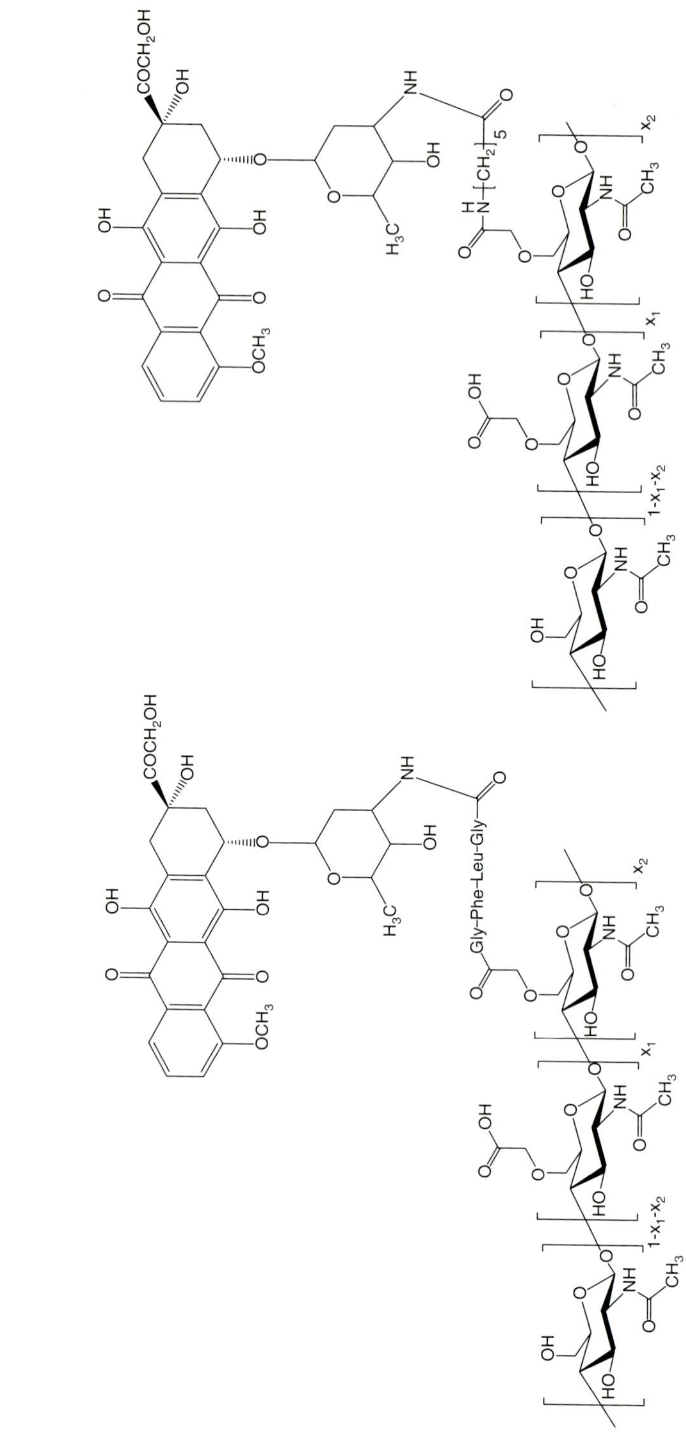

Figure 23.9 Chemical structure of chitin-based drug conjugates: (a) CM-Chit-GFLG-DOX and (b) CM-Chit-C$_5$-DOX.

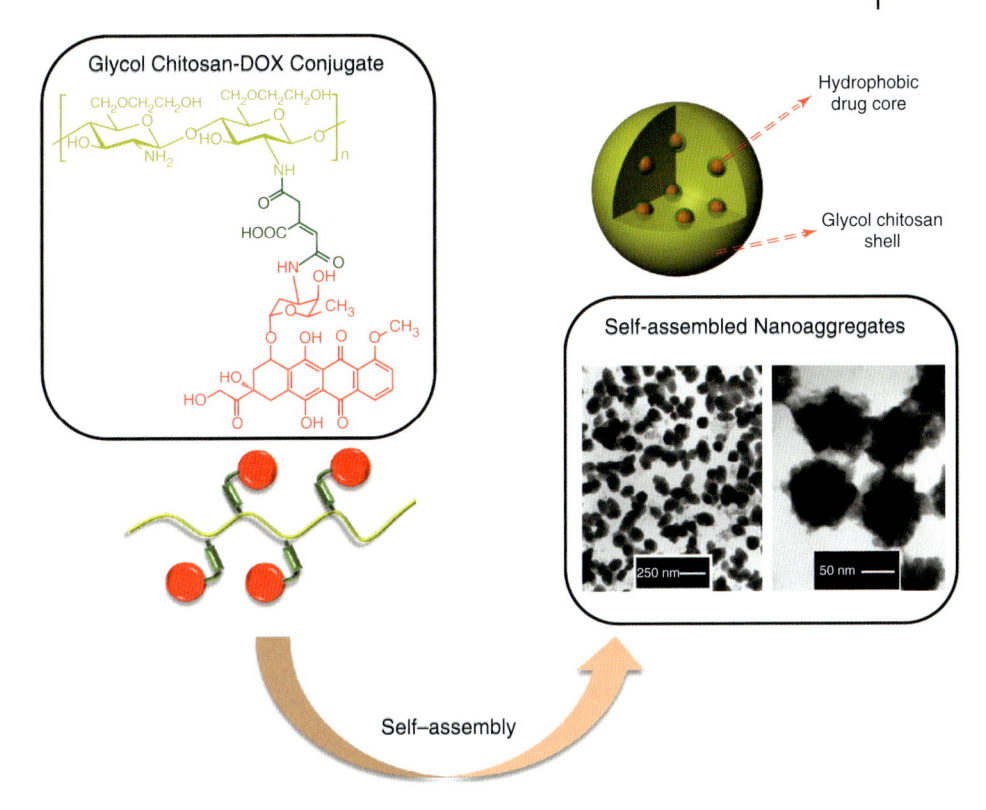

Figure 23.10 Self-assembled nanoaggregates of GC–DOX conjugate with cis-aconityl linkage. (Adapted from [53] and [54].)

with a *cis*-aconityl spacer (GC-DOX) and studied the self-assembly behavior under physiological conditions (Figure 23.10) [53, 54]. In addition, they encapsulated free DOX into the self-assembled conjugates with significantly high loading efficiency (97%). The conjugates with 2–5 wt% DOX formed self-assembled nanoparticles (250–300 nm in diameter) in aqueous conditions, whereas those with above 5.5% DOX were precipitated because of high hydrophobicity. The loading content of DOX could be increased up to 38.9% by physical encapsulation of DOX into nanoparticles. The release rate of DOX was significantly influenced by the media pH because the acid-labile *cis*-aconityl spacer was readily cleavable at the low pH. *In vivo* biodistribution study demonstrated that the distribution of nanoparticles gradually increased in tumor as blood circulation time increased, while negligible amounts of nanoparticles were found in heart and lung.

Oral delivery of anticancer drugs has often been hindered by their extremely high hydrophobicity [55]. Therefore, development of suitable formulations is of high importance to improve the bioavailability of poorly water-soluble anticancer drugs. A low-molecular-weight chitosan conjugated with PTX (LMWC–PTX) was prepared and evaluated as a carrier for the oral delivery of PTX [56].

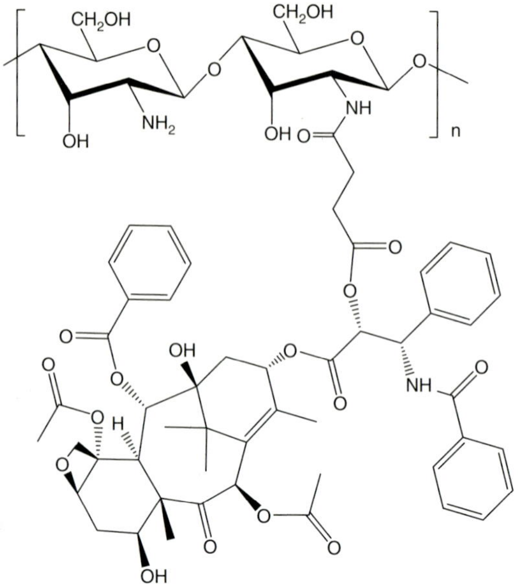

Figure 23.11 Chemical structure of LMWC–PTX conjugate with succinate linkage.

LMWC–PTX (Figure 23.11) was synthesized by chemical conjugation of low-molecular-weight chitosan and PTX through a succinate linker, which can be cleaved under physiological conditions. Compared to high-molecular-weight chitosan, low-molecular-weight chitosan (below 10 kDa) exhibits more favorable characteristics such as low toxicity and higher water solubility. Additionally, low-molecular-weight chitosan could quickly and reversibly open the tight junctions between human epithelial colorectal adenocarcinoma cells (Caco-2). Biodistribution studies performed using ^{125}I-labeled conjugates showed that LMWC–PTX was absorbed in the small intestine after oral administration and remained in its intact conjugate form until it reached the bloodstream. The main advantage of LMWC–PTX for oral delivery was the ability to bypass the P-glycoprotein-mediated barrier (efflux pump) in the gastrointestinal tract and CYP450-dependent metabolism in the intestine and liver.

N-succinyl-chitosan derivatives were conjugated with mitomycin C (MMC) in the presence of EDC as the coupling reagent [57]. However, the resulting N-succinyl-chitosan–MMC (Su-Ch–MMC) conjugates were insoluble in water due to the cross-linking reaction between the carboxyl groups and the remaining amino groups of the polymers. A soluble Su-Ch–MMC conjugate was successfully prepared by conjugating succinimidyl-activated glutaric MMC to N-succinyl-chitosan at pH 6.0 because this method avoided the use of EDC responsible for the cross-linked products. However, the drug-loading efficiency was lower (around 1.3% w/w) compared to the EDC-mediated coupling reaction (Figure 23.12) [58]. Su-Ch–MMC conjugates exhibited good antitumor activities against various tumors such as murine leukemias (L1210 and P388), B16 melanoma, Sarcoma 180

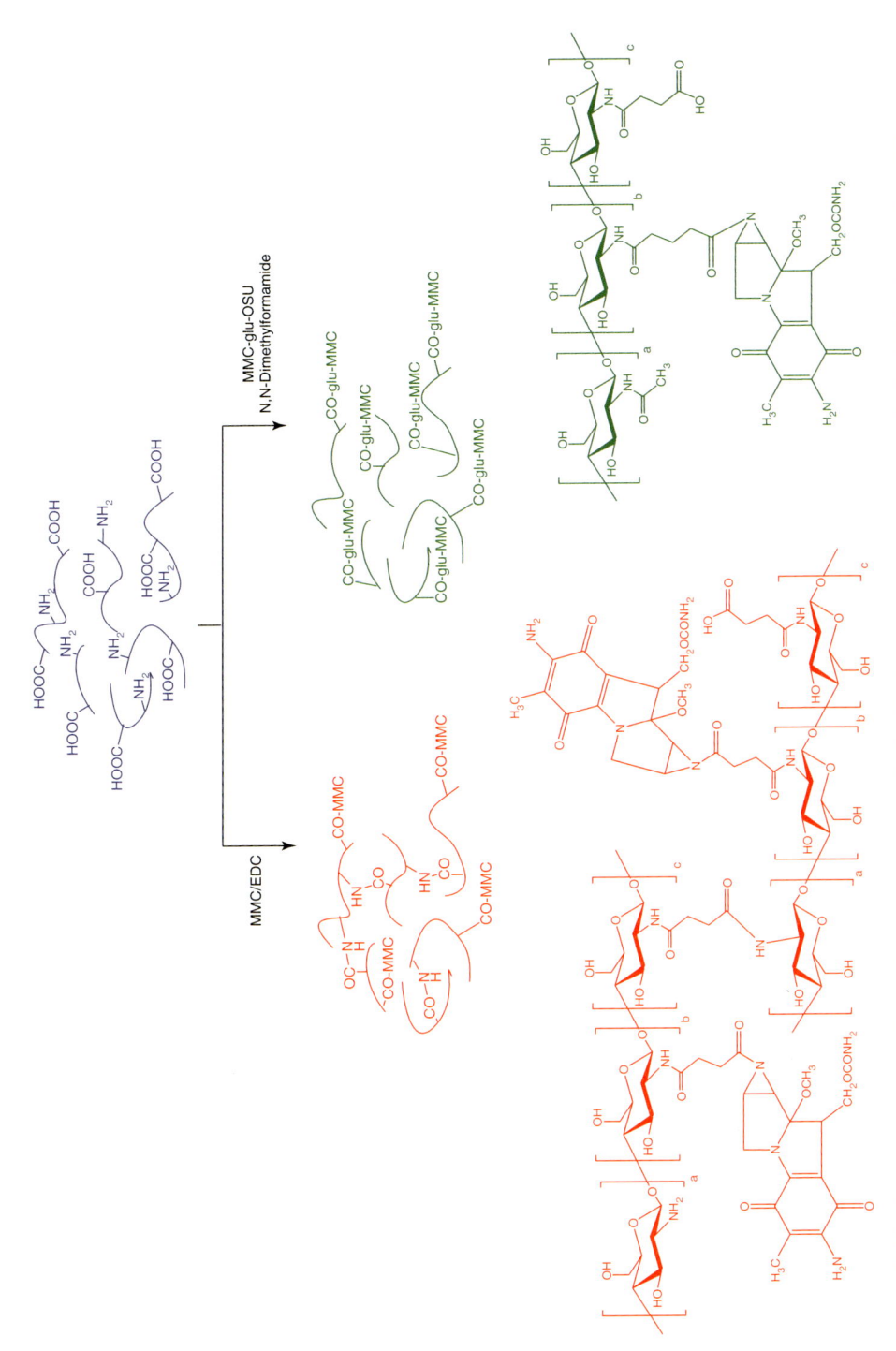

Figure 23.12 Chemical structure of cross-linked water-insoluble Su-Ch–MMC conjugate and water-soluble Su-Ch–MMC. (Adapted from [59].)

solid tumor, a murine liver metastatic tumor (M5076), and a murine hepatic cell carcinoma (MH134) [59, 60].

23.3.3
HA–Drug Conjugates

HA (also referred as hyaluronan), is a polyanionic polysaccharide found in abundance in the extracellular matrix (ECM) and synovial fluid [61, 62]. Contrary to other glycosaminoglycans, HA does not contain sulfate groups or epimerized uronic acid residues. HA plays a prominent role in the structure and organization of the ECM, and regulates various cellular functions, such as cell growth, differentiation, and migration. The chief biological function of HA is attributed to its interactions with various HA-binding receptors, such as cell surface glycoprotein CD44, a receptor for HA-mediated motility (RHAMM), HA receptor for endocytosis (HARE), and lymphatic vessel endocytic receptor (LYVE-1) [63]. Various tumors, such as epithelial, colon, and ovarian cancers, are known to overexpress HA-binding receptors (CD44 and RHAMM). Consequently, these tumor cells show enhanced binding to and effective internalization of HA. Despite the fact that the actual mechanism of the CD44–HA interaction is not fully understood, studies have shown that the CD44 receptor contains the specific binding domain (formed by 160 amino acid residues) for HA and its binding affinity increases with an increase in molecular weight of HA, due to the possibility of multiple interactions [13]. As part of our research program to explore the *in vivo* biodistribution of HA-based formulations, we recently studied the biodistribution of self-assembled HA nanoparticles using the optical imaging technique. The results obtained demonstrated that HA nanoparticles can circulate for at least 2 days in the bloodstream, and accumulate into the tumor site by a combination of passive and active targeting mechanism [64, 65].

HA has been conjugated to various drugs, including PTX, MMC, epirubicin, anthracycline antibiotics (such as DOX and DNM), and butyric acid (a short-chain fatty acid known to induce cell differentiation and inhibit the growth of various human tumor cells) [66–70]. An early synthetic approach for the preparation of HA–PTX conjugates was reported by Prestwich *et al.* [66, 71]. HA–PTX conjugates were synthesized by coupling 2′-OH PTX hydroxysuccinimide ester to adipic hydrazide-modified low-molecular-weight HA (11 kDa) (Figure 23.13). HA–PTX conjugates showed selective *in vitro* cytotoxicity against CD44-overexpressing cancer cells such as human HCT-116, SKOV-3, and HBL-100, whereas no toxicity was observed in NIH 3T3 (mouse fibroblast cell line). Competition study demonstrated that the interactions between the conjugate and the cells could be blocked by HA and anti-CD44 [71]. This strongly suggests that the selective toxicity of the conjugate is due to receptor-mediated endocytosis. The increase in cytotoxicity to cancer cells could be associated with cellular uptake of the conjugate, followed by hydrolytic release of the drugs via labile linkages (at C-2′ ester linkages). On the other hand, the conjugation of a large amount PTX to HA reduced the solubility and altered

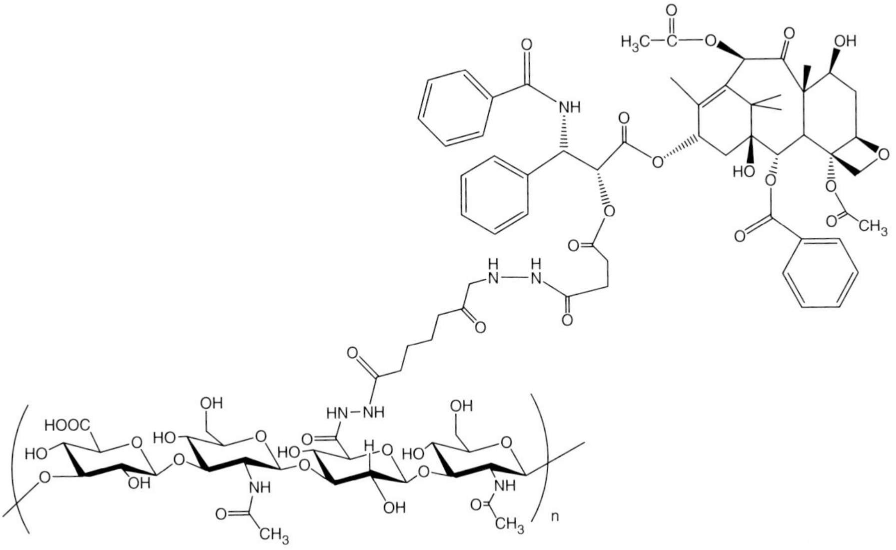

Figure 23.13 Chemical structure of HA–PTX conjugate prepared using adipic hydrazide-modified low-molecular-weight HA.

the configuration of the HA structure, which prevented binding affinity of HA to the receptor and resulted in decreased cytotoxicity [66].

Tabrizian et al. prepared a macromolecular HA–PTX prodrug by conjugating the 2′-hemisuccinate derivative of PTX to the amine-modified HA. They constructed polyelectrolyte multilayers (PEMs) by the layer-by-layer technique using the HA–PTX prodrug as polyanion and chitosan as polycation [72]. These PEMs are attractive strategies for encapsulating bioactive molecules and improving pharmacokinetics of the drug. The intrinsic hydrophilicity and poor solubility of HA in most organic solvents have limited the facile conjugation of hydrophobic drugs to the HA backbone. Recently, a simple nanocomplexing method using HA in a single organic phase was reported to prepare HA–PTX with a drug loading content of about 10.8% (w/w) [73]. When compared to the commercial available taxol formulation, HA–PTX conjugate micelles exhibited more cytotoxicity toward CD44+ cancer cells (HCT-116 and MCF-7 cells).

In recent years, a series of HA-based drug conjugates (ONCOFID™) has been developed by covalently conjugating cytotoxic drugs such as PTX, CPT, DOX, and platinum to the HA backbone directly or through spacers. The HA–PTX conjugate (referred as *ONCOFID-P*) was prepared by reacting PTX 2′-(4-bromobutanoate) with HA–thiobarbituric acid (200 kDa) in N-methyl-2-pyrrolidone (Figure 23.14a). This method resulted in a drug content of 20% (w/w) [74]. The in vitro inhibitory activity of the conjugate was much higher than free PTX against CD44 receptor-positive RT4 and RT112/84 bladder carcinoma cells. The conjugates were stable in human urine (pH 6.5), and no free drug was detected for 6 h of incubation. Similarly, the concentration of PTX in the blood was negligible after

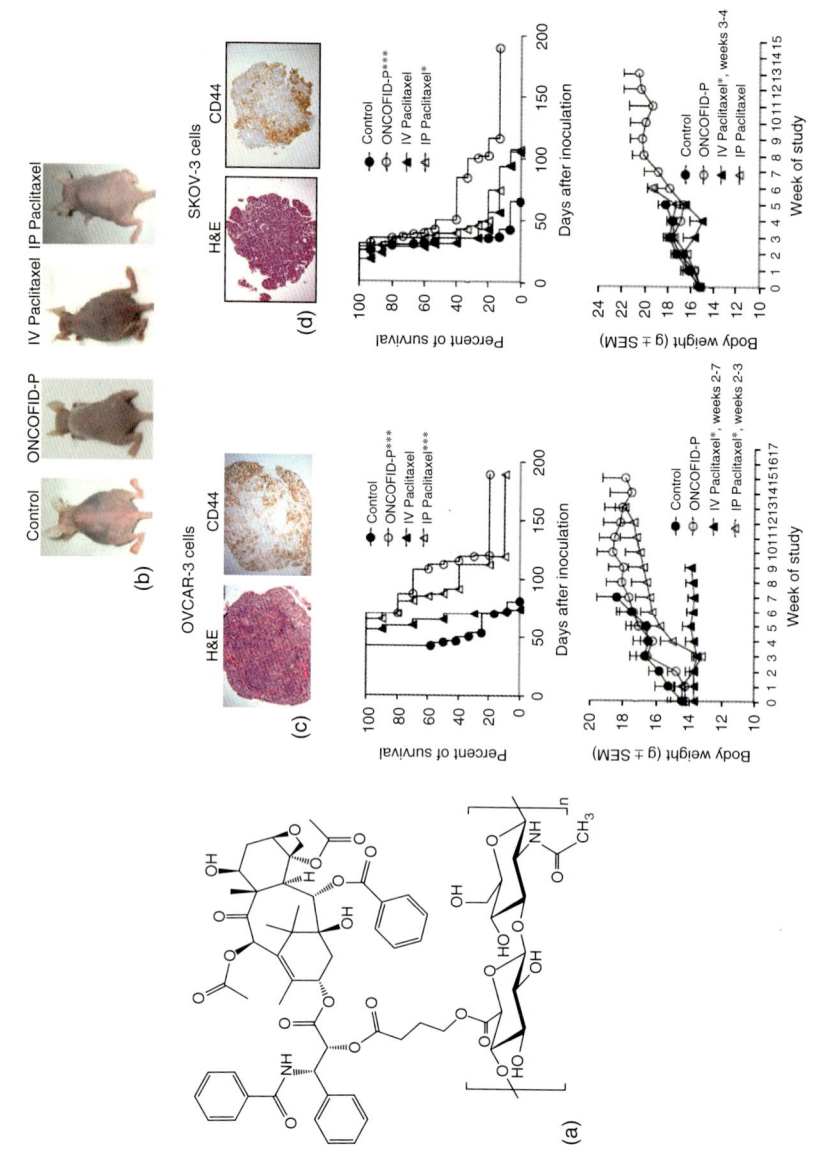

Figure 23.14 (a) Chemical structure of ONCOFID-P. (b) Representative images of mice in the different treatment groups at 6 weeks after tumor inoculation (OVCAR-3 cells). Effect of ONCOFID-P on tumor growth in female athymic mice inoculated with (c) OVCAR-3 cells and (d) SKOV-3 cells. (Adapted from [77].)

intrabladder instillation of the conjugate, indicating the conjugates were also stable under *in vivo* physiological conditions. In addition, histological examinations revealed that the conjugates were well tolerated and no significant morphological changes were observed in the urinary epithelium, while the free PTX produced notable toxic effects on the bladder. The *in vivo* antitumor therapeutic activity of the conjugate evaluated using mice-bearing RT-112/84 transitional cell carcinoma cells was comparable to that of free PTX. The results indicated that *in vivo* tumor growth inhibitory activity of ONCOFID-P against ovarian cancer cells (IGROV-1 and OVCAR-3) was higher than that of unconjugated PTX [75]. The *in vivo* biodistribution of ^{99m}Tc-labeled ONCOFID-P was evaluated after intravenous, intravesical, oral, or intraperitoneal administration in BALB/c mice. The result showed a high liver and spleen uptake for the conjugates injected intravenously, while those administered locally remained at the administration site. However, the biodistribution of free PTX was significantly different from the conjugates [76]. Recently, the bioactivity of the conjugate was evaluated by two different *in vivo* experimental models closely reflecting disease progression in human ovarian cancer with tumor dissemination throughout the peritoneum and ascites production. The results showed that for both experimental models, ONCOFID-P inhibited intra-abdominal tumor dissemination and production of ascites, resulting in prolonged survival of animals. In contrast, therapy with the maximum tolerated dose of free PTX was completely devoid of efficacy and showed toxicity, as demonstrated by loss of body weight. Notably, although administration of free PTX by the intraperitoneal route increased efficacy in comparison to free drug given by the intravenous route, the therapeutic outcome was still less than ONCOFID-P administration in both models (Figure 23.14) [77]. ONCOFID-P is under phase II evaluation for the treatment of refractory bladder cancer and a phase I study has been initiated for the treatment of peritoneal carcinosis.

23.3.4
Heparin–Drug Conjugates

Heparin, a highly sulfated polysaccharide, is composed of repeating units of 1–4-linked uronic acid and glucosamine residues. Heparin has a number of structural variations: both uronic acid and glucosamine may be substituted with sulfo groups at the pyranose ring. In addition to its anticoagulant activity, heparin has many other biological functions associated with its interaction with diverse proteins, such as inhibition of growth of smooth muscle cells, regulation of lipid metabolism, binding with acidic and basic fibroblast growth factors (FGFs), induction of apoptosis, and inhibition of angiogenesis and tumor metastasis [78–80].

Angiogenesis – the formation of new blood vessels from pre-existing vessels – is a fundamental process in a variety of physiological and pathological conditions, including tumor growth, metastasis, and inflammation. This process involves extensive interplay between cells, soluble factors, and the ECM. Cancer cells

728 *23 Polysaccharide-Based Drug Conjugates for Tumor Targeting*

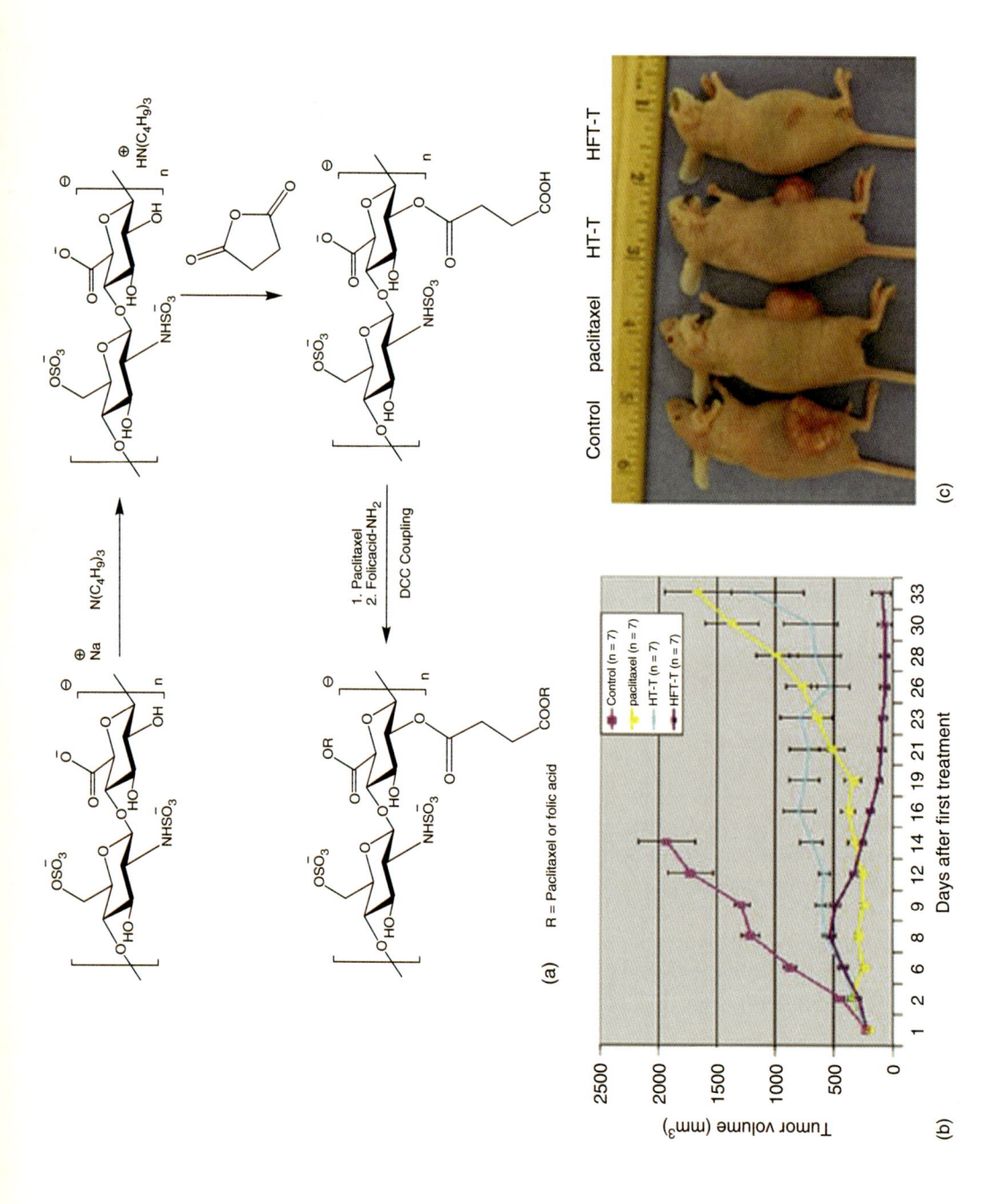

produce a number of angiogenic growth factors such as vascular endothelial growth factor (VEGF) and basic FGF. From various studies, it was demonstrated that heparin is effective for the inhibition of VEGF- and basic FGF-mediated angiogenesis [81, 82]. Despite the beneficial effect of heparin on cancer therapy, its strong anticoagulant activity limited clinical applications at high dose and for long-term treatment. Therefore, there is a great interest in the development of chemically modified heparin derivatives to reduce the anticoagulant activity, and to enhance the inhibitory effects of heparin on tumor growth and metastasis.

Xiang et al. prepared heparin–PTX conjugates by reacting PTX with the O-acetylated heparin via an ester linkage or amino acid spacer [83]. The release rate of PTX from the conjugates with the amino acid spacer increased progressively in the presence of enzyme (esterase), whereas the conjugate without the spacer was highly stable under physiological and enzymatic conditions. As a result of chemical modification, the anticoagulant activity of the heparin–PTX conjugate was significantly lower than heparin because introduction of PTX to heparin induced a conformational change in the heparin structure, thus reducing affinity to antithrombin III.

In an attempt to enhance therapeutic efficacy, heparin derivatives were modified with targeting ligands such as cyclic RGD and folic acid [84, 85]. Recently, Shin et al. synthesized a ternary conjugate comprising heparin–folic acid–PTX (HFT–PTX), to which PTX was further physically encapsulated to the self-assembled HFT nanoparticles (Figure 23.15a) [85]. For the synthesis of HFT conjugates, PTX and ethylene diamine-modified folic acid were reacted with the succinylated heparin through the formation of ester and amide bonds, respectively. The ester bond between the drug and heparin could facilitate release of the drug from the conjugate, while the amide bond between the ligand and heparin showed high stability. The conjugation reaction yielded 15% (w/w) of PTX in the carrier and the drug loading content was further increased up to 26% (w/w) by physical encapsulation of PTX into HFT nanoparticles (HFT-T). HFT-T showed higher cytotoxicity toward KB-3-1 cells expressing high levels of folate receptor compared to free PTX and the nanoparticles without folate ligand (HT-T). The *in vivo* antitumor efficacy of HFT-T, HT-T, and free PTX was also evaluated in KB-3-1 tumor-bearing mice. Compared with the control group (saline), tumor volumes in all treatment groups were significantly reduced. In particular, tumor volume in the HFT-T group was significantly smaller than in the free PTX and HT-T groups, primarily due to the active tumor targeting mechanism of HFT-T (Figure 23.15b and c).

Figure 23.15 (a) Synthetic scheme for the preparation of HFT–PTX conjugates. (b) *In vivo* antitumor activity of PTX, heparin–PTX nanoparticles, HFT nanoparticles, and control (saline). (c) Photographs of a representative mouse from each group. (Adapted from [85].)

23.3.5
Pullulan–Drug Conjugates

Pullulan is a water-soluble exopolysaccharide produced from starch by a polymorphic fungus *Aureobasidium pullulans*. Its chemical structure is composed of maltotriose (with 5–7% maltotetrose) connected by α1–4- and α1–6-glucosidic linkages in a ratio of 2 : 1 [86]. Pullulan can be chemically derivatized to impart new useful physicochemical properties for specific applications. Introduction of the carboxyl group into the backbone of pullulan increases its resistance to amylase, which allows controlling its degradation rate *in vivo* [87]. The sulfated derivative of pullulan has a similar function to anticoagulant agents such as heparin and Dex sulfate. Bioactivity of sulfated pullulan is influenced by various factors such as molecular weight and degree of substitution of the sulfate group [88]. In addition, pullulan selectively binds to the asialoglycoproteins (ASGPs) receptor, expressed exclusively on the surface of liver parenchymal cells [89]. This inherent ability of pullulan has been widely exploited for targeted delivery of drugs and genes to the liver [90, 91].

Nogusa *et al.* investigated the potential of carboxymethyl-pullulan (CM-Pul) as a carrier of anticancer drugs (Figure 23.16a) [92]. They conjugated the amino group of DOX to CM-Pul through various tetrapeptide spacers, including GGFG (CM-Pul–DOX-I), Gly–Phe–Gly–Gly (CM-Pul–DOX-II), and Gly–Gly–Gly–Gly (CM-Pul–DOX-III). Due to their amphiphilic nature, the conjugates were self-assembled in a physiological solution to form micelles. The amount of DOX released from CM-Pul–DOX-I conjugate in the presence of rat liver lysosomal enzymes was found to be 35% in 24 h, while no free DOX was released from the conjugates without the spacer. The antitumor effect of these conjugates in rats bearing Walker 256 was studied by monitoring the tumor weights after a single intravenous injection, at a dose of 0.8 mg/kg of DOX. Compared to free DOX, the conjugates CM-Pul–DOX-I and CM-Pul–DOX-II significantly suppressed tumor growth, while CM-Pul–DOX-III showed less antitumor effect than free DOX. The conjugates without the spacer showed no *in vivo* antitumor effect even at the high DOX dose of 20 mg/kg.

Similarly, a pH-sensitive pullulan–drug conjugate was prepared by covalently conjugating DOX to CM-Pul through a hydrazone bond (Figure 23.16b) [93]. The conjugates formed nanoparticles (less than 100 nm in diameter) with negatively charged surfaces, which showed low toxicity in 4T1 mouse breast cancer cells. Owing to the presence of the pH linker, the *in vitro* DOX release from the conjugates at pH 5.0 was much faster than at pH 7.4.

23.3.6
Other Natural Polymer–Drug Conjugates

23.3.6.1 Alginate–Drug Conjugates
Alginate is a linear hydrophilic natural copolymer composed of β-D-mannuronic acid and β-L-guluronic acid residues, interconnected through the

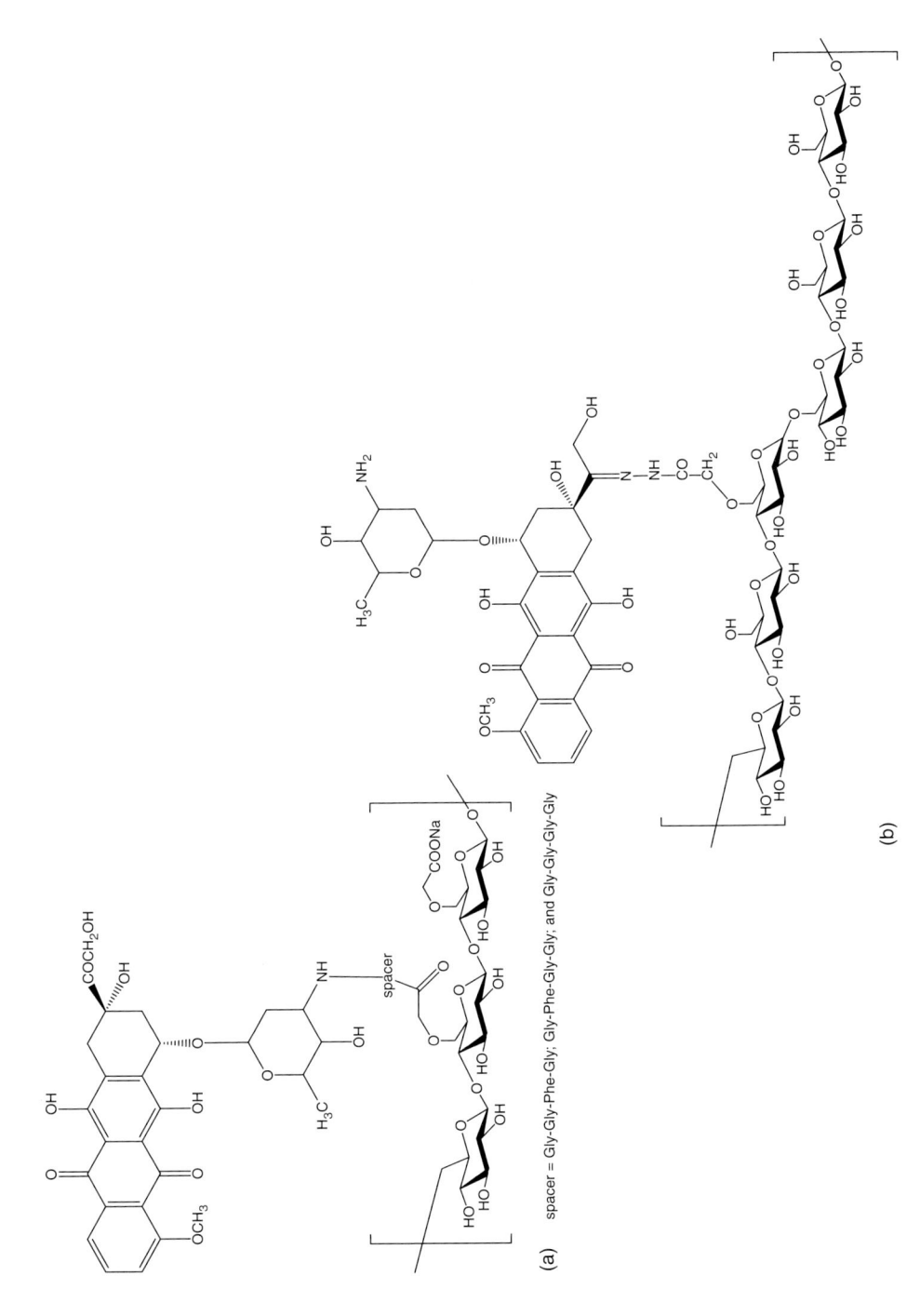

Figure 23.16 Chemical structure of (a) CM-Pul-peptide-DOX conjugate and (b) pH-sensitive pullulan–DOX conjugate.

(a) spacer = Gly-Gly-Gly; Gly-Phe-Gly-Gly; and Gly-Gly-Gly-Gly

1–4-interglycosidic linkage. It is generally extracted from marine brown algae or soil bacteria, and has a broad molecular weight distribution (10–1000 kDa) depending on the source and processing [94].

Alginate is known to exhibit inherent antitumor activity against murine tumor models because it stimulates production of cytokines such as tumor necrosis factor-α, interleukin-1, and interleukin-6 from human monocytes [95, 96]. This prompted researchers to prepare a macromolecular prodrug by covalently conjugating the antitumor agents to the alginates. Duncan et al. prepared the conjugates by the chemical reaction between alginate and 5-aminosalicyclic acid (5-ASA) or DNM [97, 98]. In particular, DNM was covalently attached to alginate via an acid-labile cis-aconityl linkage for the specific delivery of the drug into the slightly acidic extracellular fluid of solid tumors or into the endo/lysosomal compartments of tumor cells. The in vitro drug-release studies for the alginate–DNM conjugates showed a minimal release of DNM (around 2–4%) at neutral pH, whereas 22–60% of DNM was released under acidic conditions (pH 5 and 6) at 48 h. The conjugate exhibited dose-dependent cytotoxicity against B16-F10 cells, which was found to be less than free DNM. A single intraperitoneal injection of the conjugate (equivalent to 5 mg/kg DNM) into the mice effectively suppressed tumor growth, compared to mice treated with same dosage of free DNM.

23.3.6.2 Arabinogalactan–Drug Conjugates

Arabinogalactan (AG), a highly branched water-soluble polysaccharide, is isolated from plant sources such as trees of the genus *Larix* (*Larix occidentalis*) in a pure form (99.9%). AG consists of arabinose and galactose in a ratio of approximately 1 : 6 [99]. The unique feature of AG is its highly branched structure and the presence of numerous terminal galactose residues, allowing them to strongly bind to the ASGP receptor in the liver [100]. In addition, the high water solubility and ease of drug conjugation in aqueous medium makes AG an attractive macromolecular carrier option for the receptor-mediated delivery of therapeutic agents to liver parenchymal cells. In general, AG–drug conjugates can be synthesized by two methods: (i) oxidation of the polysaccharide with periodate to obtain the dialdehyde derivative, followed by conjugation to the amine-containing drug via Schiff base formation, and (ii) modification of the polysaccharide with functional leaving groups such as tosylate and mesylate on the polymer chains, followed by reaction with amine-containing drugs [101]. In recent years, MTX and folate have been conjugated into AG through a tetrapeptide linker (GFLG) (Figure 23.17) [102]. The conjugates displayed 6.3-fold higher cytotoxicity to folate receptor-overexpressing cells compared to their folate receptor-lacking counterparts. On the other hand, no significant cytotoxicity was observed for the conjugate without tetrapeptide spacer on both cell lines tested. This indicates that an intracellular release mechanism of the drug is essential to exert activity.

23.3.6.3 Pectin–Drug Conjugates

Pectins are water-soluble anionic polysaccharides found in the cell walls of plants. They are predominantly linear polymers consisting of α1–4-linked D-galacturonic

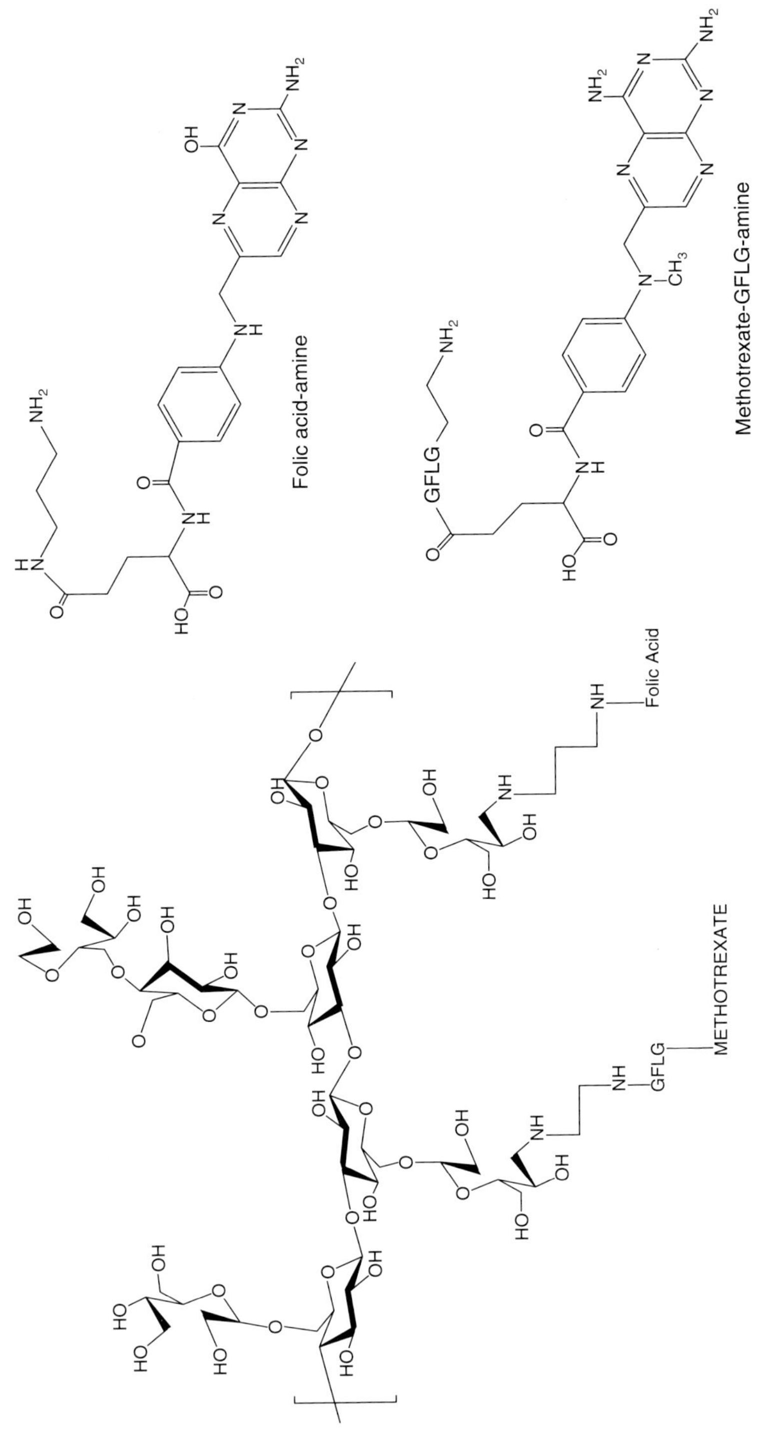

23.3 Polysaccharide-Drug Conjugates | 733

Figure 23.17 Chemical structure of AG–MTX conjugate.

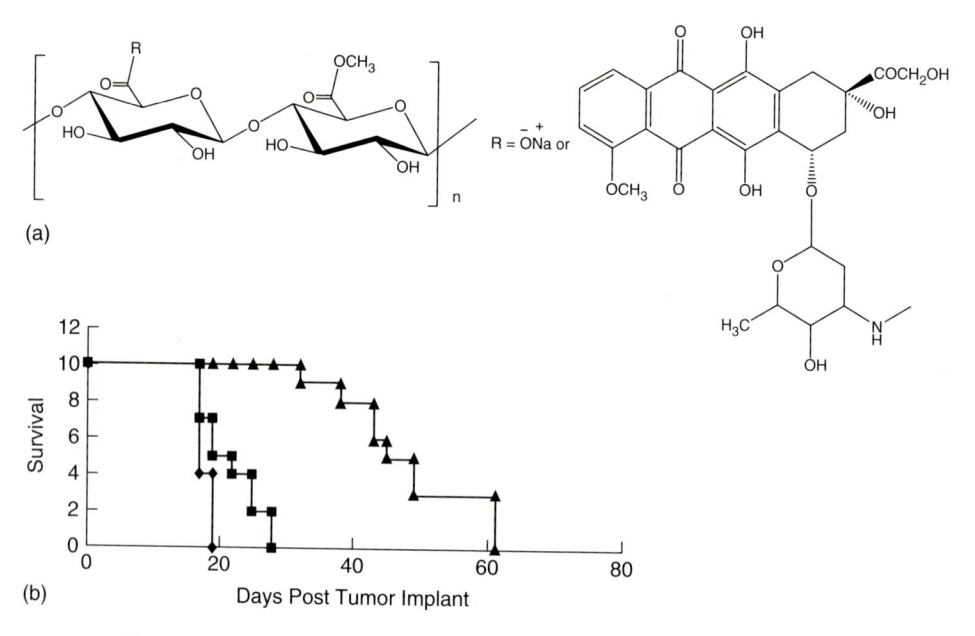

Figure 23.18 (a) Chemical structure of pectin–adriamycin conjugate. (b) Comparison of survival rate between pectin–DOX conjugate (▲), free DOX (■), and untreated group (♦) [104].

acid residues, where some of the carboxyl groups of the uronic acids are present as methyl esters. Pectin has been widely studied as a carrier for colon-specific drug delivery since pectin is resistant to protease in the upper gastrointestinal tract and is digested by a large number of microflora in the colon [103]. The carboxyl group of pectin has been utilized for the conjugation of anticancer drugs to produce pectin–drug conjugates with high loading content of the drug. A pectin–adriamycin conjugate, with a drug content of 25% (w/w), was synthesized by the chemical reaction between adriamycin and methoxylated pectin through formation of an amide linkage (Figure 23.18a) [104]. The amount of drug released from the conjugate under plasma conditions was negligible, whereas 32.2% of the drug was released from the conjugates after incubation for 30 h with lysosomes. The *in vivo* anticancer effect of the conjugates was evaluated with tumor-bearing C57BL/6 mice. Compared with free adriamycin, the conjugate suppressed tumor growth significantly and prolonged the survival time of the mice (Figure 23.18b).

23.3.6.4 Xyloglucan–Drug Conjugates

Xyloglucan (XG), a polysaccharide isolated and purified from tamarind seed, is composed of a 1–4-linked α-D-glucan backbone chain. A galactosed XG–DOX (G-XG–DOX) conjugate was synthesized by conjugating galactosamine and DOX to the carboxylic acids of XG using carbodiimide coupling reagents under aqueous conditions [105]. The conjugates with DOX content higher than 5% (w/w) exhibited low solubility and precipitated in aqueous media due to excessive hydrophobicity. However, the physical encapsulation of DOX into the G-XG–DOX nanoparticles increased the loading content up to 23.8% (w/w). G-XG–DOX nanoparticles showed similar cytotoxicity to free DOX against a human liver cancer cell line (HepG2). The *in vivo* antitumor activities of G-XG–DOX nanoparticles, XG–DOX nanoparticles, and free DOX were evaluated using male BALB/c/*nu* naked mice inoculated with HepG2 cells. The results indicated that G-XG–DOX nanoparticles exhibited the highest therapeutic effect on the tumor.

23.3.6.5 Polygalactosamine–Drug Conjugates

α1–4-Polygalactosamine (PGA) and *N*-acetyl PGA (NPGA) are biodegradable and biocompatible polysaccharides. They act as growth inhibitors of certain tumor cells through stimulation of the host immune system [106, 107]. In particular, they are expected to have high affinities to hepatocytes because they have galactosamine or *N*-acetyl galactosamine at the chain end. The prodrugs were prepared by conjugating 6-O-carboxymethyl-NPGA to DOX or 5-FU through a Gly–Phe–Leu–Gly spacer. Both the DOX conjugate and 5-FU conjugate showed cathepsin B-susceptible release of DOX. *In vitro* cytotoxicity of the 5-FU conjugate hepatoma cells was stronger than free 5-FU [106]. Further, the DOX conjugate exhibited remarkable survival effects in mice bearing MH134Y hepatoma, compared with free DOX.

23.4 Cyclodextrin–Drug Conjugates

Supramolecular architectures using cyclodextrins have received attention for delivery of genetic material, therapeutic proteins, and low molecular drugs [108–110]. Cyclodextrins are class of cyclic oligosaccharides mainly composed of six, seven, or eight D-glucopyranose units linked by α1–4 glucosidic bonds, which are referred to as α, β, and γ cyclodextrins, respectively. They have a truncated cone (toroidal) shape with a hydrophilic exterior due to the presence of hydroxyl groups at the surface of the molecules. Owing to the hydrophobic characteristics of the interior cavity, cyclodextrins can accommodate lipophilic guest molecules and form inclusion complexes with polymers [111]. This attractive feature of cyclodextrins has been exploited widely for solubilization of various lipophilic drugs, resulting in their enhanced bioavailability and reduced toxicity after systemic administration. The cyclodextrin-bearing conjugates were prepared by grafting cyclodextrin onto synthetic or natural polymers such as polyethyleneimine or chitosan. Linear cyclodextrin-containing polymers have also been synthesized for drug delivery [112]. A CPT-conjugated linear polymer containing cyclodextrin (referred to as IT-101) was reported by Davis *et al.* [113, 114]. To prepare the IT-101 conjugate, dicysteine-β-cyclodextrin was first synthesized by reacting diiodo-functionalized β-cyclodextrin with L-cysteine. Then, dicysteine-β-cyclodextrin monomer was reacted with PEG-dipropanoic succinimide to obtain a linear copolymer consisting of β-cyclodextrin and PEG. Subsequently, the pendant free carboxylic group available

(a)

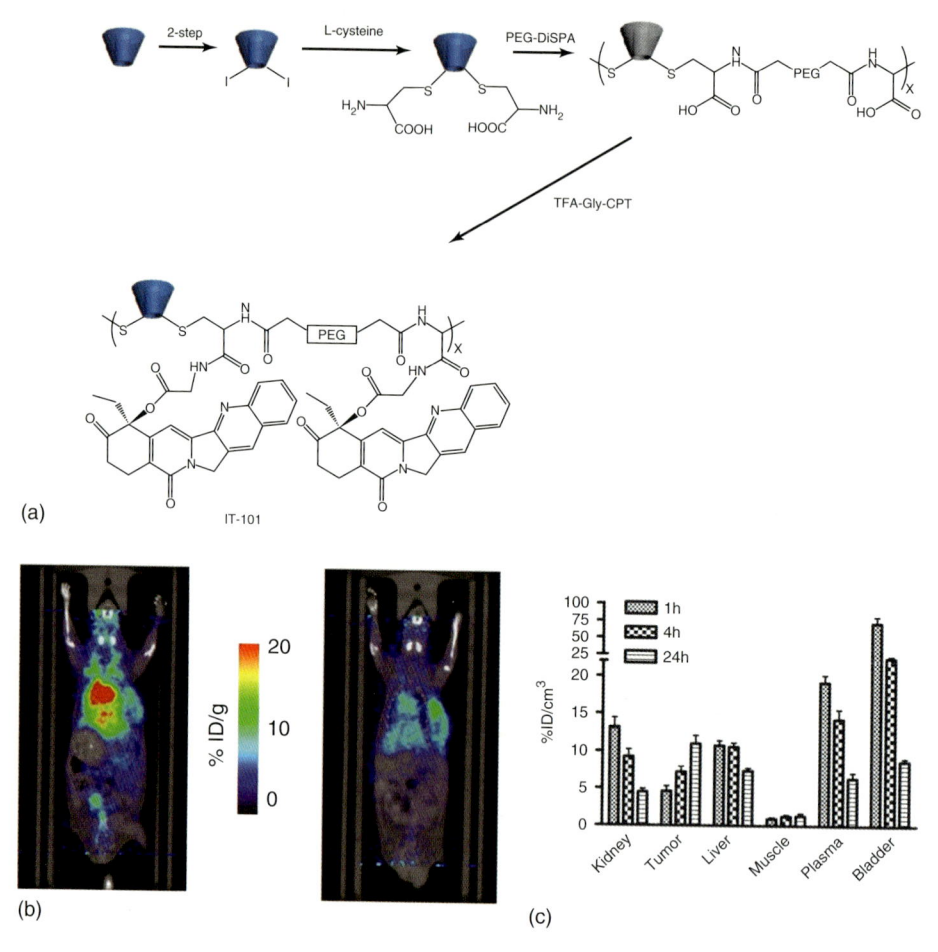

(b) (c)

Figure 23.19 (a) Schematic diagram for the synthesis of cyclodextrin-containing polymer conjugate of CPT (IT-101). In vivo biodistribution of ^{64}Cu-labeled IT-101 in mice bearing Neuro2A tumor. (b) Fused positron emission tomography/computed tomography images of tumor-bearing mouse 4 (left) and 24 h (right) after injection. (c) Tissue distribution at 1, 4, and 24 h after injection. (Adapted from [114] and [117].)

from the amino acid moiety at the main-chain was utilized for the conjugation of CPT via a biodegradable glycine-based linker (Figure 23.19a). Under aqueous conditions, the resulting conjugates formed self-assembled nanoparticles (30–40 nm in diameter) driven by interstrand CPT/β-cyclodextrin inclusion complex formation. When CPT was conjugated to the cyclodextrin-containing polymers, its solubility increased more than 3 orders of magnitudes. Intravenous administration of IT-101 nanoparticles into mice bearing LS174T colon carcinoma tumors resulted in prolonged plasma half-life (24 h) and significantly enhanced distribution to the tumors compared to CPT alone [115]. Further, the plasma half-life was significantly longer in humans (40 h) compared to mice. A single intravenous dose of IT-101

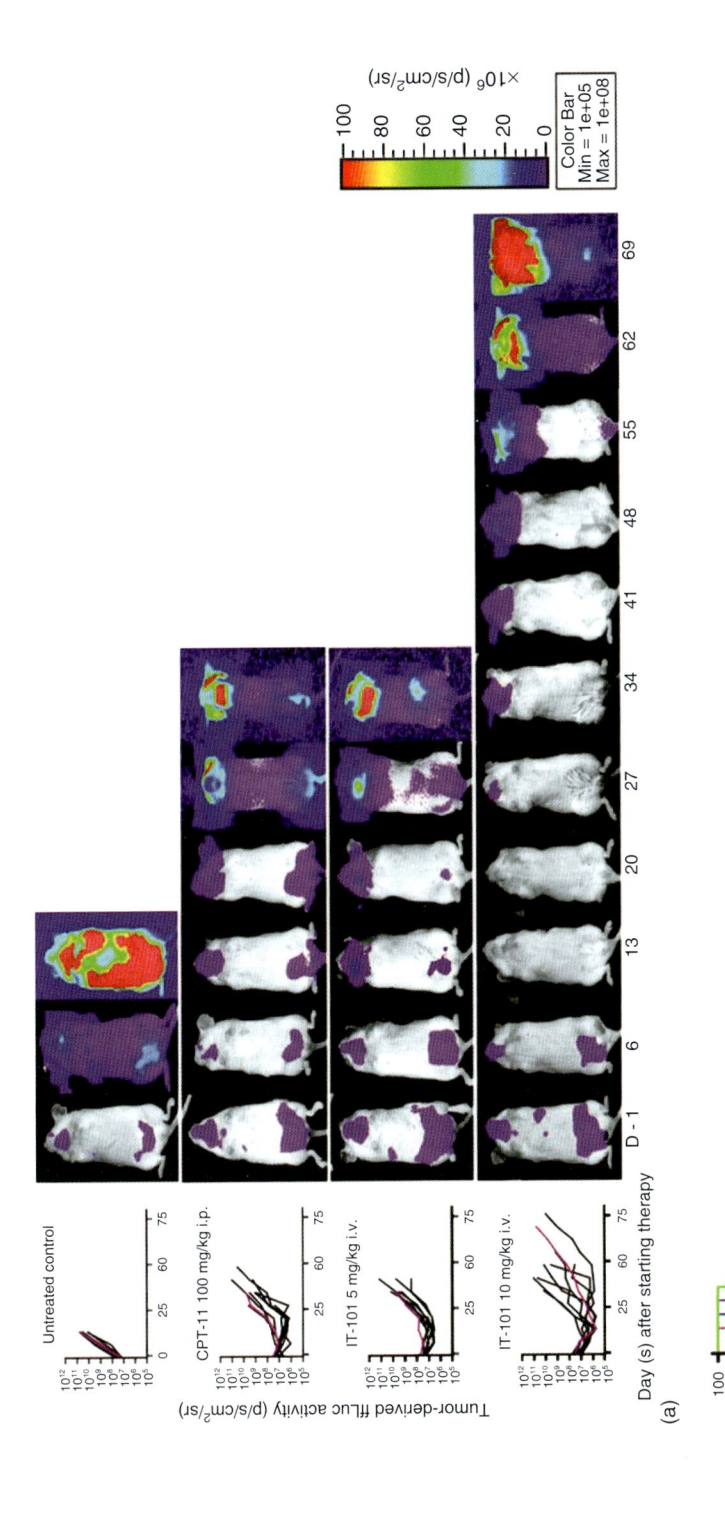

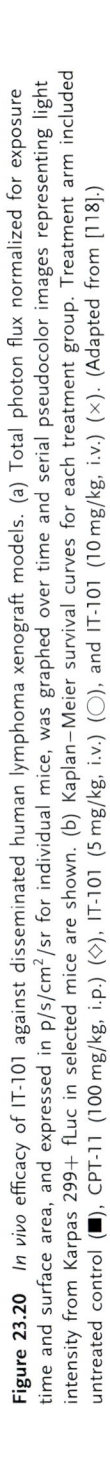

Figure 23.20 *In vivo* efficacy of IT-101 against disseminated human lymphoma xenograft models. (a) Total photon flux normalized for exposure time and surface area, and expressed in p/s/cm²/sr for individual mice, was graphed over time and serial pseudocolor images representing light intensity from Karpas 299+ fLuc in selected mice are shown. (b) Kaplan–Meier survival curves for each treatment group. Treatment arm included untreated control (■), CPT-11 (100 mg/kg, i.p.) (◊), IT-101 (5 mg/kg, i.v.) (○), and IT-101 (10 mg/kg, i.v.) (×). (Adapted from [118].)

(18.3 mg equivalent of CPT/kg) resulted in an equivalent antitumor effect to three weekly doses of irinotecan (intraperitoneal; 100 mg/kg/dose) [116]. In addition, systemic administration of IT-101 in combination with other chemotherapeutic agents such as carboplatin or CDDP exhibited greater activity than their respective monotherapies in the A2780 human carcinoma xenograft model. *In vivo* biodistribution studies using ^{64}C-labeled IT-101 in mice bearing Neuro2A tumors showed a biphasic elimination. Approximately 8% of the injected dose was rapidly cleared as a low-molecular-weight fraction through the kidneys, while the remaining circulated in plasma with a half-life of 13.3 h. At 24 h after injection, the concentration of IT-101 in the tumor steadily increased (up to 11% of injected dose/cm^3), whereas there were no significant amounts of IT-101 in other tissues (Figure 23.19b and c) [117]. In preclinical evaluation, IT-101 showed significant inhibition of tumor growth both *in vitro* and *in vivo*. In addition, administration of IT-101 to tumor-bearing mice resulted in prolonged survival of the mice. In particular, animals treated with IT-101 (10 mg/kg) showed longer survival than those with IT-101 (5 mg/kg) and CPT-11, whereas the untreated controls died within 29 days (Figure 23.20) [118]. Based on these promising results, a phase I/II clinical trial has been initiated for IT-101 to treat patients with lymphoma.

23.5
Conclusions and Perspectives

Conjugation of anticancer drugs to macromolecular carriers is an effective strategy to maximize therapeutic effects without side-effects. Natural polysaccharides hold enormous potential for the design of macromolecular drug conjugates because of their biocompatibility, biodegradability, facile chemical modification, and unique physicochemical characteristics. In this chapter, we have discussed synthetic strategies and the recent development of numerous tumor-targeted drug conjugates based on polysaccharides. Beginning with the passive targeting of anticancer drugs to the tumors by the simple conjugation of drugs to polysaccharides, in the past few years significant research efforts have been made toward the design of novel drug conjugates that could selectively deliver drug to tumors through an active targeting mechanism. Active and selective uptake of conjugates into tumors could be achieved by either conjugating a biorecognizable moiety to the backbone of the polysaccharide (e.g., folate-conjugated heparin–PTX conjugate) or directly conjugating drugs to polysaccharides that have an inherent ability to recognize specific receptors on the tumor cells (e.g., HA–drug conjugates). Also, various linkers, such as acid-sensitive linkages (e.g., *cis*-aconityl and hydrazone bonds), enzymatically cleavable linkers, and reduction-sensitive linkers, have been utilized to ensure controlled drug release at the target site.

Nevertheless, the successful clinical translation of macromolecular drug conjugates requires optimization of many distinct parameters, including characteristics of the macromolecular carrier, spacer molecule between the drug and the carrier, stability of the spacer in the vascular circulation, release of drugs within the cellular targets, and more detailed understanding of microenvironment of the tumor. Despite all the promising aspects, compared with other synthetic (biodegradable) polymers, only a few polysaccharide-based drug conjugates have entered clinical trials. Recently, the OX-Dex–DOX conjugate revealed significant toxicities in phase I studies, presumably owing to the toxicity of the OX-Dex carrier. Hence, it is important that modification of polysaccharides should not alter their physiochemical or biological characteristics. Currently, the HA–PTX conjugate (ONCOFID-P) is undergoing phase II evaluation for the treatment of refractory bladder cancer, and a phase I study has been initiated for intraperitoneal carcinosis in ovarian, breast, stomach, bladder, and colon cancer.

In recent years, combination therapy using conjugates bearing two chemotherapeutic agents has offered new hope to improve the therapeutic potential, since they can attack the tumor cells through multiple mechanisms and thus effectively inhibit tumor growth. Polymer-directed enzyme prodrug therapy by sequential administration of macromolecular drug conjugates containing enzymatically cleavable linkers and polymer–enzyme conjugates has been developed to improve the therapeutic effectiveness by generating drugs selectively at the tumor site. In conclusion, it is evident that polysaccharide-based drug conjugates have promising potential for effective therapy of tumors and they will pave the way for reducing mortality caused by tumors.

References

1. Jain, R.K. (1996) Delivery of molecular medicine to solid tumors. *Science*, **271**, 1079–1080.
2. Allen, T.M. and Cullis, P.R. (2004) Drug delivery systems: entering the mainstream. *Science*, **303**, 1818–1822.
3. Park, J.H., Lee, S., Kim, J.-H., Park, K., Kim, K., and Kwon, I.C. (2008) Polymeric nanomedicine for cancer therapy. *Prog. Polym. Sci.*, **33**, 113–137.
4. Maeda, H., Seymour, L.W., and Miyamoto, Y. (1992) Conjugates of anticancer agents and polymers: advantages of macromolecular therapeutics in vivo. *Bioconjug. Chem.*, **3**, 351–362.
5. Maeda, H., Wu, J., Sawa, T., Matsumura, Y., and Hori, K. (2000) Tumor vascular permeability and the EPR effect in macromolecular therapeutics: a review. *J. Control. Release*, **65**, 271–284.
6. Duncan, R. (2003) The dawning era of polymer therapeutics. *Nat. Rev. Drug Discov.*, **2**, 347–360.
7. Ringsdorf, H. (1975) Structure and properties of pharmacologically active polymers. *J. Polym. Sci. Polym. Symp.*, **51**, 135–153.
8. Khandare, J. and Minko, T. (2006) Polymer–drug conjugates: progress in polymeric prodrugs. *Prog. Polym. Sci.*, **31**, 359–397.
9. Larsen, C. (1989) Dextran prodrugs – structure and stability in relation to therapeutic activity. *Adv. Drug Deliv. Rev.*, **3**, 103–154.
10. Kopecek, J. and Kopecková, P. (2010) HPMA copolymers: origins, early developments, present, and future. *Adv. Drug Deliv. Rev.*, **62**, 122–149.
11. Kratz, F., Abu Ajaj, K., and Warnecke, A. (2007) Anticancer carrier-linked prodrugs in clinical trials. *Expert Opin. Invest. Drugs*, **16**, 1037–1058.
12. Pasut, G. and Veronese, F.M. (2009) PEG conjugates in clinical development or use as anticancer agents: an overview. *Adv. Drug Deliv. Rev.*, **61**, 1177–1188.

13. Platt, V.M. and Szoka, F.C. (2008) Anticancer therapeutics: Targeting macromolecules and nanocarriers to hyaluronan or CD44, a hyaluronan receptor. *Mol. Pharm.*, **5**, 474–486.
14. Soyez, H., Schacht, E., and Vanderkerken, S. (1996) The crucial role of spacer groups in macromolecular prodrug design. *Adv. Drug Deliv. Rev.*, **21**, 81–106.
15. Christie, R.J. and Grainger, D.W. (2003) Design strategies to improve soluble macromolecular delivery constructs. *Adv. Drug Deliv. Rev.*, **55**, 421–437.
16. Nichifor, M. and Mocanu, G. (2006) Polysaccharide–drug conjugates as controlled drug delivery systems, in *Polysaccharides for Drug Delivery and Pharmaceutical Applications* (eds R.H. Marchessault, F. Ravenelle, and X.X. Zhu), Oxford University Press, New York, pp. 289–303.
17. Levi-Schaffer, F., Bernstein, A., Meshorer, A., and Arnon, R. (1982) Reduced toxicity of daunorubicin by conjugation to dextran. *Cancer Treat. Rep.*, **66**, 107–114.
18. Takakura, Y., Kaneko, Y., Fujita, T., Hashida, M., Maeda, H., and Sezaki, H. (1989) Control of pharmaceutical properties of soybean trypsin inhibitor by conjugation with dextran I: synthesis and characterization. *J. Pharm. Sci.*, **78**, 117–121.
19. Mocanu, G., Constantin, M., and Carpov, A. (1996) Chemical reactions on polysaccharides, 5. Reaction of mesyl chloride with pullulan. *Angew. Makromol. Chem.*, **241**, 1–10.
20. Móra, M. and Pató, J. (1990) Polymeric prodrugs, 8. Synthesis and hydrolytic behaviour of dextran-bound anticancer agents. *Makromol. Chem.*, **191**, 1051–1056.
21. Aspinall, G. (1982) *The Polysaccharides*, Academic Press, New York.
22. Kojima, T., Hashida, M., Muranishi, S., and Sezaki, H. (1980) Mitomycin C–dextran conjugate: a novel high molecular weight pro-drug of mitomycin C. *J. Pharm. Pharmacol.*, **32**, 30–34.
23. Hashida, M., Takakura, Y., Matsumoto, S., Sasaki, H., Kato, A., Kojima, T., Muranishi, S., and Sezaki, H. (1983) Regeneration characteristics of mitomycin C–dextran conjugate in relation to its activity. *Chem. Pharm. Bull.*, **31**, 2055–2063.
24. Yoshinobu, T., Satoshi, M., Mitsuru, H., and Hitoshi, S. (1989) Physicochemical properties and antitumor activities of polymeric prodrugs of mitomycin C with different regeneration rates. *J. Control. Release*, **10**, 97–105.
25. Takakura, Y., Takagi, A., Hashida, M., and Sezaki, H. (1987) Disposition and tumor localization of mitomycin C–dextran conjugates in mice. *Pharm. Res.*, **4**, 293–300.
26. Nomura, T., Saikawa, A., Morita, S., Sakaeda, T., Yamashita, F., Honda, K., Yoshinobu, T., and Hashida, M. (1998) Pharmacokinetic characteristics and therapeutic effects of mitomycin C–dextran conjugates after intratumoural injection. *J. Control. Release*, **52**, 239–252.
27. Takakura, Y., Matsumoto, S., Hashida, M., and Sezaki, H. (1984) Enhanced lymphatic delivery of mitomycin C conjugated with dextran. *Cancer Res.*, **44**, 2505–2510.
28. Ueda, Y., Munechika, K., Kikukawa, A., Kanoh, Y., Yamanouchi, K., and Yokoyama, K. (1989) Comparison of efficacy, toxicity and pharmacokinetics of free adriamycin and adriamycin linked to oxidized dextran in rats. *Chem. Pharm. Bull.*, **37**, 1639–1641.
29. Munechika, K., Sogame, Y., Kishi, N., Kawabata, Y., Ueda, Y., Yuamanouchi, K., and Yokoyama, K. (1994) Tissue distribution of macromolecular conjugate, adriamycin linked to oxidized dextran, in rat and mouse bearing tumor cells. *Biol. Pharmacol. Bull.*, **17**, 1193–1198.
30. Lam, W., Chan, H., Yang, M., Cheng, S., and Fong, W. (1999) Synergism of energy starvation and dextran-conjugated doxorubicin in the killing of multidrug-resistant KB carcinoma cells. *Anti-Cancer Drugs*, **10**, 171–178.

31. Sheldon, K., Marks, A., and Baumal, R. (1989) Sensitivity of multidrug resistant KB-C1 cells to an antibody–dextran–adriamycin conjugate. *Anti-Cancer Res.*, **9**, 637–641.
32. Kikukawa, A., Munechika, K., Ueda, Y., Yamanouchi, K., Yokoyama, K., and Tsukagoshi, S. (1990) Tissue concentration of adriamycin and adriamycin-oxidized dextran conjugate in tumor bearing rats and mice. *Drug Deliv. Syst.*, **5**, 255–260.
33. Danhauser-Riedl, S., Hausmann, E., Schick, H.-D., Bender, R., Dietzfelbinger, H., Rastetter, J., and Hanauske, A.-R. (1993) Phase I clinical and pharmacokinetic trial of dextran conjugated doxorubicin (AD-70, DOX-OXD). *Invest. New Drugs*, **11**, 187–195.
34. Sugahara, S.-I., Kajiki, M., Kuriyama, H., and Kobayashi, T.-R. (2007) Complete regression of xenografted human carcinomas by a paclitaxel–carboxymethyl dextran conjugate (AZ10992). *J. Control. Release*, **117**, 40–50.
35. Harada, M., Sakakibara, H., Yano, T., Suzuki, T., and Okuno, S. (2000) Determinants for the drug release from T-0128, camptothecin analogue–carboxymethyl dextran conjugate. *J. Control. Release*, **69**, 399–412.
36. Okuno, S., Harada, M., Yano, T., Yano, S., Kiuchi, S., Tsuda, N., Sakamura, Y., Imai, J., Kawaguchi, T., and Tsujihara, K. (2000) Complete regression of xenografted human carcinomas by camptothecin analogue–carboxymethyl dextran conjugate (T-0128). *Cancer Res.*, **60**, 2988–2995.
37. Harada, M., Imai, J., Okuno, S., and Suzuki, T. (2000) Macrophage-mediated activation of camptothecin analogue T-2513–carboxymethyl dextran conjugate (T-0128): possible cellular mechanism for antitumor activity. *J. Control. Release*, **69**, 389–397.
38. Schechter, B., Pauzner, R., Arnon, R., and Wilchek, M. (1986) Cis-platinum(II) complexes of carboxymethyl-dextran as potential antitumor agents. I. Preparation and characterization. *Cancer Biochem. Biophys.*, **8**, 277–287.
39. Nakashima, M., Ichinose, K., Kanematsu, T., Masunaga, T., Ohya, Y., Ouchi, T., Tomiyama, N., Sasaki, H., and Ichikawa, M. (1999) In vitro characteristics and *in vivo* plasma disposition of cisplatin conjugated with oxidized and dicarboxymethylated dextrans. *Biol. Pharm. Bull.*, **22**, 756–761.
40. Ohya, Y., Oue, H., Nagatomi, K., and Ouchi, T. (2001) Design of macromolecular prodrug of cisplatin using dextran with branched galactose units as targeting moieties to hepatoma cells. *Biomacromolecules*, **2**, 927–933.
41. Chau, Y., Tan, F.E., and Langer, R. (2004) Synthesis and characterization of dextran–peptide–methotrexate conjugates for tumor targeting via mediation by matrix metalloproteinase II and matrix metalloproteinase IX. *Bioconjug. Chem.*, **15**, 931–941.
42. Kumar, M.N.V.R., Muzzarelli, R.A.A., Muzzarelli, C., Sashiwa, H., and Domb, A.J. (2004) Chitosan chemistry and pharmaceutical perspectives. *Chem. Rev.*, **104**, 6017–6084.
43. Rinaudo, M. (2006) Chitin and chitosan: properties and applications. *Prog. Polym. Sci.*, **31**, 603–632.
44. Aiba, S.-I. (1992) Studies on chitosan: 4. Lysozymic hydrolysis of partially N-acetylated chitosans. *Int. J. Biol. Macromol.*, **14**, 225–228.
45. Kim, J.H., Kim, Y.S., Kim, S., Park, J.H., Kim, K., Choi, K., Chung, H., Jeong, S.Y., Park, R.W., Kim, I.S., and Kwon, I.C. (2006) Hydrophobically modified glycol chitosan nanoparticles as carriers for paclitaxel. *J. Control. Release*, **111**, 228–234.
46. Leitner, V.M., Walker, G.F., and Bernkop-Schnürch, A. (2003) Thiolated polymers: evidence for the formation of disulphide bonds with mucus glycoproteins. *Eur. J. Pharm. Biopharm.*, **56**, 207–214.
47. Kato, Y., Onishi, H., and Machida, Y. (2000) Evaluation of N-succinyl-chitosan as a systemic long-circulating polymer. *Biomaterials*, **21**, 1579–1585.

48. Park, J.H., Saravanakumar, G., Kim, K., and Kwon, I.C. (2010) Targeted delivery of low molecular drugs using chitosan and its derivatives. *Adv. Drug Deliv. Rev.*, **62**, 28–41.
49. Amidi, M., Mastrobattista, E., Jiskoot, W., and Hennink, W.E. (2010) Chitosan-based delivery systems for protein therapeutics and antigens. *Adv. Drug Deliv. Rev.*, **62**, 59–82.
50. Ohya, Y., Nonomura, K., Hirai, K., and Ouchi, T. (1994) Synthesis of 6-*O*-carboxymethylchitin immobilizing doxorubicins through tetrapeptide spacer groups and its enzymatic release behavior of doxorubicin *in vitro*. *Macromol. Chem. Phys.*, **195**, 2839–2853.
51. Ohya, Y., Nonomura, K., and Ouchi, T. (1995) *In vivo* and *in vitro* antitumor activity of CM-chitin immobilized doxorubicins by lysosomal digestible tetrapeptide spacer groups. *J. Bioact. Compat. Polym.*, **10**, 223–234.
52. Davis, M.E., Chen, Z., and Shin, D.M. (2008) Nanoparticle therapeutics: an emerging treatment modality for cancer. *Nat. Rev. Drug Discov.*, **7**, 771–782.
53. Son, Y.J., Jang, J.S., Cho, Y.W., Chung, H., Park, R.W., Kwon, I.C., Kim, I.S., Park, J.Y., Seo, S.B., Park, C.R., and Jeong, S.Y. (2003) Biodistribution and anti-tumor efficacy of doxorubicin loaded glycol-chitosan nanoaggregates by EPR effect. *J. Control. Release*, **91**, 135–145.
54. Park, J.H., Kwon, S., Lee, M., Chung, H., Kim, J.H., Kim, Y.S., Park, R.W., Kim, I.S., Bong Seo, S., Kwon, I.C., and Young Jeong, S. (2006) Self-assembled nanoparticles based on glycol chitosan bearing hydrophobic moieties as carriers for doxorubicin: *in vivo* biodistribution and anti-tumor activity. *Biomaterials*, **27**, 119–126.
55. Lipinski, C. (2002) Poor aqueous solubility – an industry wide problem in drug discovery. *Am. Pharm. Rev.*, **5**, 82–85.
56. Lee, E., Lee, J., Lee, I.-H., Yu, M., Kim, H., Chae, S.Y., and Jon, S. (2008) Conjugated chitosan as a novel platform for oral delivery of paclitaxel. *J. Med. Chem.*, **51**, 6442–6449.
57. Song, Y., Onishi, H., and Nagai, T. (1993) Conjugate of mitomycin C with *N*-succinyl-chitosan: *in vitro* drug release properties, toxicity and antitumor activity. *Int. J. Pharm.*, **98**, 121–130.
58. Sato, M., Onishi, H., Takahara, J., Machida, Y., and Nagai, T. (1996) *In vivo* drug release and antitumor characteristics of water-soluble conjugates of mitomycin C with glycol-chitosan and *N*-succinyl-chitosan. *Biol. Pharm. Bull.*, **19**, 1170–1177.
59. Kato, Y., Onishi, H., and Machida, Y. (2004) *N*-succinyl-chitosan as a drug carrier: water-insoluble and water-soluble conjugates. *Biomaterials*, **25**, 907–915.
60. Kato, Y., Onishi, H., and Machida, Y. (2000) Biological fate of highly-succinylated *N*-succinyl-chitosan and antitumor characteristics of its water-soluble conjugate with mitomycin C at i.v. and i.p. administration into tumor-bearing mice. *Biol. Pharm. Bull.*, **23**, 1497–1503.
61. Laurent, T. and Fraser, J. (1992) Hyaluronan. *FASEB J.*, **6**, 2397–2404.
62. Lapčik, L., De Smedt, S., Demeester, J., and Chabreček, P. (1998) Hyaluronan: preparation, structure, properties, and applications. *Chem. Rev.*, **98**, 2663–2684.
63. Toole, B.P. (2004) Hyaluronan: from extracellular glue to pericellular cue. *Nat. Rev. Cancer*, **4**, 528–539.
64. Choi, K.Y., Min, K.H., Na, J.H., Choi, K., Kim, K., Park, J.H., Kwon, I.C., and Jeong, S.Y. (2009) Self-assembled hyaluronic acid nanoparticles as a potential drug carrier for cancer therapy: synthesis, characterization, and *in vivo* biodistribution. *J. Mater. Chem.*, **19**, 4102–4107.
65. Choi, K.Y., Chung, H., Min, K.H., Yoon, H.Y., Kim, K., Park, J.H., Kwon, I.C., and Jeong, S.Y. (2010) Self-assembled hyaluronic acid nanoparticles for active tumor targeting. *Biomaterials*, **31**, 106–114.
66. Luo, Y. and Prestwich, G.D. (1999) Synthesis and selective cytotoxicity of a hyaluronic acid–antitumor bioconjugate. *Bioconjug. Chem.*, **10**, 755–763.

67. Akima, K., Ito, H., Iwata, Y., Matsuo, K., Watari, N., Yanagi, M., Hagi, H., Oshima, K., Yagita, A., Atomi, Y., and Tatekawa, I. (1996) Evaluation of antitumor activities of hyaluronate binding antitumor drugs: synthesis, characterization and antitumor activity. *J. Drug Target.*, **4**, 1–8.
68. Cera, C., Palumbo, M., Stefanelli, S., Rassu, M., and Palu, G. (1992) Water-soluble polysaccharide–anthracycline conjugates: biological activity. *Anti-Cancer Drug Des.*, **7**, 141–151.
69. Coradini, D., Pellizzaro, C., Miglierini, G., Daidone, M.G., and Perbellini, A. (1999) Hyaluronic acid as drug delivery for sodium butyrate: improvement of the anti-proliferative activity on a breast-cancer cell line. *Int. J. Cancer*, **81**, 411–416.
70. Coradini, D. and Perbellini, A. (2004) Hyaluronan: a suitable carrier for an histone deacetylase inhibitor in the treatment of human solid tumors. *Cancer Ther.*, **2**, 201–216.
71. Luo, Y., Ziebell, M.R., and Prestwich, G.D. (2000) A hyaluronic acid–taxol antitumor bioconjugate targeted to cancer cells. *Biomacromolecules*, **1**, 208–218.
72. Thierry, B., Kujawa, P., Tkaczyk, C., Winnik, F.M., Bilodeau, L., and Tabrizian, M. (2005) Delivery platform for hydrophobic drugs: prodrug approach combined with self-assembled multilayers. *J. Am. Chem. Soc.*, **127**, 1626–1627.
73. Lee, H., Lee, K., and Park, T.G. (2008) Hyaluronic acid–paclitaxel conjugate micelles: synthesis, characterization, and antitumor activity. *Bioconjug. Chem.*, **19**, 1319–1325.
74. Rosato, A., Banzato, A., De Luca, G., Renier, D., Bettella, F., Pagano, C., Esposito, G., Zanovello, P., and Bassi, P. (2006) HYTAD1-p20: a new paclitaxel–hyaluronic acid hydrosoluble bioconjugate for treatment of superficial bladder cancer. *Urol. Oncol. Semin. Orig. Invest.*, **24**, 207–215.
75. Banzato, A., Bobisse, S., Rondina, M., Renier, D., Bettella, F., Esposito, G., Quintieri, L., Meléndez-Alafort, L., Mazzi, U., Zanovello, P., and Rosato, A. (2008) A paclitaxel–hyaluronan bioconjugate targeting ovarian cancer affords a potent *in vivo* therapeutic activity. *Clin. Cancer Res.*, **14**, 3598–3606.
76. Banzato, A., Rondina, M., Meléndez-Alafort, L., Zangoni, E., Nadali, A., Renier, D., Moschini, G., Mazzi, U., Zanovello, P., and Rosato, A. (2009) Biodistribution imaging of a paclitaxel–hyaluronan bioconjugate. *Nucl. Med. Biol.*, **36**, 525–533.
77. De Stefano, I., Battaglia, A., Zannoni, G., Prisco, M., Fattorossi, A., Travaglia, D., Baroni, S., Renier, D., Scambia, G., Ferlini, C., and Gallo, D. (2011) Hyaluronic acid–paclitaxel: effects of intraperitoneal administration against CD44$^+$ human ovarian cancer xenografts. *Cancer Chemother. Pharmacol.*, **68** (1), 107–116.
78. Casu, B. and Lindahl, U. (2001) Structure and biological interactions of heparin and heparan sulfate. *Adv. Carbohydr. Chem. Biochem.*, **57**, 159–206.
79. Vlodavsky, I., Abboud-Jarrous, G., Elkin, M., Naggi, A., Casu, B., Sasisekharan, R., and Ilan, N. (2006) The impact of heparanase and heparin on cancer metastasis and angiogenesis. *Pathophysiol. Haemost. Thromb.*, **35**, 116–127.
80. Garg, H.G., Thompson, B.T., and Hales, C.A. (2000) Structural determinants of antiproliferative activity of heparin on pulmonary artery smooth muscle cells. *Am. J. Physiol.*, **279**, L779–L789.
81. Norrby, K. (1993) Heparin and angiogenesis: a low-molecular-weight fraction inhibits and a high-molecular-weight fraction stimulates angiogenesis systemically. *Pathophysiol. Haemost. Thromb.*, **23** (Suppl. 1), 141–149.
82. Norrby, K. and Østergaard, P. (1996) Basic-fibroblast-growth-factor-mediated de novo angiogenesis is more effectively suppressed by low-molecular-weight than by high-molecular-weight heparin. *Int. J. Microcirc.*, **16**, 8–15.
83. Wang, Y., Xin, D., Liu, K., and Xiang, J. (2009) Heparin–paclitaxel conjugates

using mixed anhydride as intermediate: synthesis, influence of polymer structure on drug release, anticoagulant activity and *in vitro* efficiency. *Pharm. Res.*, **26**, 785–793.

84. Park, K., Kim, Y.-S., Lee, G., Park, R.-W., Kim, I.-S., Kim, S., and Byun, Y. (2008) Tumor endothelial cell targeted cyclic RGD-modified heparin derivative: inhibition of angiogenesis and tumor growth. *Pharm. Res.*, **25**, 2786–2798.

85. Wang, X., Li, J., Wang, Y., Cho, K.J., Kim, G., Gjyrezi, A., Koenig, L., Giannakakou, P., Shin, H.J.C., Tighiouart, M., Nie, S., Chen, Z., and Shin, D.M. (2009) HFT-T, a targeting nanoparticle, enhances specific delivery of paclitaxel to folate receptor-positive tumors. *ACS Nano*, **3**, 3165–3174.

86. Leathers, T.D. (2002) Pullulan, in *Biopolymers 6: Polysaccharides II: Polysaccharides from Eukaryotes* (eds A. Steinbüchel, E.J. Vandamme, and S. De Baets), Wiley-VCH Verlag GmbH, Weinheim, pp. 1–35.

87. Shingel, K.I. (2004) Current knowledge on biosynthesis, biological activity, and chemical modification of the exopolysaccharide, pullulan. *Carbohydr. Res.*, **339**, 447–460.

88. Alban, S., Schauerte, A., and Franz, G. (2002) Anticoagulant sulfated polysaccharides: part I. Synthesis and structure–activity relationships of new pullulan sulfates. *Carbohydr. Polym.*, **47**, 267–276.

89. Kaneo, Y., Tanaka, T., Nakano, T., and Yamaguchi, Y. (2001) Evidence for receptor-mediated hepatic uptake of pullulan in rats. *J. Control. Release*, **70**, 365–373.

90. Hosseinkhani, H., Aoyama, T., Ogawa, O., and Tabata, Y. (2002) Liver targeting of plasmid DNA by pullulan conjugation based on metal coordination. *J. Control. Release*, **83**, 287–302.

91. Na, K., Bum Lee, T., Park, K.-H., Shin, E.-K., Lee, Y.-B., and Choi, H.-K. (2003) Self-assembled nanoparticles of hydrophobically-modified polysaccharide bearing vitamin H as a targeted anti-cancer drug delivery system. *Eur. J. Pharm. Sci.*, **18**, 165–173.

92. Nogusa, H., Yano, T., Okuno, S., Hamana, H., and Inoue, K. (1995) Synthesis of carboxymethylpullulan–peptide–doxorubicin conjugates and their properties. *Chem. Pharm. Bull.*, **43**, 1931–1936.

93. Lu, D., Wen, X., Liang, J., Gu, Z., Zhang, X., and Fan, Y. (2009) A pH-sensitive nano drug delivery system derived from pullulan/doxorubicin conjugate. *J. Biomed. Mater. Res.*, **89B**, 177–183.

94. Priego-Jimenéz, R., Peña, C., Ramírez, O.T., and Galindo, E. (2005) Specific growth rate determines the molecular mass of the alginate produced by *Azotobacter vinelandii*. *Biochem. Eng. J.*, **25**, 187–193.

95. Otterlei, M., Østgaard, K., Skjåk-Bræk, G., Smidsrød, O., Soon-Shiong, P., and Espevik, T. (1991) Induction of cytokine production from human monocytes stimulated with alginate. *J. Immunother.*, **10**, 286–291.

96. Fujihara, M. and Nagumo, T. (1992) The effect of the content of D-mannuronic acid and L-guluronic acid blocks in alginates on antitumor activity. *Carbohydr. Res.*, **224**, 343–347.

97. Morgan, S.M., Al-Shamkhani, A., Callant, D., Schacht, E., Woodley, J.F., and Duncan, R. (1995) Alginates as drug carriers: covalent attachment of alginates to therapeutic agents containing primary amine groups. *Int. J. Pharm.*, **122**, 121–128.

98. Al-Shamkhani, A. and Duncan, R. (1995) Synthesis, controlled release properties and antitumour activity of alginate–*cis*-aconityl–daunomycin conjugates. *Int. J. Pharm.*, **122**, 107–119.

99. Adams, M.K. and Douglas, C. (1963) Arabinogalactan – a review of the literature. *Tech. Assoc. Pulp Pap. Ind.*, **46**, 544–548.

100. Groman, E.V., Enriquez, P.M., Jung, C., and Josephson, L. (1994) Arabinogalactan for hepatic drug delivery. *Bioconjug. Chem.*, **5**, 547–556.

101. Ehrenfreund-Kleinman, T., Golenser, J., and Domb, A.J. (2004) Conjugation of amino-containing drugs to

polysaccharides by tosylation: amphotericin B–arabinogalactan conjugates. *Biomaterials*, **25**, 3049–3057.

102. Pinhassi, R.I., Assaraf, Y.G., Farber, S., Stark, M., Ickowicz, D., Drori, S., Domb, A.J., and Livney, Y.D. (2009) Arabinogalactan–folic acid–drug conjugate for targeted delivery and target-activated release of anticancer drugs to folate receptor-overexpressing cells. *Biomacromolecules*, **11**, 294–303.

103. Sinha, V.R. and Kumria, R. (2001) Polysaccharides in colon-specific drug delivery. *Int. J. Pharm.*, **224**, 19–38.

104. Tang, X.-H., Xie, P., Ding, Y., Chu, L.-Y., Hou, J.-P., Yang, J.-L., Song, X., and Xie, Y.-M. (2010) Synthesis, characterization, and *in vitro* and *in vivo* evaluation of a novel pectin–adriamycin conjugate. *Bioorg. Med. Chem.*, **18**, 1599–1609.

105. Cao, Y., Gu, Y., Ma, H., Bai, J., Liu, L., Zhao, P., and He, H. (2010) Self-assembled nanoparticle drug delivery systems from galactosylated polysaccharide–doxorubicin conjugate loaded doxorubicin. *Int. J. Biol. Macromol.*, **46**, 245–249.

106. Ouchi, T., Tada, M., Matsumoto, M., Ohya, Y., Hasegawa, K., Arai, Y., Kadowaki, K., Akao, S., Matsumoto, T., Suzuki, S., and Suzuki, M. (1998) Design of macromolecular prodrug of 5-fluorouracil using N-acetylpolygalactosamine as a targeting carrier to hepatoma. *React. Funct. Polym.*, **37**, 235–244.

107. Ouchi, T., Tada, M., Matsumoto, M., Ohya, Y., Hasegawa, K., Arai, Y., Kadowaki, K., Akao, S., Matsumoto, T., Suzuki, S., and Suzuki, M. (1998) Design of lysosomotropic macromolecular prodrug of doxorubicin using N-acetyl-α-1,4-polygalactosamine as a targeting carrier to hepatoma tissue. *J. Bioact. Compat. Polym.*, **13**, 257–269.

108. Li, J. and Loh, X.J. (2008) Cyclodextrin-based supramolecular architectures: syntheses, structures, and applications for drug and gene delivery. *Adv. Drug Deliv. Rev.*, **60**, 1000–1017.

109. Davis, M.E. and Brewster, M.E. (2004) Cyclodextrin-based pharmaceutics: past, present and future. *Nat. Rev. Drug Discov.*, **3**, 1023–1035.

110. van de Manakker, F., Vermonden, T., van Nostrum, C.F., and Hennink, W.E. (2009) Cyclodextrin-based polymeric materials: synthesis, properties, and pharmaceutical/biomedical applications. *Biomacromolecules*, **10**, 3157–3175.

111. Harada, A., Takashima, Y., and Yamaguchi, H. (2009) Cyclodextrin-based supramolecular polymers. *Chem. Soc. Rev.*, **38**, 875–882.

112. Heidel, J.D. (2006) Linear cyclodextrin-containing polymers and their use as delivery agents. *Expert Opin. Drug Deliv.*, **3**, 641–646.

113. Cheng, J., Khin, K.T., Jensen, G.S., Liu, A., and Davis, M.E. (2003) Synthesis of linear, β-cyclodextrin-based polymers and their camptothecin conjugates. *Bioconjug. Chem.*, **14**, 1007–1017.

114. Davis, M.E. (2009) Design and development of IT-101, a cyclodextrin-containing polymer conjugate of camptothecin. *Adv. Drug Deliv. Rev.*, **61**, 1189–1192.

115. Schluep, T., Cheng, J., Khin, K., and Davis, M. (2006) Pharmacokinetics and biodistribution of the camptothecin–polymer conjugate IT-101 in rats and tumor-bearing mice. *Cancer Chemother. Pharmacol.*, **57**, 654–662.

116. Schluep, T., Hwang, J., Cheng, J., Heidel, J.D., Bartlett, D.W., Hollister, B., and Davis, M.E. (2006) Preclinical efficacy of the camptothecin–polymer conjugate IT-101 in multiple cancer models. *Clin. Cancer Res.*, **12**, 1606–1614.

117. Schluep, T., Hwang, J., Hildebrandt, I.J., Czernin, J., Choi, C.H.J., Alabi, C.A., Mack, B.C., and Davis, M.E. (2009) Pharmacokinetics and tumor dynamics of the nanoparticle IT-101 from PET imaging and tumor histological measurements. *Proc. Natl. Acad. Sci. USA*, **106**, 11394–11399.

118. Numbenjapon, T., Wang, J., Colcher, D., Schluep, T., Davis, M.E., Duringer, J., Kretzner, L., Yen, Y., Forman, S.J., and Raubitschek, A. (2009) Preclinical results of camptothecin–polymer conjugate (IT-101) in multiple human lymphoma xenograft models. *Clin. Cancer Res.*, **15**, 4365–4373.

24
Serum Proteins as Drug Carriers of Anticancer Agents
Felix Kratz, Andreas Wunder, and Bakheet Elsadek

24.1
Introduction

Once tumors reach a size of approximately 1 cm^3, they form an expanding network of capillaries, and rely on a continuous supply of nutrients for tumor growth and progression. It is therefore perhaps not surprising that tumor cells selectively use vitamins, growth factors, and serum proteins circulating in the bloodstream to cover their needs for enhanced cell proliferation.

Blood is a complex mixture of a multitude of cells and low- and high-molecular weight compounds (general components after centrifugation are shown in Figure 24.1).

In the blood plasma, albumin is by far the most abundant protein with a concentration of around 35–50 mg/ml. The amounts of other major plasma proteins are much lower (Figure 24.2), and concentrations of transferrin are around 2.5–3.5 mg/ml and concentrations of low-density lipoprotein (LDL) are around 5–20 mg/ml.

The complexity of the human serum proteome – comprised of approximately 100 000 proteins whose concentrations span over 12 orders of magnitude – makes the separation and identification of all plasma proteins and peptides a formidable task, and indeed the highly abundant plasma protein components (primarily albumin and immunoglobulins) have to be removed prior to the identification of plasma proteins by two-dimensional gel electrophoresis in the low nano- or picomolar range (Figure 24.2).

An enhanced uptake of major plasma proteins by tumor cells is primarily restricted to transferrin, albumin, and LDL. All three plasma proteins are important transport proteins covering the body's need for metal ions and nutrients.

Transferrin is responsible for the transfer of Fe(III) and ferries it between very different cell types, such as the intestine epithelium, where iron enters the body from the diet, the liver, where it is stored as ferritin (a protein containing iron–phosphate–hydroxide complexes), the developing erythroid cells, which require it for hemoglobin synthesis, and cells that need iron for cell growth, including tumor cells. Albumin acts as a solubilizing agent for long-chain fatty acids and

Drug Delivery in Oncology: From Basic Research to Cancer Therapy, First Edition.
Edited by Felix Kratz, Peter Senter, and Henning Steinhagen.
© 2012 Wiley-VCH Verlag GmbH & Co. KGaA. Published 2012 by Wiley-VCH Verlag GmbH & Co. KGaA.

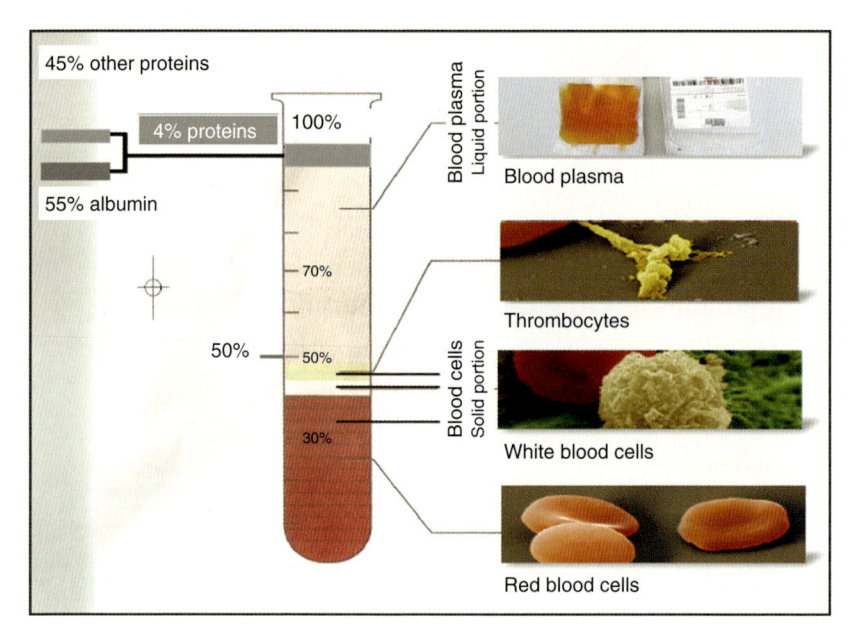

Figure 24.1 General composition of human blood.

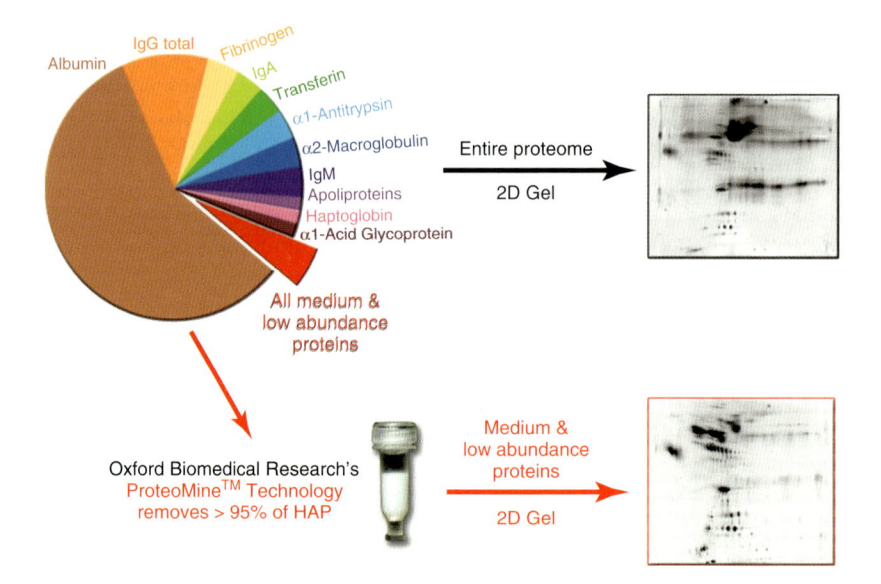

Figure 24.2 Overview of plasma proteins and the possibilities of separating those using electrophoretic techniques and additionally removing the high abundant proteins (HAPs) before analysis. (Reproduced courtesy of Oxford Biomedical Research.)

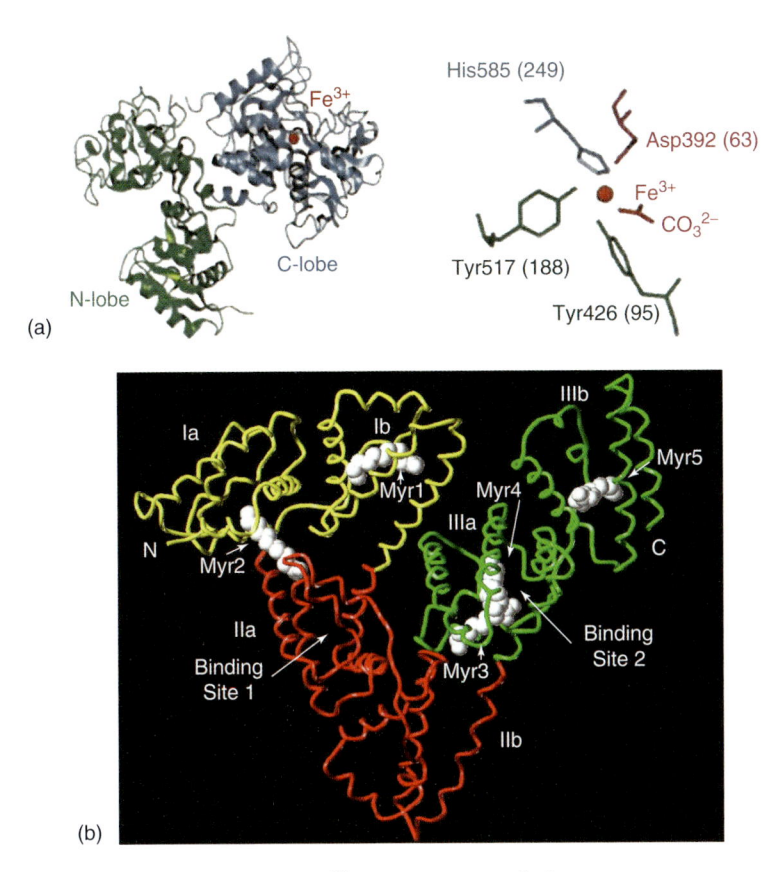

Figure 24.3 (a) X-ray structure of human serum transferrin [1]. (b) X-ray structure of HSA (pdb entry 1bj5) [2]. (Reproduced with permission from [1].)

is therefore essential for the metabolism of lipids, it binds Cu(II) and Ni(II) in a specific manner, and Ca(II) and Zn(II) in a relatively nonspecific manner, and acts as the transport vehicle for these metal ions in the blood. Following endocytosis and enzymatic degradation in lysosomes, it serves as a source of amino acids for the cell. LDL is the principal carrier of cholesterol to tissues.

Human serum albumin (HSA, 66.5 kDa) and transferrin (78 kDa) have a comparable size, and both proteins have been elucidated by X-ray structure analysis (Figure 24.3a).

Iron-free transferrin is called apotransferrin and can bind two-equivalents of Fe(III) [1]. Protein crystallographic studies show that the iron-binding sites are located within an interdomain cleft in the N- and C-terminal lobe of the protein (Figure 24.3a) where iron is octahedrally coordinated by four protein donors (i.e., two Tyr phenolates, one His imidazole, and one Asp carboxylate) and by a bidentate carbonate anion.

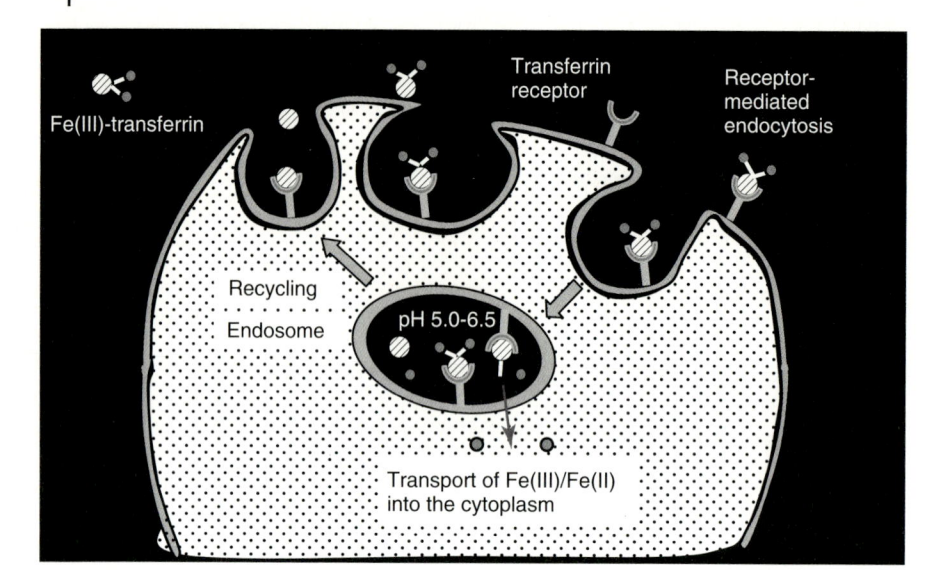

Figure 24.4 Schematic presentation of the transferrin cycle: Fe(III)-transferrin binds the transferrin receptor and the transferrin/receptor complex is taken up by endocytosis. Upon acidification in endosomes (and in part lysosomes) Fe(III) is set free and apotransferrin and the transferrin receptor is primarily recycled.

Diferric transferrin binds to the specific receptor for transferrin (a 190-kDa glycoprotein) located on the cell surface [3] and is then rapidly internalized in nonlysosomal vesicles (Figure 24.4). The acidic environment of these vesicles causes iron to dissociate from the protein while apotransferrin remains bound to the receptor. Intracellular chelates, such as ATP, might then be involved in the further uptake and transport of Fe(III) within the cell. Release of Fe(III) by reduction to Fe(II) meditated by DMT1 (divalent metal transporter 1), an endosomal membrane transfer of Fe(II) by the divalent metal transporter, has also been evoked. Subsequently, the complex of apotransferrin and its receptor is rapidly returned to the cell surface where apotransferrin dissociates from the receptor at neutral pH.

The approximate three-dimensional shape of HSA can be described as a heart-shaped macromolecule consisting of three flexible spheres in a row (domains I–III) (Figure 24.3) [2, 4].

HSA is one of the smallest proteins present in blood plasma. Both its size and abundance explain the fact that so many metabolic compounds and therapeutic drugs are transported by this protein. The numerous binding sites for metabolic substrates and therapeutic drugs have been extensively studied and reviewed [5–7]. HSA has a half-life of around 19 days in humans.

LDL is a much larger protein lipid system with a spherical particle size of approximately 220 Å, consisting of an outer coat and inner core of hydrophobic lipids (about 1500 molecules of cholesteryl esters and about 300 molecules of

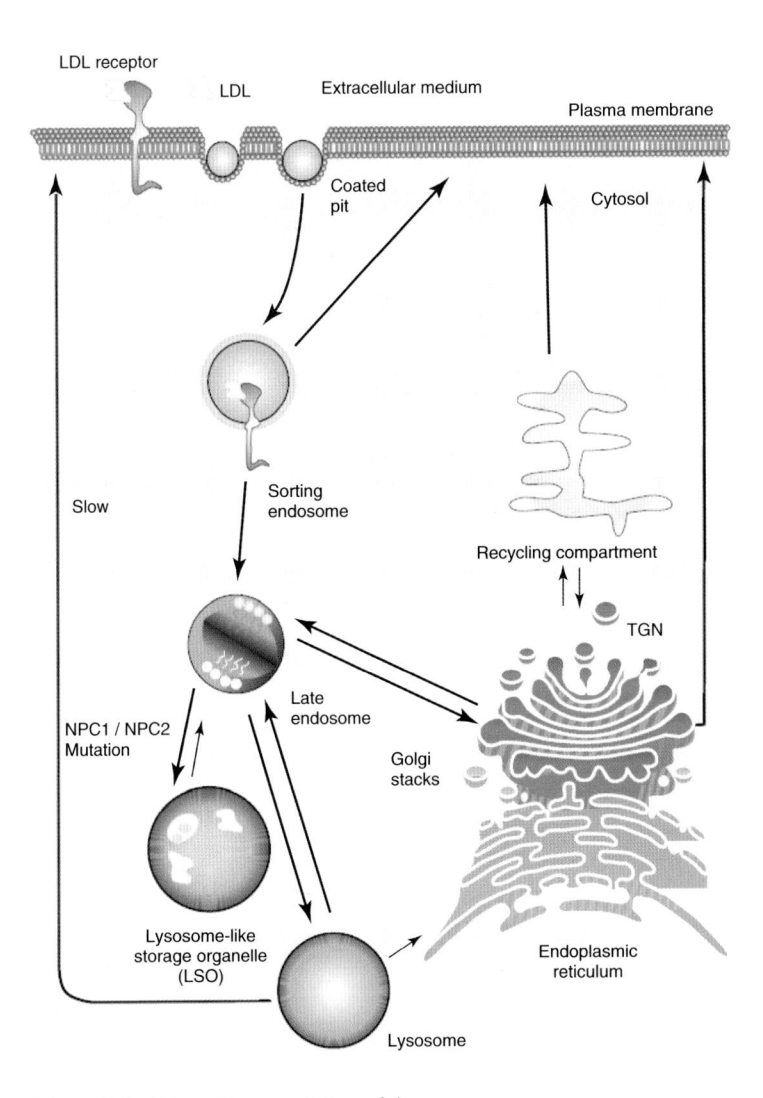

Figure 24.5 Schematic presentation of the receptor-mediated uptake of LDL by the LDL receptor, subsequent sorting in early and late endosomes, and degradation in lysosomes to release cholesterol and phospholipids.

triacylglycerol). LDL is one of the five major groups of lipoproteins (the others being chylomicrons, and very-low-density, intermediate-density, and high-density lipoprotein) that enable lipids like cholesterol and triglycerides to be transported within the water-based bloodstream. The coat of human LDL is comprised of phosphatidylcholine, sphingomyelin, unesterified cholesterol, and a single protein termed apolipoprotein B (514 kDa). This protein is responsible for the specific binding to cell surface LDL receptors where LDL is internalized by endocytosis and then transported to lysosomes in which the cholesteryl esters are hydrolyzed, making free cholesterol available for cell membrane and steroid synthesis (Figure 24.5). LDL is formed from very-low-density lipoprotein particles after lipid exchanges and lipolysis by lipoprotein and hepatic lipase. The half-life of human LDL in the blood is of the order of days (for a review, see [8]).

A major disadvantage of anticancer agents is their lack of selectivity for tumor tissue, causing severe side-effects and low cure rates. Any strategy by which a cytotoxic drug is targeted to the tumor, thus increasing the therapeutic index of the drug, is a way of improving cancer chemotherapy and minimizing systemic toxicity. Serum transferrin, albumin, and LDL are suitable as drug carriers for a number of reasons: (i) they exhibit a preferential uptake in tumor tissue [9–12]; (ii) tumor cells express high amounts of specific transferrin or LDL receptors on their cell surface [13, 14]; (iii) they are readily available in a pure and uniform form exhibiting good biological stability; and (iv) they are biodegradable, nontoxic, and nonimmunogenic.

The rationale and diagnostic evidence for using these proteins as drug carriers for tumor targeting is outlined in detail below.

24.2
Rationale for Exploiting Albumin, Transferrin, and LDL as Carriers for Drug Delivery to Solid Tumors

In the middle of the twentieth century, the first reports appeared in the literature demonstrating that tumors are able to trap serum proteins and utilize their degradation products for proliferation [15, 16]. Further clinical research identified a common feature of all the three proteins (i.e., albumin, transferrin, and LDL) in malignant diseases – a decrease in serum concentration that correlated with the degree of differentiation of the tumor cells and the stage of the cancer disease. In an elegant study, Warner et al. demonstrated that transferrin serum levels were low in rats bearing a lymphosarcoma, but increased under effective treatment with cisplatin [17]. In addition, Aulbert has shown that the serum half-life of injected ^{67}Ga-transferrin in animals and patients with different tumors can be reduced to a half or even a third of that found for healthy controls [10]. As an example, Figure 24.6a shows that transferrin serum levels decrease with the increase in malignancy when compared to transferrin serum concentrations in healthy individuals.

Hypoalbuminemia is also a characteristic feature of cancer patients and is especially prominent in patients with high tumor burden [19].

Figure 24.6b illustrates depletion of albumin as well as transferrin in a more recent study of 260 anemic tumor patients, which clearly shows that the serum levels for both proteins for the majority of patients fall below the normal range of healthy individuals.

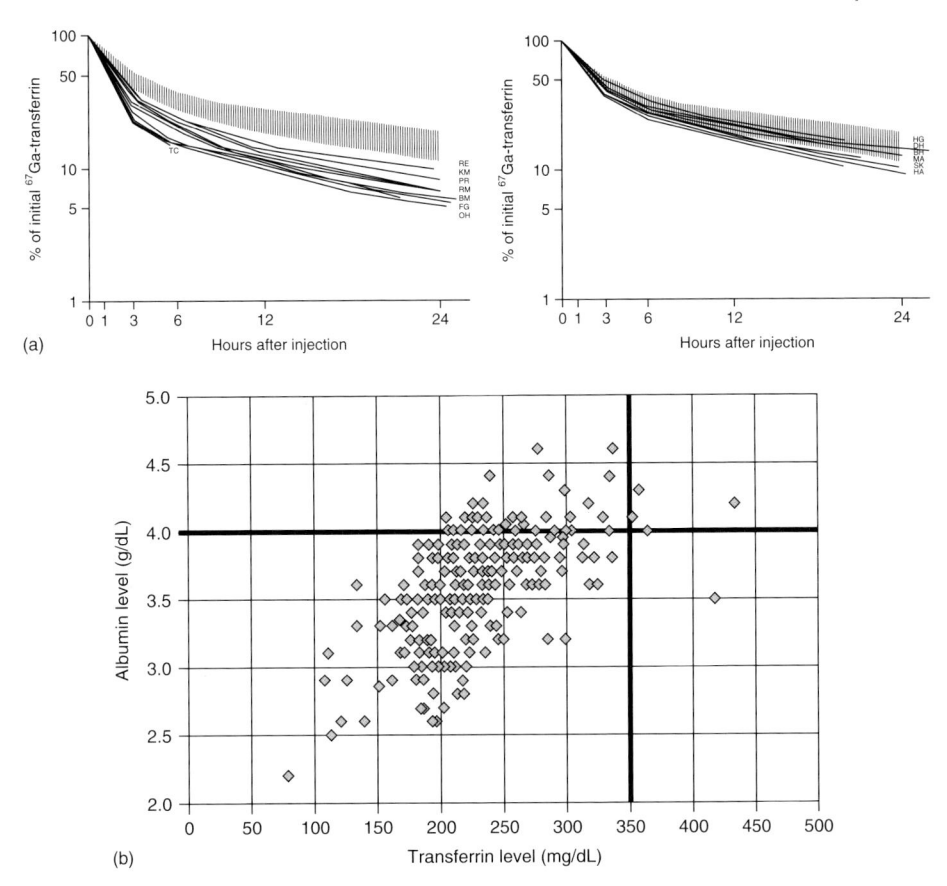

Figure 24.6 (a) Decreased levels of transferrin in tumor patients. The graph on the left shows elimination of radiolabeled ^{67}Ga-transferrin in patients with tumors of high malignancy, the graph on the right shows elimination of radiolabeled ^{67}Ga-transferrin in patients with tumors of low malignancy in comparison to the elimination profile of healthy subjects (shaded area). (Reproduced with permission from [10]). (b) Depletion of plasma levels of albumin and transferrin in tumor patients. Serum protein range in 260 tumor patients (g/l): albumin, 36 (24–46); transferrin, 2.0 (0.8–4.3). Normal range in healthy individuals 36 (g/l): albumin, 40 (35–50); transferrin 3.4 (2.4–4.5). (Reproduced with permission from [18].)

In such cases, which are generally associated with cachexia, albumin infusions are used to compensate for the overall albumin loss. As an explanation for the high albumin turnover in rodent tumors, Stehle *et al.* have proposed that plasma proteins such as albumin are the major energy and nutrition sources for tumor growth (reviewed in [20]). At the center of their hypothesis on tumor nutrition are an excessive plasma protein catabolism by the tumor itself and an active metabolic role of the liver, which seem to be important factors for the genesis of cachexia.

Following the rationale that tumor cells sequester large amounts of LDL, reduced levels of plasma cholesterol would be expected in cancer patients and a large set of data is available that demonstrates that plasma cholesterol levels in cancer patients are reduced [8, 9, 21–25]. The main reason why LDL is utilized by fast-growing tumor cells is their need for cholesterol in order to synthesize new membranes. Body cells obtain cholesterol either by *de novo* synthesis or from LDL, or both. As a great part of the tumor tissue is metabolically highly active, it is logical to expect that some types of cancer cells will have higher LDL requirements than normal cells. Indeed, a number of studies have demonstrated that especially human leukemia cells and tumor cells of gynecological origin have a higher uptake of LDL than the corresponding normal cells [21, 26–28]. The cell's need for LDL is generally associated with specific LDL receptors on the cell surface. Binding and internalization studies of LDL by tumor cells in cell culture have shown that a variety of tumor cells have a high expression of LDL cell receptors [9]. *In vitro* studies have shown that about 75% of LDL uptake by cells is mediated by the LDL receptor [29]. In contrast to the intracellular pathway of transferrin, LDL is transported to lysosomes after receptor-mediated endocytosis where the cholesterol esters of LDL are hydrolyzed.

Some tumor cells do not internalize a great amount of LDL although they express a large number of LDL cell receptors (e.g., cervical cancer EC-168 [30] or epitheloid carcinoma A-431 [31]). Firestone has therefore pointed out that it is important to show receptor binding as well as internalization of LDL before concluding that a given tumor cell type is suitable for LDL-mediated drug targeting [9].

The data from clinical studies regarding cholesterol depletion in malignant diseases have been intensively reviewed [8, 9]. The variations in plasma cholesterol levels of cancer patients are not always extreme, but plasma levels are especially low in patients with aggressive metastasizing tumors in accord with a greater LDL requirement and this fact is well documented in the literature [22–25].

In addition to the depletion of transferrin, albumin, and LDL in the blood circulation due to tumor progression and the formation of metastases, a large body of direct diagnostic evidence with the respective dye-labeled or radiolabeled proteins is available that demonstrates preferential uptake in solid tumors. The following summarizes relevant studies regarding the accumulation of these three serum proteins in tumors, beginning with transferrin.

Tumors in animals and man exhibit a high "parasitic" uptake of Fe(III) when they are fast growing. A major part of the experimental evidence has been gathered by using ^{67}Ga-, ^{68}Ga-, ^{111}In-, ^{97}Ru-, or ^{103}Ru-transferrin [10, 32, 33] as markers for iron uptake, which are very similar to Fe-transferrin in their biochemical behavior. Aulbert has reviewed the literature on this phenomenon [10] and, together with his investigations, demonstrated that fast-growing tumor cells show a much higher uptake of transferrin than the normal surrounding tissue of the affected organ. This uptake, which is directly related to the degree of differentiation of the tumor, can be 2- to even 8-fold higher than in the normal surrounding tissue as determined in tumor-bearing mice or rats.

Pioneering work by Edwards and Hayes in 1969 had shown that ^{67}Ga is concentrated in the lymph nodes in Hodgkin's disease [34] and the medical literature is rich on reports of the use of ^{67}Ga compounds to detect many

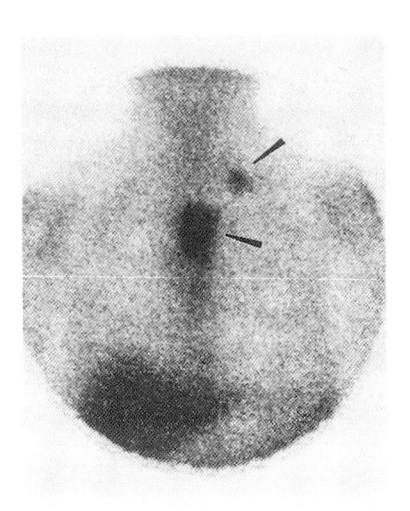

Figure 24.7 Gallium scintigram of a Hodgkin's lymphoma patient using ^{67}Ga-citrate (arrows show tumor localization around the breast bone).

types of malignancies in humans (reviewed in [35]). Some indications are lung cancer, Hodgkin's and non-Hodgkin's lymphomas, malignant melanoma, breast carcinoma, and Ewing's sarcoma. As an example, a radioscintigraphic picture of a Hodgkin's lymphoma patient treated with ^{67}Ga-citrate, which binds rapidly to apotransferrin after intravenous administration, is shown in Figure 24.7. Tumor nodes are seen at the breast bone and collar bone.

The distribution of the transferrin receptor in different cell types, the modulation of its expression, and its molecular recognition properties appear to be critical factors with regard to the physiology of iron metabolism and to the use of transferrin and its derivatives in medicine [36]. Several investigators have determined the number of transferrin receptors on a variety of human cell types and their numbers per cell range from around 40 000–2 800 000 in tumor cells as compared to approximately 45 000–400 000 present on reticulocytes [14].

Apart from transferrin, albumin is a further serum protein that is able to accumulate in tumor tissue. Tumor uptake in preclinical models can be easily visualized by injecting the dye Evans blue that binds rapidly and with high affinity to circulating albumin, and that makes subcutaneously growing tumors turn blue within a few hours postinjection (Figure 24.8).

These and other studies concerning tumor uptake, tumor blood flow, and transport of molecules in the interstitium led Maeda and Matsumura to coin the expression "enhanced permeability and retention (EPR)" ([37] and Chapter 3). The leaky defective blood vessels of tumor tissue make its vasculature permeable for macromolecules, whereas in blood vessels of healthy tissue only small molecules can pass the endothelial barrier. The pore size of tumor microvessels varies from 100 to 1200 nm in diameter [38, 39]. Macromolecules employed as carriers for the development of macromolecular prodrugs typically have hydrodynamic radii that are between 2 and 10 nm (e.g., serum albumin has an effective hydrodynamic diameter of 7.2 nm), allowing extravasation into tumor tissue, but not into normal tissue.

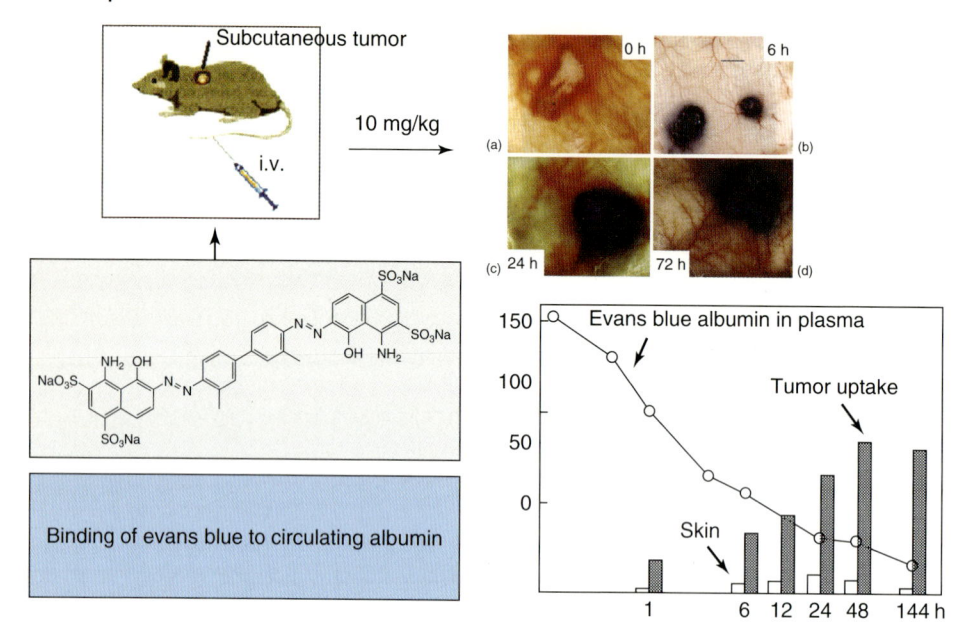

Figure 24.8 Uptake of Evans blue after intravenous injection and binding to albumin in subcutaneously growing tumors in mice. (Adapted from [11]).

The enhanced uptake of macromolecules in tumor tissue cannot be solely explained by an enhanced permeability of the vascular system since this would affect smaller molecules in a similar manner, but is also due to a reduced clearance from the tumor when the molecular weight exceeds 40 kDa [40]. Whereas smaller molecules were shown to be rapidly cleared from the tumor interstitium, large molecules are retained, thus showing high intratumor concentrations even after 100 h postapplication [40]. This enhanced retention of macromolecules in tumor tissue is primarily caused by a lack of lymphatic drainage due to an impaired or absent lymphatic system. Hence, it is the EPR effect that is responsible for the accumulation of macromolecules in solid tumors (see Chapter 3 for a detailed description).

From 1990 onwards, an increasing number of distribution studies concerning the tumor uptake of labeled albumin in animal tumor models appeared in the literature. These studies, in which albumin was either radiolabeled or conjugated with dyes, showed that between 3 and 25% of the applied dose was found in the tumor (reviewed in [41]).

In a number of studies, Sinn *et al.* have demonstrated that the amount of albumin found in the tumor is dependent on the kind and size of the tumor as well as on the labeling technique employed [42, 43]. Metabolically unstable protein labels, such as conventional radiolabeling with ^{131}I, are not suitable for long-term observation of tumor uptake and lead to apparent low uptake rates. In contrast, when residualizing protein labels are used (e.g., ^{131}I-tyramine-desoxysorbitol or ^{111}In-DTPA; DTPA =

diethylenetriamene pentaacetate, an effective chelating agent) high uptake rates of labeled albumin in rat tumors are observed. As an example, scintigraphic images of rats bearing ovarian tumors of different size or a Walker-256 carcinoma in the left hind leg 72 h after administration of ^{111}In-DTPA labeled rat serum albumin (RSA) are shown in Figure 24.9a.

As can be seen, the amounts of tracer substance increase with tumor weight and more than 20% of a single dose of radiolabeled albumin accumulates in large tumors (tumor weight around 6.24% of body weight). Only a few studies have shed light on differences between transferrin and albumin regarding tumor uptake in animal models. Using fluorescein isothiocyanate-labeled proteins, Tanaka et al. have demonstrated that transferrin uptake is approximately twice as high than for albumin in mice bearing subcutaneously growing sarcoma 180 [45]. In contrast, Sinn et al. observed little difference in the tumor uptake of serum albumin and transferrin when evaluated in the above-mentioned rat models [20].

The distribution of albumin in tumor-bearing animals was further studied by microautoradiography after injection of radiolabeled albumin and fluorescence imaging after injection of fluorescent-labeled albumin (Figure 24.9b). Both techniques impressively demonstrate the high rate of albumin uptake compared to normal tissue on the histological level.

Tumor accumulation of radiolabeled LDL has been investigated in a few studies in rodent models [46–49]. The data regarding biodistribution and tumor uptake have been conflicting, however, due to the fact that different radiolabeling techniques were used. Versluis et al. has shed light on the observed discrepancies by comparing different labeling techniques [49]. When directly iodinated LDL was used, as in the earlier studies, tumor uptake of the radiolabel was high in B16 melanoma-bearing mice, uptake being exceeded only by that in the stomach. In contrast, when ^{125}I-tyramine-cellobiose, an intracellularly accumulating label, was used, a different tissue distribution was observed. At 24 h after injection, the adrenals, liver, spleen, and intestines showed the highest tissue/serum ratios followed by uptake in the tumor. Uptake in the tumor was about a half of that found in the liver using this label. From these studies, Versluis et al. concluded that an accumulating label is needed in order to accurately determine uptake of LDL by tumor tissue [49]. As the adrenals, liver, and spleen showed high LDL uptake in these studies, various pretreatment strategies have been suggested for downregulating LDL receptors on these organs without affecting the LDL receptor status on tumor cells. Uptake of LDL by the liver can be decreased by a diet rich in cholesterol and triglycerides or by the administration of bile salts, such as cholic acid or taurocholate. Uptake of LDL by tumor cells was found to be unaffected by this treatment in mice [47]. In addition, the uptake of LDL by the adrenals was shown to be greatly reduced in rats and rabbits by the administration of corticosteroids [47, 50].

A final interesting finding from the former studies was the role of receptor-mediated and nonspecific uptake of LDL in animal models. In order to determine these effects, the tissue distribution of radiolabeled methylated LDL and radiolabeled LDL was compared in B16 melanoma bearing mice [49]. Reductive methylation of LDL is a suitable tool for the determination of nonspecific as

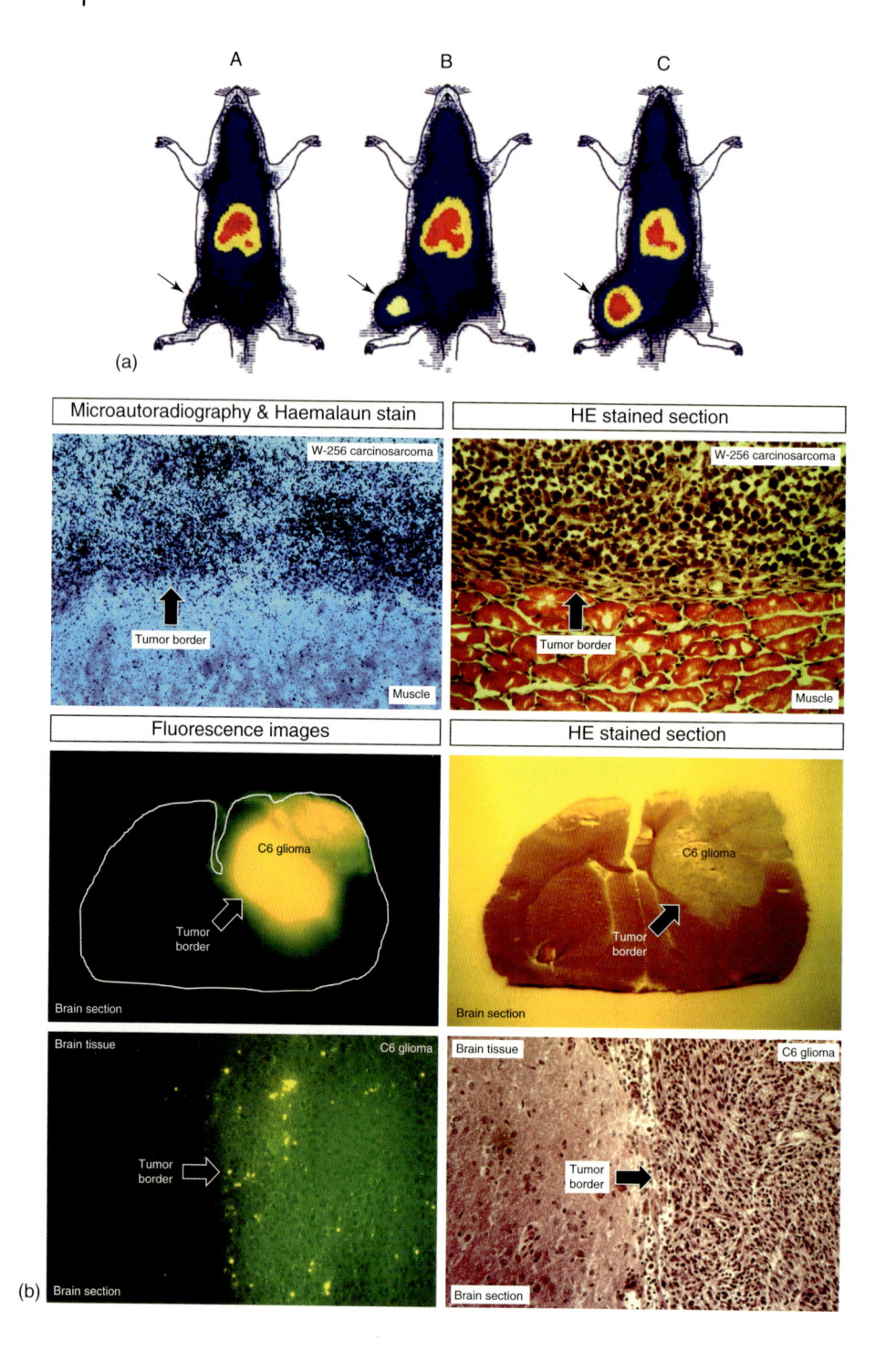

758 *24 Serum Proteins as Drug Carriers of Anticancer Agents*

A B C

(a)

Microautoradiography & Haemalaun stain

W-256 carcinosarcoma
Tumor border
Muscle

HE stained section

W-256 carcinosarcoma
Tumor border
Muscle

Fluorescence images

C6 glioma
Tumor border
Brain section

HE stained section

C6 glioma
Tumor border
Brain section

Brain tissue — C6 glioma
Tumor border
Brain section

Brain tissue — C6 glioma
Tumor border
Brain section

(b)

Figure 24.9 (a) Scintigrams 72 h after administration of ^{111}In-DTPA-RSA to a rat bearing an ovarian tumor (A and B) of varying size or a Walker-256 carcinosarcoma (C) in the left hind leg. (A) Tumor weight 0.4 g or 0.16% of the respective body weight, tracer uptake 0.23% of the injected amount; (B) tumor weight 5.9 g or 2.8% of the respective body weight, tracer uptake 4.2% of the injected amount); (C) tumor weight 15.0 g or 6.24% of the respective body weight, tracer uptake 23.1% of the injected amount). The color code for increasing amounts of radioactivity is blue, green, yellow, and red. (Reproduced with permission from [41]). (b) Microautoradiography and fluorescence images of tissue sections taken from tumor-bearing rats showing the border between tumor and normal tissue 24 h after intravenous injection of radiolabeled or fluorescently labeled albumin respectively. (A) Tissue sections of a rat implanted intramuscularly with Walker-256 carcinosarcoma cells and injected with radiolabeled albumin (left: microautoradiography stained with hemalaun; right: hematoxylin & eosin (HE)-stained adjacent section). The black dots are silver grains. Significantly more silver grains are visible in the tumor tissue, indicating the exposure to higher amounts of radioactivity. (Images courtesy of Andreas Wunder, Charité Berlin.) (B) Tissue section of a rat intracranially implanted with C6 glioma cells and injected with fluorescent albumin (left: fluorescence images; right: hematoxylin & eosin (HE) stain of the same section after fluorescence inspection). Compared to the normal brain tissue, the tumor tissue shows much higher fluorescence intensities, which is attributed to the uptake of high albumin amounts in the tumor. Note that the tumor border is clearly visible in both cases. (Reproduced with permission from [44]).

---

opposed to receptor-mediated uptake of LDL. Tissue uptake of methylated LDL was significantly lower in the major organs (2- to 6-fold lower in the adrenals, liver, and spleen) and only about a half of the dose was found in the tumor compared to LDL. Thus, there is evidence that tumor uptake of LDL is receptor-mediated, but that nonspecific uptake, presumably by fluid-phase endocytosis, also plays a role.

24.3
Examples of Drug Delivery Systems with Serum Proteins

24.3.1
Synthetic Approaches for Realizing Drug Conjugates, Drug Complexes, and Drug Nanoparticles with Albumin, Transferrin, or LDL

Before presenting an overview of drug delivery systems realized with serum proteins, it is useful to address the different coupling and complexing techniques for preparing drug conjugates, drug adducts, albumin-binding prodrugs, and nanoparticles with LDL, albumin, and transferrin.

Principally, three drug delivery technologies can be distinguished: (i) coupling of low-molecular weight drugs to exogenous or endogenous albumin or transferrin, (ii) genetically engineering or conjugation of transferrin or albumin with bioactive proteins to form targeted toxins or albumin fusion proteins, and (iii) encapsulation of drugs into LDL or albumin to produce nanoparticles and microspheres. Characteristic examples of such drug delivery systems with albumin are shown schematically in Figure 24.10.

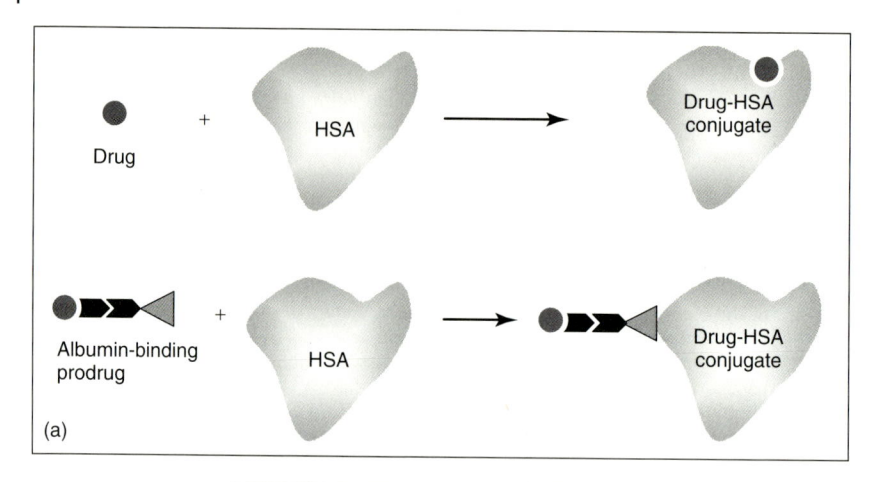

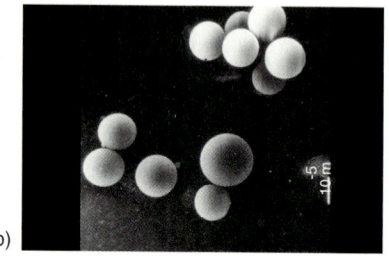

Figure 24.10 (a) Illustration of direct coupling of a drug to albumin (top) or of an albumin-binding prodrug containing a protein-binding group and a cleavable linker to albumin (HSA) (bottom). (b) Illustration of albumin microspheres.

Initially, direct coupling methods (e.g., using glutaraldehyde or carbodiimides) were employed for the preparation of dye and drug–protein conjugates. Although direct coupling methods are easy to carry out, they do have a number of drawbacks for obtaining a defined cleavable drug–protein conjugate: (i) they are limited to drugs exhibiting suitable functional groups, (ii) the bond between drug and carrier is chemically not well defined, (iii) polymeric products are likely to be formed in the coupling step, and (iv) the bond between drug and carrier is often too stable (e.g., an amide bond), so that the drug cannot be released efficiently at the tumor site.

In order to improve the coupling methods required for obtaining better defined conjugates in which the stability of the bond between the carrier and the drug could also be varied, a second generation of drug–protein conjugates was synthesized by first derivatizing the drug with a spacer group and then attaching the drug derivative to a suitable functional group on the protein. In this way the bond between the drug and the spacer can act as a cleavage site, allowing the drug to be released inside or outside of the tumor cell. Examples are peptide spacers designed to release the bound drug through cleavage by lysosomal or extracellular enzymes or acid-sensitive linkers. The significance of adjusting the chemical properties of the bond between the drug and the macromolecular carrier can then be verified experimentally through *in vitro* and *in vivo* investigations.

Another strategy for developing transferrin and albumin conjugates with therapeutically active peptides is to fuse the gene for human albumin or transferrin (or alternatively an antibody directed against the transferrin receptor) to the gene that encodes the active protein. This technology has initially been applied to plant or bacteria toxins for creating targeted protein conjugates that target the transferrin receptor (described in Chapter 45) or to cytokines such as interferons or interleukins with albumin [51].

Two principal applications of albumin as nanosized drug delivery systems are worth mentioning. The first concerns the use of albumin in microsphere formulations. Albumin microspheres are colloidal particles and are generally prepared by chemical cross-linking or by addition of an organic solvent and stabilization at elevated temperatures. The size of the albumin microspheres, which is usually in the range of 1–100 µm, is the decisive factor for the biodistribution characteristics of the albumin microsphere. Small microspheres (1–3 µm) are taken up by the reticuloendothelial system (RES), and accumulate in the liver and spleen as well as in solid tumors. Larger microspheres (greater than 15 µm) will effectively target the capillary bed of the lungs. Albumin microspheres can carry therapeutic or diagnostic agents. The therapeutic approaches with albumin microspheres will not be discussed here since there was only one preliminary report of phase I trials with a cisplatin-loaded or mitomycin C–albumin microsphere in the mid-1980s, and no candidate has currently reached an advanced preclinical stage (for details, see review articles on this topic [52, 53]).

For diagnostic applications, a ^{99m}Tc-macroaggregated albumin has been developed that has found various clinical applications. ^{99m}Tc-macroaggregated albumin is prepared by mixing a colloid solution of Sn(II) chloride with a solution of HSA and subsequent labeling with sodium pertechnetate (^{99m}TcO$_4^-$ Na$^+$). Depending on the amount and reaction time chosen, larger particles are formed in the range of 200–1000 nm (Albures; Nycomed Amersham) [54] or smaller particles with an average size of 8 nm (Nanocoll; Nycomed Amersham) [55], so the latter are nano- rather than microparticles. ^{99m}Tc-macroaggregated albumin has been used diagnostically for various indications in oncology, including lymphoscintigraphy [56], and sentinel node detection in breast cancer [57] and other solid tumors [58, 59].

The second clinically successful application of using albumin to form nanoparticles is the *nab*™ technology developed by American Bioscience (meanwhile incorporated by Celgene), that is ideal for encapsulating lipophilic drugs into nanoparticles. The technology as such appears simple: the drug is mixed with HSA in an aqueous solvent and passed under high pressure through a jet to form drug–albumin nanoparticles in the size range of 100–200 nm that is comparable to the size of small liposomes. Abraxane®, an albumin–paclitaxel nanoparticle that disperses into albumin–paclitaxel complexes after intravenous administration, was approved 2005 for treating metastasized breast cancer. *nab* technology and its current preclinical/clinical status is described in Chapter 35 of this book edition.

The design of drug carrier systems with LDL is somewhat different than for transferrin and albumin. Due to the substantial lipid content and spherical shape of LDL, it shows some resemblance to liposomes. However, in contrast to many liposomal formulations, LDL is not rapidly cleared by the RES and can be considered as a natural equivalent of the so-called "stealth" liposomes (PEGylated liposomes) [60, 61]. The principal technique to incorporate antineoplastic drugs into LDL is the so-called delipidation–reconstitution method. The cholesterol esters can be extracted from the core of LDL and the core subsequently reconstituted with other hydrophobic compounds. Successful reconstitution of LDL is achieved by attaching lipophilic groups (LDL anchors) to the drug, thus rendering the drug derivative compatible with LDL's phospholipid coat and lipophilic core. Preferred LDL anchors are oleyl, retinyl, and cholesteryl. The first published procedure of a delipidation–reconstitution method was by Krieger *et al.*, in which LDL was lyophilized on potato starch, stripped of its core by heptane extraction, and then reconstituted by adding the lipophilic drug in a nonpolar solvent, which is finally evaporated and replaced with aqueous buffer [62]. Other reconstitution methods have been described that differ in the carrier substance to which LDL is absorbed, the agent needed to disrupt LDL, and the solvent used for reconstitution [63–69]. The methods vary in drug-loading rate and the leakage of the drug from the formed LDL particles.

24.3.2
Drug Complexes and Conjugates with Albumin, Transferrin, and LDL

Table 24.1 summarizes the various transferrin, albumin, and LDL conjugates realized with anticancer drugs. When studying Table 24.1, a number of general features become apparent:

- In the early 1980s research focused on transferrin as a drug delivery system with the number of publications on anticancer drug–albumin conjugates increasing during the 1990s; work on LDL complexes with clinically relevant anticancer drugs is restricted to a handful of investigations.
- Research concerning the coupling of anticancer agents to serum proteins has concentrated primarily on those that can be conveniently detected through visible spectrophotometry, such as methotrexate (MTX), camptothecins, and anthracyclines
- Although the antitumor activity of a number of serum protein conjugates with antineoplastic agents has been extensively evaluated *in vitro*, respective *in vivo* data is limited to a few prominent examples.

Several targeted protein toxins have been developed with transferrin and these are listed at the bottom of Table 24.1. One of these, a transferrin conjugate of diphtheria toxin (Tf-CRM107), advanced to phase III clinical trails for treating malignant gliomas (see Section 24.4).

24.3 Examples of Drug Delivery Systems with Serum Proteins | 763

Table 24.1 Conjugates and complexes of anticancer agents with serum albumin, transferrin and LDL.

Cytotoxic agent	Conjugated or complexed to	Biological evaluation	Special remarks	References
Doxorubicin	transferrin	in vitro	conjugates of doxorubicin coupled to transferrin by glutaraldehyde bind to transferrin receptors on cell membranes of Daudi and HL-60 cells; their in vitro cytotoxicity correlates directly with both the time of exposure and the amount of conjugate employed	[70]
	transferrin	in vitro/ in vivo	this transferrin–doxorubicin conjugate was found to exert more efficient cytotoxicity than free drug through a mechanism other than intercalation with nuclear DNA; the transferrin–doxorubicin conjugate provides a more effective tool by inhibiting the plasma membrane electron transport than is given by the free drug	[71, 72]
	transferrin	in vitro	conjugates of doxorubicin coupled to transferrin by glutaraldehyde are cytotoxic to anthracycline-resistant human promyelocytic (HL-60) and erythroleukemic (K562) cell lines; the effect of the conjugate was dependent on its doxorubicin content (i.e., on the loading ratio)	[73]
	transferrin	patients	transferrin–doxorubicin conjugate prepared by glutaraldehyde coupling reduced the number of tumor cells in peripheral blood of patients with leukemia and bone marrow aspirates showed no evidence of disease progression	[74]
	transferrin	in vitro	in vitro studies in cell culture experiments performed with human endothelial cells and tumor cells showed that the acid-sensitive transferrin conjugates of doxorubicin possessed a high selectivity of the conjugates for tumor cells	[75]
	transferrin	in vitro/ in vivo	an acid-sensitive transferrin–doxorubicin conjugate with a comparable in vitro cytotoxicity to free doxorubicin can be administered at higher doses than free doxorubicin in nude mice models with a concomitant improvement in antitumor activity	[76]
	transferrin	in vitro	doxorubicin–gallium–transferrin conjugate demonstrated approximately the same inhibitory effect as doxorubicin and overcomes multidrug resistance in the MCF7/ADR cell line	[77]

(continued overleaf)

Table 24.1 (continued)

Cytotoxic agent	Conjugated or complexed to	Biological evaluation	Special remarks	References
	transferrin	in vitro/in vivo	N-(2-hydroxypropyl)methacrylamide (HPMA) copolymer-bound doxorubicin targeted to the transferrin receptor with transferrin exhibited promising in vitro and in vivo effect against B-cell lymphoma 38C13	[78]
	transferrin	in vitro	transferrin-conjugated liposomes coencapsulating doxorubicin were highly effective in overcoming drug resistance in K562 leukemia cells	[79]
	transferrin	in vivo	doxorubicin-loaded stealth liposomes were able to enhance the intracellular tumor uptake of doxorubicin into the tumor cells by receptor-mediated endocytosis in tumor-bearing mice	[80]
	transferrin	in vitro	doxorubicin–transferrin conjugate selectively overcomes multidrug resistance in leukemia cell lines with a very limited effect on normal tissue cells	[81]
	HSA	in vitro	doxorubicin microcapsules retain activity in vitro and appear to overcome P-glycoprotein-mediated doxorubicin resistance and their activity correlates with the rate of particle uptake	[82]
	HSA	in vitro/in vivo	an acid-sensitive albumin–doxorubicin conjugate with a comparable in vitro cytotoxicity to free doxorubicin can be administered at higher doses than free doxorubicin in nude mice models with a concomitant improvement in antitumor activity; the antitumor activity was comparable to analogously constructed transferrin–doxorubicin conjugates	[76, 83]
	HSA	in vitro	albumin-binding doxorubicin conjugate that was cleaved efficiently by activated MMP-2 and -9 showed antiproliferative activity in a murine renal cell carcinoma line in the low micromolar range	[84]
	HSA	in vivo	MMP/MMP-cleavable albumin-binding doxorubicin prodrug was superior to the parent compound doxorubicin in the A375 human melanoma xenograft, which is characterized by a high expression of MMP-2	[85]
	HSA	in vivo	albumin-binding 6-maleimidocaproyl hydrazone derivative of doxorubicin was distinctly superior to the parent compound doxorubicin in three animal tumor models with respect to antitumor efficacy and toxicity	[86]

HSA	in vitro/ in vivo	albumin-binding doxorubicin prodrug that is cleaved by prostate-specific antigen showed good activity in the CWR22 PSA-positive model that was comparable to doxorubicin	[87]
HSA	in vitro	doxorubicin-loaded HSA nanoparticle preparations showed increased anticancer effects in comparison to doxorubicin in two different neuroblastoma cell lines	[88]
HSA	in vitro/ in vivo	albumin-binding cathepsin B cleavable prodrug of doxorubicin with an excellent water solubility and comparable in vivo activity to that of free doxorubicin in the M-3366 breast carcinoma xenograft model at equimolar dose	[89]
HSA	in vitro	nanoparticles based on biodegradable HSA loaded with doxorubicin showed good cellular binding and uptake into human epidermal growth factor receptor-2 (HER2)-overexpressing breast cancer cells with improved activity versus free doxorubicin	[90]
HSA	in vitro/ in vivo	albumin-binding prodrug of doxorubicin that is cleaved by PSA showed enhanced antitumor efficacy when compared to doxorubicin in a mouse model of human prostate cancer using luciferase-transduced LNCaP cells orthotopically implanted in SCID mice	[91]
HSA	in vitro/ in vivo	albumin-binding prodrug of doxorubicin that incorporates a maleimide moiety and a PABC self-immolative spacer was cleaved by cathepsin B and exhibited superior antitumor activity in vivo compared to doxorubicin in an effective way to increase the therapeutic index of doxorubicin	[92]
HSA	in vitro	doxorubicin-loaded DI17E6 nanoparticles demonstrated increased cytotoxic activity in $\alpha_v\beta_3$-positive melanoma cells compared to free drug	[93]
HSA	in vitro/ in vivo	spray-dried doxorubicin–albumin microparticulate systems for treatment of multidrug-resistant melanomas	[94]
LDL	in vivo	N-trifluoroacetyladriamycin-14-valerate–LDL complex containing about 100 drug molecules per LDL particle is a possible way to complex cytotoxic agents with LDL without interfering with its in vivo behavior in mice	[63]

(continued overleaf)

Table 24.1 (continued)

Cytotoxic agent	Conjugated or complexed to	Biological evaluation	Special remarks	References
	LDL	in vitro/ in vivo	LDL as a promising targeted carrier for doxorubicin in nude mice bearing human hepatoma R-HepG2 cells with a higher antiproliferative effect and reduced cardiotoxicity than that of free doxorubicin in addition to circumventing multidrug resistance	[95]
Daunorubicin	transferrin	in vitro	transferrin–daunorubicin conjugates with at least 10 times more in vitro activity than the free drug against small-cell carcinoma of the lung cell line NCI-H69	[96]
	transferrin	in vitro/ in vivo	daunorubicin–transferrin conjugate is more active upon malignant cells than free daunorubicin while being less toxic for normal cells	[97]
	transferrin	in vitro	acid-sensitive transferrin–daunorubicin conjugate with a high activity in human melanoma cells using a clonogenic cell assay comparable to or exceeding that of daunorubicin	[98]
	HSA	in vitro/ in vivo	daunorubicin conjugated to succinylated serum albumin by an amide bond via tri- and tetrapeptide spacer arms is more active than daunorubicin, inducing a high percentage of long-term survivors following drug release through the action of lysosomal hydrolases in vivo	[99]
	LDL	in vitro	daunorubicin–LDL complex that exhibited an improved in vitro cytotoxic toward LDL receptor-positive Chinese hamster ovary cells than LDL receptor-negative cells	[100]
	LDL	in vitro	comparative cellular uptake and cytotoxicity of a complex of a daunomycin–LDL complex in human squamous lung tumor cell monolayers with an equal in vitro cytotoxicity and a granular distribution within the cytoplasm	[101]
MTX	HSA	in vivo	MTX that was covalently linked to HSA (MTX–HSA) showed a comparative cytotoxicity to the free drug in five cell lines from human solid tumors and five lines of human lymphocytes	[102]
	HSA	in vitro/ in vivo	HSA–MTX that was synthesized by means of 1-ethyl-3-(3′ – dimethylaminopropyl)-carbodiimide exhibited more toxicity than free MTX, but its therapeutic activity was better against Gardner lymphosarcoma with a 5 times higher efficacy compared to free MTX; in addition, HSA–MTX more efficiently inhibited the growth of B16 melanoma tumor than free MTX, and significantly reduced both the number and size of pulmonary metastatic colonies, but with no proportional difference in lifespan prolongation after therapy with these drugs	[103, 104]

	HSA	patients	In a phase I study, MTX–HSA was well tolerated with no signs of severe toxicity or drug accumulation in addition to tumor responses that were seen in three patients: (i) a partial response was seen in one patient with renal cell carcinoma; (ii) a minor response was seen in one patient with pleural mesothelioma; and (iii) a minor response was seen in one patient with renal cell carcinoma	[105]
	HSA	in vivo	promising improved therapeutic effects of MTX–HSA compared to free MTX in three xenograft models including soft-tissue sarcoma model SXF 1301, prostate cancer model PRXF PC3M, and osteosarcoma model SXF 1410	[106]
	HSA	in vitro/in vivo	albumin-binding prodrug of MTX that is cleaved by both cathepsin B and plasmin with distinct superior antitumor efficacy compared to free MTX in an OVCAR-3 xenograft model	[107]
	LDL	in vitro	LDL–MTX covalent complex with a lower activity than the free drug against L1210 murine leukemia cells in vitro	[108]
Floxuridine	LDL	in vitro/in vivo	improved in vitro cytotoxicity of dioleoyl-FdUrd–LDL complex against the hepatocellular carcinoma cell line HepG2 in addition to increased therapeutic effect of the complex in a rat tumor model with 6-fold increase in the serum half-life accompanied by enhanced tumor delivery	[69]
Chlorambucil	transferrin	in vitro	conjugation of chlorambucil to transferrin through an acid-sensitive carboxylic hydrazone bond enhanced the in vitro cytotoxicity of chlorambucil against MCF7 mammary carcinoma and MOLT4 leukemia cell line	[109]
	HSA	in vitro	enhanced in vitro cytotoxicity of chlorambucil–albumin conjugate with a carboxylic hydrazone bond against MCF7 mammary carcinoma and MOLT4 leukemia cell line with subsequent significant increase in the MTD in comparison to unbound chlorambucil	[110]
Nitrogen mustards	LDL	in vitro	two compounds that reconstituted as a LDL complex kill or arrest tumor cells at reasonably low concentrations due to their exclusive cellular delivery via the LDL pathway	[111]

(continued overleaf)

Table 24.1 (continued)

Cytotoxic agent	Conjugated or complexed to	Biological evaluation	Special remarks	References
Paclitaxel	HSA	in vitro	paclitaxel–albumin conjugates that were stable in physiological solution maintained high cytotoxicity in three different tumor cell lines with efficient cell binding and internalization followed by release of the drug inside the cell	[112]
	HSA	in vitro	PEGylated HSA–paclitaxel conjugates with improved antitumor activity in three tumor cell lines	[113]
	HSA	in vivo	nab-paclitaxel (i.e., nanoparticle albumin-bound paclitaxel; ABI-007; Abraxane) is a novel formulation of paclitaxel that does not employ Cremophor/ethanol, and demonstrates greater efficacy and a favorable safety profile compared with standard paclitaxel in patients with advanced disease (breast cancer)	[114]
	HSA	in vitro	folate-mediated targeting of albumin conjugates of paclitaxel, obtained through a heterogeneous phase system, exhibited increased selectivity and antitumor activity in an in vitro cytotoxicity study on human nasopharyngeal epidermal carcinoma KB and colorectal carcinoma HT-29 cells (as negative control)	[115]
	LDL	in vitro	synthetic nano-LDLs that incorporate paclitaxel oleate are capable of killing glioblastoma multiforme cells via the LDL receptor	[116]
	transferrin	in vitro	paclitaxel–transferrin conjugates using glutaraldehyde exhibited a slightly decreased in vitro cytotoxicity on small cell carcinoma of the lung cell line (H69)	[117]
	transferrin	in vitro	sustained release transferrin-conjugated paclitaxel-loaded biodegradable nanoparticles with improved in vitro cytotoxicity against human prostate cancer cell line (PC-3) and enhanced antitumor efficacy in a murine model of prostate cancer	[118]
	transferrin	in vitro	paclitaxel-loaded poly(lactic-co-glycolic acid) nanoparticles surface modified with transferrin exhibited a significant increase in cytotoxicity using a C6 rat glioma cell line and a better in vivo biodistribution compared to free drug in a rat model	[119]

24.3 Examples of Drug Delivery Systems with Serum Proteins | 769

Drug	Carrier	Study	Description	Ref.
Vincristine	LDL	patients	LDL delivery vehicle containing vincristine as cytotoxic drug apparently reduced the commonly seen side-effects in patients with ovarian or endometrial cancer	[120]
Cisplatin	transferrin	in vitro	transferrin could be a promising carrier protein for the transport of cisplatin to tumors with improved in vitro antiproliferative activities and improved in vivo distribution	[121]
	HSA	in vivo	cisplatin-encapsulated transferrin–PEG glycol liposomes as a more effective targeting strategy for treatment of gastric cancer with significantly higher survival rates compared with PEGylated liposomes without transferrin, bare liposomes, or free cisplatin formulations	[122]
	transferrin	in vivo	albumin microspheres and microcapsules containing cisplatin as chemotherapeutic agents for the treatment of hepatocellular carcinoma, accumulated in the liver at a higher concentration and alleviated cisplatin induced side-effects after injection into the hepatic artery of adult dogs	[123]
	HSA	in vitro/ in vivo	polymer-coated albumin microspheres as carriers for intravascular tumor targeting of cisplatin offer an improved system of administration for hepatic artery infusion or adjuvant therapy, enabling better clinical handling and the promise of a higher tumor tissue to normal tissue ratio	[124]
	HSA	in vitro	targeted immunospecific albumin microspheres loaded with cisplatin with improved in vitro cytotoxicity against a rodent ovarian carcinoma	[125]
Mitomycin C	transferrin	in vitro	receptor-mediated endocytosis and cytotoxicity of transferrin–mitomycin C conjugate in the HepG2 cell and primary cultured rat hepatocyte	[126]
	HSA	in vitro	mitomycin C-loaded albumin microspheres, prepared by chemical denaturation in a multiparticulate system, followed first-order release kinetics better than spherical matrix kinetics	[127]

(continued overleaf)

Table 24.1 (continued)

Cytotoxic agent	Conjugated or complexed to	Biological evaluation	Special remarks	References
Ru(III) complexes	HSA/ transferrin	in vitro/ in vivo	adduct formation of the Ru(III) complex NAMI-A with serum albumin and serum transferrin possessed a very encouraging preclinical profile of metastasis inhibition, but caused a drastic decrease of NAMI-A bioavailability and a subsequent reduction of its biological activity, implying that association to plasma proteins essentially represents a mechanism of drug inactivation	[128]
	transferrin	in vitro	transferrin-bound Ru(III) complexes exhibit high antiproliferative activity in a human colon cancer cell line, which exceeds that of the free complex, indicating that this protein can act as a carrier of the ruthenium complexes into the tumor cell	[129]
Neocarzinostatin	transferrin	in vitro/ in vivo	preferential uptake of transferrin–neocarzinostatin conjugate through transferrin receptor-mediated endocytosis with remarkable inhibitory effect on human colorectal cancer cell line M7609, in vitro and in vivo efficacy in inhibiting the growth of M7609 cells implanted subcutaneously into nude	[130]
	transferrin	in vitro	transferrin–neocarzinostatin conjugate with an apparent improved in vitro cytotoxicity compared to the free drug	[131]
	transferrin	in vitro	transferrin-neocarzinostatin conjugate is internalized specifically by transferrin receptors, and is at least partly transferred to and accumulated in lysosomal compartments, resulting in the inhibition of cellular DNA synthesis in the human leukemia cell line K562	[132]
Ricin A-chain	transferrin	in vitro	highly cytotoxic human transferrin–ricin A-chain conjugate incorporating a disulfide bond that exerted potent cytotoxic effects on human leukemia CEM cells	[133]
Ricin A	transferrin	in vitro	human diferric transferrin linked to ricin A demonstrated pronounced cytotoxic activity, being about 5000 times more toxic than ricin A alone against glioma cells and about 6000 times more toxic against Jurkat cells in the presence of the carboxylic ionophore monensin	[134]

Diphtheria toxin	transferrin	in vitro	AF192 cells were mildly resistant to the transferrin–diphtheria toxin conjugate, and were cross-resistant to the protein toxins modeccin, abrin, ricin, and *Pseudomonas aeruginosa* exotoxin A	[135]
CRM 107	transferrin	in vitro	Tf-CRM107 conjugate, unlike native diphtheria toxin, exhibited a high toxicity against murine cells	[136]
	transferrin	in vivo	regional perfusion with Tf-CRM107 produces tumor responses without systemic toxicity in patients with malignant brain tumors refractory to conventional therapy	[137]
	transferrin	in vivo	chloroquine treatment may be useful to reduce the toxicity of Tf-CRM107 for normal brain tissue without inhibiting the antitumor efficacy of Tf-CRM107 for brain tumor therapy	[138]
	transferrin	patients	in a phase II study, optimized Tf-CRM107 delivery to targeted brain regions resulted in complete and partial tumor responses without severe toxicity in 35% of the evaluable patients	[139]
Diphtheria toxin A-chain	transferrin	in vitro	transferrin–diphtheria toxin conjugate that binds to transferrin receptors is internalized into acidic endocytic vesicles exerting subsequent high cytotoxicity against mouse LMTK cells in culture due to reduction of protein synthesis	[140]
Saporin-6	transferrin	in vitro	conjugates between human transferrin and saporin-6 displayed an inhibitory activity on K562 cells	[141]
Abrin variant	transferrin	in vitro	human diferric transferrin–abrin variant exhibited efficient *in vitro* cytotoxicity against three malignant human cell lines, glioblastoma multiforme SNB19 and SF295 and the LOX melanoma, and a nonhuman control murine melanoma cell line B16	[142]
RNase A	transferrin	in vitro	transferrin–RNase is taken up by receptor-mediated endocytosis, and provides a new approach to selective cell killing possibly with less systemic toxicity and importantly less immunogenicity than the currently employed ligand–toxin conjugates	[143]

Important examples of serum protein conjugates realized with low-molecular weight anticancer drugs and toxins are described in the following.

24.3.2.1 Drug Conjugates with Transferrin and Albumin

Research focusing on conjugates with transferrin and clinically established agents are restricted to a limited number, including doxorubicin, daunorubicin, mitomycin, paclitaxel, and chlorambucil [71, 74, 112, 120, 133, 144–148] (Table 24.1). Direct coupling methods employing glutaraldehyde for cross-linking doxorubicin and daunorubicin to transferrin have resulted in active conjugates. Faulk *et al.* have shown that these transferrin conjugates of doxorubicin show high *in vitro* activity and that the mode of action is not due to intercalation of the drug with DNA, but probably due to interactions of the conjugate at the cell membrane [71, 74]. In a mesothelioma animal model the drug–transferrin conjugates were able to increase the lifespan compared to doxorubicin (69% for the doxorubicin transferrin conjugate versus 39% for doxorubicin compared to controls) [149].

Other research efforts have concentrated on developing drug conjugates with doxorubicin, daunorubicin, and chlorambucil that incorporate an acid-sensitive linker between the drug and transferrin [90, 112, 120, 146]. These conjugates efficiently released the drug in an acidic environment (pH 4–6), demonstrated *in vitro* activity against cancer cell lines, and the acid-sensitive doxorubicin transferrin conjugates showed an increased maximum tolerated dose (MTD) and superior antitumor efficacy over doxorubicin in a breast cancer xenograft model (Figures 24.14 and 24.15 below). However, analogously constructed doxorubicin–albumin conjugates practically demonstrated an identical activity profile (see below).

An emphasis with respect to transferrin-based drug delivery has been on gene delivery and the development of immunotoxins. These drug delivery systems comprise conjugates, protamine, or cationized nanoparticles, for example, with poly(L-lysine) or polyethylenimine, or immunoliposomes, and the general structure of these systems is depicted in Figure 24.11. Since the pioneering work of E. Wagner in Vienna, a multitude of studies have been reported that use these systems for delivering oligonucleotides or small interfering RNA (siRNA) to cells, either using transferrin or antibody constructs directed against the transferrin receptor. Several *in vitro* and some *in vivo* proof of concepts have been obtained preclinically, and we refer to comprehensive reviews that cover this field [1, 150, 151].

Due the fact that the transferrin is not solely expressed on tumor cells, it was reasoned that targeting approaches that use highly toxic agents such as neocarzinostatin or plant- or animal-derived toxins would be more successful when administered intratumorally (Table 24.1, bottom). Since conventional chemotherapy is not very effective in the treatment of brain tumors, and healthy brain cells generally do not divide and express none or only small amounts of transferrin receptors, research focused on the development of a conjugate consisting of transferrin that is bound to diphtheria toxin through a lysine cross-linker and a thioester, that was nicknamed Tf-CRM107 (later TransMID in clinical trials). Once bound to glioma cells, it is taken up by endocytosis, and the thioester is cleaved and releases the toxin which kills the malignant glioblastoma cell [139].

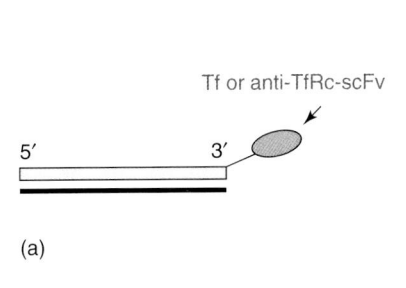

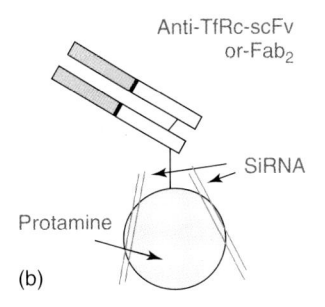

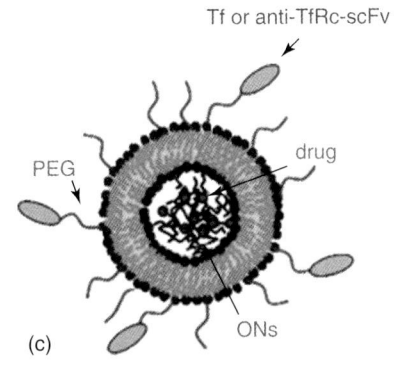

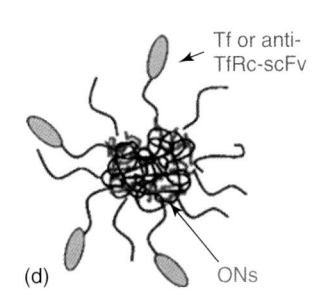

Figure 24.11 Targeting strategies in gene or drug delivery using transferrin (Tf) or antibody constructs directed against the transferrin receptor (TfRc): (a) conjugates with oligonucleotides; (b) antibody fragments conjugated to small, arginine-rich, nuclear proteins (protamine) loaded with small interfering RNA (siRNA); (c) oligonucleotides (ONs) encapsulated in immunoliposomes with transferrin or antibody constructs directed against the transferrin receptor linked to the surface of the liposome through a poly(ethylene glycol) (PEG) linker; and (d) structure of a lipoplex where transferrin is conjugated to a cationized polymer, such as poly(L-lysine) or polyethyleneimine, and negatively charged oligonucleotides are complexed with the polymer. (Adapted from [150]).

Tf-CRM107 is active in the picomolar range and is able to induce complete remissions in preclinical glioblastoma models. An example where Tf-CRM107 was administered intratumorally into subcutaneously growing U251 gliomas in nude mice is shown in Figure 24.12.

Tf-CRM107 progressed to phase III for treating glioblastoma multiforme, the most common from of brain tumors, and the clinical results are summarized in Section 24.4.

The first drug conjugates with HSA were developed in the late 1970s. Chu and Whiteley coupled the folate antagonist MTX to HSA through direct coupling with carbodiimides and have shown that MTX–albumin conjugates are more effective than the free drug in reducing the number of lung metastases in mice inoculated subcutaneously with Lewis lung carcinoma [152].

Research on MTX–HSA conjugates carried out a decade later focused on the required coupling techniques in more detail [153]. Preparation methods using

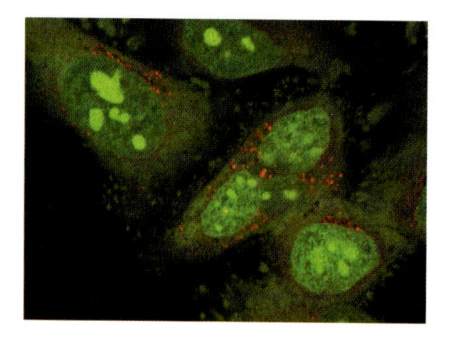

Figure 24.14 Confocal microscopy demonstrating the uptake of fluorescently labeled albumin into cultivated tumor cells. HeLa cells were incubated with albumin labeled with a red fluorescent dye (purpurin, red color). To visualize cellular compartments, the cells were also incubated with acridine orange, a green fluorescent dye (green color). High amounts of fluorescent albumin were detected in the cytoplasm of the tumor cells. (Image courtesy of Andreas Wunder, Charité Berlin.)

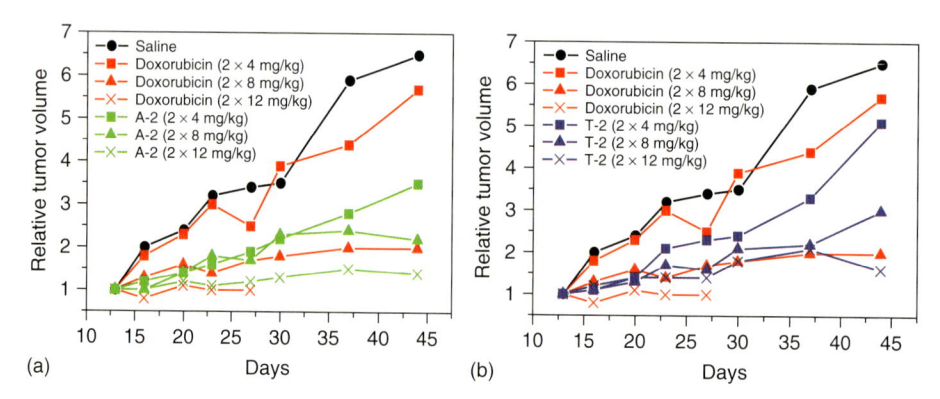

Figure 24.15 Efficacy of an acid-sensitive doxorubicin-albumin (a) and -transferrin (b) conjugate (A-2 and T-2) and doxorubicin in the xenograft MDA-MB 435 breast carcinoma model.

2- to 3-fold higher than for free doxorubicin. The conjugates showed significantly reduced toxicity (reduced lethality and body weight loss) with a concomitantly stable and improved antitumor activity compared to the free drug.

Interestingly, as observed in the *in vitro* analyses, there was no pronounced difference between identically constructed transferrin and albumin–doxorubicin conjugates with regard to *in vivo* efficacy (Figure 24.15) [76].

As a consequence, research efforts focused on the development of albumin–drug conjugates considering that the costs for obtaining albumin are 10-fold lower than for transferrin. In addition, Kratz *et al.* investigated methods of improving the coupling methods of drug derivatives to obtain better-defined drug–albumin conjugates having high purity, a constant drug loading ratio, and a minimal alteration of the three-dimensional protein structure.

Commercially available albumin is a mixture of mercaptalbumin and non-mercaptalbumin containing approximately 20–60% free sulfhydryl groups per molecule albumin due to the fact that the Cys34 position is blocked by sulfhydryl compounds, such as cysteine, homocysteine, or glutathione. Kratz *et al.* therefore developed a procedure of selectively reducing HSA with suitable agents, such as dithiothreitol (Cleland's reagent) in a first step so that approximately one sulfhydryl group (Cys34) per molecule albumin is present. In a second step, doxorubicin maleimide derivatives such as the 4-maleimidophenylacetyl hydrazone derivative of doxorubicin (DOXO-HYD) were coupled to this reduced form of albumin [147].

In subsequent biological studies, the *in vivo* efficacy and pharmacokinetic properties of the acid-sensitive doxorubicin–albumin conjugate A-DOXO-HYD were evaluated against murine metastatic renal cell carcinoma (RENCA model) in comparison to free doxorubicin at equitoxic doses [147]. A-DOXO-HYD was superior compared to free doxorubicin against murine renal carcinoma. In the RENCA model, the subcapsular renal injection of RENCA cells in a syngenic BALB/c mouse is followed by the progressive development of a primary tumor mass in the left kidney while the right kidney is not injected with murine renal cancer cells and serves as a healthy kidney. One week after application, the primary tumor is macroscopically visible in the left kidney and therapy is initiated. As shown in Figure 24.16a–c, therapy with the conjugate induced complete remissions of primary kidney tumors at a dose of 4×12 mg/kg doxorubicin-equivalents and only two metastases in the lungs were observed. In contrast, mice treated with doxorubicin at the MTD of 4×6 mg/kg manifested clearly visible kidney tumors at the end of the experiment and large numbers of lung metastases.

Inspired by these results, Kratz *et al.* focused their work on a prodrug concept that exploits endogenous albumin as a drug carrier [86, 157]. In this therapeutic strategy, the prodrug is designed to bind rapidly and selectively to the Cys34 position of circulating serum albumin after intravenous administration, thereby generating a macromolecular transport form of the drug *in situ* in the blood (Figure 24.17).

We reasoned that exploiting circulating albumin as a drug carrier would have several advantages over *ex vivo* synthesized drug–albumin conjugates: (i) the use of commercial and possibly pathogenic albumin is avoided; (ii) albumin-binding drugs are chemically well-defined and based on straightforward organic chemistry; (iii) albumin-binding drugs are fairly simple and inexpensive to manufacture; (iv) a broad range of drugs for developing albumin-binding drugs can be used; and (v) the analytical requirements for defining the pharmaceutical products are comparable to any other low-molecular-weight drug candidate.

A further important asset of using albumin for *in situ* coupling of prodrugs was the presence of a suitable and specific binding site near the protein surface. The novel macromolecular prodrug approach targets the Cys34 position of albumin that is located in subdomain IA of HSA (Figure 24.18a).

This cysteine residue is highly conserved in all mammalian species studied with the exception of salmon albumin [5]. The free HS group of Cys34 is an unusual feature of an extracellular protein. The X-ray structure of defatted albumin reveals that Cys34 is located in a hydrophobic crevice on the surface of the protein

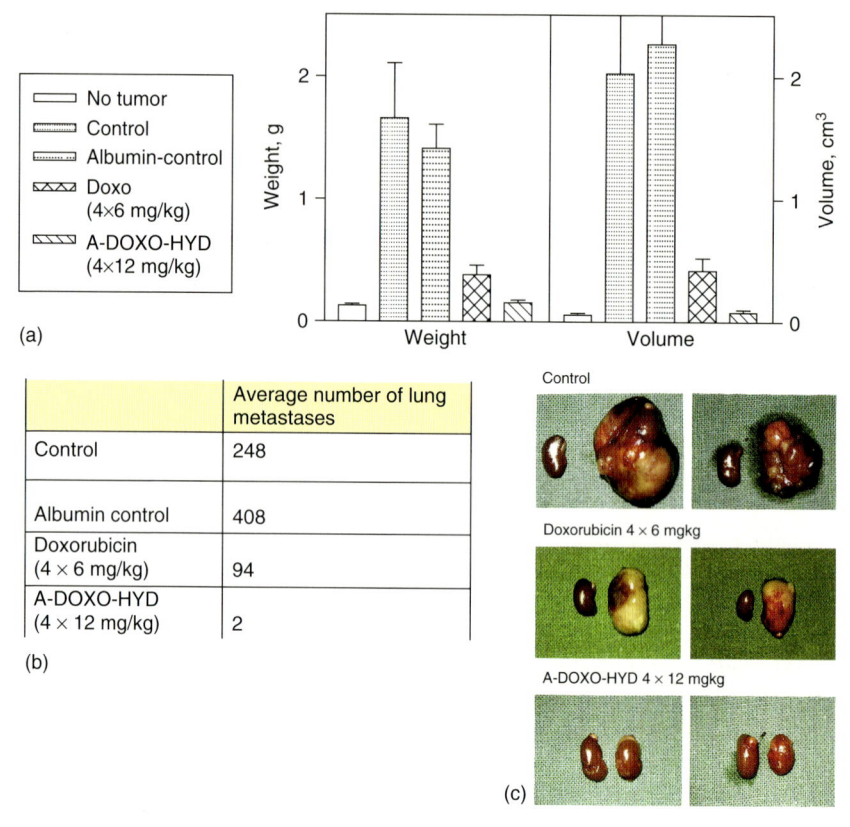

	Average number of lung metastases
Control	248
Albumin control	408
Doxorubicin (4 × 6 mg/kg)	94
A-DOXO-HYD (4 × 12 mg/kg)	2

Figure 24.16 Therapeutic effects of doxorubicin (4 × 6 mg/kg) and A-DOXO-HYD (4 × 12 mg/kg) on (right) healthy kidney (no tumor) and (left) kidney tumor weight and volume (a), and on the number of lung metastases (b). (c) Representative photographic images of control healthy kidneys (right) as well as treated kidney tumors (left) of two mice from the control group, the doxorubicin-treated group, and the A-DOXO-HYD-treated group. Body weight loss in both treatment groups was comparable (−10 and −12%, respectively).

that is approximately 10–12 Å deep (Figure 24.18b). When HSA is complexed with long-chain fatty acids, as in the X-ray structure in which five molecules of myristic acid are bound, the crevice is opened up exposing the HS group of Cys34 (Figure 24.18b).

In human plasma, circulating albumin is generally complexed with one to three molecules of long-chain fatty acids (reviewed in [41]). Approximately 70% of circulating albumin in the bloodstream is mercaptalbumin containing an accessible Cys34, which is not blocked by endogenous sulfhydryl compounds such as cysteine, homocysteine, cysteinylglycine, glutathione, or nitric oxide. Considering that free thiol groups are not found on the majority of circulating serum proteins except for albumin, Cys34 of endogenous albumin is a unique amino acid on the surface of a circulating protein.

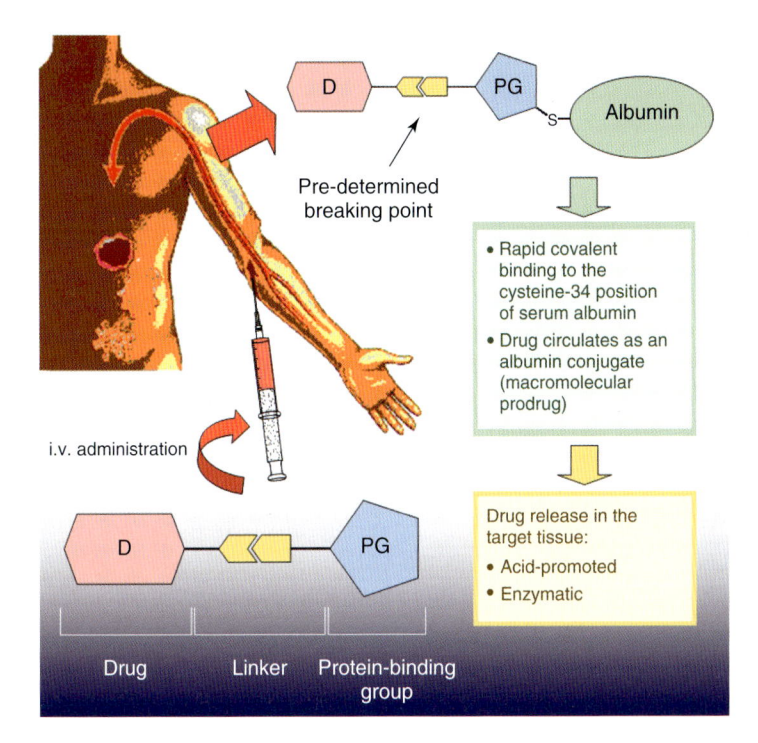

24.3 Examples of Drug Delivery Systems with Serum Proteins | 779

Figure 24.17 Illustration of the *in situ* binding of a prodrug to the Cys34 position of HSA after intravenous administration and the subsequent release of the active drug at the tumor site.

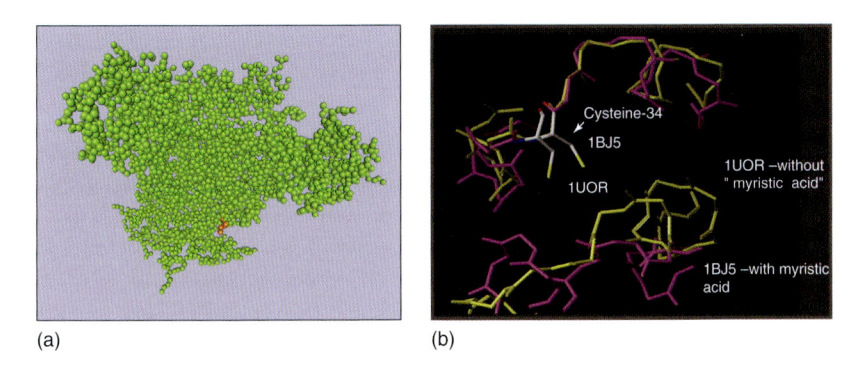

Figure 24.18 (a) X-ray structure of HSA (pdb entry 1ao6) in which the Cys34 position is highlighted orange. (b) Videographic presentation of the Cys34 binding pocket of HSA according to the X-ray structure of the defatted protein structure (pdb entry 1ao6) and the albumin structure in which five molecules of myristic acid are bound (pdb entry 1bj5).

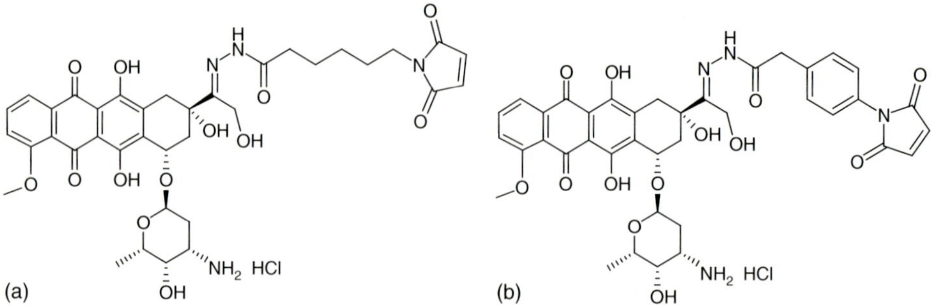

Figure 24.19 Structure (a) DOXO-EMCH and (b) DOXO-HYD that were investigated in a prodrug concept that exploits endogenous albumin as a drug carrier.

Proof of concept was obtained with two acid-sensitive doxorubicin prodrugs – DOXO-HYD and 6-maleimidocaproyl hydrazone derivative of doxorubicin (DOXO-EMCH) (Figure 24.19), which are rapidly and selectively bound to circulating albumin within a few minutes [86, 157].

Therapy with DOXO-EMCH dramatically improved the efficacy of doxorubicin in preclinical tumor models [147, 158, 159]. As an example, the antitumor efficacy of DOXO-EMCH was compared to that of doxorubicin in the MDA-MB 435 model at the following doses: doxorubicin: 2 × 8 mg/kg; and DOXO-EMCH: 2 × 8, 3 × 16, and 3 × 24 mg/kg doxorubicin-equivalents. Preliminary toxicity studies in nude mice had shown that the MTD of DOXO-EMCH was approximately 4.5 times higher than for free doxorubicin. The results of this animal experiment are shown in Figure 24.20a.

At the MTD of free doxorubicin (2 × 8 mg/kg), a moderate inhibition in tumor growth is observed with DOXO-EMCH, comparable to the effect of free doxorubicin at the same dose. At higher doses therapy with DOXO-EMCH produced good antitumor effects at 3 × 16 mg/kg doxorubicin-equivalents and complete remissions at 3 × 24 mg/kg.

The biodistribution of ^{14}C-labeled DOXO-EMCH and doxorubicin was assessed in the same xenograft model, and the results after 2, 6, 24, and 48 h are shown in Figure 24.20b for serum, tumor, heart, liver, and kidneys. As expected, there is a pronounced difference between the radioactivity levels of DOXO-EMCH and doxorubicin in the serum; whereas levels for serum doxorubicin are below 0.3% of the applied dose for all timepoints, levels for DOXO-EMCH after 2 h are around 25% and still around 6% of the applied dose after 48 h, which is a clear indication of rapid binding of DOXO-EMCH to albumin and a large area under the curve (AUC) in the blood pool. Tumor levels for DOXO-EMCH increase over 24 h, and are approximately 2-fold higher between 24 and 48 h compared to free doxorubicin levels. In contrast, the levels in heart, liver, and kidneys are significantly lower for DOXO-EMCH than for doxorubicin over several hours after intravenous administration.

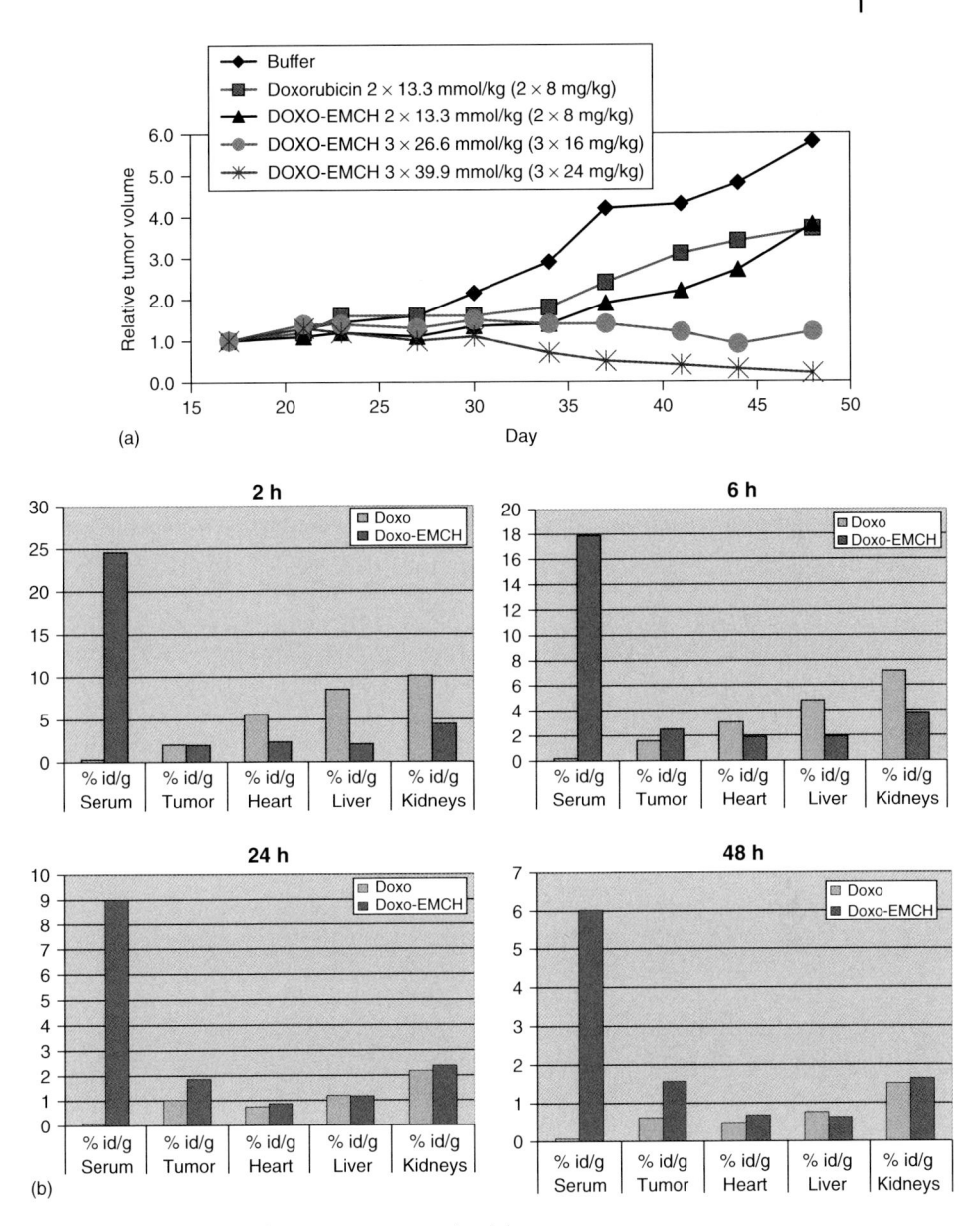

Figure 24.20 (a) Curves depicting tumor growth inhibition of subcutaneously implanted MDA-MB-435 xenografts under therapy with doxorubicin and DOXO-EMCH. (b) Biodistribution study in the MDA-MB 435 xenograft model with ^{14}C-labeled doxorubicin or ^{14}C-DOXO-EMCH (organ values were corrected for blood volume); $P < 0.05$.

When viewing such impressive antitumor responses, one would have probably expected a larger drug-targeting potential compared to a free drug, but this is obviously not the case. Rather, it is the combination of an enhanced, albeit not dramatic improvement in tumor uptake for the respective albumin-based drug delivery system over the free drug when assessed at the MTD of the free drug combined with a favorable biodistribution and significant increase in its MTD that accounts for the striking difference noted between the two drugs in preclinical tumor models. Based on the shift of the MTD of DOXO-EMCH (around 4.5-fold) over the respective free drug in mice, the overall increase in drug tumor accumulation can be estimated to be at least 6-fold at an equitoxic comparison.

The enhanced uptake of albumin-based drug delivery systems in solid tumors is mediated by the pathophysiology of tumor tissue, characterized by angiogenesis, hypervasculature, a defective vascular architecture, and an impaired lymphatic drainage. In addition, scientists at American Bioscience have collected data that accumulation of *nab*-paclitaxel is also due to transcytosis initiated by binding of albumin to a cell surface, 60-kDa glycoprotein (gp60) receptor (albondin) as well as due to binding of albumin to secreted protein acid and rich in cysteine (SPARC). Albumin binds to the gp60 receptor, which in turn results in binding of gp60 with an intracellular protein (caveolin-1) and subsequent invagination of the cell membrane to form transcytotic vesicles (i.e., caveolae) [158, 160] (see Chapter 35 for details). This uptake mechanism by transcytosis in the tumor interstitium might well occur for the albumin conjugate of DOXO-EMCH.

An interesting aspect that has received too little intention is the efficacy of macromolecular prodrugs in combination with low-molecular-weight anticancer drugs in preclinical models. As an example, the antitumor efficacy of doxorubicin at its MTD in nude mice (2×8 mg/kg, weekly schedule) and the albumin-binding doxorubicin prodrug DOXO-EMCH (3×24 mg/kg doxorubicin-equivalents, weekly schedule) at its MTD is shown in Figure 24.21a and body weight change in Figure 24.21b in the A2780 ovarian cancer xenograft model in comparison to a combination of DOXO-EMCH (3×12 mg/kg, weekly schedule) and doxorubicin (3×4 mg/kg, weekly schedule) at a dose that corresponds to half or even less than half of the respective MTDs of the compounds. DOXO-EMCH was significantly more active than doxorubicin, producing complete remissions, but also produced around 30% body weight loss. In contrast, the combination of DOXO-EMCH (3×12 mg/kg), which dosed alone would ideally show a tumorstasis in this dose schedule, combined with doxorubicin (3×4 mg/kg), which dosed alone would not show any activity, surprisingly demonstrated complete remissions (Figure 24.21a) and the best tolerability, with only around 12% body weight loss at the end of the experiment (Figure 24.21b).

These results emphasize the need to investigate macromolecular prodrugs in combination with conventional low-molecular-weight prodrugs in the preclinical as well as clinical setting in order to explore the additive and synergistic potential of such combinations.

DOXO-EMCH was selected as the investigational product for clinical evaluation after toxicology studies in mice, rats, and dogs had shown that DOXO-EMCH

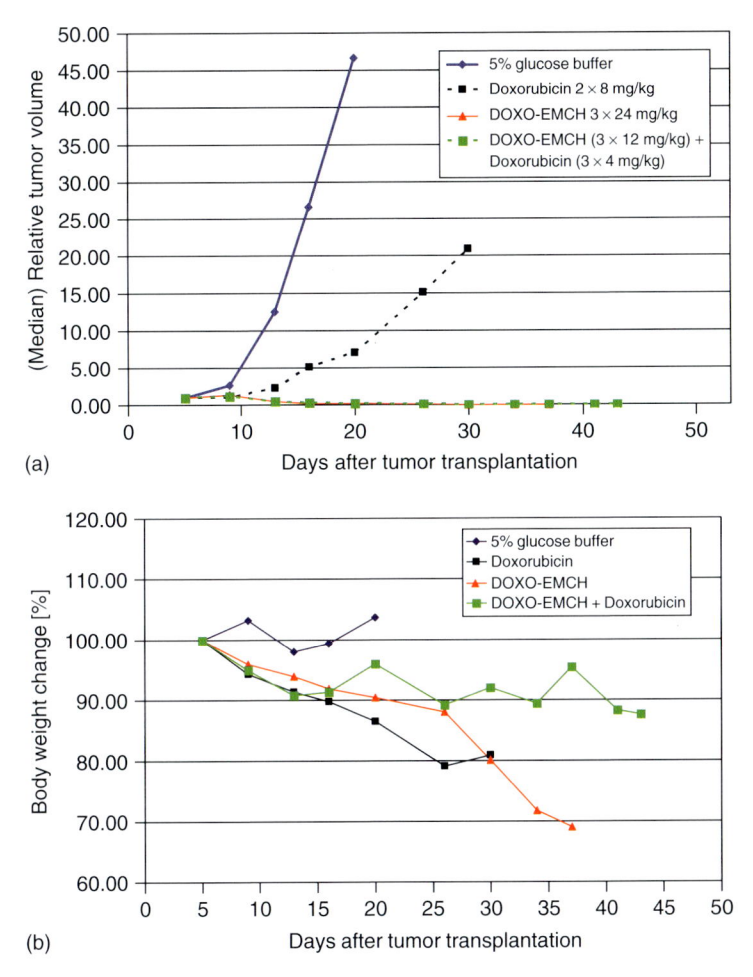

Figure 24.21 (a) Antitumor efficacy and (b) body weight changes of doxorubicin, DOXO-EMCH, and a combination of DOXO-EMCH and doxorubicin against ovarian cancer A2780 xenografts.

exhibits a 2- to 5-fold increase in the MTD in these animals when compared to conventional doxorubicin [161]. A four-cycle intravenous study with DOXO-EMCH at dose levels of 4×2.5, 4×5.0, or 4×7.5 mg/kg doxorubicin-equivalents in rats revealed approximately 3-fold less side-effects on the bone marrow system when compared to 4×2.5 mg/kg doxorubicin, whereas effects on the testes, thymus, and spleen were comparable between both drugs at equitoxic dose, but with a clear indication for recovery in the DOXO-EMCH-treated animals. A No Observable Adverse Effect Level (NOAEL) for DOXO-EMCH of 4×2.5 mg/kg doxorubicin-equivalents was established in this study. This dose is equivalent to the MTD of doxorubicin in rats.

In a two-cycle study over a period of 6 weeks in beagle dogs (intravenous administration of DOXO-EMCH at dose levels of 1.5, 3.0, or 4.5 mg/kg doxorubicin-equivalents), only temporary effects on hematology, urinary function as well as on histopathology in mid- and/or high-dose animals were observed. The low dose of 2 × 1.5 mg/kg was considered to be the NOAEL in this study, which is equivalent to twice the MTD of doxorubicin in beagle dogs [161]. DOXO-EMCH has also shown significantly less chronic cardiotoxicity at equimolar as well as equitoxic doses compared to doxorubicin in a rat model [162]. Details of the phase I study carried out with this prodrug are summarized in Section 24.4.

Inspired by the translational research with DOXO-EMCH, a broad spectrum of albumin-binding prodrugs has been developed by Kratz et al. (Figure 24.22).

The majority of these prodrugs consist of an anticancer drug, the maleimide group as the thiol-binding moiety, and an enzymatically cleavable peptide linker. Examples include doxorubicin prodrugs that are cleaved by matrix metalloprotease (MMP)-2 and -9 [85], cathepsin B [89], urokinase [163], or prostate-specific antigen (PSA) [91, 164], MTX prodrugs that are cleaved by cathepsin B and plasmin [107], and camptothecin prodrugs that are cleaved by cathepsin B or unidentified proteases [89, 165, 166]. In addition, maleimide derivatives with 5-fluorouracil analogs and Pt(II) complexes have been developed [167, 168].

An extension of the *in situ* albumin technology is the current development of novel albumin-binding prodrugs that combine passive and active targeting or act as dual-acting prodrugs (Figure 24.23).

In the first strategy, a receptor- or antigen-recognizing ligand is additionally introduced in the prodrug construct. Examples of suitable receptors are the folate receptor, integrins, or the asialoglycoprotein receptor that are overexpressed by various solid tumors, the tumor endothelium, and liver tumors or the spectrum of tumor-associated antigens. Through *in situ* binding of a ligand-based albumin-binding prodrug to endogenous or exogenous albumin a modified albumin–drug conjugate is formed that besides passive uptake in solid tumors has the potential to preferentially interact with tumor-associated receptors or antigens and improve overall tumor targeting.

The second new approach relies on binding two drugs to albumin (Figure 24.23). In its simplest form these can be two anticancer agents for a cellular combination therapy approach or a dual-acting prodrug consists of a drug such as an anticancer agent and the second drug as a modulator (e.g., an inhibitor of P-glycoprotein or an inducer of apoptosis). The goal of such prodrugs is to circumvent chemoresistance of solid tumors – a pivotal and unresolved issue in cancer chemotherapy. First prototypes of dual-acting prodrugs have been recently synthesized by Kratz et al. (Figure 24.24a and b) [169, 170].

Drug–albumin conjugates that contain an appropriate ligand for receptor targeting such as sugars [171] for liver tumor targeting (see Chapter 47 for details) or RGD peptides [172] for application in vascular targeting have already been developed. In addition, in the diagnostic field, fluorescein-labeled albumin and ^{99m}Tc-galactosyl HSA could find application in laser-induced fluorescence imaging for delineating

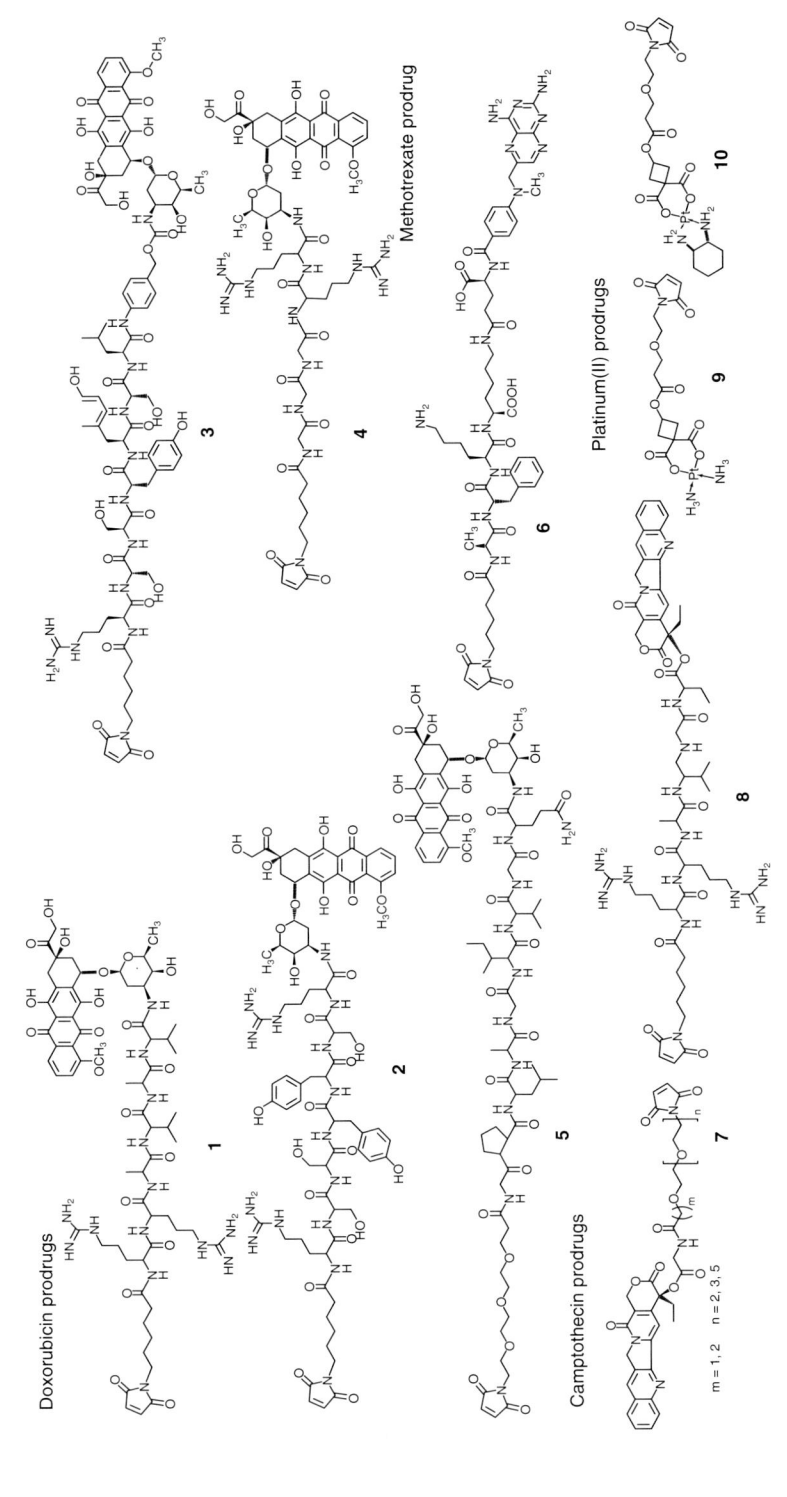

24.3 Examples of Drug Delivery Systems with Serum Proteins | 785

Figure 24.22 Structures of a selection of albumin-binding prodrugs. **1**, Doxorubicin prodrug that is cleaved by cathepsin B; **2**, **3**, doxorubicin prodrugs that are cleaved by PSA; **4**, doxorubicin prodrug that is cleaved by MMP-2; **5**, doxorubicin prodrug that is cleaved by cathepsin B and plasmin; **6**, MTX prodrug that is cleaved by urokinase; **7**, camptothecin prodrugs that are cleaved by unidentified proteases; **8**, camptothecin prodrug that is cleaved by cathepsin B; **9**, **10**, albumin-binding prodrugs with Pt(II) complexes.

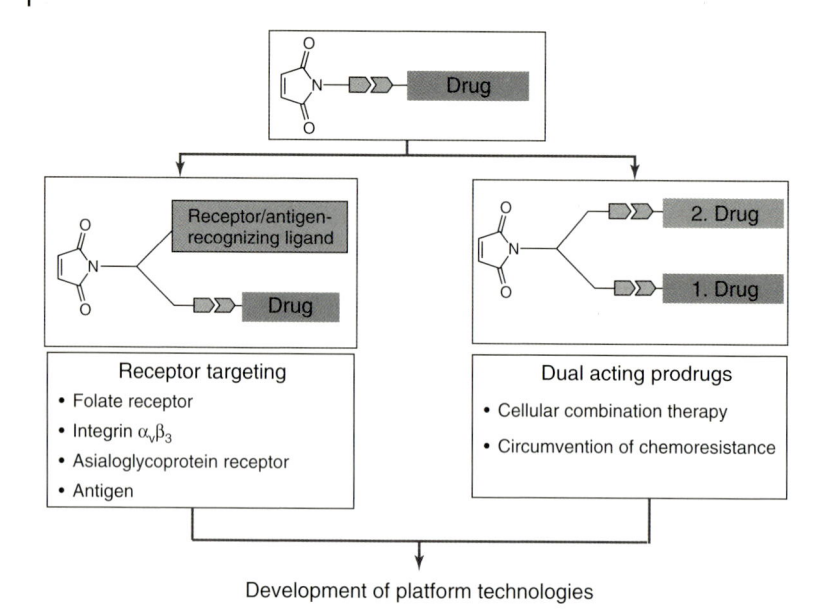

Figure 24.23 Novel prodrug concepts based on albumin as a drug carrier: receptor/antigen targeting and dual-acting prodrugs.

tumor margins under the operating microscope or for diagnosing liver disease [44, 173].

A somewhat different approach of obtaining drug–albumin conjugates is albumin fusion technology, yielding albumin protein conjugates that are genetically engineered by splicing together the genes of the two molecules and expressing the albumin fusion proteins in yeast strains. Human Genome Sciences has applied their technology to cytokines, primarily to interferon α-2b, interleukin-2, and granulocyte colony-stimulating factor, but also to bioactive peptides [51]. Of interest for the oncologist is Albuleukin® – an albumin fusion protein with recombinant interleukin-2 that has shown promising antitumor efficacy against murine renal cell carcinoma and melanoma [174].

Finally serum proteins have also been exploited as carriers for metal ions, such as Ga(III), In(III), Bi(III), Ti(III), Ru(III) [151], and anticancer metal complexes such as Pt(II) and Ru(III) complexes. A detailed description is given in Chapter 49.

24.3.2.2 LDL–Drug Complexes

LDL complexes with daunorubicin have been prepared by a simple mixing procedure [101, 175], and the cytotoxicity of these has been found to be equal to that of free daunorubicin against lung carcinoma cells. However, receptor-mediated uptake of the LDL–daunorubicin complexes was not demonstrated so that leakage of daunorubicin from the complex before cellular uptake could have occurred. A lipophilic derivative of doxorubicin, N-trifluoroacetyl-doxorubicin-14-valerate, has been incorporated into LDL with about 100 drug molecules per LDL particle.

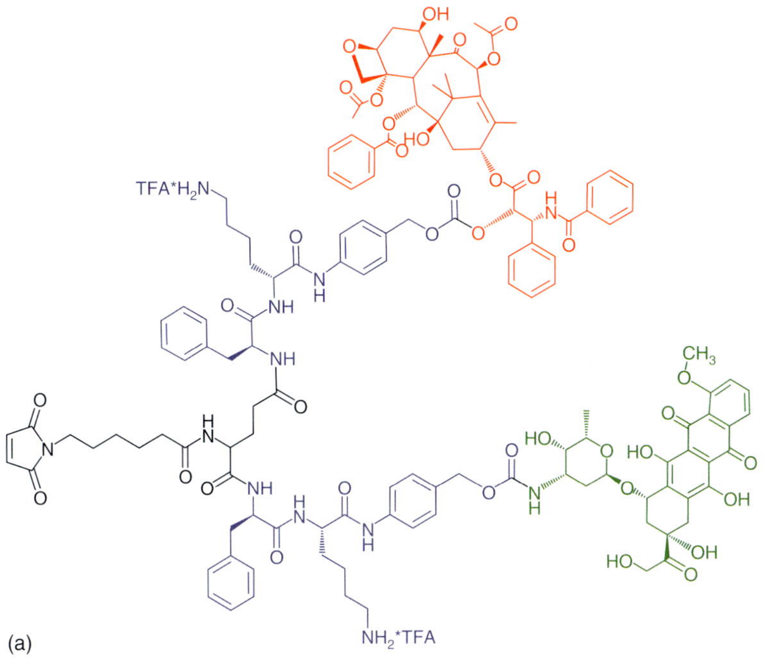

Figure 24.24 Structures of dual-acting pro-drugs containing either (a) two anticancer agents, doxorubicin (green) and paclitaxel (red), or (b) doxorubicin (green) and a P-glycoprotein inhibitor (brown). Additionally, they contain the maleimide moiety as an albumin-binding group and Phe–Lys–p-aminobenzyloxycarbony (PABC) as a cathepsin substrate.

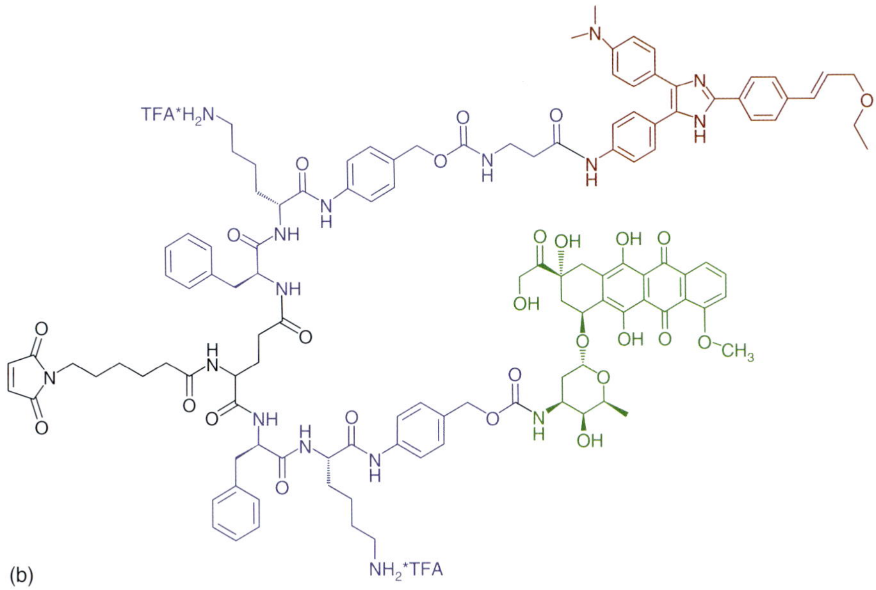

The *in vivo* fate of this complex in mice was similar to that of native LDL [63]. *In vitro* and *in vivo* activity of these doxorubicin–LDL complexes has not been reported, however.

A series of nitrogen mustards have been derivatized with one or two LDL anchors, and appropriate LDL–drug complexes studied for cytotoxicity and selectivity. Distinct LDL complexes with nitrogen mustard derivatives containing two LDL anchors (oleyl and a steroid) demonstrated selective inhibitory effects against LDL receptor-positive tumor cells [111]. Other lipophilic analogs of nitrogen mustards, such as estramustine and prednimustine, have also been incorporated into LDL particles, but they were found to be 10- to 100-fold less active than the free drug [176, 177].

24.4
Clinical Development

Primarily, clinical trials have been performed with drug conjugates and complexes with albumin, not only in oncology such as with a MTX–albumin conjugate or an albumin-binding prodrug of doxorubicin described below or the approved albumin–paclitaxel nanoparticle Abraxane®, but also albumin fusion proteins for treating hepatitis C (Albuferon®) as well as albumin-binding fatty acid derivative of insulin or glucagon-like peptides (GLPs) (Levemir® and Victoza®) for treating diabetes [178]. LDL–drug complexes have so far not entered clinical studies.

Anticancer conjugates with transferrin and conventional anticancer drugs such as doxorubicin have only been assessed in orientating phase I trials in the late 1980s, such as those by Faulk *et al.* in which glutaraldehyde cross-linked transferrin–doxorubicin conjugates were used in the treatment of patients with acute leukemia, and the results have shown diminished numbers of leukemia cells in peripheral blood and no anaphylactic reaction in the patients [74].

In contrast, following the strategy of actively targeting the transferrin receptor with highly toxic drugs, a transferrin–diphtheria drug conjugate (Tf-CRM107) reached phase III studies for treating malignant gliomas. Convection-enhanced delivery – a method for delivery of large molecules to brain tissue via continuous interstitial microinfusion – has permitted direct administration of toxins to brain tumors or to surrounding brain tissue infiltrated by tumor cells. Tf-CRM107 was studied in a phase I study against malignant glioma and produced nine partial responses in the 15 evaluable patients with malignant brain tumors refractory to conventional therapy. In addition, no severe neurologic symptoms or systemic toxicity were observed [137].

The results of a multicenter, open-label, randomized phase II study in histologically confirmed glioblastoma multiforme produced encouraging tumor responses in patients that no longer responded to standard therapy. Of 34 evaluable patients (44 patients in total who received 40 ml of 0.67 µg/ml of Tf-CRM107), five had a complete response (15%), seven a partial remission (21%), and nine a stable disease (26%) [139].

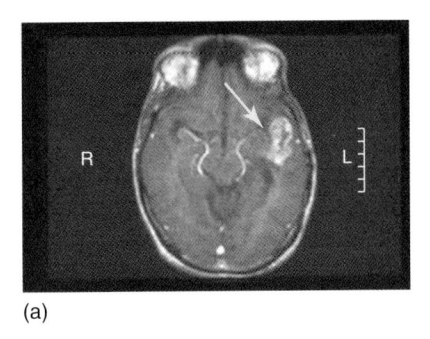

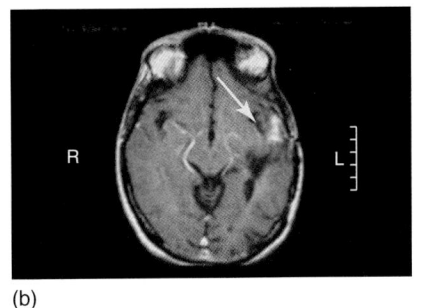

Figure 24.25 (a) Initial magnetic resonance image of the brain and brain tumor, and (b) one year after treatment with Tf-CRM107. The arrow in the image highlights the brain tumor. (Reproduced with permission from [139]).

Figure 24.25 illustrates an objective response (a partial remission) for one patient of the phase II trial as shown by magnetic resonance imaging. The survival analyses showed an overall medium and mean survival time of 37 and 45 weeks, respectively, with 13 of 44 patients surviving over 12 months after the first infusion.

These data warranted a phase III study in comparison to standard therapy with a regimen containing either a nitrosourea, a platinum complex, temozolomide, or procarbazine. However, the clinical trial was prematurely stopped since the sponsor, Xenova Biomedix, anticipated that endpoints of the study would not be reached.

The first drug–albumin conjugate that was evaluated in phase I/II clinical studies was a MTX–albumin conjugate (MTX–HSA). MTX–HSA was synthesized by directly coupling the drug to lysine residues of HSA. It was found that the drug-loading ratio significantly determined the tumor-targeting properties of MTX–albumin conjugates in rats. The MTX–HSA conjugate loaded with 1.3 equivalents of MTX has shown promising antitumor efficacy in various animal models. A clinical phase I study has been performed with 17 patients treated with weekly MTX–HSA [105]. Stomatitis proved to be dose-limiting above $50 \, mg/m^2$ MTX–HSA (MTX-equivalents). A noteworthy finding of this study was that two patients with renal cell carcinoma and one patient with mesothelioma responded to MTX–HSA therapy (one partial response and two minor responses). However, it was not possible to confirm these results in a subsequent phase II study in 17 patients with metastatic renal carcinoma in which no objective response was seen [179]. Another phase II study with MTX–HSA in combination with cisplatin was conducted for the first-line treatment of patients with advanced bladder cancer [180]. Treatment was started with a loading dose of $110 \, mg/m^2$ of MTX–HSA followed by a weekly dose of $40 \, mg/m^2$. Cisplatin was given monthly at a dose of $75 \, mg/m^2$. One complete and one partial remission were observed in seven evaluable patients. However, there is currently no indication that the clinical assessment of MTX–HSA is being further pursued.

INNO-206 (formerly DOXO-EMCH) emerged as a clinical candidate due to superior efficacy of INNO-206 in several murine tumor models, a 2- to 5-fold increase in the MTD, and a low cardiotoxic potential when compared to doxorubicin. INNO-206 avoids the use of exogenous albumin and is selectively bound to the Cys34 position of endogenous albumin within a few minutes after intravenous administration, and contains an acid-sensitive hydrazone linker that allows doxorubicin to be released either extracellularly in the slightly acidic environment often present in tumor tissue or intracellularly in acidic endosomal or lysosomal compartments after cellular uptake of the conjugate by the tumor cell.

In a phase I study, a starting dose of 20 mg/m^2 doxorubicin-equivalents was chosen and 41 patients with advanced cancer disease were treated at dose levels of 20–340 mg/m^2 doxorubicin-equivalents [181]. Treatment with DOXO-EMCH was well tolerated up to 200 mg/m^2 without manifestation of drug-related side-effects, which is an around 3-fold increase over the standard dose for doxorubicin (60 mg/kg). Myelosuppression and mucositis were the predominant adverse effects at dose levels of 260 mg/m^2 and became dose-limiting at 340 mg/m^2. Pharmacokinetically, the albumin-bound form of DOXO-EMCH has a large AUC, a small volume of distribution, and low clearance compared to doxorubicin, and there are some clear similarities but also differences to liposomal doxorubicin (Doxil®), as can be noted when comparing the data presented in Table 24.2.

Thirty of 41 patients were assessable for analysis of response. Partial responses were observed in three patients (10%, small-cell lung cancer, liposarcoma, and breast carcinoma). As an example a patient with metastatic breast cancer pretreated with adjuvant CMF (cyclophosphamide/MTX/5-fluorouracil), second-line trofosfamide, and different hormonal treatments was treated with 340 mg/m^2; INNO-206, and reached a partial remission. The significant remission regarding the large liver metastasis after four cycles of INNO-206 is shown in Figure 24.26.

Fifteen patients (50%) showed a stable disease at different dose levels and 12 patients (40%) had evidence of tumor progression. The recommended dose for phase II studies of INNO-206 is 260 mg/m^2 doxorubicin-equivalents, which is a around 4.5-fold increase over a standard dose of 60 mg/m^2 free doxorubicin.

Table 24.2 Pharmacokinetic parameters of doxorubicin, DOXO-EMCH, and Doxil in humans (values from [182]).

	$t_{1/2}$ terminal (h)	C_{max} (µM)	AUC (µM)	V_z (l)	CL (ml/min)
Doxorubicin (60 mg/m^2)	17–30	~8.6	~3.5	~2000	~1000
DOXO-EMCH (80 mg/m^2)	~18	~28	~520	~5.8	~9
DOXO-EMCH (260 mg/m^2)	~20	~235	~2550	~4.6	~8.5
Doxil (60 mg/m^2)	56–90	30–47	2340–4070	3.0–5.6	0.3–1.25

[a]$t_{1/2}$, terminal plasma half-life; C_{max}, maximum plasma concentration; V_z, volume of distribution; CL, clearance; AUC, area under the curve.

Before INNO-206 treatment

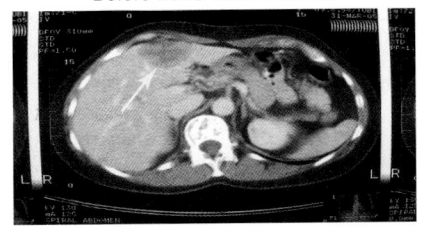

After 4-cycles INNO-206 (340 mg/m^2)

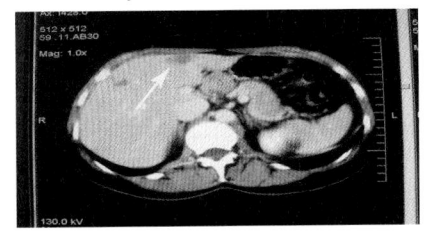

Figure 24.26 Regression of a large liver metastasis in a breast cancer patient under therapy with INNO-206 (340 mg/m^2) after four cycles; first line: cyclophosphamide, MTX, 5-FU; second line: trofosfamide (arrow indicates liver metastasis) before and after treatment; time to progression was 24 weeks.

Phase II trials at the dose of 260 mg/m^2 in patients with gastric and cancer as well as sarcoma are scheduled for 2011 with INNO-206 by CytRx (*http://www.cytrx.com*).

24.5
Conclusions and Perspectives

The uptake of the serum proteins transferrin, albumin, and LDL in tumors is well documented in the literature. A quantitative comparison between these proteins regarding their tumor accumulation in experimental animal models is limited to date, although existing diagnostic data together with the *in vitro* and *in vivo* data on anticancer transferrin and albumin conjugates with conventional anticancer agents have not revealed a significant difference between transferrin and albumin as potential drug carriers. In fact, if one of the major reasons for protein uptake by tumors is that the vasculature of viable tumor tissue is hyperpermeable to macromolecules, the tumor accumulation of the former serum proteins is mediated by passive targeting. Receptor-mediated endocytosis of transferrin and LDL is well understood, and drug conjugates or complexes with these proteins that comprise highly cytotoxic potent drugs might be more active than albumin where cellular uptake is mediated by fluid-phase or adsorptive endocytosis. Using such potent agents, drug delivery systems with transferrin and LDL might achieve the targeting potential of antibody conjugates that use agents such as auristatins, calicheamicins, or maystatins (see Chapter 10) where saturation of the transferrin or LDL receptor on tumor cells would not be a limiting factor for their targeting potential. Indeed, saturation of the transferrin receptor could be an explanation why we did not observe any major difference in the *in vitro* and *in vivo* activity between analogous transferrin and albumin conjugates with anthracyclines or chlorambucil [94, 131, 132]. Indeed, an estimation of the ratio of the number of drug–protein conjugates to the number of transferrin receptors expressed on tumor cells reveals a ratio of around 10^5–10^6 : 1 at the IC_{50} values of anthracyclines in cell culture systems, indicating that the contribution of the transferrin receptor might be small when other endocytotic pathways in tumor cells are dominant. For drug–albumin conjugates and complexes, the gp60 receptor (albondin) expressed on the tumor endothelium appears to be an important additional factor for tumor uptake and for ensuring an even distribution within the tumor besides the EPR effect which can be heterogeneous within the tumor mass (see also Chapter 35).

In any case, for designing effective drug–protein conjugates, spacers can be incorporated between the anticancer agent and the carrier protein that allow the drug to be released either extra- or intracellularly. Examples are peptide bonds, which can be cleaved by lysosomal enzymes or acid-sensitive bonds. Acid-sensitive protein conjugates can additionally liberate the bound drug extracellularly due to a slightly acidic environment often present in tumor tissue. This might prove to be an advantage over drug conjugates which need to be degraded inside the tumor cell because serum proteins are primarily trapped in the periphery of the tumor corresponding to the histologically viable regions and not in the low vascularized center of the tumor. Once released, low-molecular-weight drugs can gain access to this part of the tumor through diffusion. Most of this work has been carried out with the more robust and commercially more attractive albumin rather than with transferrin, or prodrug concepts have been developed that rely on the *in situ* binding of low-molecular-weight prodrugs to the Cys34 position of endogenous albumin following intravenous administration.

LDL complexes with anticancer agents have not been studied as intensively as anticancer drug conjugates with transferrin or albumin, and their formulation relies on attaching lipophilic groups to anticancer agents and then incorporating them into the LDL particle. Such formulations may prove to have advantages over liposomes as drug delivery systems in cancer chemotherapy considering that LDL does not bind to scavenger receptors of the RES and it is truly unfortunate that so few *in vivo* studies have addressed this issue considering the immense research efforts on liposomal formulations in the past 30 years.

For the reasons stated above it is not surprising that the majority of clinical trials have been performed with albumin–drug conjugates or complexes and albumin-binding prodrugs, not just in the field of oncology [178]. The development and market approval of the paclitaxel–albumin nanoparticle, Abraxane®, can be viewed as a landmark for albumin-based drug delivery technology. Other drug formulations based on this technology (e.g., with docetaxel or rapamycin) or an albumin-binding prodrug of doxorubicin (INNO-206) drugs are advancing to phase I or II and III trials, respectively.

In summary, transferrin, serum albumin, and LDL are potential macromolecular carriers for the delivery of anticancer agents to solid tumors. Although the tissue distribution of these serum proteins is naturally influenced by their biology and functional role, a multitude of investigations indicate that the anatomical and physiological characteristics of tumor tissue serve as a three-dimensional target and mediate the uptake of protein carriers. In our opinion, future research in the field of anticancer drug carriers using serum proteins will focus on the following issues:

- Development of tailor-made linkers adapted to release the protein-bound or encapsulated drug intra- and/or extracellularly at the tumor site. If tumor-associated protease are to be exploited for such a selective release, screening of protease expression in tumor patients prior to therapy would be a necessary prerequisite for drug–protein conjugates to exert their antitumor efficacy effectively in the form of a personalized medicine.
- Research addressing the physiological and anatomical characteristics of tumors in human patients with respect to vascularization, angiogenesis, and metastases in order to select patients with pronounced EPR effects. For this purpose suitable diagnostic probes are already available (e.g., ^{67}Ga(III)-citrate) or could be easily developed (e.g., ^{99m}Tc-labeled albumin).
- Research addressing the combination of anticancer serum protein with free anticancer drugs in order to elucidate additive and synergistic activity, respectively.
- Galenic formulation of anticancer serum protein conjugates and prodrugs for clinical trials, including the development of orally applicable prodrugs that bind to serum proteins.

In addition, there are some exciting avenues for the medical application of serum proteins that have not been fully explored, such as their use in photodynamic therapy [183, 184], as transport proteins for metal complexes [185, 186], the use of transferrin and cationized albumin as drug carriers for blood–brain barrier transport [187], for albumin and transferrin as a gene delivery vector [151, 188, 189], liposomal formulations coated with transferrin or antitransferrin receptor antibodies [151], as well as albumin microbubbles that release the drug after destruction by ultrasound [190].

References

1. Li, H. and Qian, Z.M. (2002) Transferrin/transferrin receptor-mediated drug delivery. *Med. Res. Rev.*, **22**, 225–250.
2. Carter, D.C. and Ho, J.X. (1994) Structure of serum albumin. *Adv. Protein Chem.*, **45**, 153–203.
3. Testa, U., Pelosi, E., and Peschle, C. (1993) The transferrin receptor. *Crit. Rev. Oncog.*, **4**, 241–276.
4. Carter, D.C., He, X.M., Munson, S.H., Twigg, P.D., Gernert, K.M., Broom, M.B., and Miller, T.Y. (1989) Three-dimensional structure of human serum albumin. *Science*, **244**, 1195–1198.
5. Peters, T. (1985) Serum albumin. *Adv. Protein Chem.*, **37**, 161–245.
6. Fasano, M. et al. (2005) The extraordinary ligand binding properties of

human serum albumin. *IUBMB Life*, **57**, 787–796.

7. Bertucci, C. and Domenici, E. (2002) Reversible and covalent binding of drugs to human serum albumin: methodological approaches and physiological relevance. *Curr. Med. Chem.*, **9**, 1463–1481.

8. Cantafora, A. and Blotta, I. (1996) Neutral lipids production, transport, utilization. *Anticancer Res.*, **16**, 1441–1449.

9. Firestone, R.A. (1994) Low-density lipoprotein as a vehicle for targeting antitumor compounds to cancer cells. *Bioconjug. Chem.*, **5**, 105–113.

10. Aulbert, E. (1986) *Transferrinmangelanämie bei malignen Tumorerkrankungen*, Thieme, Stuttgart.

11. Matsumura, Y. and Maeda, H. (1986) A new concept for macromolecular therapeutics in cancer chemotherapy: mechanism of tumoritropic accumulation of proteins and the antitumor agent smancs. *Cancer Res.*, **46**, 6387–6392.

12. Sinn, H., Schrenk, H.H., Friedrich, E.A., Schilling, U., and Maier-Borst, W. (1990) Design of compounds having an enhanced tumour uptake, using serum albumin as a carrier. Part I. *Int. J. Radiat. Appl. Instrum. B*, **17**, 819–827.

13. Vitols, S. (1991) Uptake of low-density lipoprotein by malignant cells--possible therapeutic applications. *Cancer Cells*, **3**, 488–495.

14. Brock, J.H. (1985) in *Metalloproteins, Part 2: Metal Proteins with Non-Redox Roles*, Verlag Chemie, Weinheim, pp. 183–263.

15. Mider, G., Tesluk, H., and Morton, J. (1948) Effects of Walker carcinoma 256 on food intake, body weight and nitrogen metabolism of growing rats. *Acta Union Int. Contra Cancrum*, **6**, 409–420.

16. Babson, A.L. and Winnick, T. (1954) Protein transfer in tumor-bearing rats. *Cancer Res.*, **14**, 606–611.

17. Warner, F.W., Demanuelle, M., Stjernholm, R., Cohn, I., and Baddley, W.H. (1977) Response to transferrin bound iron to treatment of rat lymphosarcoma with cis-dichlorodiammine-platinum(II). *J. Clin. Hematol. Oncol.*, **7**, 180–189.

18. Henry, D.H. and Dahl, N.V., on behalf of the Ferrlecit Cancer Study Group (2006) Iron or vitamin B_{12} deficiency in anemic cancer patients prior to erythropoiesis-stimulating agent therapy. *Commun. Oncol.*, **4**, 95–101.

19. Hauser, C.A., Stockler, M.R., and Tattersall, M.H. (2006) Prognostic factors in patients with recently diagnosed incurable cancer: a systematic review. *Support Care Cancer*, **14**, 999–1011.

20. Stehle, G. et al. (1997) Plasma protein (albumin) catabolism by the tumor itself – implications for tumor metabolism and the genesis of cachexia. *Crit. Rev. Oncol.*, **26**, 77–100.

21. Gal, D., Ohashi, M., MacDonald, P.C., Buchsbaum, H.J., and Simpson, E.R. (1981) Low-density lipoprotein as a potential vehicle for chemotherapeutic agents and radionucleotides in the management of gynecologic neoplasms. *Am. J. Obstet. Gynecol.*, **139**, 877–885.

22. Miller, S.R., Tartter, P.I., Papatestas, A.E., Slater, G., and Aufses, A.H. Jr. (1981) Serum cholesterol and human colon cancer. *J. Natl. Cancer Inst.*, **67**, 297–300.

23. Kritchevsky, S.B., Wilcosky, T.C., Morris, D.L., Truong, K.N., and Tyroler, H.A. (1991) Changes in plasma lipid and lipoprotein cholesterol and weight prior to the diagnosis of cancer. *Cancer Res.*, **51**, 3198–3203.

24. Porta, C., Moroni, M., Nastasi, G., Invernizzi, R., and Bobbio-Pallavicini, E. (1991) Hypocholesterolemia and acute myeloid leukemia (AML). *Haematologica*, **76**, 348.

25. Henriksson, P. et al. (1989) Hypocholesterolaemia and increased elimination of low-density lipoproteins in metastatic cancer of the prostate. *Lancet*, **2**, 1178–1180.

26. Ho, Y.K., Smith, R.G., Brown, M.S., and Goldstein, J.L. (1978) Low-density lipoprotein (LDL) receptor activity in human acute myelogenous leukemia cells. *Blood*, **52**, 1099–1114.

27. Vitols, S., Gahrton, G., Ost, A., and Peterson, C. (1984) Elevated low density lipoprotein receptor activity in

leukemic cells with monocytic differentiation. *Blood*, **63**, 1186–1193.
28. Gal, D., MacDonald, P.C., Porter, J.C., and Simpson, E.R. (1981) Cholesterol metabolism in cancer cells in monolayer culture. III. Low-density lipoprotein metabolism. *Int. J. Cancer*, **28**, 315–319.
29. Goldstein, J.L. and Brown, M.S. (1977) The low-density lipoprotein pathway and its relation to atherosclerosis. *Annu. Rev. Biochem.*, **46**, 897–930.
30. Gal, D., Simpson, E.R., Porter, J.C., and Snyder, J.M. (1982) Defective internalization of low density lipoprotein in epidermoid cervical cancer cells. *J. Cell Biol.*, **92**, 597–603.
31. Anderson, R.G., Brown, M.S., and Goldstein, J.L. (1981) Inefficient internalization of receptor-bound low density lipoprotein in human carcinoma A-431 cells. *J. Cell Biol.*, **88**, 441–452.
32. Srivastava, S., Richards, P., Meinken, G.E., Larson, S.M., and Grunbaum, Z. (1981) Tumor uptake of radioruthenium compounds in *Radiopharmaceuticals: Structure–Activity Relationship* (ed. R. Spencer), Grune & Stratton, New York, pp. 207–223.
33. Som, P. et al. (1983) ^{97}Ru-transferrin uptake in tumor and abscess. *Eur. J. Nucl. Med.*, **8**, 491–494.
34. Edwards, C.L. and Hayes, R.L. (1969) Tumor scanning with ^{67}Ga citrate. *J. Nucl. Med.*, **10**, 103–105.
35. Ward, S.G. and Taylor, R.C. (1988) in *Metal-based Antitumor Drugs* (ed. M.F. Gielen), Freund, London, pp. 1–54.
36. Cazzola, M., Bergamaschi, G., Dezza, L., and Arosio, P. (1990) Manipulations of cellular iron metabolism for modulating normal and malignant cell proliferation: achievements and prospects. *Blood*, **75**, 1903–1919.
37. Maeda, H., Wu, J., Sawa, T., Matsumura, Y., and Hori, K. (2000) Tumor vascular permeability and the EPR effect in macromolecular therapeutics: a review. *J. Control. Release*, **65**, 271–284.
38. Hobbs, S.K. et al. (1998) Regulation of transport pathways in tumor vessels: role of tumor type and microenvironment. *Proc. Natl. Acad. Sci. USA*, **95**, 4607–4612.
39. Yuan, F. et al. (1995) Vascular permeability in a human tumor xenograft: molecular size dependence and cutoff size. *Cancer Res.*, **55**, 3752–3756.
40. Noguchi, Y. et al. (1998) Early phase tumor accumulation of macromolecules: a great difference in clearance rate between tumor and normal tissues. *Jpn. J. Cancer Res.*, **89**, 307–314.
41. Kratz, F. and Beyer, U. (1998) Serum proteins as drug carriers of anticancer agents: a review. *Drug Deliv.*, **5**, 281–299.
42. Stehle, G. et al. (1997) Plasma protein (albumin) catabolism by the tumor itself – implications for tumor metabolism and the genesis of cachexia. *Crit. Rev. Oncol. Hematol.*, **26**, 77–100.
43. Wunder, A. et al. (1997) Enhanced albumin uptake by rat tumors. *Int. J. Oncol.*, **11**, 497–507.
44. Kremer, P. et al. (2000) Laser-induced fluorescence detection of malignant gliomas using fluorescein-labeled serum albumin: experimental and preliminary clinical results. *Neurol. Res.*, **22**, 481–489.
45. Tanaka, T., Kaneo, Y., Shiramoto, S., and Iguchi, S. (1993) The disposition of serum proteins as drug-carriers in mice bearing Sarcoma 180. *Biol. Pharm. Bull.*, **16**, 1270–1275.
46. Norata, G. et al. (1984) *In vivo* assimilation of low density lipoproteins by a fibrosarcoma tumour line in mice. *Cancer Lett.*, **25**, 203–208.
47. Hynds, S.A. et al. (1984) Low-density lipoprotein metabolism in mice with soft tissue tumours. *Biochim. Biophys. Acta*, **795**, 589–595.
48. Lombardi, P. et al. (1989) Assimilation of LDL by experimental tumours in mice. *Biochim. Biophys. Acta*, **1003**, 301–306.
49. Versluis, A.J., van Geel, P.J., Oppelaar, H., van Berkel, T.J., and Bijsterbosch, M.K. (1996) Receptor-mediated uptake of low-density lipoprotein by B16 melanoma cells *in vitro* and *in vivo* in mice. *Br. J. Cancer*, **74**, 525–532.

50. Isaacsohn, J.L. et al. (1986) Adrenal imaging with technetium-99m-labelled low density lipoproteins. *Metabolism*, **35**, 364–366.
51. Subramanian, G.M., Fiscella, M., Lamouse-Smith, A., Zeuzem, S., and McHutchison, J.G. (2007) Albinterferon alpha-2b: a genetic fusion protein for the treatment of chronic hepatitis C. *Nat. Biotechnol.*, **25**, 1411–1419.
52. Gupta, P.K. and Hung, C.T. (1989) Albumin microspheres. II: applications in drug delivery. *J. Microencapsul.*, **6**, 463–472.
53. Gupta, P.K. and Hung, C.T. (1989) Albumin microspheres. I: physico-chemical characteristics. *J. Microencapsul.*, **6**, 427–462.
54. Weiss, M., Gildehaus, F.J., Brinkbaumer, K., Makowski, M., and Hahn, K. (2005) Lymph kinetics with technetium-99m labeled radiopharmaceuticals: animal studies. *Nuklearmedizin*, **44**, 156–165.
55. Jimenez, I.R. et al. (2008) Particle size of colloids to be used in sentinel lymph node radiolocalization. *Nucl. Med. Commun.*, **29**, 166–172.
56. Nishiyama, Y. et al. (1998) Usefulness of technetium-99m human serum albumin lymphoscintigraphy in chyluria. *Clin. Nucl. Med.*, **23**, 429–431.
57. Rink, T. et al. (2001) Lymphoscintigraphic sentinel node imaging and gamma probe detection in breast cancer with Tc-99m nanocolloidal albumin: results of an optimized protocol. *Clin. Nucl. Med.*, **26**, 293–298.
58. Bedrosian, I. et al. (1999) ^{99m}Tc-human serum albumin: an effective radiotracer for identifying sentinel lymph nodes in melanoma. *J. Nucl. Med.*, **40**, 1143–1148.
59. Dhabuwala, A., Lamerton, P., and Stubbs, R.S. (2005) Relationship of 99m technetium labelled macroaggregated albumin (^{99m}Tc-MAA) uptake by colorectal liver metastases to response following selective internal radiation therapy (SIRT). *BMC Nucl. Med.*, **5**, 7.
60. Allen, T.M. and Chonn, A. (1987) Large unilamellar liposomes with low uptake into the reticuloendothelial system. *FEBS Lett.*, **223**, 42–46.
61. Gabizon, A. and Papahadjopoulos, D. (1988) Liposome formulations with prolonged circulation time in blood and enhanced uptake by tumors. *Proc. Natl. Acad. Sci. USA*, **85**, 6949–6953.
62. Krieger, M., Brown, M.S., Faust, J.R., and Goldstein, J.L. (1978) Replacement of endogenous cholesteryl esters of low density lipoprotein with exogenous cholesteryl linoleate. Reconstitution of a biologically active lipoprotein particle. *J. Biol. Chem.*, **253**, 4093–4101.
63. Masquelier, M., Vitols, S., and Peterson, C. (1986) Low-density lipoprotein as a carrier of antitumoral drugs: *in vivo* fate of drug-human low-density lipoprotein complexes in mice. *Cancer Res.*, **46**, 3842–3847.
64. Walsh, M.T., Ginsburg, G.S., Small, D.M., and Atkinson, D. (1982) Apo B–lecithin–cholesterol ester complexes: reassembly of low density lipoprotein. *Arteriosclerosis*, **2**, 445a.
65. Lundberg, B. (1992) Assembly of prednimustine low-density-lipoprotein complexes and their cytotoxic activity in tissue culture. *Cancer Chemother. Pharmacol.*, **29**, 241–247.
66. Chun, P.W., Brumbaugh, E.E., and Shiremann, R.B. (1986) Interaction of human low density lipoprotein and apolipoprotein B with ternary lipid microemulsion. Physical and functional properties. *Biophys. Chem.*, **25**, 223–241.
67. Lundberg, B. and Suominen, L. (1984) Preparation of biologically active analogs of serum low density lipoprotein. *J. Lipid Res.*, **25**, 550–558.
68. Ginsburg, G.S., Walsh, M.T., Small, D.M., and Atkinson, D. (1984) Reassembled plasma low density lipoproteins. Phospholipid–cholesterol ester–apoprotein B complexes. *J. Biol. Chem.*, **259**, 6667–6673.
69. de Smidt, P.C. and van Berkel, T.J. (1990) Prolonged serum half-life of antineoplastic drugs by incorporation into the low density lipoprotein. *Cancer Res.*, **50**, 7476–7482.
70. Yeh, C.J. and Faulk, W.P. (1984) Killing of human tumor cells in culture with adriamycin conjugates of

human transferrin. *Clin. Immunol. Immunopathol.*, **32**, 1–11.
71. Barabas, K., Sizensky, J.A., and Faulk, W.P. (1992) Transferrin conjugates of adriamycin are cytotoxic without intercalating nuclear DNA. *J. Biol. Chem.*, **267**, 9437–9442.
72. Sun, I.L., Sun, E.E., Crane, F.L., Morre, D.J., and Faulk, W.P. (1992) Inhibition of transplasma membrane electron transport by transferrin–adriamycin conjugates. *Biochim. Biophys. Acta*, **1105**, 84–88.
73. Fritzer, M. et al. (1992) Cytotoxicity of a transferrin–adriamycin conjugate to anthracycline-resistant cells. *Int. J. Cancer*, **52**, 619–623.
74. Faulk, W.P., Taylor, C.G., Yeh, C.J., and McIntyre, J.A. (1990) Preliminary clinical study of transferrin–adriamycin conjugate for drug delivery to acute leukemia patients. *Mol. Biother.*, **2**, 57–60.
75. Kratz, F. et al. (1998) Transferrin conjugates of doxorubicin: synthesis, characterization, cellular uptake, and in vitro efficacy. *J. Pharm. Sci.*, **87**, 338–346.
76. Kratz, F. et al. (2000) In vitro and in vivo efficacy of acid-sensitive transferrin and albumin doxorubicin conjugates in a human xenograft panel and in the MDA-MB-435 mamma carcinoma model. *J. Drug Target.*, **8**, 305–318.
77. Wang, F., Jiang, X., Yang, D.C., Elliott, R.L., and Head, J.F. (2000) Doxorubicin–gallium–transferrin conjugate overcomes multidrug resistance: evidence for drug accumulation in the nucleus of drug resistant MCF-7/ADR cells. *Anticancer Res.*, **20**, 799–808.
78. Kovar, M., Strohalm, J., Ulbrich, K., and Rihova, B. (2002) In vitro and in vivo effect of HPMA copolymer-bound doxorubicin targeted to transferrin receptor of B-cell lymphoma 38C13. *J. Drug Target.*, **10**, 23–30.
79. Wu, J. et al. (2007) Reversal of multidrug resistance by transferrin-conjugated liposomes co-encapsulating doxorubicin and verapamil. *J. Pharm. Pharm. Sci.*, **10**, 350–357.
80. Li, X., Ding, L., Xu, Y., Wang, Y., and Ping, Q. (2009) Targeted delivery of doxorubicin using stealth liposomes modified with transferrin. *Int. J. Pharm.*, **373**, 116–123.
81. Lubgan, D., Jozwiak, Z., Grabenbauer, G.G., and Distel, L.V. (2009) Doxorubicin-transferrin conjugate selectively overcomes multidrug resistance in leukaemia cells. *Cell. Mol. Biol. Lett.*, **14**, 113–127.
82. Eatock, M. et al. (1999) Activity of doxorubicin covalently bound to a novel human serum albumin microcapsule. *Invest. New Drugs*, **17**, 111–120.
83. Kratz, F. et al. (1998) Preparation, characterization and in vitro efficacy of albumin conjugates of doxorubicin. *Biol. Pharm. Bull.*, **21**, 56–61.
84. Kratz, F. et al. (2001) Development and in vitro efficacy of novel MMP2 and MMP9 specific doxorubicin albumin conjugates. *Bioorg. Med. Chem. Lett.*, **11**, 2001–2006.
85. Mansour, A.M. et al. (2003) A new approach for the treatment of malignant melanoma: enhanced antitumor efficacy of an albumin-binding doxorubicin prodrug that is cleaved by matrix metalloproteinase 2. *Cancer Res.*, **63**, 4062–4066.
86. Kratz, F. et al. (2002) Probing the cysteine-34 position of endogenous serum albumin with thiol-binding doxorubicin derivatives: improved efficacy of an acid-sensitive doxorubicin derivative with specific albumin-binding properties compared to that of the parent compound. *J. Med. Chem.*, **45**, 5523–5533.
87. Kratz, F. et al. (2005) Development of albumin-binding doxorubicin prodrugs that are cleaved by prostate-specific antigen. *Arch. Pharm.*, **338**, 462–472.
88. Dreis, S. et al. (2007) Preparation, characterisation and maintenance of drug efficacy of doxorubicin-loaded human serum albumin (HSA) nanoparticles. *Int. J. Pharm.*, **341**, 207–214.
89. Schmid, B., Chung, D.E., Warnecke, A., Fichtner, I., and Kratz, F. (2007) Albumin-binding prodrugs of camptothecin and doxorubicin with an Ala-Leu-Ala-Leu-linker that are cleaved

90. Anhorn, M.G., Wagner, S., Kreuter, J., Langer, K., and von Briesen, H. (2008) Specific targeting of HER2 overexpressing breast cancer cells with doxorubicin-loaded trastuzumab-modified human serum albumin nanoparticles. *Bioconjug. Chem.*, **19**, 2321–2331.

91. Graeser, R. et al. (2008) Synthesis and biological evaluation of an albumin-binding prodrug of doxorubicin that is cleaved by prostate-specific antigen (PSA) in a PSA-positive orthotopic prostate carcinoma model (LNCaP). *Int. J. Cancer*, **122**, 1145–1154.

92. Abu Ajaj, K., Graeser, R., Fichtner, I., and Kratz, F. (2009) *In vitro* and *in vivo* study of an albumin-binding prodrug of doxorubicin that is cleaved by cathepsin B. *Cancer Chemother. Pharmacol.*, **64**, 413–418.

93. Wagner, S. et al. (2010) Enhanced drug targeting by attachment of an anti alphav integrin antibody to doxorubicin loaded human serum albumin nanoparticles. *Biomaterials*, **31**, 2388–2398.

94. Jones, A.K., Bejugam, N.K., Nettey, H., Addo, R., D'Souza, M.J. (2011) Spray-dried doxorubicin–albumin microparticulate systems for treatment of multidrug resistant melanomas. *J. Drug Target.*, **19**(6): 427–433.

95. Lo, E.H., Ooi, V.E., and Fung, K.P. (2002) Circumvention of multidrug resistance and reduction of cardiotoxicity of doxorubicin *in vivo* by coupling it with low density lipoprotein. *Life Sci.*, **72**, 677–687.

96. Bejaoui, N., Page, M., and Noel, C. (1991) Cytotoxicity of transferrin–daunorubicin conjugates on small cell carcinoma of the lung (SCCL) cell line NCI-H69. *Anticancer Res.*, **11**, 2211–2213.

97. Lemieux, P., Page, M., and Noel, C. (1992) *In vivo* cytotoxicity and antineoplastic activity of a transferrin–daunorubicin conjugate. *In Vivo*, **6**, 621–627.

98. Kratz, F. et al. (1997) Synthesis of new maleimide derivatives of daunorubicin and biological activity of acid labile transferrin conjugates. *Bioorg. Med. Chem. Lett.*, **7**, 617–622.

99. Trouet, A., Masquelier, M., Baurain, R., and Deprez-De Campeneere, D. (1982) A covalent linkage between daunorubicin and proteins that is stable in serum and reversible by lysosomal hydrolases, as required for a lysosomotropic drug–carrier conjugate: *in vitro* and *in vivo* studies. *Proc. Natl. Acad. Sci. USA*, **79**, 626–629.

100. Masquelier, M. et al. (2000) Plasma stability and cytotoxicity of lipophilic daunorubicin derivatives incorporated into low density lipoproteins. *Eur. J. Med. Chem.*, **35**, 429–438.

101. Kerr, D.J., Hynds, S.A., Shepherd, J., Packard, C.J., and Kaye, S.B. (1988) Comparative cellular uptake and cytotoxicity of a complex of daunomycin–low density lipoprotein in human squamous lung tumour cell monolayers. *Biochem. Pharmacol.*, **37**, 3981–3986.

102. Chu, B.C. and Howell, S.B. (1981) Differential toxicity of carrier-bound methotrexate toward human lymphocytes, marrow and tumor cells. *Biochem. Pharmacol.*, **30**, 2545–2552.

103. Bures, L., Bostik, J., Motycka, K., Spundova, M., and Rehak, L. (1988) The use of protein as a carrier of methotrexate for experimental cancer chemotherapy. III. Human serum albumin–methotrexate derivative, its preparation and basic testing. *Neoplasma*, **35**, 329–342.

104. Bostik, J., Bures, L., and Spundova, M. (1988) The use of protein as a carrier of methotrexate for experimental cancer chemotherapy. IV. Therapy of murine melanoma B16 by human serum albumin–methotrexate derivative. *Neoplasma*, **35**, 343–349.

105. Hartung, G. et al. (1999) Phase I trial of a methotrexate–albumin in a weekly intravenous bolus rgimen in cancer patients. *Clin. Cancer Res.*, **5**, 753–759.

106. Burger, A.M., Hartung, G., Stehle, G., Sinn, H., and Fiebig, H.H. (2001) Pre-clinical evaluation of

106. a methotrexate–albumin conjugate (MTX–HSA) in human tumor xenografts *in vivo*. *Int. J. Cancer*, **92**, 718–724.
107. Warnecke, A., Fichtner, I., Sass, G., and Kratz, F. (2007) Synthesis, cleavage profile, and antitumor efficacy of an albumin-binding prodrug of methotrexate that is cleaved by plasmin and cathepsin B. *Arch. Pharm.*, **340**, 389–395.
108. Halbert, G.W., Stuart, J.F., and Florence, A.T. (1985) A low density lipoprotein–methotrexate covalent complex and its activity against L1210 cells *in vitro*. *Cancer Chemother. Pharmacol.*, **15**, 223–227.
109. Beyer, U. *et al.* (1998) Synthesis and *in vitro* efficacy of transferrin conjugates of the anticancer drug chlorambucil. *J. Med. Chem.*, **41**, 2701–2708.
110. Kratz, F. *et al.* (1998) Albumin conjugates of the anticancer drug chlorambucil: synthesis, characterization, and *in vitro* efficacy. *Arch. Pharm. Pharm. Med. Chem.*, **331**, 47–53.
111. Firestone, R.A., Pisano, J.M., Falck, J.R., McPhaul, M.M., and Krieger, M. (1984) Selective delivery of cytotoxic compounds to cells by the LDL pathway. *J. Med. Chem.*, **27**, 1037–1043.
112. Dosio, F., Brusa, P., Crosasso, P., Arpicco, S., and Cattel, L. (1997) Preparation, characterization and properties *in vitro* and *in vivo* of a paclitaxel–albumin conjugate. *J. Control. Release*, **47**, 293–304.
113. Dosio, F., Arpicco, S., Brusa, P., Stella, B., and Cattel, L. (2001) Poly(ethylene glycol)–human serum albumin–paclitaxel conjugates: preparation, characterization and pharmacokinetics. *J. Control. Release*, **76**, 107–117.
114. Pinder, M.C; Ibrahim, N.K., (2006) Nanoparticle albumin-bound paclitaxel for treatment of metastatic breast cancer. *Drugs Today (Barc).*, **42**(9) 599–604.
115. Dosio, F., Arpicco, S., Stella, B., Brusa, P., and Cattel, L. (2009) Folate-mediated targeting of albumin conjugates of paclitaxel obtained through a heterogeneous phase system. *Int. J. Pharm.*, **382**, 117–123.
116. Nikanjam, M., Gibbs, A.R., Hunt, C.A., Budinger, T.F., and Forte, T.M. (2007) Synthetic nano-LDL with paclitaxel oleate as a targeted drug delivery vehicle for glioblastoma multiforme. *J. Control. Release*, **124**, 163–171.
117. Bicamumpaka, C. and Page, M. (1998) *In vitro* cytotoxicity of paclitaxel–ransferrin conjugate on H69 cells. *Oncol. Rep.*, **5**, 1381–1383.
118. Sahoo, S.K., Ma, W., and Labhasetwar, V. (2004) Efficacy of transferrin-conjugated paclitaxel-loaded nanoparticles in a murine model of prostate cancer. *Int. J. Cancer*, **112**, 335–340.
119. Shah, N., Chaudhari, K., Dantuluri, P., Murthy, R.S., and Das, S. (2009) Paclitaxel-loaded PLGA nanoparticles surface modified with transferrin and Pluronic®P85, an *in vitro* cell line and *in vivo* biodistribution studies on rat model. *J. Drug Target.*, **17**, 533–542.
120. Filipowska, D. *et al.* (1992) Treatment of cancer patients with a low-density-lipoprotein delivery vehicle containing a cytotoxic drug. *Cancer Chemother. Pharmacol.*, **29**, 396–400.
121. Iinuma, H. *et al.* (2002) Intracellular targeting therapy of cisplatin-encapsulated transferrin–polyethylene glycol liposome on peritoneal dissemination of gastric cancer. *Int. J. Cancer*, **99**, 130–137.
122. Hoshino, T. *et al.* (1995) *In vitro* cytotoxicities and *in vivo* distribution of transferrin–platinum(II) complex. *J. Pharm. Sci.*, **84**, 216–221.
123. Nishioka, Y. *et al.* (1989) Preparation and evaluation of albumin microspheres and microcapsules containing cisplatin. *Chem. Pharm. Bull.*, **37**, 1399–1400.
124. Verrijk, R., Smolders, I.J., McVie, J.G., and Begg, A.C. (1991) Polymer-coated albumin microspheres as carriers for intravascular tumour targeting of cisplatin. *Cancer Chemother. Pharmacol.*, **29**, 117–121.
125. Truter, E.J., Santos, A.S., and Els, W.J. (2001) Assessment of the antitumour

125. activity of targeted immunospecific albumin microspheres loaded with cisplatin and 5-fluorouracil: toxicity against a rodent ovarian carcinoma in vitro. *Cell Biol. Int.*, **25**, 51–59.
126. Tanaka, T., Fujishima, Y., and Kaneo, Y. (2001) Receptor mediated endocytosis and cytotoxicity of transferrin–mitomycin C conjugate in the HepG2 cell and primary cultured rat hepatocyte. *Biol. Pharm. Bull.*, **24**, 268–273.
127. Natsume, H., Sugibayashi, K., and Morimoto, Y. (1991) In vitro release profile of mitomycin C from albumin microspheres: extrapolation from macrospheres to microspheres. *Pharm. Res.*, **8**, 185–190.
128. Bergamo, A., Messori, L., Piccioli, F., Cocchietto, M., and Sava, G. (2003) Biological role of adduct formation of the ruthenium(III) complex NAMI-A with serum albumin and serum transferrin. *Invest. New Drugs*, **21**, 401–411.
129. Kratz, F., Keppler, B.K., Hartmann, M., Messori, L., and Berger, M.R. (1996) Comparison of the antiproliferative activity of two antitumour ruthenium(III) complexes with their apotransferrin and transferrin-bound forms in a human colon cancer cell line. *Metal-Based Drugs*, **3**, 15–23.
130. Kohgo, Y., Kato, J., Sasaki, K., and Kondo, H. (1988) Targeting chemotherapy with transferrin–neocarzinostatin conjugate. *Gan To Kagaku Ryoho*, **15**, 1072–1076.
131. Schonlau, F., Maibucher, A., Kohnlein, W., and Garnett, M.C. (1997) Mechanism of free and conjugated neocarzinostatin activity: studies on chromophore and protein uptake using a transferrin–neocarzinostatin conjugate. *Z. Naturforsch. C*, **52**, 245–254.
132. Kohgo, Y. et al. (1990) Kinetics of internalization and cytotoxicity of transferrin–neocarzinostatin conjugate in human leukemia cell line, K562. *Jpn. J. Cancer Res.*, **81**, 91–99.
133. Raso, V. and Basala, M. (1984) A highly cytotoxic human transferrin–ricin A chain conjugate used to select receptor-modified cells. *J. Biol. Chem.*, **259**, 1143–1149.
134. Colombatti, M., Bisconti, M., Dell'Arciprete, L., Gerosa, M.A., and Tridente, G. (1988) Sensitivity of human glioma cells to cytotoxic heteroconjugates. *Int. J. Cancer*, **42**, 441–448.
135. O'Keefe, D.O. and Draper, R.K. (1988) Two pathways of transferrin recycling evident in a variant of mouse LMTK-cells. *Somat. Cell Mol. Genet.*, **14**, 473–487.
136. Johnson, V.G., Wilson, D., Greenfield, L., and Youle, R.J. (1988) The role of the diphtheria toxin receptor in cytosol translocation. *J. Biol. Chem.*, **263**, 1295–1300.
137. Laske, D.W., Youle, R.J., and Oldfield, E.H. (1997) Tumor regression with regional distribution of the targeted toxin TF-CRM107 in patients with malignant brain tumors. *Nat. Med.*, **3**, 1362–1368.
138. Neville, D.M. Jr., Srinivasachar, K., Stone, R., and Scharff, J. (1989) Enhancement of immunotoxin efficacy by acid-cleavable cross-linking agents utilizing diphtheria toxin and toxin mutants. *J. Biol. Chem.*, **264**, 14653–14661.
139. Weaver, M. and Laske, D.W. (2003) Transferrin receptor ligand-targeted toxin conjugate (Tf-CRM107) for therapy of malignant gliomas. *J. Neurooncol.*, **65**, 3–13.
140. O'Keefe, D.O. and Draper, R.K. (1985) Characterization of a transferrin–diphtheria toxin conjugate. *J. Biol. Chem.*, **260**, 932–937.
141. Bergamaschi, G. et al. (1988) Killing of K562 cells with conjugates between human transferrin and a ribosome-inactivating protein (SO-6). *Br. J. Haematol.*, **68**, 379–384.
142. Hall, W.A., Godal, A., Juell, S., and Fodstad, O. (1992) In vitro efficacy of transferrin-toxin conjugates against glioblastoma multiforme. *J. Neurosurg.*, **76**, 838–844.
143. Rybak, S.M., Saxena, S.K., Ackerman, E.J., and Youle, R.J. (1991) Cytotoxic potential of ribonuclease and ribonuclease hybrid proteins. *J. Biol. Chem.*, **266**, 21202–21207.

144. Di Stefano, G. et al. (2006) Doxorubicin coupled to lactosaminated albumin: effects on rats with liver fibrosis and cirrhosis. *Dig. Liver Dis.*, **38**, 404–448.
145. Di Stefano, G., Lanza, M., Kratz, F., Merina, L., and Fiume, L. (2004) A novel method for coupling doxorubicin to lactosaminated human albumin by an acid sensitive hydrazone bond: synthesis, characterization and preliminary biological properties of the conjugate. *Eur. J. Pharm. Sci.*, **23**, 393–397.
146. Qu, X. et al. (2010) In vitro evaluation of a folate–bovine serum albumin–doxorubicin conjugate. *J. Drug Target.*, **18**, 351–361.
147. Drevs, J., Hofmann, I., Marmé, D., Unger, C., and Kratz, F. (1999) In vivo and in vitro efficacy of an acid-sensitive albumin conjugate of adriamycin compared to the parent compound in murine renal cell carcinoma. *Drug Deliv.*, **6**, 89–95.
148. Sakhno, L.A. et al. (2006) The study of possibility to elevate antitumor activity and decrease of systemic toxic effects of cisplatin by its binding with deliganded albumin. *Exp. Oncol.*, **28**, 303–307.
149. Singh, M. (1999) Transferrin as a targeting ligand for liposomes and anticancer drugs. *Curr. Pharm. Des.*, **5**, 443–451.
150. Yu, B., Zhao, X., Lee, L.J., and Lee, R.J. (2009) Targeted delivery systems for oligonucleotide therapeutics. *AAPS J.*, **11**, 195–203.
151. Qian, Z.M., Li, H., Sun, H., and Ho, K. (2002) Targeted drug delivery via the transferrin receptor-mediated endocytosis pathway. *Pharmacol. Rev.*, **54**, 561–587.
152. Chu, B.C. and Whiteley, J.M. (1979) Control of solid tumor metastases with a high-molecular-weight derivative of methotrexate. *J. Natl. Cancer Inst.*, **62**, 79–82.
153. Bures, L., Lichy, A., Bostik, J., and Spundova, M. (1990) The use of protein as a carrier of methotrexate for experimental cancer chemotherapy. V. Alternative method for preparation of serum albumin–methotrexate derivative. *Neoplasma*, **37**, 225–231.
154. Stehle, G. et al. (1997) The loading rate determines tumor targeting properties of methotrexate–albumin conjugates in rats. *Anticancer Drugs*, **8**, 677–685.
155. Stehle, G. et al. (1997) Pharmacokinetics of methotrexate–albumin conjugates in tumor-bearing rats. *Anticancer Drugs*, **8**, 835–844.
156. Beyer, U., Rothern-Rutishauser, B., Unger, C., Wunderli-Allenspach, H., and Kratz, F. (2001) Differences in the intracellular distribution of acid-sensitive doxorubicin–protein conjugates in comparison to free and liposomal formulated doxorubicin as shown by confocal microscopy. *Pharm. Res.*, **18**, 29–38.
157. Kratz, F., Mueller-Driver, R., Hofmann, I., Drevs, J., and Unger, C. (2000) A novel macromolecular prodrug concept exploiting endogenous serum albumin as a drug carrier for cancer chemotherapy. *J. Med. Chem.*, **43**, 1253–1256.
158. John, T.A., Vogel, S.M., Tiruppathi, C., Malik, A.B., and Minshall, R.D. (2003) Quantitative analysis of albumin uptake and transport in the rat microvessel endothelial monolayer. *Am. J. Physiol.*, **284**, L187–L196.
159. Graeser, R. et al. (2010) INNO-206, the (6-maleimidocaproyl hydrazone derivative of doxorubicin), shows superior antitumor efficacy compared to doxorubicin in different tumor xenograft models and in an orthotopic pancreas carcinoma model. *Invest. New Drugs*, **28**, 14–19.
160. Desai, N. et al. (2006) Increased antitumor activity, intratumor paclitaxel concentrations, and endothelial cell transport of cremophor-free, albumin-bound paclitaxel, ABI-007, compared with cremophor-based paclitaxel. *Clin. Cancer Res.*, **12**, 1317–1324.
161. Kratz, F., Ehling, G., Kauffmann, H.M., and Unger, C. (2007) Acute and repeat-dose toxicity studies of the (6-maleimidocaproyl)hydrazone derivative of doxorubicin (DOXO-EMCH), an albumin-binding prodrug of the anticancer agent doxorubicin. *Hum. Exp. Toxicol.*, **26**, 19–35.

162. Lebrecht, D. et al. (2007) The 6-maleimidocaproyl hydrazone derivative of doxorubicin (DOXO-EMCH) is superior to free doxorubicin with respect to cardiotoxicity and mitochondrial damage. *Int. J. Cancer*, **120**, 927–934.

163. Chung, D.E. and Kratz, F. (2006) Development of a novel albumin-binding prodrug that is cleaved by urokinase-type-plasminogen activator (uPA). *Bioorg. Med. Chem. Lett.*, **16**, 5157–5163.

164. Kratz, F. et al. (2005) Development of albumin-binding doxorubicin prodrugs that are cleaved by prostate-specific antigen (PSA). *Arch. Pharm.*, **338**, 462–472.

165. Schmid, B., Warnecke, A., Fichtner, I., Jung, M., and Kratz, F. (2007) Development of albumin-binding camptothecin prodrugs using a peptide positional scanning library. *Bioconjug. Chem.*, **18**, 1786–1799.

166. Warnecke, A. and Kratz, F. (2003) Maleimide-oligo(ethylene glycol) derivatives of camptothecin as albumin-binding prodrugs: synthesis and antitumor efficacy. *Bioconjug. Chem.*, **14**, 377–387.

167. Abu Ajaj, K., Biniossek, M.L., and Kratz, F. (2009) Development of protein-binding bifunctional linkers for a new generation of dual-acting prodrugs. *Bioconjug. Chem.*, **20**, 390–396.

168. Warnecke, A., Fichtner, I., Garmann, D., Jaehde, U., and Kratz, F. (2004) Synthesis and biological activity of water-soluble maleimide derivatives of the anticancer drug carboplatin designed as albumin-binding prodrugs. *Bioconjug. Chem.*, **15**, 1349–1359.

169. Beyer, U., Schumacher, P., Unger, C., Frahm, A.W., and Kratz, F. (1996) Synthesis of maleimide derivatives of the anticancer drugs 5-fluorouracil and 5'-deoxy-5-fluorouridine for the preparation of chemoimmunoconjugates. *Pharmazie*, **52**, 480–482.

170. Abu Ajaj, K. and Kratz, F. (2009) Development of dual-acting prodrugs for circumventing multidrug resistance. *Bioorg. Med. Chem. Lett.*, **19**, 995–1000.

171. Fiume, L. et al. (2005) Doxorubicin coupled to lactosaminated albumin inhibits the growth of hepatocellular carcinomas induced in rats by diethylnitrosamine. *J. Hepatol.*, **43**, 645–652.

172. Temming, K., Schiffelers, R.M., Molema, G., and Kok, R.J. (2005) RGD-based strategies for selective delivery of therapeutics and imaging agents to the tumour vasculature. *Drug Resist. Updat.*, **8**, 381–402.

173. Kokudo, N., Vera, D.R., and Makuuchi, M. (2003) Clinical application of TcGSA. *Nucl. Med. Biol.*, **30**, 845–849.

174. Melder, R.J. et al. (2005) Pharmacokinetics and *in vitro* and *in vivo* anti-tumor response of an interleukin-2–human serum albumin fusion protein in mice. *Cancer Immunol. Immunother.*, **54**, 535–547.

175. Iwanik, M.J., Shaw, K.V., Ledwith, B.J., Yanovich, S., and Shaw, J.M. (1984) Preparation and interaction of a low-density lipoprotein:daunomycin complex with P388 leukemic cells. *Cancer Res.*, **44**, 1206–1215.

176. Eley, J.G., Halbert, G.W., and Florence, A.T. (1990) The incorporation of estramustine into low density lipoprotein and its activity in tissue culture. *Int. J. Pharm.*, **63**, 121–127.

177. Eley, J.G., Halbert, G.W., and Florence, A.T. (1990) Incorporation of prednimustine into low density lipoprotein: activity against P388 cells in tissue culture. *Int. J. Pharm.*, **65**, 219–224.

178. Kratz, F. (2008) Albumin as a drug carrier: design of prodrugs, drug conjugates and nanoparticles. *J. Control. Release*, **132**, 171–183.

179. Vis, A.N. et al. (2002) A phase II trial of methotrexate–human serum albumin (MTX–HSA) in patients with metastatic renal cell carcinoma who progressed under immunotherapy. *Cancer Chemother. Pharmacol.*, **49**, 342–345.

180. Bolling, C. et al. (2006) Phase II study of MTX–HSA in combination with cisplatin as first line treatment in patients with advanced or metastatic transitional cell carcinoma. *Invest. New Drugs*, **24**, 521–527.

181. Unger, C. et al. (2007) Phase I and pharmacokinetic study of the (6-maleimidocaproyl)hydrazone derivative of doxorubicin. *Clin. Cancer Res.*, **13**, 4858–4866.
182. Kratz, F. (2007) DOXO-EMCH (INNO-206): the first albumin-binding prodrug of doxorubicin to enter clinical trials. *Expert Opin. Invest. Drugs*, **16**, 855–866.
183. Anatelli, F. et al. (2006) Macrophage-targeted photosensitizer conjugate delivered by intratumoral injection. *Mol. Pharm.*, **3**, 654–664.
184. Brasseur, N., Langlois, R., La Madeleine, C., Ouellet, R., and van Lier, J.E. (1999) Receptor-mediated targeting of phthalocyanines to macrophages via covalent coupling to native or maleylated bovine serum albumin. *Photochem. Photobiol.*, **69**, 345–352.
185. Kratz, F. (1993) Interactions of antitumour metal complexes with serum proteins. Perspectives for anticancer drug development. A review in *Metal Complexes as Antitumour Agents* (ed. B.K. Keppler), Verlag Chemie, Weinheim, pp. 392–429.
186. Kratz, F. and Schütte, M.T. (1998) Anticancer metal complexes and tumour targeting strategies. *Cancer J.*, **11**, 60–67.
187. Pardridge, W.M. (1999) Non-invasive drug delivery to the human brain using endogenous blood–brain barrier transport systems. *Pharm. Sci. Technol. Today*, **2**, 49–59.
188. Mo, Y., Barnett, M.E., Takemoto, D., Davidson, H., and Kompella, U.B. (2007) Human serum albumin nanoparticles for efficient delivery of Cu, Zn superoxide dismutase gene. *Mol. Vis.*, **13**, 746–757.
189. Fischer, D., Bieber, T., Brusselbach, S., Elsasser, H., and Kissel, T. (2001) Cationized human serum albumin as a non-viral vector system for gene delivery? Characterization of complex formation with plasmid DNA and transfection efficiency. *Int. J. Pharm.*, **225**, 97–111.
190. Shohet, R.V. et al. (2000) Echocardiographic destruction of albumin microbubbles directs gene delivery to the myocardium. *Circulation*, **101**, 2554–2556.

25
Future Trends, Challenges, and Opportunities with Polymer-Based Combination Therapy in Cancer

Coralie Deladriere, Rut Lucas, and María J. Vicent

25.1
Introduction

The application of drug delivery systems has been mainly restricted to the delivery of single agents; however, their use to deliver "cocktails" of therapeutics is still largely unexplored. This might seem unusual since combination therapy is routinely used in cancer treatment and indeed the combination of different therapeutic agents often improves therapeutic profile [1]. In the last 5 years, a number of pioneering studies have been carried out that highlight the suitability of different drug delivery systems to deliver drug combinations. In fact, Celator Technologies (*www.celatorpharma.com*) has developed CombiPlex® technology – a novel approach that identifies a synergistic ratio of two or more drugs and locks the ratio in a drug delivery vehicle. CombiPlex is able to deliver and maintain the synergistic ratio in patients by means of a pharmacokinetic control. CombiPlex has already led to two liposome-based products in phase II clinical development: CPX-1 (irinotecan/floxuridine) [2] and CPX-351 (cytarabine/daunorubicin) [3]. Although at much earlier stages, the promising approaches offered by combination therapy has been already identified in the case of polymer–drug conjugates [4, 5].

The aim of this chapter is to systematically review these early works. We will first give an overview of the current use of combination therapy in cancer treatment. Following this, the concept of polymer–drug conjugates for combination therapy is defined, and the challenges and opportunities associated with its use are analyzed. Finally, representative examples of the field are described with particular attention to clinical studies.

25.1.1
Combination Therapy in Cancer

Combination therapy for the treatment of a disease generally refers to either the combinations of different types of therapy (e.g., chemotherapy and radiotherapy), or to the simultaneous administration of two or more pharmacologically active agents. Unlike single-agent therapy, multiagent therapy can modulate different signaling pathways in diseased cells, thus maximizing the therapeutic effect and a possibly overcoming mechanisms of resistance [1].

Within this context, combination therapy applied to cancer has a remarkable therapeutic value, as already demonstrated by its routine clinical use. Several principles are involved in the design of therapeutic combinations for cancer treatment, which include biochemical synergism, tumor cell kinetics, fractional cell kill, dose scheduling, intensity and total dose, nonoverlapping toxicity, active agents, tumor cell resistance, non-cross-resistant agents, and host rescue. In the clinics, these considerations also set up the basis for the design of adjuvant and neoadjuvant approaches [6].

Taking into account the principles mentioned above, four main types of combination therapy are currently considered of routine clinical use:

1) **Combination of different types of therapy.** Depending on the tumor class, single-type therapy could be considered sufficient. For example, in early-stage Hodgkin's disease, non-Hodgkin's lymphoma, and certain types of prostate or brain cancer, radiation therapy alone may cure the disease. However, in most cases, radiation therapy used in conjunction with surgery, chemotherapy, or both, increases survival rates over any of these therapies used alone. Therefore, the combination of surgery, radiotherapy, and chemotherapy is routinely used in the clinic as different cycle phases. More importantly, recent studies are assessing the combination of radiation therapy with new drugs and/or new therapeutic approaches. A phase II clinical study showed that the application of X-rays together with low-dose cisplatin can potentiate the effect of the radiation by means of a drug pretreatment regime [7]. The National Cancer Institute (NCI) has promoted a phase II trial to evaluate the combination of radiation with a prostate-specific antigen (PSA)-based vaccine in patients with prostate cancer [8]. The design was based on the patient's immune system stimulation, which enhances the radiotherapy effect. Indeed, based on preclinical observations, it was demonstrated that the radiation therapy can alter tumor cells and make them more susceptible to the action of the body's immune system [9].

2) **Chemotherapy combinations.** Clinical chemotherapeutic agents are described to induce DNA damage, act as topoisomerase I or II inhibitors, DNA intercalators, reactive oxygen species (ROS) inducers, or microtubule stabilizers. Since the 1940s, the combination of different chemotherapeutics has been developed, allowing for remarkable survival improvement, particularly in childhood leukemia and Hodgkin's disease [6]. As mentioned above, this progression was based on the rational impairment of several empiricism principles, such as biochemical synergy, tumor cell kinetics, nonoverlapping toxicity, non-cross-resistant agents, or tumor cell resistance [6]. Treatments resulting from these concepts are various; for instance, looking at biochemical synergy, the administration of leucovorin prior to 5-fluorouracil (5-FU) in colorectal cancer, where leucovorin markedly enhanced the fixation of the 5-FU and consequently its therapeutic effect. Another example of a complementary treatment

used for acute nonlymphocytic leukemia is the combination of anthracycline daunorubicin (DNA intercalator) with arabinofuranosylcytidine (inhibitor of DNA polymerase), achieving a simultaneous effect of blocking both the DNA repair and DNA synthesis. Other traditional drug combinations considered of routine clinical use are: anthracycline and cyclophosphamide (AC) and cyclophosphamide, adriamycin, and 5-FU (CAF) [10] based on anthracycline combinations [6, 11], cyclophosphamide, methotrexate, and 5-FU (CMF), and cyclophosphamide, methotrexate, 5-FU, vincristine, and prednisone (CMFVP) [6, 11] based on methotrexate combinations, and paclitaxel (PTX)-containing regimes, such as the combination of PTX with carboplatin for ovary and lung cancer or with vinorelbine for non-small-cell lung cancer (NSCLC) [12, 13]. Presently, new possibilities, including variations of administration patterns, are being explored in order to increase response, reduce side-effects, and maximize therapeutic benefit. For instance, a phase II study, combining PTX, 5-FU, folinic acid, and cisplatin showed promising results in patients with advanced gastric cancer [14]. In this trial, the weekly intravenous administration of the PTX cocktail as opposed to the three administrations per week of single PTX was compared and the same therapeutic effect was achieved with much fewer side-effects [14].

On the other hand, small-molecule chemotherapy combinations can also be used as palliative treatment by decreasing the symptoms and prolonging life expectancy [15]. Finally, its use has been described as adjuvant therapy pre- or postsurgery, by diminishing the tumor mass in advanced and metastatic cancer prior to surgery, and eradicating undetectable micrometastasis in a postsurgical treatment [16].

3) **Combinations based on endocrine therapy.** Hormone-dependent cancers (mainly prostate and breast) can be treated with surgery, radiotherapy, chemotherapy, or the combinations described above. However, endocrine therapy represents an additional alternative for this type of solid tumor. In breast cancer, two main types of therapies are described: (i) use of selective estrogen receptor modulators [17], which are agents mainly administered in premenopausal women trying to block the estrogen receptor and consequently the protein cascade involved in tumor cell proliferation, and (ii) inhibition of the estrogen flow by means of aromatase inhibitors [18], mainly prescribed for postmenopausal women. Indeed, in breast cancer patients clinical studies combining endocrine and chemotherapy have already been reported since the 1980s [19], and it is believed that targeted multidrug therapy is a valuable option for addressing the multiple mechanisms (side-toxicity, resistance, etc.) that may be responsible for reduced efficacy of current therapies [20]. Recently, several trials have described the use of endocrine therapy in combination with adjuvant bisphosphate therapy (zoledronic acid) to counterbalance the bone loss associated with the estrogen suppression induced by aromatase inhibitors, and therefore preventing future chronic disease and fracture in this cohort of patients [21]. In addition to bone protection, other clinical trials were carried out

to confirm the antitumor activity of zoledronic acid that had emerged in previous preclinical and clinical studies [22]. For instance, a large clinical trial was performed with 1805 premenopausal women with hormone-responsive breast cancer, comparing the effects of endocrine therapy with or without the addition of zoledronic acid [22]. Patients in this trial displayed significant prolonged disease-free survival and relapse-free survival 5 years after the beginning of the treatment with zoledronic acid and endocrine therapy. The authors attribute these positive results to the antimetastatic properties of zoledronic acid and highlight the importance of such combination [23]. Similar results were obtained in the CALGB 79809 trial [24]. With regard to prostate cancer, different types of hormonal therapy are also described in order to block the testosterone role involved in tumor growth [25]. Luteinizing hormone-releasing hormone (LHRH) analogs [26] and antiandrogens [27] are the two main families reported as hormone therapy in prostate cancer. In contrast to breast cancer, endocrine therapy in prostate cancer is commonly used in locally advanced or high-grade, high-risk disease, but always within an adjuvant scheme. The rational behind this combination is to achieve tumor confinement by reducing its volume. In particular, androgen ablation (mainly by LHRH analogs) prescribed with external irradiation increases clinical and biochemical relapse-free survival in patients with advanced prostate cancer [28].

4) **Molecularly targeted cancer therapeutic agents in combination.** In recent years, the development of agents that target specific molecular pathways, such as antibody therapies, has played important roles in cancer treatment either alone or in combination with other therapeutic agents [29]. The monoclonal antibody (mAb) trastuzumab (Herceptin®) is routinely used in combination with a chemotherapeutic agent in the treatment of HER2-positive breast cancer [30]. Other mAbs, such as rituximab (Rituxan®) [31] or bevacizumab (Avastin®) [32], are used for metastatic treatment in colorectal cancer or NSCLC and esophageal cancer, and have recently been administered with traditional chemotherapy for the treatment of advanced breast tumors [33, 34]. Currently, bevacizumab, the first antiangiogenic drug to be granted US Food and Drug Administration (FDA) approval to market (February 2004), is combined with 5-FU-based chemotherapy, carboplatin, or PTX for the treatment of metastatic colorectal cancer, NSCLC, and metastatic breast cancer, respectively [33]. In February 2008, after a phase III trial showing that metastatic breast cancer patients treated with bevacizumab in combination with PTX chemotherapy displayed prolonged progression-free survival in comparison with PTX alone [34], bevacizumab received accelerated approval from the FDA for use in metastatic breast cancer as combination. More multiagent therapies are currently in clinical trials using the same rationale, targeting different molecular pathways to maximize the efficacy and, therefore, assessing the efficacy of antiangiogenic drugs in combination with traditional chemotherapy. However, it is important to be aware that although the rationale for this type of combination is, strong, some trials failed to improve overall survival. This is the case found in phase III trials with antiangiogenic drugs in combination with traditional chemotherapy

and with inhibitors of specific molecular pathways such as erlotinib (Tarceva®) [35]. These disappointing results can at least be partially attributed to the lack of an in-depth understanding of the molecular pathways underlying cancer disease and, as a consequence, the difficulties of optimizing combination therapy.

It is clear that combination therapy already plays a key role in cancer treatment and, if supported by an understanding of the underlying molecular mechanisms, it is expected to do so even more in the future. In this context, new strategies currently under preclinical development are being considered. Adams and Weiner suggested an interesting approach to develop rationally designed drug combinations looking at identifying and targeting antigens whose expression is triggered by exposure to chemotherapy [36, 37]. In this study, a xenograft model of colorectal cancer was exposed to irinotecan (camptothecin, CPT-11) that induced LY6D/E46 antigen. A mAb against this antigen was then prepared and conjugated to monomethyl auristatin, a potent antitubulin drug, to form an immunoconjugate. CPT-11 together with the immunoconjugate yielded complete tumor regression, whereas the single agents did not [36]. Another example of combination therapy has also been described for the first time based on the attachment of two agents as prodrugs in a defined 1 : 1 ratio through one polymer or protein binding group [38, 39]. Finally, it is worth mentioning a very recent combination approach described by Sugahara *et al.* [40–42] reporting that the coadministration of a peptide named iRGD with small molecules (doxorubicin (DOX)), nanoparticles (*nab*–PTX or DOX liposomes), or mAbs (trastuzumab) enhanced the penetration of the anticancer agent and therefore their efficacy whilst reducing side-effects. From this point of view, the application of drug delivery systems for multiagent therapy to ensure that such drug cocktails are truly simultaneously delivered at the target site is of clear interest.

All conventional treatments discussed up to now, even in combination, are still responsible for side-toxicity in healthy organs as well as a decrease in the patient's quality of life. To overcome these drawbacks, the development of systems able to specifically deliver and release a bioactive drug in a controlled manner is one of the challenges in cancer research. Therefore, the use of drug delivery systems has been sought to (i) alter drug biodistribution, (ii) improve biological activity, and (iii) increase tumor specificity [4]. More importantly, using a drug delivery system for a drug combination ensures the delivery of the drugs at the adequate ratio and at the same time in the same site. The individual drugs without a drug delivery system could be metabolized independently and at different rates, and this may negatively impact their effectiveness.

In this chapter, we focus our attention on polymer conjugates as drug delivery systems and, in particular, on the design of combination therapy with polymer–drug conjugates.

25.2
Concept of Polymer–Drug Conjugates for Combination Therapy

Polymer–drug conjugates are drug delivery nanotechnologies in which the drug is covalently bound to a polymer carrier, normally via a biodegradable linker. The main benefits of polymer–drug conjugates compared to the parent free drug are: (i) passive tumor targeting by the enhanced permeability and retention (EPR) effect, which can be utilized for tumor targeting and polymer–drug conjugate accumulation [43], (ii) a decrease of toxicity [44], (iii) an increase of solubility in biological fluids [45], (iv) an ability to overcome some mechanisms of drug resistance [46], and (v) an ability to elicit immunostimulatory effects [47, 48]. At present, more than 16 polymer–drug conjugates have undergone clinical evaluation [49] and polyglutamic acid (PGA)–PTX conjugate (CT-2103, poliglumex (PPX), Opaxio® (Figure 25.1), previously known as Xyotax®) [50] is expected to enter the market in the near future as a potential treatment for various types of cancer, such

Figure 25.1 Chemical structure of PGA–PTX conjugate (Opaxio).

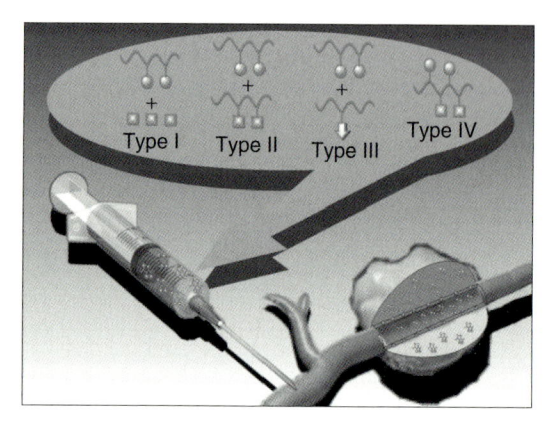

Figure 25.2 Schematic representation of the different types of polymer-based combination therapy for targeted drug delivery by the EPR effect. (Reproduced with permission from [15].)

25.2 Concept of Polymer–Drug Conjugates for Combination Therapy | 811

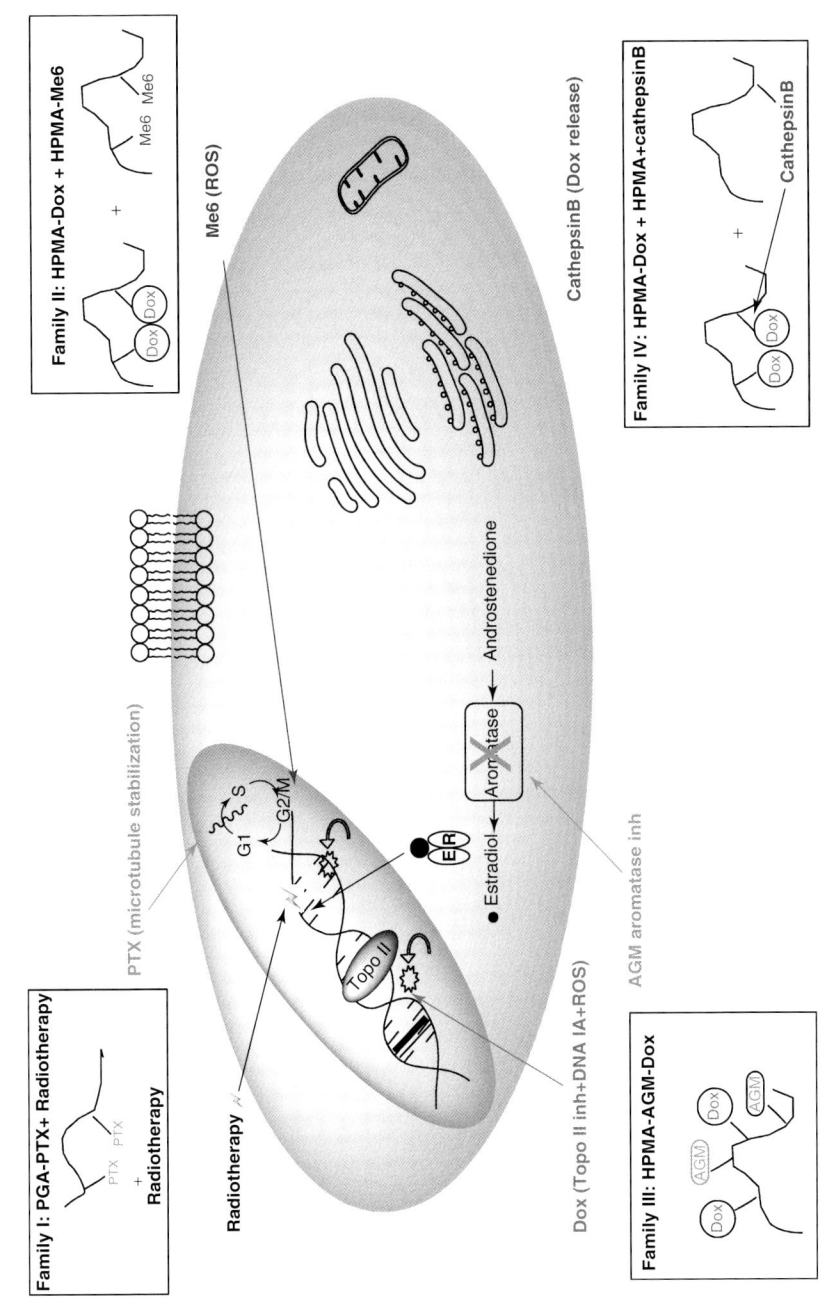

Figure 25.3 Schematic representation of the different types of polymer-based combination therapy with representative examples and their target sites. Family I: PGA–PTX conjugate + radiotherapy; Family II: HPMA copolymer–DOX conjugate + HPMA copolymer–Me6 conjugate; Family III: HPMA copolymer–AGM–DOX conjugate; Family IV: PDEPT approach, HPMA copolymer–DOX conjugate + HPMA copolymer–cathepsin B conjugate, DNA IA: DNA intercalating agent.

as NSCLC or ovarian cancer ([50–52] and *http://www.celltherapeutics.com/opaxio*). All of these compounds are built on orthodox chemotherapeutic agents; for example, DOX [53–55], CPT and their derivatives ([55–60], *www.ceruleanrx.com, and www.nektar.com/product-pipline/oncology-nktr-102.html*), PTX [45, 50, 52, 61], and platinates [62, 63]. An exhaustive review on the clinical benefits of polymer–drug conjugates as single agents is beyond the scope of this chapter; however, it is recommended to read recent revisions in this field [49, 64–67] and other relevant chapters in this volume.

The term *"polymer–drug conjugates for combination therapy"* is a general phrase that comprises at least four families of systems (Figures 25.2 and 25.3):

Family I	Polymer–drug conjugate plus free drugs. This concept is developed based on the combination of a polymer–drug conjugate carrying a single drug administered with a low-molecular-weight drug or a different type of therapy (e.g., radiotherapy).
Family II	Polymer–drug conjugate plus polymer–drug conjugate. In this approach the strategy developed is the combination of two different polymer–drug conjugates, each containing a single therapeutic agent.
Family III	Single polymeric carrier carrying a combination of drugs. In contrast to the other families, this approach involves only one polymer main-chain in which two or more drugs are conjugated.
Family IV	Polymer-directed enzyme prodrug therapy (PDEPT) (Figure 25.4) and polymer enzyme liposome therapy (PELT). PDEPT relies on the combination of a polymer–drug conjugate with a polymer–enzyme conjugate capable of the selective release of the drug at the tumor site. PELT is a comparable strategy where a polymer enzyme conjugate is administered in combination with the liposome to induce its degradation, allowing the release of the drug encapsulated inside.

25.3
Challenges and Opportunities Associated with the Use of Polymer-Based Combination Therapy

Due to the intratumor heterogeneity of the tumor tissue and the complex molecular mechanism of tumor progression, the presence of two or more therapeutic agents on a single polymeric chain opens new therapeutic possibilities, but also new challenges to overcome. Therefore, several issues should be considered in order to develop polymer–drug conjugates for combination therapy.

25.3.1
Identification of Appropriate Drug Combinations and Drug Ratios

Most drug combinations are based on the assumption that by targeting different cellular pathways there is an enhancement in the therapeutic benefit and a decrease

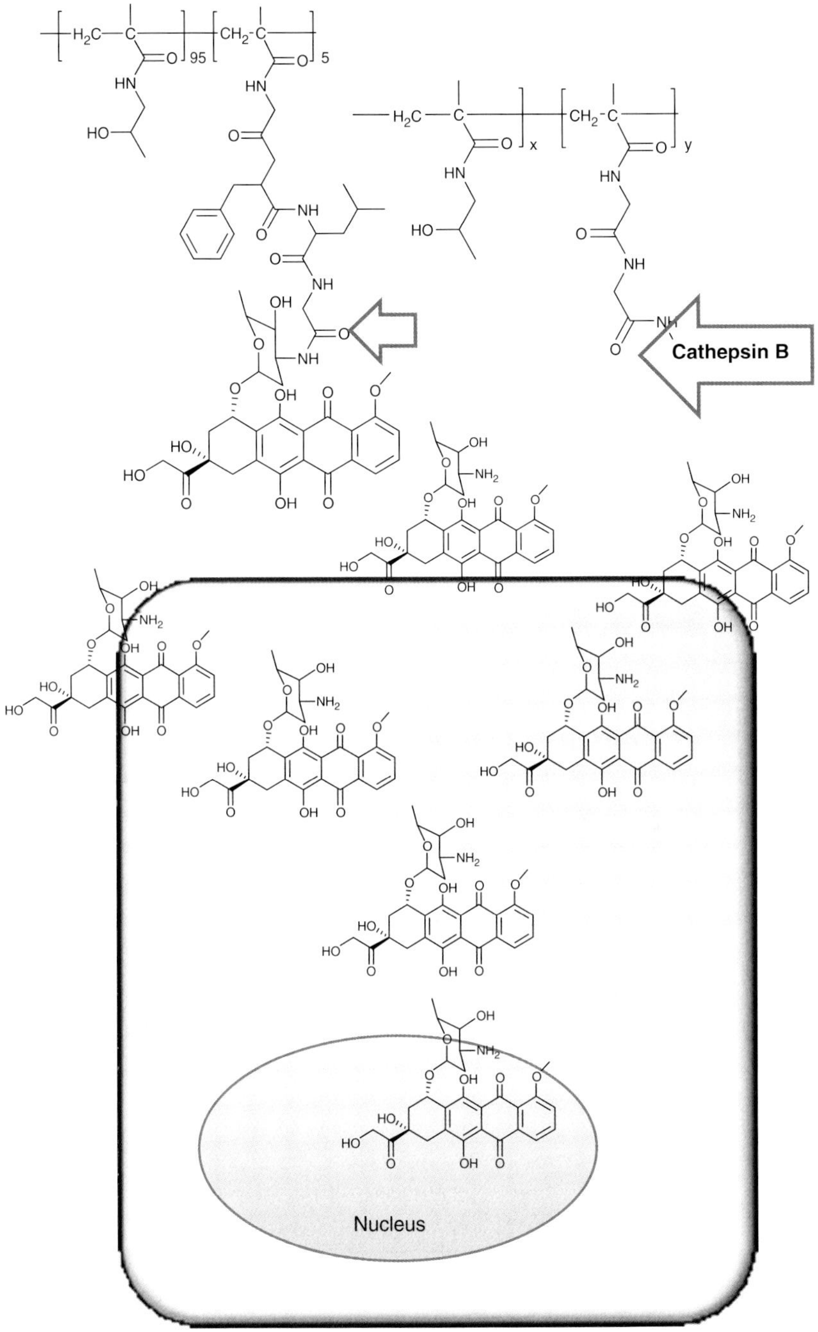

Figure 25.4 Schematic representation of PDEPT (Family IV), showing HPMA copolymer–DOX (PK1) activated by HPMA copolymer-GG-cathepsin B as an example. (Reproduced with permission from [15].)

in toxicity. Several studies confirmed this statement while others did not reach their expectations [35]. Indeed, two important and not trivial points have to be considered: (i) the identification of the drugs to be combined that will be subsequently released together and (ii) the determination of the optimal drug ratio.

In order to achieve the maximum clinical benefit in patients, clinicians usually combine drugs that do not have overlapping toxicities at their individual maximum tolerated dose (MTD). However, this assumption is not correct in many cases as a different ratio of the selected drugs may be synergistic (greater effect than the sum of the individual drugs), additive (equal activity to the sum of the individual drugs), or antagonistic (less anticancer effect than the sum of the individual drugs). Drug ratios can play a critical role when combining drugs. The results of multiple *in vitro* and preclinical studies have demonstrated that the molar ratios of drugs used can have a significant impact on the overall efficacy and safety of combination chemotherapy [68]. The full understanding of this concept has been the key to the successful technology developed by the Canadian company Celator Technologies, as explained in Section 25.1. Ideally, it is hoped that a similar approach will be applied to the development of combination polymer–drug conjugates. In this context, further studies investigating the impact of different drug ratios on biological activity of polymer–drug conjugates should be carried out.

25.3.2
Kinetics of Drug Release

This is another important parameter to control when developing combination polymer–drug conjugates that confers clear benefits to this platform technology when compared to other nanopharmaceuticals. The presence of bioresponsive polymer–drug(s) linker(s) offers the possibility of fine-tuning drug release ratio(s) that could be directly translated into the enhancement of the therapeutic output. However, achieving successful drug(s) release rates is not a trivial issue.

It is well established that the drug release rate from the polymer to the target site is an essential requirement for polymer–drug conjugates to reach its activity. Therefore, the ideal linker has to be stable in blood, but readily cleaved at the target site. Meticulous research carried out in the 1980s comparing peptidyl linkers for selective cleavage in the lysosomal compartment led to the development and clinical assessment of (*N*-(2-hydroxypropyl)methacrylamide) HPMA-GFLG-DOX (GFLG = Gly–Phe–Leu–Gly) [69]. These early studies showed that the different peptidyl linker displayed a different release rate. It was also observed that the biodegradability of the linker also depended on the conjugated drug. Indeed, the linker Gly–Gly (GG) is nonbiodegradable when it is designed in the conjugate HPMA-GG-DOX. However, when it is used in the conjugate HPMA-GG-melphalan, the drug release is achieved [70]. In addition, when more than one drug is linked to the carrier, drug release can be clearly affected by the presence of the second bioactive agent, mainly due to changes in hydrophobicity, pH, or conjugate conformation in solution. Also, for conjugates combining more than one agent, relative drug release rate (i.e., which drug is released faster) and sequential drug release (i.e., which drug is released first) can further increase the complexity of the system and become key factors for activity [71].

25.3.3
Loading Capacity

In order to design polymer-based combinations, a multifunctional carrier should be used; ideally, with a loading capacity adequate to ensure delivery of sufficient amount of drugs to the tumor site, which is particularly important if multiagent therapy is used. For instance, cyclodextrins [60], polyacetals [56], or PGA can theoretically carry one drug molecule per monomer and indeed, conjugates based on these platforms have a high drug loading (10 wt% cyclodextrin–CPT [60], 10 wt% poly(1-hydroxymethylene hydroxymethyl formal) (Fleximer®)–CPT (XMT-1001) [56], or 37 wt% PGA–PTX [44]). It is important to note that to achieve an efficient polymer combination system it is required to obtain the best drug ratio that will provide an optimal therapeutic output, whilst maintaining water solubility (www.celatorpharma.com and [50, 69, 72]). In addition to linear polymers, novel branched polymeric architectures that display a good carrying capacity together with other interesting characteristics are also being explored [73, 74].

25.3.4
Correlation of *In Vitro* Studies with Behavior *In Vivo*

The main limitation here is the lack of preclinical models of combination therapy, either *in vitro* (i.e., screening cell models to examine combinations) or *in vivo* models standardized for use with targeted combinations.

Preliminary screening of the anticancer activity of newly synthesized polymer–drug conjugates is normally carried out *in vitro* against cancer cells using standard cell-viability assays. The usefulness of such *in vitro* screening is debatable as polymer–drug conjugates rely on accumulation in the tumor tissue via the EPR effect, which can be observed only *in vivo* models. In addition, and due to the different cell trafficking mechanisms, the free drug is normally more active *in vitro* than the conjugated drug, but *in vivo* studies show the opposite trend [69]. Based on these considerations, the significance of *in vitro* tests and their relevance to predict *in vivo* behavior are difficult issues. Ethical considerations and cost are obvious reasons for favorable use of *in vitro* prescreening, but there are additional advantages, particularly in the case of polymer-based combination therapy:

- *In vitro* testing allows a comparison of the relative activity of different polymer–drug conjugates and the possible benefits of combining two agents within a single drug carrier can be highlighted at this early stage.
- An extensive evaluation of different drug ratios can be carried out, which would not be feasible at a later stage (see also Section 25.3.1).
- Specific experiments can be designed to elucidate the mechanism of action of these systems, including drug release mechanisms and their ability to trigger or block specific cell processes.

25.3.5
Physicochemical Characterization

To achieve a careful physicochemical characterization is one of the main limitations in the development process of these complex macromolecules. For this reason, there is a need to know "what do we have in the bottle" in order to secure transfer to the clinics following the regulatory authority standards. In comparison with small molecules, these systems are intrinsically heterogeneous due to the polydispersity of the polymeric carrier and the randomized conjugation process (although optimization of reaction conditions ensures a good degree of batch-to-batch reproducibility). Consequently, the attachment of a second drug to the same carrier complicates the matter even further. Deemed compulsory (from the regulatory point of view), an adequate physicochemical characterization is somewhat difficult to achieve. More importantly, knowledge of physicochemical parameters can help in understanding the conjugate biological behavior and contribute to the development of rationally designed subsequent generations. An armory of techniques can be employed to properly characterize combination polymer–drug conjugates: (i) covalent attachment of drug to the polymer could be determined by nuclear magnetic resonance (NMR), Fourier-transform IR spectroscopy, and matrix-assisted laser desorption ionization time-of-flight (MALDI-TOF); (ii) total and drug content by high-pressure liquid chromatography and UV spectroscopy; (iii) molecular weight/polydispersity by gel-permeation chromatography, MALDI-TOF, or static light scattering (quasi-elastic light scattering); and (iv) size/conformation of the conjugate in solution including aggregation or supramolecular assemblies by dynamic light scattering or by more sophisticated techniques such as small angle neutron scattering and diffusion NMR techniques [15, 73].

25.3.6
Clinical Development

Transfer of these combination products into the clinic is extremely challenging, since it calls for additional measures to unequivocally prove their clinical benefit. In particular, there is the need to demonstrate that clinical benefits are due to the advanced drug delivery strategy rather than simply the additive/synergistic effects of the parent compounds administered as separate therapeutic entities. In other words, there is the need to demonstrate that the combination of two or more agents within a single delivery system provides advantages over the simple administration of the free drugs. Due to the complexity in designing such clinical trials and the consequent ethical issues, it is envisaged that the development costs for such combination products might be significantly more than the development of current pharmaceutical preparations. However, if the therapeutic output of the developed combination is clinically valuable, it would be always possible to accelerate this process by asking the FDA to recognize the combination compound as a single entity; this is the case for CombiPlex technology (*www.celatorpharma.com*).

25.4
Representative Examples of Polymer–Drug Conjugates for Combination Therapy

Representative examples of each family system are described and classified below following their clinical status. It is important to note that the combination therapy based on polymer–drug conjugate plus free drug (Family I) is already in clinical trials, and Families II–IV are mainly in preclinical status and a few of them are still under early *in vitro* evaluation (Table 25.1 and examples in Figure 25.3).

25.4.1
Preclinical Development

25.4.1.1 *In Vitro* Status

25.4.1.1.1 Family II: Polymer–Drug Conjugate plus Polymer–Drug Conjugate
CPT–PEG–LHRH + CPT–PEG–BH3 Minko *et al.* developed a system based on the combination of a chemotherapeutic drug CPT (topoisomerase I inhibitor), hormonal therapy (LHRH, used as a targeting residue), and the proapoptotic peptide BH3 using poly(ethylene glycol) (PEG) as a carrier [80]. In order to evaluate the best combination, the authors tested free CPT, CPT–PEG, CPT–PEG–BH3, or CPT–PEG–LHRH conjugates and a mixture of CPT–PEG–LHRH and CPT–PEG–BH3 in human ovarian carcinoma cells. *In vitro* results of this study led to an increase of the proapoptotic activity when the combination was CPT–PEG–LHRH plus CPT–PEG–BH3 in the ovarian cell line [81].

25.4.1.1.2 Family III: Single Polymeric Carrier Carrying a Combination of Drugs This family should not be confused with polymer–drug conjugates bearing targeting residues [53] (as described in other chapters in this volume). Only over the last 5 years has a new generation of polymer–drug conjugates been developed based on combinations of two or more drugs covalently linked to the same polymer main-chain. In this case, both agents have a specific therapeutic action, whereas when a targeting moiety is conjugated, it is only used as active homing moiety in order to delivery the conjugate to the specific target site.

HPMA Copolymer–DOX–DEX In 2008, a combination copolymer based on HPMA carrying the anticancer agent DOX (topoisomerase II inhibitor, DNA intercalating agent, and ROS inducer) and the anti-inflammatory agent dexamethasone (DEX) linked by a hydrolytically labile pH-sensitive hydrazone bond was developed (Figure 25.5) [76]. A library of conjugates containing solely DOX, DEX, or the combination of the two with a drug loading ranging from 2 to 6 wt% for DEX and 8 to 9 wt% for DOX was synthesized. The authors studied the physicochemical properties of the newly generated two-drug containing copolymer and its stability under hydrolytic conditions, and consequently its release rates upon activation with carboxyesterases. No differences were observed between the copolymers containing only one drug and the copolymer containing both pharmacologically active agents,

Table 25.1 Summary of polymer–drug conjugates based on combination therapy classified by clinical status.

	Name	Family	Carrier	Drugs	Drug types	References
Preclinical in vitro	CPT–PEG–LHRH + CPT–PEG–BH3	II	PEG	CPT LHRH BH3	chemotherapeutic targeting residue proapoptotic protein	[80, 81]
	HPMA–DOX–DEX	III	HPMA copolymer	DOX DEX	chemotherapeutic anti-inflammatory	[76]
	HPMA–AGM–DOX	III	HPMA copolymer	AGM DOX	endocrine therapy chemotherapeutic	[71, 79]
	PEG–poly(aspartate hydrazide) block copolymer–DOX–WOR	III	PEG–poly(aspartate hydrazide)	DOX WOR	chemotherapeutic phosphotidylinositol-3 kinase inhibitor	[77]
Preclinical in vivo	HPMA copolymer–DOX + HPMA copolymer–Me$_6$	II	HPMA copolymer	DOX Me$_6$	chemotherapeutic phototherapy	[78, 82–83]
	PEG–ZnPP + PEG–DAO	II	PEG	ZnPP DAO	heme oxygenase inhibitor enzyme oxidative chemotherapeutic type	[84]
	HPMA–TNP-470–ALN	III	HPMA copolymer	ALN TNP-470	bone-targeting, antiangiogenic agent antiangiogenic agent	[86, 87–88]

25.4 Representative Examples of Polymer–Drug Conjugates for Combination Therapy

Name	Phase	Polymer	Drugs	Function	Ref.
HPMA–PTX–ALN	III	HPMA copolymer	PTX ALN	chemotherapeutic bone-targeting, antiangiogenic agent	[89–98]
HPMA–GEM–DOX	III	HPMA copolymer	GEM DOX	chemotherapeutic chemotherapeutic	[71, 93]
PEG–NO–EPI	III	PEG	NO EPI	signaling molecule chemotherapeutic	[94–96]
CPT–PEG–LHRH–BH3	III	PEG branched	CPT LHRH BH3	chemotherapeutic targeting residue proapoptotic protein	[80–81, 97]
HPMA copolymer–DOX + HPMA copolymer–cathepsin B	IV	HPMA copolymer	DOX cathepsin B	chemotherapeutic proteolytic enzyme	[75]
HPMA copolymer–DOX + HPMA copolymer–β-lactamase	IV	HPMA copolymer	DOX β-lactamase	chemotherapeutic proteolytic enzyme	[99, 95]
Clinical					
PGA–PTX + cisplatin	Phase I	PGA	PTX cisplatin	chemotherapeutic chemotherapeutic	[100]
PGA–PTX + radiotherapy	Phase I	PGA	PTX radiotherapy	chemotherapeutic radiotherapy	[103]
PGA–PTX + carboplatin	Phase III	PGA	PTX carboplatin	chemotherapeutic chemotherapeutic	[101]

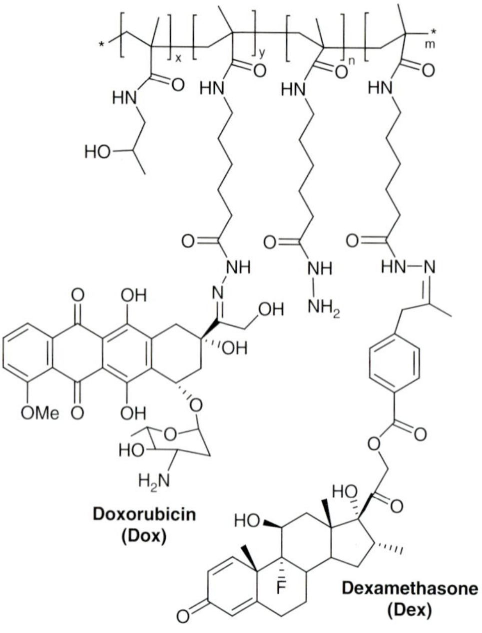

Figure 25.5 Chemical structure of HPMA copolymer–DOX–DEX conjugate (Family III).

indicating that DOX and DEX can be coconjugated to the same HPMA copolymer without affecting their release profiles [76]. Biological studies assessing the activity of the conjugate warranted the therapeutic benefit of this combination.

HPMA Copolymer–AGM–DOX A HPMA copolymer–AGM–DOX conjugate was the first conjugate that combined an endocrine therapy based on aminoglu-thetimine (AGM), which inhibits the aromatase enzyme blocking the estrogen synthesis involved in tumor cell proliferation, and the chemotherapeutic agent DOX [71] (Figure 25.6). The conjugate was determined to carry 5 wt% AGM and 7 wt% DOX, both linked to the HPMA copolymer through the cathepsin B responsive linker GFLG, achieving the uptake via endocytosis and a lysosomotropic drug release [71]. The activity of this conjugate was evaluated *in vitro* against selected breast cancer cell lines. Interestingly, the combination of both agents in the same polymer induced higher cell toxicity than the single conjugates separately or when added together (HPMA–AGM, HPMA–DOX, and HPMA–AGM + HPMA–DOX) [71]. Further studies on the possible molecular mechanisms responsible for synergy with this conjugate suggested that such increased activity of HPMA copolymer–DOX–AGM conjugate could be explained by various factors, including drug release rate, conjugate conformation in solution, and, possibly, activation of certain molecular pathways (induction of apoptosis by down regulation of BCL2 protein) [71, 79]. This conjugate is currently being investigated in an *in vivo* aromatase mouse model (Figure 25.3).

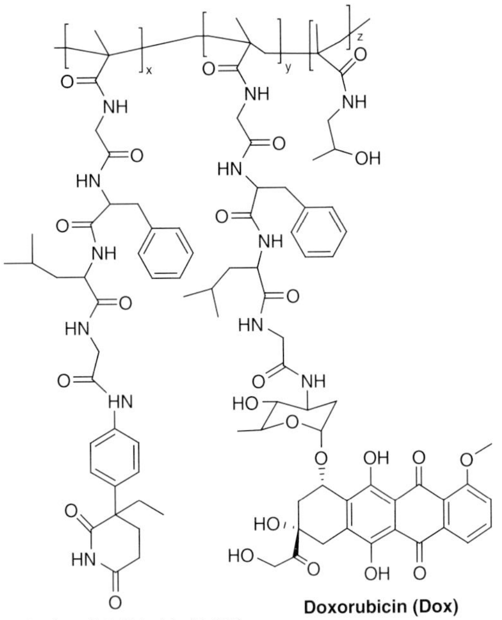

25.4 Representative Examples of Polymer–Drug Conjugates for Combination Therapy | 821

Figure 25.6 Chemical structure of HPMA copolymer–AGM–DOX conjugate (Family III).

PEG–Poly(Aspartate Hydrazide) Block Copolymers–DOX–WOR In another example, Kwon *et al.* developed an interesting system based on polymer–drug conjugates and polymeric micelles [77]. An amphiphilic block copolymer constituted of PEG–poly(aspartate hydrazide) was prepared, and DOX and the phosphatidylinositol-3 kinase inhibitor wortmannin (WOR) were attached alone or in combination, at different drug ratios (Figure 25.7). Physicochemical studies confirmed that the conjugates assembled to form micellar structures. It was observed that the delivery of both agents via the micellar system reduced the amount of drug necessary to elicit biological activity in MCF-7 breast cancer cell line [77].

25.4.1.2 *In Vivo* Status

25.4.1.2.1 Family II: Polymer–Drug Conjugate plus Polymer–Drug Conjugate
HPMA Copolymer–DOX + HPMA Copolymer–Mesochlorin e_6 In the combination of HPMA copolymer–DOX with HPMA copolymer–mesochlorin e_6 (Me$_6$), Me$_6$ acted as a photosensitizer producing ROS and showing more activity than either conjugate alone. An enhancement in the activity was also observed when the antibody OV-TL16 was added for active targeting [78] (Figures 25.3 and 25.8). The therapeutic activity was demonstrated in a N2A neuroblastoma mice model, where the conjugate combination led to a full regression of the tumor. On the contrary, neither the single conjugate or free drugs were able to achieve any effect [82]. Furthermore, in a

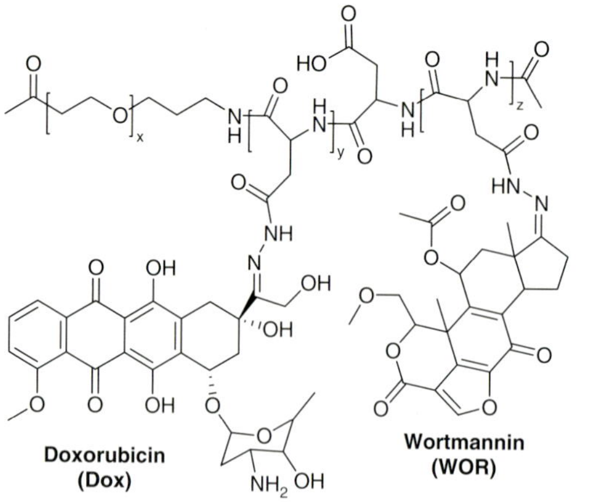

Figure 25.7 PEG–poly(aspartate hydrazide) block copolymer–DOX–WOR conjugate chemical structure (Family III).

very recent study, the same authors demonstrated the efficacy of this strategy by exposing an ovarian carcinoma cell line to sequential administration of two polymer conjugates – HPMA copolymer–SOS (2,5-bis(5-hydroxymethyl-2-thienyl)furan) followed by HPMA copolymer–Me$_6$ monoethylenediamine – and observed a synergistic effect [83].

PEG–ZnPP + PEG–DAO In another study, a new design was developed targeting the heme oxygenase-I enzyme (HO-I), which could be involved in the protection against oxidative stress in the tumor, associated to tumor proliferation (Figure 25.9). To overcome the enzyme action, a PEG–zinc protoporphyrin (ZnPP), described as a potent HO-I inhibitor, followed by PEG–D-amino acid oxidase (DAO) and D-proline acting as an oxidative chemotherapeutic agent, showed a significant inhibition in mice colon carcinoma tumor growth, contrary to each single conjugate [84].

In recent work, Lammers *et al.* demonstrated the synergistic interaction between radiotherapy and chemotherapy [85]. In an example involving two polymer–drug conjugates, HPMA copolymer–DOX and in another case HPMA copolymer–gemcitabine (GEM), the authors proved that radiotherapy can enhance the tumor accumulation of both anticancer agents and that selective drug delivery increased the therapeutic index of the active agent.

25.4.1.2.2 Family III: Single Polymeric Carrier Carrying a Combination of Drugs

HPMA Copolymer–TNP-470–ALN Satchi-Fainaro *et al.* developed the first polymer–drug conjugate containing an antiangiogenic agent, TNP-470 (caplostatin) [86, 87], which is at present under preclinical development by SinDevRx (www.syndevrx.com) for various tumor models (melanoma, glioblastoma, colon, prostate, and lung carcinomas). Building on this single-drug system, the authors subsequently developed a HPMA copolymer containing TNP-470 and the

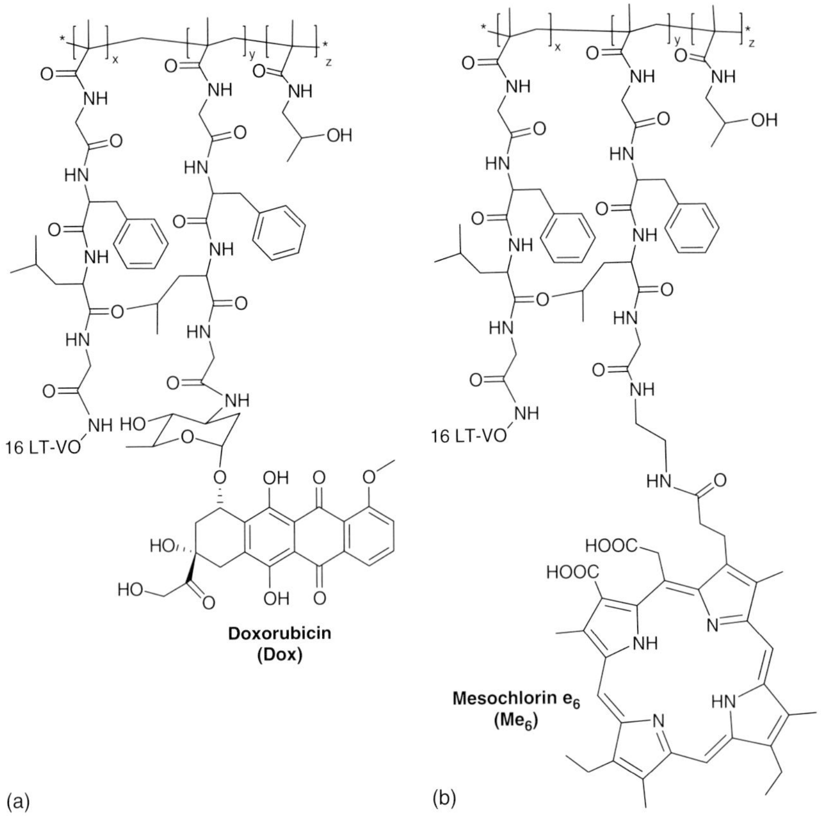

Figure 25.8 Chemical structure of (a) HPMA copolymer–DOX conjugate and (b) HPMA copolymer–Me₆ conjugate (Family II).

aminobisphosphonate alendronate (ALN) (Figure 25.10) [88] in order to establish a novel therapeutic strategy for the treatment of angiogenesis-dependent calcified neoplasms, such as osteosarcomas and bone metastases [88]. In this combination, ALN has the double function of a targeting moiety (to promote bone targeting) and a pharmacologically active agent. *In vitro* studies with this combination conjugate in endothelial cells (human umbilical vein endothelial cells) confirmed its antiangiogenic and antitumor properties, and *in vivo* assessment further strengthened these positive results with almost complete tumor regression observed in a human osteosarcoma model [88].

HPMA Copolymer–PTX–ALN Satchi-Fainaro *et al.* extended the above research by coconjugating the bone-targeting agent ALN and the chemotherapeutic agent PTX, which induces microtubule stabilization, to a single HPMA copolymer (Figure 25.11) [89]. Aside from having potential for bone targeting, ALN has

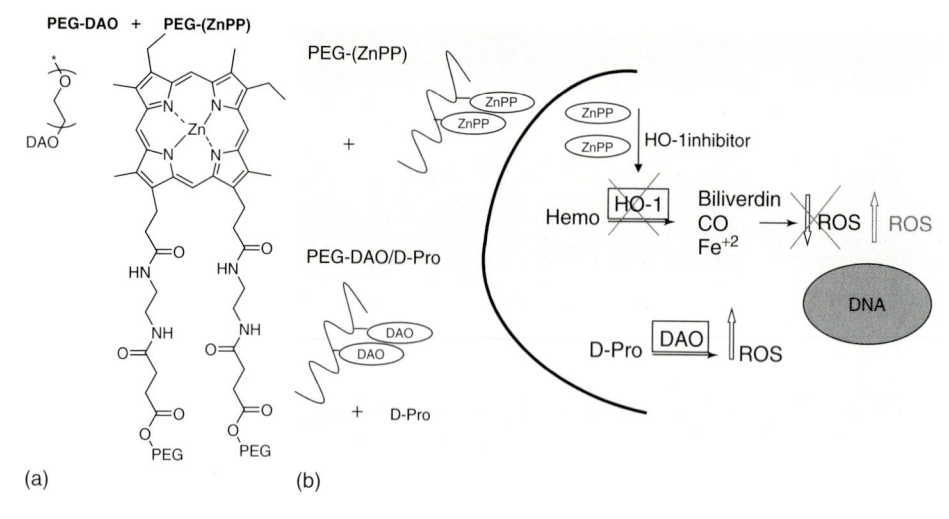

Figure 25.9 Chemical structure and mechanism of action of PEG–ZnPP conjugate + PEG–DAO conjugate (Family II). (a) Chemical structure and (b) *in vivo* mechanism of action, ZnPP inhibits HO-I, increasing ROS production triggering cell death; in addition, D-Pro is used as a substrate for the DAO enzyme in order to enhance ROS release.

also been shown to possess antitumor [90, 91] and antiangiogenic [92] activity, implying that besides being an actively targeted nanomedicine formulation, this construct in principle also delivers two different drugs to tumors simultaneously. *In vitro* evaluation of HPMA copolymer containing both drugs showed an effective binding of the conjugate to the bone mineral hydroxyapatite, along with cytotoxic and antiangiogenic properties against prostate and breast cancer cells, suggesting promising therapeutic applications for bone metastasis [89].

HPMA Copolymer–GEM–DOX Following the previous studies in regard to the potential of polymer-based multidrug targeting [71], one conjugate based on HPMA copolymer carrying two chemotherapeutic drugs – GEM (acting on DNA replication) and DOX – was assessed for the first time *in vivo* and proved able to deliver the two drugs to the tumor tissue (Figure 25.12) [93]. When tested in a tumor rat model, the combination conjugate HPMA copolymer–GEM–DOX was more active than the combination of two polymer conjugates each carrying a single drug and even more than the combination of the free drugs. The initial analyses looking for the mechanism of action of HPMA copolymer–GEM–DOX indicated that both angiogenesis and apoptosis-related processes contribute to its improved *in vivo* efficacy.

PEG–NO–EPI Branched PEG was used to combine the chemotherapeutic agent epirubicin (EPI) (topoisomerase II inhibitor, DNA intercalating agent, and ROS

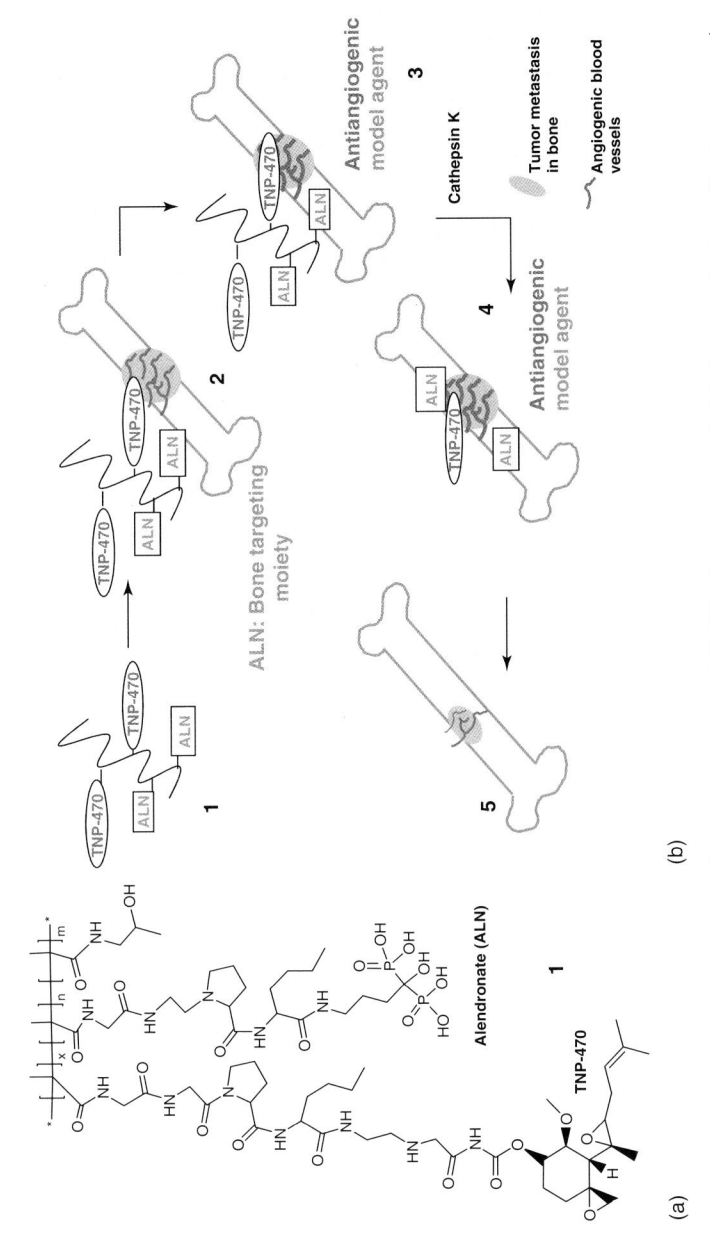

Figure 25.10 (a) Chemical structure of HPMA copolymer–TNP-470–ALN conjugate. (b) Mechanism of action: (1) intravenous administration of HPMA copolymer–TNP-470–ALN conjugate (TNP-470, antiangiogenic agent; ALN, targeting moiety and antiangiogenic agent); (2) ALN targets bone; (3) presence of cathepsin B and cathepsin K enzymes the triggers TNP-470 and ALN release; (4) TNP-470 and ALN act as antiangiogenic drugs; and, consequently, (5) angiogenic blood vessels are diminished, inducing tumor disappearance.

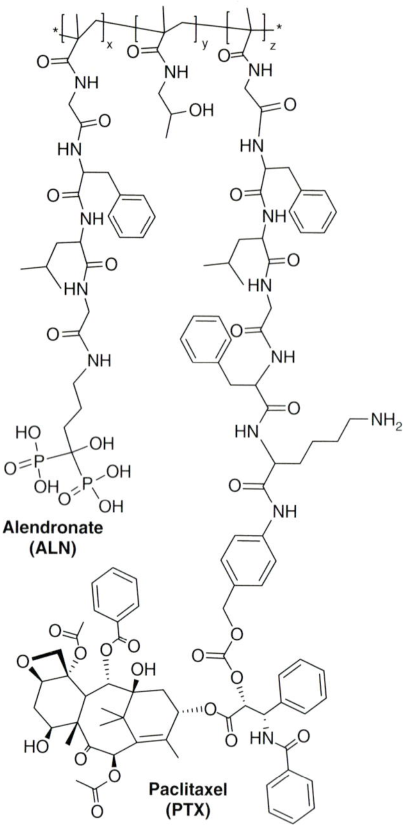

Figure 25.11 Chemical structure of HPMA copolymer–PTX–ALN conjugate (Family III).

inducer) with nitric oxide (NO) – a diffusible messenger with vasodilator properties (Figure 25.13). To enhance the classical PEG-loading capacity, the authors elegantly developed this conjugate by building a dendronized structure to one polymer chain end [94, 95]. This strategy allowed them to significantly increase NO loading (up to eight molecules per chain) as well as to obtain two chemically distinct termini (a carboxylic acid used for NO conjugation and a hydroxyl group to conjugate EPI). By modulating the presence of ROS, NO can control the pro- and antiapoptotic properties of chemotherapeutic agents. In cancer cells, anthracyclines, such as EPI, and the diffusible messenger NO can act synergistically [94]. The presence of NO in the conjugate is able to counterbalance EPI-induced cardiotoxicity, as already demonstrated in cardiomyocytes and in an *in vivo* mouse model [94, 96]. *In vivo* studies in a model for colon adenocarcinoma also confirmed that the PEG–EPI–NO conjugate displayed anticancer activity [96]. Conjugation of both agents onto a single chain ensures that they undergo the same body distribution, thus maximizing the benefits of this combination.

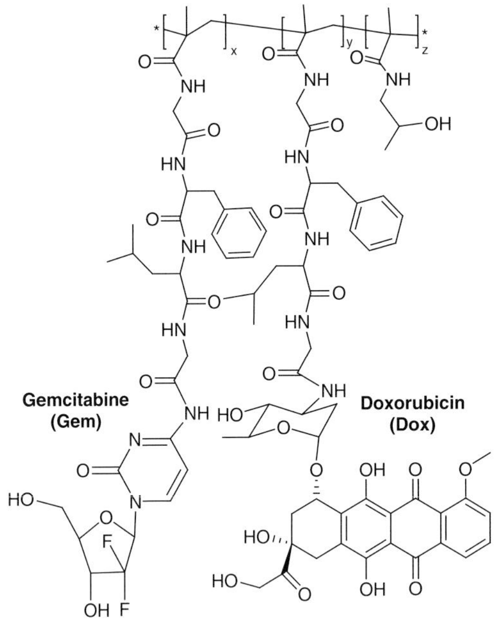

25.4 Representative Examples of Polymer–Drug Conjugates for Combination Therapy | 827

Figure 25.12 Chemical structure of HPMA copolymer–GEM–DOX conjugate (Family III).

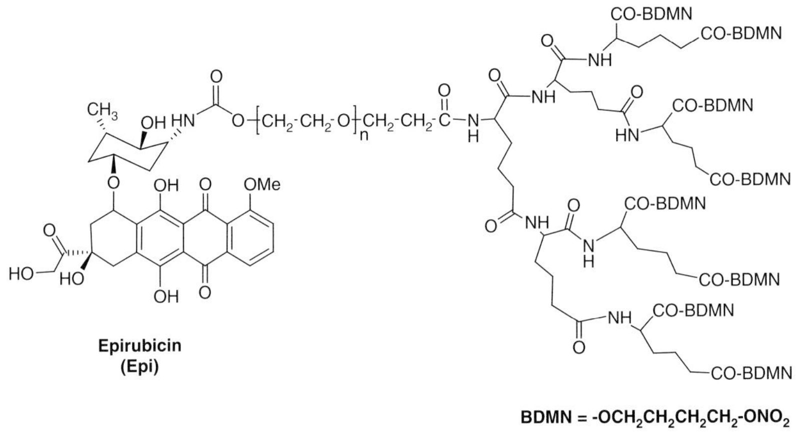

Figure 25.13 Chemical structure of PEG–(NO)$_8$–EPI conjugate (Family III).

CPT–PEG–LHRH–BH3 By means of a branched PEG carrier, Minko *et al.* moved a step further with a proapoptotic BH3-based PEG conjugate previously described by conjugating the three components in the same main-chain [80]. A six-branched PEG conjugate containing equimolecular amounts of CPT, BH3, and LHRH was therefore synthesized. *In vitro* studies showed that such multicomponent conjugate was almost 100 times more cytotoxic than the single parent compounds. Even more

CPT-PEG-LHRH-BH3

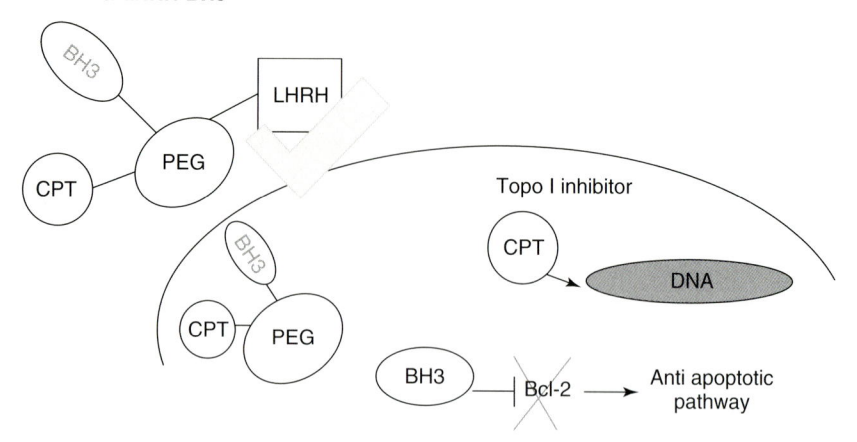

Figure 25.14 *In vivo* mechanism of action of CPT–PEG–LHRH–BH3 conjugate (Family III).

important is that the combination conjugate displayed enhanced antitumor activity *in vivo* when compared with single monotherapy (Figure 25.14) [81, 97].

25.4.1.2.3 Family IV: PDEPT and PELT

PDEPT is a two-component strategy based on polymer conjugates. In this approach, a polymer–drug conjugate is combined with a polymer–enzyme conjugate [98] with the aim of achieving selective release of the drug at the tumor site. Indeed, the linker binding the drug to the polymer in the first conjugate is designed to be degraded by the enzyme of the second conjugate. In this case, administration of a polymer–enzyme conjugate ensured appropriate drug release from the polymer–drug conjugate at the tumor site, independently from the endocytosis rate and the intracellular trafficking mechanisms (Figures 25.3 and 25.4).

HPMA Copolymer–DOX + HPMA Copolymer–Cathepsin B The idea of this combination is to ensure the cathepsin B activity requires to trigger DOX release. In this way, the constitutive lysosomal cathepsin B was enhanced by the presence of HPMA copolymer–cathepsin B, yielding a better degradation of the linker and thus drug release rate. Preclinical results confirmed that the HPMA–cathepsin B was able to trigger DOX release in animal models, with an area under the curve almost 4-fold higher than that obtained with HPMA copolymer–DOX alone (Figure 25.4) [75].

HPMA Copolymer–DOX + HPMA Copolymer–β-Lactamase With regard to the combination of HPMA copolymer–DOX with HPMA copolymer–β-lactamase, the same principle based on the PDEPT strategy was applied. Here, DOX was linked to HPMA via a GG-cephalosporin linker sensitive to the nonmammalian β-lactamase [99]. In this study, mice treated with the current combination showed an increase of survival rate and decreased tumor growth compared to the control. Whilst lower toxicity was observed, the immune response was considered to be an issue due to the use of nonhuman protein [95].

25.4.2
Clinical Development

25.4.2.1 Family I: Polymer–Drug Conjugate plus Free Drug

As anticancer schedules routinely involve the administration of drug combinations (discussed in Section 25.1.1), the evaluation in the clinics of polymer–drug conjugates in combination with free drugs or other type of therapies is a logical step to undertake.

25.4.2.1.1 PGA–PTX + Cisplatin and PGA–PTX + Carboplatin Clinical studies are being developed with PGA–PTX conjugates in combination with different platinates (DNA alkylating agent). Several phase I studies have been already performed in order to determine the toxicity, MTD, and pharmacokinetics. For instance, a phase I study was assessed on 43 patients with advanced solid tumors combining a fixed dose of cisplatin (75 mg/m^2) with increasing doses of PGA–PTX and demonstrated that this combination had good activity in refractory patients [100]. In a second phase I study carried out on 22 patients with advanced solid tumors testing the combination of Opaxio® with carboplatin [101], the previous responses were observed with the MTD of 225 mg/ml. Similarly, partial responses were observed in patients who had previously failed PTX therapy. After these promising results with phase I–II trials, a phase III clinical trial named STELLAR 3 was developed on 400 patients with NSCLC cancer. Results showed that although there was no improvement in patient survival, the combination containing the conjugate was less toxic [101]. However, the design to evaluate and compare Opaxio plus carboplatin against PTX plus carboplatin was very poor. Furthermore, based on previous results suggesting that the anticancer activity of poliglumex might be affected by estrogen levels, a new clinical trial was developed by Cell Therapeutics involving female patients with advanced NSCLC and baseline estradiol greater than 25 pg/ml, again comparing carboplatin with Opaxio or with PTX (*http://www.celltherapeutics.com/opaxio*). Nevertheless, since no comparisons were done against the conjugates alone, the added therapeutic value of such combination compared to monotherapy is difficult to quantify.

25.4.2.1.2 PGA–PTX + Estradiol As mentioned above, the anticancer effect of Opaxio could be affected by estrogen levels due to its cross-talk mechanisms with the expression of cathepsin B. Based on this observation, very recently a phase II study of PPX in combination with transdermal estradiol for the treatment of metastatic castration-resistant prostate cancer after docetaxel chemotherapy was designed. However, this regimen of low-dose transdermal estradiol induction followed by PGA–PTX did not show activity in taxane pretreated patients with castration-resistant prostate cancer [102].

25.4.2.1.3 PGA–PTX + Radiotherapy As chemotherapy and radiotherapy (DNA damage therapy) are often combined in clinical practice, a singular but promising approach in cancer therapy is the use of polymer–drug conjugates combined with radiotherapy (Figure 25.3). Polymer–drug conjugates are known to passively accumulate in the tumor tissue as a result of the leaky tumor vasculature (EPR effect) [43]. Ideally, radiotherapy impacts on tumor vasculature, possibly magnifying the EPR effect, which makes the combination of radiotherapy with a polymer–drug conjugate extremely interesting. An illustrative case could be PGA–PTX and radiotherapy, which were involved in a phase I study assessed on 21 patients with esophageal and gastric cancer. The aim of this trial was to establish the safety and MTD of this combination, which was found to be 80 mg/m^2. Additional analysis included an absolute clinical response in 33% of patients with locoregional disease [103]. Opaxio is one of the most potent radiation sensitizers reported in the literature, selectively increasing tumor sensitivity to radiation up to 8- to 10-fold in animal models and increasing activity when radiotherapy was given as a treatment before polymer–drug conjugates, and has already been reported in early clinical trials [103].

In November 2010, Cell Therapeutics announced the preliminary results of a phase II study of Opaxio combined with a chemotherapy drug called temozolomide (TMZ) and radiotherapy in patients with newly diagnosed high-grade gliomas. This combination has so far demonstrated high response rates (76%) with encouraging 6-month progression-free survival in malignant brain cancer [54]. The successful molecular mechanisms of action of this improvement are currently being explored, mainly looking at the possibility of Opaxio to bypass O^6-methylguanine-DNA methyltransferase (MGMT) tumor resistance. (MGMT is an enzyme overexpressed in most glioblastoma patients that removes alkylating agents from DNA, thus preventing their DNA-damaging effect.)

25.5
Conclusions and Perspectives

The complex genetics of cancer and the intratumor heterogeneity of the tumor tissue are considered to be major reasons for the low treatment efficacy and the development of chemoresistance when using classical approaches. The application of combination therapy has already demonstrated clinical benefits in that respect. However, there are still major issues to overcome, such as the control of individual drug metabolism that could induce the loss of the combination concept and may negatively impact the effectiveness.

The use of drug delivery systems offers the opportunity to ensure delivery of a drug combination to the same target site whilst maintaining the originally designed synergistic ratio. Moreover, the use of polymer conjugates as drug delivery systems could also offer the possibility to modulate intracellular pharmacokinetics due to the presence of rationally designed bioresponsive polymer–drug(s) linkers. This fact, together with the successful development of first-generation polymer–drug conjugates as anticancer agents, has inspired more recent studies assessing their potential as drug delivery platforms for combination therapy. These early works unveiled therapeutic benefits, but raised new challenges, in particular regarding the complex design and characterization. A better understanding of how drug combinations impact upon cellular and molecular mechanisms is required to rationally design new therapeutics.

Acknowledgments

This work was supported by grants from Ministerio de Ciencia e Innovación (CTQ-2007-60601, FPI grant BES-2008-006801) and Fundacion de la Comunidad Valenciana Centro de Investigación Príncipe Felipe. R.L. is a FIS researcher and M.J.V. is a Ramon y Cajal researcher. The authors have no other relevant affiliations or financial involvement with any organization or entity with a financial interest in or financial conflict with the subject matter or materials discussed in the manuscript apart from those disclosed.

References

1. Broxterman, H.J. and Georgopapadakou, N.H. (2005) Anticancer therapeutics: "addictive" targets, multi-targeted drugs, new drug combinations. *Drug Resist. Updat.*, **8**, 183–197.
2. Batist, G., Gelmon, K.A., Chi, K.N., Miller, W.H. Jr., Chia, S.K., Mayer, L.D., Swenson, C.E., Janoff, A.S., and Louie, A.C. (2009) Safety, pharmacokinetics, and efficacy of CPX-1 liposome injection in patients with advanced solid tumors. *Clin. Cancer Res.*, **15**, 692–700.
3. Tardi, P., Johnstone, S., Harasym, N., Xie, S., Harasym, T., Zisman, N., Harvie, P., Bermudes, D., and Mayer, L. (2009) *In vivo* maintenance of synergistic cytarabine:daunorubicin ratios greatly enhances therapeutic efficacy. *Leuk. Res.*, **33**, 129–139.
4. Greco, F. and Vicent, M.J. (2008) Polymer–drug conjugates: current status and future trends. *Front. Biosci.*, **13**, 2744–2756.
5. Lammers, T. (2010) Improving the efficacy of combined modality anticancer therapy using HPMA copolymer-based nanomedicine formulations. *Adv. Drug Deliv. Rev.*, **62**, 203–230.
6. Friedland, M.L. (1992) in *The Chemotherapy Source Book* (ed. M.E. Perry) Combination cheuotherapy, Williams & Wilkins, Baltimore, MD, pp. 90–96.
7. Rampino, M., Ricardi, U., Munoz, F., Reali, A., Barone, C., Musu, A.R., Balcet, V., Franco, P., Grillo, R., Bustreo, S., Pecorari, G., Cavalot, A., Garzino Demo, P., Ciuffreda, L., Ragona, R., and Schena, M. (2011) Concomitant adjuvant chemoradiotherapy with weekly low-dose cisplatin for high-risk squamous cell carcinoma of the head and neck: a phase II prospective trial. *Clin. Oncol. (R. Coll. Radiol.)*, **23**, 134–40.
8. Gulley, J.L., Arlen, P.M., Bastian, A., Morin, S., Marte, J., Beetham, P., Tsang, K.Y., Yokokawa, J., Hodge, J.W., Menard, C., Camphausen, K., Coleman, C.N., Sullivan, F., Steinberg, S.M., Schlom, J., and Dahut, W. (2005) Combining a recombinant cancer vaccine with standard definitive radiotherapy in patients with localized prostate cancer. *Clin. Cancer Res.*, **11**, 3353–3362.
9. Chakraborty, M., Abrams, S.I., Coleman, C.N., Camphausen, K.,

Schlom, J., and Hodge, J.W. (2004) External beam radiation of tumors alters phenotype of tumor cells to render them susceptible to vaccine-mediated T-cell killing. *Cancer Res.*, **64**, 4328–4337.

10. Hortobagyi, G.N. (2002) The status of breast cancer management: challenges and opportunities. *Breast Cancer Res. Treat.*, **75** (Suppl. 1), S57–S65.

11. Tanabe, M., Ito, Y., Tokudome, N., Sugihara, T., Miura, H., Takahashi, S., Seto, Y., Iwase, T., and Hatake, K. (2009) Possible use of combination chemotherapy with mitomycin C and methotrexate for metastatic breast cancer pretreated with anthracycline and taxanes. *Breast Cancer*, **12**, 1–6.

12. Muggia, F. (2009) Platinum compounds 30 years after the introduction of cisplatin: implications for the treatment of ovarian cancer. *Gynecol. Oncol.*, **112**, 275–281.

13. Berhoune, M., Banu, E., Scotte, F., Prognon, P., Oudard, S., and Bonan, B. (2008) Therapeutic strategy for treatment of metastatic non-small cell lung cancer. *Ann. Pharmacother.*, **42**, 1640–1652.

14. Honecker, F., Kollmannsberger, C., Quietzsch, D., Haag, C., Schroeder, M., Spott, C., Hartmann, J.T., Baronius, W., Hempel, V., Kanz, L., and Bokemeyer, C. (2002) Phase II study of weekly paclitaxel plus 24-h continuous infusion 5-fluorouracil, folinic acid and 3-weekly cisplatin for the treatment of patients with advanced gastric cancer. *Anti-Cancer Drugs*, **13**, 497–503.

15. Greco, F. and Vicent, M.J. (2009) Combination therapy: opportunities and challenges for polymer–drug conjugates as anticancer nanomedicines. *Adv. Drug Deliv. Rev.*, **61**, 1203–1213.

16. Akeson, M., Zetterqvist, B.M., Dahllof, K., Brannstrom, M., and Horvath, G. (2008) Effect of adjuvant paclitaxel and carboplatin for advanced stage epithelial ovarian cancer: a population-based cohort study of all patients in western Sweden with long-term follow-up. *Acta Obstet. Gynecol. Scand.*, **87**, 1343–1352.

17. Jordan, V.C. (2006) Tamoxifen (ICI46,474) as a targeted therapy to treat and prevent breast cancer. *Br. J. Pharmacol.*, **147**, S269–S276.

18. Jordan, V.C. and Brodie, A.M. (2007) Development and evolution of therapies targeted to the estrogen receptor for the treatment and prevention of breast cancer. *Steroids*, **72**, 7–25.

19. Pearson, O.H., Hubay, C.A., Gordon, N.H., Marshall, J.S., Crowe, J.P., Arafah, B.M., and McGuire, W. (1989) Endocrine versus endocrine plus five-drug chemotherapy in postmenopausal women with stage II estrogen receptor-positive breast cancer. *Cancer*, **64**, 1819–1823.

20. Wang, B., Rosano, J.M., Cheheltani, R., Achary, M.P., and Kiani, M.F. (2010) Towards a targeted multi-drug delivery approach to improve therapeutic efficacy in breast cancer. *Expert Opin. Drug Deliv.*, **7**, 1159–1173.

21. Logman, J.F., Heeg, B.M., Botteman, M.F., Kaura, S., and Van Hout, B.A. (2008) Economic evaluation of zoledronic acid for the prevention of fractures in postmenopausal women with early-stage breast cancer receiving aromatase inhibitors in the united kingdom. ASCO Breast Cancer Symposium, Washington, DC, p. 177.

22. Gnant, M., Mlineritsch, B., Schippinger, W., Luschin-Ebengreuth, G., Poestlberger, S., Menzel, C., Jakesz, R., Kubista, E., Marth, C., and Greil, R. (2008) Adjuvant ovarian suppression combined with tamoxifen or anastrozole, alone or in combination with zoledronic acid, in premenopausal women with hormone-responsible, stage I and II breast cancer: first efficacy results from ABCSG-12. *J. Clin. Oncol.*, **26**, (Suppl. 18 II), LBA4.

23. Gnant, M., Mlineritsch, B., Luschin-Ebengreuth, G., Kainberger, F., Kassmann, H., Piswanger-Solkner, J.C., Seifert, M., Ploner, F., Menzel, C., Dubsky, P., Fitzal, F., Bjelic-Radisic, V., Steger, G., Greil, R., Marth, C., Kubista, E., Samonigg, H., Wohlmuth, P., Mittlbock, M., and Jakesz, R. (2008) Adjuvant endocrine therapy plus zoledronic acid in premenopausal women with early-stage breast cancer: 5-year follow-up of the ABCSG-12

bone-mineral density substudy. *Lancet Oncol.*, **9**, 840–849.
24. Shapiro, C.L., Halabi, S., Gibson, G., Weckstein, D.J., Kirshner, J., Sikov, W.M., Winer, E.P., Hudis, C.A., Isaacs, C., Weckstein, D., Schilsky, R.L., and Paskett, E. (2008) Effect of zoledronic acid (ZA) on bone mineral density (BMD) in premenopausal women who develop ovarian failure (OF) due to adjuvant chemotherapy (Adc): first result from CALGB trial 79809. *J. Clin. Oncol.*, **26** (Suppl. 18 II), 512.
25. Nielson, J.B. (2007) in *Campbell Walsh – Urology*, 9th edn (eds A.J. Wein, L.R. Kavoussi, A.C. Novick, A.W. Partin, and C.A. Peters) hormone-therapy for prostate cancer. Saunders Elsevier, Philadelphia, PA, pp. 3082–3100.
26. Moul, J.W. and Chodak, G. (2004) Combination hormonal therapy: a reassessment within advanced prostate cancer. *Prostate Cancer Prostatic Dis.*, **7** (Suppl. 1), S2–7.
27. Itsieh, A.C. and Ryan, C.J. (2008) Novel concepts in androgen receptor blockade. *Cancer J.*, **14**, 11–14.
28. Bolla, M., Fourneret, P., Beneyton, V., Tessier, A., Jover, F., and Verry, C. (2010) Combination of external irradiation and androgen suppression for prostate cancer: facts and questions. *Cancer Radiother.*, **14**, 510–514.
29. Kummar, S., Chen, H.X., Wright, J., Holbeck, S., Millin, M.D., Tomaszewski, J., Zweibel, J., Collins, J., and Doroshow, J.H. (2010) Utilizing targeted cancer therapeutic agents in combination: novel approaches and urgent requirements. *Nat. Rev. Drug Discov.*, **9**, 843–856.
30. Metro, G., Mottolese, M., and Fabi, A. (2008) HER-2-positive metastatic breast cancer: trastuzumab and beyond. *Expert Opin. Pharmacother.*, **9**, 2583–2601.
31. Bharthuar, A., Egloff, L., Becker, J., George, M., Lohr, J.W., Deeb, G., and Iyer, R.V. (2009) Rituximab-based therapy for gemcitabine-induced hemolytic uremic syndrome in a patient with metastatic pancreatic adenocarcinoma: a case report. *Cancer Chemother. Pharmacol.*, **64**, 177–181.
32. Van Poppel, H. (2009) Treatment of advanced and metastatic renal cancer: a revolution? *Eur. Urol.*, Suppl. 8, 483–488.
33. Rugo, H.S. (2004) Bevacizumab in the treatment of breast cancer: rationale and current data. *Oncologist*, **9** (Suppl. 1), 43–49.
34. Miller, K., Wang, M., Gralow, J., Dickler, M., Cobleigh, M., Perez, E.A., Shenkier, T., Cella, D., and Davidson, N.E. (2007) Paclitaxel plus bevacizumab versus paclitaxel alone for metastatic breast cancer. *N. Engl. J. Med.*, **357**, 2666–2676.
35. Jones, D. (2009) Avastin–Tarceva combination fails in lung cancer. *Nat. Biotechnol.*, **27**, 108–109.
36. Lane, D. (2006) Designer combination therapy for cancer. *Nat. Biotechnol.*, **24**, 163–164.
37. Adams, G.P. and Weiner, L.M. (2005) Monoclonal antibody therapy of cancer. *Nat. Biotechnol.*, **23**, 1147–1157.
38. Abu Ajaj, K. and Kratz, F. (2009) Development of dual-acting prodrugs for circumventing multidrug resistance. *Bioorg. Med. Chem. Lett.*, **19**, 995–1000.
39. Abu Ajaj, K., Biniossek, M., and Kratz, F. (2009) Development of protein-binding bifunctional spacers for a new generation of dual-acting prodrugs. *Bioconjug. Chem.*, **20**, 390–396.
40. Teesalu, T., Sugahara, K.N., Kotamraju, V.R., and Ruoslahti, E. (2009) C-end rule peptides mediate neuropilin-1-dependent cell, vascular, and tissue penetration. *Proc. Natl. Acad. Sci. USA*, **106**, 16157–16162.
41. Sugahara, K.N., Teesalu, T., Karmali, P.P., Kotamraju, V.R., Agemy, L., Girard, O.M., Hanahan, D., Mattrey, R.F., and Ruoslahti, E. (2009) Tissue-penetrating delivery of compounds and nanoparticles into tumors. *Cancer Cell*, **16**, 510–520.
42. Sugahara, K.N., Teesalu, T., Karmali, P.P., Kotamraju, V.R., Agemy, L., Greenwald, D.R., and Ruoslahti, E. (2010) Coadministration of a

tumor-penetrating peptide enhances the efficacy of cancer drugs. *Science*, **328**, 1031–1035.
43. Maeda, H. (1994) in *Polymeric Site-Specific Pharmacotherapy*, polymers drugs in the clinical stage. John Wiley & Sons, Ltd, Chichester, pp. 96–116.
44. Vasey, P.A., Kaye, S.B., Morrison, R., Twelves, C., Wilson, P., Duncan, R., Thomson, A.H., Murray, L.S., Hilditch, T.E., Murray, T., Burtles, S., Fraier, D., Frigerio, E., and Cassidy, J. (1999) Phase I clinical and pharmacokinetic study of PK1 [N-(2-hydroxypropyl)methacrylamide copolymer doxorubicin]: first member of a new class of chemotherapeutic agents–drug–polymer conjugates. Cancer Research Campaign Phase I/II Committee. *Clin. Cancer Res.*, **5**, 83–94.
45. Meerum Terwogt, J.M., Ten Bokkel Huinink, W.W., Schellens, J.H.M., Schot, M., Mandjes, I., Zurlo, M., Rocchetti, M., Rosing, H., and Beijnen, K.J.H. (2001) Phase I clinical and pharmacokinetic study of PNU166945, a novel water soluble polymer conjugated prodrug of paclitaxel. *Anticancer Drugs Des.*, **12**, 315–323.
46. Minko, T., Kopeckova, P., Pozharov, V., and Kopecek, J. (1998) HPMA copolymer bound adriamycin overcomes MDR1 gene encoded resistance in a human ovarian carcinoma cell line. *J. Control. Release*, **54**, 223–233.
47. Rihova, B., Strohalm, J., Prausova, J., Kubackova, K., Jelinkova, M., Rozprimova, L., Sirova, M., Plocova, D., Etrych, T., Subr, V., Mrkvan, T., Kovar, M., and Ulbrich, K. (2003) Cytostatic and immunomobilizing activities of polymer-bound drugs: experimental and first clinical data. *J. Control. Release*, **91**, 1–16.
48. Sirova, M., Strohalm, J., Subr, V., Plocova, D., Rossmann, P., Mrkvan, T., Ulbrich, K., and Rihova, B. (2007) Treatment with HPMA copolymer-based doxorubicin conjugate containing human immunoglobulin induces long-lasting systemic anti-tumour immunity in mice. *Cancer Immunol. Immunother.*, **56**, 35–47.
49. Vicent, M.J., Ringsdorf, H., and Duncan, R. (2009) Polymer therapeutics: clinical applications and challenges for development. *Adv. Drug Deliv. Rev.*, **61**, 1117–1120.
50. Singer, J.W., Shaffer, S., Baker, B., Bernareggi, A., Stromatt, S., Nienstedt, D., and Besman, M. (2005) Paclitaxel poliglumex (XYOTAX; CT-2103): an intracellularly targeted taxane. *Anti-Cancer Drugs*, **16**, 243–254.
51. Darcy, K.M. and Birrer, M.J. (2010) Translational research in the Gynecologic Oncology Group: evaluation of ovarian cancer markers, profiles, and novel therapies. *Gynecol. Oncol.*, **117**, 429–439.
52. Chipman, S.D., Oldham, F.B., Pezzoni, G., and Singer, J.W. (2006) Biological and clinical characterization of paclitaxel poliglumex (PPX, CT-2103), a macromolecular polymer–drug conjugate. *Int. J. Nanomed.*, **1**, 375–383.
53. Seymour, L.W., Ferry, D.R., Anderson, D., Hesslewood, S., Julyan, P.J., Poyner, R., Doran, J., Young, A.M., Burtles, S., and Kerr, D.J. (2002) Hepatic drug targeting: phase I evaluation of polymer-bound doxorubicin. *J. Clin. Oncol.*, **20**, 1668–1676.
54. Seymour, L.W., Ferry, D.R., Kerr, D.J., Rea, D., Whitlock, M., Poyner, R., Boivin, C., Hesslewood, S., Twelves, C., Blackie, R., Schatzlein, A., Jodrell, D., Bissett, D., Calvert, H., Lind, M., Robbins, A., Burtles, S., Duncan, R., and Cassidy, J. (2009) Phase II studies of polymer–doxorubicin (PK1, FCE28068) in the treatment of breast, lung and colorectal cancer. *Int. J. Oncol.*, **34**, 1629–1636.
55. Danhauser-Riedl, S., Hausmann, E., Schick, H.D., Bender, R., Dietzfelbinger, H., Rastetter, J., and Hanauske, A.R. (1993) Phase I clinical and pharmacokinetic trial of dextran conjugated doxorubicin (AD-70, DOX-OXD). *Invest. New Drugs*, **11**, 187–195.
56. Yurkovetskiy, A.V. and Fram, R.J. (2009) XMT-1001, a novel polymeric

camptothecin pro-drug in clinical development for patients with advanced cancer. *Adv. Drug Deliv. Rev.*, **61**, 1193–1202.

57. Schluep, T., Hwang, J., Cheng, J., Heidel, J.D., Bartlett, D.W., Hollister, B., and Davis, M.E. (2006) Preclinical efficacy of the camptothecin–polymer conjugate IT-101 in multiple cancer models. *Clin. Cancer Res.*, **12**, 1606–1614.

58. Bissett, D., Cassidy, J., de Bono, J.S., Muirhead, F., Main, M., Robson, L., Fraier, D., Magne, M.L., Pellizzoni, C., Porro, M.G., Spinelli, R., Speed, W., and Twelves, C. (2004) Phase I and pharmacokinetic (PK) study of MAG–CPT (PNU 166148): a polymeric derivative of camptothecin (CPT). *Br. J. Cancer*, **91**, 50–55.

59. Soepenberg, O., de Jonge, M.J., Sparreboom, A., de Bruin, P., Eskens, F.A., de Heus, G., Wanders, J., Cheverton, P., Ducharme, M.P., and Verweij, J. (2005) Phase I and pharmacokinetic study of DE-310 in patients with advanced solid tumors. *Clin. Cancer Res.*, **11**, 703–711.

60. Davis, M.E. (2009) Design and development of IT-101, a cyclodextrin-containing polymer conjugate of camptothecin. *Adv. Drug Deliv. Rev.*, **61**, 1189–1192.

61. Li, C., Yu, D.F., Newman, R.A., Cabral, F., Stephens, L.C., Hunter, N., Milas, L., and Wallace, S. (1998) Complete regression of well-established tumors using a novel water-soluble poly(L-glutamic acid)–paclitaxel conjugate. *Cancer Res.*, **58**, 2404–2409.

62. Rademaker-Lakhai, J.M., van den Bongard, D., Pluim, D., Beijnen, J.H., and Schellens, J.H. (2004) A Phase I and pharmacological study with imidazolium-*trans*-DMSO-imidazole-tetrachlororuthenate, a novel ruthenium anticancer agent. *Clin. Cancer Res.*, **10**, 3717–3727.

63. Nowotnik, D.P. and Cvitkovic, E. (2009) ProLindac (AP5346): a review of the development of an HPMA DACH platinum polymer therapeutic. *Adv. Drug Deliv. Rev.*, **61**, 1214–1219.

64. Duncan, R. (2009) Development of HPMA copolymer–anticancer conjugates: clinical experience and lessons learnt. *Adv. Drug Deliv. Rev.*, **61**, 1131–1148.

65. Rihova, B. (2009) Clinical experience with anthracycline antibiotics–HPMA copolymer–human immunoglobulin conjugates. *Adv. Drug Deliv. Rev.*, **61**, 1149–1158.

66. Duncan, R. (2003) The dawning era of polymer therapeutics. *Nat. Rev. Drug Discov.*, **2**, 347–360.

67. Haag, R. and Kratz, F. (2006) Polymer therapeutics: concepts and applications. *Angew. Chem. Int. Ed. Engl.*, **45**, 1198–1215.

68. Mayer, L.D. and Janoff, A.S. (2007) Optimizing combination chemotherapy by controlling drug ratios. *Mol. Interv.*, **7**, 216–223.

69. Duncan, R. (2005) in *Polymeric Drug Delivery System, N-(2 hydroxypropyl) methacrylamide copolymer conjugates* (ed. G.S. Kwon), Dekker, New York, pp. 1–92.

70. Duncan, R., Hume, I.C., Yardley, H.J., Flanagan, P.A., Ulbrich, K., Subr, V., and Strohalm, J. (1991) Macromolecular prodrugs for use in targeted cancer chemotherapy: melphalan covalently coupled to N-(2-hydroxypropyl) methacrylamide copolymers. *J. Control. Release*, **16**, 121–136.

71. Vicent, M.J., Greco, F., Nicholson, R.I., Paul, A., Griffiths, P.C., and Duncan, R. (2005) Polymer therapeutics designed for a combination therapy of hormone-dependent cancer. *Angew. Chem. Int. Ed. Engl.*, **44**, 4061–4066.

72. Bhatt, R., de Vries, P., Tulinsky, J., Bellamy, G., Baker, B., Singer, J.W., and Klein, P. (2003) Synthesis and *in vivo* antitumor activity of poly(L-glutamic acid) conjugates of 20S-camptothecin. *J. Med. Chem.*, **46**, 190–193.

73. Vicent, M.J., Dieudonne, L., Carbajo, R.J., and Pineda-Lucena, A. (2008) Polymer conjugates as therapeutics: future trends, challenges and opportunities. *Expert Opin. Drug Deliv.*, **5**, 593–614.

74. Duncan, R. and Izzo, L. (2005) Dendrimer biocompatibility and toxicity. *Adv. Drug Deliv. Rev.*, **57**, 2215–2237.
75. Satchi-Fainaro, R., Hailu, H., Davies, J.W., Summerford, C., and Duncan, R. (2003) PDEPT: polymer-directed enzyme prodrug therapy. 2. HPMA copolymer–beta-lactamase and HPMA copolymer–C-Dox as a model combination. *Bioconjug. Chem.*, **14**, 797–804.
76. Krakovicova, H., Etrych, T., and Ulbrich, K. (2009) HPMA-based polymer conjugates with drug combination. *Eur. J. Pharm. Sci.*, **37**, 405–412.
77. Bae, Y., Diezi, T.A., Zhao, A., and Kwon, G.S. (2007) Mixed polymeric micelles for combination cancer chemotherapy through the concurrent delivery of multiple chemotherapeutic agents. *J. Control. Release*, **122**, 324–330.
78. Shiah, J.G., Sun, Y., Kopeckova, P., Peterson, C.M., Straight, R.C., and Kopecek, J. (2001) Combination chemotherapy and photodynamic therapy of targetable N-(2-hydroxypropyl)methacrylamide copolymer–doxorubicin/mesochlorin e_6–OV-TL 16 antibody immunoconjugates. *J. Control. Release*, **74**, 249–253.
79. Greco, F., Vicent, M.J., Gee, S., Jones, A.T., Gee, J., Nicholson, R.I., and Duncan, R. (2007) Investigating the mechanism of enhanced cytotoxicity of HPMA copolymer–Dox–AGM in breast cancer cells. *J. Control. Release*, **117**, 28–39.
80. Khandare, J.J., Chandna, P., Wang, Y., Pozharov, V.P., and Minko, T. (2006) Novel polymeric prodrug with multivalent components for cancer therapy. *J. Pharmacol. Exp. Ther.*, **317**, 929–937.
81. Khandare, J.J. and Minko, T. (2006) Polymer–drug conjugates: progress in polymeric prodrugs. *Prog. Polym. Sci.*, **31**, 359–397.
82. Krinick, N.L., Sun, Y., Joyner, D., Spikes, J.D., Straight, R.C., and Kopecek, J. (1994) A polymeric drug delivery system for the simultaneous delivery of drugs activatable by enzymes and/or light. *J. Biomater. Sci. Polym. Ed.*, **5**, 303–324.
83. Hongrapipat, J., Kopeckova, P., Liu, J., Prakongpan, S., and Kopecek, J. (2008) Combination chemotherapy and photodynamic therapy with fab' fragment targeted HPMA copolymer conjugates in human ovarian carcinoma cells. *Mol. Pharm.*, **5**, 696–709.
84. Fang, J., Sawa, T., Akaike, T., Greish, K., and Maeda, H. (2004) Enhancement of chemotherapeutic response of tumor cells by a heme oxygenase inhibitor, pegylated zinc protoporphyrin. *Int. J. Cancer*, **109**, 1–8.
85. Lammers, T., Peschke, P., Kuhnlein, R., Subr, V., Ulbrich, K., Debus, J., Huber, P., Hennink, W., and Storm, G. (2007) Effect of radiotherapy and hyperthermia on the tumor accumulation of HPMA copolymer-based drug delivery systems. *J. Control. Release*, **117**, 333–341.
86. Satchi-Fainaro, R., Puder, M., Davies, J.W., Tran, H.T., Sampson, D.A., Greene, A.K., Corfas, G., and Folkman, J. (2004) Targeting angiogenesis with a conjugate of HPMA copolymer and TNP-470. *Nat. Med.*, **10**, 255–261.
87. Satchi-Fainaro, R., Mamluk, R., Wang, L., Short, S.M., Nagy, J.A., Feng, D., Dvorak, A.M., Dvorak, H.F., Puder, M., Mukhopadhyay, D., and Folkman, J. (2005) Inhibition of vessel permeability by TNP-470 and its polymer conjugate, caplostatin. *Cancer Cell*, **7**, 251–261.
88. Segal, E., Pan, H., Ofek, P., Udagawa, T., Kopeckova, P., Kopecek, J., and Satchi-Fainaro, R. (2009) Targeting angiogenesis-dependent calcified neoplasms using combined polymer therapeutics. *PLoS ONE*, **4**, e5233.
89. Miller, K., Erez, R., Segal, E., Shabat, D., and Satchi-Fainaro, R. (2009) Targeting bone metastases with a bispecific anticancer and antiangiogenic polymer–alendronate–taxane conjugate. *Angew. Chem. Int. Ed. Engl.*, **48**, 2949–2954.
90. Tuomela, J.M., Valta, M.P., Vaananen, K., and Harkonen, P.L. (2008) Alendronate decreases orthotopic PC-3 prostate tumor growth and metastasis to prostate-draining lymph nodes in nude mice. *BMC Cancer*, **8**, 81–81.

91. Hashimoto, K., Morishige, K., Sawada, K., Tahara, M., Kawagishi, R., Ikebuchi, Y., Sakata, M., Tasaka, K., and Murata, Y. (2005) Alendronate inhibits intraperitoneal dissemination in in vivo ovarian cancer model. *Cancer Res.*, **65**, 540–545.

92. Hashimoto, K., Morishige, K., Sawada, K., Tahara, M., Shimizu, S., Ogata, S., Sakata, M., Tasaka, K., and Kimura, T. (2007) Alendronate suppresses tumor angiogenesis by inhibiting Rho activation of endothelial cells. *Biochem. Biophys. Res. Commun.*, **354**, 478–484.

93. Lammers, T., Subr, V., Ulbrich, K., Peschke, P., Huber, P.E., Hennink, W.E., and Storm, G. (2009) Simultaneous delivery of doxorubicin and gemcitabine to tumors in vivo using prototypic polymeric drug carriers. *Biomaterials*, **30**, 3466–3475.

94. Santucci, L., Mencarelli, A., Renga, B., Pasut, G., Veronese, F., Zacheo, A., Germani, A., and Fiorucci, S. (2006) Nitric oxide modulates proapoptotic and antiapoptotic properties of chemotherapy agents: the case of NO-pegylated epirubicin. *FASEB J.*, **20**, 765–767.

95. Pasut, G., Scaramuzza, S., Schiavon, O., Mendichi, R., and Veronese, F. (2005) PEG–epirubicin conjugates with high drug loading. *J. Bioact. Compat. Polym.*, **20**, 213–230.

96. Santucci, L., Mencarelli, A., Renga, B., Ceccobelli, D., Pasut, G., Veronese, F.M., Distrutti, E., and Fiorucci, S. (2007) Cardiac safety and antitumoral activity of a new nitric oxide derivative of pegylated epirubicin in mice. *Anticancer Drugs*, **18**, 1081–1091.

97. Chandna, P., Saad, M., Wang, Y., Ber, E., Khandare, J., Vetcher, A.A., Soldatenkov, V.A., and Minko, T. (2007) Targeted proapoptotic anticancer drug delivery system. *Mol. Pharm.*, **4**, 668–678.

98. Veronese, F.M. and Harris, J.M.E. (2008) Peptide protein PEGylation III: advances in chemistry and clinical applications. *Adv. Drug Deliv. Rev.*, **60**, 1–88.

99. Satchi-Fainaro, R., Wrasidlo, W., Lode, H.N., and Shabat, D. (2002) Synthesis and characterization of a catalytic antibody–HPMA copolymer conjugate as a tool for tumor selective prodrug activation. *Bioorg. Med. Chem.*, **10**, 3023–3029.

100. Verschraegen, C.F., Skubitz, K., Daud, A., Kudelka, A.P., Rabinowitz, I., Allievi, C., Eisenfeld, A., Singer, J.W., and Oldham, F.B. (2009) A phase I and pharmacokinetic study of paclitaxel poliglumex and cisplatin in patients with advanced solid tumors. *Cancer Chemother. Pharmacol.*, **63**, 903–910.

101. Langer, C.J., O'Byrne, K.J., Socinski, M.A., Mikhailov, S.M., Lesniewski-Kmak, K., Smakal, M., Ciuleanu, T.E., Orlov, S.V., Dediu, M., Heigener, D., Eisenfeld, A.J., Sandalic, L., Oldham, F.B., Singer, J.W., and Ross, H.J. (2008) Phase III trial comparing paclitaxel poliglumex (CT-2103, PPX) in combination with carboplatin versus standard paclitaxel and carboplatin in the treatment of PS 2 patients with chemotherapy-naive advanced non-small cell lung cancer. *J. Thorac. Oncol.*, **3**, 623–630.

102. Beer, T.M., Ryan, C., Alumkal, J., Ryan, C.W., Sun, J., and Eilers, K.M. (2010) A phase II study of paclitaxel poliglumex in combination with transdermal estradiol for the treatment of metastatic castration-resistant prostate cancer after docetaxel chemotherapy. *Anti-Cancer Drugs*, **21**, 433–438.

103. Dipetrillo, T., Milas, L., Evans, D., Akerman, P., Ng, T., Miner, T., Cruff, D., Chauhan, B., Iannitti, D., Harrington, D., and Safran, H. (2006) Paclitaxel poliglumex (PPX-Xyotax) and concurrent radiation for esophageal and gastric cancer: a phase I study. *Am. J. Clin. Oncol.*, **29**, 376–379.

26
Clinical Experience with Drug–Polymer Conjugates
Khalid Abu Ajaj and Felix Kratz

26.1
Introduction

In addition to the poor water solubility of many anticancer agents that limits their application, chemotherapy is accompanied by systemic toxicities. Sufficient concentrations of the anticancer drug in naive as well as resistant tumor cells are often not achieved due to a lack of accumulation of anticancer drugs in solid tumors.

In 1975, Helmut Ringsdorf proposed a general scheme of designing a drug delivery system using synthetic polymers for low-molecular weight drugs (Figure 26.1) [1, 2]. One to several drug molecules are bound to a polymeric backbone through a spacer that incorporates a predetermined breaking point to ensure release of the drug before or after cellular uptake of the conjugate. The system can also contain solubilizing groups or targeting moieties that render water solubility and targeting properties to the carrier.

Inspired by Ringsdorf's pioneering work, numerous anticancer drug–polymer conjugates with different macromolecular carriers have been developed in the last three decades. Coupling of low-molecular weight anticancer drugs to synthetic polymers or serum proteins through a cleavable linker has been an effective method for improving their therapeutic index through active and passive targeting

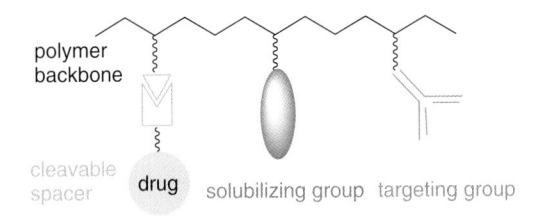

Figure 26.1 Ringsdorf's model for a polymeric drug containing the drug, solubilizing groups, and targeting groups bound to a linear polymer backbone.

Drug Delivery in Oncology: From Basic Research to Cancer Therapy, First Edition.
Edited by Felix Kratz, Peter Senter, and Henning Steinhagen.
© 2012 Wiley-VCH Verlag GmbH & Co. KGaA. Published 2012 by Wiley-VCH Verlag GmbH & Co. KGaA.

approaches, and convincing proof of concepts have been obtained preclinically for a substantial number of prodrug candidates [3].

Although great efforts are being made to develop novel polymer carriers, synthetic polymers that have been used in clinically evaluated drug conjugates have been mainly restricted to N-(2-hydroxypropyl)methacrylamide (HPMA), poly(ethylene glycol) (PEG), and poly(glutamic acid) (PGA) as water-soluble drug delivery vehicles, but there are also some recent developments worth mentioning that have focused on more sophisticated biodegradable drug carriers such as polyacetals, dextrans, or PEG–dendrimer hybrids. Table 26.1 gives an overview of different synthetic polymers that have been frequently used as macromolecular carriers.

In addition to synthetic polymers, the serum protein human serum albumin (HSA) is attracting increasing interest as a drug carrier [4].

26.2
Rationale for Developing Drug–Polymer Conjugates

The rationale for developing drug–polymer conjugates is to broaden the therapeutic window by improving drug solubility and pharmacokinetics, passively targeting the drug–polymer conjugate to the tumor, and reducing the levels of free drug in healthy tissue. The overall concept of using macromolecules as drug carriers is supported by detailed studies concerning the enhanced vascular permeability of circulating macromolecules for tumor tissue and their subsequent accumulation in solid tumors [5, 6]. This phenomenon has been termed enhanced permeability and retention (EPR) in relation to passive tumor targeting ("EPR effect") (see Chapter 3).

Coupling a low-molecular weight anticancer to a macromolecular carrier should result in a water-soluble macromolecular prodrug that passively accumulates in tumor tissue and releases the drug in its active form in the extracellular environment of tumor tissue or upon cellular uptake via the endosomal/lysosomal pathway. As shown in Figure 26.2 (www.celltherapeutics.com) for a paclitaxel–PGA conjugate (Opaxio™), unlike vessels in healthy tissue (Figure 26.2a), those in tumor tissue (Figure 26.2b) are porous and "leaky" with a diameter of up to 400 nm. Due to the larger size of the drug–polymer conjugate compared to the low-molecular weight drug, the drug–polymer conjugate leaks through the pores in tumor blood vessels, and is preferentially trapped and distributed to the tumor tissue due to an absent or defective lymphatic drainage system. Once inside the tumor tissue (Figure 26.2c), the drug–polymer conjugate is primarily taken up by the tumor cells through a cellular process called endocytosis. As the polymer is designed to contain predetermined cleavage points, it is hydrolyzed inside the endosomes and/or lysosome of the tumor cell to release the active anticancer agent (Figure 26.2d). The hydrolysis depends on the cleavable linker, which can be an enzymatically cleavable, acid-sensitive, reductive, or hydrolyzable linker.

The therapeutic properties of a drug–polymer conjugate depend on the type and molecular weight of the polymer carrier, its hydrophobicity as well as the conjugate's supramolecular structure and the type of covalent linkage between the

Table 26.1 Examples of frequently used polymeric drug carriers.

Name	Structure
N-(2-Hydroxypropyl) methacrylamide (HPMA) copolymers	
Poly(ethylene glycol) (PEG) or poly(ethylene oxide) (PEO)	
MethoxyPEG (mPEG)	
Poly(glutamic acid) (PGA)	
Dextran	
Four-arm PEG	

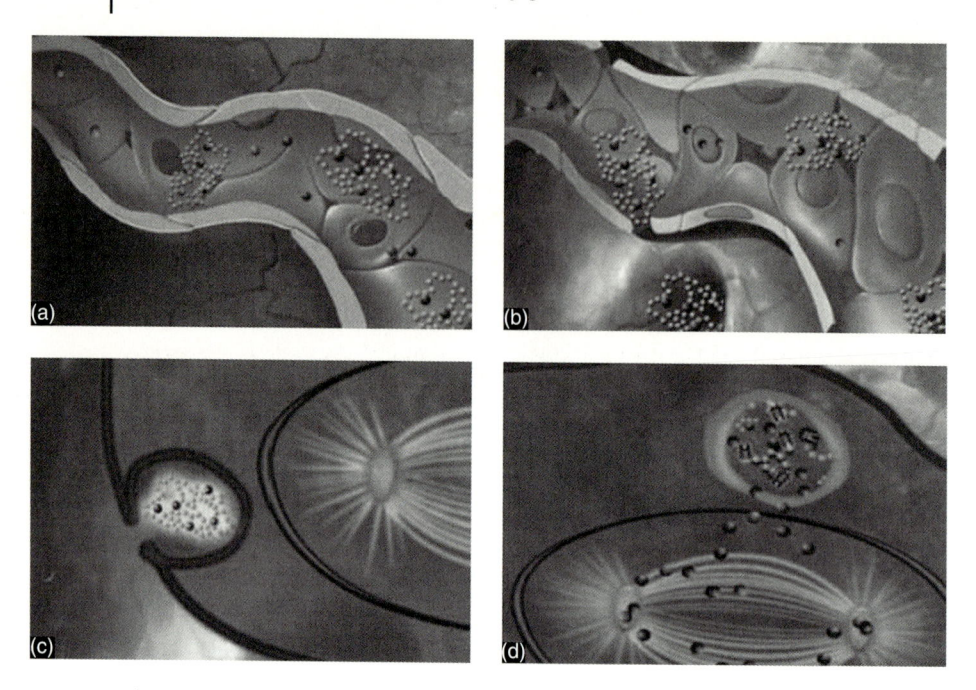

Figure 26.2 Uptake of Opaxio in tumor tissue and cells, and release of paclitaxel. Unlike vessels in healthy tissue (a), those in tumor tissue (b) are porous and "leaky". Owing to the large size of Opaxio, it leaks through the pores in tumor blood vessels and is distributed in the tumor tissue (c). Opaxio is enzymatically metabolized inside the lysosome of the tumor cell to release the active anticancer drug paclitaxel that then interacts with the microtubules of the tumor cell (d). (Reproduced courtesy of Cell Therapeutics.)

drug and the polymer. The nature of the covalent linkage defines the drug release mechanism, and markedly affects the bioavailability of active drug in the biological milieu and at the tumor site.

The first generation of drug–polymer conjugates mainly concentrated on the development of enzymatically cleavable compounds. The first clinically assessed drug–polymer conjugates were designed with the cathepsin B-cleavable tetrapeptide spacer Gly–Phe–Leu–Gly bound to HPMA, which are hydrophilic and water-soluble polymers. Biocompatible macromolecular conjugates based on HPMA preferentially accumulate in tumors and possess a higher anticancer efficacy than the low-molecular weight drugs. Since HPMA copolymers are nonbiodegradable, the relatively low molecular weight of around 28 kDa was chosen to ensure slow renal clearance, thus preventing side-effects that might result from an unwanted long-term tissue accumulation of the polymeric carrier [7]. Although most of these conjugates are no longer under clinical assessment, phase I and II studies have shown that no special toxicity can be attributed to HMPA and the drug–polymer conjugates have in most cases shown a favorable toxicity profile (Section 28.3) [8].

However, the anticipated broad antitumor efficacy of HPMA–drug conjugates such as PK1 – the first doxorubicin HPMA conjugate to enter clinical trails – was not observed in phase II studies [8]. It is possible that the cathepsin B-cleavable tetrapeptide Gly–Phe–Leu–Gly might not be the ideal linker considering that the antitumor efficacy of this conjugate in preclinical models was correlated with the expression of cathepsin B in tumor cells and tumor tissue [9]. The antitumor effect of PK1 was compared to that of doxorubicin in animals with murine colon tumor models (MAC26 and MAC15A) that have different vascularization and enzymatic properties. PK1 was not significantly more effective than doxorubicin alone against the MAC26 tumor even at doses that were 4-fold that for doxorubicin (10 mg/kg doxorubicin versus 40 mg/kg doxorubicin-equivalents for PK1) (Figure 26.3a). In contrast, when evaluated in the MAC15A xenograft model, PK1 was as effective as doxorubicin at 10 mg/kg (Figure 26.3b), but increasing the dose level to 40 mg/kg doxorubicin-equivalents (Figure 26.3c) resulted in significantly superior antitumor efficacy ($P = 0.01$) [9]. To correlate the different response to PK1 with the vascular permeability of these tumors, the EPR effect was evaluated with Evans blue dye

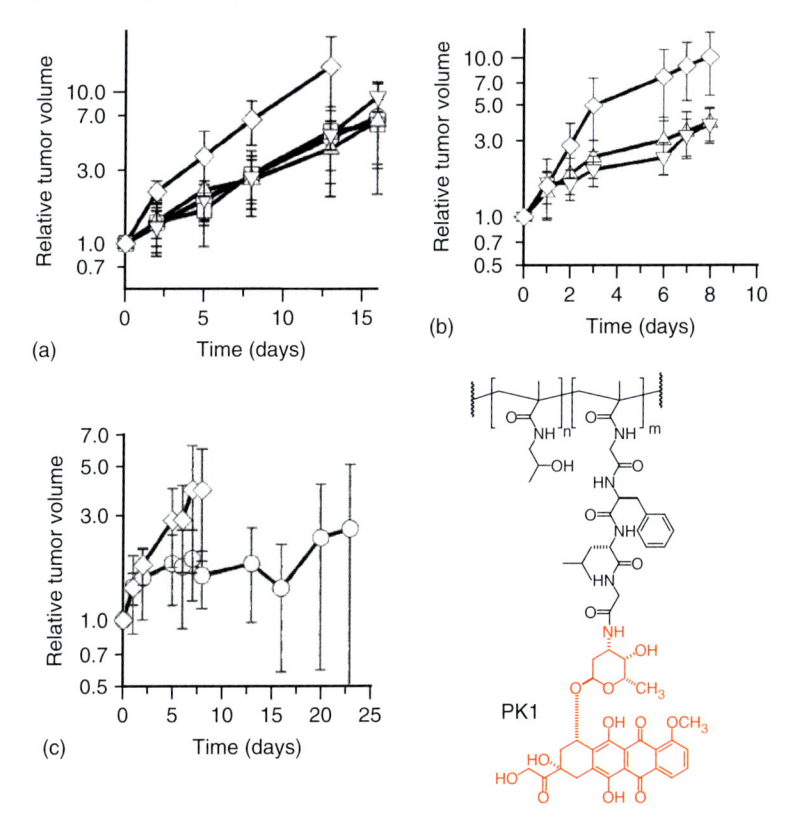

Figure 26.3 Antitumor effects of doxorubicin or PK1 against MAC26 tumors (low EPR and cathepsin B status) (a) and MAC15A tumors (high EPR and cathepsin B status) (b) and (c). Points indicate mean relative tumor volumes ($n > 5$); ○, PK1 (40 mg/kg); PK1 (20 mg/kg); △, PK1 (10 mg/kg); ▽, doxorubicin (10 mg/kg); ◇, controls. (Reproduced with permission from [7].)

and showed that the MAC15A tumors exhibited a pronounced EPR phenomenon in contrast to the MAC15A tumors. Furthermore, it was also shown that MAC15A tumors have a higher cathepsin B activity than the MAC26 tumors [9]. In summary, this study has highlighted that the activity of the drug–polymer conjugate PK1 and its drug release depend on the vascular properties and enzyme expression of the tumor.

HPMA drug–polymer conjugates have also been developed with paclitaxel [10], camptothecin (CPT) [11], and platinum complexes [12, 13].

In addition to HPMA, other polymers such as PEG have been used to develop hydrolyzable drug PEG conjugates that have been clinically evaluated. PEG – a nonbiodegradable polymer – is one of the most versatile polymers for medical applications and characterized by its outstanding chemical properties, including the chemical inertness of the polyether backbone and its excellent solubility in aqueous media. Furthermore, PEGs are nontoxic and nonimmunogenic, making them suitable for the modification of various biologically active compounds. Drug–PEG conjugates (around 40 kDa) have been realized with clinically established anticancer drugs, primarily with CPT derivatives. In addition, increased loading ratios and circulation time in the blood can be achieved by synthesizing branched, soluble PEG-based polymers with high molecular weights. Subsequent renal elimination can be achieved when using degradable backbones [14]. A new generation of polymers based on multiarm PEGs has been developed for the synthesis of new clinically assessed drug–polymer conjugates with a higher drug loading ratio than that of PEG analogs (Figure 26.4).

Further biodegradable polyacetal polymers based on as poly(1-hydroxymethylethylene hydroxymethylformal (PHF, Fleximer®; around 70 kDa) with a dual-phase release mechanism have been recently developed to address bladder as well as gastrointestinal toxicity while enhancing the efficacy of CPT. The polymer backbone of the prodrug utilizes a linkage, which releases CPT via well-defined small-molecule drug intermediates in two successive steps: a nonenzymatic intramolecular transacylation followed by hydrolysis (Figure 26.5) [15].

Other efforts in the field of drug–polymer conjugates focused on biodegradable drug carriers with higher molecular weight such as polyglutamic acid (PGA)

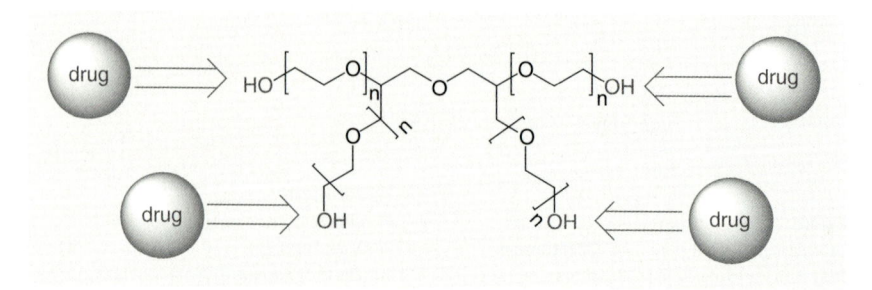

Figure 26.4 Structure of multiarm PEG.

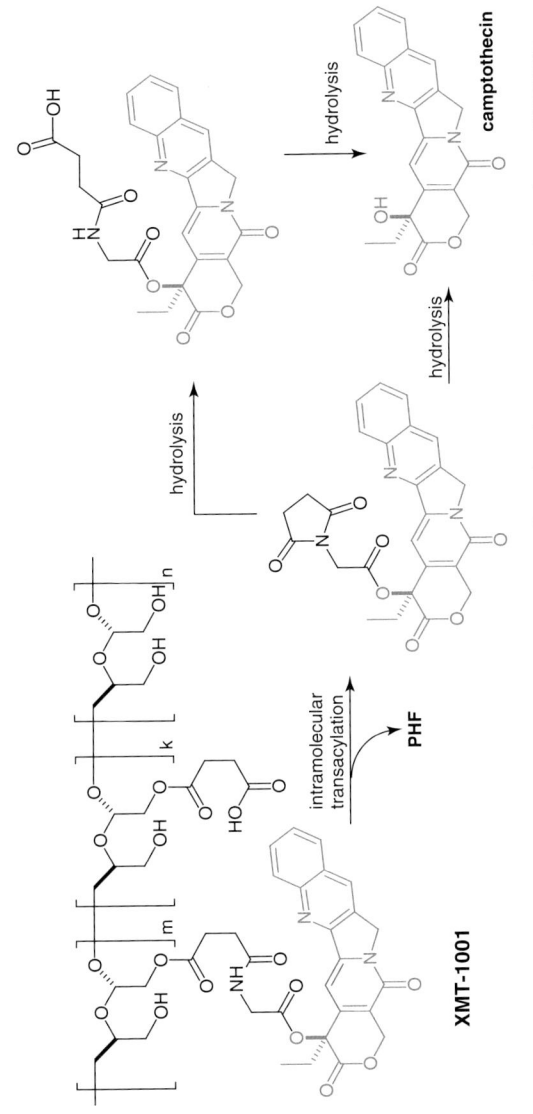

Figure 26.5 Dual-phase release mechanism for camptothecin from the Fleximer–camptothecin conjugate XMT-1001 (around 70 kDa) PHF.

(around 50 kDa) and carboxymethyldextran polyalcohol (around 340 kDa). The most widely utilized biodegradable drug carrier, PGA, is used as a water-soluble, biocompatible, nontoxic, and biodegradable drug delivery carrier.

Many other novel polymers, including biodegradable polymer backbones, dendritic architectures, block copolymer micelles, and polycyclodextrin, are being used to prepare a second generation of polymer therapeutics [16]. Although the cyclodextrin-containing polymer is nonbiodegradable, it was designed to be linear and of suitable size for renal clearance as a single molecule.

26.3
Clinical Development

With the aim of improving the therapeutic efficacy of anticancer drugs, a spectrum of drug–polymer conjugates has been developed in the last three decades. Such compounds should be water soluble, less toxic than the single drugs, and target tumor cells. During the last 15 years several carrier-linked prodrugs with anticancer drugs have been or are being evaluated in clinical trials. In addition to synthetic polymers, serum albumin has also been investigated as a drug carrier. Drug conjugates with synthetic polymers or serum proteins that have undergone clinical assessment have used clinically established agents or their active metabolites, such as doxorubicin, CPT, paclitaxel, methotrexate (MTX), and Pt(II) complexes. An overview of the development of the clinically evaluated prodrugs and the stage of development are shown in Figure 26.6 and Table 26.2.

In 2007, Kratz *et al.* reviewed the clinical studies with the first-generation macromolecular [8]. Meanwhile, several clinical trials with carrier-linked prodrugs have been discontinued, but other candidates have moved into to the clinical setting or advanced to later stages of clinical trials. In this chapter we therefore restrict our discussion to a comparative analysis of the clinical data and give an update of ongoing clinical trials with macromolecular prodrugs in cancer therapy that should serve as a timely resource for interested parties in this field of drug delivery.

The first clinically assessed drug–polymer conjugates were based on HPMA coupled to the drug through a cathepsin B-cleavable peptide. The first HPMA–drug conjugate that entered clinical evaluation in 1994 was the HPMA copolymer–doxorubicin conjugate PK1. PK1 has a molecular weight of approximately 28 kDa with around 8.5 wt% doxorubicin linked to the polymer linked through its amino sugar to the HPMA copolymer via a tetrapeptide spacer (Gly–Phe–Leu–Gly) that is cleaved by lysosomal proteases, such as cathepsin B (Figure 26.7) [17].

In a phase I study with PK1, neutropenia and mucositis were the dose-limiting factors observed in this study (Table 26.3). In terms of activity, PK1 produced two partial and two minor responses in a cohort of 36 patients enrolled, and these were in non-small-cell lung cancer (NSCLC), colorectal cancer, and anthracycline-naive and -resistant breast cancer [18].

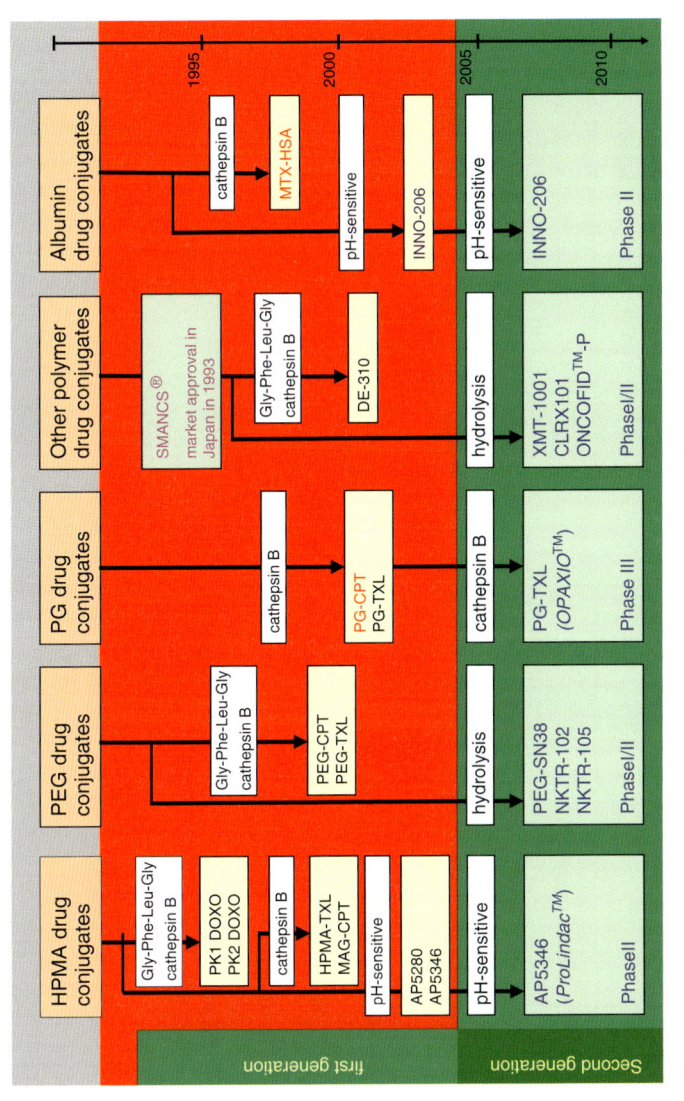

Figure 26.6 Anticancer drug conjugates with synthetic or natural polymers that have been or are being assessed in clinical trials (red: discontinued; blue: ongoing; pink: approved). PG, PGA; TXL, paclitaxel.

Table 26.2 Overview of anticancer drug conjugates with synthetic or natural polymers that have been or are being assessed in clinical trials.

Prodrug	Synonyms	Drug used	Carrier	Molecular weight (kDa)	Percent of drug (w/w)	Status of clinical development	Company
HPMA copolymer prodrugs							
PK1	FCE28068	doxorubicin	HPMA copolymer	~30	~8.5	phase II	Pharmacia/Cancer Research UK
PK2	FCE28069	doxorubicin	HPMA copolymer	25	7.5	phase II	Pharmacia/Pfizer
HPMA–paclitaxel	PNU-166945	paclitaxel	HPMA copolymer	n/a	~5	phase I	Pharmacia/Pfizer
MAG–CPT	PNU-166148	camptothecin	MAG HPMA copolymer	20	10	phase I	Pharmacia/Pfizer
AP5280	–	carboplatin	HPMA copolymer	~25	8.5 (Pt)	phase I/II	Access Pharmaceuticals
AP5346	ProLindac	oxaliplatin	HPMA copolymer	~25	10.5 (Pt)	phase II	Access Pharmaceuticals
PEG prodrugs							
PEG–CPT	EZN-246, Pegamotecan, Prothecan	camptothecin	PEG, diol	40	~1.7	phase II	Enzon
PEG–paclitaxel	–	paclitaxel	PEG	≥ 30	n/a	phase I	Enzon

Name	Code	Drug	Polymer			Phase	Company
PEG-SN-38	EZN-2208	SN-38	PEG 4-arm	40	3.7	phase I/II	Enzon
NKTR-105	–	docetaxel	PEG 4-arm	–	–	phase I	Nektar Therapeutics
NKTR-102	–	irinotecan	PEG 4-arm	40	–	phase II	Nektar Therapeutics
PGA prodrugs							
PGA–CPT	CT-2106	camptothecin	PGA	30–50	30–35	phase II	Cell Therapeutics
PGA–paclitaxel	Opaxio, Xyotax, CT-2103, paclitaxel poliglumex	paclitaxel	PGA	~52	37	phase III	Cell Therapeutics
Other polymer prodrugs							
SMANCS	–	NCS	SMA	15	78	market approval	Astellas Pharma
DE-310	–	camptothecin analog	dextran	340	5–7	phase I	Daiichi Pharmaceuticals UK
XMT-1001	polyacetal-CPT	camptothecin	biodegradable polyacetal polymer	70	5–7	phase I	Mersana Therapeutics
CRLX101	IT-101 cyclodextrin-PEG–CPT	camptothecin	cyclodextrin-PEG	62–107	~8	phase I/II	Cerulean Pharma
ONCOFID-P	–	paclitaxel	hyaluronic acid	200	20	phase I/II	Fidia Farmaceutici
Albumin-based prodrugs or conjugates							
INNO-206	DOXO-EMCH	doxorubicin	HSA	67	~1	phase I/II	CytRx
MTX–HSA	–	methotrexate	HSA	67	~1	phase II	Klinge Pharma/Fujisawa

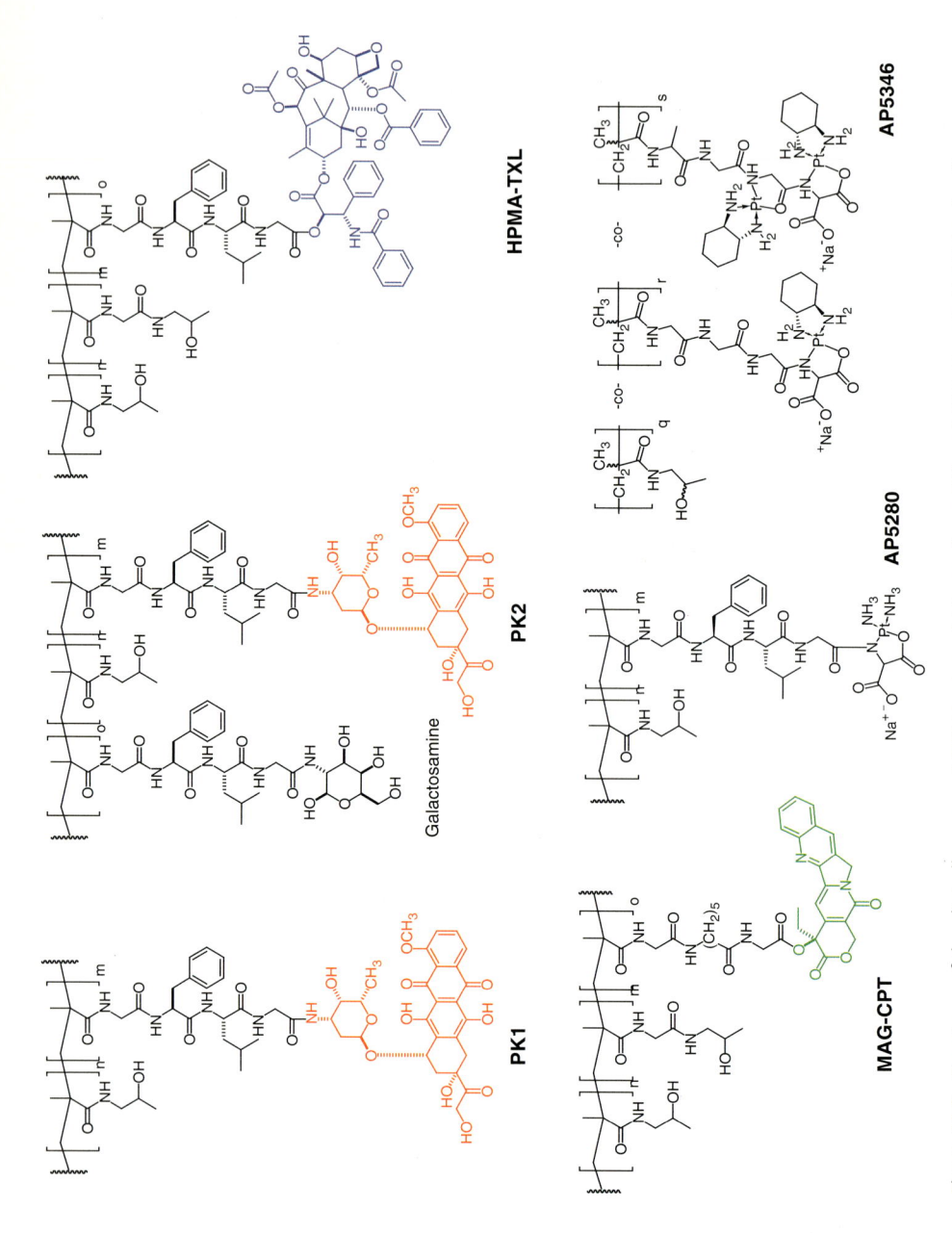

Figure 26.7 Structures of the clinically assessed HPMA–doxorubicin prodrugs PK1 and PK2 (drug is highlighted red), HPMA–paclitaxel (HPMA–TXL; drug is highlighted blue), MAG–CPT (drug highlighted in green), and the platinum-based prodrugs AP5280 and AP5346 (ProLindac).

Table 26.3 Data of phase I clinical trials with HPMA prodrugs.

Drug	Date of clinical study	References	Number of patients[a]	DLT	Tumor response[b]
PK1	<1998	[18]	36	neutropenia and mucositis	2 PR, 2 MR
PK2	<2000	[19]	31 (18)	neutropenia	2 PR, 1 MR
HPMA–paclitaxel	<2001	[10]	12	–	1 PR, 2 SD
MAG–CPT	<2002	[11]	16 (11)	cumulative bladder toxicity	1 SD
	1999–2000	[20]	23	myelosuppression, neutropenic sepsis, and diarrhea	1 MR, 2 SD
	2000–2001	[21]	9 (6)	cumulative bladder toxicity	2 SD
AP5280	<2002	[12]	29 (19)	vomiting	5 SD
AP5346	2003–2004	[13]	26 (16)	neutropenia	2 PR, 1 MR, 4 SD

[a] Values in parentheses indicate those who were able to be evaluated for tumor response.
[b] PR, partial remission; MR, minor response; SD, stable disease.

Phase II trials with PK1 initiated in 1999 at the recommended dose of 280 mg/m^2, which is almost a 5-fold increase over the standard dose of doxorubicin (60 mg/m^2), in breast, NSCLC and colon cancer appear to have been disappointing, with only a few positive responses being reported in an interim report [22]. While none of the evaluable patients with colorectal cancer showed a response, three anthracycline-naive of 14 evaluable patients with breast cancer and three of 26 evaluable patients with NSCLC had partial remissions.

In the following years, several approaches were undertaken in order to improve the PK1 system by (i) modifying the molecular mass and/or the topology of the polymer, (ii) replacing the cathepsin-cleavable peptide spacer with an acid-cleavable hydrazone bond, or (iii) employing PK1 in an antibody-directed enzyme prodrug therapy (ADEPT) strategy [3].

Furthermore, in addition to PK1 that was designed for passive targeting, another doxorubicin–HPMA conjugate, PK2, was designed for receptor-mediated targeting and made its way from the lab to the clinic. PK2 is a doxorubicin–HPMA conjugate, in which doxorubicin was coupled via the enzymatically cleavable tetrapeptide Gly–Phe–Leu–Gly to the polymer backbone that contained additional 2 wt% galactosamine as a targeting ligand that was designed to be taken up by the asialoglycoprotein receptor of liver tumor cells (Figure 26.7). PK2 was less soluble than PK1 due to the increased content of relatively hydrophobic side-chains. A phase I study of PK2 was performed in patients with primary or metastatic liver cancer (Table 26.3) [19]. Two partial responses and one minor response were observed. Comparable to PK1, neutropenia and mucositis and additionally severe fatigue were the dose-limiting toxicities (DLTs); 120 mg/m² was recommended as the dose for phase II studies. PK2 did not undergo further clinical assessment.

In spite of its very poor water solubility, paclitaxel in combination or as a single agent is the drug of choice in the treatment of various cancer diseases, such as ovarian cancer, breast cancer, and NSCLC. For intravenous administration a solution of paclitaxel in ethanol/Cremophor EL® is diluted to a final concentration of approximately 1 mg/ml. Unfortunately, Cremophor EL is known to cause hypersensitivity reactions that can only be partially prevented by premedication with corticosteroids and antihistamines. Therefore, coupling paclitaxel to synthetic macromolecules was performed primarily with the aim of improving water solubility in order to avoid the use of problematic solubilizing agents.

The first clinically assessed HMPA macromolecular paclitaxel prodrug, HMPA–paclitaxel, was developed by Pharmacia with the aim of improving drug solubility in order to enable more convenient administration with subsequent controlled release of paclitaxel [10]. Paclitaxel was linked through its 2′-OH group to the HPMA copolymer backbone via the cathepsin B-cleavable peptide linker (Gly–Phe–Leu–Gly) in analogy to the doxorubicin conjugate PK1 (Figure 26.7). HPMA–paclitaxel is a HPMA copolymer of unpublished molecular weight with a drug content of around 5 wt%. The prodrug is characterized by an enhanced water solubility (greater than 2 mg/ml conjugate compared to 0.0001 mg/ml paclitaxel). Although paclitaxel can be released from HMPA–paclitaxel by hydrolysis, enzymatic cleavage, or a combination of both mechanisms, it has been shown that drug release by hydrolysis predominates for this conjugate with its relatively low drug loading. A clinical phase I study with HMPA–paclitaxel was aborted before reaching DLT due to severe neurotoxicity observed in concurrent rat studies [10]. A reason for the occurrence of unpredictable neurotoxicity was not given. Antitumor activity was observed (one partial remission and two stable diseases) (Table 26.3).

Although CPT never gained any clinical importance, various clinically assessed macromolecular prodrugs are based on CPT. Pharmacia developed a series of HPMA copolymer conjugates to improve the clinical administration of CPT, but only one candidate, MAG–CPT, entered clinical trials. MAG–CPT is a HMPA conjugate in which two to several molecules of CPT are bound at the C-20-OH position through a glycine amino acid linker to the polymer backbone, which is a HMPA copolymer precursor composed of HMPA bound to methacryloyl-glycine (MAG) (Figure 26.7). This conjugate has a molecular weight of around 20 kDa with a total drug content of around 10 wt%. The amino acid linker is thought to be cleaved by hydrolysis or under the influence of unspecific enzymes. MAG–CPT has been evaluated in three phase I studies [11, 20, 21] (Table 26.3). These were the first phase I studies involving a HMPA copolymer conjugate where no objective responses were observed. Furthermore, serious bladder toxicity was noted. In a pilot clinical study that was conducted to investigate MAG–CPT tumor targeting, an assessment of colon tumor uptake in patients who received MAG–CPT prior to elective surgery indicated no preferential uptake of the prodrug [23]. In addition, since ester bonds can also be cleaved by esterases in the circulation, releasing the drug prematurely, this could serve as an explanation for the lack of antitumor response. The results of these studies were in marked contrast to previous experiments in xenografted animals that showed a clear benefit over CPT [24]. Due to its toxicity and the lack of an evidence of tumor targeting, Pharmacia stopped the clinical development of MAG–CPT. One can speculate whether the relative low molecular weight of MAG–CPT (around 20 kDa) or the differences in the stability of MAG–CPT in human and rodent plasma is to some extent responsible for the clinical failure of this prodrug [25].

In addition to doxorubicin, CPT, and paclitaxel, other drug–polymer conjugates are based on platinum complexes (see Chapter 49). Due to their inorganic nature, antineoplastic platinum complexes hold an exceptional position among cytotoxic drugs. Numerous platinum analogs have undergone clinical testing, but only three drugs – cisplatin, carboplatin, and oxaliplatin – have been approved for clinical use. These compounds are indicated for the treatment of testicular cancer, tumors of the head and neck, ovarian as well as lung cancer. Cisplatin and carboplatin have revolutionized the therapy of testicular cancer, achieving cure rates of greater than 90%. In order to improve their therapeutic index, a number of different synthetic polymers were used as macromolecular polymers for platinum. Access Pharmaceuticals has transferred two HPMA-based drug candidates into clinical trials: a carboplatinum analog AP5280 and an oxaliplatin (1,2-diaminocyclohexyl) (DACH) platinum analog AP5346 (ProLindac™) (Figure 26.7). Both prodrugs consist of a HPMA copolymer backbone to which the complexing aminomalonate unit is bound through the cathepsin B-cleavable tetrapeptide Gly–Phe–Leu–Gly in AP5280 or through the peptide Gly–Gly–Gly in AP5346 with subsequent release of the active platinum complex from the polymer occurring in the intra- or extracellular acidic environment [26, 27].

AP5280 was clinically assessed in a phase I study [12] (Table 26.3). Compared with cis- and carboplatin, the recommended safe dose of 3300 mg/m^2 means a remarkable increase in tolerability, approximately by a factor of 10–30. Furthermore, nephrotoxicity and myelosuppression – toxicities that are typical for low-molecular weight platinum drugs – were minimal. The start of a phase I/II clinical study with a weekly dose schedule of 3300 mg Pt/m^2 was announced for 2003 (www.accesspharma.com), but no results have been published since. It is likely that the development of AP5280 had been discontinued in favor of the structurally very similar successor AP5346 (ProLindac).

ProLindac has been studied in more than 10 tumor models. It was never inferior to oxaliplatin and was usually markedly superior, as demonstrated in BALB/c mice with subcutaneously growing B16 melanoma tumors in Figure 26.8 [27]. These tumors grow rapidly in mice that are not treated as shown by the tumor growth curve for the control ("vehicle"). When the mice were treated with oxaliplatin there was a slight reduction in the rate of growth of the tumor (open circles). However, ProLindac inhibited tumor growth to a much greater extent than oxaliplatin (www.accesspharma.com).

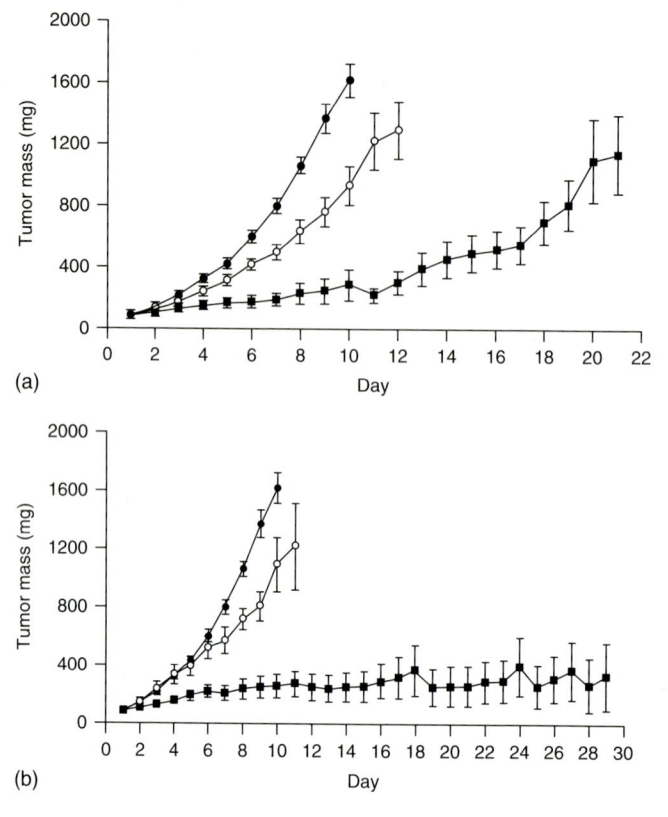

Figure 26.8 Antitumor activity of AP5346 versus oxaliplatin in the subcutaneously growing murine B16 melanoma tumor model. Each agent was administered intraperitoneally at its respective maximum tolerated dose. (a) Single dose. (b) Drugs administered weekly for three doses. ♦, Vehicle; ■, AP5346 at 100 mg Pt/kg (single) or 75 mg Pt/kg (weekly × 3); ○, oxaliplatin at 5 mg Pt/kg. Bars, standard error. (Reproduced with permission from [27].)

In a phase I study, ProLindac could be safely administered up to a 640 mg/m^2 (Pt) weekly dosage, which is approximately a 6- to 8-fold dose of weekly oxaliplatin. Antitumor activity was observed with two partial responses in metastatic melanoma and ovarian cancer, and CA-125 normalization in a suspected ovarian cancer patient [13] (Table 26.3). It is remarkable that two of the responders had platinum-resistant ovarian carcinoma, indicating that appropriate prodrug formulations of platinum drugs may circumvent platinum resistance. ProLindac has been pursued in a phase II clinical study that has now been completed in patients with recurrent platinum-sensitive ovarian cancer, and in patients with head and neck cancer. In March 2009, Access Pharmaceuticals announced positive and safety efficacy results from a phase II single-agent clinical study of ProLindac, with 66% of late-stage, heavily pretreated ovarian cancer patients achieving meaningful disease stabilization. No evidence of acute neurotoxicity was observed in any patient in the trial (www.accesspharma.com) [7]. ProLindac is the only drug conjugate with a HPMA copolymer that is currently being evaluated clinically.

As anticancer chemotherapy mostly involves the administration of drug combinations, the evaluation of drug–polymer conjugates in combination with low-molecular weight free drugs or other therapy (such as radiotherapy) was a logical step to undertake [28].

While ProLindac demonstrated good efficacy and considerable promise in clinical studies when used alone, a next step involved its clinical evaluation in combinations with other compounds. Access Pharmaceuticals has announced that a number of combination trials with other chemotherapeutic agents, such as paclitaxel, gemcitabine, (5-fluorouracil) 5-FU/leucovorin, and fluoropyrimidines, will follow in various clinical settings such as multiple solid tumor indications, including colorectal and ovarian cancer [7]. Furthermore, ProLindac has been licensed to Jiangsu Pharmaceutical and to JCOM for development in the Greater China Region and South Korea, respectively [7]. Both companies will conduct further phase II studies in specific tumor types.

Apart from HMPA, other polymers such as PEG with higher molecular weight have been investigated as drug carriers. PEG–drug conjugates that have been investigated in clinical trials are summarized in Table 26.4.

The first drug conjugate with PEG, PEG–CPT, that has been assessed clinically is based on CPT. PEG–CPT (Prothecan™ or Pegamotecan™) is obtained by coupling two molecules of CPT through an alanine spacer to a diol PEG of 40 kDa (Figure 26.9). The drug is therefore linked through an ester bond via its C-20-OH group [32–34]. This drug–polymer conjugate exhibited excellent water solubility compared to free CPT that is practically water insoluble. PEG–CPT has been evaluated in two phase I studies (Table 26.4). For PEG–CPT, at least five phase II studies were conducted in small-cell lung cancer (SCLC), pancreatic cancer, NSCLC as well as gastric and gastroesophageal junction cancers (first and second line). Preliminary results reported at the 2004 American Society of Clinical Oncology (ASCO) meeting [35] showed that the prodrug was well tolerated with a low incidence of grade 3/4 toxicities. A phase II study conducted in patients with gastric or gastroesophageal adenocarcinoma has recently shown that five out of 35 patients had a partial response [36]. However, PEG–CPT was as toxic as its native

Table 26.4 Data of phase I clinical trials with PEG prodrugs.

Drug	Date of clinical study	References	Number of patients[a]	DLT	Tumor response[b]
PEG–CPT	1999–2003	[29]	37 (36)	neutropenia	1 PR, 2 MR
	2000–2001	[30]	27	neutropenia	2 MR
PEG–paclitaxel	2001–2002	[31]	13	neutropenia	not available

[a]Values in parentheses indicate those who were able to be evaluated for tumor response.
[b]PR, partial remission; MR, minor response.

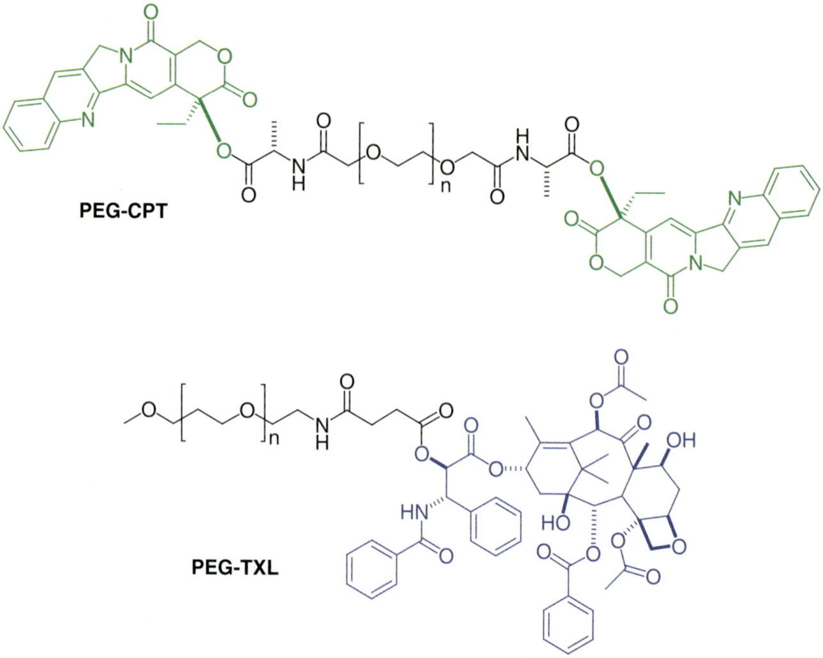

Figure 26.9 Structures of the clinically assessed PEG prodrugs PEG–CPT (drug highlighted in green) and PEG–paclitaxel (PEG–TXL; drug highlighted in blue).

drug, which is probably due to the very fast *in vivo* hydrolysis of the ester bond between the drug and the polymer with subsequent release of CPT prior to reaching the tumor. At the beginning of 2005, Enzon announced the discontinuation of the clinical development of Pegamotecan (*www.enzon.com*), while focusing on a new and promising PEG conjugate with SN-38, PEG–SN-38 (see below).

Following HPMA–paclitaxel from Pharmacia, the second macromolecular paclitaxel prodrug that entered clinical trials was PEG–paclitaxel, developed by Enzon (Figure 26.9). The Enzon researchers reported the importance of conjugation with PEGs with a molecular weight of 30 kDa or higher in order to prevent rapid elimination by the kidneys [37]. Although the exact molecular weight is not disclosed, it can be assumed that this clinically assessed macromolecular prodrug has been obtained from a direct esterification with PEG carboxylic acid (40 kDa). PEG–paclitaxel entered phase I trials in 2001 (Table 26.4). However, no more than preliminary results of this study were reported at the 2002 ASCO meeting [31]. In 2003, Enzon announced the discontinuation of further development of this product.

Drug–polymer conjugates close to the renal threshold (around 45 kDa) are cleared from the blood circulation and eliminated by glomerular filtration, and thus do not display optimal tumor targeting. Increased circulation time can be achieved by synthesizing branched, soluble polymers with high molecular weights.

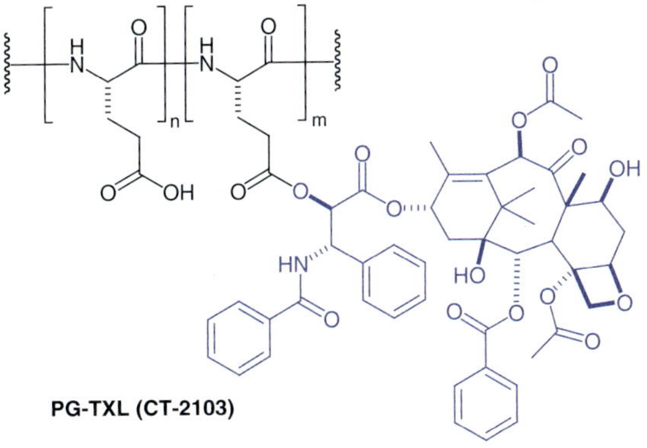

PG-TXL (CT-2103)

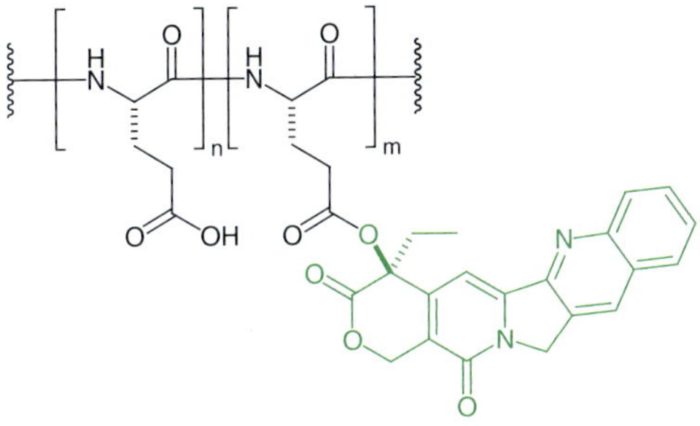

PG-CPT (CT-2106)

Figure 26.10 Structures of the clinically assessed PGA prodrugs PGA–paclitaxel (PG–TXL; drug highlighted in blue) and PGA–CPT (PG–CPT; drug highlighted in green) and.

Subsequent renal elimination can be achieved when using degradable backbones [14]. With a molecular weight of around 50 kDa, Cell Therapeutics has developed new biodegradable drug carriers based on the water-soluble, biocompatible, biodegradable, and nontoxic PGA. Two PGA carrier-linked prodrugs are being assessed clinically in phase II and III studies: PGA–CPT and PGA–paclitaxel (Figure 26.10).

PGA–CPT, a PGA conjugate with CPT, in which the 20-OH position of CPT was bound directly to the carboxylic acid groups of PGA (Figure 26.10), has been assessed in phase I studies in patients with advanced solid tumors (Table 26.5) [38, 39]. One partial response and a few stable diseases were observed. In 2006, Cell Therapeutics announced the clinical evaluation of PGA–CPT in phase I/II studies in combination with 5-FU in patients with colorectal cancer and in phase II as a single agent for second-line therapy of ovarian carcinoma (www.celltherapeutics.com). Unfortunately, there are no interim results available to date.

Opaxio (formerly known as Xyotax™; paclitaxel poliglumex, or CT-2103) – a biodegradable poly(L-glutamic acid) conjugate of paclitaxel (Figure 26.10) – is the most advanced drug–polymer conjugate to date and is currently undergoing phase

III trials. Opaxio has a high loading ratio (around 37 wt% paclitaxel) compared to HMPA–paclitaxel (around 5 wt% paclitaxel), with paclitaxel being linked through its 2'-OH group directly to the PGA backbone. Although the link between the drug and the PGA carrier is realized by an ester bond, the conjugate is sufficiently stable in plasma with less than 14% of the drug being liberated after a 24-h incubation with human plasma at 37 °C [44]. Furthermore, in contrast to HPMA or PEG, the PGA backbone of Opaxio is biodegradable; *in vitro* and *in vivo* studies have shown that paclitaxel and paclitaxel glutamic acid derivatives are released, which, in part, appears to be due to cleavage by cathepsin B [45].

Opaxio has meanwhile been evaluated in several clinical trials for several indications. Currently, Opaxio is being tested in two phase III studies in NSCLC and ovarian cancer.

In addition to the evaluation of Opaxio as a single agent, clinical studies assessed Opaxio in combination with platinum complexes (*www.celltherapeutics.com* and [46, 47]) and radiation [43]. Selected phase I data are summarized in Table 26.5. A phase I study was carried out with Opaxio in combination with carboplatin in patients with advanced solid tumors and confirmed partial responses in patients who had previously failed paclitaxel therapy [46]. A phase I study of Opaxio in combination

Table 26.5 Data of phase I clinical trials with PGA prodrugs.

Drug	Date of clinical study	References	Number of patients[a]	DLT	Tumor response[b]
PGA–CPT	<2004	[38]	24	neutropenia and thrombocytopenia	1 PR, 5 SD
	<2006	[39]	26 (25)	thrombocytopenia and fatigue	3 SD
PGA–paclitaxel, Opaxio Xyotax, or CT-2103	2000	[40]	19 (13)	neutropenia	1 PR, 8 SD
	2000	[40]	11 (8)	neuropathy	1 PR, 1 SD
	<2005	[41]	7	neutropenia and neuropathy	2 SD
	2001–2003	[42]	22 (19)	neutropenia and thrombocytopenia	3 PR, 12 SD
	<2006	[43]	21 (12)	gastris, esophagitis, neutropenia, and dehydration	4 CR, 7 PR

[a] Values in parentheses indicate those who were able to be evaluated for tumor response.
[b] PR, partial remission; SD, stable disease; CR, complete remission.
[c] Only locoregional response was evaluated.

with cisplatin in patients with solid tumors showed good activity in refractory patients [47]. Synergistic effects of Opaxio treatment and concurrent radiation have been assessed in a recently published phase I study, initiated in 2006, in patients suffering from gastric or esophageal cancer (Table 26.5) [43]. As a result, significant locoregional activity could be observed, including patients who developed systemic progression. The authors attributed the enhanced local efficacy to an increased vascular permeability evoked by radiation. Complete responses were observed in 35% of patients with locoregional disease (Table 26.5).

Phase II studies have also been initiated in patients with NSCLC combined with cisplatin and combined with Alimta™ (pemetrexed – an antimetabolite approved by the US FDA (Food and Drug Administration) for the treatment of patients with advanced nonsquamous NSCLC), and in prostate and metastatic breast cancers combined with Xeloda™ (capecitabine,– an orally applicable 5-FU prodrug) (www.celltherapeutics.com) [8].

Although phase I and II studies had shown a promising response rate, four large phase III studies (STELLAR 2, 3, and 4, and PIONEER) were conducted in a total of more than 1900 patients with advanced NSCLC [46, 48]. In the STELLAR 2 trial, Opaxio had a comparable efficacy when compared to docetaxel for second-line treatment in 849 patients (www.celltherapeutics.com).

The efficacy of Opaxio as a first-line treatment in advanced NSCLC was evaluated in STELLAR 3 and 4 trials. In STELLAR 3, therapy with PGA–paclitaxel in combination with carboplatin was compared in 400 patients to treatment with paclitaxel in combination with carboplatin. Very similar efficacy was observed in both arms of this study, resulting in similar overall survival times. However, more grade 3/4 neuropathy, thrombocytopenia, and neutropenia were seen in the Opaxio arm [49]. Slightly improved results were obtained in the STELLAR 4 study when comparing PGA–paclitaxel with a combination of gemcitabine and vinorelbine in 381 patients [49]. The STELLAR trials did not meet their endpoints of superior survival. However, these studies have primarily shown a significant survival benefit for women treated with Opaxio (198 patients) compared to the control arms, where men treated with Opaxio responded similarly to men treated with comparator agents (www.celltherapeutics.com). The largest improvement in survival with Opaxio was seen in women under the age of 55 and in women with premenopausal estrogen levels, regardless of age (51 patients). Studies showed that premenopausal women and women receiving hormone replacement therapy have a poor outcome compared to postmenopausal women. Elevated estrogen levels have an adverse effect on prognosis in advanced NSCLC even with standard chemotherapy. The retrospective analysis of clinical data suggested that the activity of the drug–polymer conjugate might be affected by estrogen levels – a trend toward improved survival was observed in female, but not in male patients [49]. Estrogens are known to induce cathepsin B activity; cathepsin B-mediated proteolysis is a key enzymatic processing step in Opaxio metabolism. Therefore, another phase III (PIONEER) open-label trial initiated in 2006 compared Opaxio to paclitaxel in first-line treatment of poor performance status (PS2) chemotherapy-naive women (450 patients) with advanced NSCLC. This study has shown improved efficacy over paclitaxel [48], but only in women with plasma free estradiol values greater than 30 pg/ml (www.celltherapeutics.com) [48]. In December 2006, Cell Therapeutics closed the PIONEER trial and took patients off both treatment arms (www.celltherapeutics.com).

Based on these results, Cell Therapeutics is now performing an additional multinational, phase III open-label study to evaluate the combination of Opaxio with carboplatin for the treatment of chemotherapy-naive advanced NSCLC in women who have premenopausal estrogen levels (above 25 pg/ml) – a patient group whose survival is significantly shorter than for postmenopausal women (www.celltherapeutics.com). This phase III trial is expected to enroll 450 patients. Each study arm of approximately 225 patients will be randomized to receive Opaxio plus carboplatin or paclitaxel plus carboplatin once every 3 weeks. Patients will be treated for up to six cycles. The primary endpoint is superior overall survival with several secondary endpoints, including progression-free survival, disease control, clinical benefit, response rate, quality of life, and the safety and tolerability of the treatment arms (www.celltherapeutics.com).

Additionally, Opaxio has been clinically evaluated for the treatment of patients with ovarian cancer. Preliminary data were reported from a phase II study of Opaxio in combination with carboplatin for first-line induction and single-agent maintenance therapy of advanced stage III/IV ovarian cancer. Of the 82 patients studied, 98% (80 patients) achieved a major tumor response, including 85% complete response and 12% partial response (www.celltherapeutics.com). Based on these results, Cell Therapeutics and the Gynecologic Oncology Group are presently evaluating Opaxio (135 mg/m^2) as monthly maintenance in a phase III clinical trial in ovarian cancer patients who have achieved a complete response following standard first-line chemotherapy. Target enrollment for the trial, which includes a third paclitaxel arm to determine safety, comprises approximately 1100 patients.

Between April 2006 and April 2007, a phase II study was conducted to examine the tolerability and efficacy of the combination of Opaxio and capecitabine (Xeloda) in 48 first-line patients with metastatic breast cancer. In August 2008, Cell Therapeutics announced that although the study did not meet its predefined endpoint of 21 or more responses in the first 41 patients, 20 patients (42%) of the 48 evaluable patients demonstrated a confirmed tumor response, including two complete responses and 18 partial responses [50]. The authors concluded the combination of Opaxio and capecitabine was well tolerated and active in metastatic breast cancer. The most common severe (grade 3/4) side-effects reported included leukopenia, neutropenia, neuro-sensory side-effects, skin reaction (hand/foot syndrome), and dyspnea. Approximately 50% of the patients (25/47) experienced a grade 3 adverse event and 13% experienced a grade 4 adverse event.

In August 2009, Cell Therapeutics announced that the combination of Opaxio with Alimta in a phase II study in 12 patients with advanced NSCLC was well tolerated and resulted in median progression-free survival of 3.3 months [51]. The best response was stable disease in nine patients. Two patients remain without evidence of disease progression. Aside from grade 3 fatigue in two patients, there were no grade 3 or greater nonhematologic toxicities. Cell Therapeutics announced that future studies of such combinations are recommended (www.celltherapeutics.com).

In June 2010, Cell Therapeutics announced an update of phase II study results of Opaxio in patients with advanced esophageal cancer demonstrating that 38% (15/40) patients receiving Opaxio in combination with cisplatin and concurrent radiation achieved a pathologic or endoscopic complete response. A pathological complete response, observed in 32% of patients, is recorded only when the esophagus is surgically removed after therapy and no tumor can be found microscopically. In historical studies, pathologic complete response has correlated with prolonged survival [52]. There were no grade 4 hematologic adverse events. Grade 3 hematologic adverse events included neutropenia, and grade 3 nonhematologic toxicities included nausea, esophagitis, allergy, and fatigue.

Based on these results, Cell Therapeutics started a randomized Phase II trial of maintenance chemotherapy comparing 12 monthly cycles of single agent paclitaxel or OPAXIO versus no treatment until documented relapse in women with advanced ovarian or primary peritoneal or fallopian tube cancer who achieve a complete clinical response to primary platinum/taxane chemotherapy (*www.celltherapeutics.com*).

These clinical studies have in part demonstrated benefits of combining a drug–polymer conjugate with another therapeutic agent, but no superior efficacy of Opaxio compared to its combination with one or more clinically established anticancer drugs has been shown. Thus, to date Opaxio in combination with an anticancer drug versus combination chemotherapy with conventional anticancer agents is difficult to assess.

Independently, in March 2008, Cell Therapeutics submitted a proposal for registration for Opaxio to the European Medicines Agency as a treatment of premenopausal women with NSCLC [53].

When reviewing the first 15 years of experience of clinical trials with drug–polymer conjugates, one realizes that not only clinically established anticancer drugs were used as the drug of choice, but also derivatives of these. In addition to CPT, irinotecan, and SN-38, other synthetic derivatives have undergone clinical development. CPT analogs reached over US$1 billion in annual global sales in 2007 (*www.mersana.com*). Exatecan mesylate (DX-8951) is a synthetic CPT analog with increased aqueous solubility (Figure 26.11). A phase I trial in patients with advanced solid tumors, all previously treated, showed that neither complete nor partial responses were observed, but four patients had stable disease [54]. To enhance its antitumor activity by exploiting the EPR effect, DX-8951 was linked through the cathepsin B-cleavable tetrapeptide Gly–Phe–Leu–Gly to the biodegradable carboxymethyldextran polyalcohol polymer yielding the drug–polymer conjugate DE-310 with a molecular weight of 340 kDa (Figure 26.11). In a phase I clinical trial, DE-310 has demonstrated antitumor activity including one complete remission, one partial remission, and 14 stable diseases. Neutropenia, thrombocytopenia, and hepatotoxicity were the DLT [55]. However, no additional clinical trials with this prodrug have been reported.

In addition to synthetic polymers, two conjugates that use albumin as a drug carrier have been assessed in clinical trials: an albumin conjugate of MTX, MTX–HSA, and an acid-sensitive albumin-binding prodrug of doxorubicin, INNO-206 (Figure 26.12).

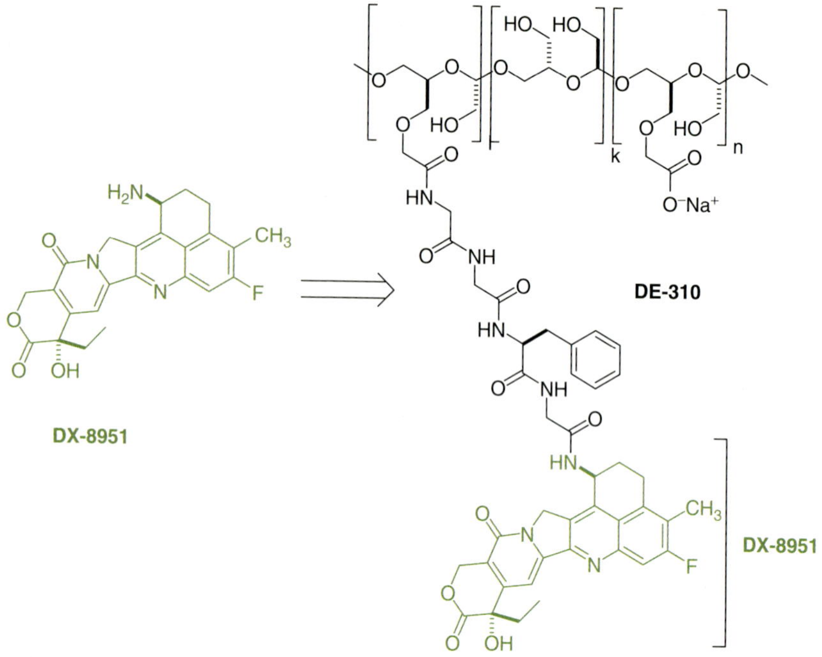

Figure 26.11 Structures of the drug DX-8951 (a camptothecin derivative) and its clinically assessed dextran polymer conjugate DE-310 (drug highlighted in green).

MTX, a folic acid antagonist, is a widely used agent for the treatment of certain human cancers and autoimmune diseases. The efficacy of MTX in anticancer chemotherapy is hampered by its very short plasma half-life. It is therefore administered in relatively high doses, causing a number of undesired side-effects such as bone marrow toxicity and mucositis. With the aim of achieving a prolonged circulatory retention and passive tumor targeting, a MTX–albumin conjugate (MTX–HSA) was synthesized by directly coupling the drug to lysine residues of HSA (Figure 26.12) [56]. It was found that the drug-loading ratio significantly determines the tumor targeting properties of MTX–albumin conjugates in rats with a drug loading ratio of around 1 exhibiting optimal tumor targeting. A clinical phase I study has been performed with patients treated with weekly MTX–HSA (Table 26.6) [57]. Stomatitis proved to be dose limiting above 50 mg/m^2 MTX–HSA (MTX-equivalents). A noteworthy finding of this study was that two patients with renal cell carcinoma and one patient with mesothelioma responded to MTX–HSA therapy (one partial response, two minor responses). However, it was not possible to confirm these results in a subsequent phase II study in patients with metastatic renal carcinoma in which no objective responses were seen [58]. Another phase II study with MTX–HSA in combination with cisplatin was initiated for the first-line treatment of patients with advanced bladder cancer [59]; however, the clinical development of MTX–HSA was then discontinued [58].

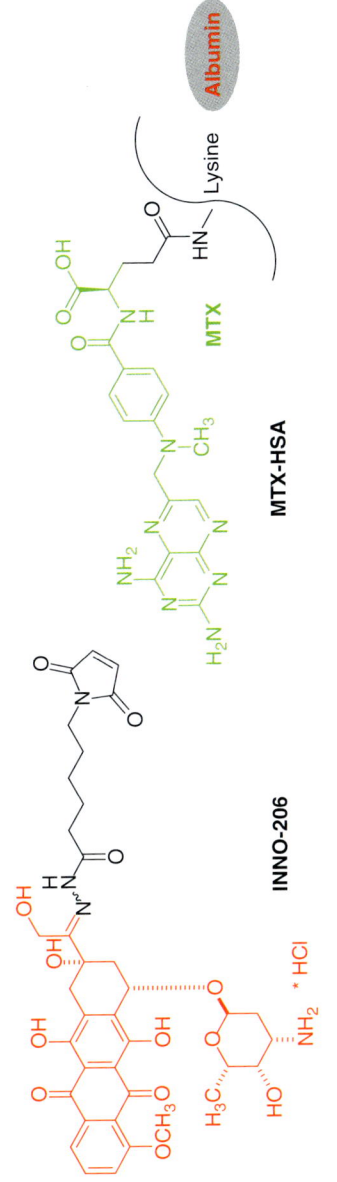

Figure 26.12 Structures of the clinically assessed albumin-binding prodrug INNO-206 (drug highlighted in red) and the albumin–MTX conjugate MTX–HSA (drug highlighted in green).

Table 26.6 Data of phase I clinical trials with a methotrexate albumin conjugate (MTX–HSA) and the albumin-binding doxorubicin prodrug (INNO-206).

Drug	Date of clinical study	References	Number of patients[a]	DLT	Tumor response[b]
MTX–HSA	<1999	[57]	17	stomatitis	1 PR, 2 MR
INNO-206	2003–2005	[60]	41 (30)	neutropenia and mucositis	3 PR, 2 MR, 15 SD

[a]Values in parentheses indicate those who were able to be evaluated for tumor response.
[b]PR, partial remission; MR, minor response; SD, stable disease.

INNO-206 (formerly DOXO-EMCH; the 6-maleimidocaproyl hydrazone derivative of doxorubicin) (Figure 26.12) is the first albumin-binding prodrug of doxorubicin to enter clinical trials [61]. INNO-206 is selectively bound to the Cys34 position of endogenous albumin within a few minutes after intravenous administration and contains an acid-sensitive hydrazone linker that allows doxorubicin to be released either extracellularly in the slightly acidic environment often present in tumor tissue or intracellularly in acidic endosomal or lysosomal compartments after cellular uptake of the conjugate by the tumor cell [61]. In a phase I study, treatment with INNO-206 was well tolerated up to 200 mg/m^2 without manifestation of drug-related side-effects. Myelosuppression and mucositis were dose limiting at 340 mg/m^2 [60, 61] (Table 26.6). No clinical signs of congestive heart failure were observed. Three partial responses (sarcoma, SCLC, and breast carcinoma) and two minor responses (sarcoma and parotis) were achieved [61]. After completion of the phase I study, INNO-206 was licensed to Innovive Pharmaceuticals and subsequently to CytRx in late 2008 (www.cytrx.com). Phase II studies at a dose of 260 mg/m^2 are scheduled for 2011 to assess the antitumor potential of INNO-206 against gastric cancer, pancreatic cancer, and sarcoma (www.cytrx.com).

From 2005 onwards, a second generation of drug–polymer conjugates was developed comprising novel polymers including biodegradable polymer backbones, dendritic architectures, block copolymer micelles, and polycyclodextrin [16]. In the last 5 years, efforts of researchers have concentrated on the development of new polymer–drug conjugates with a linkage that is not restricted to a specific enzyme (Figure 26.6).

In addition to ProLindac, Opaxio, and INNO-206, two novel CPT polymer conjugates (XMT-1001 and CLRX101), a SN-38 conjugate (EZN-2208), an irinotecan conjugate (NKTR-102), a docetaxel conjugate (NKTR-105), and a paclitaxel conjugate (ONCOFID™-P) are currently in clinical development (see Figure 26.6 and Table 26.7).

Although several CPT polymer conjugates evaluated in the clinic have shown antitumor activity in patients, these conjugates were often associated with bladder toxicity resulting from high levels of free (unconjugated) CPT in the urine [15]. While not causing hemorrhagic cystitis, conjugates of irinotecan and SN-38 commonly

Table 26.7 Overview of ongoing clinical trials with second generation drug–polymer conjugates.

Conjugate	Current status	Indication	References
Monotherapy			
XMT-1001	phase I	advanced refractory solid tumors	[62]
CLRX101	phase II	ovarian cancer	[15, 63]
	phase I/II	lymphoma	www.ceruleanrx.com
EZN-2208	phase I/II	pediatric patients with cancer	[64]
	phase II	metastatic colorectal carcinoma	–
	phase II	metastatic breast cancer	–
NKTR-102	phase II	colorectal cancer	www.nektar.com
	phase II	platinum-resistant ovarian cancer	www.nektar.com
	phase II	breast cancer	www.nektar.com
NKTR-105	phase I	refractory solid tumors	www.nektar.com
	phase I	refractory bladder carcinoma	www.nektar.com
ONCOFID-P	phase II	refractory bladder cancer	www.fidiapharma.com
	phase I	peritoneal carcinosis	www.fidiapharma.com
Combination therapy			
NKTR-102 + 5-FU	phase I	gastrointestinal and solid tumors	www.nektar.com
EZN-2208 + cetuximab	phase II	metastatic colorectal carcinoma	–

cause significant diarrhea [15, 65]. With the goal to address bladder as well as gastrointestinal toxicity while enhancing efficacy of CPT, Mersana Therapeutics has recently developed a new CPT polymeric prodrug, XMT-1001, with a dual-phase release mechanism [15]. Unlike many conjugated CPT analogs that rely upon slow hydrolysis or enzymatic cleavage of the CPT-20-*O*-ester bond to release free CPT in one step, the polymer backbone utilizes a CPT-20-*O*-(*N*-succinimidoyl-glycinate) linkage, which generates CPT via well-defined small-molecule drug intermediates in two successive steps: a non-enzymatic intramolecular transacylation followed by hydrolysis (Figure 26.5).

Based on this principle, XMT-1001 represents a system for drug release enabling CPT delivery to tumor, both in a low-molecular weight and in a macromolecular form [66]. XMT-1001 (Figure 26.13) is a biodegradable polyacetal polymer conjugate of CPT, in which CPT is chemically bound via a hydrolyzable linker to the hydrophilic, biodegradable polyacetal Fleximer. XMT-1001 (around 70 kDa) contains 5–7% of CPT by weight [15]. An open-label, dose-escalation phase I study of the safety, tolerability, and pharmacokinetics of intravenous XMT-1001 in patients with advanced, refractory solid tumors started in April 2007 [62] (Table 26.8). Early

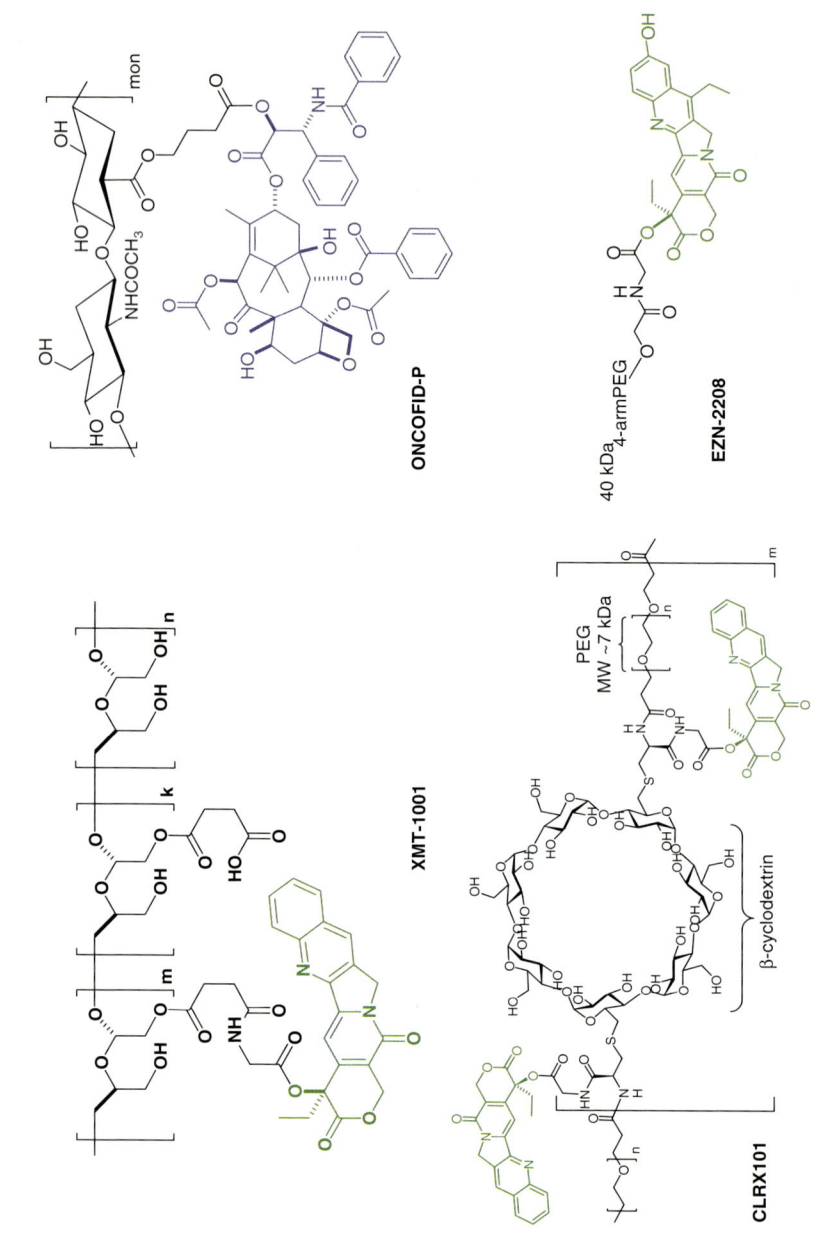

Figure 26.13 Structures of the clinically assessed second-generation polymeric prodrugs: XMT-1001, CLRX101, and EZN-2208 (drug highlighted in green), and ONCOFID (drug highlighted in blue).

Table 26.8 Data of phase I clinical trials with second-generation polymeric prodrugs.

Drug	Date of clinical study	References	Number of patients[a]	DLT	Tumor response[b]
EZN-2208	>2007	[67]	39	neutropenia	15 SD
	>2007	[68]	41	neutropenia	18 SD
XMT-1001	2007	[62]	60	neutropenia	1 PR, 10 SD
CRLX101	2006	[63, 69]	12	hematologic toxicity	6 SD
	2006	[63]	18 (4)	thrombocytopenia	4 SD
ONCOFID-P	2006	[70]	16	NA	9 CR
NKTR-102	2008	[65]	57	diarrhea and noncholinergic in nature	7 PR, 6 MR
NKTR-105	>2009	[71]	17	NA	NA

NA, not available.
[a]Values in parentheses indicate those who were able to be evaluated for tumor response.
[b]SD, stable disease; PR, partial remission; CR, complete remission; MR, minor response.

results from this ongoing study demonstrated no severe diarrhea or hemorrhagic cystitis, and confirmed the antitumor activity of the evaluated macromolecular prodrug XMT-1001 (www.mersana.com) [62]. One patient with relapsed resistant SCLC had a partial response. Numerous patients, including two patients each with metastatic pancreatic carcinoma and advanced NSCLC, had a prolonged stable disease. Further clinical development is under consideration after completion of the phase I study.

Cerulean Nanopharmaceuticals has used cyclodextrin as a drug solubilizer for the development of a cyclodextrin-containing polymer conjugate of CPT, CRLX101 (Figure 26.13). Although this polymer is nonbiodegradable, it was designed to be linear, water-soluble, highly biocompatible and of sufficient size to be cleared renally as a single molecule. As in many other CPT prodrugs, the drug is bound through a glycine linker to the carboxylate groups of the polymer [63].

Clinical studies with CRLX101 started in May 2006 for the treatment of advanced solid tumors using a 60-min intravenous infusion either at 3-weekly doses with a week of rest (phase Ia) or every other week (phase Ib) [63]. Both trials are finished and to date preliminary results confirm that six out of 12 patients enrolled in phase Ia had stable disease (Table 26.8) [63, 69]. A phase II trial was initiated in the fall of 2008 as a maintenance therapy in ovarian cancer patients in women who received second-line platinum-based chemotherapy without disease progression [15, 63]. Other phase II trials are being planned and initiation of a phase I/II trial in lymphoma has been announced (www.ceruleanrx.com).

Based on a multiarm PEG (Figure 26.4), a new generation of drug–polymer conjugates has been developed with the goal of obtaining a higher loading ratio of the anticancer drug. Three conjugates have entered clinical studies and are currently being evaluated: EZN-2208, NKTR-102, and NKTR105.

Enzon developed EZN-2208 (also known as PEG–SN-38), a 40-kDa PEG conjugate with an active metabolite of CPT, SN-38, by binding the 20-OH group of the drug via a glycine linker to the four-arm PEG (Figure 26.13). EZN-2208 showed a higher loading ratio (3.7 wt%) than that of PEG–CPT (1.7 wt%). This conjugation also enhanced the solubility of SN-38 by about 1000-fold [72].

Two phase I studies with different schedules of administration of EZN-2208 have been recently evaluated in patients with advanced malignancies (Table 26.8) [67, 68]. For both studies, the DLT of EZN-2208 was neutropenia with or without fever. In both studies, stable disease (sometimes exceeding 90 days and associated with tumor shrinkage) was observed as best response.

Additionally, a phase I/II study is being evaluated in pediatric patients with cancer [64]. A phase II study of EZN-2208 administered without (arm A) or with (arm B) cetuximab, an antibody targeting epidermal growth factor, in patients with metastatic colorectal carcinoma started in June 2009. Study treatment will be continued until evidence of disease progression, unacceptable toxicity, or withdrawal of the patient's consent for participation in the study. Additionally, a phase II, open-label study of EZN-2208 in patients with previously treated metastatic breast cancer was started in November 2009. In both studies, EZN-2208 was administered as an intravenous infusion on a weekly basis for 3 weeks within a 4-week interval.

Irinotecan is an important chemotherapeutic agent used for the treatment of solid tumors, including colorectal cancer. However, its pharmacokinetic profile and half-life are suboptimal. Irinotecan is typically cleared from the body within a few hours of dosing, resulting in a low time–concentration profile that may limit its efficacy. Nektar Therapeutics has applied the multiarm PEG architecture to develop the PEG–irinotecan conjugate, NKTR-102, which is designed to overcome these limitations. Preclinical studies of NKTR-102 have shown an increase in the half-life and exposure profiles of irinotecan, which results in improved antitumor activity in animal models (www.nektar.com). For example, preclinical studies in an irinotecan-resistant mouse colorectal tumor model showed that NKTR-102 inhibited tumor growth by 94% at the highest dose of 90 mg/kg irinotecan-equivalents on day 50. There was no significant decrease in tumor growth and no tumor regression when equivalent doses of irinotecan were administered (Figure 26.14) (www.nektar.com).

Although there is no published structure of this polymer, NKTR-102 has been evaluated clinically in a phase I open-label, dose-escalation, multicenter study in patients with advanced solid tumors such as NSCLC, breast, ovarian, and cervical cancers, who had failed prior anticancer treatments or have tumors where no standard treatment is available (Table 26.8). Interestingly, a significant antitumor activity in a broad spectrum of tumors has been reported in 13 patients out of 57 enrolled in this study [65]. Seven patients had confirmed partial responses in triple-negative breast cancer, NSCLC and SCLC, cervix, ovarian, maxillary sinus, and bladder cancer. Six patients had confirmed minor responses in ovarian and triple-negative breast cancer ($n = 2$), adrenocortical and esophageal cancer, and Hodgkin's disease. As an example, Figure 26.15 shows a partial response (tumor

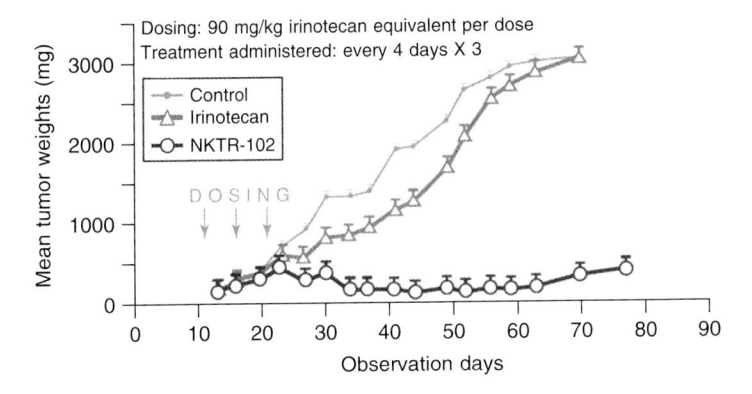

Figure 26.14 NKTR-102 inhibits growth of irinotecan-resistant human colon tumor (HT29) in a mouse xenograft model. (Reproduced courtesy of Nektar Therapeutics.)

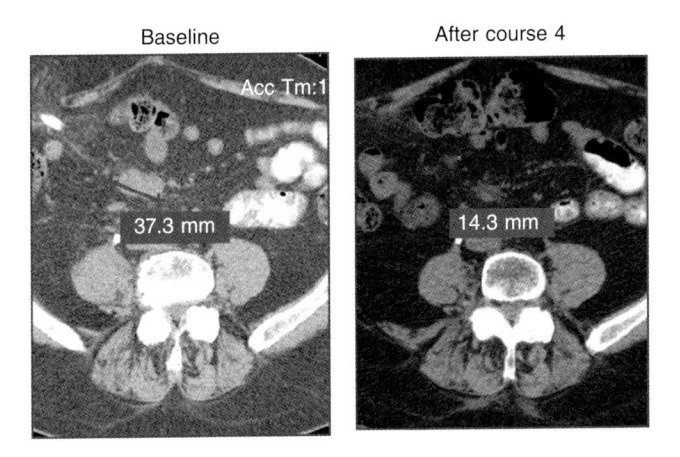

Figure 26.15 Partial response-confirmed RECIST lesions tumor reduction less than 53% in a patient with bladder cancer with small-cell component after four courses of NKTR-102 at a dose of 145 mg/m^2 irinotecan equivalent every 14 days. (Reproduced with permission from [65].)

reduction less than 53%) in a patient with bladder cancer with small cell features [65, 73].

Based on significant evidence of antitumor activity, Nektar Therapeutics has announced additional clinical phase I and phase II studies of NKTR-102, including drug combination trials [65]. A phase I clinical trial of NKTR-102 in combination with 5-FU cancer is ongoing in patients with gastrointestinal and solid tumors (www.nektar.com). In January 2008, a phase II study was started evaluating the safety and efficacy of NKTR-102 for the treatment of patients with colorectal cancer. The study is comprised of two sequential components – phases IIa and IIb. The phase IIa portion is an open-label, dose-finding trial in multiple solid tumor types

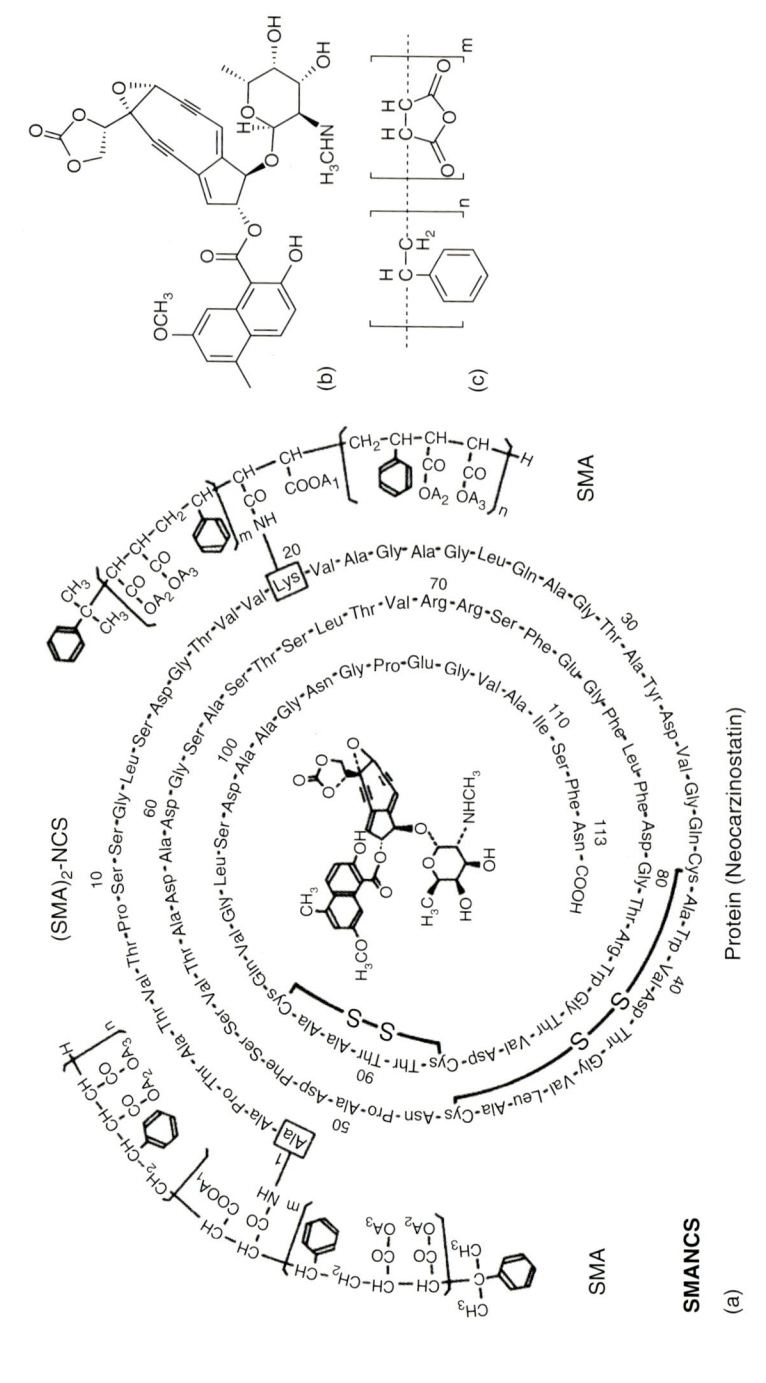

Figure 26.16 (a) Structure of SMANCS, (b) chemical structure of the highly toxic chromophore dienediyne antibiotic of NCS, and (c) schematic structure of SMA.

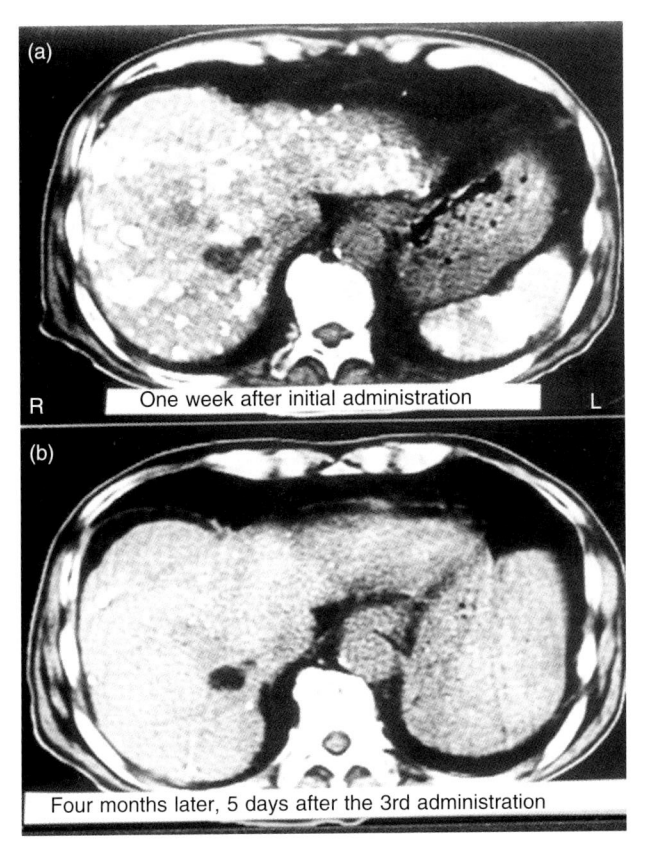

Figure 26.17 X-ray computed tomography scan images of multinodular HCC after arterial infusion of SMANCS/Lipiodol. (a) One week after the infusion under normotensive states. Note the numerous tumor nodules in the entire liver have taken up SMANCS/Lipiodol. (b) The same image after 4 months. The patient was treated with 3 infusions of the drug under normotension over 4 months.

SMANCS shows excellent targeting properties for hepatic tumors and is especially effective against solitary/massive or small multinodular HCC, and those tumors resistant against transcatheter arterial embolization therapy. Computed tomography scan images taken after infusion of SMANCS/Lipiodol confirm clearly the EPR effect and thus the tumor-selective targeting. The tumor-selective delivery of SMANCS/Lipiodol is not only observed in highly vascularized solitary HCC, but also in multinodular type HCC, as shown in Figure 26.17a, in which white areas demonstrate that SMANCS/Lipiodol is taken up effectively into small micronodules of size less than 5 mm. The majority of small nodules disappeared in 4 months (Figure 26.17b).

A postmarketing survey of SMANCS therapy for HCC in about 4000 cases shows that the drug caused very few serious adverse effects even in the advanced stages of HCC and yet a good therapeutic response was documented [90].

Furthermore, the effect on metastatic liver cancer is also encouraging when SMANCS/Lipiodol is infused into the tumor-feeding artery under angiotensin II-induced high blood pressure (e.g., 110 → 150 mmHg) [91]. The therapeutic efficacy of SMANCS/Lipiodol injected similarly into the tumor-feeding artery is also promising for cancers of the lung and other difficult-to-treat abdominal tumors, such as cancers of the kidney and the pancreas [85, 88, 89], and the bile duct and gall bladder as described earlier and recently [91].

26.4
Conclusions and Perspectives

Drug–polymer conjugates have been developed with the goal of reducing the systemic toxicity of anticancer agents and improving their antitumor efficacy. Basically, all of these macromolecular prodrugs are designed to be selectively taken up by solid tumors through passive targeting and subsequently release the active drug inside or outside of the tumor cells.

Although several anticancer polymer–drug conjugates have shown considerable promise in clinical trials over the last 15 years, only SMANCS earned market approval for the treatment of HCC in Japan in the early 1990s. In contrast to the other drug–polymer conjugates, SMANCS not only contains a highly toxic agent (i.e., NCS), but is administered together with a contrast agent (Lipiodol) intra-arterially and does not act as a prodrug.

The HMPA copolymer platinate ProLindac and the poly(L-glutamic acid) conjugate of paclitaxel Opaxio, currently in phase II and III clinical trials, are the nearest first-generation macromolecular prodrugs to obtain market approval.

Looking back on the clinical experience with 20 macromolecular prodrugs that have been assessed in the past two decades, it is worthwhile analyzing some of the lessons that have been learned and to take these into consideration when designing future clinical trials as wells as designing new drug–polymer conjugates preclinically. Figure 26.18 summarizes key issues that need to be considered in our opinion for the further clinical development of the first as well as second generation of drug–polymer conjugates.

The drug–polymer conjugates are designed to release the drug at the tumor site subsequent to uptake in the tumor or after internalization by the tumor cells. Therefore, the significance of the predetermined breaking point incorporated in the drug–polymer conjugate is a crucial issue to address not just in the preclinical setting, but also in clinical studies. The majority of the first generation of drug–polymer conjugates used the cathepsin B-cleavable tetrapeptide Gly–Phe–Leu–Gly as a predetermined breaking point. In clinical studies, however, now prescreening of patients regarding the expression of cathepsin B was performed even in advanced phase II and II trials. Considering that the activity of an enzymatically cleavable prodrug depends on the enzyme content of the tumors, a detailed knowledge of the expression of tumor-related proteases in individual tumor entities and patients would certainly be the logical step for a rational clinical design. There is a considerable amount of information in the literature suggesting

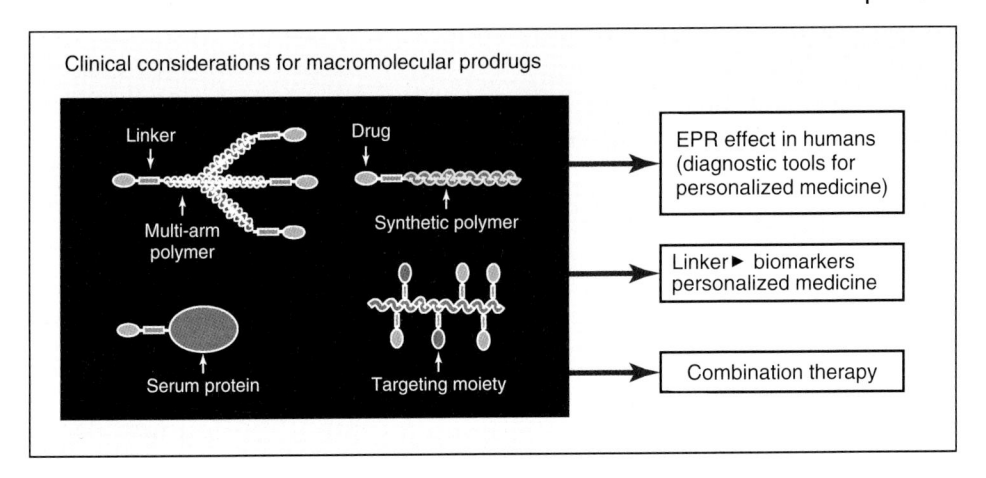

Figure 26.18 Pivotal issues that should be considered for designing clinical trials with macromolecular prodrugs.

that tumors differ greatly in their expression of proteases, particularly cysteine proteases such as cathepsin B. Therefore, for a fruitful application of enzymatically cleavable drug–polymer conjugates with conventional anticancer drugs, there is a need to personalize the cancer treatment by applying diagnostic tools to measure the activity of the respective enzyme in each patient before treatment with the drug–polymer conjugate in question. This should not only be performed with plasma from the patient, but also from tumor biopsies where possible. For example, the concentration of cathepsin B can be conveniently measured using an enzyme-linked immunosorbent assay while its activity can be measured using with a fluorogenic assay.

In a recent study, Kratz *et al.* have measured the concentration and activity of cathepsin B in 30–32 human tissues from patients with breast cancer, examining malignant tissue as well as healthy breast tissue from the same patient (Figures 26.19 and 26.20 and Table 26.9) [92]. As can be seen in Figures 26.19 and 26.20 and Table 26.9, cathepsin B concentration and activity was overexpressed in the patients' tumor tissues in comparison to the corresponding normal tissue, but there was a considerable heterogeneity in the cathepsin B content as well as activity, and there were several patients were the content and/or activity of cathepsin B was extremely low. Thus, without a preselection of patients with respect to these parameters, a cathepsin B-cleavable drug–polymer conjugate will show little activity if a critical cathepsin activity is not present in the tumors and metastases.

The retrospective analysis of clinical data with Opaxio – the cathepsin B-biodegradable poly(L-glutamic acid) conjugate of paclitaxel from Cell Therapeutics – has shed some light on this issue considering that the activity of the drug–polymer conjugate appears to be affected by estrogen levels; a trend toward improved survival was observed in female, but not in male patients [49]. Estrogens are known to induce cathepsin B activity. Therefore, a phase III (PIONEER) open-label trial compared Opaxio to paclitaxel in first-line treatment women (450

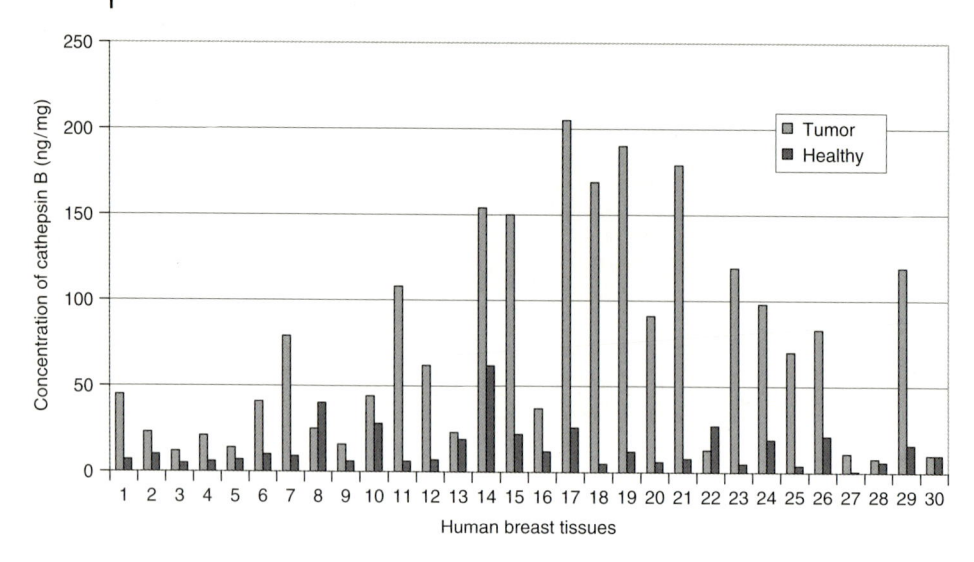

Figure 26.19 Concentration of cathepsin B in tumor and healthy tissues of 30 patients with breast cancer.

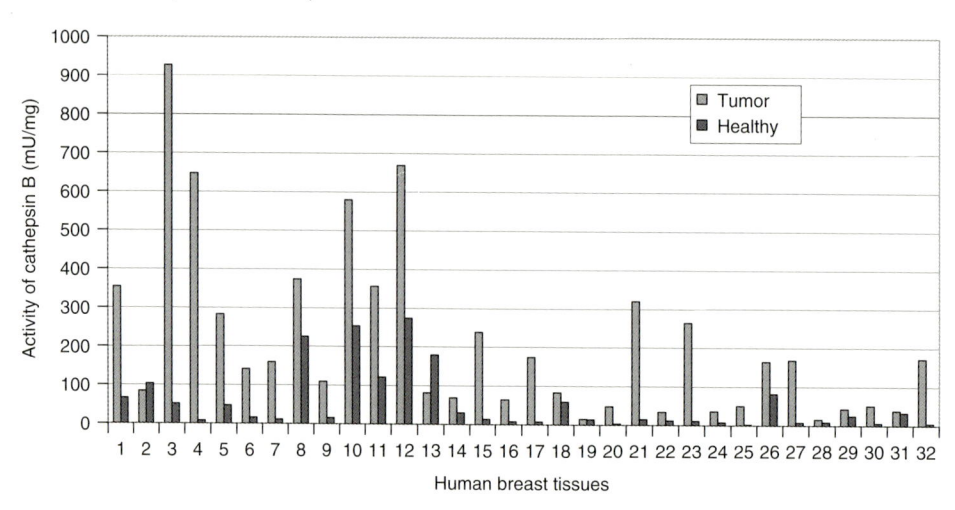

Figure 26.20 Activity of cathepsin B in tumor and healthy tissues of 32 patients with breast cancer.

patients) with advanced NSCLC. This study has shown improved efficacy over paclitaxel [48], but only in women with plasma free estradiol values greater than 30 pg/ml (*www.celltherapeutics.com*) [48].

As a consequence, if the protease expression of cancer patients is not addressed, drug–polymer conjugates with conventional anticancer drugs might not achieve the anticipated antitumor response rates. In this context it is important to note that this issue is not so critical for drug–antibody conjugates, which use highly potent drugs where much smaller amounts of the drug have to be cleaved.

Table 26.9 Concentration and activity of cathepsin B in human breast tissues.

Human breast tissues	Activity (mU/mg) of cathepsin B in tissues of 32 patients with cancer			Concentration (ng/mg) of cathepsin B in tissues of 30 patients with cancer		
	Lowest value	Highest value	Mean value	Lowest value	Highest value	Mean value
Healthy tissues	2	274	52	0.75	62	14
Tumor tissues	15	928	213	8	205	74

Ongoing clinical trials with drug–polymer conjugates that are based on nonenzymatic hydrolyzable or acid-sensitive linkers might therefore be more universally applicable if a prescreening of tumor patients with respect to their tumor expression is not performed.

The second important issue for the success of a drug–polymer conjugate based on passive targeting will depend mainly on the vascular properties of the tumor and metastases. Variation in the response of solid tumors may be explained by the extent of vascular permeability of the tumor lesions *per se* as well the heterogeneity of the EPR effect within a tumor. In fact, none of the clinical trials with macromolecular prodrugs have prescreened their patients regarding the extent of the EPR effect of the individual tumor burden and although there is a wealth of information on the EPR effect in animal tumor models, we unfortunately have acquired only sparse information on the situation in tumor patients. This is quite surprising since methods such as ^{99m}Tc-albumin aggregates, ^{67}Ga scintigraphy or magnetic resonance imaging gadolinium contrast agents such as the albumin-binding gadolectic acid B22956/1 (Bracco Imaging) could serve this purpose. Such diagnostic results would greatly help the clinical sponsor in selecting the patients that are most likely to profit from passive targeting strategies.

The third issue that has not been sufficiently addressed is the potential of delivering two drugs to the tumor, either by attaching both to the drug carrier or by combining the free anticancer drug with a drug–polymer conjugate. This could be realized by designing polymer-binding dual-acting prodrugs [93, 94] (Figure 26.21) that consist of different active agents coupled through cleavable linkers to a binding moiety. Different linkers can additionally control the sequential release of the drugs.

Alternatively, optimized combinations of free drug with drug–polymer conjugates could have the advantage that the combination achieves a more uniform drug distribution within the tumor due to its inherent heterogeneity and/or synergistic or additive affects that can be exploited on the cellular level.

A fourth issue is to intensify the research on synthetic and natural polymers with a molecular weight above 50 kDa since this seems to be the minimal size that is necessary for optimal tumor targeting. If such carriers are to be used, they should be biodegradable to avoid the potential risk of cumulative toxicity.

In summary, the era of drug–polymer conjugates in oncology that basically aims to circumvent the inadequate biodistribution of conventional low-molecular weight

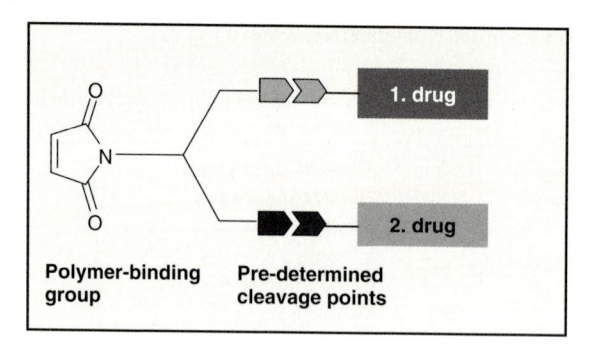

Figure 26.21 Dual-acting prodrug.

anticancer drugs by coupling these to macromolecules is in full stride. Ongoing efforts of adapting linker chemistry, optimizing combination approaches that draw on additive and synergistic affects, and foremost addressing the EPR effect and protease expression in tumor patients within the scope of a personalized medicine will form a sound rationale for the first macromolecular prodrug candidates to obtain market approval.

References

1. Ringsdorf, H. (1975) Structure and properties of pharmacologically active polymers. *J. Polym. Sci. Polym. Symp.*, **51**, 135–153.
2. Gros, L., Ringsdorf, H., and Schupp, H. (1981) Polymere antitumormittel auf molekularer und zellulärer basis? *Angew. Che.*, **93**, 311–322.
3. Kratz, F., Muller, I.A., Ryppa, C., and Warnecke, A. (2008) Prodrug strategies in anticancer chemotherapy. *ChemMedChem*, **3**, 20–53.
4. Kratz, F. (2008) Albumin as a drug carrier: design of prodrugs, drug conjugates and nanoparticles. *J. Control. Release*, **132**, 171–183.
5. Jain, R.K. (1999) Transport of molecules, particles, and cells in solid tumors. *Annu. Rev. Biomed. Eng.*, **1**, 241–263.
6. Jain, R.K. (1987) Transport of molecules across tumor vasculature. *Cancer Metastasis Rev.*, **6**, 559–593.
7. Duncan, R. (2009) Development of HPMA copolymer–anticancer conjugates: clinical experience and lessons learnt. *Adv. Drug Deliv. Rev.*, **61**, 1131–1148.
8. Kratz, F., Abu Ajaj, K., and Warnecke, A. (2007) Anticancer carrier-linked prodrugs in clinical trials. *Expert. Opin. Investig. Drugs*, **16**, 1037–1058.
9. Loadman, P.M., Bibby, M.C., Double, J.A., Al-Shakhaa, W.M., and Duncan, R. (1999) Pharmacokinetics of PK1 and doxorubicin in experimental colon tumor models with differing responses to PK1. *Clin. Cancer Res.*, **5**, 3682–3688.
10. Meerum Terwogt, J.M., ten Bokkel Huinink, W.W., Schellens, J.H., Schot, M., Mandjes, I.A., Zurlo, M.G., Rocchetti, M., Rosing, H., Koopman, F.J., and Beijnen, J.H. (2001) Phase I clinical and pharmacokinetic study of PNU166945, a novel water-soluble polymer-conjugated prodrug of paclitaxel. *Anti-Cancer Drugs*, **12**, 315–323.
11. Schoemaker, N.E. van Kesteren, C., Rosing, H., Jansen, S., Swart, M., Lieverst, J., Fraier, D., Breda, M., Pellizzoni, C., Spinelli, R., Grazia Porro, M., Beijnen, J.H., Schellens, J.H., ten Bokkel Huinink, W.W. (2002) A phase I and pharmacokinetic study of MAG–CPT, a water-soluble polymer conjugate

of camptothecin. *Br. J. Cancer*, **87**, 608–614.

12. Rademaker-Lakhai, J.M., Terret, C., Howell, S.B., Baud, C.M., De Boer, R.F., Pluim, D., Beijnen, J.H., Schellens, J.H., and Droz, J.P. (2004) A Phase I and pharmacological study of the platinum polymer AP5280 given as an intravenous infusion once every 3 weeks in patients with solid tumors. *Clin. Cancer Res.*, **10**, 3386–3395.

13. Campone, M., Rademaker-Lakhai, J.M., Bennouna, J., Howell, S.B., Nowotnik, D.P., Beijnen, J.H., and Schellens, J.H. (2007) Phase I and pharmacokinetic trial of AP5346, a DACH-platinum–polymer conjugate, administered weekly for three out of every 4 weeks to advanced solid tumor patients. *Cancer Chemother. Pharmacol.*, **60**, 523–533.

14. Segal, E. and Satchi-Fainaro, R. (2009) Design and development of polymer conjugates as anti-angiogenic agents. *Adv. Drug Deliv. Rev.*, **61**, 1159–1176.

15. Yurkovetskiy, A.V. and Fram, R.J. (2009) XMT-1001, a novel polymeric camptothecin pro-drug in clinical development for patients with advanced cancer. *Adv. Drug Deliv. Rev.*, **61**, 1193–1202.

16. Duncan, R. (2006) Polymer conjugates as anticancer nanomedicines. *Nat. Rev. Cancer*, **6**, 688–701.

17. Duncan, R., Seymour, L.W., O'Hare, K.B., Flanagan, P.A., Wedge, S., Hume, I.C., Ulbrich, K., Strohalm, J., Subr, V., Spreafico, F., Grandi, M., Ripamonti, M., Farao, M., and Suarato, A. (1992) Preclinical evaluation of polymer-bound doxorubicin. *J. Control. Release*, **19**, 331–346.

18. Vasey, P.A., Kaye, S.B., Morrison, R., Twelves, C., Wilson, P., Duncan, R., Thomson, A.H., Murray, L.S., Hilditch, T.E., Murray, T., Burtles, S., Fraier, D., Frigerio, E., and Cassidy, J. (1999) Phase I clinical and pharmacokinetic study of PK1 [N-(2-hydroxypropyl)methacrylamide copolymer doxorubicin]: first member of a new class of chemotherapeutic agents – drug–polymer conjugates. *Clin. Cancer Res.*, **5**, 83–94.

19. Seymour, L.W., Ferry, D.R., Anderson, D., Hesslewood, S., Julyan, P.J., Poyner, R., Doran, J., Young, A.M., Burtles, S., and Kerr, D.J. (2002) Hepatic drug targeting: phase I evaluation of polymer-bound doxorubicin. *J. Clin. Oncol.*, **20**, 1668–1676.

20. Bissett, D., Cassidy, J., de Bono, J.S., Muirhead, F., Main, M., Robson, L., Fraier, D., Magne, M.L., Pellizzoni, C., Porro, M.G., Spinelli, R., Speed, W., and Twelves, C. (2004) Phase I and pharmacokinetic (PK) study of MAG–CPT (PNU 166148): a polymeric derivative of camptothecin (CPT). *Br. J. Cancer*, **91**, 50–55.

21. Wachters, F.M., Groen, H.J., Maring, J.G., Gietema, J.A., Porro, M., Dumez, H., de Vries, E.G., and van Oosterom, A.T. (2004) A phase I study with MAG–camptothecin intravenously administered weekly for 3 weeks in a 4-week cycle in adult patients with solid tumours. *Br. J. Cancer*, **90**, 2261–2267.

22. Bilim, V. (2003) Technology evaluation: PK1, Pfizer/Cancer Research UK. *Curr. Opin. Mol. Ther.*, **5**, 326–330.

23. Sarapa, N., Britto, M.R., Speed, W., Jannuzzo, M., Breda, M., James, C.A., Porro, M., Rocchetti, M., Wanders, A., Mahteme, H., and Nygren, P. (2003) Assessment of normal and tumor tissue uptake of MAG–CPT, a polymer-bound prodrug of camptothecin, in patients undergoing elective surgery for colorectal carcinoma. *Cancer Chemother. Pharmacol.*, **52**, 424–430.

24. Zamai, M., VandeVen, M., Farao, M., Gratton, E., Ghiglieri, A., Castelli, M.G., Fontana, E., D'Argy, R., Fiorino, A., Pesenti, E., Suarato, A., and Caiolfa, V.R. (2003) Camptothecin poly[N-(2-hydroxypropyl) methacrylamide] copolymers in antitopoisomerase-I tumor therapy: intratumor release and antitumor efficacy. *Mol. Cancer Ther.*, **2**, 29–40.

25. Noguchi, Y., Wu, J., Duncan, R., Strohalm, J., Ulbrich, K., Akaike, T., and Maeda, H. (1998) Early phase tumor accumulation of macromolecules:

a great difference in clearance rate between tumor and normal tissues. *Jpn. J. Cancer Res.*, **89**, 307–314.

26. Sood, P., Thurmond, K. B. 2nd, Jacob, J.E., Waller, L.K., Silva, G.O., Stewart, D.R., and Nowotnik, D.P. (2006) Synthesis and characterization of AP5346, a novel polymer-linked diaminocyclohexyl platinum chemotherapeutic agent. *Bioconjug. Chem.*, **17**, 1270–1279.

27. Rice, J.R., Gerberich, J.L., Nowotnik, D.P., and Howell, S.B. (2006) Preclinical efficacy and pharmacokinetics of AP5346, a novel diaminocyclohexane-platinum tumor-targeting drug delivery system. *Clin. Cancer Res.*, **12**, 2248–2254.

28. Greco, F. and Vicent, M.J. (2009) Combination therapy: opportunities and challenges for polymer–drug conjugates as anticancer nanomedicines. *Adv. Drug Deliv. Rev.*, **61**, 1203–1213.

29. Rowinsky, E.K., Rizzo, J., Ochoa, L., Takimoto, C.H., Forouzesh, B., Schwartz, G., Hammond, L.A., Patnaik, A., Kwiatek, J., Goetz, A., Denis, L., McGuire, J., and Tolcher, A.W. (2003) A phase I and pharmacokinetic study of pegylated camptothecin as a 1-hour infusion every 3 weeks in patients with advanced solid malignancies. *J. Clin. Oncol.*, **21**, 148–157.

30. Posey, J.A. 3rd, Saif, M.W., Carlisle, R., Goetz, A., Rzzo, J., Stevenson, S., Rudoltz, M.S., Kwiatek, J., Simmons, P., Rowinsky, E.K., Takimoto, C.H., and Tolcher, A.W. (2005) Phase 1 study of weekly polyethylene glycol–camptothecin in patients with advanced solid tumors and lymphomas. *Clin. Cancer Res.*, **11**, 7866–7871.

31. Beeram, M., Rowinsky, E.K., Hammond, L.A., Patnaik, A., Schwartz, G.H., de Bono, J.S., Forero, L., Forouzesh, B., Berg, K.E., Rubin, E.H., Beers, S., Killian, A., Kwiatek, J., McGuire, J., Spivey, L., Takimoto, C.H., and Army, B. (2002) A phase I and pharmacokinetic (PK) study of PEG–paclitaxel in patients with advanced solid tumors. *Proc. Am. Soc. Clin. Oncol.*, **21**, 405.

32. Greenwald, Richard B., Pendri, Annapurna, Conover, Charles D., Lee, Chyi, Choe, Yun H., Gilbert, Carl, Martinez, Anthony, Xia, Ying, Wu, Dechun, and Hsue, M. (1998) Camptothecin-20-PEG ester transport forms: the effect of spacer groups on antitumor activity. *Bioorg. Med. Chem.*, **6**, 551–562.

33. Greenwald, R.B., Conover, C.D., and Choe, Y.H. (2000) Poly(ethylene glycol) conjugated drugs and prodrugs: a comprehensive review. *Crit. Rev. Ther. Drug Carrier Syst.*, **17**, 101–161.

34. Conover, C.D., Greenwald, R.B., Pendri, A., and Shum, K.L. (1999) Camptothecin delivery systems: the utility of amino acid spacers for the conjugation of camptothecin with polyethylene glycol to create prodrugs. *Anti-Cancer Drug Des.*, **14**, 499–506.

35. Scott, L.C., Evans, T., Yao, J.C., Benson, A.I., Mulcahy, M., Thomas, A., Decatris, M., Falk, S., Rudoltz, M., and Ajani, J.A. (2004) Pegamotecan (EZ-246), a novel PEGylated camptothecin conjugate, for treatment of adenocarcinomas of the stomach and gastroesophageal (GE) junction: preliminary results of a single-agent phase II study. *J. Clin. Oncol.*, **22**, 4030.

36. Scott, L.C., Yao, J.C., Benson, A. B., 3rd, Thomas, A.L., Falk, S., Mena, R.R., Picus, J., Wright, J., Mulcahy, M.F., Ajani, J.A., and Evans, T.R. (2009) A phase II study of pegylated-camptothecin (pegamotecan) in the treatment of locally advanced and metastatic gastric and gastro-oesophageal junction adenocarcinoma. *Cancer Chemother. Pharmacol.*, **63**, 363–370.

37. Greenwald, R.B., Gilbert, C.W., Pendri, A., Conover, C.D., Xia, J., and Martinez, A. (1996) Drug delivery systems: water soluble taxol 2′-poly(ethylene glycol) ester prodrugs – design and *in vivo* effectiveness. *J. Med. Chem.*, **39**, 424–431.

38. McNamara, M.V., Doroshow, J.H., Dupont, J., Spriggs, D., Eastham, E., Pezzulli, S., Syed, S., Bernareggi, A., and Takimoto, C. (2004) Preliminary

pharmacokinetics of CT-2106 (polyglutamate camptothecin) in patients with advanced malignancies. *J. Clin. Oncol.*, **22** (Suppl. 14), 2073.

39. Daud, A., Garrett, C., Simon, G.R., Munster, P., Sullivan, D., Stromatt, S., Allevi, C., and Bernareggi, B. (2006) Phase I trial of CT-2106 (polyglutamated camptothecin) administered weekly in patients (pts) with advanced solid tumors. *J. Clin. Oncol.*, **24** (Suppl. 18), 2015.

40. Boddy, A.V., Plummer, E.R., Todd, R., Sludden, J., Griffin, M., Robson, L., Cassidy, J., Bissett, D., Bernareggi, A., Verrill, M.W., and Calvert, A.H. (2005) A phase I and pharmacokinetic study of paclitaxel poliglumex (XYOTAX), investigating both 3-weekly and 2-weekly schedules. *Clin. Cancer Res.*, **11**, 7834–7840.

41. Veronese, M.L., Flaherty, K., Kramer, A., Konkle, B.A., Morgan, M., Stevenson, J.P., and O'Dwyer, P.J. (2005) Phase I study of the novel taxane CT-2103 in patients with advanced solid tumors. *Cancer Chemother. Pharmacol.*, **55**, 497–501.

42. Nemunaitis, J., Cunningham, C., Senzer, N., Gray, M., Oldham, F., Pippen, J., Mennel, R., and Eisenfeld, A. (2005) Phase I study of CT-2103, a polymer-conjugated paclitaxel, and carboplatin in patients with advanced solid tumors. *Cancer Invest.*, **23**, 671–676.

43. Dipetrillo, T., Milas, L., Evans, D., Akerman, P., Ng, T., Miner, T., Cruff, D., Chauhan, B., Iannitti, D., Harrington, D., and Safran, H. (2006) Paclitaxel poliglumex (PPX-Xyotax) and concurrent radiation for esophageal and gastric cancer: a phase I study. *Am. J. Clin. Oncol.*, **29**, 376–379.

44. Singer, J.W., Shaffer, S., Baker, B., Bernareggi, A., Stromatt, S., Nienstedt, D., and Besman, M. (2005) Paclitaxel poliglumex (XYOTAX; CT-2103): an intracellularly targeted taxane. *Anti-Cancer Drugs*, **16**, 243–254.

45. Auzenne, E., Donato, N.J., Li, C., Leroux, E., Price, R.E., Farquhar, D., and Klostergaard, J. (2002) Superior therapeutic profile of poly-L-glutamic acid–paclitaxel copolymer compared with taxol in xenogeneic compartmental models of human ovarian carcinoma. *Clin. Cancer Res.*, **8**, 573–581.

46. Langer, C.J., O'Byrne, K.J., Socinski, M.A., Mikhailov, S.M., Lesniewski-Kmak, K., Smakal, M., Ciuleanu, T.E., Orlov, S.V., Dediu, M., Heigener, D., Eisenfeld, A.J., Sandalic, L., Oldham, F.B., Singer, J.W., and Ross, H.J. (2008) Phase III trial comparing paclitaxel poliglumex (CT-2103, PPX) in combination with carboplatin versus standard paclitaxel and carboplatin in the treatment of PS 2 patients with chemotherapy-naive advanced non-small cell lung cancer. *J. Thorac. Oncol.*, **3**, 623–630.

47. Verschraegen, C.F., Skubitz, K., Daud, A., Kudelka, A.P., Rabinowitz, I., Allievi, C., Eisenfeld, A., Singer, J.W., and Oldham, F.B. (2009) A phase I and pharmacokinetic study of paclitaxel poliglumex and cisplatin in patients with advanced solid tumors. *Cancer Chemother. Pharmacol.*, **63**, 903–910.

48. Albain, K.S., Belani, C.P., Bonomi, P., O'Byrne K, J., Schiller, J.H., and Socinski, M. (2006) PIONEER: a phase III randomized trial of paclitaxel poliglumex versus paclitaxel in chemotherapy-naive women with advanced-stage non-small-cell lung cancer and performance status of 2. *Clin. Lung Cancer*, **7**, 417–419.

49. Chipman, S.D., Oldham, F.B., Pezzoni, G., and Singer, J.W. (2006) Biological and clinical characterization of paclitaxel poliglumex (PPX, CT-2103), a macromolecular polymer–drug conjugate. *Int. J. Nanomed.*, **1**, 375–383.

50. Northfelt, D.W., Allred, J.B., Liu, H., Hobday, T.J., Rodacker, M.W., Lyss, A.P., Fitch, T.R., and Perez, E.A. (2008) Phase II trial of paclitaxel polyglumex (PPX) with capecitabine (C) for metastatic breast cancer (MBC). *J. Clin. Oncol.*, **26** (Suppl.), 1063.

51. Rigas, J.R., Slagle, B.M., Dragnev, K.H., Williams, I., DiSalvo, W., Engman, C., Lipe, B., and Simeone, S. (2009) Dose-ranging study of the combination of paclitaxel poliglumex and pemetrexed in advanced nonsmall

cell lung cancer (NSCLC). International Association for the Study of Lung Cancer 13th World Conference on Lung Cancer, San Francisco, CA.

52. NG, T., Fontaine, J., Suntharalingam, M., Dipetrillo, T., Horiba, N., Oldenburg, N., Perez, K., Chen, W., Khuri, F., and Sarfan, H. (2010) Neoadjuvant paclitaxel Poligumex (PPX), cisplatin, and radiation (RT) for esophageal cancer. American Society of Clinical Oncology Annual Meeting, Chicago, IL.

53. Vicent, M.J., Ringsdorf, H., and Duncan, R. (2009) Polymer therapeutics: clinical applications and challenges for development. *Adv. Drug. Deliv. Rev.*, **61**, 1117–1120.

54. Royce, M.E., Hoff, P.M., Dumas, P., Lassere, Y., Lee, J.J., Coyle, J., Ducharme, M.P., De Jager, R., and Pazdur, R. (2001) Phase I and pharmacokinetic study of exatecan mesylate (DX-8951f): a novel camptothecin analog. *J. Clin. Oncol.*, **19**, 1493–1500.

55. Soepenberg, O., de Jonge, M.J., Sparreboom, A., de Bruin, P., Eskens, F.A., de Heus, G., Wanders, J., Cheverton, P., Ducharme, M.P., and Verweij, J., (2005) Phase I and pharmacokinetic study of DE-310 in patients with advanced solid tumors. *Clin. Cancer Res.*, **11**, 703–711.

56. Burger, A.M., Hartung, G., Stehle, G., Sinn, H., and Fiebig, H.H. (2001) Pre-clinical evaluation of a methotrexate–albumin conjugate (MTX–HSA) in human tumor xenografts in vivo. *Int. J. Cancer*, **92**, 718–724.

57. Hartung, G., Stehle, G., Sinn, H., Wunder, A., Schrenk, H.H., Heeger, S., Kränzle, L., Fiebig, H.H., Maier-Borst, W., Heene, D.L., and Queißer, W. (1999) Phase I trial of a methotrexate–albumin in a weekly intravenous bolus rgimen in cancer patients. *Clin. Cancer Res.*, **5**, 753–759.

58. Vis, A.N., van der Gaast, A., van Rhijn, B.W., Catsburg, T.K., Schmidt, C., and Mickisch, G.H. (2002) A phase II trial of methotrexate–human serum albumin (MTX–HSA) in patients with metastatic renal cell carcinoma who progressed under immunotherapy. *Cancer Chemother. Pharmacol.*, **49**, 342–345.

59. Bolling, C., Graefe, T., Lubbing, C., Jankevicius, F., Uktveris, S., Cesas, A., Meyer-Moldenhauer, W.H., Starkmann, H., Weigel, M., Burk, K., and Hanauske, A.R. (2006) Phase II study of MTX–HSA in combination with cisplatin as first line treatment in patients with advanced or metastatic transitional cell carcinoma. *Invest. New Drugs*, **24**, 521–527.

60. Unger, C., Haring, B., Medinger, M., Drevs, J., Steinbild, S., Kratz, F., and Mross, K. (2007) Phase I and pharmacokinetic study of the (6-maleimidocaproyl)hydrazone derivative of doxorubicin (DOXO-EMCH), an albumin-binding prodrug of the anticancer agent doxorubicin. *Clin. Cancer Res.*, **13**, 4858–4866.

61. Kratz, F. (2007) DOXO-EMCH (INNO-206), the first albumin-binding prodrug of doxorubicin to enter clinical trials. *Expert Opin. Investig. Drugs,*, **16**, 855–866.

62. Sausville, E.A., Garbo, L., Weiss, G.J., Shkolny, D., Yurkovetskiy, A.V., Bethune, C., Ramanathan, R.K., and Fram, R.J. (2009) Phase 1 study of XMT-1001, a novel water soluble camptothecin conjugate, given as an intravenous infusion once every three weeks to patients with advanced solid tumors. *Mol. Cancer Ther.*, **8** (Suppl. 1), B52.

63. Davis, M.E. (2009) Design and development of IT-101, a cyclodextrin-containing polymer conjugate of camptothecin. *Adv. Drug Deliv. Rev.*, **61**, 1189–1192.

64. Pastorino, F., Loi, M., Sapra, P., Becherini, P., Cilli, M., Emionite, L., Ribatti, D., Greenberger, L.M., Horak, I.D., and Ponzoni, M. (2010) Tumor regression and curability of preclinical neuroblastoma models by PEGylated SN-38 (EZN-2208), a novel topoisomerase I inhibitor. *Clin. Cancer Res.*, **16**, 4809–4821.

65. Von Hoff, D.D., Jameson, G., Board, M.J., Rosen, L.S., Utz, J., Dhar, S., Acosta, L., Barker, T., Walling, J., and

Hamm, J.T. (2008) First phase I trial of NKTR-102 (PEG–irinotecan) reveals early evidence of broad anti-tumor activity in three schedules. *Eur. J. Cancer*, **6**, (Suppl.), 595.

66. Yurkovetskiy, A.V., Hiller, A., Syed, S., Yin, M., Lu, X.M., Fischman, A.J., and Papisov, M.I. (2004) Synthesis of a macromolecular camptothecin conjugate with dual phase drug release. *Mol. Pharm.*, **1**, 375–382.

67. Kurzrock, R., Wheler, J., Hong, D.S., Guo, Z., Mulcahy, M.F., Benson III, A.B., Goel, S., Swami, U., Mani, S., and Buchbinder, A. (2009) Phase 1, first-in-human, dose-escalation study of EZN-2208, a novel anticancer agent, in patients (pts) with advanced malignancies. *Mol. Cancer Ther.*, **8**, C216.

68. Patnaik, A., Papadopoulos, K.P., Beeram, M., Kee, D., Tolcher, A.W., Schaaf, L.J., Tahiri, S., Bekaii-Saab, T., and Buchbinder, A., (2009) EZN-2208, a novel anticancer agent, in patients (pts) with advanced malignancies: a phase 1 dose-escalation study. *Mol. Cancer Ther.*, **8**, C221.

69. Oliver, J.C., Yen, Y., Synold, T.W., Schluep, T., and Davis, M. (2008) A dose-finding pharmacokinetic study of IT-101, the first de novo designed nanoparticle therapeutic, in refractory solid tumors. *J. Clin. Oncol.*, **26** (Suppl.), 14538.

70. Bassi, P., Volpe, A., D'Agostino, D., Cappa, E., Sacco, E., Miglioranza, E., Passaro, G., and Racioppi, M. (2010) Paclitaxel plus hyaluronic acid bioconiugated for intravesical therapy of BCG-refractory carcinoma *in situ* of the bladder: results of a phase I study. Genitourinary Cancers Symposium, San Francisco, CA, abstract 302.

71. Calvo, E., Hoch, U., Maslyar, D.J., and Tolcher, A.W. (2010) Dose-escalation phase I study of NKTR-105, a novel pegylated form of docetaxel. *J. Clin. Oncol.*, **28** (Suppl. 7s), TPS160.

72. Pasut, G. and Veronese, F.M. (2009) PEG conjugates in clinical development or use as anticancer agents: an overview. *Adv. Drug Deliv. Rev.*, **61**, 1177–1188.

73. Hoch, U., Masuoka, L., Maslyar, D., and Von Hoff, D. (2009) NKTR-102 demonstrates nonclinical and phase 1 clinical anti-tumor activity in ovarian cancer. Joint 15th Congress of the European Cancer Organization and 34th Congress of the European Society for Medical Oncology, Berlin, abstract 8015.

74. Hamm, J.T., Richards, D., Ramanathan, R.K., Becerra, C., Jameson, G., Walling, J., Gribben, D., Dhar, S., Eldon, M., and Von Hoff, D. (2009) Dose-finding study of NKTR-102 in combination with cetuximab. *J. Clin. Oncol.*, **27** (Suppl.), e13503.

75. Vergote, I.B., Micha, J.P. Jr., Pippitt, C. H. , Rao, G.G., Spitz, D.L., Reed, N., Dark, G.G., Garcia, A., Maslyar, D.J., and Rustin, G.J. (2010) P2 study of NKTR-102 in women with platinum resistant/refractory ovarian cancer. *J. Clin. Oncol.*, **28**, (Suppl.), 5013).

76. Wolff, R., Routt, S., Hartsook, R., Riggs, J., Zhang, W., Persson, H., and Johnson, R. (2008) NKTR-105, a novel pegylated-docetaxel, demonstrates superior anti-tumor activity versus docetaxel in human non-small cell lung and colon mouse xenograft models. 20th EORTC–NCI–AACR Symposium on Molecular Targets and Cancer Therapeutics, Geneva, poster 448.

77. Rosato, A., Banzato, A., De Luca, G., Renier, D., Bettella, F., Pagano, C., Esposito, G., Zanovello, P., and Bassi, P. (2006) HYTAD1-p20: a new paclitaxel–hyaluronic acid hydrosoluble bioconjugate for treatment of superficial bladder cancer. *Urol. Oncol.*, **24**, 207–215.

78. Banzato, A., Bobisse, S., Rondina, M., Renier, D., Bettella, F., Esposito, G., Quintieri, L., Melendez-Alafort, L., Mazzi, U., Zanovello, P., and Rosato, A. (2008) A paclitaxel–hyaluronan bioconjugate targeting ovarian cancer affords a potent *in vivo* therapeutic activity. *Clin. Cancer Res.*, **14**, 3598–3606.

79. Gardner, M.J., Catterall, J.B., Jones, L.M., and Turner, G.A. (1996) Human ovarian tumour cells can bind hyaluronic acid via membrane CD44: a

possible step in peritoneal metastasis. *Clin. Exp. Metastasis*, **14**, 325–334.

80. Maeda, H., Sawa, T., and Konno, T. (2001) Mechanism of tumor-targeted delivery of macromolecular drugs, including the EPR effect in solid tumor and clinical overview of the prototype polymeric drug SMANCS. *J. Control. Release*, **74**, 47–61.

81. Maeda, H., Takeshita, J., and Kanamaru, R. (1979) A lipophilic derivative of neocarzinostatin: a polymer conjugation of an antitumor protein antibiotic. *Int. J. Peptide Protein Res.*, **14**, 81–87.

82. Maeda, H., Ueda, M., Morinaga, T., and Matsumoto, T. (1985) Conjugation of poly(styrene-*co*-maleic acid) derivatives to the antitumor protein neocarzinostatin: pronounced improvements in pharmacological properties. *J. Med. Chem.*, **28**, 455–461.

83. Maeda, H., Edo, K., and Ishida, N. (1997) *Neocarzinostatin: The Past, Present, and Future on an Anticancer Drug*, Springer, Tokyo, pp. 227–267.

84. Iwai, K., Maeda, H., and Konno, T. (1984) Use of oily contrast medium for selective drug targeting to tumor: enhanced therapeutic effect and X-ray image. *Cancer Res.*, **44**, 2115–2121.

85. Konno, T., Maeda, H., Iwai, K., Tashiro, S., Maki, S., Morinaga, T., Mochinaga, M., Hiraoka, T., and Yokoyama, I. (1983) Effect of arterial administration of high-molecular-weight anticancer agent SMANCS with lipid lymphographic agent on hepatoma: a preliminary report. *Eur. J. Cancer Clin. Oncol.*, **19**, 1053–1065.

86. Konno, T., Maeda, H., Iwai, K., Maki, S., Tashiro, S., Uchida, M., and Miyauchi, Y. (1984) Selective targeting of anticancer drug and simultaneous image enhancement in solid tumors by arterially administered lipid contrast medium. *Cancer*, **54**, 2367–2374.

87. Konno, T., Maeda, H., Yokoyama, I., Iwai, K., Ogata, K., Tashiro, S., Uemura, K., Mochinaga, M., Watanabe, E., Nakakuma, K., Morinaga, T., and Miyauchi, Y. (1982) Use of a lipid lymphographic agent, lipiodol, as a carrier of high molecular weight antitumor agent, SMANCS, for hepatocellular carcinoma. *Jpn. J. Cancer Chemother.*, **9**, 2005–2015.

88. Seymour, L.W., Olliff, S.P., Poole, C.J., De Takats, P.G., Orme, R., Ferry, D.R., Maeda, H., Konno, T., and Kerr, D.J. (1998) A novel dosage approach for evaluation of SMANCS [poly-(styrene-*co*-maleyl-half-*n*-butylate)–neocarzinostatin] in the treatment of primary hepatocellular carcinoma. *Int. J. Oncol.*, **12**, 1217–1223.

89. Maki, S., Konno, T., and Maeda, H. (1985) Image enhancement in computerized tomography for sensitive diagnosis of liver cancer and semi-quantitation of tumor selective drug targeting with oily contrast medium. *Cancer*, **56**, 751–757.

90. Greish, K., Fang, J., Inuzuka, T., Nagamitsu, A., and Maeda, H. (2003) Macromolecular anticancer therapeutics for effective solid tumor targeting: advantages and prospects. *Clin. Pharmacokinet.*, **42**, 1089–1105.

91. Nagamitsu, A., Greish, K., and Maeda, H. (2009) Elevating blood pressure as a strategy to increase tumor targeted delivery of macromolecular drug SMANCS: cases of advanced solid tumors. *Jpn. J. Clin. Oncol.*, **39**, 756–766.

92. Markert, S. (2006) Cathepsin B und der α-Folsäurerezeptor zielstrukturen einer gerichteten chemotherapie des ovarial- und mammakarzinoms. PhD thesis. University of Freiburg.

93. Abu Ajaj, K. and Kratz, F. (2009) Development of dual-acting prodrugs for circumventing multidrug resistance. *Bioorg. Med. Chem. Lett.*, **19**, 955–1000.

94. Abu Ajaj, K., Biniossek, M.L., and Kratz, F. (2009) Development of protein-binding bifunctional linkers for the development of dual-acting prodrugs. *Bioconjug. Chem.*, **20**, 390–396.

Part IV
Nano- and Microparticulate Drug Delivery Systems

Lipid-Based Systems

27
Overview on Nanocarriers as Delivery Systems

Haifa Shen, Elvin Blanco, Biana Godin, Rita E. Serda,
Agathe K. Streiff, and Mauro Ferrari

27.1
Introduction

Despite significant achievements and milestones in the areas of cancer imaging and therapy over the last several decades, cancer has recently surpassed heart disease as the leading cause of death in patients under the age of 85 [1]. Multiple advances in the discovery and development of novel anticancer agents have not been translated into improvements in cancer management. While no doubt remains concerning the *in vitro* curative potential of these drugs, several factors limit their clinical success. First, the majority of drugs have low aqueous solubility, preventing their intravenous administration [2]. Second, these agents suffer from nonspecific drug distribution upon injection, with only $1:10\,000-100\,000$ molecules reaching the intended site [3]. Last, but not least, and as a direct result of the diffusive nature of present drug formulations, the therapeutic window of these drugs is narrow, leading to issues regarding tolerability and considerable mortality [4].

Application of nanotechnology to medical sciences has brought a major breakthrough for cancer therapy. Nanotechnological devices are defined by the following criteria: they are manmade, are in the 1- to 100-nm range in at least one dimension, and possess properties that only arise because of their nanoscopic dimensions [5, 6]. Nanomedicine, or the use of nanoscale constructs for diagnostic and therapeutic applications, represents a revolutionary field with the potential to facilitate drug stability and site-specific delivery [3, 7]. It is important to highlight the advantages afforded by nanoscale drug delivery devices. Nanocarriers have the potential to significantly improve the pharmacokinetics of drugs by enhancing solubilization, all the while guarding against enzymatic degradation and inactivation [8]. Encapsulation within nanoparticles also allows for longer circulation times, enhancements in tolerability, and site-specific delivery to tumors, all translating into improved therapeutic outcomes. Nanoparticles may passively and preferentially accumulate at tumor sites due to the enhanced permeability and retention (EPR) effect – a result of tumor blood vessel leakiness due to a state of ongoing angiogenesis [9, 10]. The accumulation of these nanoparticles at the diseased site significantly lowers collection in healthy organs and ensuing toxic side-effects. The advantages of nanoparticle-mediated delivery of therapeutic and imaging agents are easily appreciable, and as a result, several nanotherapeutic platforms based on the passive targeting mechanism have been successfully translated to the clinic. Doxorubicin (DOX)-containing liposomes were the first drug-carrying nanoparticles to reach cancer patients. Other novel nanoscale drug delivery strategies are currently finding their way into the clinical arena, with several micelle formulations currently in phase I and II trials [11, 12].

Presently, there is a significant emphasis on the optimization of nanocarriers to ensure adequate drug delivery to tumors, all with the hope of achieving maximal antitumor efficacy and minimal toxic side-effects. This includes fashioning the outer surface of the nanoparticles with high-affinity targeting ligands for receptors overexpressed on tumor surfaces and their associated vasculature [13, 14], as well as modifying the geometry and size to further enhance site-specific uptake and cellular internalization [15–17].

However, it is now becoming painstakingly obvious that these modifications do not address all of the biological barriers that prevent adequate transport of these nanocarriers to tumors, biological barriers that include enzymatic degradation, phagocytosis, and the inability to marginate and adhere to the vessel wall due to hemodynamic forces [7]. In an effort to address these biological barriers and effectively transport nanoparticles to the site of action, research in our laboratory has led us to the design of a multistage vector (MSV) nanocarrier for drug delivery [18]. The strategy involves using a mesoporous silicon delivery system (the first stage) loaded with one or more types of nanoparticles (the second stage), which in turn encapsulate therapeutic agents and/or imaging agents. This novel platform will be discussed in further detail below, following discussions of various examples of innovative science and platforms within the burgeoning field of nanotechnology for cancer treatment, which has immense potential to revolutionize cancer care by providing for personalized medicine.

In this chapter we provide an overview of nanocarriers in use and under investigation for cancer therapy. We introduce nanosized carriers such as liposomes [19] and polymer micelles [20] that enhance drug accumulation in the tumor based on EPR effect or active targeting. These carriers will be discussed in extensive detail in the chapters that follow. Based on some classifications [21, 22], macromolecular aggregates such as polymeric drug conjugates [23] and dendrimers [24] are included in the nanocarrier category. Since these systems were previously discussed in the current volume, they will not be in the focus of this chapter. We further describe chitosan, protein-based, and carbon-based carriers, and conclude with a review of the literature on multistage delivery carriers.

27.2
Overview on Liposome-Based Systems

Lipid-based systems possess a variety of attractive features for drug delivery. Among these characteristics are versatility in their entrapment capacity and general biocompatibility. Moreover, the physicochemical properties of lipid carriers (e.g., size and surface characteristics) are relatively easy to modify based on their composition and manufacturing process. A prominent example of a lipid-based delivery system is the liposome, which represents a nanotherapeutic modality that showed immense clinical potential for drug delivery in cancer care [25–28]. Other examples include solid lipid nanoparticles [29], microemulsions [30], and lipid micelles [31]. Liposomes are currently approved by regulatory authorities as carriers for drugs in various malignancies (Table 27.1) and thus we further focus on introducing this delivery system as an example of the lipid-based nanovectors belonging to the first and second generations.

Since Bangham's surprising discovery of highly purified phospholipid dispersions, currently called liposomes, in 1965 [32], a variety of liposomal formulations encapsulating cytotoxic chemotherapeutic agents have been studied, with several drugs approved for clinical use. The systems that are currently approved for clinical use belong to the first generation of nanovectors that use passive targeting as the main mechanism for drug localization in the tumor. These are either plain liposomes or "stealth" poly(ethylene glycol) (PEG)-conjugated (PEGylated) liposomes. These systems will be discussed subsequently as well as the liposomes pertaining to the second-generation nanovectors bearing additional functionalities (e.g., targeting or triggered drug release components).

Generally, liposomes are spherical vesicles in which the aqueous core is encircled by lipid bilayers mainly composed of phospholipids and cholesterol. The phospholipids used for the preparation of liposomes are derived from or based on the structure of biological membranes lipids in which a glycerol backbone is linked to two fatty acids [33]. The lipid head-groups of naturally occurring phospholipids can be either zwitterionic (e.g., phosphatidylcholine, phosphatidylethanolamine) or negatively charged (e.g., phosphatidic acid, phosphatidylglycerol, phosphatidylserine, phosphatidylinositol). Positively charged lipids (e.g., N-(1-(2,3-dioleoyloxy)propyl)-N,N,N-trimethylammonium (DOTAP) and N-(1-(2,3-dioleyloxy) propyl)-N,N,N-trimethylammonium chloride (DOTMA)) are not naturally occurring and do not contain a glycerol backbone. These molecules were designed and synthesized to incorporate genetic materials and to bind to negatively charged biological membranes. Saturated acyl chains typically vary in length from 10 carbons (lauryl), 12 (myristoyl), 14 (palmitoyl) to 16 (stearoyl), and the longer 18-carbon chains are usually unsaturated with one (oleoyl), two (linoleyl), or three (linolenyl) *cis* double bonds. Cholesterol is readily incorporated into liposomal structures up to 50% of the total lipid content. Liposomes may vary significantly in terms of size (from tens of nanometers to microns) and structure. Depending on the preparation method and their chemical composition, small unilamellar vesicles (SUVs), large unilamellar vesicles (LUVs)

Table 27.1 Examples of liposomal drugs currently in clinical use and in advanced clinical trials.

Active ingredient	Examples of tradename(s)	Indication
Doxorubicin-HCl	Doxil®, Caelyx®, Myocet® (approved)	ovarian cancer, AIDS-related Kaposi's sarcoma, multiple myeloma, and breast cancer
Daunorubicin citrate	DaunoXome® (approved)	first-line cytotoxic therapy for advanced HIV-associated Kaposi's sarcoma
Amphotericin	AmBiosome® (approved)	visceral leishmaniasis and fungal infections
Vincristine sulfate	Marqibo® (phase II clinical trial)	Hodgkin's lymphoma, B-cell lymphoma, non-Hodgkin's lymphoma, small-cell lung cancer, lymphoblastic leukemia, and pediatric malignancies
Cisplatin	SPI-77, liposomal cisplatin (phase III multicenter trials)	ovarian germ cell malignant tumor, hereditary breast and ovarian cancer syndrome, ovarian malignant tumor of sex cord-stromal origin, and osteosarcoma in dogs
Annamycine	phase I/II trials	acute lymphocytic leukemia
Cytarabine, Ara-C	DepoCyt® (approved)	leukemia and lymphoma that are in the fluid surrounding the brain
Amikacin	MiKaspme™ (approved), Arikase™ (pulmonary for cystic fibrosis – phase I/II trials)	bacterial septicemia, serious infections of deep tissues, and organs

or multilamellar vesicles (MLVs) are generated, the latter containing one or several concentric bilayers, respectively. Given that in liposomes one or more phospholipid bilayers surround the aqueous core, hydrophilic molecules are entrapped in the aqueous environment of the vesicles, while the entrapment of lipophilic molecules is restricted to lipid bilayers. The ζ potential of liposomal membranes is an important factor that can affect drug attachment as well as binding of vesicles to biological membranes. The membrane charge of liposomes can be modified using positively or negatively charged phospholipids or, alternatively, charged species such as stearylamine or diacetyl phosphate [33].

Due to the relatively long history of their clinical development and use, liposomal systems exemplify very well the rationale, challenges, and solutions in the design and development of nanomedicine. As an example, in order to prolong their circulation time, the surface of liposomal systems are generally decorated with a "stealth" layer (e.g., PEG) that prevents their uptake by phagocytic blood cells and organs of the reticuloendothelial (RES) system. PEGylation also decreases the binding of hydrophobic serum proteins that can act as opsonins, which can potentiate uptake of liposomes by phagocytes, thus resulting in the "stealth" effect. PEGylated liposomes were shown to have an enhanced circulation time, bioavailability, and tumor accumulation in comparison with their unPEGylated counterparts [34–39]. Several studies, however, have shown that PEGylation does not provide enhanced therapeutic efficacy [40, 41]. There are also non-PEGylated liposomes in the clinic, such as liposomal daunorubicin (DaunoXome) (80–90 nm in diameter), that have been reported to exhibit enhanced drug circulation times, although to a lesser degree than PEGylated liposomes such as liposomal DOX (Doxil/Caelyx). To illustrate the pronounced advantages of liposomally encapsulated drugs, the elimination half-life is only 0.2 h for free DOX; but it increases to 2.5 and 55 h, respectively, when non-PEGylated and PEGylated liposomal formulations are administered. Moreover, the area under the time–plasma concentration curve (AUC), which indicates the bioavailability of an agent following its administration, is increased by 11- and 200-fold for Myocet and Doxil, respectively, compared to the free drug [35, 40, 42, 43]. Encapsulation into the liposomal carrier also causes a significant reduction in the most severe adverse side-effect related to DOX, namely cardiotoxicity, as demonstrated in clinical trials [43]. Liposomal DOX is currently approved for the treatment of various malignancies, including Kaposi's sarcoma, metastatic breast cancer, advanced ovarian cancer, and multiple myeloma. Examples of other liposomal drugs that are either currently in use or are being evaluated in clinical trials include liposomal daunorubicin (DaunoXome) and vincristine (Marqibo, formerly referred to as Onco TCS) (Table 27.1).

With these first-generation nanovector systems, an enhanced accumulation of the drug into the target tissue is generally achieved through a pronounced extravasation of the carrier-associated therapeutic agent into the interstitial fluid at the tumor site, exploiting the locally increased vascular permeability or the previously mentioned EPR effect [44, 45]. An additional physiological factor that contributes to the EPR effect is that of impaired lymphatic function impeding clearance of the nanocarriers from their site of action. The localization in this case is driven only by the particles' nanodimensions and is not related to any specific recognition of tumor or neovascular targets.

Unfortunately, liposomes belonging to the second generation of nanovectors still have not made it to the clinic. Nanocarriers belonging to this category are, for example, immunoliposomes and thermosensitive liposomes [46–50]. These systems, possessing an additional degree of complexity and functionality, will be extensively discussed later in this book.

27.3
Overview on Polymer Micelle-Based Systems

Initially developed by Ringsdorf et al. in the early 1980s for use as drug delivery vehicles [51], polymer micelles comprise a promising nanoparticle strategy, with formulations currently being explored in different stages of clinical trials. The platform consists of spherical, supramolecular constructs, with sizes ranging from 10 to 100 nm, formed from the self-assembly of biocompatible amphiphilic block copolymers in aqueous environments [52]. As a result of this self-assembly, the hydrophobic portion of the polymer forms a semi-solid core that effectively entraps the hydrophobic drug. Examples of the hydrophobic polymer components include poly(D,L-lactic acid) (PDLLA), poly(ε-caprolactone) (PCL), and poly(propylene oxide) (PPO), to name a few, with sizes ranging from 2 to 15 kDa [53]. Concomitantly, the hydrophilic block of the polymer forms a hydrating layer that protects against opsonization and RES clearance [54]. The polymer of choice for the hydrophilic block is PEG, while polymers such as poly(N-vinyl pyrrolidone) (PVP) and poly(N-isopropylacrylamide) (PNIPAM) have recently been explored [20].

Polymer micelles allow for the delivery of drugs that are otherwise deemed too toxic, providing numerous advantages that are immediately appreciable, with their chief benefit consisting of their ability to solubilize hydrophobic drugs within the cores. Paclitaxel is one of these examples, as it has a water solubility of 0.0015 mg/ml. Encapsulation of the drug within the micellar core effectively increases the solubility by more than a 1000-fold to 2 mg/ml [55]. Drug encapsulation within the core also protects against degradation, conferring an extra degree of drug stability. While the hydrophobic core is of paramount importance for micellar drug delivery, the hydrophilic portion proves equally essential. As mentioned previously, the corona of the micelles provides a hydrating layer that hinders plasma protein interactions and opsonization that would otherwise result in phagocytic clearance [56]. Additionally, polymer micelles possess a very low critical micelle concentration (CMC; the concentration at which monomers form micelles), resulting in stable constructs that do not easily destabilize upon injection [57]. Innate chemistry aside, another unique property of polymer micelles is their small size, which also prevents RES uptake [58]. The small size and the PEGylated corona contribute to longer circulation times in the blood, which in turn results in an increase in the preferential accumulation of micelles in tumor tissue – a result of the EPR effect.

Wooley et al. have constructed shell cross-linked knedel (SCK)-like nanoparticles that have a hydrophobic core and a cross-linked shell domain that stabilizes the structure (Figure 27.1), allowing for higher loading [59]. The cationic micelles are approximately 14 nm and are able to complex with plasmid DNA. The ratio of polymer amines to DNA phosphates (N/P) determines the size of the complex and the degree of DNA binding. Cellular uptake was greatest for particles with an N/P ratio of 6:1. A variety of amphiphilic block polymers can be used in the assembly process, providing particles that vary by functionality of the cores and shell domains, degree of polymerization, and hydrophobic/hydrophilic ratio [60].

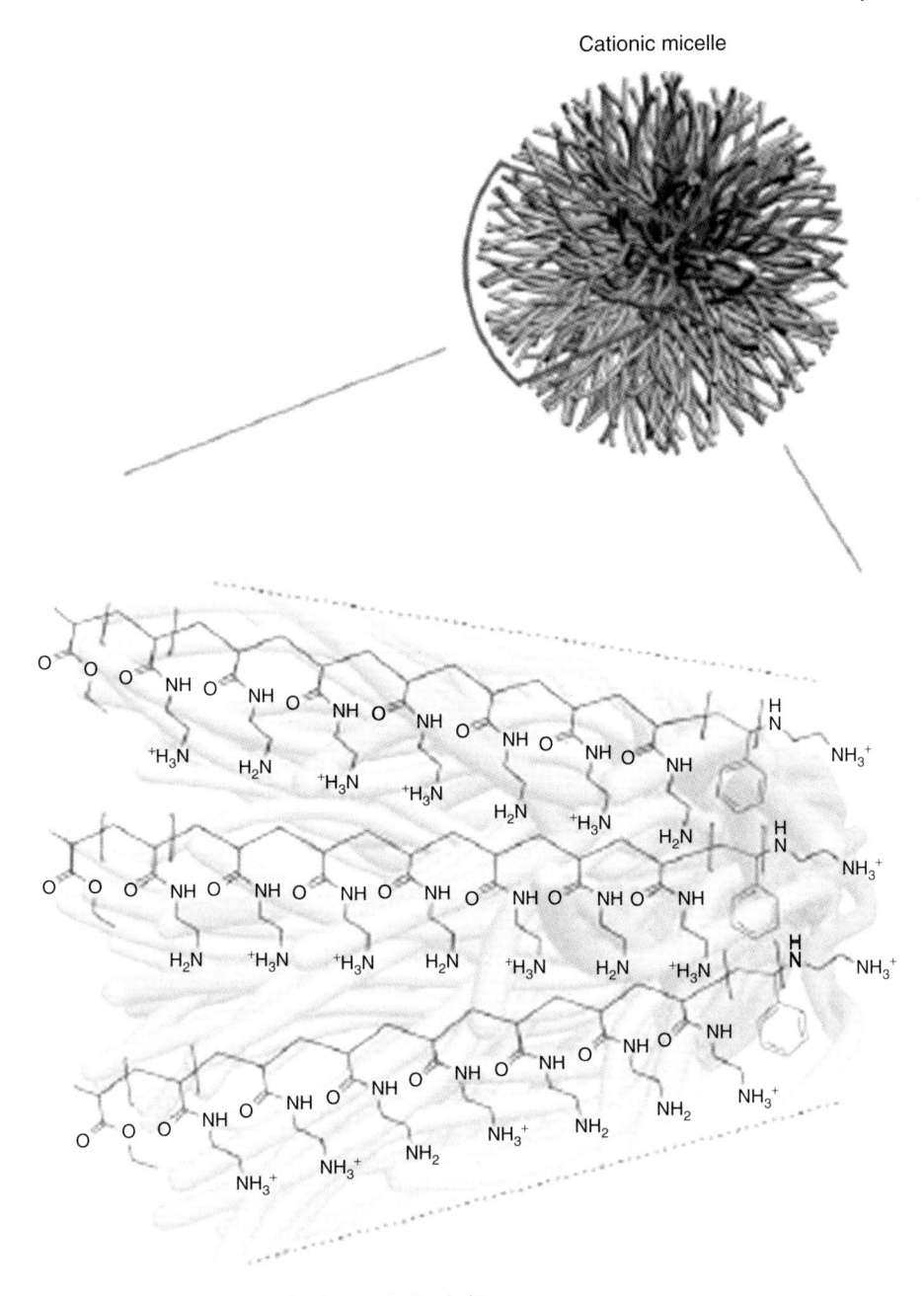

Figure 27.1 SCK nanoparticles have a hydrophobic core and a cross-linked shell domain. Use of a diacid-derivatized cross-linker provides a cationic shell, able to complex with DNA. (Reproduced with permission from [59]. Courtesy of Elsevier.)

Targeting moieties, imaging contrast agents, and therapeutics can all be integrated into the SCK nanoparticles, creating targeted theranostics.

Polymer micelles have matured into a viable drug delivery platform with various formulations being explored in clinical trials. Kataoka et al. developed PEG–poly(L-aspartic acid) micelles containing DOX, showing impressive preclinical antitumor efficacy [61]. The formulation, known as, has a longer half-life, and a much reduced drug clearance [62]. Genexol-PM, another micellar formulation in clinical trials, consists of a paclitaxel-containing PEG-*b*-poly(D,L-lactide) micellar platform. This formulation of paclitaxel has proven to be much more tolerable than Taxol®, the currently available paclitaxel formulation in the clinic consisting of Cremophor® EL – an excipient shown to result in hypersensitivity reactions [63]. Antitumor activities were reported in previously unresponsive patients simply because the dose of the micelles could be escalated significantly as compared to traditional formulations of paclitaxel [64].

27.4
Other Nanoparticulate Drug Delivery Systems

27.4.1
Chitosan and Chitosan-Coated Nanoparticles

Delivery of chemotherapeutic agents in a lipid, polymer, or polysaccharide coating enhances stability and provides a means for targeted delivery to the lesion, and potentially, sustained or triggered release of therapeutic agents. Chitosan, derived from chitin, is a biodegradable, biocompatible polysaccharide composed of random β1–4-linked D-glucosamine and *N*-acetyl-D-glucosamine units. It has been used to both coat and create novel nanoparticles. For example, iron oxide nanoparticles coated with chitosan have been shown to be nontoxic at 200 μg/ml, and internalization of these nanoparticles by mesenchymal stem cells neither alters expression of surface markers nor impacts their differentiation potential [65]. The positively charged chitosan gives the coated nanoparticles an overall positive charge.

Based on the high charge density of *N*-acetyl histidine-conjugated glycol chitosan, it is reported to aid in tissue penetration and membrane translocation, potentially leading to intracytoplasmic delivery of drugs and nanoparticles [66, 67]. Our group has demonstrated that coating iron oxide nanoparticles in chitosan and loading them into a porous silicon microparticle creates a drug delivery vector that is capable of being internalized by cells and is able to escape the endosome [68]. Both chitosan nanoparticles and chitosan-coated nanoparticles (iron oxide) are internalized by cells, and do not alter cell survival and viability [68, 69]. Chitosan-coated nanoparticles and free chitosan are reported to inhibit the production of pro-inflammatory cytokines [70]. Additionally, chitosan, with molecular weights of 50, 150, and 300 kDa, significantly inhibits expression of cyclooxygenase-2 and the production of prostaglandin E_2, which benefits both cancer therapy and wound healing [71]. Moreover, hydrophilic glycol chitosan can be derivatized with 5β-cholanic acid, creating hydrophobic chitosan nanoparticles [72]. These particles, which were shown to have a globular shape, average diameter of 359 nm, and a ζ potential of 22 mV, were internalized by cells and demonstrated low toxicity.

Bisht and Maitra have shown that DOX cardiotoxicity can be minimized by coupling the drug with dextran and encapsulating it within chitosan [73]. Chitosan has also been shown to be a safe material for nonviral gene delivery compared to other reagents such as polyethylenimine (PEI) [74]. Chitosan and PEI are both able to associate with plasmid DNA and protect the nucleic acid from serum degradation, and both chitosan- and PEI-mediated gene delivery results in similar levels of gene expression. However, unlike chitosan, PEI-mediated delivery of nucleic acids proves toxic to cells.

27.4.2
Albumin Nanoparticles

Nanoparticle albumin-bound (*nab*®) technologies are an emerging generation of drug delivery systems that have been shown to reduce toxicity and improve therapeutic efficacy in cancer treatment. One class of drugs that has benefited from this new drug delivery method is the taxanes, which cause mitotic arrest by hyperstabilizing microtubules [75]. Since these anticancer agents are hydrophobic, they depend on solvent-based delivery vehicles for intravenous administration. As described previously, paclitaxel is rendered more soluble using Cremophor EL, which is itself toxic [75]. The administration of the drug is also further complicated by the requirement of further dilution with either normal saline or 5% dextrose solutions, contributing to increased infusion times and volumes [76]. These infusions often result in toxicities such as hypersensitivity reactions and neutropenia [77]. In addition to toxicities, solvent-based drug delivery methods are associated with reduced efficacy. It has been postulated that this is due to the formation of large polar micelles that reduces the amount of unbound drug [77]. This drug entrapment mechanism may explain why efficacy, or more specifically, response rate, survival, and quality of life, does not improve with increased dose of Cremophor EL–paclitaxel [75]. Abraxane®, the 130-nm albumin-bound form of paclitaxel, allows for a 50% dose increase compared to solvent-based paclitaxel, despite more frequent sensory neuropathy, which is easily manageable in the clinic [78].

The *nab* technologies can serve as an improved delivery method by exploiting endogenous pathways in the body for albumin – a natural carrier of hydrophobic molecules. Albumin binds substances in a noncovalent fashion, allowing release at a target site, and has been shown to facilitate endothelial transcytosis of its cargo via a 60-kDa glycoprotein (gp60) receptor-mediated mechanism [79]. In the case of paclitaxel, Abraxane has been shown to allow for more efficacious doses of a therapeutic agent to be tolerated by the patient and hence improve clinical outcomes in the treatment of metastatic breast cancer [80]. In addition, since *nab* technology does not require increased dilutions and toxicity management medications of the solvent-based drug delivery systems, infusion times are reduced and administration of the nanoparticle is simplified [75].

Currently, albumin nanoparticles are being investigated as carrier systems for other water-insoluble anti-cancer agents in various cancers as well as in combination therapy [75]. For instance, *nab*-docetaxel, a solvent-free nanoparticle alternative to docetaxel in polysorbate 80, is being studied in various solid tumors [75].

27.4.3
Carbon Nanotubes

Carbon nanotubes (CNTs) are tube-shaped allotropes of carbon in the sp^2 configuration. They can make up a plain cylinder, also known as single-walled CNTs (single-walled carbon nanotubeSWNTs), or have layers of walls, also known as multiwalled CNTs (multiwalled carbon nanotubeMWNTs). Their diameters can vary, with the smallest being the SWNTs, and the largest varying among the MWNTs. They have a needle-like shape and have been likened to asbestos in this aspect. CNTs are a valuable drug delivery system since they can encapsulate covalently and noncovalently bound compounds, with their aspect ratio and geometry allowing for penetration into the cell [81]. It is this high aspect ratio that allows for a high loading capacity of the carried drug [82]. CNTs can deliver various therapeutic agents efficiently including anticancer drugs, DNA, and small interfering RNA (siRNA) [83].

Release of drug molecules from CNTs is dependent not only on diameter, but also on water solubility and other characteristics of nanotubes [84]. Synthetic and natural polymers such as polyphenylacetylene and polysaccharides have been used to encase SWNTs to improve their water solubility and to reduce the formation of poorly dispersing bundles [85, 86]. Certain CNT-based drug delivery systems also take advantage of the reduced pH of tumor environments to control the release of their contents. For instance, SWNTs loaded with the anticancer drug DOX have been shown *in vitro* to contain bound drug at physiological pH (7.4), which then is subsequently unbound at the site of the tumor [87]. This characteristic is imparted on the SWNTs by modifying the surface polysaccharides and effectively changing the surface potentials of the nanotube [87]. As with other types of nanoparticles, tumor targeting of carbon nanoparticles can be enhanced by surface modification with affinity moieties, including antibodies and low-molecular-weight targeting agents such as folic acid [59].

Future work involves studies regarding the toxicity of CNTs as they become more frequently used as drug delivery methods, since their role in occupational hazards has been well characterized [88]. Even though CNTs have been well studied in the context of engineering, they are relatively new in the field of nanomedicine and have a promising role in oncology.

27.5
MSV Drug Delivery Systems

Successful cancer treatment demands that drugs are delivered to the right place at the right time, without causing significant collateral damage in order to achieve a sufficient therapeutic index. Many systems are being developed as intravascular carriers to enhance tissue-specific drug delivery [21, 89]. However, the biological barriers inside the body pose a great challenge to achieve this goal [7]. En route to their target after entering the circulation, nanoparticle drugs encounter many biobarriers, such as enzymatic degradation, sequestration by monocytes and macrophages of the RES, the vascular endothelium, and the tumor interstitium [7, 90].

The MSV drug delivery platform pioneered by our laboratory represents a synergistic combination of different nanocarrier systems to attain the goal of overcoming a multiplicity of biological barriers to achieve site-specific delivery [3, 18]. In this system, each stage performs part of the journey from the site of administration toward the tumor lesion (Figure 27.2). The first-stage silicon nanocarriers can be loaded with second-stage nanoparticles, such as liposomes and micelles containing different types of payloads or imaging agents. Figure 27.3 shows images of a silicon nanocarrier loaded with iron oxide nanoparticles. The first-stage particle is designed to navigate within the circulatory system and target the tumor neovasculature. The second-stage nanoparticles within the pores of the first stage are then released toward the tumor mass from the site of vascular adhesion. These nanoparticles are sufficiently small, undergo passive extravasation from tumor vasculature, and diffuse within the extravascular compartment (Figure 27.2).

We have applied multiscale modeling in the design of drug delivery vectors to maximize particle distribution in tumor tissues [17, 92]. By using combinatorial nanomanufacturing methodologies within the framework of photolithography, we can manufacture MSV silicon particles of any desired size, shape, and porosity. Porosification of silicon creates material that is biodegradable, biocompatible, and a carrier for second-stage nanoparticles. By loading second-stage nanoparticles into the pores of the first-stage silicon particles, the enzymatic degradation and RES uptake are prevented in circulation. At tumor tissues, porous silicon is degraded into orthosilicic acid over time, which is readily excreted from the body. The rate of degradation is partially determined by the porosity of the silicon particles. The second-stage nanoparticles are gradually released from the pores of the silicon particles during the process, creating a system for sustained and controlled release. The ability to form particles of different sizes and shapes is crucial for tissue distribution, and consequently, improved clinical outcomes. We have used mathematical models to design multistage particles with optimal properties to increase margination to the vascular endothelium. In a recent study, we demonstrated that small spherical particles (with diameters 1 μm or less) had a more uniform tissue distribution than larger ones, with more diskoidal particles accumulating in tumor tissues than spherical, hemispherical, or cylindrical particles [17]. Surface modification of the silicon particles is another major determinant on tissue distribution of the MSVs and subcellular partitioning of the second-stage nanoparticles. Aminopropyltriethoxylsilane-modified silicon particles are selectively internalized by vascular endothelial cells, while macrophages prefer negatively charged oxidized particles [68, 93]. Nanoparticles with different surface modifications go through

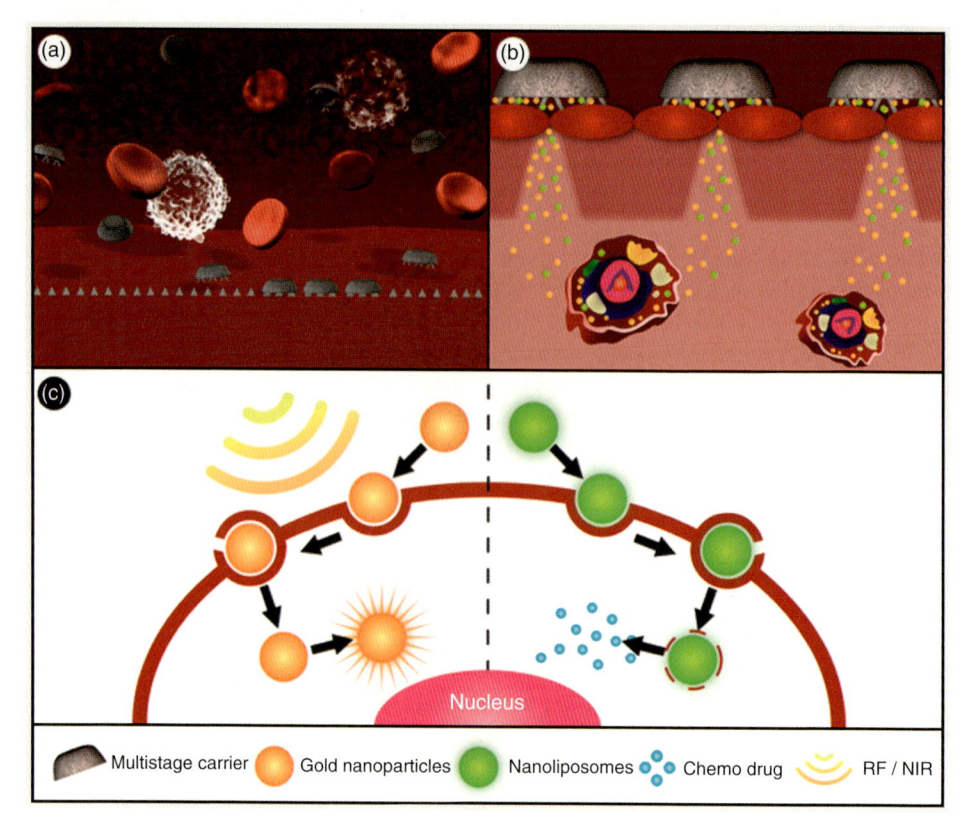

Figure 27.2 Schematic illustration of the action of a multistage vector. (a) A nontoxic, biodegradable first-stage carrier is optimally designed to evade RES, and has margination, adhesion, and internalization properties that allow it to attain preferential concentration on the target tumor vascular endothelium. (b) The first-stage particle coreleases second-stage carrier nanoparticles with agents that facilitate their permeation through the vascular endothelium into the tumor tissues. (c) The second-stage nanoparticles penetrate the cellular membrane and deploy different, synergistic therapeutic agents into the cytoplasm, the nucleus, or to the subcellular targets. The particles themselves can serve as a means of physical therapy, for example, by converting external radiation (light, radiofrequency, ultrasound) into heat, for a localized form of thermal ablation. (Reproduced from [7]. Courtesy of the Cell Press.)

different routes of intracellular trafficking (Figure 27.4). These results will guide us in the design of particles with advantageous margination, adhesion, and rheological properties, resulting in improved performance for endothelial antigen recognition and cell internalization probabilities, and ultimately the biodistribution of the MSVs and therapeutic index of the cytotoxic payload delivered by the MSVs. It is important to note that silicon-based MSVs do not appear to cause obvious toxicities to the body. Mice administered with silicon vectors had no obvious changes in plasma levels of renal (blood urea nitrogen and creatinine) and hepatic

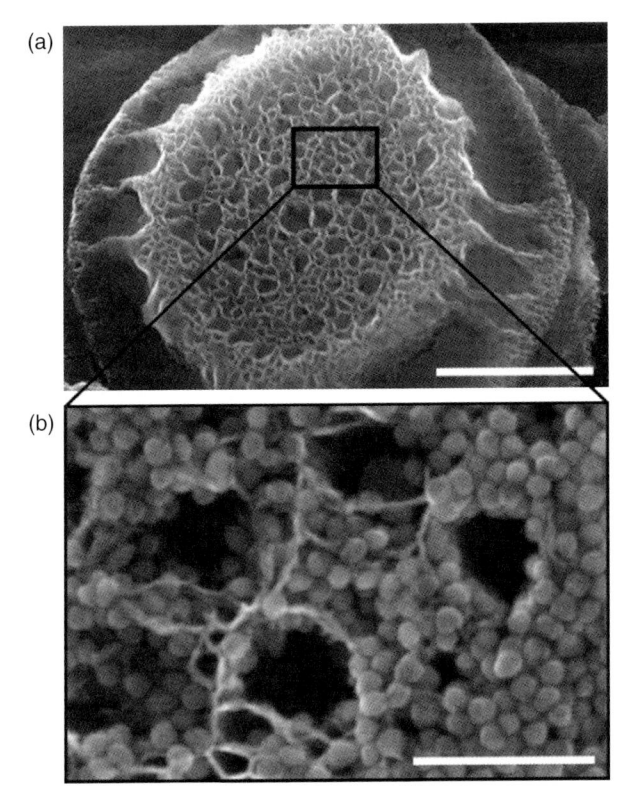

Figure 27.3 High-resolution scanning electron microscopy images of MSVs. Diskoidal porous silicon microparticles were loaded with superparamagnetic iron oxide nanoparticles (SPIONs) at increasing magnifications. (a) Diskoidal porous silicon microparticle ($\times 25\,000$, bar $= 1$ μm) and (b) silicon microparticle loaded with 30-nm SPIONs ($\times 450\,000$, bar $= 100$ nm). (Reproduced from [91]. Courtesy of Wiley Interscience.)

(lactate dehydrogenase) biomarkers, 23 plasma cytokines, or pathological infiltration of leukocytes in major organs [94].

The MSV platform has been successfully applied for experimental cancer therapeutics with animal tumor models. One of the first therapeutic agents tested in this system belongs to the class of siRNA therapeutics [94]. The discovery of RNA interference by Fire *et al.* [95] opened up an exciting field of cancer therapeutics with vast clinical application by theoretically being able to silence any cancer-related gene pathway. However, the safe and effective delivery of siRNA therapeutics has been the major bottleneck in the translation of this technology to clinical application. "Naked" siRNAs have an extremely high degradation rate, and are subjected to the immune system activation and recognition. Liposomes were intensely investigated as an attractive delivery system for siRNA therapeutics, as they can protect siRNA from extensive degradation and inhibit harmful nonspecific binding to normal tissues. *In vitro* and *in vivo* studies have demonstrated the improvement of siRNA delivery to melanomas, lung cancer, breast cancer, and ovarian cancer

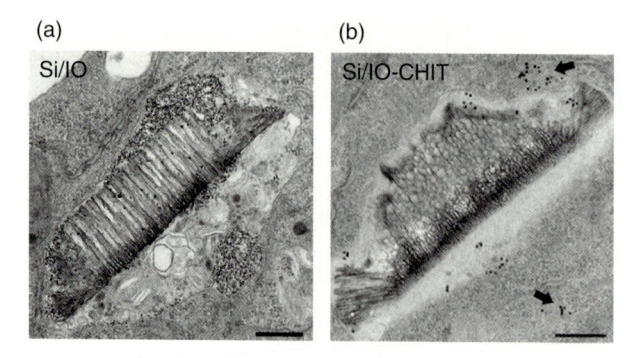

Figure 27.4 Intracellular trafficking of multistage vectors. Macrophages were incubated with either PEGylated amine (a) or chitosan (CHIT)-coated (b) iron oxide (IO) nanoparticles (30 nm diameter) loaded into porous silicon microparticles (Si). Twenty-four hours after cellular internalization, released PEGylated amine nanoparticles clustered into specific areas of the endosome, which were found to pinch off and form unique vesicles. Released chitosan-coated nanoparticles escaped the endosome and resided in the cytosol.

when liposomal carriers were used [96, 97]. In our recent study, we evaluated MSVs loaded with neutral dioleoyl phosphatidylcholine nanoliposomes containing EphA2-specific siRNA. The EphA2 oncoprotein is absent in normal tissues, but overexpressed in most malignancies, including ovarian cancer. In this study, conducted in two independent orthotopic mouse models of ovarian cancer, a single intravenous injection of the multistage siRNA system caused gene silencing for at least 3 weeks, which resulted in significantly reduced tumor burden, angiogenesis, and cell proliferation. This effect of a single, once-in-3-weeks dose was equivalent to six doses of liposomal siRNA administered twice a week [94]. The mechanism of the efficient and sustained liposomal siRNA delivery is likely a result of surface modification, tissue distribution, and slow biodegradation of the first-stage mesoporous silicon particles. The first-stage particles not only served as a storage depot for liposomal siRNA, but also shielded siRNA oligos from degradation by enzymes inside the body. We used positively charged silicon particles to enhance entrapment of the negatively charged liposomal siRNA. Silicon particles were apparent in the spleen 2 weeks after administration. Up to 25% of the first-stage silicon particles stilled remained in the liver 3 weeks after injection. Analysis of blood samples did not reveal any toxicity to the liver, kidney, and spleen. Moreover, no significant levels of inflammatory cytokines were induced by the silicon particles, validating the MSV as a safe and efficient delivery system for nanoparticle drugs.

27.6
Conclusions and Perspectives

In this chapter, we gave a brief introduction of nanocarriers used in oncology, most of which will be highlighted in the chapters to follow. While all of these platforms have clear advantages on administration over unencapsulated drugs, a general consensus is that these systems are in a constant state of evolution, wherein the versatility and multifunctionality are the key elements for enhancements in tumor therapy. Programming the nanocarrier to perform several tasks, such as synergizing its controlled delivery of drugs with tumor imaging and targeting, will most likely result in better management of the disease. Indeed, current research involves novel strategies to attach targeting ligands with high affinity for receptors overexpressed on tumors or ways to utilize the tumor's own microenvironment as a stimulus for drug release. More recent approaches involve a synergistic combination of various nanofabricated systems to overcome a multiplicity of biological barriers aiming to bring the drug to the right place at the right time. An example of such a system is a multistage carrier, where rationally designed porous degradable particles are used as primary delivery cargo for nanoscale drugs and/or imaging agents.

To conclude, advances in cancer nanomedicine can revolutionize current medical practice through the introduction of highly specific agents, ushering us closer to an era of personalized medicine in oncology.

References

1. Jemal, A. et al. (2009) Cancer statistics. CA Cancer J. Clin., 59, 225–249.
2. Hatefi, A. and Amsden, B. (2002) Camptothecin delivery methods. Pharm. Res., 19, 1389–1399.
3. Ferrari, M. (2005) Cancer nanotechnology: opportunities and challenges. Nat. Rev. Cancer, 5, 161–171.
4. Canal, P., Gamelin, E., Vassal, G., and Robert, J. (1998) Benefits of pharmacological knowledge in the design and monitoring of cancer chemotherapy. Pathol. Oncol. Res., 4, 171–178.
5. Theis, T. et al. (2006) nan'o.tech.nol'o.gy n. Nat. Nanotechnol., 1, 8–10.
6. Ferrari, M., Philibert, M.A., and Sanhai, W.R. (2009) Nanomedicine and society. Clin. Pharmacol. Ther., 85, 466–467.
7. Ferrari, M. (2010) Frontiers in cancer nanomedicine: directing mass transport through biological barriers. Trends Biotechnol., 28, 181–188.
8. Jones, M. and Leroux, J. (1999) Polymeric micelles – a new generation of colloidal drug carriers. Eur. J. Pharm. Biopharm., 48, 101–111.
9. Hashizume, H. et al. (2000) Openings between defective endothelial cells explain tumor vessel leakiness. Am. J. Pathol., 156, 1363–1380.
10. Maeda, H. (2001) The enhanced permeability and retention (EPR) effect in tumor vasculature: the key role of tumor-selective macromolecular drug targeting. Adv. Enzyme Regul., 41, 189–207.
11. Matsumura, Y. and Kataoka, K. (2009) Preclinical and clinical studies of anticancer agent-incorporating polymer micelles. Cancer Sci., 100, 572–579.
12. Saif, M.W. et al. (2010) Phase II clinical trial of paclitaxel loaded polymeric micelle in patients with advanced pancreatic cancer. Cancer Invest., 28, 186–194.
13. Pasqualini, R., Koivunen, E., and Ruoslahti, E. (1997) Alpha v integrins as receptors for tumor targeting by circulating ligands. Nat. Biotechnol., 15, 542–546.
14. Torchilin, V. (2008) Antibody-modified liposomes for cancer chemotherapy. Expert Opin. Drug Deliv., 5, 1003–1025.
15. Lee, S.Y., Ferrari, M., and Decuzzi, P. (2009) Shaping nano-/micro-particles for enhanced vascular interaction in laminar flows. Nanotechnology, 20, 495101.
16. Sakamoto, J., Annapragada, A., Decuzzi, P., and Ferrari, M. (2007) Antibiological barrier nanovector

17. Decuzzi, P. et al. (2010) Size and shape effects in the biodistribution of intravascularly injected particles. *J Control. Release*, **141**, 320–327.
18. Tasciotti, E. et al. (2008) Mesoporous silicon particles as a multistage delivery system for imaging and therapeutic applications. *Nat. Nanotechnol.*, **3**, 151–157.
19. Torchilin, V.P. (2005) Recent advances with liposomes as pharmaceutical carriers. *Nat. Rev. Drug Discov.*, **4**, 145–160.
20. Sutton, D., Nasongkla, N., Blanco, E., and Gao, J. (2007) Functionalized micellar systems for cancer targeted drug delivery. *Pharm. Res.*, **24**, 1029–1046.
21. Peer, D. et al. (2007) Nanocarriers as an emerging platform for cancer therapy. *Nat. Nanotechnol.*, **2**, 751–760.
22. Sakamoto, J.H. et al. (2010) Enabling individualized therapy through nanotechnology. *Pharmacol. Res.*, **62**, 57–89.
23. Duncan, R. (2003) The dawning era of polymer therapeutics. *Nat. Rev. Drug Discov.*, **2**, 347–360.
24. Lee, C.C., MacKay, J.A., Frechet, J.M., and Szoka, F.C. (2005) Designing dendrimers for biological applications. *Nat. Biotechnol.*, **23**, 1517–1526.
25. Malam, Y., Loizidou, M., and Seifalian, A.M. (2009) Liposomes and nanoparticles: nanosized vehicles for drug delivery in cancer. *Trends Pharmacol. Sci.*, **30**, 592–599.
26. Fanciullino, R. and Ciccolini, J. (2009) Liposome-encapsulated anticancer drugs: still waiting for the magic bullet? *Curr. Med. Chem.*, **16**, 4361–4371.
27. Tan, M.L., Choong, P.F., and Dass, C.R. (2010) Recent developments in liposomes, microparticles and nanoparticles for protein and peptide drug delivery. *Peptides*, **31**, 184–193.
28. Kaasgaard, T. and Andresen, T.L. (2010) Liposomal cancer therapy: exploiting tumor characteristics. *Expert Opin. Drug Deliv.*, **7**, 225–243.
29. Lee, M.K., Lim, S.J., and Kim, C.K. (2007) Preparation, characterization and *in vitro* cytotoxicity of paclitaxel-loaded sterically stabilized solid lipid nanoparticles. *Biomaterials*, **28**, 2137–2146.
30. Nornoo, A.O., Osborne, D.W., and Chow, D.S. (2008) Cremophor-free intravenous microemulsions for paclitaxel I: formulation, cytotoxicity and hemolysis. *Int. J. Pharm.*, **349**, 108–116.
31. Wu, Y., Sefah, K., Liu, H., Wang, R., and Tan, W. (2010) DNA aptamer-micelle as an efficient detection/delivery vehicle toward cancer cells. *Proc. Natl. Acad. Sci. USA*, **107**, 5–10.
32. Deamer, D.W. (2010) From "banghasomes" to liposomes: a memoir of Alec Bangham, 1921–2010. *FASEB J.*, **24**, 1308–1310.
33. New, R.R.C., (1990) *Liposomes: A Practical Approach*, Oxford University Press, New York.
34. Hamidi, M., Azadi, A., and Rafiei, P. (2006) Pharmacokinetic consequences of pegylation. *Drug Deliv.*, **13**, 399–409.
35. Marina, N.M. et al. (2002) Dose escalation and pharmacokinetics of pegylated liposomal doxorubicin (Doxil) in children with solid tumors: a pediatric oncology group study. *Clin. Cancer Res.*, **8**, 413–418.
36. Litzinger, D.C., Buiting, A.M., van Rooijen, N., and Huang, L. (1994) Effect of liposome size on the circulation time and intraorgan distribution of amphipathic poly(ethylene glycol)-containing liposomes. *Biochim. Biophys. Acta*, **1190**, 99–107.
37. Papahadjopoulos, D. et al. (1991) Sterically stabilized liposomes: improvements in pharmacokinetics and antitumor therapeutic efficacy. *Proc. Natl. Acad. Sci. USA*, **88**, 11460–11464.
38. Kamaly, N. et al. (2008) Bimodal paramagnetic and fluorescent liposomes for cellular and tumor magnetic resonance imaging. *Bioconjug. Chem.*, **19**, 118–129.
39. Zalipsky, S. et al. (2007) Antitumor activity of new liposomal prodrug of mitomycin C in multidrug resistant solid tumor: insights of the mechanism of action. *J. Drug Target.*, **15**, 518–530.
40. Hong, R.L. et al. (1999) Direct comparison of liposomal doxorubicin with or without polyethylene glycol coating in C-26 tumor-bearing mice: is surface coating with polyethylene glycol beneficial? *Clin. Cancer Res.*, **5**, 3645–3652.

41. Parr, M.J., Masin, D., Cullis, P.R., and Bally, M.B. (1997) Accumulation of liposomal lipid and encapsulated doxorubicin in murine Lewis lung carcinoma: the lack of beneficial effects by coating liposomes with poly(ethylene glycol). *J. Pharmacol. Exp. Ther.*, **280**, 1319–1327.
42. Rahman, A. et al. (1990) A phase I clinical trial and pharmacokinetic evaluation of liposome-encapsulated doxorubicin. *J. Clin. Oncol.*, **8**, 1093–1100.
43. Hofheinz, R.D., Gnad-Vogt, S.U., Beyer, U., and Hochhaus, A. (2005) Liposomal encapsulated anti-cancer drugs. *Anti-Cancer Drugs*, **16**, 691–707.
44. Fang, J., Nakamura, H., and Maeda, H. (2011) The EPR effect: unique features of tumor blood vessels for drug delivery, factors involved, and limitations and augmentation of the effect. *Adv. Drug Deliv. Rev.*, **63** (3), 136–151.
45. Maeda, H., Wu, J., Sawa, T., Matsumura, Y., and Hori, K. (2000) Tumor vascular permeability and the EPR effect in macromolecular therapeutics: a review. *J. Control. Release*, **65**, 271–284.
46. Torchilin, V. (2009) Multifunctional and stimuli-sensitive pharmaceutical nanocarriers. *Eur. J. Pharm. Biopharm.*, **71**, 431–444.
47. Torchilin, V.P. (2006) Multifunctional nanocarriers. *Adv. Drug Deliv. Rev.*, **58**, 1532–1555.
48. Auguste, D.T. et al. (2008) Triggered release of siRNA from poly(ethylene glycol)-protected, pH-dependent liposomes. *J. Control. Release*, **130**, 266–274.
49. Moses, M.A., Brem, H., and Langer, R. (2003) Advancing the field of drug delivery: taking aim at cancer. *Cancer Cell*, **4**, 337–341.
50. McNeeley, K.M., Karathanasis, E., Annapragada, A.V., and Bellamkonda, R.V. (2009) Masking and triggered unmasking of targeting ligands on nanocarriers to improve drug delivery to brain tumors. *Biomaterials*, **30**, 3986–3995.
51. Gros, L., Ringsdorf, H., and Schupp, H. (1981) Polymeric anti-tumor agents on a molecular and on a cellular-level. *Angew. Chem. Int. Ed.*, **20**, 305–325.
52. Savic, R., Luo, L., Eisenberg, A., and Maysinger, D. (2003) Micellar nanocontainers distribute to defined cytoplasmic organelles. *Science*, **300**, 615–618.
53. Blanco, E., Kessinger, C.W., Sumer, B.D., and Gao, J. (2009) Multifunctional micellar nanomedicine for cancer therapy. *Exp. Biol. Med.*, **234**, 123–131.
54. Torchilin, V.P. (2001) Structure and design of polymeric surfactant-based drug delivery systems. *J. Control. Release*, **73**, 137–172.
55. Soga, O. et al. (2005) Thermosensitive and biodegradable polymeric micelles for paclitaxel delivery. *J. Control. Release*, **103**, 341–353.
56. Torchilin, V.P. (2002) PEG-based micelles as carriers of contrast agents for different imaging modalities. *Adv. Drug Deliv. Rev.*, **54**, 235–252.
57. Torchilin, V.P., Lukyanov, A.N., Gao, Z., and Papahadjopoulos-Sternberg, B. (2003) Immunomicelles: targeted pharmaceutical carriers for poorly soluble drugs. *Proc. Natl. Acad. Sci. USA*, **100**, 6039–6044.
58. Haag, R. (2004) Supramolecular drug-delivery systems based on polymeric core-shell architectures. *Angew. Chem. Int. Ed.*, **43**, 278–282.
59. Zhang, K., Fang, H., Wang, Z., Taylor, J.S., and Wooley, K.L. (2009) Cationic shell-crosslinked knedel-like nanoparticles for highly efficient gene and oligonucleotide transfection of mammalian cells. *Biomaterials*, **30**, 968–977.
60. Nystrom, A.M., Bartels, J.W., Du, W., and Wooley, K.L. (2009) Perfluorocarbon-loaded shell crosslinked knedel-like nanoparticles: lessons regarding polymer mobility and self assembly. *J. Polym. Sci. A*, **47**, 1023–1037.
61. Nakanishi, T. et al. (2001) Development of the polymer micelle carrier system for doxorubicin. *J. Control. Release*, **74**, 295–302.
62. Matsumura, Y. et al. (2004) Phase I clinical trial and pharmacokinetic evaluation of NK911, a micelle-encapsulated doxorubicin. *Br. J. Cancer*, **91**, 1775–1781.
63. Wiernik, P.H. et al. (1987) Phase I clinical and pharmacokinetic study of taxol. *Cancer Res.*, **47**, 2486–2493.

64. Kim, T.Y. et al. (2004) Phase I and pharmacokinetic study of Genexol-PM, a cremophor-free, polymeric micelle-formulated paclitaxel, in patients with advanced malignancies. *Clin. Cancer Res.*, **10**, 3708–3716.

65. Reddy, A.M. et al. (2010) *In vivo* tracking of mesenchymal stem cells labeled with a novel chitosan-coated superparamagnetic iron oxide nanoparticles using 3.0T MRI. *J. Korean Med. Sci.*, **25**, 211–219.

66. Ghosn, B. et al. (2010) Efficient mucosal delivery of optical contrast agents using imidazole-modified chitosan. *J. Biomed. Opt.*, **15**, 015003.

67. Park, J.S. et al. (2006) N-acetyl histidine-conjugated glycol chitosan self-assembled nanoparticles for intracytoplasmic delivery of drugs: endocytosis, exocytosis and drug release. *J. Control. Release*, **115**, 37–45.

68. Serda, R., Mack, A., van de Ven, A., Ferrati, S., Dunner, K. Jr., Godin, B., Chiappini, C., Landry, M., Brousseau, L., Liu, X., Bean, A.J., and Ferrari, M. (2010) Logic-embedded vectors for intracellular partitioning and exocytosis of nanoparticles. *Small*, **6**, 2691–2700.

69. Enriquez de Salamanca, A. et al. (2006) Chitosan nanoparticles as a potential drug delivery system for the ocular surface: toxicity, uptake mechanism and *in vivo* tolerance. *Invest. Ophthalmol. Vis Sci.*, **47**, 1416–1425.

70. Kim, M.S. et al. (2002) Water-soluble chitosan inhibits the production of pro-inflammatory cytokine in human astrocytoma cells activated by amyloid beta peptide and interleukin-1beta. *Neurosci. Lett.*, **321**, 105–109.

71. Chou, T.C., Fu, E., and Shen, E.C. (2003) Chitosan inhibits prostaglandin E2 formation and cyclooxygenase-2 induction in lipopolysaccharide-treated RAW 264.7 macrophages. *Biochem. Biophys. Res. Commun.*, **308**, 403–407.

72. Nam, H.Y. et al. (2009) Cellular uptake mechanism and intracellular fate of hydrophobically modified glycol chitosan nanoparticles. *J. Control. Release*, **135**, 259–267.

73. Bisht, S. and Maitra, A. (2009) Dextran–doxorubicin/chitosan nanoparticles for solid tumor therapy. *Wiley Interdiscipl. Rev. Nanomed. Nanobiotechnol.*, **1**, 415–425.

74. Koping-Hoggard, M. et al. (2001) Chitosan as a nonviral gene delivery system. Structure–property relationships and characteristics compared with polyethylenimine *in vitro* and after lung administration *in vivo*. *Gene Ther.*, **8**, 1108–1121.

75. Hawkins, M.J., Soon-Shiong, P., and Desai, N. (2008) Protein nanoparticles as drug carriers in clinical medicine. *Adv. Drug Deliv. Rev.*, **60**, 876–885.

76. Singla, A.K., Garg, A., and Aggarwal, D. (2002) Paclitaxel and its formulations. *Int. J. Pharm.*, **235**, 179–192.

77. ten Tije, A.J., Verweij, J., Loos, W.J., and Sparreboom, A. (2003) Pharmacological effects of formulation vehicles: implications for cancer chemotherapy. *Clin. Pharmacokinet.*, **42**, 665–685.

78. Gelderblom, H., Verweij, J., Nooter, K., and Sparreboom, A. (2001) Cremophor EL: the drawbacks and advantages of vehicle selection for drug formulation. *Eur. J. Cancer*, **37**, 1590–1598.

79. Vogel, S.M., Minshall, R.D., Pilipovic, M., Tiruppathi, C., and Malik, A.B. (2001) Albumin uptake and transcytosis in endothelial cells *in vivo* induced by albumin-binding protein. *Am. J. Physiol.*, **281**, L1512–L1522.

80. Gradishar, W.J. et al. (2005) Phase III trial of nanoparticle albumin-bound paclitaxel compared with polyethylated castor oil-based paclitaxel in women with breast cancer. *J. Clin. Oncol.*, **23**, 7794–7803.

81. Firme, C.P. III and Bandaru, P.R. (2010) Toxicity issues in the application of carbon nanotubes to biological systems. *Nanomedicine*, **6**, 245–256.

82. Heister, E. et al. (2009) Triple functionalisation of single-walled carbon nanotubes with doxorubicin, a monoclonal antibody, and a fluorescent marker for targeted cancer therapy. *Carbon*, **47**, 2152–2160.

83. Cheung, W., Pontoriero, F., Taratula, O., Chen, A.M., and He, H. (2010) DNA and carbon nanotubes as medicine. *Adv. Drug Deliv. Rev.*, **62**, 633–649.

84. Liu, Z., Sun, X., Nakayama-Ratchford, N., and Dai, H. (2007) Supramolecular

chemistry on water-soluble carbon nanotubes for drug loading and delivery. *ACS Nano*, **1**, 50–56.

85. Numata, M. et al. (2004) Curdlan and Schizophyllan (β-1,3-glucans) can entrap single-wall carbon nanotubes in their helical superstructure. *Chem. Lett.*, **33**, 232–233.

86. Yuan, W. et al. (2006) Wrapping carbon nanotubes in pyrene-containing poly (phenylacetylene) chains: solubility, stability, light emission, and surface photovoltaic properties. *Macromolecules*, **39**, 8011–8020.

87. Zhang, X., Meng, L., Lu, Q., Fei, Z., and Dyson, P.J. (2009) Targeted delivery and controlled release of doxorubicin to cancer cells using modified single wall carbon nanotubes. *Biomaterials*, **30**, 6041–6047.

88. Koyama, S. et al. (2006) Role of systemic T-cells and histopathological aspects after subcutaneous implantation of various carbon nanotubes in mice. *Carbon*, **44**, 1079–1092.

89. Brannon-Peppas, L. and Blanchette, J.O. (2004) Nanoparticle and targeted systems for cancer therapy. *Adv. Drug Deliv. Rev.*, **56**, 1649–1659.

90. Minchinton, A.I. and Tannock, I.F. (2006) Drug penetration in solid tumours. *Nat. Rev. Cancer*, **6**, 583–592.

91. Serda, R.E. et al. (2010) Cellular association and assembly of a multistage delivery system. *Small*, **6**, 1329–1340.

92. Decuzzi, P. and Ferrari, M. (2008) Design maps for nanoparticles targeting the diseased microvasculature. *Biomaterials*, **29**, 377–384.

93. Serda, R.E. et al. (2009) The association of silicon microparticles with endothelial cells in drug delivery to the vasculature. *Biomaterials*, **30**, 2440–2448.

94. Tanaka, T. et al. (2010) Sustained small interfering RNA delivery by mesoporous silicon particles. *Cancer Res.*, **70**, 3687–3696.

95. Fire, A. et al. (1998) Potent and specific genetic interference by double-stranded RNA in *Caenorhabditis elegans*. *Nature*, **391**, 806–811.

96. Mangala, L.S., Han, H.D., Lopez-Berestein, G., and Sood, A.K. (2009) Liposomal siRNA for ovarian cancer. *Methods Mol. Biol.*, **555**, 29–42.

97. Whitehead, K.A., Langer, R., and Anderson, D.G. (2009) Knocking down barriers: advances in siRNA delivery. *Nat. Rev. Drug Discov.*, **8**, 129–138.

28
Development of PEGylated Liposomes

I. Craig Henderson

28.1
Introduction and Rationale

The original stimulus for using liposomes as a delivery system may have been the desire to better administer water-insoluble drugs intravenously. In fact, the drugs that have most successfully been packaged in a liposome are water soluble, and the advantages for liposomes have derived from their impact on drug pharmacokinetics and tissue distribution. Liposomal, and especially PEGylated liposomal, delivery systems have the potential for increasing the amount of drug delivered to a target and thus increasing efficacy while at the same time reducing drug delivered to normal tissues and thus decreasing toxicity.

28.2
Structure, Formation, and Characteristics of Liposomes

28.2.1
Non-PEGylated Liposomes

The basic structure of most liposomes is shown in Figure 28.1. Common to all of them is a lipid bilayer surrounding an inner aqueous compartment in which drug is dissolved or suspended. (In some liposomal formulations water-insoluble drugs are carried totally or partially in the lipid membrane.) The ideal characteristics of a liposome may vary with the drug being delivered and the condition under treatment. In most situations desirable liposomes are those that preferentially deliver more of the administered drug to the target (e.g., the tumor) and less to normal, healthy tissues. To achieve this the ideal liposome will retain most of its payload while circulating in the blood, but release it when the target is reached. Numerous factors affect liposome characteristics; some of these are shown in Table 28.1. Often the factors that increase retention of drug within the liposome will lead to poor release on reaching the target and vice versa.

Drug Delivery in Oncology: From Basic Research to Cancer Therapy, First Edition.
Edited by Felix Kratz, Peter Senter, and Henning Steinhagen.
© 2012 Wiley-VCH Verlag GmbH & Co. KGaA. Published 2012 by Wiley-VCH Verlag GmbH & Co. KGaA.

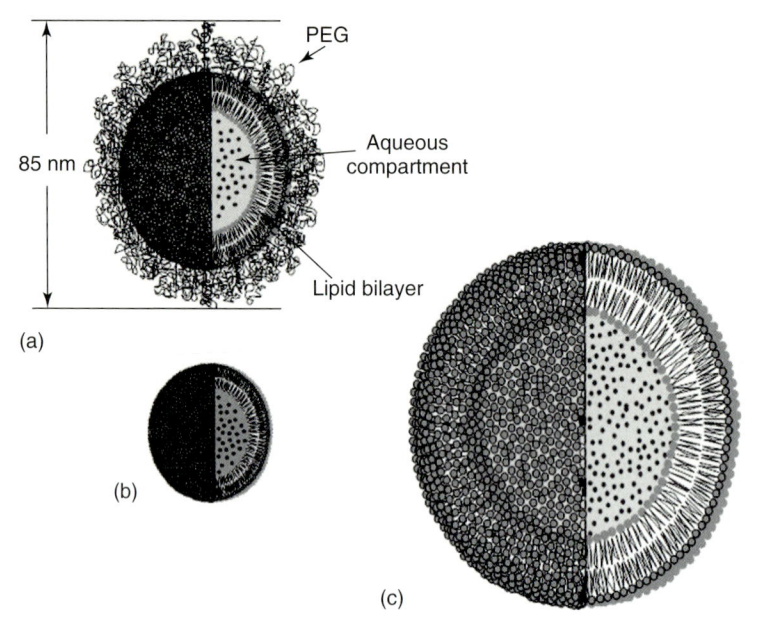

Figure 28.1 General structure of a liposome showing the proportional size of three different types of liposome. (a) Stealth liposome composed of HSPC/cholesterol/PEG-distearoylphosphatidylethanolamine (DSPE) (56 : 39 : 5) measuring 85–100 nm, such as PLD (Doxil/Caelyx). (b) Conventional liposome composed of HSPC/cholesterol (2 : 1) measuring around 45 nm, such as liposomal daunorubicin (DaunoXome). (c) Conventional liposome composed of egg phosphatidylcholine/cholesterol (55 : 45) measuring around 150 nm, such as non-PEGylated doxorubicin (Evacet).

Table 28.1 Factors affecting liposomal behavior [1, 2].

Lipid composition; degree of lipid unsaturation
Lipid ratios
Liposome size
Surface charge
Osmolarity during loading
Water and lipid solubility of drug
Method for loading drug
Surface pegylation
Ligand targeting

The lipids used most commonly are phosphatidylcholine (e.g., hydrogenated soy phosphatidylcholine (HSPC) or distearoylphosphatidylcholine (DSPC)) [1]. The precise lipids chosen and the ratios of phosphatidylcholine to cholesterol affect various pharmacokinetic parameters, including circulation time, penetration of the target, and leakage of drug from the liposome. For example, cholesterol is critical for retaining drug in the aqueous interior of the liposome and liposomes composed of DSPC/cholesterol or sphingomyelin/cholesterol have longer half-lives ($t_{1/2}$) in circulation than those containing egg phosphatidylcholine or 1,2-dipalmitoyl-3-sn-phosphatidylcholine [1].

Liposomes are formed by extruding a lipid suspension through filters; the lipid composition and the size of the pores in these filters will determine the size of the liposome, which in turn will affect the pharmacokinetics of the liposome. In general larger liposomes are more quickly taken up the reticuloendothelial system (RES), and this results in a breakdown of the liposome and release of free drug. Conventional (non-PEGylated) liposomes of 400 nm in diameter are cleared 7.5 times faster than 200-nm liposomes, which are cleared 5 times faster than small unilamellar vesicles. The relative size of two conventional liposomes (liposomal daunorubicin (DaunoXome®) and non-PEGylated liposomal doxorubicin (Evacet®)) and a pegylated liposomal doxorubicin (PLD) (Doxil®/Caelyx®) are shown in Figure 28.1.

The potential of drugs to be encapsulated will vary with their water solubility [3]. Drugs that are very water soluble, such as cytarabine and methotrexate ("hydrophilic drugs"), are easily taken up into the aqueous compartment of the liposome, but may not be easily released when the liposomes reach the tumor. Drugs that are relatively water insoluble, such as the taxanes ("hydrophobic drugs"), are more likely to be associated with the bilayer than the aqueous compartment, and when they enter the bloodstream they may be readily released and become associated with lipophilic components in the blood. Solubilizing these drugs in a liposome may ease intravenous administration, but will not provide pharmacokinetic advantages that are achieved with other drugs. Drugs in between these two extremes, such as the anthracyclines and the vinca alkaloids ("amphipathic drugs"), are readily solubilized in the aqueous chamber of the liposome and readily released when they reach the tumor.

Drugs may be loaded into the liposome against a concentration gradient. For conventional liposomes this is more often a pH gradient, while for PEGylated liposomes it is usually an ammonium sulfate gradient. Liposomes that are unstable may be stored empty and loaded with a pH gradient just prior to administration. When the ammonium sulfate gradient is used to load doxorubicin it becomes entrapped in the liposome interior, forming an insoluble salt with the entrapped sulfate anions. This results in a luminal doxorubicin concentration in excess of the aqueous solubility of doxorubicin, and enhances both the stability of drug during circulation and the dose of drug delivered to the target. Passive encapsulation is used for very water-soluble drugs and then water volume in the liposome interior limits the maximum amount of drug that can be delivered. The relative concentrations for daunorubicin are 0.079, 0.250, and 0.125 µg drug/µg lipid for passive encapsulation, a pH gradient, and an ammonium sulfate gradient, respectively [1]. There are 10 000–15 000 molecules of doxorubicin in a liposome loaded with an ammonium sulfate gradient [2].

28.2.2
Sterically Stabilized or "Stealth" Liposomes

If encapsulated drug is released from the liposome into the circulation before the liposome reaches its target, much or all of the advantage of the liposome is lost since most of the drug is distributed to the same organs with the same pharmacokinetics as free drug. Factors that accelerate liposome breakdown and/or drug release without breakdown include flocculation and aggregation of liposomes, the attachment of plasma proteins to the liposome surface, and liposomal destruction by the macrophages in the RES. Plasma proteins attached to the liposomal surface have a direct effect on permeability as well as serve as opsonins for uptake into the RES. Alterations in the lipid composition and changes in the surface charge of the liposome may also alter both aggregation and RES uptake.

The addition of surface polymers, such as the gangliosides GM1 or polyethylene glycol (PEG), will ameliorate this premature liposome breakdown and loss of drug (Figure 28.1). The attachment of these polymers to the surface of the liposome limits the access of plasma proteins and other macromolecules to the liposomal surface, hence the term "steric stabilization." Liposomes with surface polymers are also frequently referred to as "stealth" liposome because without opsonins on the surface liposomes are less easily recognized by the immune system and uptake into RES macrophages is reduced. PEG is the polymer on stealth liposomes that are currently approved in the United States (Doxil) and Europe (Caelyx), and these liposomes are frequently referred to generically as PLD to distinguish them from conventional liposomes encapsulating doxorubicin.

28.2.3
Tumor Targeting

The physical characteristics of liposomes, especially PLDs, enable tumor targeting. Blood vessels in healthy tissues have relatively tight junctions, estimated to be 20 and 60 Å (2–6 nm) between endothelial cells [4]. Liposomes such as PLD, which are 85–100 nm, are too large to pass through these spaces and as long as the liposome remains stable it will continue to circulate until it can exit through a larger space. Intercellular junctions in tumors (as well as in other disease processes, such as wound healing) are much larger. Although they may vary with tumor size and tumor growth rate (and can be increased with epidermal growth factor (EGF)), intratumoral intercellular junctions have been measured to be between 400 and 600 nm in a xenograft model system [5]. The relative size of endothelial cell junctions ("leaky junctions"), PLD, platelets and red cells, and the mechanism for tumor targeting with PLD, are illustrated in Figure 28.2.

That such tumor targeting happens *in vivo* has been shown in both preclinical models and in the clinic. Using a prostate tumor model, PC-3, Vaage *et al.* showed that the tissue area under the curve (AUC) for doxorubicin was increased by 25-fold when it was delivered in a PEGylated liposome rather than as free doxorubicin [6] (Figure 28.3). Doxorubicin could be detected in tumor tissue for only 24 h when

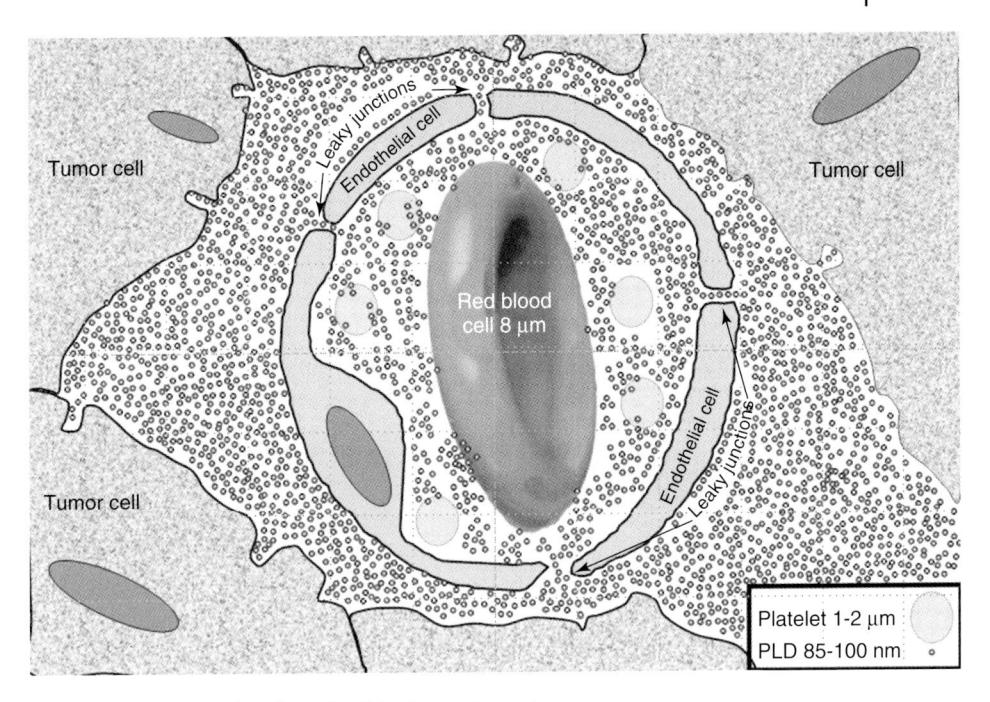

Figure 28.2 Cross-section through a blood vessel coursing through tumor tissue showing the relative size of the blood vessel, red blood cells, platelets, and PEGylated liposomes (PLD).

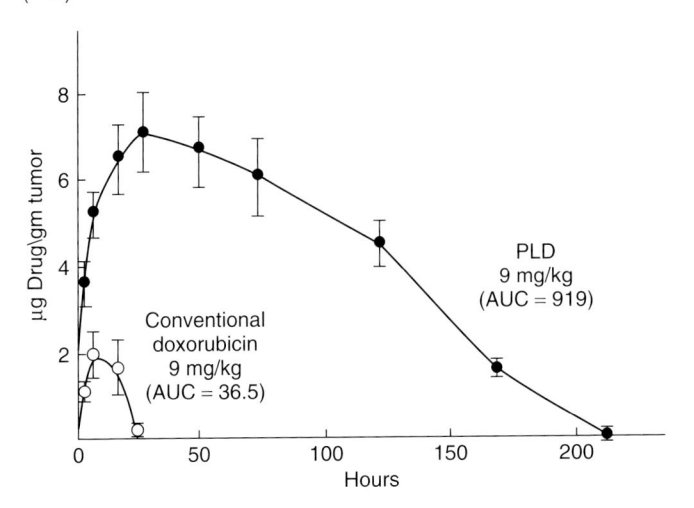

Figure 28.3 Comparison of tissue levels (AUC) of doxorubicin after a single injection of 9 mg/kg of either conventional doxorubicin or PLD to athymic nude Swiss mice 30 days after implantation of 9–10 mm in diameter PC-3 prostate tumors, a tumor cell line derived from human tumors. (Reproduced with permission from [6]. © 1994 American Cancer Society.)

administered as free drug compared to 216 h for PLD and the tissue C_{max} for PLD was almost 4 times higher than for conventional drug. With repeated doses of PLD or doxorubicin on days 1, 8, 15, and 22 after implantation, there was significantly greater suppression of tumor growth with PLD as well as significantly less toxicity. At the end of the experiment 18 of 19 mice treated with PLD compared to one of 20 treated with conventional doxorubicin were alive; the median survival of each group was 62.5 and 32.4 days, respectively ($P < 0.00005$).

Tumor targeting with PLD was demonstrated in patients with breast, lung, and head and neck cancers, gliomas, and AIDS-related Kaposi's sarcoma using ^{111}In-labeled PLD and γ-camera imaging [7]. In the first hours after injection of PLD to a patient with Kaposi's sarcoma most of the label is in the blood pool, but some can be seen in Kaposi's sarcoma lesions that were readily identifiable on physical examination of the patient (see Section 28.4.2 and Figure 28.6). Over 72 h liposomes continue to accumulate and the intensity of the radiolabel increased in the Kaposi's sarcoma lesions and decreased in the blood pool, as evidenced by the absence of labeled liposomes in the heart at 72 h. (The average plasma half-life of the labeled PLD was approximately 3 days, similar to that of pharmacokinetic studies of PLD routinely used in the various clinical applications.) Persistent uptake in the Kaposi's sarcoma lesions is seen at 7 days after much of the label has been cleared from plasma. Similar results were obtained with all of the other tumor types studied; 15 of 17 patients had evidence of tumor targeting with PLD. The avidity of smaller tumors was greater than larger tumors and even greater than well vascularized organs such as liver, lung, and kidney.

28.2.4
Implication of Tumor Targeting for Dosing PLD

The pharmacokinetics and tissue distribution of PLD suggest two distinct ways in which it might prove advantageous compared to conventional doxorubicin in the clinic: the same dose of PLD might result in greater efficacy if there is a dose effect of doxorubicin on tumor growth *or* a smaller dose of PLD might be equally effective against the tumor but less toxic to nontumorous tissues, especially the heart. The increase potency of PLD has been demonstrated in a number preclinical tumor models [10]. In the Lewis lung and C26 colon carcinoma mouse models the relative of potency of PLD was 4.5 times that of conventional doxorubicin, and with human breast cancer xenografts BT474 and MCF7 in nude mice the relative potency was 2-fold greater for PLD. In the Lewis lung study the effect of conventional doxorubicin administered at its maximum tolerated dose (9 mg/kg) was compared to a range of PLD doses (0.5–9 mg/kg) [10]. The conventional doxorubicin and PLD at 1 mg/kg had a modest effect on tumor growth, while the lowest dose of PLD had none (Figure 28.4). The highest dose of PLD (9 mg/kg) not only inhibited tumor growth significantly better than conventional doxorubicin, it caused tumors to decrease in size. PLD at 2 mg/kg was about equal to or a little more effective than 9 mg/kg of conventional doxorubicin. In the saline treated animals there were more than eight gross metastases per animal compared to two

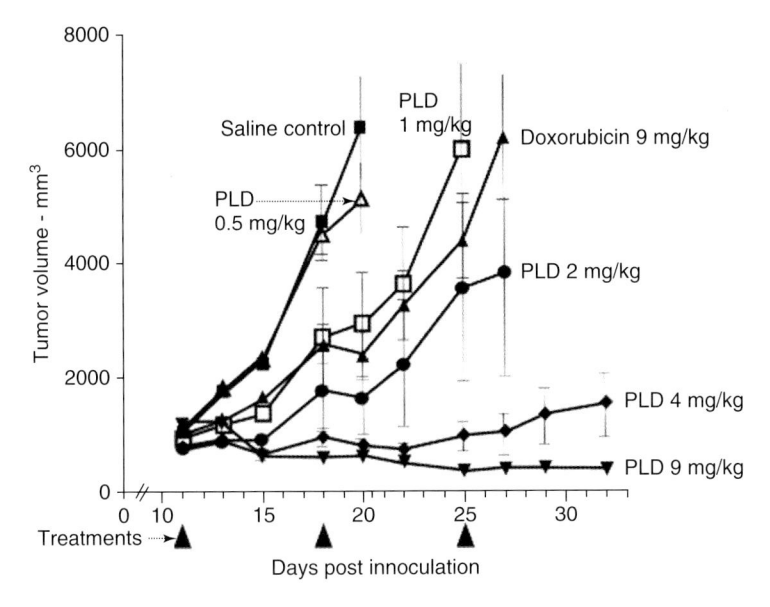

Figure 28.4 Effect on tumor volume of various doses of saline, conventional doxorubicin, or PLD on volume of Lewis lung tumors implanted in B6C2-F1 mice, and treated on days 11, 18, and 25 after implantation. (Reproduced with permission from [10]. © 1999 Marcel Dekker.)

per animal for those treated with conventional doxorubicin or 4 mg/kg PLD and none in those treated with 9 mg/kg PLD. These data suggest that the maximum tolerated dose of PLD might not be required in the clinic to obtain the same benefit as that usually obtained with doxorubicin. However, the relative efficacy of conventional dose doxorubicin and PLD may vary from one tumor type to another, thus limiting generalizations about dose across the spectrum of human tumor types and patients.

28.3
Pharmacokinetics of Stealth Liposomes

PLD has a plasma half-life in humans of 45–55 h [8, 11]. This is at least 4 times the half-life of free doxorubicin and twice that of a conventional liposomal preparation of doxorubicin. The kinetics of PLD are little affected by the drug dose. The clearance of free doxorubicin from plasma is characterized by a biphasic exponential curve (Figure 28.5). Most of the free drug disappears within minutes following administration due to rapid and widespread distribution of drug to body tissues. PLD also has a biphasic distribution, but less than 30% of the drug disappears in the first (α) phase because the drug leaves the vascular compartment very slowly. This is reflected in the volumes of distribution: depending on dose,

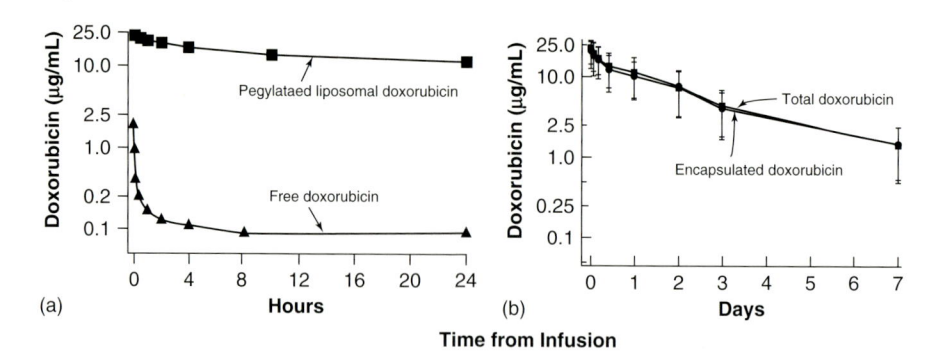

Figure 28.5 (a) Plasma doxorubicin levels over the first 24 h following a single 50 mg/m² dose of either PLD ($N = 14$) or free doxorubicin ($N = 4$) in patients with solid tumors. The doxorubicin levels represent total doxorubicin: free plus encapsulated doxorubicin. (Reproduced with permission from [8].) (b) Plasma doxorubicin levels broken down for total doxorubicin and encapsulated doxorubicin over 7 days following a single injection of PLD at a dose of 50 mg/m² ($N = 14$). A Dowel column capable of measuring 7% or more free drug in the plasma was used to estimate the amounts of total measured doxorubicin that was free or encapsulated. (Reproduced with permission from [9].)

Table 28.2 Comparative pharmacokinetics in humans of free doxorubicin or doxorubicin encapsulated in either a PEGylated liposome (PLD; e.g., Doxil/Caelyx) or a conventional liposome (TLC D-99, Evacet®).

Drug (reference)	Dose (mg/m²)	$t_{1/2}$ (h)		V_d (l)	AUC (mg · h/l)
		α	β		
Free doxorubicin [8]	50	0.06 (0.06–0.08)	10.4 (5.4–26.8)	365 (131–501)	3.5 (2.6–6.0)
PLD [8]	50	1.4 (0.2–7.3)	45.9 (29.3–74.0)	5.9 (2.3–10.1)	902 (335–2497)
Conventional liposome [1, 12]	30	0.37 ± 0.16	25.0 ± 22.5	8.2 ± 3.0	50.5 ± 44.9

V_d, volume of distribution; $t_{1/2\alpha}$, initial distribution phase; $T_{1/2\beta}$, elimination phase of doxorubicin clearance.

254–365 l for free doxorubicin compared to only 4.1–5.9 l for PLD and 8.2–21.4 l for a non-PLD [1, 8, 12]. PLD can be detected in plasma as long as 2–3 weeks after an injection. This prolonged intravascular circulation results in as much as a 300-fold greater AUC for PLD than for free doxorubicin (Table 28.2). Owing to the stability of the drug in plasma and the lack of breakdown in RES macrophages, around 98% of the doxorubicin in PLD remains encapsulated throughout the time it is in circulation (Figure 28.5).

28.4
Clinical Development

28.4.1
Toxicity Profile

Two cytotoxics, 5-fluorouracil and doxorubicin, have commonly been administered intravenously both as a bolus and continuous infusion [13–15]. The toxicities from bolus and continuous infusion are strikingly different. Bolus infusion results in greater myelosuppression and nausea/vomiting than continuous infusion. Doxorubicin as a continuous infusion results in significantly less cardiotoxicity. Continuous infusion of either drug results in palmar–plantar erythrodysesthesia (PPE, hand–foot syndrome), which is rarely seen when these drugs are given as a bolus infusion. Not surprisingly in light of our understanding about the pharmacokinetics of PLD, which are similar to that of continuous infusion doxorubicin, the toxicity profile for PLD is also similar to that of continuous infusion doxorubicin (Table 28.3).

When PLD is given as a single agent the most commonly used dose schedule is 50 mg/m^2 every 4 weeks. In a randomized breast cancer trial this dose schedule was compared to one of the most commonly used doxorubicin dose schedules, 60 mg/m^2 every 3 weeks [16]. The toxicities observed on each arm are shown in Table 28.4. As predicted by the comparison with continuous infusion doxorubicin, the PLD patients had less nausea, vomiting, alopecia, and neutropenia than those given doxorubicin. They had more PPE, mucositis, and infusion reactions. Differences in the frequency of alopecia with these two drugs are often underestimated in large, multicenter randomized trials. Most women treated with an anthracycline have sufficient hair loss within 3 weeks of the first dose that they will begin wearing a wig soon after that. This is unusual with PLD. In this direct comparison the authors noted that "pronounced or total hair loss" was reported for 54% of the doxorubicin but only 7% of the PLD patients.

Table 28.3 Predominant toxicities associated with administration of bolus, continuous infusion, and liposomal doxorubicin.

Adverse effect	Doxorubicin bolus	Doxorubicin continuous infusion	PLD
PPE	0	+++	+++
Cardiotoxicity	+++	+	+
Alopecia	+++	+++	+
Myelosuppression	+++	+	+
Mucositis/stomatitis	++	++	+
Nausea/vomiting	+++	+	+
Infusion reaction	0	±	+

Table 28.4 Adverse events in two breast cancer studies of PLD as a single agent, one in which patients were randomized to either PLD or doxorubicin and the other to PLD or observation.

Trial	PLD versus doxorubicin [16]				PLD versus observation [17]	
Drug and dose schedule	Doxorubicin 60 mg/m² every 3 weeks		PLD 50 mg/m² every 4 weeks		PLD 40 mg/m² every 4 weeks	
	Percentage of patients affected					
	All grades	Grade 3	All grades	Grade 3	All grades	Grades 3/4
PPE	2	0	48	17	33	4
Nausea	53[a]	5[a]	37[a]	3[a]	21	0
Vomiting	31[a]	4[a]	19[a]	<1[a]		
Mucositis	13	2	23	4	37	5
Alopecia	66	0	20	0	29	0
Pronounced hair loss	–	7	–	54	–	–
Infusion reaction	3	–	13	–	2	1
Neutropenia	10	8[b]	4	2[c]	44	12
Cardiac event	18.8[d]	–	3.9[d]	–	9[e]	–
+ CHF	4.4	–	0	–	0	–

[a]Antiemetic use was allowed on both arms but given more commonly with doxorubicin (83%) than with PLD (72%).
[b]Half were grade 4.
[c]One out of four 4 were grade 4.
[d]Decrease of 20% or more from baseline LVEF if resting LVEF was in the normal range or decrease of 10% or more if LVEF fell into the abnormal range.
[e]Decrease in LVEF 10% or more regardless of normal range (5/78 patients) or decrease in LVEF to below 50% (2/78).

Lower doses of PLD are less commonly used except in combination with other cytotoxics and there are no data from randomized trials to allow robust comparisons of the toxicity of different dose schedules of PLD. An indirect comparison is made in Table 28.4 by showing the results of a randomized comparison of 40 mg/m² every 4 weeks next to 50 mg/m² [17]. This comparison between these two trials with somewhat different patient populations in different countries suggests that with the lower dose the incidence of PPE, nausea/vomiting, and infusions reactions may be less. Although the incidence of mucositis and neutropenia is higher, there is no easy explanation for this other than possibly different criteria used by the two sets of investigators.

28.4.1.1 PPE

PPE is the single most important toxicity associated with PLD treatment and the most common reason patients discontinue this therapy. PPE is seen with a number of other cytotoxic anticancer drugs, most notably continuous infusion 5-fluororuacil and the long-acting congener of fluorouracil, capecitabine. It is seen with continuous infusion doxorubicin, but only rarely with the non-PEGylated, shorter-circulating liposomal formulations of doxorubicin [18].

The first symptoms of PPE are usually tingling or a feeling of warmth in the hands and feet 2–12 days after the administration of drug. This progresses to symmetrical edema and erythema, but it is not limited to the hands and feet in spite of the commonly used name for the phenomenon. It occurs predominantly in areas of pressure or heat, including the soles of the feet, buttocks, groin, axillae, or undersurface of the breast. With time it will begin to itch and violaceous plaques will appear. In most cases this will resolve after 1–2 weeks, but in some patients, especially those treated with high doses of PLD or when PLD is combined with other drugs, such as the taxanes that seem to synergize with PLD in causing this syndrome, the edema will become painful and skin may blister or ulcerate.

Preclinical studies suggest there is a correlation between the density of PLD administration and both the frequency and severity of the condition [19]. From studies in dogs, the dose rate predicted to induce symptomatically important PPE in patients was anything greater than 10–12 mg/m^2/week. Clinical studies have confirmed these predictions. PLD was first administered to patients using 20 mg/m^2 every 2–3 weeks (below 10 mg/m^2/week) in Kaposi's sarcoma studies (see below) and the incidence of PPE was less than 5%. An early phase I/II trial in patients with breast cancer used 60 mg/m^2 (20 mg/m^2/week) as a starting dose [20]. Fifty-four percent of the patients developed grade 3/4 PPE. The incidence of this severe PPE fell only slightly when PLD was given at 45 mg/m^2 every 3 weeks, but fell much further to 16% with 45 mg/m^2 every 4 weeks (11 mg/m^2/week). Presumably this is related to the long half-life of PPE and is supported by the observation that PPE often appears for the first time after the second or third dose of drug. Differences in toxicity related to PLD dose schedule were also demonstrated in a trial that randomized breast cancer patients to receive either 60 mg/m^2 every 6 weeks or 50 mg/m^2 every 4 weeks [21]. The delivered dose intensity for the two study arms was 9.8 and 11.9 mg/m^2/week. The incidence of grade 3/4 PPE was 2 and 16% for the lower- and higher-dose-intensity schedules, respectively. The relative incidence of grade 3/4 mucositis was reversed: 35% in the low-intensity arm and 14% in the high-intensity arm. There was no significant difference in response rate.

The pathophysiology of PPE is not well understood. Its high incidence with continuous infusion of drugs, including doxorubicin, suggests that it is related to the long dwell time in the capillaries of the skin. Presumably pressure or heat increases release of drug from the circulation into the epidermis. The most important element in managing the syndrome is early identification of the symptoms by routinely asking patients about burning or tingling, and delaying the next drug dose until these symptoms and any signs have cleared entirely. A number of prevention strategies, such as regional cooling with ice packs, the application of dimethylsulfoxide, or the use of pyridoxine, amifostine, and dexamethasone, have been tried [22]. Multiple myeloma patients treated with the vincristine and doxorubicin (VAD) or the VAd combination that includes dexamethasone have a lower frequency and less severe PLD than those given PLD alone or in other combinations (see Section 28.4.3.3). However, a recently reported randomized trial failed to demonstrate any decrease in symptoms from using pyridoxine [23]. Various creams and lotions have been used to ameliorate symptoms after progression to a more advanced state [24].

28.4.1.2 Infusion Reactions

A relatively small percentage of patients will develop acute infusion reactions (Table 28.4) during their first dose of drug, but not with subsequent doses. These have the hallmarks of a hypersensitivity reaction and are often labeled as such when reported in clinical trials, but unlike hypersensitivity reactions the symptoms do not recur with repeated exposure to the drug [18]. Dyspnea, flushing, palpitations, facial swelling, headache, tightness in the chest or throat, and hypotension may appear within a few minutes of the first dose, but these symptoms will disappear quickly once the drug infusion is discontinued. When the symptoms have cleared, treatment may be started again at a slower rate of infusion. As many as 10% of patients may have a reaction when PLD is infused at rates exceeding 1 mg/min (the recommended starting dose). The reaction is likely related to the liposome and maybe to the diameter of the liposome since this reaction is seen with other liposomal formulations as well as PLD. Based on preclinical studies it is thought that the reaction may occur because of transient plugging of pulmonary capillaries.

28.4.1.3 Cardiotoxicity

Both weekly and continuous infusions of doxorubicin are associated with less cardiotoxicity than 3-weekly dosing, possibly because the peak plasma drug level is lower [14, 25]. Not surprisingly, there is less cardiotoxicity from PLD, which mimics continuous infusion. The best demonstration of this came from a randomized trial in which 509 patients with metastatic breast cancer were randomized to receive either doxorubicin 60 mg/m^2 every 3 weeks or PLD 50 mg/m^2 every 4 weeks [16] (see Section 28.4.3.2, and Table 28.4). Cardiac function was monitored with (MUGA) scans that measured left ventricular ejection fraction (LVEF) before the start of treatment, after a cumulative anthracycline dose of 300 mg/m^2 and then after each additional 100 mg/m^2 of PLD or 120 mg/m^2 of conventional doxorubicin. A cardiac event was defined as a decrease of 20% or greater from baseline LVEF if the resting LVEF remained in the normal range or a decrease of 10% or greater if the LVEF fell below the normal range. The hazard rate for developing cardiotoxicity on doxorubicin compared to PLD was 3.16, $P < 0.001$. A cardiac event was observed in 18.8% of the patients on doxorubicin compared with only 3.9% of those on PLD. Among the patients with a cardiac event, 10/48 on doxorubicin but none of those on PLD developed signs and symptoms of congestive heart failure (CHF). Two patients on each arm had signs and symptoms on CHF without abnormalities in LVEF. The rate of cardiac events occurring relative to the cumulative doxorubicin dose administered is shown in Figure 28.8b. This is not an ideal evaluation of the cardiotoxicity of PLD relative to doxorubicin because the dose rate of doxorubicin administration as PLD is necessarily lower than that usually used for nonliposomal doxorubicin. However, it is unavoidable because many/most physicians are reluctant to use a lower doxorubicin dose because of concern about compromising efficacy or a higher dose rate of PLD because of unacceptable PPE.

There are anecdotal reports of patients receiving cumulative doses of PLD in excess of 550 mg/m^2, but no studies sufficiently robust to provide estimates on the probability of cardiac dysfunction or CHF above this level. In an observational study, 14 patients with ovarian cancer were given PLD, 30 mg/m^2 at 3- to 6-week intervals along with a taxane and platinum, to cumulative doses in excess of 550 mg/m^2 [26]. The cumulative doses of PLD ranged from 552 to 1015 mg/m^2; 11 patients received more than 600 mg/m^2 and 6 patients received more than 700 mg/m^2. All patients had LVEF determined by echocardiography at the end of treatment and 10 of the 14 had baseline LVEF as well. None of the patients had signs or symptoms of heart failure, or a clinically significant decrease in LVEF. One patient with metastases to the pericardium with fibrinous peritonitis had an LVEF of 40 at the end of treatment.

There are three clinical scenarios where the lower cardiotoxicity of PLD might be particularly advantageous and ongoing studies have been designed to assess each. One is combining PLD with trastuzumab, which is synergistic with nonliposomal doxorubicin in causing cardiotoxicity. Another is in elderly patients with increased risk of heart disease. The third is the readministration of an anthracycline sometime after a patient has been previously successfully treated, such as following adjuvant chemotherapy. Many of the patients in the trials described below are in this category. In a prospective trial, 70 breast cancer patients with metastases diagnosed more than a year after completing an adjuvant anthracycline regimen were given PLD, 35 mg/m^2, plus cyclophosphamide, 600 mg/m^2, every 3 weeks [27]. The patients in this study received a lifetime cumulative doxorubicin dose (median, maximum, and minimum) of 453, 720, and 258 mg/m^2 or cumulative epirubicin doses of 700, 1280, and 286 mg/m^2. No patient had symptoms of cardiotoxicity. Five patients had an LVEF decrease of 10% or more and one of 15% or more. All abnormal LVEF values returned to normal.

28.4.2
First Clinical Indication: AIDS-Related Kaposi's Sarcoma

AIDS-related Kaposi's sarcoma was selected as the first tumor type in which to evaluate the clinical benefits of PLD because these patients are particularly sensitive to cytotoxics and anxious to avoid the toxicities, especially hair loss, associated with commonly used chemotherapy agents. Kaposi's sarcoma lesions have been shown to have a network of dilated vessels interlacing tumor cells, suggesting that these tumors might be particularly susceptible to a delivery system dependent on a leaky vascular plexus. Finally, when PLD was introduced no treatment had been approved for Kaposi's sarcoma by regulatory bodies, so it was classified as an "unmet medical need" and could be evaluated by the US Food and Drug Administration (FDA) under what were then newly approved regulations for an accelerated approval under subpart H.

Preclinical and correlative laboratory studies of clinical trials demonstrated the potential advantage of PLD in Kaposi's sarcoma. Transgenic mice bearing the HIV *tat* gene have dermal lesions similar to those seen in patients with Kaposi's sarcoma. In preclinical evaluations of PLD using this model it was shown that liposomes encapsulating colloidal gold preferentially concentrated in these lesions and in tumor-like cells within the lesions [28]. In a phase I/II study patients with Kaposi's sarcoma were randomized to receive either PLD or conventional doxorubicin and lesions were biopsied 72 h after drug administration. Intralesional doxorubicin concentration after treatment with PLD was 5.2–11.4 times that obtained after administration of the same dose of conventional doxorubicin [29]. Selective distribution of ^{111}In-labeled radiolabeled PLD to Kaposi's sarcoma lesions was subsequently demonstrated in gamma camera images (Figure 28.6).

In Kaposi's sarcoma clinical trials the dose of PLD most commonly has been 20 mg/m^2 every 3 weeks. (This is a substantially smaller dose than subsequently used for other tumor types.) In 14 published studies utilizing doses of 10–40 mg/m^2, usually in patients with prior exposure to a cytotoxic agent, the response rates ranged from 38% to 100% [30]. In the study submitted to the FDA for initial approval of the drug, 19 of 53 (38%) treated patients had a partial response and one patient a complete response [31]. Among 28 patients whose tumors had progressed while receiving a combination that contained doxorubicin, nine (32%)

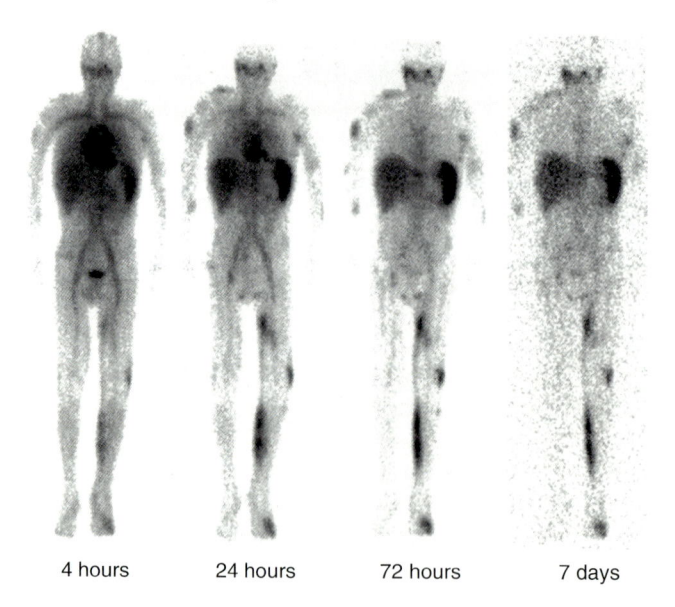

Figure 28.6 Distribution of ^{111}In-labeled radiolabeled PEGylated liposomes (26 MBq, 0.7 mCi) from γ-camera images obtained 4, 24, and 72 h, and 7 days after a single injection to a 45-year-old man with AIDS-related Kaposi's sarcoma. Circulating liposomes are evident in blood pools in the heart and liver. Uptake in Kaposi's sarcoma lesions that were also clinically apparent on physical examination can be seen in the left foot, left leg, right arm, and the right side of the face. (Reproduced with permission from [7]. © 2001 American Association for Cancer Research.)

had a partial response. Clinical benefits included flatting of lesions in 48% of patients, lessening of the intensity of the lesion color that made them less apparent in 56%, pain relief in 45%, and loss of edema in 83%. The most common side-effect was leukopenia; this occurred in 40% of patients and was severe in 17%. Nineteen percent of patients had nausea and vomiting, and 9% had alopecia, but these symptoms were not severe in any patients. Two of the 53 patients discontinued treatment due to intolerance of PLD. None died of PLD toxicity.

PLD has been evaluated in three randomized trials – two comparing PLD with a cytotoxic combination of drugs commonly used to treat AIDS-related Kaposi's sarcoma [32, 33] and one comparing PLD with liposomal daunorubicin [34]. The design and results of these trials are summarized in Table 28.5. The trials comparing PLD with chemotherapy used control regimens then considered standard for AIDS-related Kaposi's sarcoma. Both utilized bleomycin and vincristine (BV), and one trial used doxorubicin (ABV) as well. The PLD dose schedule was 20 mg/m^2 every 3 weeks in one and every 2 weeks in the other trial, both for six cycles. The patients had very advanced disease, including visceral involvement in a substantial portion of each patient cohort, a large number of Kaposi's sarcoma lesions, and low CD4 counts. In both cases the percentage of lesions that responded to PLD was about twice the percentage responding to combination chemotherapy. The time to response to PLD was shorter, but there were no significant differences in either the duration of response or the overall survival (OS) of these patients. In one but not the other study leukopenia was significantly greater for PLD, but in both studies peripheral neuropathy was greater for the BV or ABV combination. The comparison of PLD with ABV is especially interesting because this is the only comparison of PLD with conventional doxorubicin at the same dose in a phase III trial. Nausea/vomiting and alopecia were significantly less with PLD while the incidence of mucositis was significantly greater. The cumulative doses of anthracycline were too small and the duration of follow-up too short in these studies to provide meaningful information on cardiotoxicity from PLD or comparative cardiotoxicity from PLD and doxorubicin.

The third randomized trial of PLD in patients with Kaposi's sarcoma was to evaluate clinical benefits using a patient self-assessment questionnaire [34]. Owing to potential placebo effects, the trial was randomized and double-blind with liposomal daunorubicin as the control. Randomization was 3 : 1. The trial is very small because the incidence of AIDS-related Kaposi's sarcoma decreased rapidly following the introduction of effective antiviral drugs for AIDS soon after the approval of PLD. This was confounded by the fact that many physicians preferred either PLD or liposomal daunorubicin and were not willing to randomize patients to the less-preferred drug. Eventually the liposomal anthracyclines were routinely combined with "highly active antiretroviral therapy" (HAART), but this had not been anticipated in the original protocol design. Nonetheless this study does support the principle that either a liposomal anthracycline alone or in combination with HAART will reduce symptoms such as lymphedema, shortness of breath, or coughing in patients with Kaposi's sarcoma in the lung, difficulty swallowing or eating for patients with Kaposi's sarcoma involving the gastrointestinal track, and

Table 28.5 Randomized trials comparing PLD with other systemic therapies in patients with AIDS-related Kaposi's sarcoma.

	PLD versus BV [32]			PLD versus ABV [33]			PLD versus liposomal daunorubicin[a] [34]	
	PLD	BV	P value	PLD	ABV	P value	PLD	Liposomal daunorubicin
Drug dose (mg/m^2)	20	15[b]/2	–	20	20/10/1	–	20	40
Treatment interval (weeks)	3	3	–	2	2	–	2	2
Number of cycles	6	6	–	6	6	–	6	6
Number of patients	121	120	–	133	125	–	60	19
Patient characteristics								
Prior chemotherapy (%)	ND	ND	–	78	77	–	9	23
Median CD4 count (cells/μl)	30	30	–	12.5	13	–	131	168
More than 50 lesions (% of patients)	25	17	–	19	20	–	57	58
Responses								
Overall response rate (%)	59	23	<0.001	46	25	<0.001	55	32
Complete response (%)	5.8	0.8	–	0.8	0	–	–	–
Median time to response (days)	44	64	<0.025	39	50	0.014	30	27
Median duration response (days)	142	123	<0.572	90	92	0.234	129	NR
Median survival (days)	239	160	–	160	160	NS	NR	NR
Clinical benefit (%)	–	–	–	–	–	–	80	63
Duration clinical benefit (days)[c]	–	–	–	–	–	–	62	55
Toxicity								
Leukopenia (%)	72	51	<0.001	36	42	NS	5	11

Nausea and/or vomiting (%)	16	25	–	15	34	<0.001	28	26
Alopecia (%)	3	8	–	1	19	<0.001	ND	ND
Peripheral neuropathy (%)	3	14	<0.005	6	14	0.002	12	11
Mucositis/stomatitis (%)	7	5	–	5	2	0.026	ND	ND
Skin rash (%)	12	9	0.67	4	1	–	7	11

ND = not published, NR = median not reached, NS = not significant, B = bleomycin, V = vincristine, A = doxorubicin.
[a] Patients in this study were randomized in a ratio of 3 : 1. The study was not designed to compare the two treatment arms.
[b] IU = international units.
[c] Clinical benefit in this study was based on an 11-item patient questionnaire that was corroborated by objective measurements. The Kaposi's sarcoma symptom categories on the questionnaire included lymphedema, shortness of breath or cough, difficulty swallowing or eating, disfiguring Kaposi's sarcoma lesions, and Kaposi's sarcoma-associated pain.

pain from Kaposi's sarcoma lesions. They will also improve cosmesis when lesions are in locations that cause disfigurement. The observed objective response rate, time to response, and duration of response to PLD in this trial are similar to that seen in the two earlier randomized trials.

In all three of these comparative trials, as well as in most phase II trials, the incidence of skin rash and PPE are low. In the comparison of PLD with ABV, one patient had PPE. None was observed in the comparison of PLD with BV. In the comparison of PLD with liposomal daunorubicin, five patients on the PLD arm but none on the liposomal daunorubicin arm had PPE.

28.4.3
Activity in Solid Tumors and Hematological Malignancies

Conventional doxorubicin is active in almost all tumor types with the notable exception of nongastric gastrointestinal cancers, renal cancer, and cancers of the head and neck. PLD has been evaluated in almost all of the cancers for which doxorubicin is commonly used and it has appears to be active in all of them (Table 28.6). PLD has been approved by regulatory agencies in the United States and/or Europe for the treatment of ovarian cancer, breast cancer, and multiple myeloma, but increasingly it is being used to treat other cancers, such as soft-tissue sarcomas, as well.

Table 28.6 Phase II/III evaluations of PLD in solid tumors and hematological malignancies other than Kaposi's sarcoma.

Tumor type	PLD dose schedule		N	Range of overall response rates (%)	Combinations evaluated
	Dose (mg/m^2)	Interval (weeks)			
Ovarian cancer [35–46]	50	3	50	6–29	+ topotecan
	50	4	1027		+ gemcitabine
	40–45	4	111		+ oxaliplatin
	20	2	70		+ paclitaxel
					+ carboplatin
					+ cyclophosphamide
					+ vinorelbine
					+ ifosfamide
Breast cancer [16, 17, 20, 21, 47–53]	60–70	6	77	0–50	+ cyclophosphamide
	50	4	481		+ taxanes
	45	4	62		+ vinorelbine
	40	4	219		+ gemcitabine
	60	3	13		+ trastuzumab
	45	3	26		+ pemetrexed

(continued overleaf)

Table 28.6 (continued)

Tumor type	PLD dose schedule		N	Range of overall response rates (%)	Combinations evaluated
	Dose (mg/m^2)	Interval (weeks)			
	30	3	25		+ ixabepilone
	20	2	59		
Multiple myeloma combined with vincristine and dexamethasone [54]	40	4	89	39–72	+ dexamethasone + bortezomib + lenalidomide + thalidomide + cyclophosphamide
Soft-tissue sarcoma [18, 55–57]	50–60	4	128	0–55	+ ifosfamide
	40–60	4	11		+ radiotherapy
	50	3	25		+ paclitaxel
	35	3	22		–
Leiomyosarcoma [58]	50	4	32	15	+ paclitaxel
Angiosarcoma [59–61]	45-50	4	6	50	+ interferon
Pediatric sarcomas [62]	50	4	8	38	–
Aggressive fibromatosis [63]	50	4	11	36	–
Mesothelioma [18]	55	4	14	7–29	–
	45	4	31	–	–
Lymphoma [18, 64]	30	3	32	31	+ cyclophosphamide + vincristine + prednisone + gemcitabine + vinorelbine + rituximab
Lymphoma T-cell cutaneous [65]	20–50	2–6	34	88	–
Head and neck cancers	40	3	18	24–50%	+ radiotherapy
	35–45	3	45		
	25	3	32		

Most of the response rates shown here are from studies in patients previously treated with cytotoxic therapy, including many with prior exposure to anthracyclines. Only the tumor types studied most intensively are shown here.
N = the sum of the number of patients treated at that dose level in all reported studies for that tumor type.

28.4.3.1 Ovarian Cancer

Although doxorubicin is an active agent against ovarian cancer, it is not considered to be as active as either cisplatin or paclitaxel [35]. When added to a combination of these drugs doxorubicin significantly improves survival, but this benefit has generally been considered too modest to justify the added toxicity it imparts to a three-drug combination. Most phase II and phase III trials of PLD have been performed in ovarian patients who have recurred after treatment with a platinum combination. The first dose schedule utilized was 50 mg/m^2 every 3 weeks [36]. Although the response rate was high in a group of heavily pretreated patients, the incidence of PPE was unacceptable. Subsequently, most studies in ovarian cancer patients have utilized a dose schedule of 50 mg/m^2 every 4 weeks with responses ranging from 6 to 29% [35, 37–39] (Table 28.6). Two studies used 20 mg/m^2 every 2 weeks. One of these enrolled 50 patients (40 of them resistant to platinum) and an overall response rate of 40% was observed [37]. However, the incidence of PPE was similar to that seen in other studies even if it might have been less severe.

In the pivotal trial leading to regulatory approval of PLD for ovarian cancer, 474 patients, all of whom had received prior platinum therapy and 53% of whom were considered refractory to platinum because they had relapsed while receiving this therapy or within 6 months of completing a course, were randomized to receive PLD 50 mg/m^2 every 4 weeks or topotecan 1.5 mg/m^2 daily for 5 days at the beginning of each 3 week cycle [40]. Progression-free survival (PFS) – the primary endpoint for the study – was slightly longer for PLD than topotecan ($P = 0.095$) (Table 28.7). This PFS advantage for PLD was significant in the platinum-sensitive group (median PFS 28.9 and 23.3 weeks for PLD and topotecan, respectively; $P = 0.037$). OS was also significantly longer for patients randomized to PLD and this advantage was statistically significant for those with platinum-sensitive tumors, too [41] (Figure 28.7). More adverse events were reported with topotecan, especially grade 4 events, which occurred in 71.1% of the topotecan and 17.2% of the PLD patients. The most important toxicities associated with PLD were PPE (all grades 49% of patients, grade 3 = 22%, grade 4 = 0.8%) and stomatitis (40%). Ninety percent of topotecan patients had hematologic toxicity and two-thirds of these were grade 3 or 4. More patients on topotecan required blood transfusions (58 versus 15% on PLD), hematopoietic growth factors (29 versus 5%) and erythropoietin (23 versus 6%). Nine patients on topotecan and none on PLD had treatment related sepsis and three of these nine died as a result.

Subsequent to this trial comparing PLD with topotecan, PLD has been compared to paclitaxel, gemcitabine, topotecan, and a combination of PLD and trabectedin in patients who have recurred following initial treatment with a platinum combination [42–46] (Table 28.7). These results consistently demonstrate the efficacy of PLD in this patient population. Owing to this and its relatively favorable toxicity profile, PLD is one of the agents used most frequently in patients with recurrent ovarian cancer.

Evaluation of PLD in combination with a platinum in place of the current standard, paclitaxel, has only recently been done, but early results of two studies and mature results of a very small trial have been published [66–69]. These studies combined PLD at 30 mg/m^2 with carboplatin AUC 5, but one administered this combination every 3 weeks and the other two every 4 weeks. Two trials used the same control group: paclitaxel 175 mg/m^2 and carboplatin AUC every 3 weeks (Table 28.7). The MITO-2 trial plans for an accrual of 820 patients with stage 1c-IV ovarian cancer that had not been previously treated with chemotherapy. At the time of an interim activity analysis, only 137 patients had been enrolled on the PLD arm and 50 of these had measurable disease [66]. The response rate in these 50 was

Table 28.7 Randomized trials in which PLD, alone or in combination, was compared with another drug or drug combination in patients with ovarian cancer.

Trial	Drug dose schedule (dose (mg/m^2)/cycle length (weeks))				Number of patients	Platinum sensitive (%)	Response rate (%)		PFS (months)		Survival (months)	
	PLD		Non-PLD				PLD arm	Non-PLD	PLD	Non-PLD	PLD	Non-PLD
Comparison of PLD alone and either another single agent or drug combination in patients with recurrent ovarian cancer												
30-49 [40, 41]	50	4	topotecan 1.5 days 1–5	3	474	47	20 $P = 0.390$	17	PLD > topotecan $P = 0.095$		16 $p = 0.05$	15
30-57 [42]	50	4	paclitaxel 175	4	216	39	18	22	ND		12 $P = 0.062$	14
Mutch [43]	50	4	gemcitabine 1000 days 1,8	3	195	0	8 $P = 0.589$	6	3 $P = 0.87$	4	14 $P = 0.997$	13
Italian [44]	40	4	gemcitabine 1000 days 1,8,15	4	153	57	16 $P = 0.056$	29	4^a $P = 0.411$	5^a	14 $P = 0.048$	13
Telik [45]	50	4	topotecan^b 1.5 days 1–5	3	461	25	ND	ND	ND		14 $P = $ NS	11
J&J [46]	50	4	PLD + trabectedin^c		672	65	19 $P = 0.008$	28	6 $P = 0.019$	7	19 $P = 0.1506$	21
Comparison of PLD in combination with either another single agent or drug combination in previously untreated patients												
MITO-2 [66]	PLD + carboplatin 30/AUC 5	3	paclitaxel + carboplatin 175/AUC 5	3	137^d	100	68	ND	ND		ND	
SWOG [67, 68]	PLD + carboplatin 30/AUC 5	4	carboplatin AUC 5	4	61	100	67 $P = 0.02$	32	12 $P = 0.03$	8	31 $P = 0.2$	18
GICG [69]	PLD + carboplatin 30/AUC 5	4	paclitaxel + carboplatin 175/AUC 5	3	976	100	ND		11 $P = 0.005$	9	ND	

NS, not significant.
^{a}Time to treatment failure instead of PFS.
^{b}Three-arm trial comparing canfosfamide with either PLD or topotecan in patients who previously had platinum in an initial therapy and either PLD or topotecan as second line. Only comparison between PLD and topotecan shown.
^{c}Trabectin is a new unapproved drug previously shown to be synergistic with PLD.
^{d}50 were evaluable for response on the PLD + carboplatin arm only.

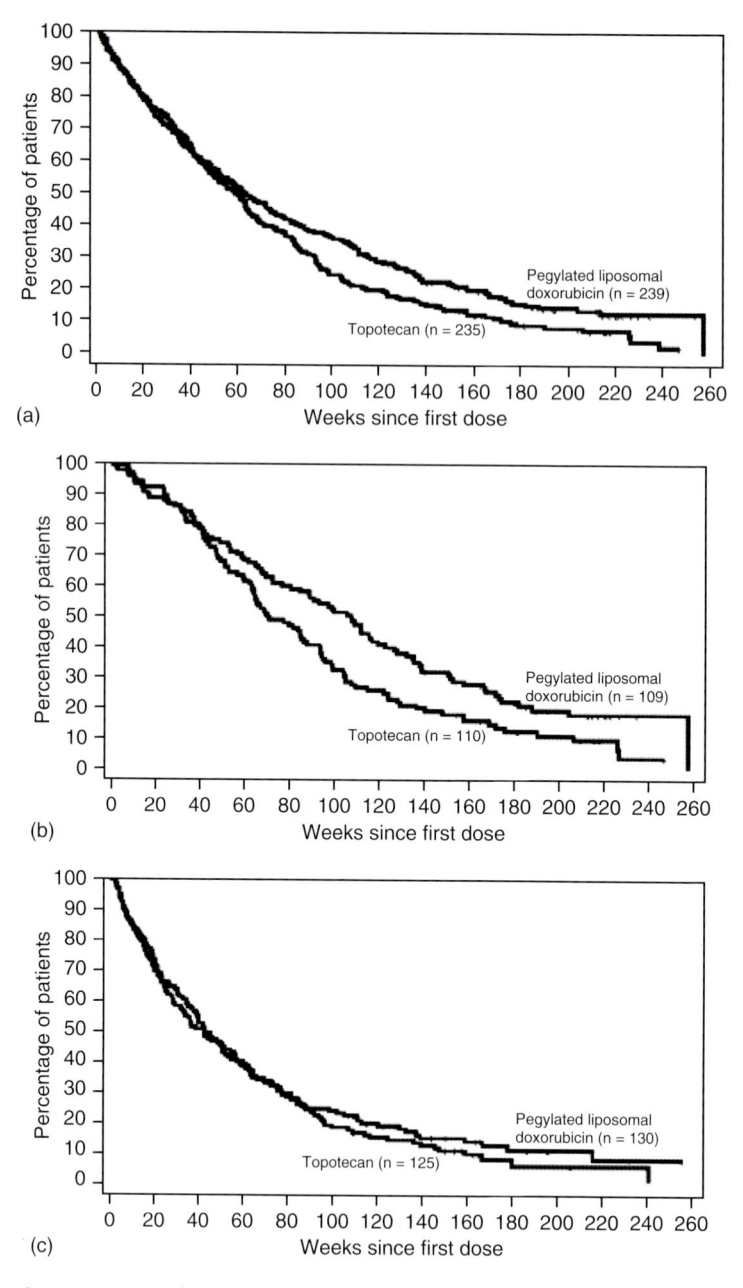

Figure 28.7 OS of patients randomized to either PLD or topotecan (see text for details). (a) All treated patients (N = 474; hazard ratio = 1.216; 95% confidence interval 1.000–1.478; P = 0.050), (b) patients with platinum-sensitive tumors (N = 219; hazard ratio = 1.432; 95% confidence interval 1.066–1.923; P = 0.017), and (c) patients with platinum-refractory tumors (N = 255; hazard ratio = 1.069; 95% confidence interval 0.823–1.387; P = 0.618). (Reproduced with permission from [41]. © 2004 Elsevier.)

68%; the complete response rate was 28%. No comparisons with the control arm have been made yet, but the authors felt that this demonstrated sufficient activity for the PLD combination to complete accrual. The Gynecologic Cancer Intergroup (GCIG) study enrolled 976 patients with platinum-sensitive tumors (all greater than 6 months and 65% greater than 12 months since their last chemotherapy) who had also received a taxane [69]. The trial had a noninferiority design with PFS and OS as its primary endpoints. There was a 2-month difference in the median PFS favoring the PLD arm ($P = 0.005$), but the OS data are not sufficiently mature for analysis (Table 28.7). Grade 3/4 nonhematologic toxicity occurred in 28 and 37% ($P = 0.01$) of the patients on the PLD and non-PLD arms, respectively. Patients on PLD experienced grade 2 or greater alopecia (7 versus 84%) and neuropathies less frequently, and grade 2 or 3 PPE (12 versus 2%), nausea and mucositis more frequently than those on the non-PLD arm. The authors concluded that in patients with prior taxane exposure, a combination of PLD with carboplatin had a superior PFS and therapeutic index.

There is no advantage from adding PLD or any other drug to the standard platinum/taxane combination in patients with no prior chemotherapy. The Gynecologic Cancer Intergroup randomized 4312 women to either a standard doublet of carboplatin and paclitaxel or one of four other regimens that incorporated one other drug into the combination: PLD, gemcitabine, or topotecan [70]. None of the triplets proved advantageous in either PFS or OS.

28.4.3.2 Breast Cancer

Anthracyclines, either doxorubicin or epirubicin, are central to the treatment of breast cancers in both the adjuvant and metastatic setting. PLD appears to be about as effective, but with a very different toxicity profile. More than 1000 women with metastatic breast cancer have been enrolled in studies that employed PLD as a single agent in a wide range of dose schedules [47–52] (Table 28.6). There is no evidence that one of these is more effective than another.

PLD and doxorubicin were compared directly in a randomized trial that served as the basis for regulatory approval of PLD in Europe [16]. In this study 509 patients without prior chemotherapy for recurrent disease were randomly treated with either PLD 50 mg/m^2 every 4 weeks or doxorubicin 60 mg/m^2 every 3 weeks. About 15% of the patients had previously been treated with an adjuvant regimen that included an anthracycline. This trial was designed as a noninferiority trial with 80% power to determine if the PFS of PLD was noninferior to that of doxorubicin. Small differences in response rate, PFS, and OS were not statistically significant (Table 28.8 and Figure 28.8a). Patients in the PLD group had less alopecia, nausea, vomiting, and neutropenia, and more PPE, mucositis, stomatitis, and infusion reactions (Table 28.4). Adverse events thought to cause death occurred in two PLD and three doxorubicin patients. Twenty-four percent of patients on each arm discontinued because of either an adverse event (22% for PLD versus 9.4% for doxorubicin) or cardiotoxicity (2.4 versus 14.1%).

In another randomized trial PLD was used as maintenance therapy after induction doxorubicin and was shown to improve PFS without increasing cardiotoxicity [17].

Table 28.8 Randomized trials evaluating PLD alone or with a taxane in patients with metastatic breast cancer.

Trial	PLD dose (mg/m^2)	PLD cycle (weeks)	N	Response rate (%) PLD	Response rate (%) Non-PLD	PFS (months) PLD	PFS (months) Non-PLD	OS (months) PLD	OS (months) Non-PLD
PLD versus doxorubicin[a] For metastatic disease without prior chemotherapy[b] [16]	50	4	509	33	38	7 P = NS	8	21 P = NS	22
PLD versus "comparator"[c] In taxane-refractory patients [53]	50	4	301	10	12	2.4 P = 0.11	2.7	11 P = 0.71	9
PLD versus nil as maintenance therapy After induction of response with A -> D[e] [17]	40	4	155	ND		8[d] P = 0.0002	5[d]	25 P = 0.435	22
PLD + paclitaxel versus doxorubicin + paclitaxel[f] For metastatic disease without prior chemotherapy [71]	30	3	23	70	70	ND		ND	
PLD + docetaxel versus docetaxel[g] After adjuvant anthracycline 12 or more months earlier [72]	30	3	751	35 P = 0.0085	26	10 P = 0.000001	7	21 P = 0.81	21

N = number of patients enrolled in study; NS = not significant; ND = no data.
[a]Doxorubicin 60 mg/m every 3 weeks.
[b]Patients could have had prior adjuvant therapy including prior anthracyclines as long as there was 12 months or longer interval.
[c]Vinorelbine 20 mg/m^2 weekly, or a combination of mitomycin C 20 mg/m^2 on day 1 and vinblastine 5 mg/m^2 on days 1 and 21 in a 6-week cycle.
[d]TTP.
[e]Induction therapy was doxorubicin 75 mg/m^2 every 3 weeks for three cycles followed by docetaxel 100 mg/m^2 every 3 weeks for three cycles.
[f]Paclitaxel 200 mg/m^2 every 3 weeks in both arms and doxorubicin 60 mg/m^2 every 3 weeks.
[g]Docetaxel alone 75 mg/m^2 every 3 weeks or when in combination with PLD 60 mg/m^2.

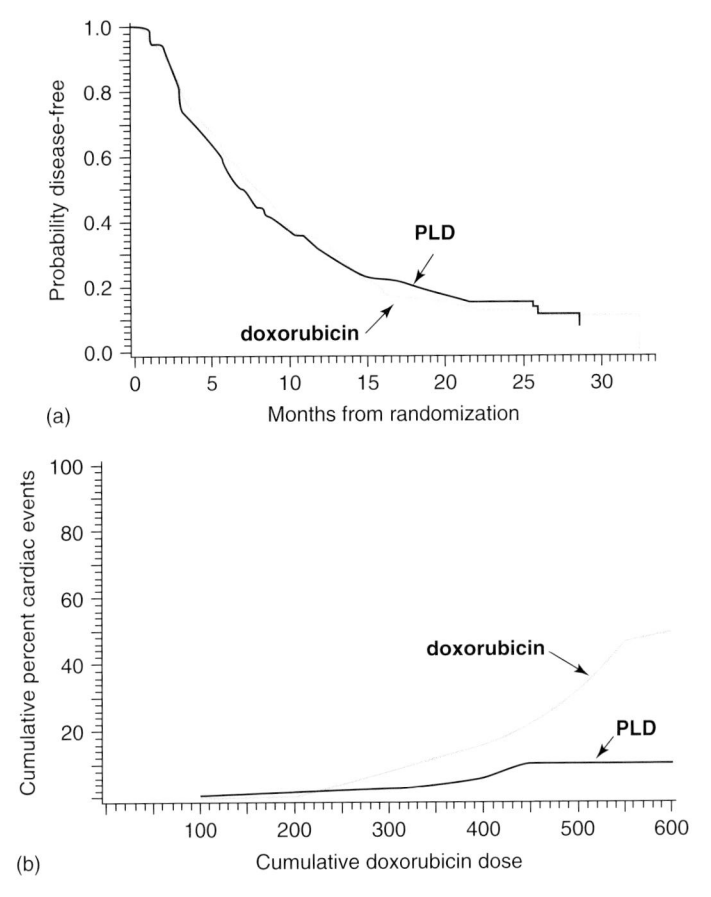

Figure 28.8 Randomized comparison of PLD, 50 mg/m^2 every 4 weeks, and conventional doxorubicin, 60 mg/m^2 every 3 weeks, in patients with metastatic breast cancer. (a) PFS (hazard ratio = 1.00; 95% confidence interval 0.82–1.22). (b) Rate of protocol-defined cardiac events occurring in each treatment group relative to the cumulative doxorubicin dose administered among the patients in the study who had both a baseline and at least one additional MUGA scan while on treatment. PLD, $n = 254$; doxorubicin, $n = 255$. Hazard ratio = 3.16; 95% confidence interval 1.58–6.31; $P < 0.001$. (Reproduced with permission from [16]. © 2004 European Society for Medical Oncology.)

Patients with newly diagnosed breast cancer ($N = 288$) were initially treated with three cycles of doxorubicin, 75 mg/m^2, followed by three cycles of docetaxel, 100 mg/m^2, each at 3-weekly intervals. Patients who responded or were stable at the end of this treatment ($N = 155$) were randomized to PLD, 40 mg/m^2, every 4 weeks for six cycles or observation. Time to progression (TTP) was significantly improved (hazard ratio = 0.54, 95% confidence interval 0.39–0.76, $P = 0.0002$) and OS nonsignificantly improved from the maintenance PLD (Table 28.8). LVEF measurements were made after completion of the induction therapy, during the maintenance period after 3 and 6 months, and every 6 months subsequent to the completion of the maintenance therapy. There was no significant difference in LVEF after 3 and 6 months. Other toxicities associated with PLD at this lower dose schedule occurred less frequently and were less severe than that described above in the comparison of PLD with doxorubicin (Table 28.4).

Although the benefit of any form of cytotoxic treatment in patients with advanced breast cancer after many previous forms of chemotherapy is modest, at best, PLD does appear to be as effective as other options used in this setting. In a randomized trial with 509 patients PLD performed as well as but no better than either vinorelbine or a combination of mitomycin C and vinblastine [53] (Table 28.8). The response rate to PLD is usually higher in patients without prior exposure to anthracyclines. For example, in a retrospective assessment of 125 patients treated with PLD (usually 40 mg/m^2 every 4 weeks) at multiple centers in Germany, 43% of the patients had a partial or complete response [49]. The response rate in those with prior anthracycline exposure was 34% and without prior anthracyclines 53%. In a pooled analysis of four studies (two randomized), 274 patients with metastatic breast cancer treated with PLD after prior exposure to anthracycline treatment were identified among 935 treated patients [73]. The primary endpoint of the study was the clinical benefit rate (CBR), which was defined as a complete response, partial response, or stable disease for at least 6 months. The CBR was 37.2% (95% confidence interval 32.4–42.0) for all patients previously exposed to an anthracycline, 36.1% for those treated with anthracyclines only as adjuvant, 42.1% for those given prior anthracyclines only in the metastatic disease setting, and 32.7% for those given anthracyclines in both settings ($P = 0.332$). For those whose prior anthracycline exposure was 0–12 months the CBR was 29.2% compared with 40.7% if that interval was more than 12 months ($P = 0.078$).

In recent years PLD, usually 30–35 mg/m^2 every 3 weeks or 40 mg/m^2 every 4 weeks, has been combined with a large number of other cytotoxic agents (Table 28.6). The combination of PLD and cyclophosphamide has produced response rates of 29–35% and clinical benefit rates of 59–86% in single-arm studies enrolling patients with metastatic disease previously untreated with chemotherapy for metastases but often with prior adjuvant chemotherapy that included anthracyclines [27, 74, 75].

PLD in combination with taxanes has been evaluated as first-line therapy of breast cancer metastases in randomized trials [71, 72] (Table 28.8). A combination of PLD plus docetaxel was compared to docetaxel alone in 751 patients with measurable metastatic disease that had been previously treated with a conventional anthracycline at least 12 months earlier [72]. Only 3% of patients had prior cytotoxic treatment for metastases. The risk of disease progression with PLD plus docetaxel was decreased by 35% (hazard ratio = 0.65, 95% confidence interval 0.55–0.77, $P = 0.000001$) (Table 28.8). There was no difference in median survival. Therapy was discontinued due to toxicity by 34% of the PLD plus docetaxel patients (20% due to PPE) and only 9% of the patients on docetaxel alone. The PLD arm had a high incidence of grade 3/4 PPE (24 versus 0%) and mucositis/stomatitis

(12 versus 1%). There were no significant differences in cardiotoxicity on the two study arms.

Anthracyclines and trastuzumab are synergistic in causing heart damage. For this reason a number of phase II trials have been performed to evaluate PLD in place of conventional anthracyclines in this combination because of the lower cardiotoxicity associated with PLD [76–80]. One trial was designed and sized to determine if the rate of CHF exceeded 3% when trastuzumab (4 mg/kg once, then 2 mg/kg weekly) was added to PLD, 30 mg/m^2, and docetaxel, 60 mg/m^2, every 3 weeks [80]. Patients with HER2/*neu*-positive tumors ($N = 46$) received the combination with trastuzumab while those with HER2/*neu*-negative tumors ($N = 38$) served as a control group and received PLD plus docetaxel without trastuzumab. The incidence of CHF was less than 3% on both arms. An unexpected finding in this trial was an increased incidence of PPE on the trastuzumab compared to the PLD plus docetaxel arm: grade 3 PPE 38 versus 22%, $P = 0.16$ and all grades PPE 75 versus 51%, $P = 0.03$.

Local recurrence on the chest wall following mastectomy is a common problem in the management of breast cancer. These lesions are often refractory to both local and systemic therapy. Hyperthermia has been shown to increase vascular leakiness in tumors. It has been demonstrated in preclinical models that pretreatment hyperthermia will increase intratumoral doxorubicin levels following PLD treatment by as much as 3-fold [81]. In a clinical study of 22 patients, the response in sites treated with hyperthermia plus PLD ($N = 20$, complete and partial response rate 60%) was significantly better than in sites treated with PLD alone ($N = 17, 35\%$) [82].

A new and unusual use for PLD is direct intraductal installation. In spontaneous HER2/*neu* transgenic mouse (neu-N) models of breast cancer intraductal administration of PLD was more effective than intravenous injection in causing regression of established tumor and prevention of tumor development ($P < 0.0001$) [83]. There was no systemic toxicity or evidence of damage to the mammary gland. This approach is now being evaluated in the clinic [84].

28.4.3.3 Multiple Myeloma

Cytotoxics long established as standard for the treatment of multiple myeloma are melphalan (usually given with prednisone) as initial treatment and a doxorubicin combination following melphalan failure. Since PLD had already been shown to be active as a single agent in other tumor types, no single-agent trials of PLD were undertaken in multiple myeloma. Instead, PLD was substituted for doxorubicin in established regimens, especially VAD (vincristine and doxorubicin given repeated as a bolus or by continuous infusion over days 1–4 plus intermittent oral dexamethasone given over a 4-week cycle) and VAd (the same vincristine and doxorubicin with dexamethasone given only in the first 4 days of the cycle). The DVD and DVd regimens substituted PLD, 40 mg/m^2 on day 1, for doxorubicin in the VAD and VAd combinations without changing the dose schedule of either dexamethasone or vincristine. In single-arm studies the response rates to DVD or DVd, generally defined as a 25% or greater decrease in the M-component, varied from 39 to 72% depending on the precise definition of response and the extent of treatment given prior to entry into the study [54] (Table 28.6).

Two randomized trials comparing DVD with VAD and DVd with VAd provide more compelling evidence that in multiple myeloma without prior treatment PLD is as effective as doxorubicin [85, 86] (Table 28.9). In both trials the response rates, TTP or PFS, and OS were not significantly different for the two study arms. The design of the studies differed in that in the DVd/VAd trial patients could undergo stem cell transplantation after a minimum of four cycles and a little over one-third of the patients on each study arm did so. The investigators felt that this might have resulted in a lower response rate since the duration on standard-dose chemotherapy was shortened, thus decreasing the time interval in which a response could be measured [86]. The DVd/VAd study was designed as a noninferiority trial with the primary endpoint being overall response. This was defined as the sum of complete remission (disappearance of all evidence of serum and urine M-components on electrophoresis and by immunofixation studies), remission (75–99% reduction in quantitative immunoglobulins and, if present, a 90–99% reduction in urine M-components or urine M-components less than 0.2 g/day), and partial remission (50–74% reduction in quantitative immunoglobulin and (if present) a 50–89% reduction in urine M-components). DVd and AVd were to be considered "therapeutically equivalent" if the two-sided 95% confidence interval for the *difference* in the objective response rates of the two treatment arms was ±20%. The observed difference in response rate was 3.3% with a 95% confidence interval of −17.3 and +10.7%. Thus, this trial met its primary endpoint.

With the notable exception of PPE, the DVD and DVd arms of these studies were considered less toxic. The PLD combination induced less neutropenia and less alopecia in both studies, significantly so in DVd/AVd. There was significantly more PPE with PLD, but none was grade 4 in either study and only 4% was grade 3. The overall incidence of PPE was 29 and 37% for DVd and DVD, respectively. This incidence is lower than that observed in many other PLD trials, plausibly because of either the dose schedule of PLD (40 mg/m^2 every 4 weeks) or the frequent use of a steroid in these regimens. Mucositis/stomatitis was nonsignificantly higher with PLD in both trials. There were also practical advantages to DVd. Significantly fewer patients required growth factors for either neutropenia or anemia (46 versus 61%, $P = 0.03$) [86]. Decreased neutropenia resulted in decreased antibiotic use and hospitalizations. Decreased frequency of drug administration resulted in fewer clinic visits. Together, these result in substantially and significantly lower costs of drug administration (Table 28.10). However, these were counter-balanced by the substantially greater cost of PLD compared to the generic doxorubicin [88].

In recent years the treatment of multiple myeloma has undergone rapid change with the introduction of new, relatively nontoxic, targeted drugs as well as increased use of stem cell transplant, especially in younger patients. These new drugs have been combined with PLD. Single-arm studies of PLD in combination with thalidomide [89–91], lenalidomide [91–93], and bortezomib [94–99] have been published. In a large randomized trial PLD, 30 mg/m^2, on day 4 plus bortezomib 1.3 mg/m^2, on days 1, 4, 8, and 11 of a 3-weekly cycle was compared to bortezomib

Table 28.9 Randomized trials in which PLD in combination with other drugs was compared to a non-PLD combination or single agent in patients with multiple myeloma.

Trial	PLD dose (mg/m^2)	PLD cycle (weeks)	Number of patients	Response rate (%) PLD	Response rate (%) Non-PLD	Hazard ratio for TTP	Hazard ratio for OS
DVD versus VAD[a] For previously untreated patients [85]	40	4	259	61	61	ND $P = 0.58$	"no difference" [85]
DVd versus VAd[b] noninferiority trial For previously untreated patient [86]	40	4	192	44 $P = 0.66$	39	1.11[c] $P = 0.69$	0.88 $P = 0.67$
PLD + bortezomib versus bortezomib[d] For patients progressing after prior therapy [87]	30	3	646	44 $P = 0.43$	41	1.82 $P = 0.00004$	1.41 $P = 0.0476$

[a]DVD, PLD 40 40 mg/m^2 + vincristine 2 mg on day 1, dexamethasone 40 mg days 1–4 alternating with days 1–4, 9–12, 17–20 on alternate cycles in a 28-day cycle. VAD, vincristine 0.4 mg/m^2 + doxorubicin bolus 9 mg/m^2 daily on days 1–4, dexamethasone as in DVD regimen.
[b]DVd, PLD 40 mg/m^2 + vincristine 1.4 mg/m^2 (maximum 2 mg) on day 1, dexamethasone 40 mg days 1–4. VAd, Vincristine 0.4 mg/m^2 + doxorubicin continuous infusion 9 mg/m^2 days 1–4, dexamethasone 40 mg days 1–4.
[c]PFS instead of TTP.
[d]PLD 30 mg/m^2 day 4, bortezomib 1.3 mg/m^2 on days 1,4,8 and 11

Table 28.10 Economic analysis of randomized trials comparing DVd and VAd for the treatment of previously untreated multiple myeloma [88].

	DVd	VAd	P value
Days in clinic	4.75	14.4	<0.01
Days in hospital	1.52	8.46	<0.01
Cost of drug (US$)	16181	788	<0.01
Costs associated with hospitalization (US$)	3311	18492	<0.01
Clinic visit costs (US$)	797	2412	<0.01
Total cost of drug, hospitalization, and treatment visits (US$)	20289	21692	0.64
Total costs including drug acquisition, cost of administration, tests, transfusions, concomitant medications, and hospitalization for adverse events (US$)	34442	35846	0.76

alone on the same dose schedule [87] (Table 28.9). Eligible patients had progressed after a response to one or more lines of therapy or had been refractory to initial therapy. There was no significant difference in response rate, but other endpoints favored the combination. The median TTP was 9.3 and 6.5 months ($P = 0.000004$) (Figure 28.9) for PLD plus bortezomib and bortezomib alone. The hazard ratio for PFS was 1.69 (95% confidence interval 1.32–2.16; $P = 0.000026$). At 15 months the OS for patients on the combination was 76% and on bortezomib alone 65% ($P = 0.03$) (Figure 28.9). The advantage for the combination was apparent in almost all patient subgroups. Sixty-seven percent of the enrolled patients had previously been treated with an anthracycline. The hazard ratio favoring PLD plus bortezomib in this subgroup of 436 patients was 1.88 (95% confidence interval

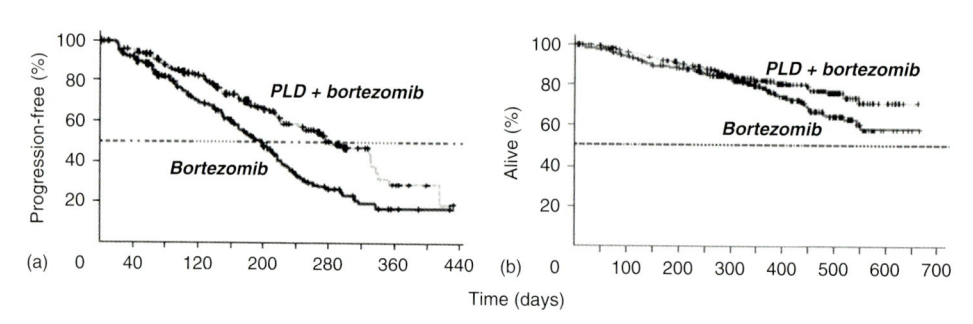

Figure 28.9 Randomized comparison of PLD + bortezomib with bortezomib alone in patients with multiple myeloma that has progressed after a response to one or more lines of therapy or was refractory to original therapy. (a) TTP (hazard ratio 1.82; 95% confidence interval 1.41–2.35; $P = 0.000004$). (b) OS (hazard ratio 1.406; 95% confidence interval 1.002–1.972; $P = 0.0476$). (Reproduced with permission from [87]. © 2007 American Society of Clinical Oncology.)

1.38–2.55); this was not different from the hazard ratio in the 210 patients without prior anthracycline: 1.83 (95% confidence interval 1.12–3.0). Drug-related adverse events and serious adverse event occurred more often among patients on the PLD arm: 94 versus 86%, $P < 0.001$ and 22 versus 15%, $P = 0.031$. Adverse events leading to discontinuation of bortezomib was not significantly different on the two arms (30 versus 24%), but 36% of patients discontinued PLD because of adverse events. There were two drug related deaths on each arm. PPE occurred in 16% of the PLD patients; 5% of these were grade 3. There was no grade 4 PPE and no PPE on the bortezomib-alone arm. Stomatitis occurred significantly more often with PLD (18%) than with bortezomib alone (3%). Neutropenia, nausea, and vomiting also occurred more often with the combination. CHF occurred in 3% of patients on both arms.

Owing to the significant improvement in TTP and OS for the combination of PLD and bortezomib in patients with relapsed or refractory multiple myeloma, this combination is now being tested in patients with previously untreated disease [96], and is being used as a scaffolding to add both new drugs and immunomodulatory drugs, such as thalidomide and lenalidomide [87].

28.4.3.4 Soft-Tissue Sarcomas

The results of trials evaluating PLD in patients with soft-tissue sarcomas are quite variable, with response rates ranging from 0 to 55% [18, 55–57] (Table 28.6). In the most recently published of these studies, which was by investigators with extensive experience in the use of PLDs, six of 11 patients with soft-tissue sarcoma had a well-document partial response [57]. The sarcoma histologies included malignant hemangio-endothelioma, malignant fibrous histiocytoma, uterine leiomyosarcoma, angiosarcoma, pleomorphic sarcoma, and a high grade-sarcoma. Response durations were 66+, 36, 16, 15+, 15, and 7+ months. It is reasonable to conclude from all of the evidence taken together that PLD is active in this tumor type, but it is unclear how active it is.

The European Organization for Research and Treatment of Cancer (EORTC) conducted a randomized trial comparing PLD, 50 mg/m² every 4 weeks, with doxorubicin, 75 mg/m², in 94 sarcoma patients. The histologies included leiomyosarcoma (33%), angiosarcoma (12%), synovial sarcoma, liposarcoma, malignant fibrous histiocytoma, and a small number of other types. Ninety-eight percent of the patients had not previously been treated with any cytotoxic drug. The differences in response rate (PLD 10%, doxorubicin 9%), TTP (median PLD 65, doxorubicin 82 days) and OS (median PLD 320, doxorubicin 245 days) were not statistically significant. In a retrospective analysis of the histologic types it was found that 28% were gastrointestinal stromal tumors. When these were removed from the analysis because they are considered a relatively chemoresistant group of tumors the response rates to PLD and doxorubicin were 14 and 12%, respectively. The response rate to doxorubicin is commonly considered to be about 20% based on literature surveys, so the relatively low response rate to doxorubicin in this EORTC study raises a question as to whether these results can be generalized to everyday practice. However, the results are likely within the lower limits of results from other trials, might be explained by the particular mix of sarcomas included in this study, and/or could be a result of more stringent response criteria used in EORTC randomized, prospective studies [100].

The histologies shown to respond include leiomyosarcomas, which were specifically evaluated by the Gynecologic Oncology Group as well as included in broader phase II trials of sarcomas [57, 58], angiosarcomas [59–61], various pediatric sarcomas [62], and fibromatosis [63].

28.4.3.5 Other Tumors

Although PLD is currently used most frequently and is being evaluated in clinical trials in new combinations as first-line therapy for ovarian and breast cancers, multiple myeloma, AIDS-related Kaposi's, and various soft-tissue sarcomas, there are other tumors where it has been shown to have at least limited activity including lymphoma [64, 65], head and neck cancer, prostate cancer, transitional cell bladder cancer, hepatoma, gastric cancer, high-grade gliomas, prostate cancer, endometrial cancer, and both small-cell and non-small-cell lung cancer [18].

28.4.4
Optimal Dose Schedule for PLD

Although there is evidence of a dose response to doxorubicin in preclinical models, it has proven difficult to demonstrate much of a dose response in the clinic. The only large, randomized clinical trials evaluating dose were in breast cancer. In one study 1550 patients were randomized to one of three doses of cyclophosphamide/doxorubicin/5-fluorouracil: $600/60/600 \times 2$ mg/m^2 every 4 weeks for four cycles, $300/30/300 \times 2$ mg/m^2 for four cycles or $400/40/400 \times 2$ mg/m^2 for six cycles. There were no differences in outcomes between the 600/60/600 and 400/40/400 dosage groups, but patients randomized to 300/30/300 had a significantly worse disease-free and OS than either of the other two groups. This study does not address simply the issue of doxorubicin dose since the doses of the three drugs in the regimen were altered as well as the duration of treatment and the results are compatible with the idea of a threshold dose (i.e., a dose below which there is no or little benefit) rather than a true dose response [101]. In a cleaner evaluation of doxorubicin dose, 3121 women were randomized to receive 600 mg/m^2 with doxorubicin at either 60, 75, or 90 mg/m^2 [102]. There was absolutely no evidence of a dose effect. Taken together there is no basis from properly controlled trials for using doxorubicin doses in excess of 40 mg/m^2 every 4 weeks.

Based on the experience with conventional doxorubicin it is reasonable to anticipate that there is some dose of PLD below which activity falls off rapidly, but it will take a very large trial to define that point. It has been argued, largely on the basis of evidence from animal models, that reduction in PLD dose even when it is combined with other cytotoxics may reduce efficacy [103]. While this position is compelling, it must be kept in mind that the preclinical argument for a dose response with conventional doxorubicin was also compelling, but not substantiated by substantial data from randomized clinical trials.

There is one randomized trial comparing two different dose schedules of PLD in patients with metastatic breast cancer: 60 mg/m^2 every 6 weeks versus 50 mg/m^2 every 4 weeks [21]. This study enrolled 115 women. While there was a significant difference in toxicity between the two arms, there was no difference in efficacy (see above).

Owing to PPE, cycle durations of less than 3 weeks and doses greater than 50 mg/m^2 cannot be recommended. Doses of 40 mg/m^2 every 4 weeks when PLD is used alone or 30 mg/m^2 when used in combination have been shown to be effective, but until more clinical data are available from randomized trials that include dose as a variable, it is uncertain that these doses are as effective as 50 mg/m^2 every 4 weeks – the dose schedule used in the vast majority of the PLD studies completed to date.

28.5
Newer Applications of PEGylated Liposomes

Theoretically stealth liposomes can serve as a delivery system for a number of drugs, especially those with amphipathic characteristics. The ideal drug for a stealth liposome might be one that has already been shown to be more effective or less toxic when given as repeated (e.g., weekly or daily) doses or by continuous infusion. The camptothecins, topoisomerase I inhibitors, meet this requirement. GG211 had been shown in phase II trials to be as effective or even more effective than other drugs in this class, but because two topoisomerase I inhibitors had already received regulatory approval the drug was not developed further [104]. Two liposomal formulations were created, one PEGylated and the other non-PEGylated [104, 105]. For business reasons only the non-PEGylated formulation (lurtotecan, NX211, OSI-211) was taken into the clinic, where it was shown be active in ovarian cancer [106, 107]. It has been evaluated in several other tumor types [108], but patients have not been accrued to new trials in several years. A relatively toxic combined topoisomerase I and II inhibitor, GKD-602, was formulated in a stealth liposome and has had limited evaluation in the clinic [109]. More recently SN-38, a metabolite of irinotecan, as well as topotecan itself have been formulated as PEGylated liposomes as well [110, 111]. This extensive effort to encapsulate camptothecins suggests that there is wide agreement that these are good candidates for a stealth delivery system and they can be encapsulated. It remains to be demonstrated that they have a clear advantage over nonliposomal formulations.

Two PEGylated liposomal formulations of cisplatin have been created. The first, SPI-77, was shown to be both more efficacious and less toxic than conventional cisplatin in animal models, and in phase I clinical trials it had remarkably little toxicity [112, 113]. It was eventually shown that this was because the drug was not released from the liposome. The lipid composition of the second liposomal cisplatin, lipoplatin, results in less dependence on lipases for drug release, and biopsies of tumor and adjacent normal tissue suggest there is considerable targeting of drug to tumor [114]. The drug has been extensively evaluated in the clinic, but all of the published response data are from trials in which it was combined with other active cytotoxic agents. As a result it is difficult to assess its antitumor activity in patients. In combination with paclitaxel and at doses well below the maximum tolerated dose, lipoplatin has been shown in a randomized trial to have significantly less toxicity, including less nephrotoxicity, than a cisplatin/paclitaxel combination while at the same time inducing a significantly higher response rate (59 versus 43%, $P = 0.036$) and no difference in survival [115, 116].

Vinca alkaloids have been successfully encapsulated, and a vincristine formulation was evaluated in the clinic but not fully developed [117, 118]. More recently a PEGylated liposomal vinorelbine has been evaluated in preclinical models and shown to be active. Clinical studies of this agent are just beginning [119].

The possibility of coencapsulation of several cytotoxic agents is under investigation in preclinical models. One of these is a combination of a vincristine and topotecan in a PEGylated liposome, which was shown in animal models to be more effective than either of the free drugs alone, either of the drugs in a liposomal formulation or the free drugs administered together [120]. In this system the ratio of the two drugs thought to be optimal when the drugs are used freely was loaded into the liposomes remotely. The ratio actually delivered to the tumor was shown to be the same as that loaded into the liposome.

An even more futuristic use of PEGylated liposomes is the development of immunoliposome achieved by attaching Fab' fragments from monoclonal antibodies targeted to tumor cells to the PEG on the surface of these liposomes [121]. This was first accomplished using antibodies to HER2/*neu*. In vitro these immunoliposomes both bind to and internalize in cells that overexpress HER2/*neu*. Using HER2/*neu*-positive tumor xenograft models it was possible to demonstrate superior efficacy of these anti-HER2/PLD immunoliposomes compared to PLD alone, doxorubicin alone, free doxorubicin plus trastuzumab, and PLD plus trastuzumab [122]. Cures were obtained in the mice treated with immunoliposomes but not in any of the mice treated with free doxorubicin or PLD. More recently, similar results have been obtained with Fab' fragments of monoclonal antibodies to EGF receptor (EGFR) [123]. The EGFR liposomes carried one of three drugs: doxorubicin, epirubicin, or vinorelbine. With each of the drugs, the immunoliposomes were superior to free drug, the PEGylated liposomal formation of the drug with attached Fab fragment, or a combination of either of these with free antibody. The pharmacokinetics and the distribution of both the anti-HER2/*neu* and anti-EGFR immunoliposomes were nearly identical to that of the PEGylated liposomal drug alone, but the internalization of drug was significantly higher with the immunoliposome. It is likely that this increase in internalization accounts for the superior efficacy.

28.6
Conclusions and Perspective

Proof of principle for the PEGylated liposome platform has been established in both preclinical models and in the clinic. In animal systems, it has been shown that the potency of the drug is increased. In the clinic, PLD use is associated with a substantial reduction in important toxicities, such as cardiotoxicity and alopecia, but at the cost of an increased incidence of PPE. Doses higher than 50 mg/m^2 or administration more often than every 4 weeks is associated with intolerable PPE, but at a dose of 50 mg/m^2 every 4 weeks PPE is manageable and usually relatively mild. PLD is now used routinely for the treatment of breast and ovarian cancers and multiple myeloma after failure of other cytotoxic drugs, including prior treatment with doxorubicin. Increasingly investigators are evaluating PLD alone or, more often, in combination regimens as initial treatment for metastatic cancer.

Although not all drugs can be encapsulated in a PEGylated liposome, this platform holds promise for amphipathic drugs that are most effective when administered more continuously. The topoisomerase I inhibitors appear to be particularly promising in this regard. Proof of principle for immunoliposomes has been established in preclinical models, but not yet in clinical trials.

References

1. Drummond, D.C., Meyer, O., Hong, K., Kirpotin, D.B. *et al.* (1999) Optimizing liposomes for delivery of chemotherapeutic agents to solid tumors. *Pharmacol. Rev.*, **51**, 691–743.
2. Allen, T.M. and Martin, F.J. (2004) Advantages of liposomal delivery systems for anthracyclines. *Semin. Oncol.*, **31** (Suppl. 13), 5–15.
3. Barenholz, Y. (2003) Relevancy of drug loading to liposomal formulation therapeutic efficacy. *J. Liposome Res.*, **13**, 1–8.
4. Jain, R.K. (1987) Transport of molecules in the tumor interstitium: a review. *Cancer Res.*, **47**, 3039–3051.
5. Yuan, F., Dellian, M., Fukumura, D., Leunig, M. *et al.* (1995) Vascular permeability in a human tumor xenograft: molecular size dependence and cutoff size. *Cancer Res.*, **55**, 3752–3756.
6. Vaage, J., Barbera-Guillem, E., Abra, R., Huang, A. *et al.* (1994) Tissue distribution and therapeutic effect of intravenous free or encapsulated liposomal doxorubicin on human prostate carcinoma xenografts. *Cancer*, **73**, 1478–1484.
7. Harrington, K.J., Mohammadtaghi, S., Uster, P.S., Glass, D. *et al.* (2001) Effective targeting of solid tumors in patients with locally advanced cancers by radiolabeled pegylated liposomes. *Clin. Cancer Res.*, **7**, 243–254.
8. Gabizon, A., Catane, R., Uziely, B., Kaufman, B. *et al.* (1994) Prolonged circulation time and enhanced accumulation in malignant exudates of doxorubicin encapsulated in polyethylene glycol coated liposomes. *Cancer Res.*, **54**, 987–992.
9. Martin, F.J. (1997) Pegylated liposomal doxorubicin: scientific rationale and preclinical pharmacology. *Oncology*, **11** (Suppl. 11), 11–20.
10. Colbern, G., Hiller, A., Musterer, R., Pegg, E. *et al.* (1999) Significant increase in antitumor potency of doxorubicin HCl by its encapsulation in pegylated liposomes (Doxil). *J. Liposome Res.*, **9**, 523–538.
11. Working, P.K. and Dayan, A.D. (1996) Pharmacological–toxicological expert

report. CAELYX (stealth liposomal doxorubicin HCl). *Hum. Exp. Toxicol.*, **15**, 751–785.
12. Cowens, J.W., Creaven, P.J., Greco, W.R., Brenner, D.E. et al. (1993) Initial clinical (phase I) trial of TLC D-99 (doxorubicin encapsulated in liposomes). *Cancer Res.*, **53**, 2796–2802.
13. Garnick, M.B., Weiss, G.R., Steele, G.D., Israel, M. Jr. et al. (1983) Clinical evaluation of long-term, continuous-infusion doxorubicin. *Cancer Treat. Rep.*, **67**, 133–142.
14. Casper, E.S., Gaynor, J.J., Hajdu, S.I., Magill, G.B. et al. (1991) A prospective randomized trial of adjuvant chemotherapy with bolus versus continuous infusion of doxorubicin in patients with high-grade extremity soft tissue sarcoma and an analysis of prognostic factors. *Cancer*, **68**, 1221–1229.
15. Meta-analysis Group in Cancer (1998) Efficacy of intravenous continuous infusion of fluorouracil compared with bolus administration in advanced colorectal cancer. *J. Clin. Oncol.*, **16**, 301–308.
16. O'Brien, M.E., Wigler, N., Inbar, M., Rosso, R. et al. (2004) Reduced cardiotoxicity and comparable efficacy in a phase III trial of pegylated liposomal doxorubicin HCl (CAELYX/Doxil) versus conventional doxorubicin for first-line treatment of metastatic breast cancer. *Ann. Oncol.*, **15**, 440–449.
17. Alba, E., Ruiz-Borrego, M., Margeli, M., Rodriguez-Lescure, A. et al. (2010) Maintenance treatment with pegylated liposomal doxorubicin versus observation following induction chemotherapy for metastatic breast cancer: GEICAM 2001-01 study. *Breast Cancer Res. Treat.*, **122**, 169–176.
18. Alberts, D.S., Muggia, F.M., Carmichael, J., Winer, E.P. et al. (2004) Efficacy and safety of liposomal anthracyclines in phase I/II clinical trials. *Semin. Oncol.*, **31** (Suppl. 13), 53–90.
19. Amantea, M., Newman, M.S., Sullivan, T.M., Forrest, A. et al. (1999) Relationship of dose intensity to the induction of palmar-plantar erythrodysesthia by pegylated liposomal doxorubicin in dogs. *Hum. Exp. Toxicol.*, **18**, 17–26.
20. Ranson, M.R., Carmichael, J., O'Byrne, K., Stewart, S. et al. (1997) Treatment of advanced breast cancer with sterically stabilized liposomal doxorubicin: results of a multicenter phase II trial. *J. Clin. Oncol.*, **15**, 3185–3191.
21. Coleman, R.E., Biganzoli, L., Canney, P., Dirix, L. et al. (2006) A randomised phase II study of two different schedules of pegylated liposomal doxorubicin in metastatic breast cancer (EORTC-10993). *Eur. J. Cancer*, **42**, 882–887.
22. Lorusso, D., Di Stefano, A., Carone, V., Fagotti, A. et al. (2007) Pegylated liposomal doxorubicin-related palmar–plantar erythrodysesthesia ("hand–foot" syndrome). *Ann. Oncol.*, **18**, 1159–1164.
23. von Gruenigen, V., Frasure, H., Fusco, N., Debernardo, R. et al. (2010) A double-blind, randomized trial of pyridoxine versus placebo for the prevention of pegylated liposomal doxorubicin-related hand–foot syndrome in gynecologic oncology patients. *Cancer*, **116**, 4735–4743.
24. Wood, L.S. (2004) Liposomal anthracycline administration and toxicity management: a nursing perspective. *Semin. Oncol.*, **31** (Suppl. 13), 182–190.
25. Chlebowski, R.T., Paroly, W.S., Pugh, R.P., Hueser, J. et al. (1980) Adriamycin given as a weekly schedule without a loading course: clinically effective with reduced incidence of cardiotoxicity. *Cancer Treat. Rep.*, **64**, 47–51.
26. Yildirim, Y., Gultekin, E., Avci, M.E., Inal, M.M. et al. (2008) Cardiac safety profile of pegylated liposomal doxorubicin reaching or exceeding lifetime cumulative doses of 550 mg/m^2 in patients with recurrent ovarian and peritoneal cancer. *Int. J. Gynecol. Cancer*, **18**, 223–227.
27. Trudeau, M.E., Clemons, M.J., Provencher, L., Panasci, L. et al. (2009) Phase II multicenter trial of anthracycline rechallenge with pegylated liposomal doxorubicin plus

cyclophosphamide for first-line therapy of metastatic breast cancer previously treated with adjuvant anthracyclines. *J. Clin. Oncol.*, **27**, 5906–5910.
28. Huang, S.K., Martin, F.J., Jay, G., Vogel, J. et al. (1993) Extravasation and transcytosis of liposomes in Kaposi's sarcoma-like dermal lesions of transgenic mice bearing the HIV *tat* gene. *Am. J. Pathol.*, **143**, 10–14.
29. Northfelt, D.W., Martin, F.J., Working, P., Volberding, P.A. et al. (1996) Doxorubicin encapsulated in liposomes containing surface-bound polyethylene glycol: pharmacokinetics, tumor localization, and safety in patients with AIDS-related Kaposi's sarcoma. *J. Clin. Pharmacol.*, **36**, 55–63.
30. Krown, S.E., Northfelt, D.W., Osoba, D., and Stewart, J.S. (2004) Use of liposomal anthracyclines in Kaposi's sarcoma. *Semin. Oncol.*, **31** (Suppl. 13), 36–52.
31. Northfelt, D.W., Dezube, B.J., Thommes, J.A., Levine, R. et al. (1997) Efficacy of pegylated-liposomal doxorubicin in the treatment of AIDS-related Kaposi's sarcoma after failure of standard chemotherapy. *J. Clin. Oncol.*, **15**, 653–659.
32. Stewart, S., Jablonowski, H., Goebel, F.D., Arasteh, K. et al. (1998) Randomized comparative trial of pegylated liposomal doxorubicin versus bleomycin and vincristine in the treatment of AIDS-related Kaposi's sarcoma. International Pegylated Liposomal Doxorubicin Study Group. *J. Clin. Oncol.*, **16**, 683–691.
33. Northfelt, D.W., Dezube, B.J., Thommes, J.A., Miller, B.J. et al. (1998) Pegylated-liposomal doxorubicin versus doxorubicin, bleomycin, and vincristine in the treatment of AIDS-related Kaposi's sarcoma: results of a randomized phase III clinical trial. *J. Clin. Oncol.*, **16**, 2445–2451.
34. Cooley, T., Henry, D., Tonda, M., Sun, S. et al. (2007) A randomized, double-blind study of pegylated liposomal doxorubicin for the treatment of AIDS-related Kaposi's sarcoma. *Oncologist*, **12**, 114–123.
35. Markman, M., Gordon, A.N., McGuire, W.P., and Muggia, F.M. (2004) Liposomal anthracycline treatment for ovarian cancer. *Semin. Oncol.*, **31** (Suppl. 13), 91–105.
36. Muggia, F.M., Hainsworth, J.D., Jeffers, S., Miller, P. et al. (1997) Phase II study of liposomal doxorubicin in refractory ovarian cancer: antitumor activity and toxicity modification by liposomal encapsulation. *J. Clin. Oncol.*, **15**, 987–993.
37. Strauss, H.G., Hemsen, A., Karbe, I., Lautenschlager, C. et al. (2008) Phase II trial of biweekly pegylated liposomal doxorubicin in recurrent platinum-refractory ovarian and peritoneal cancer. *Anti-Cancer Drugs*, **19**, 541–545.
38. Forbes, C., Wilby, J., Richardson, G., Sculpher, M. et al. (2002) A systematic review and economic evaluation of pegylated liposomal doxorubicin hydrochloride for ovarian cancer. *Health Technol. Assess.*, **6**, 1–119.
39. Oskay-Oezcelik, G., Koensgen, D., Hindenburg, H.J., Klare, P. et al. (2008) Biweekly pegylated liposomal doxorubicin as second-line treatment in patients with relapsed ovarian cancer after failure of platinum and paclitaxel: results from a multi-center phase II study of the NOGGO. *Anticancer Res.*, **28**, 1329–1334.
40. Gordon, A.N., Fleagle, J.T., Guthrie, D., Parkin, D.E. et al. (2001) Recurrent epithelial ovarian carcinoma: a randomized phase III study of pegylated liposomal doxorubicin versus topotecan. *J. Clin. Oncol.*, **19**, 3312–3322.
41. Gordon, A.N., Tonda, M., Sun, S., and Rackoff, W. (2004) Long-term survival advantage for women treated with pegylated liposomal doxorubicin compared with topotecan in a phase 3 randomized study of recurrent and refractory epithelial ovarian cancer. *Gynecol. Oncol.*, **95**, 1–8.
42. Main, C., Bojke, L., Griffin, S., Norman, G. et al. (2006) Topotecan, pegylated liposomal doxorubicin hydrochloride and paclitaxel for second-line or subsequent treatment of advanced ovarian cancer: a systematic

review and economic evaluation. *Health Technol. Assess.*, **10**, 1–132, iii–iv.
43. Mutch, D.G., Orlando, M., Goss, T., Teneriello, M.G. et al. (2007) Randomized phase III trial of gemcitabine compared with pegylated liposomal doxorubicin in patients with platinum-resistant ovarian cancer. *J. Clin. Oncol.*, **25**, 2811–2818.
44. Ferrandina, G., Ludovisi, M., Lorusso, D., Pignata, S. et al. (2008) Phase III trial of gemcitabine compared with pegylated liposomal doxorubicin in progressive or recurrent ovarian cancer. *J. Clin. Oncol.*, **26**, 890–896.
45. Vergote, I., Finkler, N., del Campo, J., Lohr, A. et al. (2009) Phase 3 randomised study of canfosfamide (Telcyta, TLK286) versus pegylated liposomal doxorubicin or topotecan as third-line therapy in patients with platinum-refractory or -resistant ovarian cancer. *Eur. J. Cancer*, **45**, 2324–2332.
46. Monk, B.J., Herzog, T.J., Kaye, S.B., Krasner, C.N. et al. (2010) Trabectedin plus pegylated liposomal doxorubicin in recurrent ovarian cancer. *J. Clin. Oncol.*, **28**, 3107–3114.
47. Robert, N.J., Vogel, C.L., Henderson, I.C., Sparano, J.A. et al. (2004) The role of the liposomal anthracyclines and other systemic therapies in the management of advanced breast cancer. *Semin. Oncol.*, **31** (Suppl. 13), 106–146.
48. Hamilton, A., Biganzoli, L., Coleman, R., Mauriac, L. et al. (2002) EORTC 10968: a phase I clinical and pharmacokinetic study of polyethylene glycol liposomal doxorubicin (Caelyx, Doxil) at a 6-week interval in patients with metastatic breast cancer. *Ann. Oncol.*, **13**, 910–918.
49. Huober, J., Fett, W., Nusch, A., Neise, M. et al. (2010) A multicentric observational trial of pegylated liposomal doxorubicin for metastatic breast cancer. *BMC Cancer*, **10**, 2.
50. Mlineritsch, B., Mayer, P., Rass, C., Reiter, E. et al. (2004) Phase II study of single-agent pegylated liposomal doxorubicin HCl (PLD) in metastatic breast cancer after first-line treatment failure. *Onkologie*, **27**, 441–446.
51. Al-Batran, S.E., Bischoff, J., von Minckwitz, G., Atmaca, A. et al. (2006) The clinical benefit of pegylated liposomal doxorubicin in patients with metastatic breast cancer previously treated with conventional anthracyclines: a multicentre phase II trial. *Br. J. Cancer*, **94**, 1615–1620.
52. Munzone, E., Di Pietro, A., Goldhirsch, A., Minchella, I. et al. (2010) Metronomic administration of pegylated liposomal-doxorubicin in extensively pre-treated metastatic breast cancer patients: a mono-institutional case-series report. *Breast*, **19**, 33–37.
53. Keller, A.M., Mennel, R.G., Georgoulias, V.A., Nabholtz, J.M. et al. (2004) Randomized phase III trial of pegylated liposomal doxorubicin versus vinorelbine or mitomycin C plus vinblastine in women with taxane-refractory advanced breast cancer. *J. Clin. Oncol.*, **22**, 3893–3901.
54. Hussein, M.A. and Anderson, K.C. (2004) Role of liposomal anthracyclines in the treatment of multiple myeloma. *Semin. Oncol.*, **31** (Suppl. 13), 147–160.
55. Judson, I., Radford, J.A., Harris, M., Blay, J.Y. et al. (2001) Randomised phase II trial of pegylated liposomal doxorubicin (DOXIL/CAELYX) versus doxorubicin in the treatment of advanced or metastatic soft tissue sarcoma: a study by the EORTC Soft Tissue and Bone Sarcoma Group. *Eur. J. Cancer*, **37**, 870–877.
56. Poveda, A., Lopez-Pousa, A., Martin, J., Del Muro, J.G. et al. (2005) Phase II clinical trial with pegylated liposomal doxorubicin (CAELYX®/Doxil®) and quality of life evaluation (EORTC QLQ-C30) in Adult patients with advanced soft tissue sarcomas: a study of the Spanish Group for Research in Sarcomas (GEIS). *Sarcoma*, **9**, 127–132.
57. Grenader, T., Goldberg, A., Hadas-Halperin, I., and Gabizon, A. (2009) Long-term response to pegylated liposomal doxorubicin in patients with metastatic soft tissue sarcomas. *Anti-Cancer Drugs*, **20**, 15–20.

58. Sutton, G., Blessing, J., Hanjani, P., and Kramer, P. (2005) Phase II evaluation of liposomal doxorubicin (Doxil) in recurrent or advanced leiomyosarcoma of the uterus: a Gynecologic Oncology Group study. *Gynecol. Oncol.*, **96**, 749–752.
59. Skubitz, K.M. and Haddad, P.A. (2005) Paclitaxel and pegylated-liposomal doxorubicin are both active in angiosarcoma. *Cancer*, **104**, 361–366.
60. Kodali, D. and Seetharaman, K. (2006) Primary cardiac angiosarcoma. *Sarcoma*, **2006**, 39130.
61. Wollina, U., Hansel, G., Schonlebe, J., Averbeck, M. et al. (2011) Cutaneous angiosarcoma is a rare aggressive malignant vascular tumour of the skin. *J. Eur. Acad. Dermatol. Venereol.*, **25**, 964–968.
62. Munoz, A., Maldonado, M., Pardo, N., Fernandez, J.M. et al. (2004) Pegylated liposomal doxorubicin hydrochloride (PLD) for advanced sarcomas in children: preliminary results. *Pediatr. Blood Cancer*, **43**, 152–155.
63. Constantinidou, A., Jones, R.L., Scurr, M., Al-Muderis, O. et al. (2009) Pegylated liposomal doxorubicin, an effective, well-tolerated treatment for refractory aggressive fibromatosis. *Eur. J. Cancer*, **45**, 2930–2934.
64. Di Bella, N.J., Khan, M.M., Dakhil, S.R., Logie, K.W. et al. (2003) Pegylated liposomal doxorubicin as single-agent treatment of low-grade non-Hodgkin's lymphoma: a phase II multicenter study. *Clin. Lymphoma*, **3**, 235–240.
65. Wollina, U., Dummer, R., Brockmeyer, N.H., Konrad, H. et al. (2003) Multicenter study of pegylated liposomal doxorubicin in patients with cutaneous T-cell lymphoma. *Cancer*, **98**, 993–1001.
66. Pignata, S., Scambia, G., Savarese, A., Breda, E. et al. (2009) Carboplatin and pegylated liposomal doxorubicin for advanced ovarian cancer: preliminary activity results of the MITO-2 phase III trial. *Oncology*, **76**, 49–54.
67. Alberts, D.S., Liu, P.Y., Wilczynski, S.P., Clouser, M.C. et al. (2008) Randomized trial of pegylated liposomal doxorubicin (PLD) plus carboplatin versus carboplatin in platinum-sensitive (PS) patients with recurrent epithelial ovarian or peritoneal carcinoma after failure of initial platinum-based chemotherapy (Southwest Oncology Group Protocol S0200). *Gynecol. Oncol.*, **108**, 90–94.
68. Markman, M., Moon, J., Wilczynski, S., Lopez, A.M. et al. (2010) Single agent carboplatin versus carboplatin plus pegylated liposomal doxorubicin in recurrent ovarian cancer: final survival results of a SWOG (S0200) phase 3 randomized trial. *Gynecol. Oncol.*, **116**, 323–325.
69. Pujade-Lauraine, E., Wagner, U., Aavall-Lundqvist, E., Gebski, V. et al. (2010) Pegylated liposomal doxorubicin and carboplatin compared with paclitaxel and carboplatin for patients with platinum-sensitive ovarian cancer in late relapse. *J. Clin. Oncol.*, **28**, 3323–3329.
70. Bookman, M.A., Brady, M.F., McGuire, W.P., Harper, P.G. et al. (2009) Evaluation of new platinum-based treatment regimens in advanced-stage ovarian cancer: a phase III trial of the Gynecologic Cancer Intergroup. *J. Clin. Oncol.*, **27**, 1419–1425.
71. Moore, M.R., Srinivasiah, J., Feinberg, B.A., Bordoni, R.E. et al. (1998) Phase II randomized trial of doxorubicin plus paclitaxel (AT) versus dosorubicin HC liposome injection (Doxil) plus paclitaxel (DT) in metastatic breast cancer. *Proc. Am. Soc. Clin. Oncol.*, **16**, 160a.
72. Sparano, J.A., Makhson, A.N., Semiglazov, V.F., Tjulandin, S.A. et al. (2009) Pegylated liposomal doxorubicin plus docetaxel significantly improves time to progression without additive cardiotoxicity compared with docetaxel monotherapy in patients with advanced breast cancer previously treated with neoadjuvant-adjuvant anthracycline therapy: results from a randomized phase III study. *J. Clin. Oncol.*, **27**, 4522–4529.
73. Al-Batran, S.E., Guntner, M., Pauligk, C., Scholz, M. et al. (2010) Anthracycline rechallenge using pegylated liposomal doxorubicin in patients with metastatic breast cancer: a pooled

analysis using individual data from four prospective trials. *Br. J. Cancer*, **103**, 1518–1523.
74. Overmoyer, B., Silverman, P., Holder, L.W., Tripathy, D. *et al.* (2005) Pegylated liposomal doxorubicin and cyclophosphamide as first-line therapy for patients with metastatic or recurrent breast cancer. *Clin. Breast Cancer*, **6**, 150–157.
75. Kurtz, J.E., Rousseau, F., Meyer, N., Delozier, T. *et al.* (2007) Phase II trial of pegylated liposomal doxorubicin–cyclophosphamide combination as first-line chemotherapy in older metastatic breast cancer patients. *Oncology*, **73**, 210–214.
76. Chia, S., Clemons, M., Martin, L.A., Rodgers, A. *et al.* (2006) Pegylated liposomal doxorubicin and trastuzumab in HER-2 overexpressing metastatic breast cancer: a multicenter phase II trial. *J. Clin. Oncol.*, **24**, 2773–2778.
77. Andreopoulou, E., Gaiotti, D., Kim, E., Volm, M. *et al.* (2007) Feasibility and cardiac safety of pegylated liposomal doxorubicin plus trastuzumab in heavily pretreated patients with recurrent HER2-overexpressing metastatic breast cancer. *Clin. Breast Cancer*, **7**, 690–696.
78. Christodoulou, C., Kostopoulos, I., Kalofonos, H.P., Lianos, E. *et al.* (2009) Trastuzumab combined with pegylated liposomal doxorubicin in patients with metastatic breast cancer. Phase II Study of the Hellenic Cooperative Oncology Group (HeCOG) with biomarker evaluation. *Oncology*, **76**, 275–285.
79. Stickeler, E., Klar, M., Watermann, D., Geibel, A. *et al.* (2009) Pegylated liposomal doxorubicin and trastuzumab as 1st and 2nd line therapy in HER2/neu positive metastatic breast cancer: a multicenter phase II trial. *Breast Cancer Res. Treat.*, **117**, 591–598.
80. Wolff, A.C., Wang, M., Li, H., Pins, M.R. *et al.* (2010) Phase II trial of pegylated liposomal doxorubicin plus docetaxel with and without trastuzumab in metastatic breast cancer: Eastern Cooperative Oncology Group trial E3198. *Breast Cancer Res. Treat.*, **121**, 111–120.
81. Park, J., Valente, N., Stauffer, P., Diederich, C. *et al.* (2000) Phase I/II study of sequential hyperthermia + doxil for the treatment of breast cancer metastatic to the chest wall. *Proc. Am. Soc. Clin. Oncol.*, **19**, 390a.
82. Park, J.W., Stauffer, P., Diederich, C., Colbern, G. *et al.* (2001) Hyperthermia (HT) + doxil significantly enhances drug delivery and efficacy in metastatic breast cancer of the chest wall (CW): a phase I/II study. *Proc. Am. Soc. Clin. Oncol.*, **20**, 47a.
83. Murata, S., Kominsky, S.L., Vali, M., Zhang, Z. *et al.* (2006) Ductal access for prevention and therapy of mammary tumors. *Cancer Res.*, **66**, 638–645.
84. Flanagan, M., Love, S., and Hwang, E.S. (2010) Status of intraductal therapy for ductal carcinoma *in situ*. *Curr. Breast Cancer Rep.*, **2**, 75–82.
85. Dimopoulos, M.A., Pouli, A., Zervas, K., Grigoraki, V. *et al.* (2003) Prospective randomized comparison of vincristine, doxorubicin and dexamethasone (VAD) administered as intravenous bolus injection and VAD with liposomal doxorubicin as first-line treatment in multiple myeloma. *Ann. Oncol.*, **14**, 1039–1044.
86. Rifkin, R.M., Gregory, S.A., Mohrbacher, A., and Hussein, M.A. (2006) Pegylated liposomal doxorubicin, vincristine, and dexamethasone provide significant reduction in toxicity compared with doxorubicin, vincristine, and dexamethasone in patients with newly diagnosed multiple myeloma: a phase III multicenter randomized trial. *Cancer*, **106**, 848–858.
87. Orlowski, R.Z., Nagler, A., Sonneveld, P., Blade, J. *et al.* (2007) Randomized phase III study of pegylated liposomal doxorubicin plus bortezomib compared with bortezomib alone in relapsed or refractory multiple myeloma: combination therapy improves time to progression. *J. Clin. Oncol.*, **25**, 3892–3901.
88. Porter, C.A. and Rifkin, R.M. (2007) Clinical benefits and economic analysis of pegylated liposomal doxorubicin/vincristine/dexamethasone versus

doxorubicin/vincristine/dexamethasone in patients with newly diagnosed multiple myeloma. *Clin. Lymphoma Myeloma*, **7** (Suppl. 4), S150–S155.

89. Hussein, M.A., Baz, R., Srkalovic, G., Agrawal, N. *et al.* (2006) Phase 2 study of pegylated liposomal doxorubicin, vincristine, decreased-frequency dexamethasone, and thalidomide in newly diagnosed and relapsed-refractory multiple myeloma. *Mayo Clin. Proc.*, **81**, 889–895.

90. Offidani, M., Bringhen, S., Corvatta, L., Falco, P. *et al.* (2007) Thalidomide-dexamethasone plus pegylated liposomal doxorubicin vs. thalidomide-dexamethasone: a case-matched study in advanced multiple myeloma. *Eur. J. Haematol.*, **78**, 297–302.

91. Chanan-Khan, A.A. and Lee, K. (2007) Pegylated liposomal doxorubicin and immunomodulatory drug combinations in multiple myeloma: rationale and clinical experience. *Clin. Lymphoma Myeloma*, **7** (Suppl. 4), S163–S169.

92. Baz, R., Walker, E., Karam, M.A., Choueiri, T.K. *et al.* (2006) Lenalidomide and pegylated liposomal doxorubicin-based chemotherapy for relapsed or refractory multiple myeloma: safety and efficacy. *Ann. Oncol.*, **17**, 1766–1771.

93. Buda, G., Orciuolo, E., Galimberti, S., Pelosini, M. *et al.* (2010) Pegylated liposomal doxorubicin in combination with dexamethasone and bortezomib (VMD) or lenalidomide (RMD) in multiple myeloma pretreated patients. *Ann. Hematol.* DOI: 10.1007/s00277-010-1136-5.

94. Biehn, S.E., Moore, D.T., Voorhees, P.M., Garcia, R.A. *et al.* (2007) Extended follow-up of outcome measures in multiple myeloma patients treated on a phase I study with bortezomib and pegylated liposomal doxorubicin. *Ann. Hematol.*, **86**, 211–216.

95. Voorhees, P.M. and Orlowski, R.Z. (2007) Emerging data on the use of anthracyclines in combination with bortezomib in multiple myeloma. *Clin. Lymphoma Myeloma*, **7** (Suppl. 4), S156–S162.

96. Jakubowiak, A.J., Kendall, T., Al-Zoubi, A., Khaled, Y. *et al.* (2009) Phase II trial of combination therapy with bortezomib, pegylated liposomal doxorubicin, and dexamethasone in patients with newly diagnosed myeloma. *J. Clin. Oncol.*, **27**, 5015–5022.

97. Gozzetti, A., Fabbri, A., Oliva, S., Marchini, E. *et al.* (2010) Weekly bortezomib, pegylated liposomal doxorubicin, and dexamethasone is a safe and effective therapy for elderly patients with relapsed/refractory multiple myeloma. *Clin. Lymphoma Myeloma Leuk.*, **10**, 68–72.

98. Waterman, G.N., Yellin, O., Swift, R.A., Mapes, R. *et al.* (2011) A modified regimen of pegylated liposomal doxorubicin, bortezomib, and dexamethasone is effective and well tolerated in the treatment of relapsed or refractory multiple myeloma. *Ann. Hematol.*, **90**, 193–200.

99. Palumbo, A., Gay, F., Bringhen, S., Falcone, A. *et al.* (2008) Bortezomib, doxorubicin and dexamethasone in advanced multiple myeloma. *Ann. Oncol.*, **19**, 1160–1165.

100. Wagner, A. (2007) Treatment of advanced soft tissue sarcoma: conventional agents and promising new drugs. *J. Natl. Compr. Cancer Netw.*, **5**, 401–410.

101. Budman, D.R., Berry, D.A., Cirrincione, C.T., Henderson, I.C. *et al.* (1998) Dose and dose intensity as determinants of outcome in the adjuvant treatment of breast cancer. *J. Natl. Cancer Inst.*, **90**, 1205–1211.

102. Henderson, I.C., Berry, D.A., Demetri, G.D., Cirrincione, C.T. *et al.* (2003) Improved outcomes from adding sequential paclitaxel but not from escalating doxorubicin dose in an adjuvant chemotherapy regimen for patients with node-positive primary breast cancer. *J. Clin. Oncol.*, **21**, 976–983.

103. Grenader, T. and Gabizon, A. (2010) What is the right way to administer pegylated liposomal doxorubicin in breast cancer therapy? *J. Clin. Oncol.*, **28**, e193–e194; author reply e195–e196.

104. Emerson, D.L., Bendele, R., Brown, E., Chiang, S. *et al.* (2000) Antitumor

efficacy, pharmacokinetics, and biodistribution of NX 211: a low-clearance liposomal formulation of lurtotecan. *Clin. Cancer Res.*, **6**, 2903–2912.

105. Colbern, G.T., Dykes, D.J., Engbers, C., Musterer, R. et al. (1998) Encapsulation of the topoisomerase I inhibitor GL147211C in pegylated (STEALTH) liposomes: pharmacokinetics and antitumor activity in HT29 colon tumor xenografts. *Clin. Cancer Res.*, **4**, 3077–3082.

106. Dark, G.G., Calvert, A.H., Grimshaw, R., Poole, C. et al. (2005) Randomized trial of two intravenous schedules of the topoisomerase I inhibitor liposomal lurtotecan in women with relapsed epithelial ovarian cancer: a trial of the National Cancer Institute of Canada Clinical Trials Group. *J. Clin. Oncol.*, **23**, 1859–1866.

107. Seiden, M.V., Muggia, F., Astrow, A., Matulonis, U. et al. (2004) A phase II study of liposomal lurtotecan (OSI-211) in patients with topotecan resistant ovarian cancer. *Gynecol. Oncol.*, **93**, 229–232.

108. Duffaud, F., Borner, M., Chollet, P., Vermorken, J.B. et al. (2004) Phase II study of OSI-211 (liposomal lurtotecan) in patients with metastatic or loco-regional recurrent squamous cell carcinoma of the head and neck. *Eur. J. Cancer*, **40**, 2748–2752.

109. Zamboni, W.C., Ramalingam, S., Friedland, D.M., Edwards, R.P. et al. (2009) Phase I and pharmacokinetic study of pegylated liposomal CKD-602 in patients with advanced malignancies. *Clin. Cancer Res.*, **15**, 1466–1472.

110. Atyabi, F., Farkhondehfai, A., Esmaeili, F., and Dinarvand, R. (2009) Preparation of pegylated nano-liposomal formulation containing SN-38: in vitro characterization and in vivo biodistribution in mice. *Acta. Pharm.*, **59**, 133–144.

111. Drummond, D.C., Noble, C.O., Guo, Z., Hayes, M.E. et al. (2010) Development of a highly stable and targetable nanoliposomal formulation of topotecan. *J. Control. Release*, **141**, 13–21.

112. Newman, M.S., Colbern, G.T., Working, P.K., Engbers, C. et al. (1999) Comparative pharmacokinetics, tissue distribution, and therapeutic effectiveness of cisplatin encapsulated in long-circulating, pegylated liposomes (SPI-077) in tumor-bearing mice. *Cancer Chemother. Pharmacol.*, **43**, 1–7.

113. Meerum Terwogt, J.M., Groenewegen, G., Pluim, D., Maliepaard, M. et al. (2002) Phase I and pharmacokinetic study of SPI-77, a liposomal encapsulated dosage form of cisplatin. *Cancer Chemother. Pharmacol.*, **49**, 201–210.

114. Stathopoulos, G.P. (2010) Liposomal cisplatin: a new cisplatin formulation. *Anti-Cancer Drugs*, **21**, 732–736.

115. Stathopoulos, G.P., Antoniou, D., Dimitroulis, J., Michalopoulou, P. et al. (2010) Liposomal cisplatin combined with paclitaxel versus cisplatin and paclitaxel in non-small-cell lung cancer: a randomized phase III multicenter trial. *Ann. Oncol.*, **21**, 2227–2232.

116. Stathopoulos, G., Antoniou, D., Dimitroulis, J., Stathopoulos, J. et al. (2010) Comparison of response rate of advanced non-small lung cancer patients to liposomal cisplatin versus cisplatin both combined with paclitaxel: a phase III trial. *J. Clin. Oncol.*, **28** (Suppl.), 7579.

117. Sarris, A.H., Hagemeister, F., Romaguera, J., Rodriguez, M.A. et al. (2000) Liposomal vincristine in relapsed non-Hodgkin's lymphomas: early results of an ongoing phase II trial. *Ann. Oncol.*, **11**, 69–72.

118. Thomas, D.A., Sarris, A.H., Cortes, J., Faderl, S. et al. (2006) Phase II study of sphingosomal vincristine in patients with recurrent or refractory adult acute lymphocytic leukemia. *Cancer*, **106**, 120–127.

119. Drummond, D.C., Noble, C.O., Guo, Z., Hayes, M.E. et al. (2009) Improved pharmacokinetics and efficacy of a highly stable nanoliposomal vinorelbine. *J. Pharmacol. Exp. Ther.*, **328**, 321–330.

120. Zucker, D. and Barenholz, Y. (2010) Optimization of vincristine–topotecan combination – paving the way for

improved chemotherapy regimens by nanoliposomes. *J. Control. Release*, **146**, 326–333.
121. Park, J.W., Benz, C.C., and Martin, F.J. (2004) Future directions of liposome- and immunoliposome-based cancer therapeutics. *Semin. Oncol.*, **31** (Suppl. 13), 196–205.
122. Park, J.W., Hong, K., Kirpotin, D.B., Colbern, G. *et al.* (2002) Anti-HER2 immunoliposomes: enhanced efficacy attributable to targeted delivery. *Clin. Cancer Res.*, **8**, 1172–1181.
123. Mamot, C., Drummond, D.C., Noble, C.O., Kallab, V. *et al.* (2005) Epidermal growth factor receptor-targeted immunoliposomes significantly enhance the efficacy of multiple anticancer drugs *in vivo. Cancer Res.*, **65**, 11631–11638.

29
Immunoliposomes
Vladimir P. Torchilin

29.1
Introduction: Drug Targeting and Liposomes as Drug Carriers

29.1.1
Drug Targeting

For the majority of drugs currently in use, their specificity and activity toward disease sites or individual diseases is usually based on the drug's ability to interfere with local pathological processes or with defective biological pathways, but not on its selective accumulation in the specific intracellular compartment or in the target cell, organ, or tissue. Usually, pharmaceutical agents are distributed within the body proportionally to the regional blood flow. As a result, to achieve a required therapeutic concentration of a drug in a certain body compartment (tumor), one has to administer the drug in large quantities, wasting a great part of it in normal tissues and provoking negative side-effects.

Drug targeting using site-specific pharmaceutical carriers can provide a solution to these problems, providing the following advantages: simplification of drug administration protocols; reduction in the drug quantity required to achieve a therapeutic effect and in the cost of therapy; increase of drug concentration in the required sites without negative effects on nontarget compartments. Currently, numerous approaches for drug targeting have been described permitting the specific delivery of therapeutic and diagnostic pharmaceutical agents to the variety of tissues and organs; some of them are discussed in many review-type publications (e.g., [1–4]).

Fast developing nanotechnology, among other areas, is expected to have an important impact on medicine. The application of nanotechnology for the treatment, diagnosis, monitoring, and control of live systems is now often referred to as nanomedicine. Among many possible applications of nanotechnology in medicine, the use of various nanomaterials as pharmaceutical delivery systems for drugs, DNA, and imaging agents is receiving increasing attention. Many varieties of nanoparticles are available [5], such as different polymeric and metal nanoparticles,

Drug Delivery in Oncology: From Basic Research to Cancer Therapy, First Edition.
Edited by Felix Kratz, Peter Senter, and Henning Steinhagen.
© 2012 Wiley-VCH Verlag GmbH & Co. KGaA. Published 2012 by Wiley-VCH Verlag GmbH & Co. KGaA.

liposomes, niosomes, solid lipid particles, micelles, quantum dots, dendrimers, microcapsules, cells, cell ghosts, lipoproteins, and others.

The paradigm of using nanoparticulate pharmaceutical carriers to enhance the *in vivo* efficiency of many drugs, anticancer drugs first of all, has well established itself both in pharmaceutical research and the clinical setting. There already exists a great number of important review articles and monographs on this subject. Recent publications summarize the most important developments in this area, and specifically address the issues of nanocarriers designed to deliver drugs into certain individual sites of disease (cancer first of all) and to perform various functions in the body simultaneously [5–17]. The use of various nanoparticulate drug carriers aims, first of all, to minimize drug degradation and inactivation upon administration, prevent undesirable side-effects, and increase drug bioavailability and the fraction of the drug delivered in the pathological area.

29.1.2
Longevity of Pharmaceutical Nanocarriers in the Blood and the Enhanced Permeability and Retention Effect

It is now a well-established phenomenon that under certain pathological circumstances (inflammation or tumor growth) the endothelial lining of the blood vessel wall becomes more permeable than in the normal state. This was clearly demonstrated in many tumors [18, 19]. As a result, in such areas, large molecules and even relatively large particles ranging from 10 to 500 nm in size can leave the vascular bed and accumulate inside the interstitial space. Being loaded with pharmaceutical agents, these particles (pharmaceutical carriers) bring these agents into the area with the increased vascular permeability, where the drug is eventually released from a carrier. Since the cutoff size of the permeabilized vasculature varies from case to case [19, 20], the size of a drug carrying particle may be used to control the efficacy of such spontaneous "passive" drug delivery – the enhanced permeability and retention (EPR) effect [21, 22].

The surface of pharmaceutical carriers, including liposomes, can be modified by different moieties to impart them certain properties and functionalities, such as prolonged circulation in the blood [23, 24], allowing for their accumulation in various pathological areas (such as solid tumors) via the EPR effect (protective polymeric coating with poly(ethylene glycol) (PEG) is frequently used for this purpose) [21, 25]; ability to specifically recognize and bind target tissues or cells via the surface-attached specific ligand (monoclonal antibodies mAbs) as well as their Fab fragments and some other moieties, such as folate or transferrin (Tf), are used for this purpose) [26, 27–31]; ability to respond local stimuli characteristic of the pathological site by, for example, releasing an entrapped drug or specifically acting on cellular membranes under the abnormal pH or temperature in disease sites [32, 33]; ability to penetrate inside cells bypassing the lysosomal degradation for efficient targeting of intracellular drug targets (for this purpose, the surface of nanocarriers is additionally modified by cell-penetrating peptides) [34, 35].

One of the most important properties of a pharmaceutical nanocarrier loaded with any anticancer drug is its blood circulation longevity, and long-circulating pharmaceuticals and pharmaceutical carriers represent currently an important and still growing area of biomedical research (e.g., [23, 26, 36–38]). The longevity allows maintaining a required level of a pharmaceutical agent in the blood for extended time periods. Long-circulating drug-containing pharmaceutical carriers can provide better accumulation in pathological sites via the EPR effect [21, 39, 40]. In addition, the prolonged circulation can also help to achieve a better targeting effect for targeted drugs and drug carriers, allowing more time for their interaction with the target [38].

Surface modification of pharmaceutical nanocarriers including liposomes with certain synthetic polymers, such as PEG, is the most frequent way to impart the *in vivo* longevity to drug carriers, as was first suggested for liposomes [41–45]. At the biological level, coating nanoparticles with PEG sterically hinders interactions of blood components with their surface and reduces the binding of plasma proteins with PEGylated nanoparticles, as was demonstrated for liposomes [43, 46–50]. The mechanisms of preventing opsonization by PEG include the shielding of the surface charge, increased surface hydrophilicity [51], enhanced repulsive interaction between polymer-coated nanocarriers and blood components [52], and formation of the polymeric layer over the particle surface, which is impermeable for large molecules of opsonins even at relatively low polymer concentrations [51, 53]. Currently, there exist many chemical approaches to synthesize activated derivatives of PEG and to couple these derivatives with a variety of drugs and drug carriers, first of all with liposomes (reviewed in [54–56]).

29.1.3
Liposomes

Clinical applications of liposomes in cancer are well known (see some examples in Table 29.1). Doxorubicin in PEG-coated liposomes is successfully used for the treatment of solid tumors in patients with breast carcinoma metastases with subsequent survival improvement [57–59]. The same set of indications was targeted by the combination therapy involving liposomal doxorubicin and paclitaxel [60] or Doxil/Caelyx (doxorubicin in PEG-liposomes) and carboplatin [61]. Caelyx was also tested for patients with squamous cell cancer of the head and neck [62] and ovarian cancer [63, 64]. Clinical data showed the effect of doxorubicin in PEG-liposomes against unresectable hepatocellular carcinoma [65], cutaneous T-cell lymphoma [66], and sarcoma [67]. A review of the successful use of Caelyx in the treatment of ovarian cancer can be found in Perez-Lopez *et al.* [64]. It should be noted here, however, that recent evidence showed that PEG-liposomes, previously considered as biologically inert, still could induce certain side-reactions via activation of the complement system [68, 69].

Current development of the liposomal carriers often involves the attempt to combine the properties of long-circulating liposomes and targeted liposomes in one preparation [29, 85, 86]. To achieve better selectivity of PEG-coated liposomes,

Table 29.1 Some clinically tested anticancer liposomal drugs.

Active drug in liposomes	Disease	References
Daunorubicin (DaunoXome®)	Kaposi's sarcoma	[70]
Doxorubicin (Mycet®)	combinational therapy of recurrent breast cancer	[71, 72]
Doxorubicin in PEG-liposomes (Doxil®/Caelyx®)	refractory Kaposi's sarcoma, ovarian cancer, recurrent breast cancer, prostate cancer	[70, 73]
Annamycin	doxorubicin-resistant tumors	[74]
Vincristine (Marqibo®, formerly referred to as Onco TCS)	non-Hodgkin's lymphoma	[75]
Lurtotecan (NX211)	ovarian cancer	[76]
Platinum compounds (cisplatin, platar)	germ cell cancers, small-cell lung carcinoma, head and neck cancer	[77–79]
All-*trans* retinoic acid (Altragen®)	acute promyelocytic leukemia, non-Hodgkin's lymphoma, renal cell carcinoma, Kaposi's sarcoma	[80, 81]
DNA plasmid encoding HLA-B7 and β_2-microglobulin (Allovectin-7®)	metastatic melanoma	[82]
BLP 25 vaccine Stimuvax®	non-small-cell lung cancer vaccine	[83]
E1A gene	various tumors	[84]

it is advantageous to attach the targeting ligand via a PEG spacer arm, so that the ligand is extended outside of the dense PEG brush, excluding steric hindrances for the ligand binding to the target. Various advanced technologies are used for this purpose and the targeting moiety is usually attached above the protecting polymer layer, by coupling it with the distal water-exposed terminus of activated liposome-grafted polymer molecule [85, 87] (Figure 29.1).

Multiple original papers and reviews on antibody-targeted drug-loaded liposomes in cancer are available [31, 88–93]. The binding chemistry for antibody attachment to drug carriers involved the use of bifunctional reagents to couple carrier-incorporated reactive groups with a protein [94, 95]; antibody modification with hydrophobic residues providing efficient adsorption/incorporation of the modified proteins onto/into the drug carrier surface [96–99]; and a few other approaches [100–102]. The development of long-circulating liposomes coated with "sterically protecting" polymers eventually led to the development of multiple methods to attach targeting antibodies onto the surface of PEG. In general, antibody attachment can decrease the circulating time of nanopreparations because of their increased uptake via Fc receptors of circulating or liver macrophages, or opsonization of the nanocarrier-tagged antibody molecules [103, 104]. Whole antibodies can also trigger complement-mediated cytotoxicity and antibody-dependent cellular cytotoxicity (ADCC) [31]. These effects could be minimized by using antibody Fab fragments instead of whole antibodies [105].

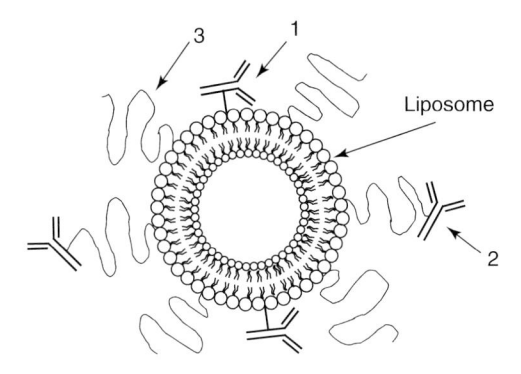

Figure 29.1 Antibody-mediated long-circulating liposome. Antibody can be attached directly to the liposome surface (1) or to the solution-exposed tips of polymeric chains used to impart longevity to liposomes (2). Protective polymer (usually PEG) (3).

29.2
Tumor-Targeted Liposomes in Cancer Chemotherapy

29.2.1
Derivatization of PEGylated Liposomes

Since PEG–lipid conjugates used for the steric protection of liposomes and other pharmaceutical nanocarriers are derived from methoxy-PEG (mPEG) and carry nonreactive methoxy terminal groups, several attempts have been made to functionalize PEG tips in PEG–lipid conjugates in order to additionally attach a targeting moiety to long-circulating drug delivery systems (liposomes). For this purpose several types of end-group-functionalized PEG–lipid conjugates of general formula X–PEG–PE [54, 106], where X represents a reactive functional group-containing moiety, while PEG–PE represents the conjugate of phosphatidyl ethanolamine (PE) and PEG, were introduced. Most of the end-group functionalized PEG–lipids were synthesized from heterobifunctional PEG derivatives containing hydroxyl and carboxyl or amino groups. Typically, the hydroxyl end-group of PEG was derivatized to form a urethane attachment with the hydrophobic lipid anchor, PE, while the amino or carboxyl groups were utilized for further functionalization. To simplify the coupling procedure and to make it applicable for single-step binding of a large variety of amino group-containing ligands (including antibodies, proteins, and small molecules) to the distal end of nanocarrier-attached polymeric chains, amphiphilic PEG derivative, p-nitrophenylcarbonyl (pNP)-PEG–PE, was introduced [87, 107, 108]. pNP-PEG–PE readily adsorbs on hydrophobic nanoparticles or incorporates into liposomes and micelles via its phospholipid residue, and easily binds any amino group-containing compound via its water-exposed pNP group forming stable and nontoxic urethane (carbamate) bonds. Other methods that could be used for the coupling of ligands to the distal tips of PEG chains include

PEG activation with hydrazine groups (in the case of antibody attachment, hydrazine reacts with the oxidized carbohydrate groups in the oligosaccharide moiety of the antibody), pyridyldithiopropionate (PDP) group (after conversion of the PDP into the thiol, it reacts with maleimide groups of the premodified ligand), or maleimide group (reacts with thiol groups in prethiolated ligand) [109–114]. The ligand (antibody) binding to PEGylated liposomes was also performed via PEG terminus modified with cyanuric chloride [115]. See reviews on various coupling techniques in [116, 117].

An additional way to couple various ligands, such as antibodies, to liposomes, including PEGylated liposomes, is based on a so-called "postinsertion" technique [118]. This technique is based on the preliminary activation of ligands with any reactive PEG–PE derivative and subsequent coincubation of unstable micelles formed by the modified ligand–PEG–PE conjugates with preformed drug-loaded plain or PEGylated liposomes. Eventually, modified ligands spontaneously incorporate from their micelles into more thermodynamically favorable surrounding of the liposome membrane.

29.2.2
Antibody-Targeted Liposomes

Antibodies (mainly of the IgG class) are the most diverse and broadly used specific ligands for experimental targeted chemotherapy of various tumors with drug-loaded liposomes. There are multiple original papers and reviews on antibody-targeted drug-loaded liposomes in cancer (reviewed in [31, 88–93]).

Early attempts to attach antibodies to liposomes for their targeting to certain cells and tissues in the body go back 40 years, when antibody molecules and some model proteins were coupled to the surface of plain, non-PEGylated liposomes. The binding chemistry involved the use of bifunctional reagents to couple liposome-incorporated reactive groups with a protein [94, 95]; protein modification with hydrophobic residues providing and efficient incorporation of the modified proteins into the liposomal membrane [96], with N-glutarylphosphatidyl ethanolamine (NGPE) becoming the most frequent modifier [97–99]; protein attachment to liposome via activated liposome-incorporated sugar moieties or via activated sugar moieties in the antibody molecule [100]; and a few other approaches [101, 102] (reviewed in [119]).

Recent reviews on the use of antibody-targeted liposomes for cancer show that there is a specific interest in using such preparations for the treatment of lung metastases [120], for targeting central nervous system tumors, such as neuroblastoma [121], and for gene delivery in the therapy of the liver cancer [122]. A significant interest is also expressed toward the use of single-chain Fv as a targeting moiety for immunoliposomes intended for cancer treatment [123]. In general, targeted liposome-encapsulated drugs are still considered as magic bullets for treating cancer [124].

In general, antibody attachment can decrease the circulating time of liposomes because of increased uptake of the modified liposomes via Fc receptors of circulating or liver macrophages, or opsonization of the liposome-tagged antibody molecules [103, 104]. Whole antibodies can also trigger complement-mediated cytotoxicity and ADCC [31]. These effects could be minimized by using antibody Fab fragments instead of whole antibodies [105]. In case of antibody-modified PEGylated liposomes, even a certain decrease in the circulation time for antibody-modified PEG-liposomes still allows for their sufficiently long circulation, permitting good target accumulation.

Although in some cases tumor accumulation of antibody-modified long-circulating liposomes is comparable with the accumulation of long-circulating antibody-free liposomes [125–128], therapeutic activity is higher for antibody-targeted liposomes because antibody-modified preparations are much better internalized by tumor cells, which allows for higher drug doses delivered inside cancer cells (i.e., for more efficient cancer cell killing) [129]. In some other cases, however, the liposome internalization seems not important. Thus, it was shown [130] that PEGylated liposomes modified (or nonmodified) with antibodies against internalizing CD19 antigen or noninternalizing CD20 antigen demonstrate therapeutic effects that depended more on the type of the drug used (vincristine or doxorubicin) than on the ability to be internalized. The authors of [131] have demonstrated that while nontargeted doxorubicin-containing liposomes were toxic to various cancer cells to the extent reflecting cell sensitivity to the drug, the cytotoxicity of antibody-targeted liposomes was proportional to the surface density of the corresponding surface antigen with similar observations made in [126, 132]. Since cancer cells are often rather heterogeneous with respect to the antigens they express, it was suggested [31] to use a combination of antibodies against different antigens on a single liposome to provide better and more uniform targeting of all cells within the tumor.

The first systematic studies on antibody-modified liposomes were performed using both non-PEGylated and PEGylated liposomes modified with the 34A mAb specific toward murine pulmonary endothelial cells [111, 133–137]. Immunoliposomes with 3′,5′-O-dipalmitoyl-5-fluoro-2′-deoxyuridine have been shown to effectively target lung metastases in a murine model [136].

The mAb against HER2, the antigen frequently overexpressed on various cancer cells, is widely used in cancer targeting. Monoclonal anti-HER2 antibodies including the humanized ones as well as currently clinically used Herceptin® antibodies have been used to render drug-loaded liposomes (long-circulating liposomes) specific for HER2-positive cancer cells [113, 125, 128, 129, 138, 139]. This antibody was successfully used to deliver doxorubicin, both in plain and long-circulating liposomes, to breast tumors xenografts in mice, which resulted in significantly enhanced therapeutic activity of the drug. PEGylated liposomes decorated with anti-HER2 antibody were shown to undergo effective endocytosis by HER2-positive cancer cells, allowing for better drug (doxorubicin) accumulation inside tumor cells with better therapeutic outcome. Compared to doxorubicin in plain PEGylated liposomes (Doxil), which normally accumulates in the tumor interstitial space, in the case of antibody-targeted Doxil, more drugs molecules were discovered inside cancer cells (i.e., targeting with the antibody increases drug internalization by target cells). Another example of therapeutic efficacy of doxorubicin in HER2-targeted liposomes against HER2-overexpressing tumors in mice was described in [140].

Recently, drug-loaded liposomes modified with antibodies against HER2 have been considered for targeted intraperitoneal therapy of micrometastatic cancer [141]. Anti-HER2-liposomes (Fab' fragments were used) have also been tested for the tumor-targeted delivery of PE38KDEL to breast cancer cells, demonstrating an increased cytotoxicity [142]. Vincristine and vinblastine in anti-HER2-liposomes were shown to specifically target breast tumors in experimental rats [143]. The combination of listeriolysin O and anti-HER2 antibody on the surface of the same drug-loaded liposomes was suggested to facilitate the endosomal escape of liposomes after their internalization by target cancer cells [144].

Another antibody to target tumors with drug-loaded liposomes is the mAb against CD19 antigen, which is also frequently overexpressed on various cancer cells. Anti-CD19 antibody-modified liposomes loaded with doxorubicin demonstrated clearly enhanced targeting and therapeutic efficacy both *in vitro* and *in vivo* in mice with human $CD19^+$ B lymphoma cells [132]. Similar results have also been obtained with doxorubicin-loaded liposomes modified with antibodies against internalizable CD19 antigen and against noninternalizable CD20 antigen [130]. Anti-CD19 antibodies have also been used to target doxorubicin-loaded liposomes with variable drug release rates to experimental tumors [145]. Recently, a successful attempt was made to target doxorubicin-loaded long-circulating liposomes to CD19-expressing cancer cells with single-chain Fv fragments of CD19 antibodies [146, 147]. $CD33^+$ tumor cells (acute myeloid leukemia cells) have been successfully targeted with immunoliposomes loaded with small interfering RNA (as a complex with polyethylenimine) [148]. CD22 antigen typical for B-cell lymphomas was targeted with doxorubicin-loaded liposomes modified with CD22-single-chain Fv [149].

Since neuroblastoma cells usually overexpress disialoganglioside GD2, antibodies against GD2 and their Fab' fragments have been suggested to target drug-loaded liposomes to corresponding tumors [150–152]. Fab' fragments of anti-GD2 antibodies covalently coupled to long-circulating liposomes loaded with doxorubicin allowed for increased binding and higher cytotoxicity against target cells both *in vitro* and *in vivo*, including in models of human tumors in nude mice and in metastatic models. GD2-targeted immunoliposomes with the novel anticancer drug, fenretinide, inducing apoptosis in neuroblastoma and melanoma cell lines, have also demonstrated strong antineuroblastoma activity both *in vitro* and *in vivo* in mice [153]. The combination of doxorubicin-loaded PEGylated liposomes targeted with anti-GD2 and with NGR peptides specifically binding with the tumor vasculature produced an improved therapeutic effect by acting on both tumor cells and tumor blood vessels [152].

Epidermal growth factor receptor (EGFR) and its variant EGFRvIII can serve as valuable targets for intracellular drug delivery into tumor cells overexpressing these receptors. Fab' fragments of the mAb C225, which binds both EGFR and EGFRvIII, and single-chain Fv fragment of the mAb, which binds only to EGFR, were coupled to drug-loaded liposomes and allowed for substantially enhanced binding of targeted liposomes with cancer cell overexpressing corresponding receptors (glioma cells U87 and carcinoma cells A0431 and MDA-MB-468). The better binding resulted in enhanced internalization and increased cytotoxicity [154]. *In vivo* therapy with such targeted drug-loaded liposomes (doxorubicin, epirubicin, and vinorelbine were used as drugs) always resulted in better tumor growth inhibition than therapy with non-targeted liposomal drugs [155]. Fab' fragment derived from the humanized anti-EGFR mAb EMD72000 was shown to provide efficient intracellular delivery of the liposomal drugs into colorectal tumor cells [156]. The authors of this study have also shown that the attachment of the targeting moiety to PEGylated liposomes requires the length of the spacer arm sufficient to overcome possible steric shielding of antibody fragments by sterically protecting PEG chains. An interesting method to construct anti-EGFR-targeted liposomes was suggested in [157], where the anti-EGFR antibody (cetuximab or C225) was covalently linked to the folate-binding protein via a thioester bond and then coupled to the preformed folate-containing liposomes. Cetuximab-liposomes loaded with boron derivatives for boron neutron capture therapy were also prepared using the cholesterol-based anchor and micelle-transfer technology [158]. Antitumor activity of EGFR-targeted pH-sensitive immunoliposomes loaded with gemcitabine was also demonstrated in A549 xenograft model in nude mice [159]. EGFR-expressing tumor cells have also been successfully targeted with sterically stabilized affibody liposomes [160].

An interesting target for antitumor drug delivery by targeted liposomes is the membrane type-1 matrix metalloproteinase (MT1-MMP), playing an important role in tumor neoangiogenesis and overexpressed both on tumor cells and on neoangiogenic endothelium. The modification of doxorubicin-loaded long-circulating liposomes with anti-MT1-MMP antibody resulted in an increased uptake of the targeted liposomes by MT1-MMP-overexpressing HT1080 fibrosarcoma cells *in vitro* and in more effective inhibition of tumor growth *in vivo* compared to antibody-free doxorubicin-loaded PEGylated liposomes [161]. It was demonstrated that anti-MM1-MMP antibody enhances the endocytic internalization of drug-loaded liposomes increasing thus their cytotoxicity [162]. Strong action of such preparation on tumor endothelial cells was noted.

Various proteins of the extracellular matrix expressed on the surface of cancer cells have also been used as targets for the antibody-mediated delivery of the liposomal drugs. Thus, β_1 integrins expressed on the surface of human non-small-cell lung carcinomas were targeted by doxorubicin-loaded liposomes modified with Fab' fragments of anti-β_1 integrin mAbs [163]. Treatment of SCID mice with lung tumor xenografts with such liposomes resulted in significant suppression of tumor growth compared to all controls and also inhibited metastases. The idea of targeting various antigens (preferably, the internalizable ones) on the endothelial cells by antibody–liposome conjugates was tested long ago [164]. However, the approach attracted a real attention only in the last few years. Thus, liposomes modified with anti-E-selectin antibodies were successfully internalized by activated endothelial cells *in vitro* through E-selectin-mediated endocytosis [165]. Another possible target for antibody-mediated cancer therapy with drug-loaded liposomes is the epithelial cell adhesion molecule (EpCAM), which is expressed in many tumors, but not in normal cells [166]. EpCAM-targeted immunoliposomes were generated by covalent attachment of the humanized single-chain Fv fragment of the 4D5MOCB mAb to the surface of PEGylated doxorubicin-loaded liposomes and demonstrated, significantly improved binding, internalization, and cytotoxicity with EpCAM-positive cancer cells. Similarly, liposomes coupled with antibodies against vascular cell adhesion molecule (VCAM)-1 can be effectively targeted to activated endothelial cells overexpressing VCAM-1 [167]. Liposomes loaded with cytotoxic drugs were also targeted to ED-B fibronectin using single-chain Fv fragment of the corresponding antibody [168]. Proliferating endothelial cells have been targeted with doxorubicin-loaded liposomes modified with single-chain Fv fragments of the antibody against endoglin overexpressed on such cells [169].

Lipid-based drug carriers have also been conjugated with antibodies (or their fragments) against Tf receptor (TfR) frequently overexpressed on the surface of various cancer cells. Thus, liposomes modified with the OX26 mAb against TfR via liposome-incorporated maleimide-modified PEG2000–PE molecules demonstrated strong binding with cells overexpressing TfR [170]. The same antibody was attached to daunomycin-loaded liposomes noncovalently via the avidin–biotin couple, and the modified liposomes demonstrated good accumulation in multidrug-resistant RBE4 brain capillary endothelial cells both *in vitro* and *in vivo* [171]. Liposomes loaded with a lipophilic prodrug 5-fluorodeoxyuridine and modified with the mAb CC531 against rat colon carcinoma demonstrated good binding with target cells [172] and effective intracellular drug delivery compared to all controls [173]. Antibody CC52 against rat colon adenocarcinoma CC531 attached to PEGylated liposomes provided specific accumulation of liposomes in a rat model of metastatic CC531 tumors [174].

Doxorubicin-loaded PEGylated liposomes were also modified with Fab' fragments of an anti-CD74 antibody via a PEG-based heterobifunctional coupling reagent and demonstrated a significantly accelerated and enhanced accumulation in Raji human B-lymphoma cells *in vitro* [175]. Anti-CD166 single-chain Fv attached to drug-loaded liposomes facilitated doxorubicin internalization by several prostate cancer cell lines (DU-145, PC-3, LNCaP) [176]. Single-chain F fragments of antibodies against leukemia stem cells and oncogenic molecules participating in acute myeloid leukemia pathogenesis were used to target acute leukemia stem cells [177]. Doxorubicin-loaded liposomes were successfully targeted to the kidney by using Fab' fragments of the monoclonal OX7 antibody directed against Thy-1.1 antigen in rats [178]. Since fibroblast activation protein (FAP) represents a cell surface antigen expressed by the tumor stromal fibroblasts in different cancers, single-chain Fv from the antibody cross-reacting with human and mouse FAP was used to target PEGylated liposomes to tumor stromal cells [179]. Tumor necrotic zones were effectively targeted by doxorubicin-loaded liposomes modified with chimeric TNT-3 mAb specific toward degenerating cells located in necrotic regions of tumors and demonstrated enhanced therapeutic efficacy in nude mice bearing H460 tumors [180]. Combination of immunoliposome and endosome-disruptive peptide improves cytosolic delivery of liposomal drug, increases cytotoxicity, and opens new approaches to constructing targeted liposomal systems as shown with diphtheria toxin A chain incorporated together with pH-dependent fusogenic peptide diINF-7 into liposomes specific toward ovarian carcinoma [181]. Anti-IL-10R (interleukin-10 receptor) antibody was shown to improve the therapeutic activity of targeted liposomal nucleotides, which is important for potential treatment of high-risk neuroblastoma [182]. Prostate cancer-specific 5D4 mAb enhanced cytotoxicity of doxorubicin-loaded liposomes against target cells *in vitro* [183].

Early clinical trials of antibody-targeted drug-loaded liposomes have already demonstrated some promising results. Thus, doxorubicin-loaded PEGylated liposomes modified with F(ab')$_2$ fragments of the GAH mAb specific for stomach cancer were tested in a phase I clinical studies and demonstrated the pharmacokinetics similar to that of Doxil [184].

Some antibodies or their fragments used for targeting liposomal anticancer drugs to tumors are listed in Table 29.2.

29.2.3
Liposomes Modified with Nucleosome-Specific Antibodies

Natural autoantibodies, including antinuclear autoantibodies (ANAs), represent a substantial part of the natural antibody repertoire, which is present throughout the lifespan of higher mammals [195–199] (and reviewed in [200]). It was found that the natural autoantibody repertoire of aged mice is drastically different from that of newborns and healthy adults [199, 201], with antinuclear specificity being more frequent in the aged [199, 202]. Autoantibodies, such as ANAs, have repeatedly been found at significantly higher titers in older humans and laboratory animals without overt disease than in younger controls (reviewed in [203, 204]).

Based on their binding specificity, we have earlier hypothesized that ANAs could participate in antitumor immunosurveillance [205]. Some ANAs with anti-DNA or antihistone specificity recognize the surface of both tumor cells and normal cells [206–208]. An ability to recognize tumor cells but not normal cells was found to be characteristic of monoclonal ANAs of the aged with nucleosome-restricted specificity and cancer cell surface-bound nucleosomes (well-characterized constituents of nuclear material consisting of DNA and four pairs of histones arranged in a characteristic pattern) have been identified as their targets [205, 209]. One can conclude that intact nucleosomes are specifically associated with tumor cells and represent a universal molecular target on their surface, whereas free DNA, individual histones, or cross-reactive determinants are associated with the surface of normal cells as well.

Thus, it was found that nucleosome-restricted mAbs recognize many different tumor cells (including those freshly isolated from *in vivo* tumors) and do not interact with normal tissues, including those enriched with proliferating cells, such as freshly isolated rodent bone marrow, thymocytes, and spermatocytes. In a dexamethasone-sensitive S49 T cell lymphoma, in which the apoptotic death was initiated among some of the cells, nucleosomes released from apoptotic cells were able to attach to the surface of surviving tumor cells, converting them into better

Table 29.2 Some drugs targeted to tumors by antibody-modified liposomes.

Drug	Targeted tumor agent	Antibody (or fragment)	Model	References
Doxorubicin	CD19	anti-CD19	Namala hu-B-cell lymphoma	[130, 132, 145]
Doxorubicin	CD19	anti-CD19	human multiple myeloma, ARH cell line	[146, 147, 185]
Doxorubicin	CD19	anti-CD19, single-chain Fv recombinant human	Raji human B-lymphoma	[146]
Doxorubicin	HER2	anti-HER2-Fab' or single-chain Fv C6.5	HER2-overexpressing human breast cancer	[126]
Paclitaxel	HER2	anti-HER2	HER2-overexpressing human breast cancer	[139]
Doxorubicin	human β_1-integrins	anti-β_1-integrin Fab	human non-small-cell lung carcinoma	[163]
Floxuridine (analog)	CC531	CC52	rat colon carcinoma	[186]
Doxorubicin	GD2	anti-GD$_2$ and anti-GD2-Fab'	human neuroblastoma	[151]
Fenretinide	disialoganglioside, GD2	anti-GD2	human melanoma	[187]
Doxorubicin	38C13 carbohydrate, ganglioside	anti-idiotype mAb, S5A8	murine D-cell lymphoma	[188]
Doxorubicin	ganglioside	anti-ganglioside GM3 (DH2)	B16BL6 mouse melanoma	[189]
Fluorodeoxyuridylate analog	B-fibronectin (ED-B domain)	anti-ED-B single-chain Fv	in vitro Caco-2 cells and in vivo murine F9 teratocarcinoma	[190]

Doxorubicin	tumor necrosis treatment (TNT)	chimeric TNT-3	human non-small-cell lung carcinoma H460	[180]
Doxorubicin	MT1-MMP	anti-MT1-MMP-Fab'	human HT1080 fibrosarcoma	[161, 162]
Doxorubicin	CD74	anti-CD74 LL1	Raji human B-lymphoma	[175]
Doxorubicin	nucleosome	anti-nucleosome 2C5 mAb	human BT-20, MCF-7, PC-3	[191, 192]
Doxorubicin	nucleosome	anti-nucleosome 2C5 mAb	murine LLC, 4T1, C26; human BT-20, MCF-7, PC-3	[193]
Doxorubicin	EGFR	C225 mAb or Fab'	human MDA-MB-468 adenocarcinoma, U87 glioblastoma	[155]
Daunomycin	rat TfR	OX26 mAb	RBE4 brain capillary cells, rat biodistribution	[171]
Doxorubicin	Thy-1.1	anti-Thy-1.1 OX7 mAb	rat mesangial cells, biodistribution	[178]
Doxorubicin	endothelin, human umbilical vein endothelial cells, human dermal microvascular endothelial cells	single-chain Fv A5	endothelial cells	[169]
Doxorubicin	parasite-specific 51-kDa protein	anti-51-kDa Fab'	mouse model of visceral leishmaniasis	[194]

inhibition as well as in the number of lung metastases. The average post-mortem tumor weight in 2C5-Doxil-treated animals was 3 times less than in Doxil-treated animals (0.5 versus 1.5 g), while lung metastases were discovered in 2 times smaller number of animals and their average number was 11 against 24 (in 2C5-Doxil and Doxil-treated animals, respectively). A similar pattern was also observed for liver metastases.

The broad study of 2C5-Doxil in various tumor models in mice produced similar results [228]. This study included primary murine tumors 4T1 and C26, and human PC-3 tumor in nude mice. In all three cases 2C5-Doxil demonstrated enhanced accumulation in tumors and resulted in final tumor weights of only 25–40% compared with control treatments with unmodified Doxil. 2C5-modified immunoliposomes demonstrated also a significantly enhanced accumulation in a subcutaneous model of U87 astrocytoma in mice [218].

To demonstrate the applicability of this approach for targeted delivery of imaging agent into tumors, mAb 2C5-modified PEGylated liposomes have been loaded with heavy metal contrast agents for γ-scintigraphy and magnetic resonance imaging (MRI; ^{111}In and Gd, respectively) via the liposome-membrane-incorporated synthetic polymers containing a large number of chelating side-groups, and allowed for significantly enhanced and accelerated tumor visualization *in vivo* compared to nontargeted contrast-loaded liposomes [229–231]. As a result, 2C5-modified gadolinium-chelating polymer-containing PEGylated liposomes allowed for fast and specific tumor MRI as early as 4 h postinjection. In control animals injected with antibody-free liposomes the corresponding R1 values at all investigated timepoints were significantly smaller.

mAb 2C5 was also used to prepare "smart" pH-responsive liposomes simultaneously carrying a targeting moiety and a cell-penetrating moiety in such a way that the antibody mediates the specific accumulation of the nanocarrier in the tumor, while cell-penetrating function activates only inside the tumor and allows for an enhanced delivery of drug-loaded pharmaceutical nanocarrier inside cancer cells for more effective therapeutic action [33].

29.2.4
Other Targeting Ligands

Several other ligands different from antibodies have also been used to target drug-loaded liposomes to tumors (Table 29.4). Thus, since TfRs are overexpressed on the surface of certain tumor cells, antibodies against TfR as well as Tf itself are among the popular ligands for liposome targeting to tumors and inside tumor cells [232]. Recent studies involve the coupling of Tf to PEG on PEGylated liposomes in order to combine longevity and targetability for drug delivery into solid tumors [233]. A similar approach was applied to deliver into tumors agents for photodynamic therapy including hypericin [234, 235] and for intracellular delivery of cisplatin into gastric cancer [236]. Tf-coupled doxorubicin-loaded liposomes demonstrate increased binding and toxicity against C6 glioma [237].

Table 29.4 Some nonantibody ligands for liposome targeting.

Targeting ligand	Cell surface antigen	Drug	Model	References
Transferrin	TfR	hypericin	HeLa cells	[238]
Transferrin	TfR	photocytotoxic AlPcS4	HeLa cells	[239]
Transferrin	TfR	cisplatin	MKN45P tumor-bearing mice	[240]
Transferrin	TfR	doxorubicin	C6 glioma cells	[241]
Folate	folate receptor	daunorubicin	KB cells, CHO-FR-β, KG-1	[242]
Folate	folate receptor	doxorubicin	KB cells	[243]
Folate	folate receptor	5-fluorouracil	B16F10 tumor-bearing mice	[244]
Folate	folate receptor	doxorubicin	mouse ascites leukemia models	[245]
Folate	folate receptor	$Na_3(B_{20}H_{17}NH_3)$	KB tumor-bearing mice	[246]
Folate	folate receptor	plasmid DNA	L1210A tumor model	[247]
Folate	folate receptor	oligonucleotide	KB tumor-bearing mice	[248]
VIP	VIP receptor	^{99m}Tc-HMPAO	rat breast cancer	[249]
RGD peptide	$\alpha_v\beta_3$ integrin	doxorubicin	C26 colon tumor-bearing mice	[250]
APRPG peptide	angiogenic vessels	nucleoside CNDAC	tumor-bearing mice	[251]
Hyaluronan	hyaluronan receptor	mitomycin C	tumor-bearing mice	[252]
TRX-20 (cationic lipid 3,5-dipentadecycloxy-benzamidine hydrochloride)	chondroitin sulfate	cisplatin	LM8G5 tumor-bearing mice	[253]

Targeting tumors with folate-modified liposomes represents another popular approach, since folate receptor expression is frequently overexpressed in many tumor cells. After early studies demonstrated the possibility of delivery of liposomes [254] into living cells utilizing folate receptor-mediated endocytosis, which could bypass multidrug resistance, the interest in folate-targeted drug delivery by liposomes grew fast (reviewed in [255, 256]). Liposomal daunorubicin [257], doxorubicin [258], and 5-fluorouracil [259] were delivered into various tumor cells both *in vitro* and *in vivo* via folate receptor and demonstrated increased cytotoxicity. The application of folate-modified doxorubicin-loaded liposomes for the treatment of acute myelogenous leukemia was combined with the induction of folate receptor using all-*trans* retinoic acid [260]. Folate-targeted liposomes have been suggested as delivery vehicles for boron neutron capture therapy [238] and used also for targeting tumors with haptens for tumor immunotherapy [239]. Within the frame of gene therapy, folate-targeted liposomes were utilized for both gene targeting to tumor cells [240] as well as for targeting tumors with antisense oligonucleotides [241].

Additionally, liposome targeting to tumors has been achieved by using vitamin and growth factor receptors [261]. Vasoactive intestinal peptide (VIP) was used to target PEG-liposomes with radionuclides to VIP receptors of the tumor, which resulted in an enhanced breast cancer inhibition in rats [262]. PEG-liposomes were also targeted by RGD peptides to integrins of the tumor vasculature and, being loaded with doxorubicin, demonstrated increased efficiency against C26 colon carcinoma in murine model [263]. Similar angiogenic homing peptides were used for targeted delivery to vascular endothelium of drug-loaded liposomes in the experimental treatment of tumors in mice [242]. Mitomycin C in long-circulating hyaluronan-targeted liposomes increases its activity against tumors overexpressing hyaluronan receptors [243]. Cisplatin-loaded liposomes specifically binding chondroitin sulfate overexpressed in many tumor cells were used for successful suppression of tumor growth and metastases *in vivo* [244]. Tumor-selective targeting of PEGylated liposomes was also achieved by grafting these liposomes with basic fibroblast growth factor-binding peptide [245].

29.3
Preparation and Administration of Antibody-Targeted Liposomal Drugs

Preparing various functional liposomes with controlled properties (targeting) requires the conjugation of certain moieties (proteins, peptides, polymers) to the liposome surface. This attachment can proceed noncovalently, via the hydrophobic adsorption of certain intrinsic or specially inserted hydrophobic groups in the ligands to be attached onto or into the surface of the nanocarrier. Thus, hydrophobically modified proteins can incorporate into the phospholipid membrane of liposomes [26] or the hydrophobic core of micelles [246]. More frequently, the attachment is performed chemically, via the interaction of reactive groups generated on the carrier surface and certain groups in the molecule to be attached. In the case of liposomes, the most popular drug delivery system and convenient example of techniques used, the conjugation methodology is based on three main reactions, which are quite efficient and selective: reaction between activated carboxyl groups and amino groups yielding an amide bond; reaction between pyridyldithiols and thiols yielding disulfide bonds; and reaction between maleimide derivatives and thiols yielding thioether bonds [264]. Some other approaches also exist, for example, yielding the carbamate bond via the reaction of the pNP groups introduced onto the surface of nanocarriers with the amino group of various ligands [247]. Detailed reviews of numerous coupling procedures and protocols used for attaching the whole variety of surface modifiers to drug carriers can be found in [116, 117].

Thus, carboxylic groups of immunoglobulins can be activated by water-soluble carbodiimide; activated protein then can be bound to free amino-group-containing surfaces, such as PE-containing liposomes [248]. For further ligand attachment, the corresponding reactive groups on the surface of nanocarriers can be pre-modified with the aid of heterobifunctional cross-linking reagents, such as the popular N-succinimidyl-3(2-pyridyldithio)propionate (SPDP) used to synthesize a PE derivative further used for the coupling to SH-containing proteins [265]. Another possibility is to rely on the reaction of the thiol groups on a ligand (protein) with the maleimide-carrying surfaces (phospholipid molecules, in the case of liposomes). This approach [249] is now one of the most widely used in research and practical applications. Different commercially available maleimide reagents can be used for the preparation of maleimide-carrying phospholipids in a simple single-step procedure. Various high- and low-molecular-weight compounds have been attached to liposomes by using pyridyldithiopropionyl-PE or maleimide reagents [116, 117]. The application of free thiol groups located on immunoglobulin Fab fragments are also used for attachment, since it is believed that these SH groups are positioned far from the antigen-binding sites.

Some ligands including antibodies carry carbohydrate residues, which can be easily oxidized to yield aldehyde groups that can react with surface amino groups with the formation of the Schiff bases [250]. On the other hand, liposomes containing surface-exposed carboxylic groups were used for the attachment of different ligands [251]. Such liposomes can be prepared by various techniques and activated with water-soluble carbodiimide directly prior to ligand addition. The same chemical reactions can be used to attach nonmodified proteins and peptides to various nanocarriers, including preformed liposomes, containing membrane-incorporated reactive lipid derivatives, such as NGPE or glutaryl-cardiolipin [98, 252, 253].

There are several clear aims one wants to achieve with antibody-mediated tumor targeting of drug-loaded liposomes: fast and effective accumulation of such liposomes in the target tumor; high concentration of the drug in the tumor; liposome internalization by target cells. To achieve these goals, the target should be identified, which is present (overexpressed) on the surface of tumor cells [131]; the specific ligand (antibody or its fragment) should be attached to the surface of the drug-loaded liposome in a way, that does not affect its specific binding properties and in sufficient quantity to provide the multipoint binding with the target (50–100 antibody molecules should be coupled to the surface of a 100 nm liposome); and in the case of PEGylated long-circulating liposomes the quantity of the attached antibodies should not be excessive in order not to compromise the liposome longevity too much [191, 266]. As already noted, it is highly desirable that the targeting antibody is internalizable and facilitates the internalization of the liposome and liposome-incorporated anticancer drug [129, 155]. Further, drug release from the liposome inside the tumor or inside the tumor cell should provide the therapeutic concentration of the drug in the target and maintain it within a reasonable period of time (few hours) [130, 145].

One can expect certain changes in the normal pharmacokinetics and biodistribution of plain and long-circulating liposomes after their modification with antibodies. Although some early studies did not reveal big differences in the biodistribution of antibody-free and antibody-modified liposomes [135, 267], in general, antibody attachment can decrease the circulating time of liposomes because of increased uptake of the modified liposomes via Fc receptors of circulating or liver macrophages, or opsonization of the liposome-tagged antibody molecules [103, 104]. Whole antibodies can also trigger complement-mediated cytotoxicity and ADCC [31]. These effects could be minimized by using antibody Fab fragments instead of whole antibodies [105]. Although Fab fragments can also accelerate liposome clearance [268], in general, Fab-liposomes circulate significantly longer than full antibody-modified liposomes [268]. In the case of antibody-modified PEGylated liposomes, even a certain decrease in the circulation time for antibody-modified PEG-liposomes still allows for their sufficiently long circulation, permitting good target accumulation. Clearly, attention should be paid not to overmodify PEG-liposomes with the antibody to the level where their longevity is seriously compromised.

The presence of proteins (antibodies) on liposomes can also result in increased immunogenicity of such preparations. Thus, it was shown that the administration in mice of liposomes (including PEG-liposomes) modified with IgG2a resulted in an increased production of anti-IgG2a antibodies in experimental animals [269]. This observation was later confirmed [270].

The addition of the surface-attached antibody to the liposomal preparation will certainly result in a cost increase of the final product because of the high cost of antibodies and additional preparation steps. At the moment, it is rather difficult to say how serious this problem could become; however, it clearly may be addressed by minimizing the quantity of the attached antibody and by using the technologies allowing for the minimal loss of the antibody during the attachment procedure.

Liposomes as a dosage form allow for a broad variety of administration routes. In addition to the most traditional and frequent parenteral (intravenous) route of administration, some alternative approaches have also been developed or are under development. After liposome freeze-drying was developed [271], aerosolized liposomal preparations become possible for lung delivery. A combined aerosol of liposomal paclitaxel and cyclosporin A gives better results in the treatment of pulmonary metastases of renal cell carcinoma in mice than each drug given alone [272]. Aerosols of liposomal 9-nitrocamptothecin were nontoxic, and efficiently treated melanoma and osteosarcoma lung metastases in mice [273]. Aerosolized liposomal paclitaxel effectively treated pulmonary metastases in murine renal carcinoma model [274]. Liposomes for drug delivery to the lungs by nebulization have also been described [275].

Since subcutaneous administration of liposomes results in their uptake by draining lymphatic capillaries at the injection site and active capture of liposomes by macrophages in regional lymph nodes, plain and ligand-targeted liposomes were suggested as a good means to target lymphatics for therapeutic and diagnostic applications after subcutaneous administration [276]. Liposomes have been used for lymphatic delivery of methotrexate [277] and for MRI with gadolinium-loaded liposomes [278].

An interesting example of a new approach is a combination of radiofrequency tumor ablation (tumor cell killing by applying high-frequency irradiation resulting in a local increase in the temperature) with intravenous liposomal doxorubicin, which resulted in better tumor accumulation of liposomes and increased necrosis in tumors [279, 280].

29.4
Conclusions

A significant number of mAbs have now been identified and obtained also as chimeric or humanized antibodies, or as Fab' or single-chain Fv fragments, and several simple and effective methods to couple these ligands fragments to the surface of plain or PEGylated drug-loaded liposomes have been developed. In many cases, antibody-targeted liposomes demonstrate better internalization by cancer cells and more effective intracellular drug delivery than other preparations, which could assist in overcoming multidrug resistance. Convincing data have been accumulated demonstrating significant benefits of antibody-targeted liposomal drugs in numerous animal models (accelerated target accumulation, increased quantity of the drug delivered to the target, decreased side-effects, and enhanced therapeutic efficacy). Early clinical trials with antibody-targeted liposomal drugs have already been initiated, yielding promising results. At the same time, modification of drug-loaded long-circulating liposomes with proteins (antibodies) could change their biodistribution compared to nonmodified liposomes and increase their uptake by the monocytes. In addition, liposome-attached proteins can elicit undesirable immune responses. These problems, however, could be relatively easily addressed by minimizing the quantity of the liposome-attached target protein and by using less-immunogenic antibody fragments instead of whole antibodies.

As a result, antibody-targeted drug-loaded liposomes are generally considered as promising candidates for cancer chemotherapy and we can expect their extensive clinical evaluation in the near future, especially in the treatment of breast cancer and lung cancer, which have been used as targets in many of the initial experimental studies.

References

1. Gregoriadis, G. (1977) Targeting of drugs. *Nature*, **265**, 407–411.
2. Torchilin, V.P. (1995) *Handbook of Targeted Delivery of Imaging Agents*, CRC Press, Boca Raton, FL.
3. Francis, G.E. and Delgado, C. (2000) *Drug Targeting: Strategies, Principles, and Applications*, Humana Press, Totowa, NJ.
4. Muzykantov, V.R. and Torchilin, V. (eds) (2003) *Biomedical Aspects of Drug Targeting*, Kluwer, Boston, MA.
5. Torchilin, V.P. (ed.) (2006) *Nanoparticulates as Pharmaceutical*

Carriers, Imperial College Press, London.
6. Torchilin, V. P. (ed.) (2006) *Nanoparticulates as Pharmaceutical Carriers*. Imperial College Press, London.
7. Torchilin, V.P. (ed.) (2008) *Multifunctional Pharmaceutical Nanocarriers*, Springer.
8. Torchilin, V.P. (2007) Tumor-targeted delivery of sparingly-soluble anti-cancer drugs with polymeric lipid-core micelles in *Nanotechnology for Cancer Therapy* (ed. M. Amiji), CRS Press, Boca Raton, FL, pp. 409–420.
9. Peppas, N.A., Hilt, J.Z., and Thomas, J.B. (eds) (2007) *Nanotechnology in Therapeutics*, Horizon Bioscience, Wymondham.
10. Thassu, D., Deleers, M., and Pathak, M. (eds) (2007) *Nanoparticulate Drug Delivery Systems*, Informa Healthcare, New York, NY.
11. Jabr-Milane, L., van Vlerken, L., Devalapally, H., Shenoy, D., Komareddy, S., Bhavsar, M., and Amiji, M. (2008) Multi-functional nanocarriers for targeted delivery of drugs and genes. *J. Control. Release*, **30**, 121–128.
12. Rytting, E., Nguyen, J., Wang, X., and Kissel, T. (2008) Biodegradable polymeric nanocarriers for pulmonary drug delivery. *Expert Opin. Drug Deliv.*, **5**, 629–639.
13. Sanvicens, N. and Marco, M.P. (2008) Multifunctional nanoparticles – properties and prospects for their use in human medicine. *Trends Biotechnol.*, **26**, 425–433.
14. Chiellini, F., Piras, A.M., Errico, C., and Chiellini, E. (2008) Micro/nanostructured polymeric systems for biomedical and pharmaceutical applications. *Nanomedicine*, **3**, 367–393.
15. Cho, K., Wang, X., Nie, S., Chen, Z.G., and Shin, D.M. (2008) Therapeutic nanoparticles for drug delivery in cancer. *Clin. Cancer Res.*, **14**, 1310–1316.
16. Torchilin, V.P. (2007) Targeted pharmaceutical nanocarriers for cancer therapy and imaging. *AAPS J.*, **9**, E128–E147.
17. Torchilin, V.P. (2006) Multifunctional nanocarriers. *Adv. Drug Deliv. Rev.*, **58**, 1532–1555.
18. Jain, R.K. (1999) Transport of molecules, particles, and cells in solid tumors. *Annu. Rev. Biomed. Eng.*, **1**, 241–263.
19. Hobbs, S.K., Monsky, W.L., Yuan, F., Roberts, W.G., Griffith, L., Torchilin, V.P., and Jain, R.K. (1998) Regulation of transport pathways in tumor vessels: role of tumor type and microenvironment. *Proc. Natl. Acad. Sci. USA*, **95**, 4607–4612.
20. Yuan, F., Dellian, M., Fukumura, D., Leunig, M., Berk, D.A., Torchilin, V.P., and Jain, R.K. (1995) Vascular permeability in a human tumor xenograft: molecular size dependence and cutoff size. *Cancer Res.*, **55**, 3752–3756.
21. Maeda, H., Wu, J., Sawa, T., Matsumura, Y., and Hori, K. (2000) Tumor vascular permeability and the EPR effect in macromolecular therapeutics: a review. *J. Control. Release*, **65**, 271–284.
22. Maeda, H. (2003) in Enhanced permeability and retention (EPR) effect: Basis for drug targeting to tumors. *Biomedical Aspects of Drug Targeting* (eds V. Muzykantov and V.P. Torchilin), Kluwer, Boston, MA, pp. 211–228.
23. Lasic, D.D. and Martin, F.J. (eds) (1995) *Stealth Liposomes*, CRC Press, Boca Raton, FL.
24. Torchilin, V.P. and Trubetskoy, V.S. (1995) Which polymers can make nanoparticulate drug carriers long-circulating? *Adv. Drug Deliv. Rev.*, **16**, 141–155.
25. Lukyanov, A.N., Hartner, W.C., and Torchilin, V.P. (2004) Increased accumulation of PEG–PE micelles in the area of experimental myocardial infarction in rabbits. *J. Control. Release*, **94**, 187–193.
26. Torchilin, V.P. (1998) Polymer-coated long-circulating microparticulate pharmaceuticals. *J. Microencapsul.*, **15**, 1–19.
27. Weinstein, J.N., Blumenthal, R., Sharrow, S.O., and Henkart, P.A. (1978) Antibody-mediated targeting of liposomes. Binding to lymphocytes does not ensure incorporation of vesicle contents into the cells. *Biochim. Biophys. Acta*, **509**, 272–288.

28. Heath, T.D., Fraley, R.T., and Papahdjopoulos, D. (1980) Antibody targeting of liposomes: cell specificity obtained by conjugation of F(ab′)₂ to vesicle surface. *Science*, **210**, 539–541.
29. Torchilin, V.P., Klibanov, A.L., Huang, L., O'Donnell, S., Nossiff, N.D., and Khaw, B.A. (1992) Targeted accumulation of polyethylene glycol-coated immunoliposomes in infarcted rabbit myocardium. *FASEB J.*, **6**, 2716–2719.
30. Torchilin, V.P., Narula, J., Halpern, E., and Khaw, B.A. (1996) Poly(ethylene glycol)-coated anti-cardiac myosin immunoliposomes: factors influencing targeted accumulation in the infarcted myocardium. *Biochim. Biophys. Acta*, **1279**, 75–83.
31. Sapra, P. and Allen, T.M. (2003) Ligand-targeted liposomal anticancer drugs. *Prog. Lipid Res.*, **42**, 439–462.
32. Na, K., Sethuraman, V.T., and Bae, Y.H. (2006) Stimuli-sensitive polymeric micelles as anticancer drug carriers. *Anticancer Agents Med. Chem.*, **6**, 525–535.
33. Sawant, R.M., Hurley, J.P., Salmaso, S., Kale, A., Tolcheva, E., Levchenko, T.S., and Torchilin, V.P. (2006) "SMART" drug delivery systems: double-targeted pH-responsive pharmaceutical nanocarriers. *Bioconjug. Chem.*, **17**, 943–949.
34. Torchilin, V.P. (2005) Fluorescence microscopy to follow the targeting of liposomes and micelles to cells and their intracellular fate. *Adv. Drug Deliv. Rev.*, **57**, 95–109.
35. Torchilin, V.P. (2008) Tat peptide-mediated intracellular delivery of pharmaceutical nanocarriers. *Adv. Drug Deliv. Rev.*, **60**, 548–558.
36. Cohen, S. and Bernstein, H. (eds) (1996) *Microparticulate Systems for the Delivery of Proteins and Vaccines*, Dekker, New York.
37. Trubetskoy, V.S. and Torchilin, V.P. (1995) Use of polyoxyethylene–lipid conjugates as long-circulating carriers for delivery of therapeutic and diagnostic agents. *Adv. Drug Deliv. Rev.*, **16**, 311–320.
38. Torchilin, V.P. (1996) How do polymers prolong circulation times of liposomes. *J. Liposome Res.*, **9**, 99–116.
39. Maeda, H. (2001) The enhanced permeability and retention (EPR) effect in tumor vasculature: the key role of tumor-selective macromolecular drug targeting. *Adv. Enzyme Regul.*, **41**, 189–207.
40. Gabizon, A.A. (1995) Liposome circulation time and tumor targeting: Implications for cancer chemotherapy. *Adv. Drug Deliv. Rev.*, **16**, 285–294.
41. Klibanov, A.L., Maruyama, K., Torchilin, V.P., and Huang, L. (1990) Amphipathic polyethyleneglycols effectively prolong the circulation time of liposomes. *FEBS Lett.*, **268**, 235–237.
42. Maruyama, K., Yuda, T., Okamoto, A., Ishikura, C., Kojima, S., and Iwatsuru, M. (1991) Effect of molecular weight in amphipathic polyethyleneglycol on prolonging the circulation time of large unilamellar liposomes. *Chem. Pharm. Bull.*, **39**, 1620–1622.
43. Senior, J., Delgado, C., Fisher, D., Tilcock, C., and Gregoriadis, G. (1991) Influence of surface hydrophilicity of liposomes on their interaction with plasma protein and clearance from the circulation: studies with poly(ethylene glycol)-coated vesicles. *Biochim. Biophys. Acta*, **1062**, 77–82.
44. Allen, T.M., Hansen, C., Martin, F., Redemann, C., and Yau-Young, A. (1991) Liposomes containing synthetic lipid derivatives of poly(ethylene glycol) show prolonged circulation half-lives in vivo. *Biochim. Biophys. Acta*, **1066**, 29–36.
45. Papahadjopoulos, D., Allen, T.M., Gabizon, A., Mayhew, E., Matthay, K., Huang, S.K., Lee, K.D., Woodle, M.C., Lasic, D.D., Redemann, C. et al. (1991) Sterically stabilized liposomes: improvements in pharmacokinetics and antitumor therapeutic efficacy. *Proc. Natl. Acad. Sci. USA*, **88**, 11460–11464.
46. Woodle, M.C. (1993) Surface-modified liposomes: assessment and characterization for increased stability and prolonged blood circulation. *Chem. Phys. Lipids*, **64**, 249–262.
47. Allen, T.M. (1994) The use of glycolipids and hydrophilic polymers in avoiding rapid uptake of liposomes by

the mononuclear phagocyte system. *Adv. Drug Deliv. Rev.*, **13**, 285–309.

48. Chonn, A., Semple, S.C., and Cullis, P.R. (1991) Separation of large unilamellar liposomes from blood components by a spin column procedure: towards identifying plasma proteins which mediate liposome clearance in vivo. *Biochim. Biophys. Acta*, **1070**, 215–222.

49. Chonn, A., Semple, S.C., and Cullis, P.R. (1992) Association of blood proteins with large unilamellar liposomes *in vivo*. Relation to circulation lifetimes. *J. Biol. Chem.*, **267**, 18759–18765.

50. Lasic, D.D., Martin, F.J., Gabizon, A., Huang, S.K., and Papahadjopoulos, D. (1991) Sterically stabilized liposomes: a hypothesis on the molecular origin of the extended circulation times. *Biochim. Biophys. Acta*, **1070**, 187–192.

51. Gabizon, A. and Papahadjopoulos, D. (1992) The role of surface charge and hydrophilic groups on liposome clearance *in vivo*. *Biochim. Biophys. Acta*, **1103**, 94–100.

52. Needham, D., McIntosh, T.J., and Lasic, D.D. (1992) Repulsive interactions and mechanical stability of polymer-grafted lipid membranes. *Biochim. Biophys. Acta*, **1108**, 40–48.

53. Torchilin, V.P., Omelyanenko, V.G., Papisov, M.I., Bogdanov, A.A., Trubetskoy, V.S., Herron, J.N., and Gentry, C.A. Jr. (1994) Poly(ethylene glycol) on the liposome surface: on the mechanism of polymer-coated liposome longevity. *Biochim. Biophys. Acta*, **1195**, 11–20.

54. Zalipsky, S. (1995) Chemistry of polyethylene glycol conjugates with biologically active molecules. *Adv. Drug Deliv. Rev.*, **16**, 157–182.

55. Veronese, F.M. (2001) Peptide and protein PEGylation: a review of problems and solutions. *Biomaterials*, **22**, 405–417.

56. Torchilin, V.P. (2002) Strategies and means for drug targeting: An overview in *Biomedical Aspects of Drug Targeting* (eds V. Muzykantov and V.P. Torchilin), Kluwer, Boston, MA, pp. 3–26.

57. Symon, Z., Peyser, A., Tzemach, D., Lyass, O., Sucher, E., Shezen, E., and Gabizon, A. (1999) Selective delivery of doxorubicin to patients with breast carcinoma metastases by stealth liposomes. *Cancer*, **86**, 72–78.

58. Perez, A.T., Domenech, G.H., Frankel, C., and Vogel, C.L. (2002) Pegylated liposomal doxorubicin (Doxil) for metastatic breast cancer: the Cancer Research Network, Inc., experience. *Cancer Invest.*, **20** (Suppl. 2), 22–29.

59. O'Shaughnessy, J.A. (2003) Pegylated liposomal doxorubicin in the treatment of breast cancer. *Clin. Breast Cancer*, **4**, 318–328.

60. Schwonzen, M., Kurbacher, C.M., and Mallmann, P. (2000) Liposomal doxorubicin and weekly paclitaxel in the treatment of metastatic breast cancer. *Anti-Cancer Drugs*, **11**, 681–685.

61. Goncalves, A., Braud, A.C., Viret, F., Genre, D., Gravis, G., Tarpin, C., Giovannini, M., Maraninchi, D., and Viens, P. (2003) Phase I study of pegylated liposomal doxorubicin (Caelyx) in combination with carboplatin in patients with advanced solid tumors. *Anticancer Res.*, **23**, 3543–3548.

62. Harrington, K.J., Lewanski, C., Northcote, A.D., Whittaker, J., Peters, A.M., Vile, R.G., and Stewart, J.S. (2001) Phase II study of pegylated liposomal doxorubicin (Caelyx) as induction chemotherapy for patients with squamous cell cancer of the head and neck. *Eur. J. Cancer*, **37**, 2015–2022.

63. Johnston, S.R. and Gore, M.E. (2001) Caelyx: phase II studies in ovarian cancer. *Eur. J. Cancer*, **37** (Suppl. 9), S8–14.

64. Perez-Lopez, M.E., Curiel, T., Gomez, J.G., and Jorge, M. (2007) Role of pegylated liposomal doxorubicin (Caelyx) in the treatment of relapsing ovarian cancer. *Anti-Cancer Drugs*, **18**, 611–617.

65. Schmidinger, M., Wenzel, C., Locker, G.J., Muehlbacher, F., Steininger, R., Gnant, M., Crevenna, R., and Budinsky, A.C. (2001) Pilot study with pegylated liposomal doxorubicin for

advanced or unresectable hepatocellular carcinoma. *Br. J. Cancer*, **85**, 1850–1852.

66. Wollina, U., Dummer, R., Brockmeyer, N.H., Konrad, H., Busch, J.O., Kaatz, M., Knopf, B., Koch, H.J., and Hauschild, A. (2003) Multicenter study of pegylated liposomal doxorubicin in patients with cutaneous T-cell lymphoma. *Cancer*, **98**, 993–1001.

67. Skubitz, K.M. (2003) Phase II trial of pegylated-liposomal doxorubicin (Doxil) in sarcoma. *Cancer Invest.*, **21**, 167–176.

68. Moghimi, S.M. and Szebeni, J. (2003) Stealth liposomes and long circulating nanoparticles: critical issues in pharmacokinetics, opsonization and protein-binding properties. *Prog. Lipid Res.*, **42**, 463–478.

69. Moein Moghimi, S., Hamad, I., Bunger, R., Andresen, T.L., Jorgensen, K., Hunter, A.C., Baranji, L., Rosivall, L., and Szebeni, J. (2006) Activation of the human complement system by cholesterol-rich and PEGylated liposomes – modulation of cholesterol-rich liposome-mediated complement activation by elevated serum LDL and HDL levels. *J. Liposome Res.*, **16**, 167–174.

70. Cooley, T., Henry, D., Tonda, M., Sun, S., O'Connell, M., and Rackoff, W. (2007) A randomized, double-blind study of pegylated liposomal doxorubicin for the treatment of AIDS-related Kaposi's sarcoma. *Oncologist*, **12**, 114–123.

71. Balbi, G., Visconti, S., Monteverde, A., Manganaro, M.A., and Cardone, A. (2007) Liposomal doxorubicin: a phase II trial. *Acta Biomed.*, **78**, 210–213.

72. Adamo, V., Lorusso, V., Rossello, R., Adamo, B., Ferraro, G., Lorusso, D., Condemi, G., Priolo, D., Di Lullo, L., Paglia, A., Pisconti, S., Scambia, G., and Ferrandina, G. (2008) Pegylated liposomal doxorubicin and gemcitabine in the front-line treatment of recurrent/metastatic breast cancer: a multicentre phase II study. *Br. J. Cancer*, **98**, 1916–1921.

73. Ferrandina, G., Ludovisi, M., Lorusso, D., Pignata, S., Breda, E., Savarese, A., Del Medico, P., Scaltriti, L., Katsaros, D., Priolo, D., and Scambia, G. (2008) Phase III trial of gemcitabine compared with pegylated liposomal doxorubicin in progressive or recurrent ovarian cancer. *J. Clin. Oncol.*, **26**, 890–896.

74. Booser, D.J., Esteva, F.J., Rivera, E., Valero, V., Esparza-Guerra, L., Priebe, W., and Hortobagyi, G.N. (2002) Phase II study of liposomal annamycin in the treatment of doxorubicin-resistant breast cancer. *Cancer Chemother. Pharmacol.*, **50**, 6–8.

75. Sarris, A.H., Hagemeister, F., Romaguera, J., Rodriguez, M.A., McLaughlin, P., Tsimberidou, A.M., Medeiros, L.J., Samuels, B., Pate, O., Oholendt, M., Kantarjian, H., Burge, C., and Cabanillas, F. (2000) Liposomal vincristine in relapsed non-Hodgkin's lymphomas: early results of an ongoing phase II trial. *Ann. Oncol.*, **11**, 69–72.

76. Dark, G.G., Calvert, A.H., Grimshaw, R., Poole, C., Swenerton, K., Kaye, S., Coleman, R., Jayson, G., Le, T., Ellard, S., Trudeau, M., Vasey, P., Hamilton, M., Cameron, T., Barrett, E., Walsh, W., McIntosh, L., and Eisenhauer, E.A. (2005) Randomized trial of two intravenous schedules of the topoisomerase I inhibitor liposomal lurtotecan in women with relapsed epithelial ovarian cancer: a trial of the National Cancer Institute of Canada Clinical Trials Group. *J. Clin. Oncol.*, **23**, 1859–1866.

77. Kim, E.S., Lu, C., Khuri, F.R., Tonda, M., Glisson, B.S., Liu, D., Jung, M., Hong, W.K., and Herbst, R.S. (2001) A phase II study of STEALTH cisplatin (SPI-77) in patients with advanced non-small cell lung cancer. *Lung Cancer*, **34**, 427–432.

78. Jehn, C.F., Boulikas, T., Kourvetaris, A., Possinger, K., and Luftner, D. (2007) Pharmacokinetics of liposomal cisplatin (lipoplatin) in combination with 5-FU in patients with advanced head and neck cancer: first results of a phase III study. *Anticancer Res.*, **27**, 471–475.

79. Kelland, L. (2007) Broadening the clinical use of platinum drug-based chemotherapy with new analogues.

Satraplatin and picoplatin. *Expert Opin. Invest. Drugs*, **16**, 1009–1021.

80. Boorjian, S.A., Milowsky, M.I., Kaplan, J., Albert, M., Cobham, M.V., Coll, D.M., Mongan, N.P., Shelton, G., Petrylak, D., Gudas, L.J., and Nanus, D.M. (2007) Phase 1/2 clinical trial of interferon alpha2b and weekly liposome-encapsulated all-*trans* retinoic acid in patients with advanced renal cell carcinoma. *J. Immunother.*, **30**, 655–662.

81. Tsimberidou, A.M., Tirado-Gomez, M., Andreeff, M., O'Brien, S., Kantarjian, H., Keating, M., Lopez-Berestein, G., and Estey, E. (2006) Single-agent liposomal all-*trans* retinoic acid can cure some patients with untreated acute promyelocytic leukemia: an update of The University of Texas M. D. Anderson Cancer Center Series. *Leuk. Lymphoma*, **47**, 1062–1068.

82. Gonzalez, R., Hutchins, L., Nemunaitis, J., Atkins, M., and Schwarzenberger, P.O. (2006) Phase 2 trial of Allovectin-7 in advanced metastatic melanoma. *Melanoma Res.*, **16**, 521–526.

83. Sangha, R. and Butts, C. (2007) L-BLP25: a peptide vaccine strategy in non small cell lung cancer. *Clin. Cancer Res.*, **13**, s4652–s4654.

84. Yoo, G.H., Hung, M.C., Lopez-Berestein, G., LaFollette, S., Ensley, J.F., Carey, M., Batson, E., Reynolds, T.C., and Murray, J.L. (2001) Phase I trial of intratumoral liposome E1A gene therapy in patients with recurrent breast and head and neck cancer. *Clin. Cancer Res.*, **7**, 1237–1245.

85. Blume, G., Cevc, G., Crommelin, M.D., Bakker-Woudenberg, I.A., Kluft, C., and Storm, G. (1993) Specific targeting with poly(ethylene glycol)-modified liposomes: coupling of homing devices to the ends of the polymeric chains combines effective target binding with long circulation times. *Biochim. Biophys. Acta*, **1149**, 180–184.

86. Abra, R.M., Bankert, R.B., Chen, F., Egilmez, N.K., Huang, K., Saville, R., Slater, J.L., Sugano, M., and Yokota, S.J. (2002) The next generation of liposome delivery systems: recent experience with tumor-targeted, sterically-stabilized immunoliposomes and active-loading gradients. *J. Liposome Res.*, **12**, 1–3.

87. Torchilin, V.P., Levchenko, T.S., Lukyanov, A.N., Khaw, B.A., Klibanov, A.L., Rammohan, R., Samokhin, G.P., and Whiteman, K.R. (2001) p-Nitrophenylcarbonyl-PEG–PE-liposomes: fast and simple attachment of specific ligands, including monoclonal antibodies, to distal ends of PEG chains via p-nitrophenylcarbonyl groups. *Biochim. Biophys. Acta*, **1511**, 397–411.

88. Vingerhoeds, M.H., Storm, G., and Crommelin, D.J. (1994) Immunoliposomes *in vivo*. *Immunomethods*, **4**, 259–272.

89. Torchilin, V.P. (1996) Affinity liposomes *in vivo*: factors influencing target accumulation. *J. Mol. Recognit.*, **9**, 335–346.

90. Torchilin, V.P. (2000) Drug targeting. *Eur. J. Pharm. Sci.*, **11** (Suppl. 2), S81–S91.

91. Park, J.W., Benz, C.C., and Martin, F.J. (2004) Future directions of liposome- and immunoliposome-based cancer therapeutics. *Semin. Oncol.*, **31**, 196–205.

92. Kontermann, R.E. (2006) Immunoliposomes for cancer therapy. *Curr. Opin. Mol. Ther.*, **8**, 39–45.

93. Sofou, S. and Sgouros, G. (2008) Antibody-targeted liposomes in cancer therapy and imaging. *Expert Opin. Drug Deliv.*, **5**, 189–204.

94. Torchilin, V.P., Goldmacher, V.S., and Smirnov, V.N. (1978) Comparative studies on covalent and noncovalent immobilization of protein molecules on the surface of liposomes. *Biochem. Biophys. Res. Commun.*, **85**, 983–990.

95. Torchilin, V.P., Khaw, B.A., Smirnov, V.N., and Haber, E. (1979) Preservation of antimyosin antibody activity after covalent coupling to liposomes. *Biochem. Biophys. Res. Commun.*, **89**, 1114–1119.

96. Torchilin, V.P., Omel'yanenko, V.G., Klibanov, A.L., Mikhailov, A.I., Gol'danskii, V.I., and Smirnov, V.N.

(1980) Incorporation of hydrophilic protein modified with hydrophobic agent into liposome membrane. *Biochim. Biophys. Acta*, **602**, 511–521.
97. Weissig, V., Lasch, J., Klibanov, A.L., and Torchilin, V.P. (1986) A new hydrophobic anchor for the attachment of proteins to liposomal membranes. *FEBS Lett.*, **202**, 86–90.
98. Bogdanov, A.A., Klibanov, A.L., and Torchilin, V.P. Jr. (1988) Protein immobilization on the surface of liposomes via carbodiimide activation in the presence of N-hydroxysulfosuccinimide. *FEBS Lett.*, **231**, 381–384.
99. Holmberg, E., Maruyama, K., Litzinger, D.C., Wright, S., Davis, M., Kabalka, G.W., Kennel, S.J., and Huang, L. (1989) Highly efficient immunoliposomes prepared with a method which is compatible with various lipid compositions. *Biochem. Biophys. Res. Commun.*, **165**, 1272–1278.
100. Bogdanov, A.A., Klibanov, A.L., and Torchilin, V.P. (1984) Immobilization of alpha chymotrypsin on sucrose stearate-palmitate containing liposomes. *FEBS Lett.*, **175**, 178–182.
101. Lasch, J., Niedermann, G., Bogdanov, A.A., and Torchilin, V.P. (1987) Thiolation of preformed liposomes with iminothiolane. *FEBS Lett.*, **214**, 13–16.
102. Niedermann, G., Weissig, V., Sternberg, B., and Lasch, J. (1991) Carboxyacyl derivatives of cardiolipin as four-tailed hydrophobic anchors for the covalent coupling of hydrophilic proteins to liposomes. *Biochim. Biophys. Acta*, **1070**, 401–408.
103. Allen, T.M., Brandeis, E., Hansen, C.B., Kao, G.Y., and Zalipsky, S. (1995) A new strategy for attachment of antibodies to sterically stabilized liposomes resulting in efficient targeting to cancer cells. *Biochim. Biophys. Acta*, **1237**, 99–108.
104. Kamps, J.A. and Scherphof, G.L. (1998) Receptor versus non-receptor mediated clearance of liposomes. *Adv. Drug Deliv. Rev.*, **32**, 81–97.
105. Flavell, D.J., Noss, A., Pulford, K.A., Ling, N., and Flavell, S.U. (1997) Systemic therapy with 3BIT, a triple combination cocktail of anti-CD19, -CD22, and -CD38-saporin immunotoxins, is curative of human B-cell lymphoma in severe combined immunodeficient mice. *Cancer Res.*, **57**, 4824–4829.
106. Zalipsky, S., Gittelman, J., Mullah, N., Qazen, M.M., and Harding, J.A. (1998) Biologically active ligand-bearing polymer-grafted liposomes in *Targeting of Drugs 6: Strategies for Stealth Therapeutic Systems* (ed. G. Gregoriadis), Plenum, New York, pp. 131–139.
107. Torchilin, V.P., Rammohan, R., Weissig, V., Khaw, B.A., Klibanov, A., and Samokhin, G.P. (2000) 27th International Symposium on Controlled Release of Bioactive Materials, Paris, pp. 217–218.
108. Torchilin, V.P., Lukyanov, A.N., Gao, Z., and Papahadjopoulos-Sternberg, B. (2003) Immunomicelles: targeted pharmaceutical carriers for poorly soluble drugs. *Proc. Natl. Acad. Sci. USA*, **100**, 6039–6044.
109. Sapra, P., Tyagi, P., and Allen, T.M. (2005) Ligand-targeted liposomes for cancer treatment. *Curr. Drug Deliv.*, **2**, 369–381.
110. Blume, G. and Cevc, G. (1993) Molecular mechanism of the lipid vesicle longevity *in vivo*. *Biochim. Biophys. Acta*, **1146**, 157–168.
111. Maruyama, K., Takizawa, T., Yuda, T., Kennel, S.J., Huang, L., and Iwatsuru, M. (1995) Targetability of novel immunoliposomes modified with amphipathic poly(ethylene glycol)s conjugated at their distal terminals to monoclonal antibodies. *Biochim. Biophys. Acta*, **1234**, 74–80.
112. Zalipsky, S. (1993) Synthesis of an end-group functionalized polyethylene glycol–lipid conjugate for preparation of polymer-grafted liposomes. *Bioconjug. Chem.*, **4**, 296–299.
113. Kirpotin, D., Park, J.W., Hong, K., Zalipsky, S., Li, W.L., Carter, P., Benz, C.C., and Papahadjopoulos, D. (1997) Sterically stabilized anti-HER2 immunoliposomes: design and targeting to human breast cancer cells *in vitro*. *Biochemistry*, **36**, 66–75.

114. Hansen, C.B., Kao, G.Y., Moase, E.H., Zalipsky, S., and Allen, T.M. (1995) Attachment of antibodies to sterically stabilized liposomes: evaluation, comparison and optimization of coupling procedures. *Biochim. Biophys. Acta*, **1239**, 133–144.
115. Bendas, G., Krause, A., Bakowsky, U., Vogel, J., and Rothe, U. (1999) Targetability of novel immunoliposomes prepared by a new antibody conjugation technique. *Int. J. Pharm.*, **181**, 79–93.
116. Torchilin, V.P., Weissig, V., Martin, F.J., Heath, T.D., and New, R.R.C. (2003) Surface modification of liposomes in *Liposomes: A Practical Approach* (eds V.P. Torchilin and V. Weissig), Oxford University Press, Oxford, pp. 193–229.
117. Klibanov, A.L., Torchilin, V.P., and Zalipsky, S. (2003) Long-circulating sterically protected liposomes in *Liposomes: A Practical Approach* (eds V.P. Torchilin and V. Weissig), Oxford University Press, Oxford, pp. 231–265.
118. Ishida, T., Iden, D.L., and Allen, T.M. (1999) A combinatorial approach to producing sterically stabilized (Stealth) immunoliposomal drugs. *FEBS Lett.*, **460**, 129–133.
119. Torchilin, V.P. (1985) Liposomes as targetable drug carriers. *Crit. Rev. Ther. Drug Carrier Syst.*, **2**, 65–115.
120. Bar, J., Herbst, R.S., and Onn, A. (2009) Targeted drug delivery strategies to treat lung metastasis. *Expert Opin. Drug Deliv.*, **6**, 1003–1016.
121. Di Paolo, D., Loi, M., Pastorino, F., Brignole, C., Marimpietri, D., Becherini, P., Caffa, I., Zorzoli, A., Longhi, R., Gagliani, C., Tacchetti, C., Corti, A., Allen, T.M., Ponzoni, M., and Pagnan, G. (2009) Liposome-mediated therapy of neuroblastoma. *Methods Enzymol.*, **465**, 225–249.
122. Hu, Y., Li, K., Wang, L., Yin, S., Zhang, Z., and Zhang, Y. (2010) Pegylated immuno-lipopolyplexes: a novel non-viral gene delivery system for liver cancer therapy. *J. Control. Release*, **144**, 75–81.
123. Cheng, W.W. and Allen, T.M. (2010) The use of single chain Fv as targeting agents for immunoliposomes: an update on immunoliposomal drugs for cancer treatment. *Expert Opin. Drug Deliv.*, **7**, 461–478.
124. Fanciullino, R. and Ciccolini, J. (2009) Liposome-encapsulated anticancer drugs: still waiting for the magic bullet? *Curr. Med. Chem.*, **16**, 4361–4371.
125. Park, J.W., Hong, K., Kirpotin, D.B., Meyer, O., Papahadjopoulos, D., and Benz, C.C. (1997) Anti-HER2 immunoliposomes for targeted therapy of human tumors. *Cancer Lett.*, **118**, 153–160.
126. Park, J.W., Hong, K., Kirpotin, D.B., Colbern, G., Shalaby, R., Baselga, J., Shao, Y., Nielsen, U.B., Marks, J.D., Moore, D., Papahadjopoulos, D., and Benz, C.C. (2002) Anti-HER2 immunoliposomes: enhanced efficacy attributable to targeted delivery. *Clin. Cancer Res.*, **8**, 1172–1181.
127. Moreira, J.N., Gaspar, R., and Allen, T.M. (2001) Targeting Stealth liposomes in a murine model of human small cell lung cancer. *Biochim. Biophys. Acta*, **1515**, 167–176.
128. Park, J.W., Kirpotin, D.B., Hong, K., Shalaby, R., Shao, Y., Nielsen, U.B., Marks, J.D., Papahadjopoulos, D., and Benz, C.C. (2001) Tumor targeting using anti-HER2 immunoliposomes. *J. Control. Release*, **74**, 95–113.
129. Kirpotin, D.B., Drummond, D.C., Shao, Y., Shalaby, M.R., Hong, K., Nielsen, U.B., Marks, J.D., Benz, C.C., and Park, J.W. (2006) Antibody targeting of long-circulating lipidic nanoparticles does not increase tumor localization but does increase internalization in animal models. *Cancer Res.*, **66**, 6732–6740.
130. Sapra, P. and Allen, T.M. (2004) Improved outcome when B-cell lymphoma is treated with combinations of immunoliposomal anticancer drugs targeted to both the CD19 and CD20 epitopes. *Clin. Cancer Res.*, **10**, 2530–2537.
131. Hosokawa, S., Tagawa, T., Niki, H., Hirakawa, Y., Nohga, K., and

Nagaike, K. (2003) Efficacy of immunoliposomes on cancer models in a cell-surface-antigen-density-dependent manner. *Br. J. Cancer*, **89**, 1545–1551.

132. Lopes de Menezes, D.E., Pilarski, L.M., and Allen, T.M. (1998) In vitro and in vivo targeting of immunoliposomal doxorubicin to human B-cell lymphoma. *Cancer Res.*, **58**, 3320–3330.

133. Maruyama, K., Kennel, S.J., and Huang, L. (1990) Lipid composition is important for highly efficient target binding and retention of immunoliposomes. *Proc. Natl. Acad. Sci. USA*, **87**, 5744–5748.

134. Maruyama, K., Holmberg, E., Kennel, S.J., Klibanov, A., Torchilin, V.P., and Huang, L. (1990) Characterization of in vivo immunoliposome targeting to pulmonary endothelium. *J. Pharm. Sci.*, **79**, 978–984.

135. Litzinger, D.C. and Huang, L. (1992) Biodistribution and immunotargetability of ganglioside-stabilized dioleoylphosphatidylethanolamine liposomes. *Biochim. Biophys. Acta*, **1104**, 179–187.

136. Mori, A., Kennel, S.J., van Borssum Waalkes, M., Scherphof, G.L., and Huang, L. (1995) Characterization of organ-specific immunoliposomes for delivery of 3′,5′-O-dipalmitoyl-5-fluoro-2′-deoxyuridine in a mouse lung-metastasis model. *Cancer Chemother. Pharmacol.*, **35**, 447–456.

137. Maruyama, K. (2002) PEG–immunoliposome. *Biosci. Rep.*, **22**, 251–266.

138. Park, J.W., Hong, K., Carter, P., Asgari, H., Guo, L.Y., Keller, G.A., Wirth, C., Shalaby, R., Kotts, C., Wood, W.I. et al. (1995) Development of anti-p185HER2 immunoliposomes for cancer therapy. *Proc. Natl. Acad. Sci. USA*, **92**, 1327–1331.

139. Yang, T., Choi, M.K., Cui, F.D., Kim, J.S., Chung, S.J., Shim, C.K., and Kim, D.D. (2007) Preparation and evaluation of paclitaxel-loaded PEGylated immunoliposome. *J. Control. Release*, **120**, 169–177.

140. Laginha, K.M., Moase, E.H., Yu, N., Huang, A., and Allen, T.M. (2008) Bioavailability and therapeutic efficacy of HER2 scFv-targeted liposomal doxorubicin in a murine model of HER2-overexpressing breast cancer. *J. Drug Target.*, **16**, 605–610.

141. Sofou, S., Enmon, R., Palm, S., Kappel, B., Zanzonico, P., McDevitt, M.R., Scheinberg, D.A., and Sgouros, G. (2010) Large anti-HER2/neu liposomes for potential targeted intraperitoneal therapy of micrometastatic cancer. *J. Liposome Res.*, **20**, 330–340.

142. Gao, J., Zhong, W., He, J., Li, H., Zhang, H., Zhou, G., Li, B., Lu, Y., Zou, H., Kou, G., Zhang, D., Wang, H., Guo, Y., and Zhong, Y. (2009) Tumor-targeted PE38KDEL delivery via PEGylated anti-HER2 immunoliposomes. *Int. J. Pharm.*, **374**, 145–152.

143. Noble, C.O., Guo, Z., Hayes, M.E., Marks, J.D., Park, J.W., Benz, C.C., Kirpotin, D.B., and Drummond, D.C. (2009) Characterization of highly stable liposomal and immunoliposomal formulations of vincristine and vinblastine. *Cancer Chemother. Pharmacol.*, **64**, 741–751.

144. Kullberg, M., Owens, J.L., and Mann, K. (2010) Listeriolysin O enhances cytoplasmic delivery by Her-2 targeting liposomes. *J. Drug Target.*, **18**, 313–320.

145. Allen, T.M., Mumbengegwi, D.R., and Charrois, G.J. (2005) Anti-CD19-targeted liposomal doxorubicin improves the therapeutic efficacy in murine B-cell lymphoma and ameliorates the toxicity of liposomes with varying drug release rates. *Clin. Cancer Res.*, **11**, 3567–3573.

146. Cheng, W.W., Das, D., Suresh, M., and Allen, T.M. (2007) Expression and purification of two anti-CD19 single chain Fv fragments for targeting of liposomes to CD19-expressing cells. *Biochim. Biophys. Acta*, **1768**, 21–29.

147. Cheng, W.W. and Allen, T.M. (2008) Targeted delivery of anti-CD19 liposomal doxorubicin in B-cell lymphoma: a comparison of whole monoclonal antibody, Fab′ fragments and single chain Fv. *J. Control. Release*, **126**, 50–58.

148. Rothdiener, M., Muller, D., Castro, P.G., Scholz, A., Schwemmlein,

M., Fey, G., Heidenreich, O., and Kontermann, R.E. (2010) Targeted delivery of SiRNA to CD33-positive tumor cells with liposomal carrier systems. *J. Control. Release*, **144**, 251–258.
149. Loomis, K., Smith, B., Feng, Y., Garg, H., Yavlovich, A., Campbell-Massa, R., Dimitrov, D.S., Blumenthal, R., Xiao, X., and Puri, A. (2010) Specific targeting to B cells by lipid-based nanoparticles conjugated with a novel CD22-ScFv. *Expert Mol. Pathol.*, **88**, 238–249.
150. Brignole, C., Marimpietri, D., Gambini, C., Allen, T.M., Ponzoni, M., and Pastorino, F. (2003) Development of Fab' fragments of anti-GD$_2$ immunoliposomes entrapping doxorubicin for experimental therapy of human neuroblastoma. *Cancer Lett.*, **197**, 199–204.
151. Pastorino, F., Brignole, C., Marimpietri, D., Sapra, P., Moase, E.H., Allen, T.M., and Ponzoni, M. (2003) Doxorubicin-loaded Fab' fragments of anti-disialoganglioside immunoliposomes selectively inhibit the growth and dissemination of human neuroblastoma in nude mice. *Cancer Res.*, **63**, 86–92.
152. Pastorino, F., Brignole, C., Di Paolo, D., Nico, B., Pezzolo, A., Marimpietri, D., Pagnan, G., Piccardi, F., Cilli, M., Longhi, R., Ribatti, D., Corti, A., Allen, T.M., and Ponzoni, M. (2006) Targeting liposomal chemotherapy via both tumor cell-specific and tumor vasculature-specific ligands potentiates therapeutic efficacy. *Cancer Res.*, **66**, 10073–10082.
153. Raffaghello, L., Pagnan, G., Pastorino, F., Cosimo, E., Brignole, C., Marimpietri, D., Bogenmann, E., Ponzoni, M., and Montaldo, P.G. (2003) Immunoliposomal fenretinide: a novel antitumoral drug for human neuroblastoma. *Cancer Lett.*, **197**, 151–155.
154. Mamot, C., Drummond, D.C., Greiser, U., Hong, K., Kirpotin, D.B., Marks, J.D., and Park, J.W. (2003) Epidermal growth factor receptor (EGFR)-targeted immunoliposomes mediate specific and efficient drug delivery to EGFR- and EGFRvIII-overexpressing tumor cells. *Cancer Res.*, **63**, 3154–3161.
155. Mamot, C., Drummond, D.C., Noble, C.O., Kallab, V., Guo, Z., Hong, K., Kirpotin, D.B., and Park, J.W. (2005) Epidermal growth factor receptor-targeted immunoliposomes significantly enhance the efficacy of multiple anticancer drugs *in vivo*. *Cancer Res.*, **65**, 11631–11638.
156. Mamot, C., Ritschard, R., Kung, W., Park, J.W., Herrmann, R., and Rochlitz, C.F. (2006) EGFR-targeted immunoliposomes derived from the monoclonal antibody EMD72000 mediate specific and efficient drug delivery to a variety of colorectal cancer cells. *J. Drug Target.*, **14**, 215–223.
157. Pan, X. and Lee, R.J. (2007) Construction of anti-EGFR immunoliposomes via folate–folate binding protein affinity. *Int. J. Pharm.*, **336**, 276–283.
158. Pan, X., Wu, G., Yang, W., Barth, R.F., Tjarks, W., and Lee, R.J. (2007) Synthesis of cetuximab-immunoliposomes via a cholesterol-based membrane anchor for targeting of EGFR. *Bioconjug. Chem.*, **18**, 101–108.
159. Kim, I.Y., Kang, Y.S., Lee, D.S., Park, H.J., Choi, E.K., Oh, Y.K., Son, H.J., and Kim, J.S. (2009) Antitumor activity of EGFR targeted pH-sensitive immunoliposomes encapsulating gemcitabine in A549 xenograft nude mice. *J. Control. Release*, **140**, 55–60.
160. Beuttler, J., Rothdiener, M., Muller, D., Frejd, F.Y., and Kontermann, R.E. (2009) Targeting of epidermal growth factor receptor (EGFR)-expressing tumor cells with sterically stabilized affibody liposomes (SAL). *Bioconjug. Chem.*, **20**, 1201–1208.
161. Hatakeyama, H., Akita, H., Ishida, E., Hashimoto, K., Kobayashi, H., Aoki, T., Yasuda, J., Obata, K., Kikuchi, H., Ishida, T., Kiwada, H., and Harashima, H. (2007) Tumor targeting of doxorubicin by anti-MT1-MMP antibody-modified PEG liposomes. *Int. J. Pharm.*, **342**, 194–200.
162. Atobe, K., Ishida, T., Ishida, E., Hashimoto, K., Kobayashi, H., Yasuda, J., Aoki, T., Obata, K., Kikuchi, H., Akita, H., Asai, T., Harashima, H.,

Oku, N., and Kiwada, H. (2007) *In vitro* efficacy of a sterically stabilized immunoliposomes targeted to membrane type 1 matrix metalloproteinase (MT1-MMP). *Biol. Pharm. Bull.*, **30**, 972–978.

163. Sugano, M., Egilmez, N.K., Yokota, S.J., Chen, F.A., Harding, J., Huang, S.K., and Bankert, R.B. (2000) Antibody targeting of doxorubicin-loaded liposomes suppresses the growth and metastatic spread of established human lung tumor xenografts in severe combined immunodeficient mice. *Cancer Res.*, **60**, 6942–6949.

164. Trubetskaya, O.V., Trubetskoy, V.S., Domogatsky, S.P., Rudin, A.V., Popov, N.V., Danilov, S.M., Nikolayeva, M.N., Klibanov, A.L., and Torchilin, V.P. (1988) Monoclonal antibody to human endothelial cell surface internalization and liposome delivery in cell culture. *FEBS Lett.*, **228**, 131–134.

165. Asgeirsdottir, S.A., Zwiers, P.J., Morselt, H.W., Moorlag, H.E., Bakker, H.I., Heeringa, P., Kok, J.W., Kallenberg, C.G., Molema, G., and Kamps, J.A. (2008) Inhibition of proinflammatory genes in anti-GBM glomerulonephritis by targeted dexamethasone-loaded AbEsel liposomes. *Am. J. Physiol.*, **294**, F554–F561.

166. Hussain, S., Pluckthun, A., Allen, T.M., and Zangemeister-Wittke, U. (2007) Antitumor activity of an epithelial cell adhesion molecule targeted nanovesicular drug delivery system. *Mol. Cancer. Ther.*, **6**, 3019–3027.

167. Voinea, M., Manduteanu, I., Dragomir, E., Capraru, M., and Simionescu, M. (2005) Immunoliposomes directed toward VCAM-1 interact specifically with activated endothelial cells – a potential tool for specific drug delivery. *Pharm. Res.*, **22**, 1906–1917.

168. Marty, C., and Schwendener, R.A. (2005) Cytotoxic tumor targeting with scFv antibody-modified liposomes. *Methods Mol. Med.*, **109**, 389–402.

169. Volkel, T., Holig, P., Merdan, T., Muller, R., and Kontermann, R.E. (2004) Targeting of immunoliposomes to endothelial cells using a single-chain Fv fragment directed against human endoglin (CD105). *Biochim. Biophys. Acta*, **1663**, 158–166.

170. Beduneau, A., Saulnier, P., Hindre, F., Clavreul, A., Leroux, J.C., and Benoit, J.P. (2007) Design of targeted lipid nanocapsules by conjugation of whole antibodies and antibody Fab′ fragments. *Biomaterials*, **28**, 4978–4990.

171. Schnyder, A., Krahenbuhl, S., Drewe, J., and Huwyler, J. (2005) Targeting of daunomycin using biotinylated immunoliposomes: pharmacokinetics, tissue distribution and *in vitro* pharmacological effects. *J. Drug Target.*, **13**, 325–335.

172. Koning, G.A., Morselt, H.W., Velinova, M.J., Donga, J., Gorter, A., Allen, T.M., Zalipsky, S., Kamps, J.A., and Scherphof, G.L. (1999) Selective transfer of a lipophilic prodrug of 5-fluorodeoxyuridine from immunoliposomes to colon cancer cells. *Biochim. Biophys. Acta*, **1420**, 153–167.

173. Koning, G.A., Kamps, J.A., and Scherphof, G.L. (2002) Efficient intracellular delivery of 5-fluorodeoxyuridine into colon cancer cells by targeted immunoliposomes. *Cancer Detect. Prev.*, **26**, 299–307.

174. Kamps, J.A., Koning, G.A., Velinova, M.J., Morselt, H.W., Wilkens, M., Gorter, A., Donga, J., and Scherphof, G.L. (2000) Uptake of long-circulating immunoliposomes, directed against colon adenocarcinoma cells, by liver metastases of colon cancer. *J. Drug Target.*, **8**, 235–245.

175. Lundberg, B.B., Griffiths, G., and Hansen, H.J. (2007) Cellular association and cytotoxicity of doxorubicin-loaded immunoliposomes targeted via Fab′ fragments of an anti-CD74 antibody. *Drug Deliv.*, **14**, 171–175.

176. Roth, A., Drummond, D.C., Conrad, F., Hayes, M.E., Kirpotin, D.B., Benz, C.C., Marks, J.D., and Liu, B. (2007) Anti-CD166 single chain antibody-mediated intracellular delivery of liposomal drugs to prostate cancer cells. *Mol. Cancer. Ther.*, **6**, 2737–2746.

177. Wang, G.P., Qi, Z.H., and Chen, F.P. (2008) Treatment of acute

myeloid leukemia by directly targeting both leukemia stem cells and oncogenic molecule with specific scFv-immunoliploplexes as a deliverer. *Med. Hypotheses*, **70**, 122–127.

178. Tuffin, G., Waelti, E., Huwyler, J., Hammer, C., and Marti, H.P. (2005) Immunoliposome targeting to mesangial cells: a promising strategy for specific drug delivery to the kidney. *J. Am. Soc. Nephrol.*, **16**, 3295–3305.

179. Baum, P., Muller, D., Ruger, R., and Kontermann, R.E. (2007) Single-chain Fv immunoliposomes for the targeting of fibroblast activation protein-expressing tumor stromal cells. *J. Drug Target.*, **15**, 399–406.

180. Pan, H., Han, L., Chen, W., Yao, M., and Lu, W. (2008) Targeting to tumor necrotic regions with biotinylated antibody and streptavidin modified liposomes. *J. Control. Release*, **125**, 228–235.

181. Mastrobattista, E., Koning, G.A., van Bloois, L., Filipe, A.C., Jiskoot, W., and Storm, G. (2002) Functional characterization of an endosome-disruptive peptide and its application in cytosolic delivery of immunoliposome-entrapped proteins. *J. Biol. Chem.*, **277**, 27135–27143.

182. Brignole, C., Marimpietri, D., Pastorino, F., Di Paolo, D., Pagnan, G., Loi, M., Piccardi, F., Cilli, M., Tradori-Cappai, A., Arrigoni, G., Pistoia, V., and Ponzoni, M. (2009) Anti-IL-10R antibody improves the therapeutic efficacy of targeted liposomal oligonucleotides. *J. Control. Release*, **138**, 122–127.

183. Sawant, R.M., Cohen, M.B., Torchilin, V.P., and Rokhlin, O.W. (2008) Prostate cancer-specific monoclonal antibody 5D4 significantly enhances the cytotoxicity of doxorubicin-loaded liposomes against target cells *in vitro*. *J. Drug Target.*, **16**, 601–604.

184. Matsumura, Y., Hamaguchi, T., Ura, T., Muro, K., Yamada, Y., Shimada, Y., Shirao, K., Okusaka, T., Ueno, H., Ikeda, M., and Watanabe, N. (2004) Phase I clinical trial and pharmacokinetic evaluation of NK911, a micelle-encapsulated doxorubicin. *Br. J. Cancer*, **91**, 1775–1781.

185. Lopes de Menezes, D.E., Pilarski, L.M., Belch, A.R., and Allen, T.M. (2000) Selective targeting of immunoliposomal doxorubicin against human multiple myeloma *in vitro* and *ex vivo*. *Biochim. Biophys. Acta*, **1466**, 205–220.

186. Koning, G.A., Gorter, A., Scherphof, G.L., and Kamps, J.A. (1999) Antiproliferative effect of immunoliposomes containing 5-fluorodeoxyuridine-dipalmitate on colon cancer cells. *Br. J. Cancer*, **80**, 1718–1725.

187. Pagnan, G., Montaldo, P.G., Pastorino, F., Raffaghello, L., Kirchmeier, M., Allen, T.M., and Ponzoni, M. (1999) GD2-mediated melanoma cell targeting and cytotoxicity of liposome-entrapped fenretinide. *Int. J. Cancer*, **81**, 268–274.

188. Tseng, Y.L., Hong, R.L., Tao, M.H., and Chang, F.H. (1999) Sterically stabilized anti-idiotype immunoliposomes improve the therapeutic efficacy of doxorubicin in a murine B-cell lymphoma model. *Int. J. Cancer*, **80**, 723–730.

189. Nam, S.M., Kim, H.S., Ahn, W.S., and Park, Y.S. (1999) Sterically stabilized anti-G_{M3}, anti-Le^x immunoliposomes: targeting to B16BL6, HRT-18 cancer cells. *Oncol. Res.*, **11**, 9–16.

190. Marty, C., Odermatt, B., Schott, H., Neri, D., Ballmer-Hofer, K., Klemenz, R., and Schwendener, R.A. (2002) Cytotoxic targeting of F9 teratocarcinoma tumours with anti-ED-B fibronectin scFv antibody modified liposomes. *Br. J. Cancer*, **87**, 106–112.

191. Lukyanov, A.N., Elbayoumi, T.A., Chakilam, A.R., and Torchilin, V.P. (2004) Tumor-targeted liposomes: doxorubicin-loaded long-circulating liposomes modified with anti-cancer antibody. *J. Control. Release*, **100**, 135–144.

192. Elbayoumi, T.A. and Torchilin, V.P. (2007) Enhanced cytotoxicity of monoclonal anticancer antibody 2C5-modified doxorubicin-loaded PEGylated liposomes against various tumor cell lines. *Eur. J. Pharm. Sci.*, **32**, 159–168.

193. Elbayoumi, T.A. and Torchilin, V.P. (2008) Tumor-specific antibody-mediated targeted delivery of Doxil® reduces the manifestation of auricular erythema side effect in mice. *Int. J. Pharm.*, **357**, 272–279.
194. Mukherjee, S., Das, L., Kole, L., Karmakar, S., Datta, N., and Das, P.K. (2004) Targeting of parasite-specific immunoliposome-encapsulated doxorubicin in the treatment of experimental visceral leishmaniasis. *J. Infect. Dis.*, **189**, 1024–1034.
195. Cote, R.J., Morrissey, D.M., Houghton, A.N., Beattie, E.J., Oettgen, H.F., and Old, L.J. Jr. (1983) Generation of human monoclonal antibodies reactive with cellular antigens. *Proc. Natl. Acad. Sci. USA*, **80**, 2026–2030.
196. Daar, A.S. and Fabre, J.W. (1981) Organ-specific IgM autoantibodies to liver, heart and brain in man: generalized occurrence and possible functional significance in normal individuals, and studies in patients with multiple sclerosis. *Clin. Exp. Immunol.*, **45**, 37–47.
197. Guilbert, B., Dighiero, G., and Avrameas, S. (1982) Naturally occurring antibodies against nine common antigens in human sera. I. Detection, isolation and characterization. *J. Immunol.*, **128**, 2779–2787.
198. Dighiero, G., Lymberi, P., Mazie, J.C., Rouyre, S., Butler-Browne, G.S., Whalen, R.G., and Avrameas, S. (1983) Murine hybridomas secreting natural monoclonal antibodies reacting with self antigens. *J. Immunol.*, **131**, 2267–2272.
199. Iakoubov, L.Z., Zakharova, A.V., Romanova, N.V., Cherepakhin, V.V., and Rokhlin, O.V. (1988) Natural autoantibodies of neonatal rats detectable by the hybridoma technique. *Bull. Exp. Biol. Med.*, **106**, 200–202.
200. Avrameas, S. (1991) Natural autoantibodies: from "horror autotoxicus" to "gnothi seauton". *Immunol. Today*, **12**, 154–159.
201. Sakharova, A.V., Iakubov, L.Z., Grivennikov, I.A., Romanova, N.V., and Lobazina, N. (1986) Ontogenetic changes in the spectrum of specificities of natural monoclonal autoantibodies reacting with nerve tissue antigens. *Zh. Obshch. Biol.*, **47**, 625–630.
202. Xavier, R.M., Yamauchi, Y., Nakamura, M., Tanigawa, Y., Ishikura, H., Tsunematsu, T., and Kobayashi, S. (1995) Antinuclear antibodies in healthy aging people: a prospective study. *Mech. Ageing Dev.*, **78**, 145–154.
203. Walford, R.L. (1974) Immunologic theory of aging: current status. *Fed. Proc.*, **33**, 2020–2027.
204. Globerson, A., Tomer, Y., and Shoenfeld, Y. (1993) Aging, natural autoantibodies, and autoimmunity in *Natural Autoantibodies: Their Physiological Role and Regulatory Significance* (eds Y. Shoenfeld and D.A. Isenberg), CRC Press, London, pp. 59–79.
205. Iakoubov, L.Z. and Torchilin, V.P. (1997) A novel class of antitumor antibodies: nucleosome-restricted antinuclear autoantibodies (ANA) from healthy aged nonautoimmune mice. *Oncol. Res.*, **9**, 439–446.
206. Rekvig, O.P. and Hannestad, K. (1977) Certain polyclonal antinuclear antibodies cross-react with the surface membrane of human lymphocytes and granulocytes. *Scand. J. Immunol.*, **6**, 1041–1054.
207. Mecheri, S., Dannecker, G., Dennig, D., Poncet, P., and Hoffmann, M.K. (1993) Anti-histone autoantibodies react specifically with the B cell surface. *Mol. Immunol.*, **30**, 549–557.
208. Raz, E., Ben-Bassat, H., Davidi, T., Shlomai, Z., and Eilat, D. (1993) Cross-reactions of anti-DNA autoantibodies with cell surface proteins. *Eur. J. Immunol.*, **23**, 383–390.
209. Iakoubov, L.Z. and Torchilin, V.P. (1998) Nucleosome-releasing treatment makes surviving tumor cells better targets for nucleosome-specific anticancer antibodies. *Cancer Detect. Prev.*, **22**, 470–475.
210. Jacob, L. and Viard, J.P. (1992) Anti-DNA antibodies and their relationships with anti-histone and anti-nucleosome specificities. *Eur. J. Med.*, **1**, 425–431.
211. Koutouzov, S., Cabrespines, A., Amoura, Z., Chabre, H., Lotton, C.,

and Bach, J.F. (1996) Binding of nucleosomes to a cell surface receptor: redistribution and endocytosis in the presence of lupus antibodies. *Eur. J. Immunol.*, **26**, 472–486.

212. Seddiki, N., Nato, F., Lafaye, P., Amoura, Z., Piette, J.C., and Mazie, J.C. (2001) Calreticulin, a potential cell surface receptor involved in cell penetration of anti-DNA antibodies. *J. Immunol.*, **166**, 6423–6429.

213. Emlen, W., Holers, V.M., Arend, W.P., and Kotzin, B. (1992) Regulation of nuclear antigen expression on the cell surface of human monocytes. *J. Immunol.*, **148**, 3042–3048.

214. Bell, D.A. and Morrison, B. (1991) The spontaneous apoptotic cell death of normal human lymphocytes *in vitro*: the release of, and immunoproliferative response to, nucleosomes *in vitro*. *Clin. Immunol. Immunopathol.*, **60**, 13–26.

215. Hefeneider, S.H., Cornell, K.A., Brown, L.E., Bakke, A.C., McCoy, S.L., and Bennett, R.M. (1992) Nucleosomes and DNA bind to specific cell-surface molecules on murine cells and induce cytokine production. *Clin. Immunol. Immunopathol.*, **63**, 245–251.

216. Le Lann, A.D., Fournie, G.J., Boissier, L., Toutain, P.L., and Benoist, H. (1994) *In vitro* inhibition of natural-killer-mediated lysis by chromatin fragments. *Cancer Immunol. Immunother.*, **39**, 185–192.

217. Watson, K., Gooderham, N.J., Davies, D.S., and Edwards, R.J. (1999) Nucleosomes bind to cell surface proteoglycans. *J. Biol. Chem.*, **274**, 21707–21713.

218. Gupta, B., Levchenko, T.S., Mongayt, D.A., and Torchilin, V.P. (2005) Monoclonal antibody 2C5-mediated binding of liposomes to brain tumor cells *in vitro* and in subcutaneous tumor model *in vivo*. *J. Drug Target.*, **13**, 337–343.

219. Chakilam, A.R., Pabba, S., Mongayt, D., Iakoubov, L.Z., and Torchilin, V.P. (2004) A single monoclonal antinuclear autoantibody with nucleosome-restricted specificity inhibits growth of diverse human tumors in nude mice. *Cancer Ther.*, **2**, 353–364.

220. Elbayoumi, T.A. and Torchilin, V.P. (2006) Enhanced accumulation of long-circulating liposomes modified with the nucleosome-specific monoclonal antibody 2C5 in various tumours in mice: gamma-imaging studies. *Eur. J. Nucl. Med. Mol. Imaging*, **33**, 1196–1205.

221. Eliaz, R.E. and Szoka, F.C. Jr. (2001) Liposome-encapsulated doxorubicin targeted to CD44: a strategy to kill CD44-overexpressing tumor cells. *Cancer Res.*, **61**, 2592–2601.

222. Sapra, P. and Allen, T.M. (2002) Internalizing antibodies are necessary for improved therapeutic efficacy of antibody-targeted liposomal drugs. *Cancer Res.*, **62**, 7190–7194.

223. Goren, D., Horowitz, A.T., Tzemach, D., Tarshish, M., Zalipsky, S., and Gabizon, A. (2000) Nuclear delivery of doxorubicin via folate-targeted liposomes with bypass of multidrug-resistance efflux pump. *Clin. Cancer Res.*, **6**, 1949–1957.

224. Xiong, X.B., Huang, Y., Lu, W.L., Zhang, X., Zhang, H., Nagai, T., and Zhang, Q. (2005) Intracellular delivery of doxorubicin with RGD-modified sterically stabilized liposomes for an improved antitumor efficacy: in vitro and in vivo. *J. Pharm. Sci.*, **94**, 1782–1793.

225. Xiong, X.B., Huang, Y., Lu, W.L., Zhang, H., Zhang, X., and Zhang, Q. (2005) Enhanced intracellular uptake of sterically stabilized liposomal Doxorubicin *in vitro* resulting in improved antitumor activity *in vivo*. *Pharm. Res.*, **22**, 933–939.

226. Huang, S.K., Stauffer, P.R., Hong, K., Guo, J.W., Phillips, T.L., Huang, A., and Papahadjopoulos, D. (1994) Liposomes and hyperthermia in mice: increased tumor uptake and therapeutic efficacy of doxorubicin in sterically stabilized liposomes. *Cancer Res.*, **54**, 2186–2191.

227. Elbayoumi, T.A. and Torchilin, V.P. (2009) Tumor-specific anti-nucleosome antibody improves therapeutic efficacy of doxorubicin-loaded long-circulating liposomes against primary and

228. ElBayoumi, T.A. and Torchilin, V.P. (2009) Tumor-targeted nanomedicines: enhanced antitumor efficacy in vivo of doxorubicin-loaded, long-circulating liposomes modified with cancer-specific monoclonal antibody. Clin. Cancer Res., 15, 1973–1980.
229. Erdogan, S., Roby, A., and Torchilin, V.P. (2006) Enhanced tumor visualization by gamma-scintigraphy with ^{111}In-labeled polychelating-polymer-containing immunoliposomes. Mol. Pharm., 3, 525–530.
230. Erdogan, S., Roby, A., Sawant, R., Hurley, J., and Torchilin, V.P. (2006) Gadolinium-loaded polychelating polymer-containing cancer cell-specific immunoliposomes. J. Liposome Res., 16, 45–55.
231. Erdogan, S., Medarova, Z.O., Roby, A., Moore, A., and Torchilin, V.P. (2008) Enhanced tumor MR imaging with gadolinium-loaded polychelating polymer-containing tumor-targeted liposomes. J. Magn. Reson. Imaging, 27, 574–580.
232. Hatakeyama, H., Akita, H., Maruyama, K., Suhara, T., and Harashima, H. (2004) Factors governing the in vivo tissue uptake of transferrin-coupled polyethylene glycol liposomes in vivo. Int. J. Pharm., 281, 25–33.
233. Ishida, O., Maruyama, K., Tanahashi, H., Iwatsuru, M., Sasaki, K., Eriguchi, M., and Yanagie, H. (2001) Liposomes bearing polyethyleneglycol-coupled transferrin with intracellular targeting property to the solid tumors in vivo. Pharm. Res., 18, 1042–1048.
234. Derycke, A.S. and De Witte, P.A. (2002) Transferrin-mediated targeting of hypericin embedded in sterically stabilized PEG-liposomes. Int. J. Oncol., 20, 181–187.
235. Gijsens, A., Derycke, A., Missiaen, L., De Vos, D., Huwyler, J., Eberle, A., and de Witte, P. (2002) Targeting of the photocytotoxic compound AlPcS4 to Hela cells by transferrin conjugated PEG-liposomes. Int. J. Cancer, 101, 78–85.
236. Iinuma, H., Maruyama, K., Okinaga, K., Sasaki, K., Sekine, T., Ishida, O., Ogiwara, N., Johkura, K., and Yonemura, Y. (2002) Intracellular targeting therapy of cisplatin-encapsulated transferrin–polyethylene glycol liposome on peritoneal dissemination of gastric cancer. Int. J. Cancer, 99, 130–137.
237. Eavarone, D.A., Yu, X., and Bellamkonda, R.V. (2000) Targeted drug delivery to C6 glioma by transferrin-coupled liposomes. J. Biomed. Mater. Res., 51, 10–14.
238. Stephenson, S.M., Yang, W., Stevens, P.J., Tjarks, W., Barth, R.F., and Lee, R.J. (2003) Folate receptor-targeted liposomes as possible delivery vehicles for boron neutron capture therapy. Anticancer Res., 23, 3341–3345.
239. Lu, Y. and Low, P.S. (2002) Folate targeting of haptens to cancer cell surfaces mediates immunotherapy of syngeneic murine tumors. Cancer Immunol. Immunother., 51, 153–162.
240. Reddy, J.A., Abburi, C., Hofland, H., Howard, S.J., Vlahov, I., Wils, P., and Leamon, C.P. (2002) Folate-targeted, cationic liposome-mediated gene transfer into disseminated peritoneal tumors. Gene Ther., 9, 1542–1550.
241. Leamon, C.P., Cooper, S.R., and Hardee, G.E. (2003) Folate-liposome-mediated antisense oligodeoxynucleotide targeting to cancer cells: evaluation in vitro and in vivo. Bioconjug. Chem., 14, 738–747.
242. Asai, T., Shimizu, K., Kondo, M., Kuromi, K., Watanabe, K., Ogino, K., Taki, T., Shuto, S., Matsuda, A., and Oku, N. (2002) Anti-neovascular therapy by liposomal DPP-CNDAC targeted to angiogenic vessels. FEBS Lett., 520, 167–170.
243. Peer, D. and Margalit, R. (2004) Loading mitomycin C inside long circulating hyaluronan targeted nano-liposomes increases its antitumor activity in three mice tumor models. Int. J. Cancer, 108, 780–789.
244. Lee, C.M., Tanaka, T., Murai, T., Kondo, M., Kimura, J., Su, W., Kitagawa, T., Ito, T., Matsuda, H., and Miyasaka, M. (2002) Novel

chondroitin sulfate-binding cationic liposomes loaded with cisplatin efficiently suppress the local growth and liver metastasis of tumor cells in vivo. *Cancer Res.*, **62**, 4282–4288.
245. Terada, T., Mizobata, M., Kawakami, S., Yamashita, F., and Hashida, M. (2007) Optimization of tumor-selective targeting by basic fibroblast growth factor-binding peptide grafted PEGylated liposomes. *J. Control. Release*, **119**, 262–270.
246. Torchilin, V.P. (2001) Structure and design of polymeric surfactant-based drug delivery systems. *J. Control. Release*, **73**, 137–172.
247. Torchilin, V.P., Levchenko, T.S., Whiteman, K.R., Yaroslavov, A.A., Tsatsakis, A.M., Rizos, A.K., Michailova, E.V., and Shtilman, M.I. (2001) Amphiphilic poly-N-vinylpyrrolidones: synthesis, properties and liposome surface modification. *Biomaterials*, **22**, 3035–3044.
248. Dunnick, J.K., McDougall, I.R., Aragon, S., Goris, M.L., and Kriss, J.P. (1975) Vesicle interactions with polyamino acids and antibody: in vitro and in vivo studies. *J. Nucl. Med.*, **16**, 483–487.
249. Martin, F.J. and Papahadjopoulos, D. (1982) Irreversible coupling of immunoglobulin fragments to preformed vesicles. An improved method for liposome targeting. *J. Biol. Chem.*, **257**, 286–288.
250. Heath, T.D., Robertson, D., Birbeck, M.S., and Davies, A.J. (1980) Covalent attachment of horseradish peroxidase to the outer surface of liposomes. *Biochim. Biophys. Acta*, **599**, 42–62.
251. Kung, V.T. and Redemann, C.T. (1986) Synthesis of carboxyacyl derivatives of phosphatidylethanolamine and use as an efficient method for conjugation of protein to liposomes. *Biochim. Biophys. Acta*, **862**, 435–439.
252. Weissig, V. and Gregoriadis, G. (1992) Coupling of aminogroup bearing ligands to liposomes in *Liposome Technology* (ed. G. Gregoriadis), CRC Press, Boca Raton, FL, pp. 231–248.
253. Weissig, V., Lasch, J., and Gregoriadis, G. (1990) Covalent binding of peptides at liposome surfaces. *Die Pharmazie*, **45**, 849–850.
254. Lee, R.J. and Low, P.S. (1994) Delivery of liposomes into cultured KB cells via folate receptor-mediated endocytosis. *J. Biol. Chem.*, **269**, 3198–3204.
255. Lu, Y. and Low, P.S. (2002) Folate-mediated delivery of macromolecular anticancer therapeutic agents. *Adv. Drug Deliv. Rev.*, **54**, 675–693.
256. Gabizon, A., Shmeeda, H., Horowitz, A.T., and Zalipsky, S. (2004) Tumor cell targeting of liposome-entrapped drugs with phospholipid-anchored folic acid-PEG conjugates. *Adv. Drug Deliv. Rev.*, **56**, 1177–1192.
257. Ni, S., Stephenson, S.M., and Lee, R.J. (2002) Folate receptor targeted delivery of liposomal daunorubicin into tumor cells. *Anticancer Res.*, **22**, 2131–2135.
258. Pan, X.Q., Wang, H., and Lee, R.J. (2003) Antitumor activity of folate receptor-targeted liposomal doxorubicin in a KB oral carcinoma murine xenograft model. *Pharm. Res.*, **20**, 417–422.
259. Gupta, Y., Jain, A., Jain, P., and Jain, S.K. (2007) Design and development of folate appended liposomes for enhanced delivery of 5-FU to tumor cells. *J. Drug Target.*, **15**, 231–240.
260. Pan, X.Q., Zheng, X., Shi, G., Wang, H., Ratnam, M., and Lee, R.J. (2002) Strategy for the treatment of acute myelogenous leukemia based on folate receptor beta-targeted liposomal doxorubicin combined with receptor induction using all-*trans* retinoic acid. *Blood*, **100**, 594–602.
261. Drummond, D.C., Hong, K., Park, J.W., Benz, C.C., and Kirpotin, D.B. (2000) Liposome targeting to tumors using vitamin and growth factor receptors. *Vitam. Horm.*, **60**, 285–332.
262. Dagar, S., Krishnadas, A., Rubinstein, I., Blend, M.J., and Onyuksel, H. (2003) VIP grafted sterically stabilized liposomes for targeted imaging of breast cancer: in vivo studies. *J. Control. Release*, **91**, 123–133.
263. Schiffelers, R.M., Koning, G.A., ten Hagen, T.L., Fens, M.H., Schraa, A.J., Janssen, A.P., Kok, R.J., Molema,

G., and Storm, G. (2003) Anti-tumor efficacy of tumor vasculature-targeted liposomal doxorubicin. *J. Control. Release*, **91**, 115–122.
264. Torchilin, V. and Klibanov, A. (1993) Coupling and labeling of phospholipids in *Phospholipid Handbook* (ed. G. Cevc), Dekker, New York, pp. 293–322.
265. Leserman, L.D., Barbet, J., Kourilsky, F., and Weinstein, J.N. (1980) Targeting to cells of fluorescent liposomes covalently coupled with monoclonal antibody or protein A. *Nature*, **288**, 602–604.
266. Moreira, J.N., Ishida, T., Gaspar, R., and Allen, T.M. (2002) Use of the post-insertion technique to insert peptide ligands into pre-formed stealth liposomes with retention of binding activity and cytotoxicity. *Pharm. Res.*, **19**, 265–269.
267. Emanuel, N., Kedar, E., Bolotin, E.M., Smorodinsky, N.I., and Barenholz, Y. (1996) Targeted delivery of doxorubicin via sterically stabilized immunoliposomes: pharmacokinetics and biodistribution in tumor-bearing mice. *Pharm. Res.*, **13**, 861–868.
268. Maruyama, K., Takahashi, N., Tagawa, T., Nagaike, K., and Iwatsuru, M. (1997) Immunoliposomes bearing polyethyleneglycol-coupled Fab' fragment show prolonged circulation time and high extravasation into targeted solid tumors *in vivo*. *FEBS Lett.*, **413**, 177–180.
269. Phillips, N.C. and Dahman, J. (1995) Immunogenicity of immunoliposomes: reactivity against species-specific IgG and liposomal phospholipids. *Immunol. Lett.*, **45**, 149–152.
270. Harding, J.A., Engbers, C.M., Newman, M.S., Goldstein, N.I., and Zalipsky, S. (1997) Immunogenicity and pharmacokinetic attributes of poly(ethylene glycol)-grafted immunoliposomes. *Biochim. Biophys. Acta*, **1327**, 181–192.
271. van Winden, E.C. (2003) Freeze-drying of liposomes: theory and practice. *Methods Enzymol.*, **367**, 99–110.
272. Koshkina, N.V., Golunski, E., Roberts, L.E., Gilbert, B.E., and Knight, V. (2004) Cyclosporin A aerosol improves the anticancer effect of paclitaxel aerosol in mice. *J. Aerosol Med.*, **17**, 7–14.
273. Gilbert, B.E., Seryshev, A., Knight, V., and Brayton, C. (2002) 9-nitrocamptothecin liposome aerosol: lack of subacute toxicity in dogs. *Inhal. Toxicol.*, **14**, 185–197.
274. Koshkina, N.V., Kleinerman, E.S., Waidrep, C., Jia, S.F., Worth, L.L., Gilbert, B.E., and Knight, V. (2000) 9-Nitrocamptothecin liposome aerosol treatment of melanoma and osteosarcoma lung metastases in mice. *Clin. Cancer Res.*, **6**, 2876–2880.
275. Zaru, M., Mourtas, S., Klepetsanis, P., Fadda, A.M., and Antimisiaris, S.G. (2007) Liposomes for drug delivery to the lungs by nebulization. *Eur. J. Pharm. Biopharm.*, **67**, 655–666.
276. Oussoren, C. and Storm, G. (2001) Liposomes to target the lymphatics by subcutaneous administration. *Adv. Drug Deliv. Rev.*, **50**, 143–156.
277. Kim, C.K. and Han, J.H. (1995) Lymphatic delivery and pharmacokinetics of methotrexate after intramuscular injection of differently charged liposome-entrapped methotrexate to rats. *J. Microencapsul.*, **12**, 437–446.
278. Fujimoto, Y., Okuhata, Y., Tyngi, S., Namba, Y., and Oku, N. (2000) Magnetic resonance lymphography of profundus lymph nodes with liposomal gadolinium-diethylenetriamine pentaacetic acid. *Biol. Pharm. Bull.*, **23**, 97–100.
279. Ahmed, M., Lukyanov, A.N., Torchilin, V., Tournier, H., Schneider, A.N., and Goldberg, S.N. (2005) Combined radiofrequency ablation and adjuvant liposomal chemotherapy: effect of chemotherapeutic agent, nanoparticle size, and circulation time. *J. Vasc. Interv. Radiol.*, **16**, 1365–1371.
280. Ahmed, M., Liu, Z., Lukyanov, A.N., Signoretti, S., Horkan, C., Monsky, W.L., Torchilin, V.P., and Goldberg, S.N. (2005) Combination radiofrequency ablation with intratumoral liposomal doxorubicin: effect on drug accumulation and coagulation in multiple tissues and tumor types in animals. *Radiology*, **235**, 469–477.

30
Responsive Liposomes (for Solid Tumor Therapy)
Stavroula Sofou

30.1
Introduction

Liposomes are closed bilayer membrane structures composed of self-assembled lipids (Figure 30.1). Liposomes are generally nontoxic nanocarriers because their constituent molecules – the amphiphilic lipids – are of natural origin and, therefore, they do not constitute a source of toxicity at any usually administered doses [1]. This is in contrast to some currently explored nanoparticles, composed of a variety of materials, whose toxicity is yet unclear [2–4]. In addition, liposomes have high drug/carrier ratios, which is particularly significant for targeted delivery to cancer cells with low levels of surface molecular targets [5]; finally, therapeutic agents are delivered in their free active form by using physical encapsulation, thus minimizing complications related to cleavage of the therapeutic agent in an active form.

Liposomes have been explored as drug delivery carriers for several years [1, 6]. A difference between the first designed liposome compositions and the structures engineered nowadays is the increasing understanding of the behavior of materials components at the molecular level. This understanding enables the engineering of new rationally designed self-assembled structures with controlled intermolecular interactions resulting, therefore, in desired materials properties and behaviors in the biological milieu.

This chapter deals with lipid membrane constructs that aim to attribute responsive properties to the lipid bilayer, affecting the liposome surface architecture – and its targeting activity – and the liposome membrane permeability and drug bioavailability.

30.2
Rationale: Uniformity in Delivery and Actual Delivery

Solid tumors still account for more than 85% of cancer mortality. For effective killing, therapeutic agents should be delivered uniformly and at lethal doses to

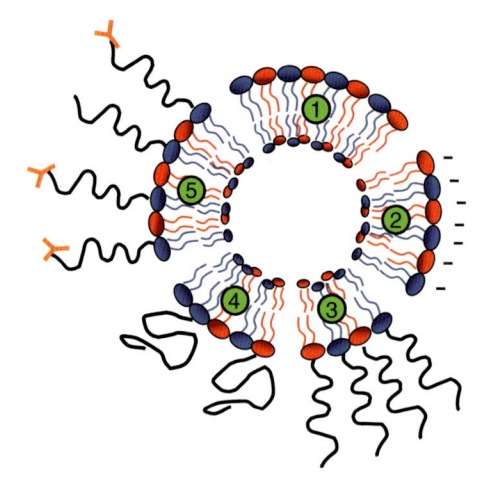

Figure 30.1 (1) Liposomes are closed bilayer membrane structures composed of self-assembled lipids. (2) Exposed electrostatic charge on liposome membranes interferes with their interactions with the biological milieu and affects their circulation times. (3) PEGylated liposomes: relatively high grafting densities of PEGylated lipids (brush regime). (4) PEGylated liposomes: relatively low grafting densities of PEGylated lipids (mushroom regime). (5) "Conventionally" targeted liposomes with the targeting moieties attached on the free ends of PEG chains.

all cancer cells comprising the tumors, while keeping normal organ toxicities to a minimum. This requirement sets two of the major challenges in drug delivery to solid cancers: uniformity in delivery and actual delivery of at least a minimum amount of therapeutics per cancer cell. Drug delivery to advanced solid cancers is a multiscale and multivariable transport problem. To improve the therapeutic outcome, therapeutic agents and their delivery carriers need to exhibit optimal performance in diverse environments ranging from the subtumor scale (transcellular and intracellular trafficking) to macroscale pharmacokinetic transport (whole-body scale). Given the different nature of challenges in transport and trafficking of therapeutic agents – and their carriers – at the various scales, the requirement for diverse responsiveness in drug delivery comes as an inherent prerequisite.

In particular, in delivery to vascularized tumors, a clear distinction may be assumed among the phases following the circulation of carriers in the blood: (i) extravasation, penetration, and accumulation of nanocarriers (liposomes) in the tumor interstitium (Figure 30.2), (ii) (possibly) cancer (or other) cell targeting by the tumor-accumulated lipid nanoparticles, and (iii) either endocytosis of liposomes followed by intracellular release of encapsulated drug or release of delivered therapeutics directly into the tumor interstitial space. Common stimuli that are intrinsic to solid tumors and are being exploited to trigger responsiveness in drug delivery carriers are: (i) the acidification of the tumor interstitium and (ii) the presence of particular enzymes. The interstitial space in solid tumors exhibits a decrease in pH and – toward the tumor core – pH values as low as 6.0 have been

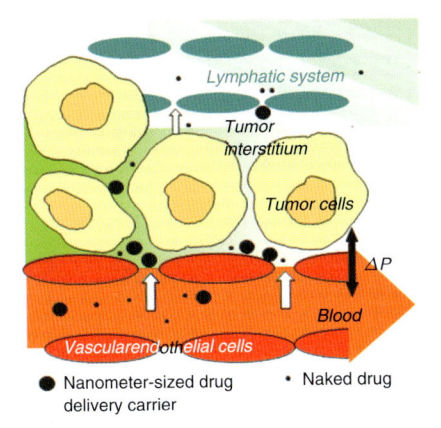

Figure 30.2 Following the circulation of nanometer-sized drug carriers in the blood, extravasation, penetration, and accumulation of nanocarriers (liposomes) in the tumor interstitium may occur. The EPR affect has been observed for nanometer-sized drug delivery carriers by solid tumors, and has been attributed to the combination of the tumor's "leaky" neovasculature, malfunctioning lymphatics, and high interstitial pressures.

reported [7, 8]. Another pH-related trigger is the progressive acidification of the endocytic vesicles (with reported values ranging from 6.5 to 5.0 [9]) that is an excellent stimulus for triggering responsiveness on delivery carriers. In addition, the levels of secretory phospholipase A2 (sPLA2) [10] have been reported to be particularly upregulated in certain solid tumors [11] and, accordingly, exploited to trigger responsiveness to liposomes.

The designs of liposomes, independent of being responsive or not, are engineered to address one or more of the challenges arising in each of the above phases during transport. Extravasation and selective accumulation at the tumors of nanometer-sized particles compared to smaller compounds have been extensively reported and attributed to the combination of the tumor's "leaky" neovasculature [12, 13], malfunctioning lymphatics, and high interstitial pressures. The enhanced permeability and retention (EPR) effect that describes this mechanism has been verified experimentally by several groups (Figure 30.2) [13, 14]. Nanometer-sized liposomes are ideal for selective tumor accumulation that is a passive process and, for tumor accretion to become clinically compelling, blood circulation of these lipid nanoparticles needs to be extensively sustained so as to increase the probability that the carrier will encounter the tumor. Practically, a significant fraction of administered liposomes is still removed relatively early from circulation and accumulated in organs, such as liver, bone marrow, and spleen, potentially increasing toxicity. This translates into the "dose-limiting toxicity" that is still a major challenge and a critical determinant of the potential success of a therapeutic strategy. The significant accumulation of drug carriers in vital organs prohibits administration of higher doses that could reach lethal absorbed levels at the tumor sites. In principle, increasing the circulation time of drug carriers could favorably impact therapeutic efficacy to solid tumors.

Regarding the factors affecting the circulation life of liposomes in the bloodstream, studies suggest that the lipid membrane is attacked via several mechanisms all aiming to eventually remove them from circulation. These mechanisms involve insertion into or adsorption of proteins on the membrane, or recognition of tumor-targeting antibodies on the liposome surface (Figure 30.1) [15, 16]. Experimental evidence shows that rigid (gel-phase) membranes consisting of high-melting temperature lipids [17] or grafted polymers on the surface of liposomes (Figure 30.1) alter the interfacial interactions of the carrier surfaces with proteins and increase blood circulation times [16]. In addition, explicit electrostatic charge on the liposome surface and the presence of surface-conjugated targeting antibodies or other ligands are shown to affect the circulation times of liposomes.

In particular, gel-phase membranes possibly delay the interactions involving protein insertion in the bilayer and, therefore, the extent the circulation times – such adsorbed proteins on the liposome surface have been suggested to be identified by circulating cells of the reticuloendothelial system (RES), resulting in liposomal uptake and removal from circulation [6].

Surface-grafted poly(ethylene glycol) (PEG) chains, due to their high mobility and extent of hydration, are thought to "sterically" stabilize the liposome surface as is demonstrated by the increase of the circulation times of liposomes [18] regardless of the liposome surface charge or the presence of cholesterol in the liposome membrane [15]. The molecular mechanism(s) explaining the effects of PEGylation on extending the circulation times of liposomes is not entirely clear. According to the steric barrier approach, undulation of PEG chains is suggested to interfere with protein adsorption on the liposome surface, altering the liposome interactions with cells (including cells of the RES) or interactions with other liposomes, thus reducing their aggregation *in vivo* [15, 16, 19]. Adsorption of total protein from plasma [20] has been reported not to be affected by the level of PEGylation (PEG grafting density on liposome membranes) that, however, seems to delay the adsorption kinetics and the type (sizes) of particular proteins that adsorb on the liposome surface [21]. Within this framework, it has also been proposed that although adsorption of serum proteins in the presence of PEG may still occur on the liposome surface [21], due to PEG's role as a steric barrier to approaching macrophages, liposome uptake by these cells is delayed, resulting in slower liposome clearance. A recent study supports the suggestion that a major mechanism by which PEGylation extends the circulation life of liposomes is by prohibiting the apposition and aggregation of liposomes while in circulation into larger liposomal structures [20] that are well known to exhibit short circulation times. Commercial formulations (e.g., stealth liposomes) contain grafted PEG at moderate-to-high surface densities (5% mol for PEG2000) that should result in extended brush conformations [22] with lengths that may extend beyond the surface of adsorbed proteins, providing the above-mentioned steric barrier. PEGylation, however, enhances accumulation of liposomes to the skin and, in the case of liposomal formulations containing doxorubicin, it may increase the incidence of palmar–plantar erythrodysesthesia.

For small liposomes (of the order of 100 nm diameter), it is the lipid composition that most probably determines the extent and types of surface-adsorbed plasma proteins. These, in turn, affect specific liposome–cell interactions, therefore determining the types of macrophages (hepatic, splenic, or from the bone marrow) or hepatocytes that will take up liposomes to a greater extent [23]. Even in negatively charged liposomes, incorporation of PEGylated lipids within the bilayer decreases complement activation to various levels determined by the fraction of PEGylation and by the linkage chemistry of PEG chains on lipids [24].

Targeted liposomes are designed with the rationale that, typically, in cancer cells the extracellular leaflet of the plasma membrane overexpresses antigens that are relatively downregulated in healthy cells [25–27]. In other words, cancer cells are not characterized by unique molecular targets. Consequently, during circulation in the blood, "conventional" targeted drug delivery carriers with "exposed" targeting ligands may specifically bind to receptors expressed by noncancerous cells, ultimately increasing toxicities [27]. Toxicities may also increase due to uptake of carriers by reticuloendothelial cells identifying the targeting ligands [5].

To summarize, these considerations on the effects of the extent and type of PEGylation, membrane rigidity, and introduction on the liposomal surface of charge or targeting ligands ultimately provide major guiding directions on the design of responsive liposomes for *in vivo* applications, as will be illustrated by several examples that follow.

30.2.1
Rationale for Responsive Targeting

Cell-targeting reactivity is required for enhanced cancer cell uptake, but only after extravasation of carriers into the solid tumor's interstitium. Extravasated nontargeted nanocarriers would not associate extensively with the cancer cells that constitute the tumor [28], unless they are positively charged [29]. Positively charged nanoparticles, however, would result in increased toxicities *in vivo*, since they will equally interact with normal tissues [30, 31]. In addition, the cancer cell surface does not have unique molecular targets. Consequently, as explained above, circulation of "conventional" targeted drug carriers could still result in binding to healthy cells or cells of the RES, increasing toxicities [27]. Improvement of selectivity in targeting is one of the challenges aimed to be addressed by various responsive targeting strategies as described in Section 30.3.1.1.1.

Lack of specific cell targeting may affect the extent of retention of carriers within the tumor's interstitial space. Targeting may provide strong association of extravasated liposomes with the cancer cells comprising the tumors, potentially resulting in slower clearance of liposomes from tumors compared to nontargeted liposomes. The implications of a targeted versus a nontargeted liposomal approach depend on several parameters. For example, studies *in vivo* on targeted noninternalizing liposomal doxorubicin – mediated by the noninternalizing ErB2 N-12A5 antibody – showed almost no additional efficacy over sterically stabilized liposomal doxorubicin without conjugated antibodies [32]. In these studies, doxorubicin was slowly released by lipid vesicles [32]. A significant detail in this study is the physicochemical nature of the delivered therapeutic agent and the mechanism of its cellular trafficking: in both approaches, doxorubicin that is released from liposomes – residing in the tumor interstitial space – passively diffuses across the plasma membranes and enters cancer cells. The release kinetics of doxorubicin from liposomes relative to the timeframe of liposome retention by the solid tumors, if significantly different, could explain such an observation. In addition, a complication is introduced in this case by doxorubicin's increasing ionization and, therefore, decreasing cell permeability as it penetrates deeper into the increasingly acidic tumor interstitium [33, 34].

Liposomal strategies that include targeting of cells followed by internalization versus targeting without internalization have been examined and compared, and their relative efficacy depends mainly on the type of delivered therapeutic agent. The mechanism of action of "conventional" therapeutic agents such as chemotherapeutics – that need to physically be in close proximity to their molecular target, for an adequate time in order to act – is different from α- or β-particle emitters – for which the critical distance from their molecular target (nuclear DNA) depends on the range in tissue traveled by the high-energy particles [35].

30.2.2
Rationale for Responsive Release

Triggered burst release improves the therapeutic effect. The fundamental rationale for responsive release of therapeutic contents is based on the obvious observation that during, for example, circulation of the delivery carrier in the blood, the encapsulated therapeutic agents should be stably retained and should be released only after the carrier localizes at the target. The main reason for this approach is that the action of most anticancer therapeutics usually does not differentiate between healthy and malignant cells. In addition, fast and extensive release of certain chemotherapeutics from their liposomal carriers has been shown to result in enhanced therapeutic efficacy. This effect was related to the expedited intracellular trafficking of the delivered therapeutic agents; doxorubicin is a characteristic example of a therapeutic agent that has been extensively studied [36, 37]. Efficient and fast (burst) release from the delivery carriers could occur either next to the plasma membrane of cancer cells while the carrier is in the tumor interstitial space (pH > 6.0) [7, 8] or during the endosomal uptake by cancer cells after internalization of targeted liposomes ($5.0 \leq$ pH ≤ 5.5) [9].

30.3
Examples

30.3.1
Preclinical Development

30.3.1.1 Activation by Tumor-Intrinsic Stimuli
The progressively acidic pH toward the core of the interstitial space of tumors and the increased concentration of enzymes such as sPLA2 have been extensively

used as intrinsic stimuli of the tumor space to trigger both targeting of cancer cells and release of therapeutic agents. Below, several different approaches are described.

30.3.1.1.1 Triggered Cell Targeting or Cell Penetration Torchilin's group [38] designed PEGylated liposomes with two functionalities. (i) A conventionally conjugated cancer-specific antibody – attached on the free ends of PEG chains – was utilized with the aim to result in binding to tumor cancer cells after liposome extravasation into the tumor interstitial space. (ii) A "cell internalization" functionality (the fusion 11mer TAT peptide) was also included in the liposome architecture in the following way: under neutral pH, this functionality – the peptide – was shielded by the corona of the protecting grafted polymer or polymer–antibody conjugate on the liposome surface. After extravasation in an acidic environment that could correspond to the tumor interstitial space, degradation of the pH-sensitive hydrazone bond that was used between the PEG chains and the lipid head-group would cause cleavage of the nonfunctionalized PEG chains, resulting in unmasking of the TAT peptide. The latter was conjugated on the liposome surface via a noncleavable anchor shorter than the cleavable PEG chains (see Figure 30.3). *In vitro*, this work demonstrated a significant increase in cell penetration due to unmasking of the TAT peptide after incubation of the functionalized nanoconstructs for 15–30 min in acidic pH conditions [39]. *In vivo* studies following intratumoral injection of TAT-functionalized plasmids encoding Green Fluorescence Protein (pEGFP)-loaded liposomes demonstrated at least 3 times more efficient transfection compared to identical liposomes containing nondegradable PEG chains [40].

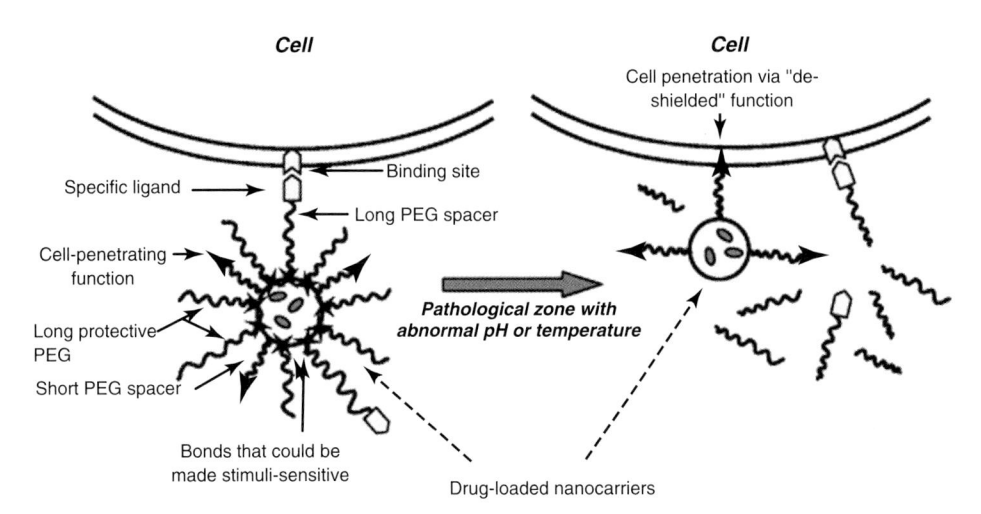

Figure 30.3 Triggerable cell penetration. Local stimuli-dependent removal of protecting PEG chains allows for the direct interaction of the TAT moiety with the cell membrane. (Reproduced from [39].)

In a different approach, to enable selective cell kill, Karve et al. [41] designed functionalized lipid vesicles with pH-triggered heterogeneous membranes and encapsulated doxorubicin that exhibit tunable surface topography. These liposomes were designed to "hide" (mask) the targeting ligands from their surface during circulation in the blood (pH 7.4–7.0) and only to progressively "expose" these ligands as they gradually penetrate deeper into the tumor interstitium (pH 6.7–6.5). Figure 30.4 provides a suggested mechanism by which a change in pH triggers self-assembly, thereby altering the membrane's surface topography and effective reactivity [41, 42]. In particular, these lipid membranes are composed of four types of lipids: (i) a "domain"-forming lipid with titratable anionic head-groups (lipid A, brown), (ii) lipids with grafted polymer chains (PEGylated lipid) and hydrocarbon tails identical to lipid A, (iii) a nonionizable lipid – such as phosphatidylcholine (PC) – with hydrocarbon tails of different length than those in lipid A (lipid B, gray), and (iv) lipids with grafted functional groups (green, representing the targeting ligands) and hydrocarbon tails identical to lipid B (ligand-labeled lipid). At high pH values (Figure 30.4, left), the lipid A head-groups are charged; repulsion between the head-groups makes the lipid energetically less likely to crystallize. The membrane appears spatially homogeneous and the functional groups (targeting antibody fragments) are obstructed by surrounding polymer chains. As the pH value is lowered (Figure 30.4, right), the anionic A head-groups become protonated, reducing electrostatic repulsion while increasing hydrogen bonding between the newly protonated A head-groups. These conditions favor phase separation in which the polymer-conjugated lipids with hydrocarbon tails identical to lipid A partition into the newly protonated lipid domains, driven by the dispersive attractive forces between hydrocarbon tails of the same length. The functionalized lipids, B, that are conjugated to functional groups preferentially partition to areas that are depleted of A; PEG is absent in these areas. The functionalized lipids thus become exposed and available to interact with their targets, increasing the effective reactivity/binding of the membranes [42]. In a proof-of-concept study where binding reactivity was introduced by biotinylated lipid head-groups and avidin "targets" were introduced to SKOV-3 ovarian cancer cells following a two-step targeting – biotinylated anti-HER2/*neu* antibody followed by avidin – these tunable functionalized vesicles when loaded with doxorubicin exhibited environmentally dependent (pH-dependent) association with cancer cells, resulting in high cell kill selectivity. Lowering the extracellular pH from 7.4 to 6.5 resulted in delivery of doxorubicin to cancer cells by the tunable functionalized vesicles that increased from 41 to 93% of maximum. This also caused cancer cell killing that increased from 23 to 71% of maximum [41].

30.3.1.1.2 Triggered Release

pH Activated The design of lipid membranes that are triggered to release their contents at acidic pH values aims to either introduce within the lipid membrane new interfaces at which the molecular packing among lipids is defective, therefore increasing the membrane permeability, or to create pore-like or other structures spanning the membrane (see the informative review by Drummond et al. [43]).

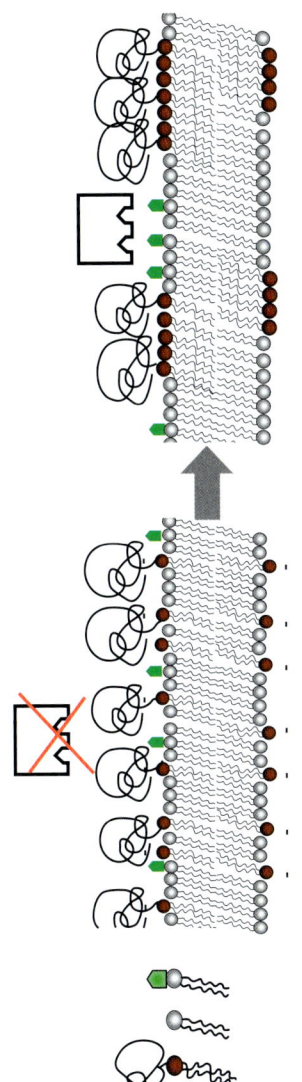

Figure 30.4 Triggerable targeting. The upper lipid leaflet represents the outer lipid leaflet of liposomes; the lower lipid leaflet represents the inner lipid leaflet of liposomes. The targeting ligand is shown in green and its exposure is dependent on the extent of phase separation of the underlying lipid membrane. Squares represent the targeting receptor with the cavities indicating the binding sites for the membrane grafted functional groups which are shown in green. (Reproduced from [41].)

Several different strategies have been reported that follow the first approach. These include pH-triggered interfacial defects formed by: (i) lateral phase separation of lipids forming gel–fluid interfacial boundaries that cross the bilayer, (ii) lateral phase separation of lipid mixtures in which some components preferentially form structures other than lamellar, and (iii) lateral phase separation on membranes composed only of lamellar-forming gel–gel interfacial boundaries.

Interfacial boundaries between lipid domains in heterogeneous membranes may contain areas of defective molecular packing, resulting in increased membrane permeability [44]. Such interfaces have been reported in membranes of single lipids or of lipid mixtures at the transition temperatures where regions of gel domains and fluid domains coexist (Figure 30.5) [45–47]. The potential of these defective interfacial boundaries in controlling drug release in biomedical and drug delivery applications has been suggested and pursued with successful outcomes (e.g., "thermosomes").

One of the first attempts of using nonlamellar lipid structures includes liposomes composed of the inverted hexagonal-phase-forming lipid 1,2-dioleoyl-sn-glycero-3-phosphoethanolamine (DOPE) and cholesteryl hemisuccinate (CHEMS), which acts as the pH-responsive component [49, 50]. At neutral pH, electrostatic repulsion among CHEMS maintains the membrane as a homogeneous bilayer. At acidic pH values, mostly corresponding to average endosomal values (pH 5.5), protonation of CHEMS allows for phase separation of DOPE. This in turn results in areas of high curvature, in lipid mixing (fusion) with apposing membranes, and, ultimately, in content release [49, 50]. PEGylation has been explored to increase the blood circulation time of these fluid membrane liposomes. Although addition of PEGylated lipids results in slower clearance, it also interferes with the pH character of these membranes by compromising their ability to release encapsulated contents at pH 5.5 in model conditions [51]. However, in studies with cells, the pH-dependent content release was reported to become restored – a result

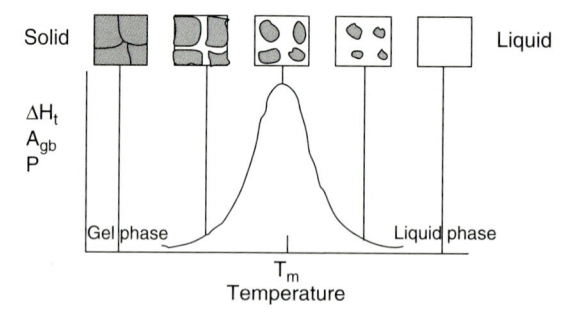

Figure 30.5 Gel–solid transition region for the lipid bilayer. Several physical properties and characteristics like specific heat, membrane permeability, and interphase boundary (between the melted liquid phase and still solid gel phase) are all at a maximum at T_m, and thus define the T_m. However, premelting at grain boundaries on the low temperature shoulder could in principal provide significant membrane permeability to release drugs entrapped in a liposome. (Reproduced from [48].)

that was attributed to a potential PEG–lipid phase separation or to dissociation of PEG chains from the membrane. Alternative approaches aiming to address the issue of steric hindrance to lipid membrane apposition and fusion due to the presence of surface-grafted polymer chains involve liposomes composed of DOPE or DOPE/CHEMS that also include PEGylated lipids that are cleaved at acidic pH values [51–53].

The formation of defective interfaces due to lateral phase separation on membranes composed only of lamellar forming lipid pairs in the gel state was exploited by Karve et al. [54] to cause burst release of encapsulated therapeutic contents. In particular, the same molecular mechanism was used as that described in Section 30.3.1.1 to develop liposomes designed to be triggered during the acidification of the endosomal pathway (pH 5.5–5.0) [55] or during penetration in the increasingly acidic tumor interstitium (pH 6.7–6.5) [41]. At low pH values, elimination of electrostatic repulsion and enhancement of hydrogen bonding among the protonated lipids takes place, resulting in lipid phase separation. At the interfacial boundaries between the different lipid domains (Figure 30.6), the extent of transient packing defects among the acyl tails of lipids is controlled by the relative acyl tail lengths of lipid pairs and the lipid acyl tail dynamics (lipid fluidity). Different acyl tail lengths of lipid pairs combined with slow lipid acyl tail dynamics (gel-phase lipids) enhance the pH-dependent bilayer membrane permeability, which translates into triggered release of encapsulated contents [54]. In addition, lipid vesicles composed of lipids in the gel phase are expected to exhibit relatively long circulation times in the blood, increasing the tumor uptake [56].

Several strategies have been reported that follow the second approach of formation of transmembrane pore-like or other structures with the aim to disrupt the continuity of the lipid bilayer. These include: (i) (poly)peptides and (ii) titratable polymers that change conformation with lowering pH, resulting in destabilization of the lipid membrane [43]. In particular, the polypeptide GALA (WEAALAEALAEALAEHLAEALAEALEALAA) was shown to change conformation from random coil at pH 7.4 to amphipathic α-helix at acidic pH. This change in

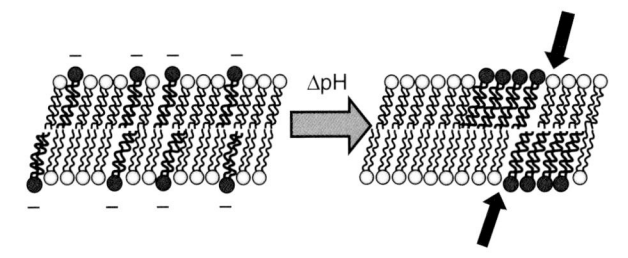

Figure 30.6 Triggered content release. Increased permeability (content release) with decreasing pH is exhibited by lipid bilayer membranes in the form of liposomes composed of lipid pairs in the gel state with nonmatching chain lengths. Permeability rates correlate strongly with the predicted extent of interfacial boundaries of these heterogeneities, suggesting defective packing among nonmatching acyl chains of lipids. (Reproduced from [54].)

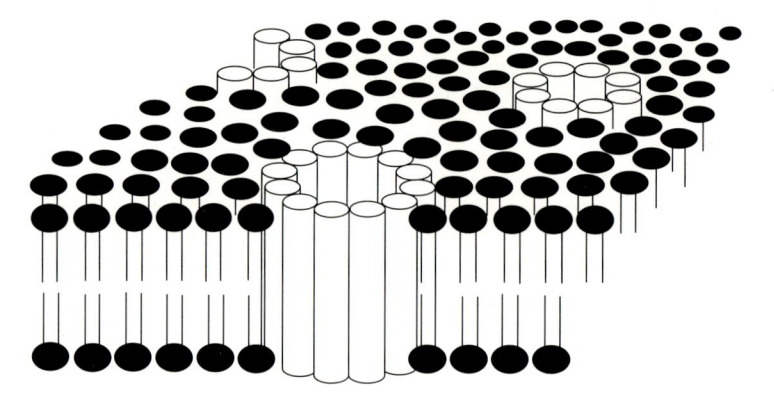

Figure 30.7 Formation of transbilayer pores at low pH by GALA peptide helices, which are depicted as cylinders. (From [57].)

conformation was shown to result in specific organization of helices forming transmembrane pores (Figure 30.7) [57].

Polyelectrolyte polymers, such as poly(2-ethylacrylic acid), have also been reported due to their conformational ability to change from hydrophilic coils at neutral pH to globular hydrophobic structures at decreasing pH [58]. The increased hydrophobicity was suggested to result in enhanced partition into the hydrophobic component of the lipid membrane, causing structural destabilization and increased membrane permeability.

Activated by Innate Enzymes The levels of sPLA2 [10] are reported to be particularly upregulated in certain solid tumors [11] and, therefore, their enzymatic action on phospholipids has been exploited to trigger release of encapsulated therapeutic contents from liposomes. sPLA2 catalyzes the cleavage of 1-acyl-lysolipid fatty acids and of free fatty acids from the *sn*-2 position of phospholipids. The cleaved products are non-lamellar-forming amphiphiles whose lateral aggregation could result locally in high curvature areas, usually affecting the permeability of the membrane [59]. It has also been shown that the enzymatic action – as demonstrated by faster release of encapsulated contents from liposomes – of the positively charged sPLA2 is stimulated in the presence of negatively charged lipids. Several byproducts of sPLA2's enzymatic activity have been suggested to additionally function as enhancers of membrane permeability, further improving the delivery of released therapeutic agents [60].

30.3.1.2 Activation at the Tumor by External Stimuli

The external stimuli that have been reported to activate targeting and content release from liposomes are diverse, and include application of heat, UV light, IR, or ultrasound. A short description of reported mechanisms is given below.

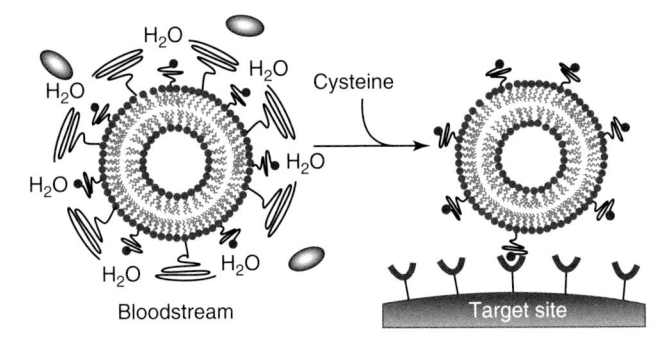

Figure 30.8 Folate receptor-targeted liposomes with long cleavable PEG–phospholipid conjugates that mask folate during circulation of liposomes in the bloodstream to enable passive targeting to tumor. Upon cysteine administration, exposure of folates enables targeting to cells overexpressing the folate receptor (Reproduced from [62].)

30.3.1.2.1 Externally Activated Targeting
Due to precision and reproducibility in cleavage of thiol-reducible cross-linkers [61] simply by addition of cysteine – a cleaving agent that is safe at the required administered doses – the disulfide bond has been explored to mask and unmask targeting/internalization ligands on the surface of liposomes. To address the issues of reduced circulation and, therefore, of decreased passive dosing of targeted liposomes to vascularized tumors, McNeeley *et al.* [62] have developed folate-targeted liposomes containing cysteine-cleavable phospholipid–PEG coronas. The aim is to remove the cleavable polymer coating and to unmask the targeting ligands only upon extravasation of liposomes into the tumor interstitium by exogenous administration of cysteine (Figure 30.8). The authors show feasibility of the design *in vitro* and promising results *in vivo* in a rat glioma model.

Cysteine has also been used by Maeda and Fujumoto [63] to reduce the disulfide linker of PEG chains to lipids and to remove the PEGylated corona, therefore unmasking the surface-conjugated membrane-permeable ligand – an arginine octamer (Figure 30.9). Liposomes were composed of DOPE and CHEMS – a membrane composition with pH-responsive permeability as discussed above – on which the cleavable PEG chains were attached. *In vitro* evaluation of these constructs encapsulating plasmids encoding enhanced GFP (plasmids encoding enhanced Green Fluorescence ProteinpEGFP) on epidermoid carcinoma resulted in promising levels of expression of EGFP observed in almost 100% of the cells.

30.3.1.2.2 Externally Activated Drug Release
Heat Activated As mentioned above, to affect the membrane permeability and, therefore, to trigger content release, the presence of defective interfacial boundaries that cross the membrane is necessary. Except for using pH gradients, another mechanism to alter the interlipid interactions is the change in temperature. Even for single-component membranes the membrane permeability close to the phase

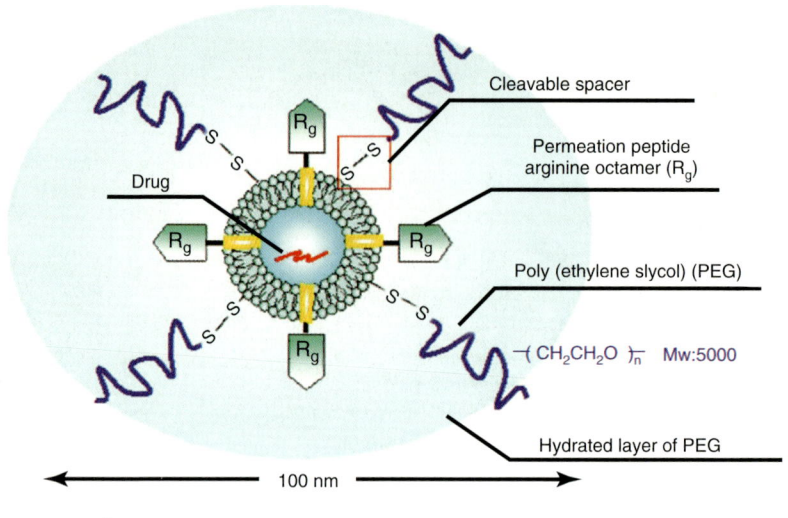

Figure 30.9 Cysteine triggers reduction of disulfide bonds enabling these liposomal carriers with detachable PEG coating to expose membrane-permeable ligands (R_g). (Reproduced from [63].)

transition temperature has been reported to increase. This property is generally attributed to the coexistence of fluid and solid (gel) domains with interfacial boundaries acting as the source of molecular defects enabling permeability to small solutes [64].

Heat-activated liposomes for localized release of therapeutic contents – activated by local hyperthermia – have been pursued since the 1970s. In a first successful study, on lipid membranes composed of a 7 : 3 mass ratio of 1,2-dipalmitoyl-sn-glycero-3-phosphocholine (DPPC) ($T_m = 41\,°C$) and 1,2-distearoyl-sn-glycero-3-phosphocholine (DSPC) ($T_m = 54\,°C$), the onset temperature for rapid release of contents was shown that can be tuned in model conditions to be as low as $40\,°C$ [65]. Murine tumors heated to 42 °C, compared to unheated tumor controls, demonstrated 4 times as much methotrexate delivered by heat-activated liposomes. In addition, the delivered methotrexate appeared to be intracellularly accumulated and bound to its enzyme target.

More recently, Needham et al. [48] used a different approach to further amplify the extent of content release from thermosensitive liposomes. These liposomes are composed of DPPC lipids and the single acyl chain lysolipid monopalmitoylphosphatidylcholine or 1-palmitoyl-2-hydroxy-sn-glycero-3-phosphocholine (MPPC). The rationale for identical acyl tail lengths on both DPPC and MPPC lipids is to promote good lipid mixing within the membrane even at low temperatures at the gel phase. Upon increase of temperature to 39–40 °C, melting of grain boundaries introduces fluid–gel interfaces. Due to their high critical micelle concentration, any MPPC lipids partitioning in the fluid–gel interfaces could also partition

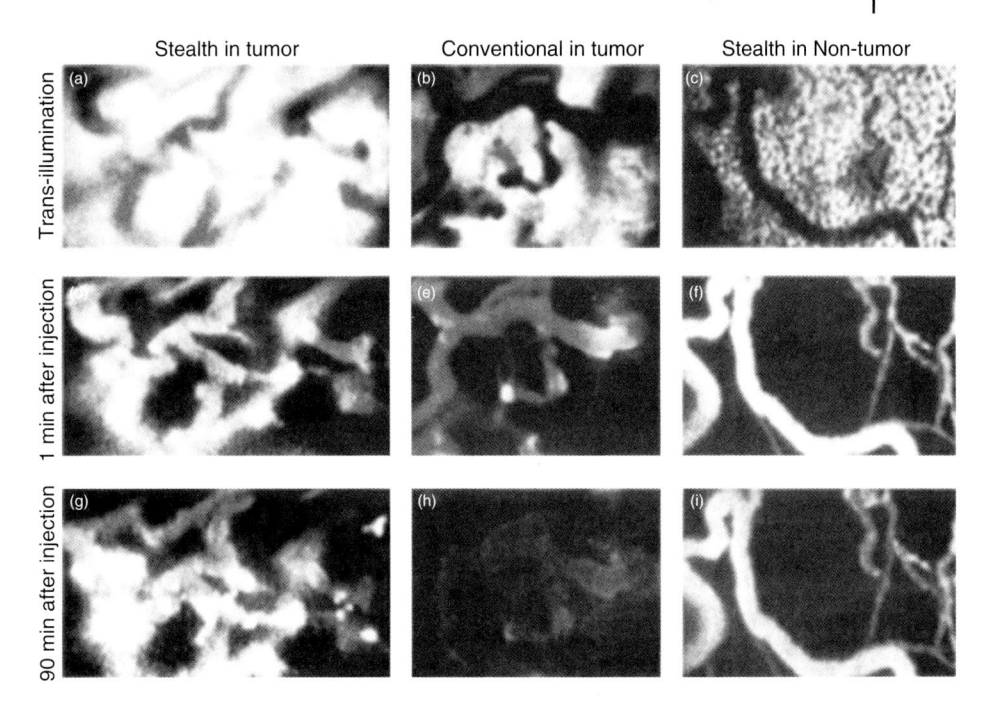

Figure 30.10 Transillumination and epifluorescent video images of fluorescent liposomes in microvascular networks in tumor tissue. (Top row) Transilluminated images of three separate experiments: (left) stealth liposomes in tumor, (middle) conventional liposomes in tumor, and (right) stealth liposomes in a nontumor preparation (healthy tissue). (Middle row) Epifluorescent images of these three experiments at 1 min after liposome injection. (Bottom row) Same preparations 90 min after liposome injection (Reproduced from [48].)

as micelles in the aqueous phase, therefore causing lysolipid depletion of the bilayer membrane and potentially formation of additional packing discontinuities accelerating content release (Figure 30.10). The potential of this approach has been demonstrated *in vivo* in a human squamous cell carcinoma xenograft line using thermosensitive liposomes encapsulating doxorubicin [66]. *In vivo*, the tumor is locally heated and liposomes circulating in the blood are designed to release their contents when reaching the tumor environment. It is an intravascular approach that aims to bypass the extravasation step of liposomes into the tumor interstitium. With this approach, doxorubicin has been shown to become delivered both in tumor cells and the tumor vascular cells.

Release Activated by UV and IR Light In several studies UV light has been used on photosensitive liposomes to induce content release in model conditions. In most studies, the main idea is the incorporation – within the lipid bilayer – of molecules that usually change conformation or structure upon irradiation, thus inducing discontinuities in the molecular packing within the bilayer and altering its permeability.

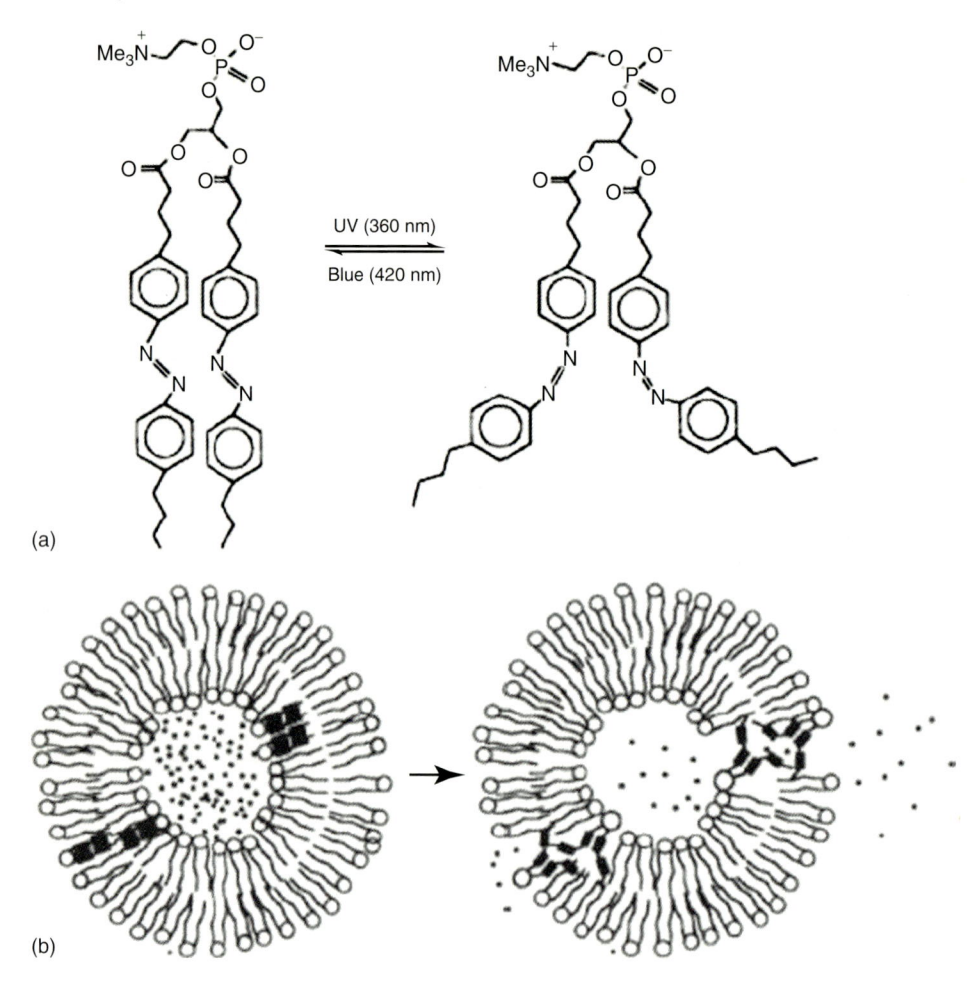

Figure 30.11 (a) Structure of Bis-AzoPC and change in structure on *cis–trans* isomerization. (b) Diagrammatic representation of the disruption of a liposome and leakage of its contents following exposure to UV light and conversion of Bis-AzoPC to the *cis*-enriched photostationary state. (Reproduced from [67].)

In one study, the photoisomerizable phospholipid Bis-AzoPC was designed. Upon UV irradiation, this lipid changes its conformation from a *trans*- to a *cis*-enriched photostationary state. As a result, the more bulky structure of the *cis* isomer causes lipid dislocations and, therefore, release of encapsulated contents (Figure 30.11) [67].

In a different approach, Thompson et al. have designed liposomes containing plasmalogens. Upon irradiation in the presence of sensitizers, cleavage of the plasmalogen vinyl ether linkage results in the formation of single-chain surfactants

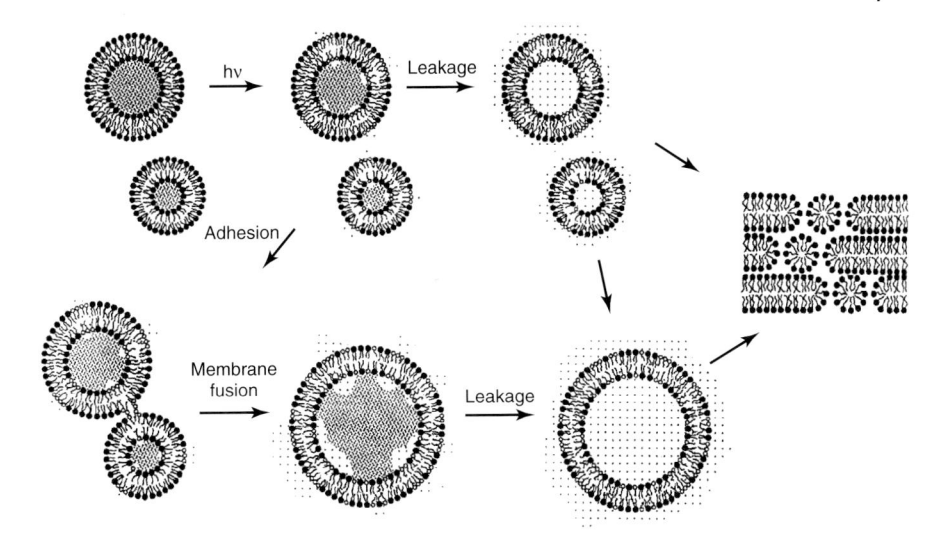

Figure 30.12 Conceptual model for liposome aggregation, interlipidic particle formation, and membrane fusion. Amphiphile notation: solid circles with two alkyl tails = intact plasmalogens; open circles with one alkyl tail = single-chain plasmenylcholine photoproduct. Densely shaded areas = intraliposomal contents at high concentration; lightly shaded areas = released liposomal contents at lower concentration. (From [68].)

that are suggested to form lipid bilayer defects due to aggregation and membrane fusion, causing significant changes in membrane permeability (Figure 30.12) [68]. Lastly, cleavage of charged amino acid head-groups from their stearyl amine hydrophobic tails has been demonstrated by irradiation of the phototriggerable linkage of o-nitrobenzyl derivatives. Photocleavage of the polar head-groups was shown to lead to lipid-packing discontinuities within the membrane that was demonstrated by increased content release [69].

Remote triggering of content release from liposomes has also been explored using near-IR light and an indirect mechanism. In particular, Moehwald *et al.* [70] have designed a liposome–gold nanoparticle composite that absorbs near-IR light. As a result, these nanoparticles locally generate heat that ultimately causes content release from the DPPC-based thermosensitive liposomes discussed above. A key point in the design of this composite is the local concentration of nanoparticles because it affects the extent of generated heat. In particular, when the interparticle distances are comparable to their size, then the generated thermal effects are additive and there is enhancement of absorption at lower energies (red shift).

Release Activated by Ultrasound Ultrasound as a release activation trigger for liposomes has been applied to generate heat (hyperthermia), to induce displacements (radiation force), or to result in activation of gas-filled bubbles (cavitation). Ultrasound is a noninvasive technique, can be focused on local areas of the body, and has the potential of deep tissue penetration.

The use of ultrasound to cause content release from PEGylated liposomes composed of DPPC-based lipid mixtures close to their transition temperature has been examined by applying 20-kHz ultrasound and an incident power of 2 W/cm^2 [71]. In model conditions, initial fast release of encapsulated contents was observed to be followed by first-order kinetics. The mechanism of release was attributed to formation of transiently formed membrane packing defects at fluid–gel interfacial boundaries, rather than pore formation or membrane tearing. In a different study, liposomes composed of hydrogenated soy L-α-phosphatidylcholine (HSPC) and cholesterol exhibit release of up to 80% of encapsulated anticancer agents such as doxorubicin, methylprednisolone hemisuccinate, and cisplatin upon short (less than 3 min) exposure to low-frequency ultrasound radiation (20 kHz) [72]. The observed release was suggested to be caused by formation of transient pore-like defects in the liposome membrane affecting its permeability.

In a different approach, acoustically active liposomes have been developed. These are structures that contain air compartments in addition to the aqueous cavity where the encapsulated therapeutic agents usually reside. In model studies, ultrasound triggered release has been demonstrated on such liposomes, exhibiting release of 33% of encapsulated contents within 10 s of application of 1 MHz at 2 W/cm^2 [73].

Release Activated by a Magnetic Field Studies on the direct interaction of magnetic fields with lipid membranes aiming to alter the membrane permeability are not particularly common. In this respect studies on lipid bilayers in the form of liposomes close to their transition temperature show an increase in membrane permeability upon introduction of liposomes in a uniform static magnetic field. The potential effect has been attributed to the orientation of lipids or lipid domains in the bilayer with the possible formation of interfacial boundaries with lipid-packing defects [74].

Alternating magnetic fields have also been explored to trigger content release from liposomes in indirect ways. In these studies, liposomes are designed to coencapsulate a therapeutic agent and another moiety, usually paramagnetic, through which hyperthermia is induced. In one approach, the interaction of a magnetic field with paramagnetic iron oxide nanoparticles encapsulated in thermosensitive liposomes was shown to result in local generation of heat that, in turn, causes release of encapsulated therapeutic agents from liposomes. The liposome composition used in this study is similar to the first reported thermosensitive liposomal composition of DPPC and DSPC developed by Yatvin *et al.* [75]. In a similar approach, thermosensitive PEGylated liposomes composed mainly of DPPC and coencapsulating magnetic nanoparticles also exhibited triggered content release in the presence of a magnetic field [76].

30.3.2
Clinical Development

Commercial liposome formulations (Table 30.1) for doxorubicin (Doxil/Caelyx), a DNA intercalating chemotherapeutic agent of the anthracycline family, are already

Table 30.1 Examples of currently marketed or pipeline liposomal anticancer formulations.

Commercial name	Composition (mole ratio)	Size (nm)	Anticancer agent
Doxil®	MPEG2000–DSPE/HSPC/cholesterol (1 : 10.7 : 7.2)	90	doxorubicin
DaunoXome®	DSPC/cholesterol (2 : 1)	45	daunorubicin
Thermodox®	saturated PC, lysolipid, cholesterol (proprietary)	100	doxorubicin

MPEG2000-DSPE: N-carbonyl-methoxy poly(ethylene glycol 2000)–1,2-distearoyl-sn-glycero-3-phosphoethanolamine.

approved for ovarian cancer, metastatic breast cancer, and AIDS-related Kaposi's sarcoma. Liposomal daunorubicin (DaunoXome), another anthracycline, has also been approved as first-line chemotherapy for patients with advanced HIV-related Kaposi's sarcoma. None of these lipid membranes are responsive. They have been designed to result in relatively long circulation times and to act as depots of the encapsulated therapeutic agents. Currently, several clinical trials are in progress where still nonresponsive liposomes encapsulating anticancer therapeutics are being evaluated in combination with other agents.

The only responsive liposome formulation currently in trials is Thermodox, the thermally responsive liposomal doxorubicin structure that was developed by Needham et al. [48]. In particular, a phase I clinical trial evaluating Thermodox combined with radiofrequency ablation for primary liver cancer has been completed and a phase III clinical trial is currently recruiting participants. The same approach is being evaluated in a phase I/II trial on patients with recurrent/metastatic adenocarcinoma of the breast with a recurrence on the chest wall.

30.4
Conclusions and Perspectives

Despite progress in the field, limited penetration of the tumor and heterogeneities in drug/drug carrier distribution within tumors still represents a major challenge. Inadequate penetration depth affects the efficacy to deliver therapeutic agents in a homogeneous way to as many cells comprising the solid tumor as possible and poor penetration is associated with low tumor kill efficacy [77]. Functionalization of liposomes to specifically target cancer cells within solid tumors is expected to decrease penetration even further in a similar way as has been shown for antibodies [78, 79] and micelles [80]. The penetration depth of targeted carriers into the tumor could be limited by several factors: the high affinity of targeted liposomes for cancer cells within tumors, the fast recycling of targeted antigens, and the slow liposome intratumoral diffusion combined with fast blood clearance of circulating liposomes. As a result, "consumption" of the targeted liposomes within only the first few cell layers of the solid tumor would be observed. The challenges of limited penetration of targeted liposomes may – to some extent – be addressed by the responsive targeting of liposomes reviewed in Section 30.3.1.1. The progressive exposure of targeting ligands on the surface of these liposomes may result in their deeper penetration into tumors.

Also, in order to address the issues of poor tumor penetration and the heterogeneous delivery to cancer cells in tumors, depending on the types of delivered therapeutic agents, it may be more logical and effective to exploit triggering the release of encapsulated contents, from extravasated liposomes, directly in the tumor interstitial space. Small therapeutic agents are expected to exhibit greater diffusivities within the tumor interstitium compared to nanometer-sized liposomal carriers, potentially resulting in deeper penetration and more homogeneous delivery. Stimuli both innate and external to cancerous tumors are being exploited toward this goal.

Although not reviewed in this chapter, targeting both the tumor (using the above approaches) and the tumor microenvironment – such as its vasculature – could potentially provide efficient treatment strategies. These tumor components may in principle not be treated with the same therapeutic agents or modalities. Ultimately, successful evolution and maturation of any of these approaches may also minimize toxicities to normal organs since lower administered doses may be required with any of these modalities, if successful.

Acknowledgments

Supported by the Susan G. Komen Breast Cancer Foundation (Career Catalyst Award), Coulter Foundation (Young Investigator Award), and NYSTAR (J.D. Watson Award).

References

1. Drummond, D.D., Meyer, O., Hong, K., Kirpotin, D.B., and Papahadjopoulos, D. (1999) Optimizing liposomes for delivery of chemotherapeutic agents to solid tumors. *Pharmacol. Rev.*, **51**, 691–743.
2. Duncan, R. and Izzo, L. (2005) Dendrimer biocompatibility and toxicity. *Adv. Drug Deliv. Rev.*, **57**, 2215–2237.
3. Nel, A., Xia, T., Madler, L., and Li, N. (2006) Toxic potential of materials at the nanolevel. *Science*, **311**, 622–627.
4. Service, R.F. (2005) Nanotechnology takes aim at cancer. *Science*, **310**, 1132–1134.
5. Allen, T.M. (2002) Ligand-targeted therapeutics in anticancer therapy. *Nat. Cancer Rev.*, **2**, 750–763.
6. Lasic, D.D. and Papahadjopoulos, D. (eds) (1997) *Medical Applications of Liposomes*, Elsevier, Amsterdam.
7. Helmlinger, G., Yuan, F., Dellian, M., and Jain, R.K. (1997) Interstitial pH and pO_2 gradients in solid tumors *in vivo*: high-resolution measurements reveal a lack of correlation. *Nat. Med.*, **3**, 177–182.
8. Vaupel, P., Kallinowski, F., and Okunieff, P. (1989) Blood flow, oxygen and nutrient supply, and metabolic

microenvironment of human tumors: a review. *Cancer Res.*, **49**, 6449–6465.

9. Mellman, I. (1992) The importance of being acid: the role of acidification in intracellular membrane traffic. *J. Exp. Biol.*, **172**, 39–45.

10. Berg, O.G., Gelb, M.H., Tsai, M.-D., and Jain, M.K. (2001) Interfacial enzymology: the secreted phospholipase A2 paradigm. *Chem. Rev.*, **101**, 2613–2654.

11. Rillema, J.A., Osmialowski, E.C., and Linebaugh, B.E. (1980) Phospholipase A2 activity in 9,10-dimethyl-1,2-benzanthracene-induced mammary tumors of rats. *Biochim. Biophys. Acta*, **617**, 150–155.

12. Jain, R.K., Munn, L.L., and Fukumura, D. (2002) Dissecting tumor pathophysiology using intravital microscopy. *Nat. Rev. Cancer*, **2**, 266–276.

13. Hobbs, S.K., Monsky, W.L., Yuan, F., Roberts, W.G., Griffith, L., Torchilin, V.P., and Jain, R.K. (1998) Regulation of transport pathways in tumor vessels: role of tumor type and microenvironment. *Proc. Natl. Acad. Sci. USA*, **95**, 4607–4612.

14. Noguchi, Y., Wu, J., Duncan, R., Strohalm, J., Ulbrich, K., Akaike, T., and Maeda, H. (1998) Early phase tumor accumulation of macromolecules: a great difference between the tumor vs.normal tissue in their clearance rate. *Jpn. J. Cancer Res.*, **89**, 307–314.

15. Allen, C., Dos Santos, N., Gallagher, R., Chiu, G.N.C., Shu, Y., Li, W.M., Johnstone, S.A., Janoff, A.S., Mayer, L.D., Webb, M.S., and Bally, M.B. (2002) Controlling the physical behavior and biological performance of liposome formulations through use of surface grafted poly(ethylene glycol). *Biosci. Rep.*, **22**, 225–250.

16. Lasic, D.D. and Martin, F. (eds) (1995) *Stealth Liposomes*, CRC Press, Boca Raton, FL.

17. Mayer, L.D., Nayar, R., Thies, R.L., Boman, N.L., Cullis, P.R., and Bally, M.B. (1993) Identification of vesicle properties that enhance the antitumour activity of liposomal vincristine against murine L1210 leukemia. *Cancer Chemother. Pharmacol.*, **33**, 17–24.

18. Klibanov, A.L., Maruyama, K., Beckerleg, A.M., Torchilin, V.P., and Huang, L. (1991) Activity of amphipathic poly(ethylene glycol) 5000 to prolong the circulation time of liposomes depends on the liposome size and is unfavorable for immunoliposome binding to target. *Biochim. Biophys. Acta*, **1062**, 142–148.

19. Lee, J.H., Lee, H.B., and Andrade, J.D. (1995) Blood compatibility of polyethylene oxide surfaces. *Prog. Polym. Sci.*, **20**, 1043–1079.

20. Dos Santos, N., Allen, C., Doppen, A.-M., Anantha, M., Cox, K.A.K., Gallagher, R.C., Karlsson, G., Edwards, K., Kenner, G., Samuels, L., Webb, M.S., and Bally, M.B. (2007) Influence of poly(ethylene glycol) grafting density and polymer length on liposomes: relating plasma circulation lifetimes to protein binding. *Biochim. Biophys. Acta*, **1768**, 1367–1377.

21. Efremova, N.V., Bondurant, B., O'Brien, D.F., and Leckband, D.E. (2000) Measurements of interbilayer forces and protein adsorption on uncharged lipid bilayers displaying poly(ethylene glycol) chains. *Biochemistry*, **39**, 3441–3451.

22. de Gennes, P.G. (1980) Conformations of polymers attached to an interface. *Macromolecules*, **13**, 1069–1075.

23. Scherphof, G.L. and Kamps, J.A.A.M. (1998) Receptor versus non-receptor mediated clearance of liposomes. *Adv. Drug Deliv. Rev.*, **32**, 81–97.

24. Moghimi, S.M., Hamad, I., Andresen, T.L., Jorgensen, K., and Szebeni, J. (2006) Methylation of the phosphate oxygen moiety of phospholipid-methoxy(polyethylene glycol) conjugate prevents PEGylated liposome-mediated complement activation and anaphylatoxin production. *FASEB J.*, **20**, 2591–2593.

25. deFazio, A., Chiew, Y.E., Sini, R.L., Janes, P.W., and Sutherland, R.L. (2000) Expression of c-*erb*B receptors, heregulin and oestrogen receptor in human breast cell lines. *Int. J. Cancer*, **87**, 487–498.

26. Kirpotin, D.B., Park, J.W., Hong, S.K., Zalipsky, S., Li, W.-L., Carter, P., Benz, C.C., and Papahadjopoulos, D. (1997) Sterically stabilized anti-HER2 immunoliposomes: design and targeting

to human breast cancer cells *in vitro*. *Biochemistry*, **36**, 66–75.

27. Yarden, Y. (2000) *HER2: Basic Research, Prognosis and Therapy – Breast Disease 11*, IOS Press, Amsterdam.

28. Kirpotin, D.B., Drummond, D.C., Shao, Y., Shalaby, M.R., Hong, K., Nielsen, U.B., Marks, J.D., Benz, C.C., and Park, J.W. (2006) Antibody targeting of long-circulating lipidic nanoparticles does not increase tumor localization but does increase internalization in animal models. *Cancer Res.*, **66**, 6732–6740.

29. Miller, C.R., Bondurant, B., McLean, S.D., McGovern, K.A., and O'Brien, D.F. (1998) Liposome–cell interactions *in vitro*: effect of liposome surface charge on the binding and endocytosis of conventional and sterically stabilized liposomes. *Biochemistry*, **37**, 12875–12883.

30. Zhang, J.-S., Liu, F., and Huang, L. (2005) Implications of pharmacokinetic behavior of lipoplex for its inflammatory toxicity. *Adv. Drug Deliv. Rev.*, **57**, 689–698.

31. Liu, F. and Liu, D. (1996) Serum independent liposome uptake by mouse liver. *Biochim. Biophys. Acta*, **1278**, 5–11.

32. Goren, D., Horowitz, A.T., Zalipsky, S., Woodle, M.C., Yarden, Y., and Gabizon, A. (1996) Targeting of stealth liposomes to erbB-2 (Her/2) receptor: *in vitro* and *in vivo* studies. *Br. J. Cancer*, **74**, 1749–1756.

33. Born, R. and Eicholtz-Wirth, H. (1981) Effect of different physiological conditions on the actions of adriamycin on Chinese hamster cells *in vitro*. *Br. J. Cancer*, **44**, 241.

34. Groos, E., Walker, L., and Masters, R.W. (1986) Intravesical chemotherapy. Studies on the relationship between pH and cytotoxicity. *Cancer*, **58**, 1199.

35. Sofou, S. (2008) Radionuclide carriers for targeting of cancer. *Int. J. Nanomed.*, **3**, 181–199.

36. Eliaz, R.E., Nir, S., Marty, C., and Szoka, F.C. Jr. (2004) Determination and modeling of kinetics of cancer cell killing by doxorubicin and doxorubicin encapsulated in targeted liposomes. *Cancer Res.*, **64**, 711–718.

37. Ishida, T., Kirchmeier, M.J., Moase, E.H., Zalipsky, S., and Allen, T.M. (2001) Targeted delivery and triggered release of liposomal doxorubicin enhances cytotoxicity against human B lymphoma cells. *Biochim. Biophys. Acta*, **1515**, 144–158.

38. Torchilin, V.P. (2008) Tat peptide-mediated intracellular delivery of pharmaceutical nanocarriers. *Adv. Drug Deliv. Rev.*, **60**, 548–558.

39. Sawant, R.M., Hurley, J.P., Salmaso, S., Kale, A., Tolcheva, E., Levchenko, T.S., and Torchilin, V.P. (2006) "SMART" drug delivery systems: double-targeted pH-responsive pharmaceutical nanocarriers. *Bioconjug. Chem.*, **17**, 943–949.

40. Kale, A.A. and Torchilin, V.P. (2007) Enhanced transfection of tumor cells *in vivo* using "Smart" pH-sensitive TAT-modified pegylated liposomes. *J. Drug Target.*, **15**, 538–545.

41. Karve, S., Bandekar, A., Ali, M.R., and Sofou, S. (2010) The pH-dependent association with cancer cells of tunable functionalized lipid vesicles with encapsulated doxorubicin for high cell-kill selectivity. *Biomaterials*, **31**, 4409–4416.

42. Bajagur Kempegowda, G., Karve, S., Bandekar, A., Adhikari, A., Khaimchayev, T., and Sofou, S. (2009) pH-dependent formation of lipid heterogeneities controls surface topography and binding reactivity in functionalized bilayers. *Langmuir*, **25**, 8144–8151.

43. Drummond, D.D., Zignani, M., and Leroux, J.C. (2000) Current status of pH-sensitive liposomes in drug delivery. *Prog. Lipid Res.*, **39**, 409–460.

44. Mouritsen, O.G. and Zucherman, M.J. (1987) Model of interfacial melting. *Phys. Rev. Lett.*, **58**, 389–392.

45. Carruthers, A. and Melchior, D.L. (1983) Study of the relationship between bilayer water permeability and bilayer physical state. *Biochemistry*, **22**, 5797–5807.

46. Clerc, S.G. and Thompson, T.E. (1995) Permeability of dimyristoyl phosphatidylcholine/dipalmitoyl phosphatidylcholine bilayer membranes with coexisting gel and liquid-crystalline phases. *Biophys. J.*, **68**, 2333–2341.

47. Papahadjopoulos, D., Jacobson, K., Nir, S., and Isac, T. (1973) Phase transitions

in phospholipid vesicles: fluorescence polarization and permeability measurements concerning the effect of temperature and cholesterol. *Biochim. Biophys. Acta*, **311**, 330–348.

48. Needham, D. and Dewhirst, M.W. (2001) The development and testing of a new temperature-sensitive drug delivery system for the treatment of solid tumors. *Adv. Drug Deliv. Rev.*, **53**, 285–305.

49. Bergstrand, N., Arfvidsson, M.C., Kim, J.M., Thompson, D.H., and Edwards, K. (2003) Interactions between pH-sensitive liposomes and model membranes. *Biophys. Chem.*, **104**, 361–379.

50. Ellens, H., Bentz, J., and Szoka, F.C. (1984) pH-induced destabilization of phosphatidylethanolamine-containing liposomes: role of bilayer contact. *Biochemistry*, **23**, 1532–1538.

51. Slepushkin, V.A., Simoes, S., Dazin, P., Newman, M.S., Guo, L.S., Pedroso de Lima, M., and Düzgünes, N. (1997) Sterically stabilized pH-sensitive liposomes. *J. Biol. Chem.*, **272**, 2382–2388.

52. Guo, X., Andrew MacKay, J., and Szoka, F.C. Jr. (2003) Mechanism of pH-triggered collapse of phosphatidylethanolamine liposomes stabilized by an ortho ester polyethyleneglycol lipid. *Biophys. J.*, **84**, 1784–1795.

53. Kirpotin, D., Hong, K., Mullah, N., Papahadjopoulos, D., and Zalipsky, S. (1996) Liposomes with detachable polymer coating: destabilization and fusion of dioleoylphosphatidylethanolamine vesicles triggered by cleavage of surface-grafted poly(ethylene glycol). *FEBS Lett.*, **388**, 115–118.

54. Karve, S., Bajagur Kempegowda, G., and Sofou, S. (2008) Heterogeneous domains and membrane permeability in phosphatidylcholine– phosphatidic acid rigid vesicles as a function of pH and lipid chain mismatch. *Langmuir*, **24**, 5679–5688.

55. Karve, S., Alaouie, A., Zhou, Y., Rotolo, J., and Sofou, S. (2009) The use of pH-triggered leaky heterogeneities on rigid lipid bilayers to improve intracellular trafficking and therapeutic potential of targeted liposomal immunochemotherapy. *Biomaterials*, **30**, 6055–6064.

56. Sofou, S. (2007) Surface-active liposomes for targeted cancer therapy. *Nanomedicine*, **2**, 711–724.

57. Parente, R.A., Nir, S., and Szoka, F.C. (1990) Mechanism of leakage of phospholipid vesicle contents induced by the peptide GALA. *Biochemistry*, **29**, 8720–8728.

58. Thomas, J.L. and Tirrell, D.A. (1992) Polyelectrolyte-sensitized phospholipid vesicles. *Acc. Chem. Res.*, **25**, 336–342.

59. Mouritsen, O.G., Andresen, T.L., Halperin, A., Jansen, P.L., Jacobsen, A.F., Jensen, U.B., and Weiss, M. (2006) Activation of interfacial enzymes at membrane surfaces. *J. Phys. Cond. Mat.*, **18**, S1293.

60. Andresen, T.L., Jensen, S.S., Kaasgaard, T., and Jørgensen, K. (2005) Triggered activation and release of liposomal prodrugs and drugs in cancer tissue by secretory phospholipase A2. *Curr. Drug Deliv.*, **2**, 353–362.

61. Zalipsky, S., Qazen, M., Walker, J.A., Mullah, N., Quinn, Y.P., and Huang, S.K. (1999) New detachable poly(ethylene glycol) conjugates: cysteine-cleavable lipopolymers regenerating natural phospholipid, diacyl phosphatidylethanolamine. *Bioconjug. Chem.*, **10**, 703–707.

62. McNeeley, K.M., Karathanasis, E., Annapragada, A.V., and Bellamkonda, R.V. (2009) Masking and triggered unmasking of targeting ligands on nanocarriers to improve drug delivery to brain tumors. *Biomaterials*, **30**, 3986–3995.

63. Maeda, T. and Fujimoto, K. (2006) A reduction-triggered delivery by a liposomal carrier possessing membrane-permeable ligands and a detachable coating. *Colloids Surf. B*, **49**, 15–21.

64. Papahadjopoulos, D., Jacobson, K., Nir, S., and Isac, I. (1973) Phase transitions in phospholipid vesicles Fluorescence polarization and permeability measurements concerning the effect of temperature and cholesterol. *Biochim. Biophys. Acta*, **311**, 330–348.

65. Weinstein, J., Magin, R., Yatvin, M., and Zaharko, D. (1979) Liposomes and local hyperthermia: selective delivery of methotrexate to heated tumors. *Science*, **204**, 188–191.
66. Kong, G., Anyarambhatla, G., Petros, W.P., Braun, R.D., Colvin, O.M., Needham, D., and Dewhirst, M.W. (2000) Efficacy of liposomes and hyperthermia in a human tumor xenograft model: importance of triggered drug release. *Cancer Res.*, **60**, 6950–6957.
67. Morgan, C.G., Bisby, R.H., Johnson, S.A., and Mitchell, A.C. (1995) Fast solute release from photosensitive liposomes: an alternative to "caged" reagents for use in biological systems. *FEBS Lett.*, **375**, 113–116.
68. Thompson, D.H., Gerasimov, O.V., Wheeler, J.J., Rui, Y., and Anderson, V.C. (1996) Triggerable plasmalogen liposomes: improvement of system efficiency. *Biochim. Biophys. Acta*, **1279**, 25–34.
69. Chandra, B., Subramaniam, R., Mallik, S., and Srivastava, D.K. (2006) Formulation of photocleavable liposomes and the mechanism of their content release. *Org. Biomol. Chem.*, **4**, 1730–1740.
70. Volodkin, D.V., Skirtach, A.G., and Möhwald, H. (2009) Near-IR remote release from assemblies of liposomes and nanoparticles. *Angew. Chem. Int. Ed.*, **48**, 1807–1809.
71. Lin, H.Y. and Thomas, J.L. (2004) Factors affecting responsivity of unilamellar liposomes to 20 kHz ultrasound. *Langmuir*, **20**, 6100–6106.
72. Schroeder, A., Avnir, Y., Weisman, S., Tzemach, D., Najajreh, Y., Gabizon, A., Talmon, Y., Kost, J., and Barenholz, Y. (2007) Controlling liposomal drug release with low frequency ultrasound: mechanism and feasibility. *Langmuir*, **23**, 4019–4025.
73. Huang, S.-L. and MacDonald, R.C. (2004) Acoustically active liposomes for drug encapsulation and ultrasound-triggered release. *Biochim. Biophys. Acta*, **1665**, 134–141.
74. Liburdy, R.P., Tenforde, T.S., and Magin, R.L. (1986) Magnetic field-induced drug permeability in liposome vesicles. *Radiat. Res.*, **108**, 102–111.
75. Tai, L.A., Tsai, P.J., Wang, Y.C., Wang, Y.J., Lo, L.W., and Yang, C.S. (2009) Thermosensitive liposomes entrapping iron oxide nanoparticles for controllable drug release. *Nanotechnology*, **20**, 135101.
76. Pradhan, P., Giri, J., Rieken, F., Koch, C., Mykhaylyk, O., Döblinger, M., Banerjee, R., Bahadur, D., and Plank, C. (2010) Targeted temperature sensitive magnetic liposomes for thermo-chemotherapy. *J. Control. Release*, **142**, 108–121.
77. Zaidi, H. and Sgouros, G. (2003) *Therapeutic Applications of Monte Carlo Calculations in Nuclear Medicine*, IOP, Bristol.
78. Thurber, G.M., Schmidt, M.M., and Wittrup, K.D. (2008) Antibody tumor penetration: transport opposed by systemic and antigen-mediated clearance. *Adv. Drug Deliv. Rev.*, **60**, 1421–1434.
79. Thurber, G.M., Zajic, S.C., and Wittrup, K.D. (2007) Theoretic criteria for antibody penetration into solid tumors and micrometastases. *J. Nucl. Med.*, **48**, 995–999.
80. Lee, H., Fonge, H., Hoang, B., Reilly, R.M., Allen, C. The effects of particle size and molecular targeting on the intratumoral and subcellular distribution of polymeric nanoparticles. *Mol. Pharm.*, **7**, 1195–1208.

31
Nanoscale Delivery Systems for Combination Chemotherapy

Barry D. Liboiron, Paul G. Tardi, Troy O. Harasym, and Lawrence D. Mayer

31.1
Introduction

Combination chemotherapy treatments for cancer continue to be developed in a manner largely unchanged since the inception of this approach over 50 years ago, where agents with nonoverlapping toxicities were typically escalated to the highest dose possible. This was done with the expectation that maximum efficacy would be achieved at the maximum tolerated doses (MTDs) of the individual drugs. Emerging evidence indicates that this approach underestimates the critical role that drug ratios play in dictating whether drug combinations interact synergistically, additively, or antagonistically. The implication of this drug ratio dependency is that the most active drug combination may require administration of one agent at sub-MTD doses. However, the ability to take advantage of this relationship *in vivo* requires that drug ratios be controlled after administration so that optimal ratios are exposed to tumor cells while avoiding antagonistic ratios. Nanoscale drug delivery vehicles such as liposomes and nanoparticles are well suited for this application since they can be designed to coordinate the release of drug combinations after injection so that synergistic drug ratios can be maintained and delivered to tumors. This "ratiometric dosing" approach can lead to dramatic increases in preclinical efficacy and is showing promising signs of activity in the clinic.

In this chapter, we review the rationale for ratiometric dosing of anticancer drug combinations, and present preclinical and clinical results for the liposome-based formulations CPX-351 (cytarabine/daunorubicin) and CPX-1 (irinotecan/floxuridine) that demonstrate the therapeutic benefits associated with locking in the synergistic ratio of two anticancer drugs within a nanoscale particulate drug carrier. This strategy can be applied to a wide range of therapeutic agents: we discuss its application to drug combinations that are reactive (e.g., cisplatin and irinotecan) as well as for those in which markedly disparate physicochemical properties between the two free agents (e.g., hydrophobic paclitaxel and hydrophilic gemcitabine) can be ameliorated through the use of prodrug nanoparticles. Ratiometric dosing opens new possibilities to prospectively

Drug Delivery in Oncology: From Basic Research to Cancer Therapy, First Edition.
Edited by Felix Kratz, Peter Senter, and Henning Steinhagen.
© 2012 Wiley-VCH Verlag GmbH & Co. KGaA. Published 2012 by Wiley-VCH Verlag GmbH & Co. KGaA.

develop drug combinations based on optimized efficacy through pharmacokinetic control of drug ratios rather than selecting drug doses based on tolerability.

31.2
Rationale for Fixed Ratio Anticancer Combination Therapy

31.2.1
Biological Basis for the Importance of Drug Ratios

The development of combination chemotherapy for the treatment of cancer arose from the pioneering work of Frei and Freireich in the 1960s [1, 2]. Seminal clinical trials in childhood leukemia demonstrated that dramatic improvements in therapeutic response could be achieved by increasing the number of drugs administered during a course of treatment. Specifically, response rates in the range of 40% and no cures with methotrexate alone increased to more than 95% complete response and 35% cure rates with the inclusion of 6-mercaptopurine, prednisone, and vincristine into the treatment regimen. Eventually, cure rates increased to 75–80% with the inclusion of asparaginase, daunorubicin, and cytarabine. The principle underlying this approach was to administer combinations of chemotherapeutic drugs with nonoverlapping toxicities in full doses as early as possible in the disease [3]. By simultaneously attacking multiple features associated with tumor progression it was expected that damage to basic cellular functions could be increased while decreasing the number of protective responses available to tumor cells, thereby enhancing the susceptibility to chemotherapy-induced cell death and minimizing the emergence of drug resistance. However, in this model the individual agents of a combination regimen were often selected empirically based on toxicity considerations. Furthermore, the expectation was that while the components of a chemotherapy "cocktail" may exhibit complementary modes of action, the ultimate therapeutic effect of the combination was an aggregate effect of independent antitumor activities.

Over the past two decades the genes, proteins, and pathways involved in most cellular functions have been elucidated, and key components have been identified that, when altered due to mutation or changes in expression levels, appear to be associated with the initiation and/or progression of specific types of cancers. This increased understanding has spawned a new wave of "targeted" cancer therapeutics where potent and highly selective molecules directed against a specific protein can be generated and optimized using combinatorial chemical libraries and structure–function analyses. As the number of targeted anticancer agents progressing into clinical testing has increased, it has become apparent for many of these drugs that their therapeutic activity as single agents is limited despite the ability to demonstrate effective inhibition of the intended target protein in patients [4–6]. However, many of these targeted antineoplastics have been able to significantly augment therapeutic activity when used in combination with other anticancer drugs (most commonly approved cytotoxic agents), resulting in improved survival outcomes compared to chemotherapy alone. Consequently, approvals of targeted anticancer agents such as bevacizumab [7], cetuximab [8, 9], bortezomib [10], lapatinib [11], and erlotinib [12, 13] have been based on increased efficacy for the targeted agent plus standard-of-care chemotherapy obtained in pivotal clinical trials.

As we have learned more about the mechanisms underlying the antitumor activity of drug combination treatments, it has become increasingly clear that individual agents often do not act independently, but rather significant interaction occurs between the various pathways affected and these interactions likely contribute considerably to the improvement in efficacy. This may not be surprising given the high degree of cross-talk between various pathways as well as the redundancies and feedback loops associated with key regulating proteins [14]. Targeted therapeutics have helped to identify and characterize such interactions due to their specificity of action, and have facilitated a more "systems biology" approach where the effects of drug combinations on networks of associated pathways can be examined and correlated with therapeutic outcomes [15–17]. This approach has (i) opened opportunities to identify unexpected drug combinations with effective antitumor activity [18], (ii) enabled researchers to prospectively test the benefits of utilizing drug combinations that target proteins in parallel or sequential pathway orientations [19], and (iii) allows a better understanding of the interactions involving combinations of conventional cytotoxic agents, many of which exhibit multiple pharmacological effects.

If one accepts the position that the majority of drug combinations will induce alterations of multiple cellular pathways that have the potential to interact, it then follows that the impact of such interactions on the ability to trigger tumor cell death and induce a therapeutic response can be favorable (synergistic), neutral (additive), or unfavorable (antagonistic). For the purposes of this chapter, it is important to note that synergistic drug activity results in tumor cell kill that is greater than the combined effect of the two drugs, as predicted from the sum of quantitative effects of the individual components [20–22]. Unfortunately, many reports refer to antitumor activity of a drug combination as being synergistic if it is merely more effective than either individual drug. When developing cancer drug combinations, one would clearly want to identify those that maximize synergistic interactions and those that avoid antagonism. These relationships are typically examined *in vitro* using any one of a number of available experimental designs to quantify the antitumor activity of drug combinations and mathematical algorithms for analyzing the results to determine whether the extent of tumor growth inhibition reflects synergy, additivity, or antagonism [21, 23–27]. However, despite the widely varying conditions (drug concentrations, drug ratios, and exposure times) under which drug–drug interactions are evaluated, combinations are typically concluded to be simply synergistic or antagonistic without reference to the testing parameters. Rarely have investigations into drug–drug interactions taken into account that, without exception, existing anticancer drug combination treatments result in widely varying concentrations of the individual agents due to (i) independent and dissimilar pharmacokinetics of the individual agents, and

(ii) different administration schedules. These factors lead to highly fluctuating drug–drug ratios *in vivo*. Consequently, it may not be surprising that the clinical development of drug combinations, including those employing targeted agents, continues to follow the same process established in the 1960s where the doses of the individual drugs are escalated until aggregate effects of toxicity are considered to be limiting. This approach assumes, perhaps incorrectly, that maximum therapeutic activity will be achieved with maximum dose intensity for all drugs in the combination and ignores the possibility that more subtle concentration-dependent drug interactions could impact the nature of specific drug–drug interactions that influence antitumor activity. In fact, evidence supporting this concept can be found with existing therapeutic agents. For example, DNA methyltransferase inhibitors such as azacytidine and decitabine when used in combination with other agents have been found to provide improved therapeutic results when administered at sub-MTD doses where their hypomethylation activity is increased [28, 29].

Recent literature has provided several examples of studies with new and existing chemotherapy combinations where the effects of drug concentrations and drug/drug ratios have been examined. The evidence emerging from these investigations indicates that anticancer drug combinations can interact synergistically, additively, or antagonistically depending on the ratio of the agents being combined [30–33] and these interactions can change as a function of absolute drug concentration. Such interactions have been observed for a variety of drug combinations comprised of a wide range of drug classes (see Table 31.1). Although the patterns of drug ratio-dependent synergy for these combinations span the full gamut of possibilities (e.g., synergy at either ratio extreme; $A \gg B$ or $A \ll B$, both extremes, or only at comparable molar ratios; $A \sim B$), the fact that drug ratio-dependent synergy is observed for such widely disparate combinations of anticancer agents suggests that this phenomenon is of widespread importance. In this context, it is important to point out that drug ratio-dependent synergy analysis should be performed at absolute drug concentrations that are pharmacologically meaningful (all results in Table 31.1 reflect analyses at concentrations that induce 50% or more cell growth inhibition); synergy results obtained at drug exposures resulting in less than 50% tumor cell growth inhibition are unlikely to be relevant to *in vivo* therapeutic applications. For example, when paclitaxel and azacytidine were tested *in vitro*, synergy was observed at 20% cell growth inhibition concentrations; however, the combination at concentrations producing 50% cell growth inhibition was merely additive [34].

The clinical relevance of drug ratio-dependent synergy is strengthened by studies where up to 20 different tumor cell lines have been used to assess the drug ratio dependency for the combination of irinotecan and cisplatin [35]. This is due to the fact that variability of drug ratio-dependent synergy may be expected to occur clinically where tumor heterogeneity between patients is high. Therefore, drug ratio-dependent synergy trends observed in a limited number of tumor cell lines may not be representative of patient populations and are unlikely to be predictive of outcomes in a clinical setting. However, in the case of the irinotecan/cisplatin investigation, a remarkably consistent drug ratio dependency

31.2 Rationale for Fixed Ratio Anticancer Combination Therapy

Table 31.1 In vitro evidence of drug ratio-dependent synergy.

No.	Drug combination	Drug classes	No. tumor lines tested	Drug ratio relationships[a]			Method	References
				A ≫ B	A ~ B	A ≪ B		
1	AZT/paclitaxel	telomerase inhibitor/microtubule inhibitor	1	+	ND	ND	combination index	[34]
2	camptothecin/doxorubicin	topoisomerase I/topoisomerase II inhibitors	1	− −	+ +	ND	median effect	[32]
3	camptothecin/etoposide	topoisomerase I/topoisomerase II inhibitors	1	+ +	±	±	median effect	[32]
4	cisplatin/daunorubicin	DNA cross-linker/topoisomerase II inhibitor	1	+	− −	ND	median effect	[31]
5	cisplatin/taxane[b]	DNA cross-linker/microtubule inhibitor	5–7	+	ND	ND	area under curve statistical analysis	[36, 37]
6	CP-4055/cloretazine	Pyr antimetabolite/DNA alkylator	2	ND	ND	±	median effect	[38]
7	CP-4055/gemcitabine	Pyr antimetabolites	2	+ +	ND	ND	median effect	[38]

(continued overleaf)

Table 31.1 (continued)

No.	Drug combination	Drug classes	No. tumor lines tested	Drug ratio relationships[a]			Method	References
				A ≫ B	A ~ B	A ≪ B		
8	CP-4055/idarubicin	Pyr antimetabolite/topoisomerase II inhibitor	2	±	ND	ND	median effect	[38]
9	cytarabine/daunorubicin	Pyr antimetabolite/topoisomerase II inhibitor	15	++	±	– –	median effect	[35, 39]
10	cytarabine/gemcitabine	Pyr antimetabolite/topoisomerase I inhibitor	2	++	±	ND	median effect	[38]
11	gefitinib/oxaliplatin	anti-EGFR TK1/DNA cross-linker	2	– –	±	ND	median effect	[40]
12	gemcitabine/fludarabine	Pyr antimetabolite/Pur antimetabolite	1	±	±	++	median effect, surface response	[41]
13	gemcitabine/mitomycin C	Pyr antimetabolite/DNA alkylator	1	+	++	±	median effect	[42]
14	gemcitabine/mitoxantrone	antimetabolite/topoisomerase II inhibitor	1	±	.	– –	median effect, surface response	[41]

#	Drugs	Category	Ratio				Notes	Refs
15	gemcitabine/SN-38	antimetabolite/topoisomerase I inhibitor	1	.	±	--	median effect, surface response	[41]
16	irinotecan/floxuridine	topoisomerase I inhibitor/Pyr antimetabolite	11	+	++	.	median effect	[30, 43]
17	nedaplatin/irinotecan	DNA cross-linker/topoisomerase I inhibitor	1	±	+	.	median effect, surface response	[44]
18	pemetrexed/docetaxel	folate antimetabolite/microtubule inhibitor	3	--	±	--	median effect	[45]
19	pemetrexed/gemcitabine	folate antimetabolite/Pyr antimetabolite	3	--	±	±	median effect	[45]
20	pemetrexed/irinotecan	folate antimetabolite/topoisomerase I inhibitor	3	±	±	+	median effect	[45]

[a] Refers to the degree of drug interaction between the drug pair: ++, strongly synergistic; +, synergistic; ±, additive; −, antagonistic; −−, strongly antagonistic.
[b] Both paclitaxel and docetaxel were tested and each yielded similar results.
AZT, 3′-azido-3′-deoxythymidine; CP-4055, cytarabine-elaidate; Pur, purine; Pyr, pyrimidine; EGFR TK1, epidermal growth factor receptor tyrosine kinase-1; ND, not determined.

trend arose in a 20-cell-line panel composed of a wide range of tumor types and molecular phenotypes where strong antagonism was observed when the two drugs were exposed at approximately equimolar concentrations and consistent synergy occurred when the irinotecan/cisplatin molar ratio was in excess of 4 : 1 (Table 31.2). The robustness of the drug ratio-dependent trend in such a diverse panel of tumor cell lines increases the likelihood that such relationships may be relevant in patients and highlights the importance of assessing drug ratio-dependent synergy in multiple tumor lines.

The potential *in vivo* implications of drug ratio-dependent synergy may be profound, particularly in cases where certain ratios exhibit significant antagonism. As described above, virtually all drug combinations used currently in the clinic will result in patients being exposed to varying drug/drug ratios due to disparate dosing schedules and pharmacokinetic properties of the individual agents. Given this lack of ability to control drug ratios exposed to tumor cells *in vivo* with conventional aqueous drug formulations, it is possible, if not highly probable, that antagonistic drug ratios may ensue after administration of such combinations and this would no doubt lead to compromised therapeutic activity. This creates a dilemma in that *in vitro* informatics on drug ratio-dependent synergy cannot be exploited *in vivo* without the ability to control drug ratios after administration. Injecting a chemotherapy combination at drug ratios identified as synergistic *in vitro* would most certainly lead to rapid divergence of the circulating ratio as the agents are metabolized and eliminated differentially and independently [22]. Furthermore, although infusional administration of drug combinations could potentially control and achieve a desired drug ratio at steady state, tissue drug levels and ratios would most likely not reflect those in the circulation due to the very high distribution phase of most anticancer agents.

An ideal solution to this problem would be a method by which the disparate pharmacokinetics of the individual agents of a combination could be controlled and matched to maintain the synergistic drug ratio for prolonged periods post *in vivo* administration. As shown in Figure 31.1a, injection of two agents as a free drug cocktail at a defined drug ratio generally leads to rapid deviation from the injected drug/drug ratio shortly after administration, due to inherent pharmacokinetic differences between the two agents. Nanoscale particulate drug delivery vehicles (Figure 31.1b) are well suited for this purpose since drug pharmacokinetic properties are dictated by the delivery system such that drug elimination can be controlled by manipulating the rate of drug release from the drug carrier. Therefore, the drug/drug ratio can be maintained *in vivo* as it becomes a function of the carrier pharmacokinetics and the release rates of the encapsulated agents. A wide range of particulate delivery systems, such as liposomes and polymer nanoparticles, are able to control and in some cases tune the pharmacokinetics of the encapsulated drug to desired characteristics. Consequently, application of these drug delivery vehicles to anticancer drug combinations represents an approach to control and maintain synergistic drug ratios *in vivo*, thereby allowing the translation of *in vitro* informatics on drug ratio-dependent synergy to preclinical and eventually clinical settings with the possibility of meaningful improvements in cancer therapies.

Table 31.2 *In vitro* synergy heat map of irinotecan/cisplatin in 20 cell lines reporting CI values at $f_a = 0.8$ (green: synergistic (<0.9); yellow: additive (0.9–1.1); red: antagonistic (>1.1)) (from [35, 39], reprinted with permission).

Cell lines screened	Tumor	1:64	1:32	1:16	1:8	1:4	1:2	1:1	2:1	4:1	8:1	16:1	32:1	64:1
LCC6	breast	0.69	0.58	0.71	0.89	0.83	1.01	1.57	1.03	0.85	0.63	0.52	0.54	0.76
MCF-7	breast	0.71	0.67	0.86	0.88	0.95	1.15	0.71	0.82	0.70	1.00	0.87	0.83	0.88
MB 231	breast	1.02	1.01	0.90	0.90	0.70	0.87	1.54	1.34	0.90	1.10	0.76	1.40	0.61
HCT-116	colon	0.38	0.36	0.37	0.33	0.62	0.84	1.50	1.73	9.40	0.71	0.76	0.82	1.06
Colon-26	colon	1.22	1.67	1.40	1.16	1.00	1.21	1.04	1.38	1.10	1.03	1.31	1.25	0.82
HT-29	colon	1.05	0.88	0.90	0.86	1.21	1.09	1.57	1.17	0.90	0.76	0.82	0.97	1.05
A549	lung	0.67	0.61	0.67	0.56	0.44	0.39	0.44	1.65	1.31	0.49	0.37	0.41	0.49
H460	lung	0.92	0.81	0.84	0.80	0.75	0.73	0.94	1.14	2.03	0.53	0.36	0.80	0.48
H322	lung	0.47	0.52	0.68	0.96	0.57	1.28	1.24	0.95	0.73	0.54	0.44	0.52	0.54
H1299	lung	1.07	1.08	1.12	1.09	0.76	0.98	3.01	2.57	1.83	0.65	0.64	1.49	0.82
H522	lung	1.15	0.62	1.09	0.84	0.82	0.92	2.26	1.80	0.89	0.48	0.39	0.73	0.47
Ovcar-3	ovarian	1.33	1.35	1.08	1.10	0.80	0.78	0.89	0.89	1.84	0.53	0.28	0.33	0.35
Ovcar-5	ovarian	1.29	1.65	1.55	1.34	1.30	1.42	1.51	1.30	1.15	0.80	1.05	0.99	1.17
SK-OV-3	ovarian	1.33	1.16	1.30	1.51	1.49	1.70	1.75	1.28	1.17	0.55	0.70	0.79	0.76
IGROV-1	ovarian	1.16	1.16	1.16	1.00	0.95	0.95	1.23	1.20	1.16	0.77	0.78	0.71	0.75
A2780	ovarian	0.93	0.94	0.81	0.75	0.80	0.81	0.87	0.70	0.81	0.81	1.20	1.03	1.25
Capan-1	pancreatic	1.46	1.22	1.11	1.25	0.86	0.89	1.12	1.17	0.69	0.89	0.83	0.71	0.99
BXPC-3	pancreatic	1.00	1.02	0.91	1.10	0.81	0.99	1.04	0.88	0.70	0.60	0.49	0.64	0.61
N87	gastric	1.76	1.87	1.35	1.55	1.65	1.09	1.05	0.68	0.51	0.18	0.11	0.06	0.04
A253	head and neck	0.85	0.84	0.81	0.92	0.76	0.63	0.79	0.78	0.86	0.83	0.90	0.82	0.84

f_a: fraction affected.

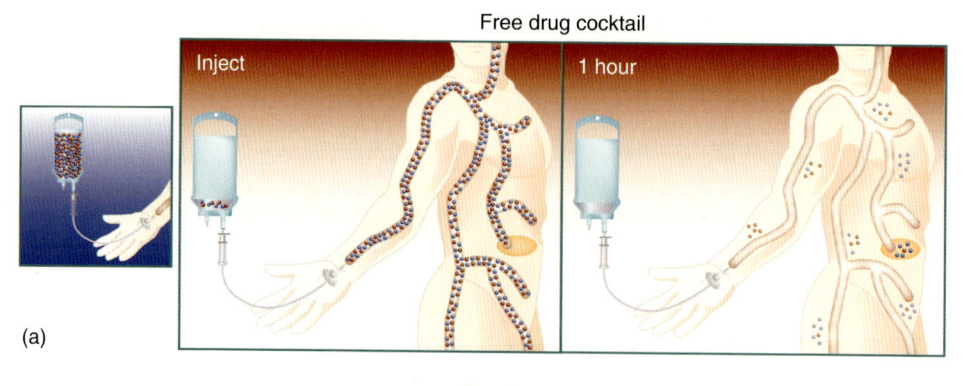

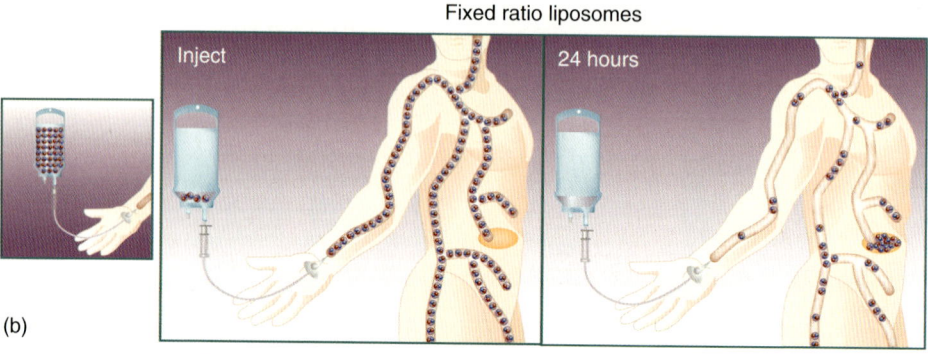

Figure 31.1 Combination chemotherapy administration strategies. (a) Administered as a free drug cocktail, no attempt is made to control the drug/drug ratio *in vivo*. The drug/drug ratio is therefore rapidly disrupted (generally less than 1 h) due to the disparate pharmacokinetic properties of the two agents. (b) When the drugs are administered in a carefully formulated drug carrier, such as a liposome, the drug/drug ratio can be fixed within the vehicle, providing a means to normalize the pharmacokinetics of each agent and maintain the drug/drug ratio *in vivo*, generally for far greater periods of time postinjection (up to 24 h and beyond) compared to free cocktail administration.

31.3
Application of Drug Delivery Systems to Develop Fixed-Ratio Drug Combination Formulations

31.3.1
Formulation Strategies for Multiagent Drug Delivery Vehicles

Given the prominent use of drug combinations in the treatment of cancer, increasing drug delivery efforts have focused on encapsulating anticancer drug combinations (typically doublets) and evaluating such formulations for therapeutic activity *in vitro* and *in vivo*. Two basic strategies can be employed for delivery of multiple agents via a particulate carrier, as shown in Figure 31.2 [30]. The first (Figure 31.2a) involves the coencapsulation of the two agents within a single carrier – a strategy referred to in Table 31.3 as dual formulation. The second

31.3 Application of Drug Delivery Systems to Develop Fixed-Ratio Drug Combination Formulations

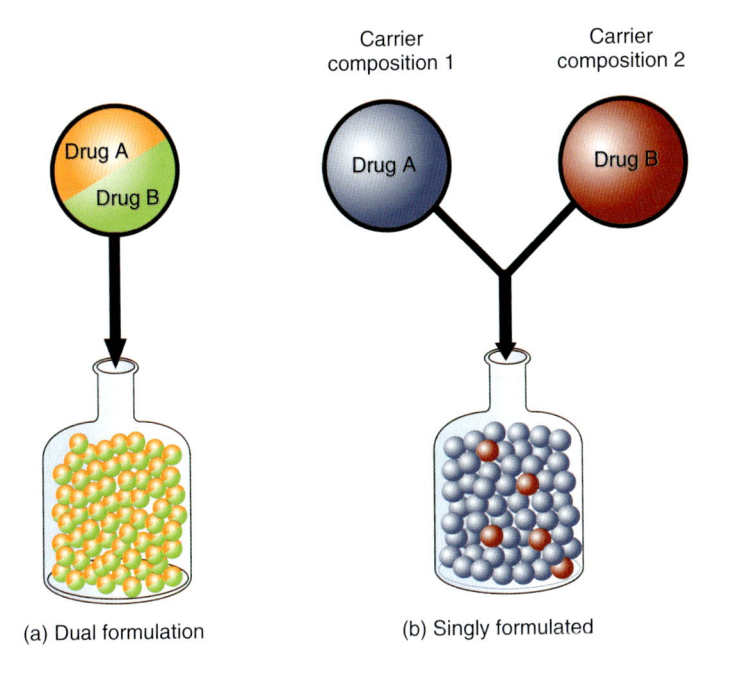

Figure 31.2 Two main strategies for administration of two or more agents within drug particulate carriers. (a) Dual formulation. Each agent is encapsulated within the same particle to the desired drug/drug ratio. (b) Singly formulated. Each agent is encapsulated within its own carrier. The individual drug-loaded carriers are then combined at the desired ratio.

strategy focuses on the development of a drug carrier system for each drug, with subsequent mixing of the two drug-loaded carriers prior to administration – an approach in which the drugs are referred to as singly formulated (Figure 31.2b).

Both methods have distinct advantages. In the first case, with both drugs encapsulated in the same carrier, the biodistribution properties of the drug-loaded particle are normalized for both drugs. This advantage assumes that the biodistribution is unaffected by *in vivo* drug leakage (both coordinated or uncontrolled), although experience with the most successful carriers indicates that this assumption is valid [31, 39]. Dual formulation also requires meticulous and typically iterative formulation activities if the plasma elimination kinetics of the two drugs are to be coordinated (i.e., the two drugs leak from the carrier at similar rates such that the drug/drug ratio within the particle is maintained). It is possible that changes in drug loading procedures, excipient, or drug concentrations, or a combination of factors can lead to the improvement of one drug's retention properties at the expense of the other. Several papers have reported changes in *in vitro* and *in vivo* release properties of a particular agent upon addition of a second agent to the same carrier [51, 53, 56, 57]. Subtle adjustments in carrier composition [58], excipient

Table 31.3 Single- and dual-drug particulate drug delivery systems for combination chemotherapy.

No.	Drug A	Drug B	Particle and composition	Release characteristics	Drug ratio considered	References
1	cytarabine	daunorubicin	liposome, dual formulation	in vivo assay: coordinated plasma elimination profiles	yes: five ratios prescreened in 11 cell lines; 1 : 1 ratio selected as optimal	[31, 39]
2	doxorubicin	gemcitabine	HMPA-based polymer–drug conjugate, dual formulation	enzymatic release assay: uncoordinated release from polymer backbone	no	[46]
3	doxorubicin	paclitaxel	GEG and LE polymer micelle, singly formulated	in vitro assay: singly formulated particles had similar release properties	no	[47]
4	doxorubicin	verapamil	liposome, dual formulation	in vitro assay: coordinated release	no	[48]
5	doxorubicin	verapamil	PEGylated liposome, dual formulation	in vitro assay: slightly faster doxorubicin release in plasma	used previously identified synergistic ratio	[49]
6	doxorubicin	vincristine	liposome, dual formulation	in vivo assay: vincristine readily released, leading to antagonistic drug ratio within liposome	yes: three ratios tested; 20 : 1 doxorubicin/vincristine ratio showed strong antagonism	[50]
7	fludarabine	mitoxantrone	PEGylated liposome, dual formulation	in vitro assay: coordinated release, only 40% of total drugs released	3.7 : 1 ratio shown to be synergistic	[51]

8	irinotecan	cisplatin	liposome, singly formulated	in vivo assay: coordinated plasma elimination profiles	yes: 13 ratios prescreened in 20 cell lines	[35]
9	irinotecan	floxuridine	liposome, dual formulation	in vivo assay: coordinated plasma elimination profiles	yes: five ratios prescreened in 11 cell lines; 1 : 1 ratio selected as optimal	[30, 31]
10	paclitaxel	ceramide	PEG–PCL nanoparticle, singly formulated	not reported	no	[59]
11	paclitaxel	curcumin	flaxseed oil nanoemulsion ± DSPE–PEG, dual formulation	not reported	no	[60]
12	topotecan	amlodipine	PEGylated liposome, dual formulation	not reported	no	[52]
13	topotecan	tamoxifen	PEGylated liposome, dual formulation	in vitro assay reported for topotecan only	no	[53]
14	vincristine	quercetin	PLGA nanoparticles, dual formulation	in vitro assay: quercetin release slower than vincristine	very high quercetin/vincristine ratio: 1000 : 1	[54]
15	vinorelbine	parthenolide	PEGylated liposome, singly formulated	not reported	no	[55]

[a] GEG, poly(γ-benzyl-L-glutamate) and PEG; LE, poly(L-lactide)-b-block copolymer.

concentration [61], and drug loading conditions [62, 63] can be used to achieve coordinated *in vitro* and/or *in vivo* drug retention properties.

Singly formulated delivery strategies for combination chemotherapy can take advantage of the fact that each drug carrier can be individually optimized to maximize encapsulation efficiency, chemical stability, and drug retention without concern for another agent present in the same carrier. For chemically incompatible agents, combining single formulations may be the only suitable solution to avoid drug–drug reactivity. Lastly, mixing of two singly formulated drugs greatly simplifies locking in of a desired drug/drug ratio. In this case, the biodistribution of disparate particles must also be carefully measured to ensure that each drug is delivered to the tumor site in amounts that maintain the desired drug ratio.

31.3.2
Examples of Dual-Drug Delivery Systems

Recent efforts to stably encapsulate multiple agents in particulate drug vehicles for the purpose of combination chemotherapy are summarized in Table 31.3. Immediately evident in Table 31.3 is both the wide disparity of drugs and their pharmacodynamic properties (ranging from the highly hydrophilic cytarabine to the strongly hydrophobic paclitaxel) and the varying strategies attempted to enable generation of stable particles that lead to improved efficacy (liposomes, PEGylated liposomes, nanoparticles, conjugated nanoparticles, and nanoemulsions).

The examples in Table 31.3 encompass a broad range of particle types to achieve the codelivery of multiple chemotherapy agents to tumors. Currently, liposomes, both PEGylated "stealth" type (entries 5, 7, 12, 13, and 15, Table 31.3) and conventional (entries 1, 4, 6, 8, and 9, Table 31.3) are the most common, although some examples of polymer nanoparticles and micelles (entries 2, 3, 10, and 14, Table 31.3) and a nanoemulsion (entry 11, Table 31.3) are reported. The type of particle used is chiefly dictated by the physicochemical properties of the encapsulated agents, with hydrophilic, water-soluble drugs (e.g., cytarabine, fludarabine, topotecan) generally employed with liposome-based carriers, while more hydrophobic agents (e.g., paclitaxel, ceramide, quercetin) are more easily incorporated into nanoparticles stabilized by amphipathic diblock copolymers.

Several groups have exploited the long blood circulation lifetime of PEGylated liposomes (colloquially known as "stealth" liposomes [64]) to deliver multiple agents to multidrug-resistant (MDR) tumors. Wang *et al.* [49] (entry 5, Table 31.3) encapsulated doxorubicin and verapamil (a P-glycoprotein inhibitor) in liposomes, while Wu *et al.* [48] extended this combination by encapsulating the two drugs in liposomes that were functionalized with transferrin for targeting of transferrin-positive K562 leukemia cells. Similarly, Li *et al.* (entry 12, Table 31.3) encapsulated another cytotoxic agent (topotecan) and the anti-MDR agent amlodipine to augment the cytotoxic activity of topotecan in resistant HL-60 cells [52]. Liu *et al.* [55] prepared single formulations of vinorelbine and parthenolide (entry 15, Table 31.3) in egg phosphatidylcholine–cholesterol–PEG2000–DSPE (PEG = poly(ethylene glycol)) liposomes and evaluated their combined efficacy against MCF-7 breast cancer xenografts. Lastly, topotecan was again encapsulated in PEGylated liposomes previously loaded with tamoxifen (entry 13, Table 31.3), which was hypothesized to reside in the lipid bilayer [53].

Retention of the two encapsulated drugs was not extensively studied by either *in vitro* or *in vivo* assays for many of the studies reported in Table 31.3. For the combination of topotecan and tamoxifen, only the *in vitro* release properties of topotecan were reported under nonsink conditions, while the stability of the hydrophobic tamoxifen in the membrane was not assessed [53]. In two reports, drug retention was not reported at all [52, 55]. The release characteristics of the two doxorubicin/verapamil combinations, however, were measured by *in vitro* assays and in both cases the release profiles of the two drugs were similar, such that the ratio of the two drugs within the carrier would be expected to be maintained during the *in vitro* assay [48, 49].

The use of polymer micelles and nanoemulsions for delivery of combination chemotherapeutics allows for combinations that contain a hydrophobic drug, which are generally unsuitable for liposomal delivery. Devalapally *et al.* (2007) reported a simple example of paclitaxel and ceramide each singly formulated in PEG-*b*-PCL (PCL = poly(ε-caprolactone)) nanoparticles, but did not study the drug stability or retention. A recent report described the generation of a nanoemulsion of flaxseed oil stabilized with DSPE–PEG, to encapsulate paclitaxel and curcumin [65]. Both drugs were found to be chemically stable in the emulsion for over 3 months, but it was not clear whether the drugs were in fact slowly leaking out of the hydrophobic phase of the emulsion.

Other examples reported in Table 31.3 highlight the difficulty encountered in normalizing drug release rates to maintain a desired drug/drug ratio. In the case of vincristine/quercetin, poly(D,L-lactide-*co*-glycolide) (PLGA) nanoparticles could be used to successful encapsulate both drugs; however, an *in vitro* release assay revealed that quercetin release was considerably slower than the more hydrophilic vincristine [54]. This disparity may be ameliorated by the very high quercetin/vincristine ratio of 1000 : 1, such that a large proportion of the quercetin could be released *in vivo* relative to vincristine yet the particle would still manage to maintain a high ratio.

Lammers *et al.* [46] and Na *et al.* [47] (entries 2 and 3, Table 31.3) demonstrate two possible means to achieve similar drug retention in a polymer micelle. Lammers *et al.* utilized a *N*-(2-hydroxypropyl)methacrylamide (HMPA)-based polymer backbone with doxorubicin and gemcitabine covalently tethered via a hydrolyzable amide linkage to the polymer chain. Subsequent study of the enzymatic release of the parent drugs from the backbone indicated that the hydrolysis rate was likely dependent on the drug structure, as shown by the very rapid hydrolysis of the conjugated gemcitabine from the backbone (virtually 100% in 10 h) compared to the sluggish cleavage of doxorubicin (around 10% at 10 h) [46].

Na *et al.* chose to formulate two separate particles, each using a different polymer to encapsulate doxorubicin (poly(γ-benzyl-L-glutamate) and poly(ethylene oxide)) and paclitaxel (poly(L-lactide)-*b*-PEG). The admixture of the two polymer micelles showed similar release rates for both drugs. As noted earlier, however, due to the use of two different polymers, it would be critical to investigate the biodistribution of both particles to ensure the active agents are delivered to the tumor site at the desired ratio [47].

While the example formulations listed in Table 31.3 illustrate the progress made in the development of drug carriers as vehicles for combination chemotherapy, it is clear that few formulations fully address the criteria for an ideal drug delivery vehicle previously described. In most of the examples, some attention has been paid to the normalization of retention/release rates of the encapsulated drugs to ensure that appreciable amounts of each drug arrive at the tumor site. Few reports, however, consider the established importance (see Table 31.1) of the drug/drug ratio within the carrier. These two criteria are closely linked. Prior to development of a nanoscale drug carrier for combination chemotherapy, the ratio and concentration dependence of the drug pair should be thoroughly investigated since by virtue of encapsulating the two drugs within a liposome or nanoparticle, one is intrinsically choosing a drug/drug ratio. Therefore, it is critical to clearly establish at which ratios the two drugs may have synergistic, antagonistic, or additive interactions. Once an appropriate drug/drug ratio is identified (see Table 31.1), the formulation goal is to develop a particulate carrier system(s) that can maintain the desired ratio *in vivo*.

To illustrate the interplay between the *in vitro/in vivo* informatics of drug interactions and formulation of particulate carrier systems, we consider the example of a liposomal dual formulation of doxorubicin and vincristine reported by Abraham *et al.* [50]. The formulation was developed using a 55 : 45 blend of 1,2-distearoyl-sn-glycero-3-phosphatidylcholine (DSPC) and cholesterol, and utilized a manganese sulfate gradient to facilitate the encapsulation of doxorubicin to a drug/lipid ratio of 0.2 : 1. Vincristine proved to be more difficult to encapsulate and required the addition of an ionophore (A23187) to achieve a drug/lipid ratio of 0.05 : 1 and a final doxorubicin/vincristine ratio of 4 : 1. Plasma elimination studies showed that doxorubicin was well retained with the liposomes as shown by maintenance of a roughly 0.2 : 1 drug/lipid ratio in mouse plasma. Vincristine, however, would leak to approximately 33% of its original concentration over 24 h. This drug leakage lead to a change in the drug/drug ratio from the original 4 : 1 doxorubicin/vincristine to nearly 20 : 1 over 24 h [50].

When administered to mice inoculated with MDA435/LCC6 tumors, the greatest growth delay of 16 days was observed with free doxorubicin administered at 10 mg/kg (time to reach 0.2 g tumor weight: 55 ± 3 days). The coencapsulated doxorubicin/vincristine liposome administered at 10 : 2.5 mg/kg was less effective, with a tumor growth delay of 12.5 days (time to reach 0.2 g tumor weight: 52 ± 2 days), despite the *addition* of 2.5 mg/kg vincristine.

To rationalize this result, *in vitro* cytotoxicity studies (using MDA435/LCC6 human breast cancer cells) were conducted on 4 : 1, 7 : 1, and 20 : 1 doxorubicin/vincristine ratios (Figure 31.3), and analyzed by the median effect method for drug synergy. As the ratios increased, the concentration required to kill 90% of the tumor cells (IC_{90} values) for vincristine were significantly higher when given in combination with doxorubicin compared to free vincristine. This result

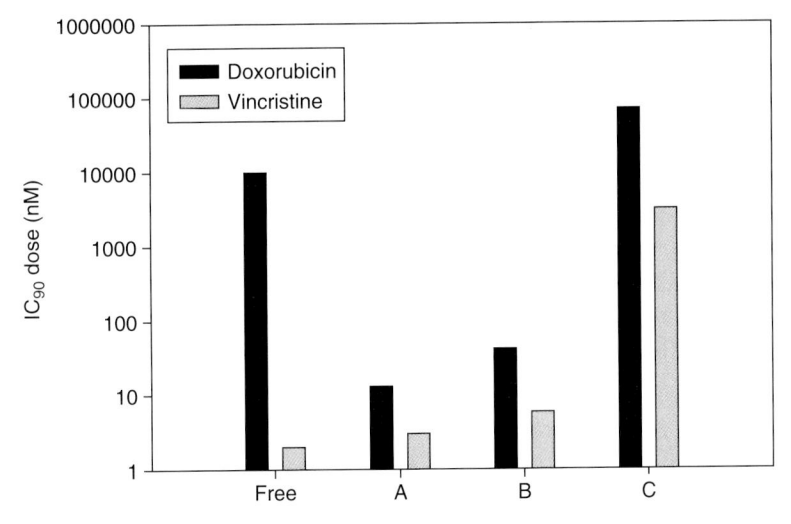

Figure 31.3 Cytotoxicity (IC_{90}) of doxorubicin and vincristine combinations in MDA435/LCC6 human breast cancer cells (Free: IC_{90} values of doxorubicin and vincristine individually; (A) 4 : 1 doxorubicin/vincristine; (B) 7 : 1 doxorubicin/vincristine; (C) 20 : 1 doxorubicin/vincristine). All drug ratios are reported as mol/mol. (Reprinted with permission from [50].)

was indicative of an antagonistic drug interaction at the ratios studied. This antagonism peaked at 20 : 1 ratio of doxorubicin/vincristine in which the IC_{90} values for both drugs given as a combination were much higher than for the free individual drugs (doxorubicin: more than 10 µM versus 10 µM for the free drug; vincristine: around 3 µM for the combination versus around 2 nM for the free drug). Therefore, the reduced *in vivo* efficacy of the liposomal combination compared to free doxorubicin is likely a result of generation of antagonistic drug/drug ratios within the liposome. It is unadvisable, therefore, to generate nanoscale carriers for combination chemotherapy without first considering drug/drug ratios at which they may interact antagonistically. Equally important is to generate particle systems that can maintain the desired ratio *in vivo* such that tumor cells are exposed to synergistic drug/drug ratios while avoiding antagonistic interactions [50].

31.4
Liposome-Based CombiPlex® Formulations

Formulations developed using the CombiPlex approach (entries 1, 8, and 9, Table 31.3) have been reported that do account for the ratio and concentration dependence of drug interactions and utilize a carrier system that allow for *in vivo* maintenance of synergistic drug ratios [31, 35–43]. These formulations, listed in Table 31.4, encompass a wide variety of drug classes from topoisomerase I inhibitors

Table 31.4 Combination chemotherapy drug delivery systems developed using the CombiPlex approach.

Formulation	Drugs		Ratio	Formulation	Indication	Development
	A	B				
CPX-1	irinotecan	floxuridine	1 : 1	dual	colorectal	phase II
CPX-351	cytarabine	daunorubicin	5 : 1	dual	AML	phase II
CPX-571	irinotecan	cisplatin	7 : 1	singly	NSCLC	preclinical

to DNA-reactive species, and have been developed using both the dual and singly formulated strategies discussed previously. The improved preclinical and clinical efficacy of these formulations over the equivalent free drug cocktails demonstrate that importance of these two criteria in the development of a nanoscale delivery vehicle for combination chemotherapy. The following sections will describe the application of the CombiPlex approach to several clinically utilized chemotherapy combinations, with the resultant improvements observed in both preclinical and clinical studies.

31.4.1
Preclinical Development of CombiPlex Formulations

31.4.1.1 CPX-351 (Cytarabine/Daunorubicin) Liposome Injection

Despite the widespread use of cytarabine/daunorubicin combination treatment for acute myelogenous leukemia (AML), there has been little research focused on understanding the interactions between these two drugs on a cellular level. Maintenance of drug ratios is likely to be relevant to this combination, since the standard first-line induction regimen for AML patients administers cytarabine as a 7-day continuous infusion while daunorubicin is provided as a bolus injection on days 1–3 [66], resulting in exposure of leukemia cells to this chemotherapy doublet at constantly changing ratios.

31.4.1.1.1 Preclinical Pharmacology of CPX-351
When tested for drug ratio-dependent synergy in a panel of 15 tumor lines *in vitro*, the combination of cytarabine and daunorubicin displayed drug ratio-dependent synergy where favorable interactions were most frequently observed when cytarabine was in excess of daunorubicin [39], with synergy maximized at a 5 : 1 ratio. Nanoscale (100 nm) liposomes were engineered that coencapsulated and maintained the two agents at the synergistic 5 : 1 molar ratio through the use of a Cu(II)-mediated drug loading mechanism [67], a technology based on the known interactions of cytarabine and daunorubicin with Cu(II) [68–70]. In addition, the CPX-351 liposomes employed low cholesterol liposomes composed of DSPC/1,2-distearoyl-*sn*-glycero-3-phosphatidylglycerol (DSPG)/cholesterol (7 : 2 : 1 molar

ratio) which have been shown to exhibit unique properties for controlling the release rates of nucleoside analogs such as cytarabine [58], thereby facilitating the coordination of cytarabine retention kinetics with daunorubicin. When administered to mice, rats, and dogs, the formulated 5 : 1 molar ratio of cytarabine/daunorubicin was maintained in plasma for up to 48 h [31, 71, 72]. In addition, the plasma drug/lipid ratio decayed over time and metabolites of both drugs could be detected in plasma, indicating that the drugs were released from the liposomes and made bioavailable over time.

The drug ratio dependency and superiority of the 5 : 1 molar ratio *in vivo* was confirmed with these delivery systems in preclinical leukemia efficacy studies. Specifically, the drug ratio-dependent synergy trends observed *in vitro* mirrored the maximum efficacy achievable in a P388 leukemia model when the two drugs where administered in liposomes at cytarabine/daunorubicin molar ratios ranging from 1 : 1 to 10 : 1 (Figure 31.4). Of particular interest was the observation that administration of the liposomal combination at a 5 : 1 ratio (CPX-351) produced 100% long-term survival, whereas the drugs delivered at a 3 : 1 molar ratio of cytarabine/daunorubicin provided only 50% long-term survival despite administering nearly twice as much daunorubicin compared to CPX-351. CPX-351 exhibited markedly superior therapeutic activity compared to the free-drug cocktail

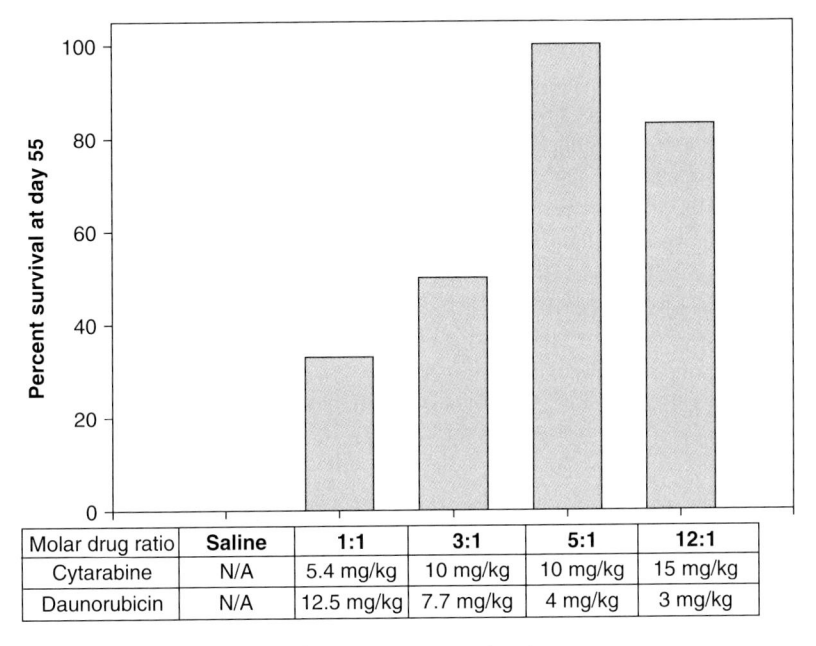

Molar drug ratio	Saline	1:1	3:1	5:1	12:1
Cytarabine	N/A	5.4 mg/kg	10 mg/kg	10 mg/kg	15 mg/kg
Daunorubicin	N/A	12.5 mg/kg	7.7 mg/kg	4 mg/kg	3 mg/kg

Figure 31.4 Percent survival of P388 ascites tumor-bearing BDF-1 mice at day 55 following intravenous treatment with saline or liposomal cytarabine/daunorubicin (day 1, 4, and 7) at different drug molar ratios ($n = 6$, all formulations dosed at MTD, except CPX-351 (5 : 1) at 0.8 MTD). (Reprinted with permission from [39].)

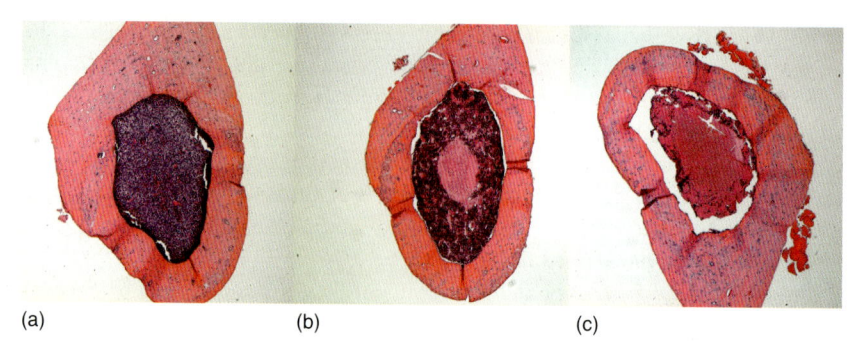

Figure 31.5 Cross-section images of hematoxylin and eosin-stained femurs engrafted with CCRF-CEM human leukemia cells taken from mice treated intravenously (day 21, 23, and 25) with saline (a), cytarabine/daunorubicin free drug cocktail (MTD, b), and CPX-351 (MTD, c). All images were acquired at 1 day post-treatment. The CCRF-CEM cells are stained blue in the above images. (Adapted from data presented in [75].)

in all leukemia models tested, with high proportions of long-term survivors, and evidence of *in vivo* synergy under conditions where the free drug cocktail provided minimal efficacy [39]. Importantly, this increased activity was selective for leukemia cells as an increase in toxicity to normal bone marrow was not observed for CPX-351 [73].

An example of the increased efficacy with CPX-351 is shown in Figure 31.5 (bone marrow cross-section) where its therapeutic effects are compared with free drug cocktail treatment at MTD in mice bearing bone marrow-engrafted human leukemia. In the absence of treatment, the bone marrow is completely overrun with human leukemia cells within 21 days of intravenous tumor inoculation. Free cytarabine/daunorubicin administered at its MTD caused a modest reduction of leukemia cells in the bone marrow as evidenced by the femur cross-sections and these mice succumbed to their leukemia shortly after treatment terminated. In contrast, the bone marrows of mice treated with CPX-351 were completely ablated of tumor cells and survival of the mice was extended by multiple weeks. It has also been demonstrated that CPX-351 persists in the bone marrow for days and there is evidence that the liposome-encapsulated drugs are taken up directly by leukemia cells [73, 74]. These results clearly demonstrate that liposomes are able to translate drug ratio informatics from *in vitro* to *in vivo* where synergistic interactions can be exploited to maximize efficacy for cytarabine/daunorubicin combinations.

31.4.1.2 CPX-1 (Floxuridine/Irinotecan) Liposome Injection

The combination of irinotecan plus fluorinated pyrimidine, typically 5-fluorouracil (5-FU), is a standard chemotherapy combination for the treatment of metastatic colorectal cancer. This combination was developed in a manner typical for most chemotherapy regimens where escalating doses of irinotecan were added to existing 5-FU regimens until dose-limiting toxicities (DLTs) were observed [76]. Subsequent trials demonstrated that the therapeutic effects of the combination were superior to that for 5-FU plus leucovorin alone [77]. In the FOLFIRI regimen used today, irinotecan is administered biweekly as a 90-min infusion of 180 mg/m^2 on day 1 and 5-FU is administered starting with a bolus loading dose of 400 mg/m^2 followed by a continuous infusion of 2.4–3 g/m^2 over 46 h starting on day 1. Consequently, irinotecan/fluoropyrimidine ratios are continuously changing during the course of therapy, with the possibility of tumor cells being exposed to antagonistic drug ratios should this combination exhibit drug ratio-dependent synergy. It should be noted that for the application of CombiPlex technology to maintain drug ratios with liposomal delivery vehicles, floxuridine rather than 5-FU was selected for evaluation of drug ratio-dependent synergy due to the fact that floxuridine displayed enhanced retention in liposomes. In addition, previous studies have demonstrated the clinical equivalency of floxuridine with 5-FU in comparative clinical trials [78].

31.4.1.2.1 Preclinical Pharmacology of CPX-1 Combinations of irinotecan and floxuridine were examined for drug ratio-dependent synergy *in vitro* in a panel of tumor cell lines with molar drug ratios ranging from 10 : 1 to 1 : 10. The 1 : 1 molar ratio of irinotecan/floxuridine was frequently synergistic and avoided antagonism, whereas other ratios exhibited a loss of synergy and in some cases the appearance of strong antagonism (e.g., 10 : 1 ratio). Similar to the case of cytarabine and daunorubicin, irinotecan and floxuridine were coencapsulated into 100-nm DSPC/DSPG/cholesterol (7 : 2 : 1 molar ratio) liposomes containing copper gluconate [43]. Not only did this formulation maintain the 1 : 1 molar ratio of the two drugs for prolonged times in the plasma, but CPX-1 selectively delivered the 1 : 1 irinotecan/floxuridine ratio to solid tumors [43]. When tested in a range of murine and human xenograft solid tumor models, CPX-1 consistently provided dramatic improvements in therapeutic efficacy over the unencapsulated free irinotecan/floxuridine "cocktail." An example of this enhanced efficacy is shown in Figure 31.6a where the efficacy of CPX-1 against the Capan-1 solid tumor model was compared to that achievable with the MTD dose of the free drug cocktail. CPX-1 produced 100% tumor regression and long-term cures, whereas the free drug cocktail provided only modest inhibition of tumor growth. Figure 31.6b demonstrates that this result was related to drug ratio-dependent synergy rather than simply liposome-mediated altered pharmacokinetics, as the efficacy of a liposome-encapsulated antagonistic ratio is compared to the individual liposomal agents. Adding floxuridine to irinotecan at a ratio shown to be antagonistic *in vitro* resulted in a significant reduction of antitumor activity such that the combination was actually markedly less efficacious than liposomal irinotecan alone.

31.4.1.3 CombiPlex Systems for Reactive Agents: CPX-571
Coencapsulation of two drugs within a single liposome can pose problems in cases where one or both of the agents are sufficiently reactive to cause or be susceptible to degradation due to drug–drug chemical interactions. In such cases, separate liposomes can be utilized to compartmentalize each drug separately, thereby eliminating deleterious drug–drug interactions while maintaining (or in some

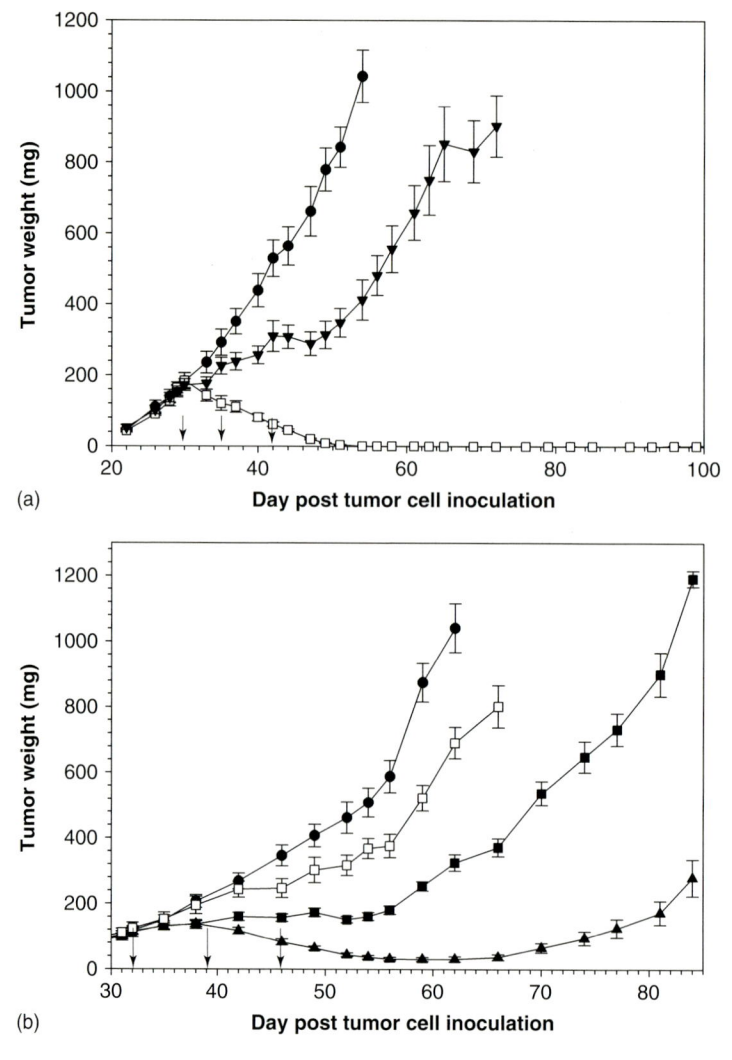

Figure 31.6 (a) Efficacy of CPX-1 (□, 25 : 9.25 mg/kg irinotecan/floxuridine) versus free drug cocktail (▼, 100 : 37 mg/kg irinotecan/floxuridine) in the Capan-1 human pancreatic tumor xenograft model. (b) Efficacy of liposome-encapsulated antagonistic ratio versus individual drugs in the Capan-1 pancreatic tumor xenograft model (□, liposomal floxuridine, 18.5 mg/kg; ■, antagonistic liposomal irinotecan/floxuridine (1 : 10 mol/mol) 5 : 18.5 mg/kg; ▲, liposomal irinotecan, 5 mg/kg); (●, saline). (Reprinted with permission from [79].)

cases increasing) the flexibility of controlling drug ratios *in vivo* by manipulating the composition of the individual liposome carriers.

Cisplatin and irinotecan are an active drug combination that has demonstrated equivalent to superior efficacy in treating extensive stage small-cell lung cancer patients compared to the current standard of care, cisplatin plus etoposide [80].

In vitro evaluation of this drug combination for drug ratio-dependent synergy in an expanded 20 tumor cell line panel revealed an "island" of antagonism for irinotecan/cisplatin molar ratios between 1 : 2 and 4 : 1 (see Table 31.2). In contrast, drug ratios above 4 : 1 consistently displayed synergy and no antagonism was observed. When cisplatin and irinotecan were coencapsulated at synergistic ratios inside low cholesterol liposomes; however, significant degradation of irinotecan was observed over short (e.g., 24 h) time periods. Cisplatin is an anticancer drug whose antitumor activity is mediated by DNA damage induced by platinum–DNA adducts formed via the reactive dichloro/diaquo coordination ligands. Consequently, it may not be surprising that it is not suitable for coencapsulation with other agents containing reactive chemical moieties such as those within irinotecan. Despite its reactivity, cisplatin has been successfully encapsulated in liposomes as a single agent and a sterically stabilized liposome formulation has been evaluated in the clinic [81–83]. Unfortunately, despite being well tolerated, this formulation did not exhibit significant therapeutic activity in patients. The lack of efficacy of this formulation was speculated to be due to the very slow release rate and associated low bioavailability of cisplatin from the liposome [84].

31.4.1.3.1 Preclinical Pharmacology of CPX-571 In view of the adverse drug–drug chemical interactions between cisplatin and irinotecan and the ability to stably encapsulate cisplatin alone in liposomes, the approach taken to generate a CombiPlex formulation of this combination was to encapsulate each agent separately in liposomes that would release both drugs at the same rate, thereby maintaining and exposing the desired drug ratio after *in vivo* administration while avoiding drug degradation reactions. Iterative manipulations of the lipid composition and internal aqueous buffer components were performed in order to identify a liposome composition into which cisplatin and irinotecan could be individually encapsulated while achieving coordinated plasma pharmacokinetic properties utilizing a drug release rate that would optimize cisplatin's therapeutic activity. This was accomplished employing a "blended acyl chain" version of 100 nm low cholesterol liposomes composed of DSPC/1,2-dipalmitoyl-*sn*-glycero-3-phosphatidylcholine (DPPC)/1,2-dipalmitoyl-*sn*-glycero-3-phosphatidylglycerol (DPPG)/cholesterol at a molar ratio of 35 : 35 : 20 : 10 [35]. The approach of utilizing separate liposomes also facilitated the evaluation of drug ratio dependency *in vivo* since alterations in the drug ratio merely required the addition of different amounts of the individual liposomal cisplatin and liposomal irinotecan components. Pharmacokinetic analysis in mice demonstrated that the injected drug ratio could be maintained in plasma for up to 24 h postinjection regardless of the starting irinotecan/cisplatin ratio and efficacy studies demonstrated that the drug ratio-dependent therapeutic activity *in vivo* correlated with the trends observed *in vitro* [35]. This led to a dramatic increase in efficacy compared to the free drug cocktail in a range of solid tumor models and evidence of strong synergy *in vivo* as presented in Figure 31.7.

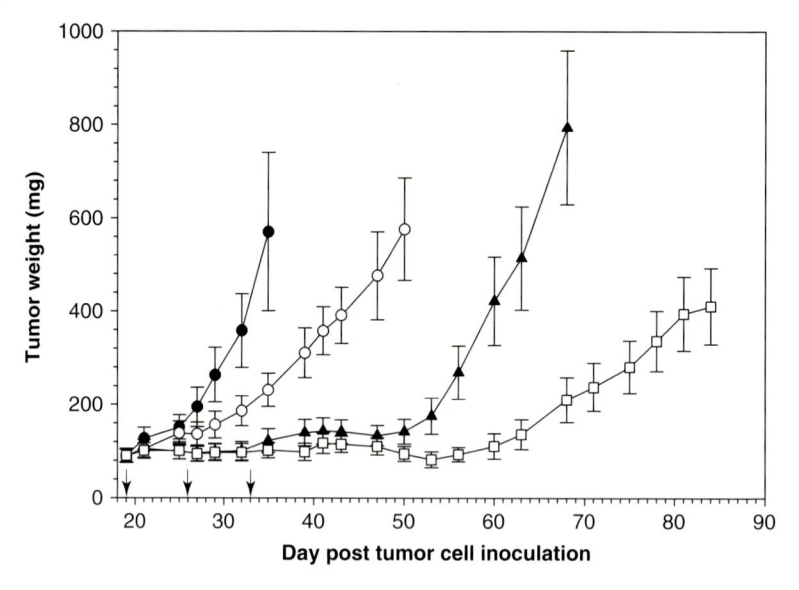

Figure 31.7 Antitumor efficacy of free drug cocktail and CPX-571 in the irinotecan-resistant HCT-116IR colon tumor xenograft model (q7d × 3 injection schedule, arrows denote injection days). Mice received injections of (●) saline, (○) liposomal cisplatin at 3 mg/kg, (▲) liposomal irinotecan at 47 mg/kg, or (□) liposomal irinotecan/cisplatin (7 : 1 molar ratio) at 47 : 3 mg/kg. (Reprinted with permission from [35].)

31.5
Clinical Studies of CombiPlex Formulations

31.5.1
Clinical Activity of CPX-351

Based on the promising preclinical results described above, CPX-351 was advanced into a phase I dose-escalation clinical trial in advanced leukemia patients [85, 86]. The toxicity profile of CPX-351 was expected to be similar to that of conventional cytarabine and daunorubicin based on results from Good Laboratory Practice (GLP) toxicology studies. Of the 48 patients entered on the study, 43 had AML. The starting dose for the phase I trial was 3 units/m², where 1 unit of CPX-351 = 1 mg cytarabine plus 0.44 mg daunorubicin, which was 1/10th the LD_{10} for the most sensitive species in GLP toxicology studies. Single-patient cohorts and dose doublings were permitted until evidence of a pharmacodynamic effect was observed. At the 24 unit/m² dose level decreases in bone marrow cellularity were observed in three of five patients, triggering a switch to three patients per cohort and 33% dose escalations for the remainder of the study. A single induction course was three doses to be given on days 1, 3, and 5, with each dose administered as a 90-min infusion, a design to mimic conventional 7 + 3 cytarabine/daunorubicin therapy. Patients were to have AML (multiply relapsed, refractory or with first complete response (CR) duration of 6 months or less); however, patients with advanced acute lymphoblastic leukemia and high-risk myelodysplastic syndrome were also eligible.

DLTs were observed at the 10th dose level: 134 units/m^2 (134 mg cytarabine plus 59 mg daunorubicin), which included hypertensive crisis, reduced cardiac function, shortness of breath, and persistent cytopenia. Some of the DLTs responded well to medical intervention; however, the prolonged cytopenia was considered dose limiting and consequently the MTD of CPX-351 was declared at 101 units/m^2 (101 mg cytarabine, 44 mg daunorubicin). The dose level of CPX-351 is comparable to the current standard of care for newly diagnosed AML patients, the "7 + 3" treatment regimen of 100 mg/m^2/day cytarabine infusion for 7 days with 60 mg/m^2 of daunorubicin administered once a day for 3 days. To minimize the risk of cardiac toxicity the phase II protocols exclude patients with significant pre-existing cardiac disease and extensive prior exposure to anthracyclines.

Gastrointestinal toxicities appeared to be less frequent and less severe than expected for conventional 7 + 3 cytarabine/daunorubicin therapy. Safety data has been tabulated for the 37 patients treated on the escalation phase of the study, 15 of whom were treated at doses of 101 units/m^2 or above. No gastrointestinal DLTs have been observed at doses of 101 units/m^2 and below, and only a single patient suffered grade 3 mucositis. Approximately half the patients suffered no gastrointestinal toxicity of any grade. Alopecia has been infrequent. Final conclusions concerning relative toxicities await completion of data collection from the extension phase of the phase I study where every patient was treated with 101 units/m^2 (MTD). It is also important to note that pharmacokinetic analysis has confirmed that the 5 : 1 molar ratio of cytarabine/daunorubicin is maintained for over 24 h in the plasma of patients treated with CPX-351. In addition, the absolute plasma concentrations of both drugs are significantly higher than expected for conventional 7 + 3 cytarabine/daunorubicin treatment where readily measurable drug levels are present 7 days after the last injection of CPX-351.

Once the MTD was identified, additional AML patients in first relapse were added as an extension cohort to provide further information on the safety of CPX-351 as well as early indications of antileukemic activity. Of the 43 AML patients entering the study, 22 patients were treated with CPX-351 after multiple relapses or multiple treatment regimens, 17 after relapse from a first CR, and 5 after no response to initial induction treatment. For the AML patients that were in second to fourth salvage treatment, CPX-351 induced CR in two patients and in a third, a complete response with incomplete platelet recovery (CRp) was obtained. In the refractory patient group, one subject treated at 134 units/m^2 achieved CR. This patient was initially treated with 7 + 3 cytarabine/daunorubicin, but did not respond. This provided early evidence that ratiometric dosing of cytarabine/daunorubicin may significantly improve therapeutic activity since CPX-351 may be effective against AML patients for which the same two drugs administered in conventional format were ineffective.

Seventeen patients on the phase I trial were treated with CPX-351 in first relapse. Seven of these were aged 60 years or under, while 10 were over 60 years old. Of the patients in the younger group, aplasia was achieved in all seven patients and CR was achieved in four patients. When compared with historical databases for AML patients in which the likelihood of achieving a CR were correlated with treatment history [87], the number of CRs achieved with CPX-351 in the total phase I patient population (9 CR + 1 CRp) was higher than predicted for these AML patients from the database (5.6 CR) despite the fact that over half of the patients were treated with CPX-351 below the MTD. Clearly, the current database with CPX-351 is very small and hence such comparisons must be put in context. However, taken together, the CRs observed with CPX-351 are very promising and suggestive that it may provide meaningful improvements over conventional cytarabine/daunorubicin therapy. These results have supported the initiation of two 120-patient randomized phase II trials with CPX-351; one in newly diagnosed elderly AML patients [88] and the second in AML patients 65 years and under in first relapse. In both trials CPX-351 is being compared to standard-of-care treatment, which for the newly diagnosed patients is conventional 7 + 3 cytarabine/daunorubicin. The results of these trials will provide important confirmation of the promising results obtained to date and establish clinical proof-of-principle for the benefits associated with drug delivery vehicle-mediated ratiometric dosing.

31.5.2
Clinical Activity of CPX-1

31.5.2.1 Phase I Clinical Trial of CPX-1

The promising preclinical results described above supported testing of CPX-1 in a phase I dose escalation clinical trial in patients with advanced solid tumors [89]. Circulating drug levels (irinotecan, SN-38, floxuridine, and 5-FU) were measured in the plasma of all patients following CPX-1 treatment, indicating that the target 1 : 1 molar ratio of irinotecan/floxuridine was maintained in the plasma of all patients for 8–12 h and in many cases up to 24 h [89].

The toxicity profile of CPX-1 was expected to be similar to that of conventional irinotecan and floxuridine based on results from GLP toxicology studies. The starting dose for the phase I trial was 30 units/m^2, where 1 unit of CPX-1 = 1 mg irinotecan plus 0.37 mg floxuridine, which was 1/10th the LD$_{10}$ for the most sensitive species in GLP toxicology studies. Dose escalation followed a modified Fibonacci design with four patients per cohort. CPX-1 was dosed as a 90-min infusion on days 1 and 15 of a 28-day cycle.

As DLTs occurred in four patients in Cycle 1 of Cohort 6 (270 units/m^2), the MTD was considered to have been exceeded. Thus, an additional two patients were enrolled at the next lowest dose level (Cohort 5, 210 units/m^2). None of the six patients at the 210 units/m^2 dose level had DLTs; this dose level was declared the MTD. The MTD of CPX-1 (210 mg/m^2 irinotecan, 77 mg/m^2 floxuridine) is similar to that of the commonly used FOLFIRI regimen (folinic acid (leucovorin) (200 mg/m^2) with 5-FU (400 mg/m^2 bolus followed by 46 h continuous infusion of 4600 mg/m^2) and irinotecan (180 mg/m^2)). Subsequently, seven patients with colorectal cancer were enrolled at 210 units/m^2 to obtain additional safety and efficacy data. Severe adverse events that were dose related included grade 3 or 4 diarrhea (24.2%), neutropenia (12.1%), and hypokalemia (12.1%). Gastrointestinal toxicities were present at all dose levels, but severity and duration increased with higher doses. Selected grade 3/4 events (diarrhea, neutropenia, nausea/vomiting, or fatigue) occurred in nine of 24 patients with no prior irinotecan therapy and five of nine patients with prior irinotecan therapy.

CR, partial response (PR), stable disease (SD), and progressive disease (PD) were evaluable in 30 of 33 patients. Three patients achieved a PR, 21 patients achieved SD, and six patients had PD. PR occurred in three of 25 (12%) subjects evaluable by RECIST criteria. Disease control (CR, PR, or SD) was observed in 11 of 15 (73.3%) patients with colorectal cancer. Among the 18 subjects with other tumor types, 1 PR (non-small-cell lung cancer (NSCLC)) and 11 SD were observed. Progression-free survival (PFS) lasting greater than 6 months was observed in six patients with colorectal cancer, and one patient each with pancreatic, ovarian, and NSCLC. The median PFS among colorectal cancer patients was 5.4 months. Surprisingly, colorectal cancer patients with prior exposure to irinotecan had no reduction in PFS compared to patients who were irinotecan-naive. These PFS results were greater than may be expected based on the literature for conventional FOLFIRI (folinic acid (leucovorin) with 5-FU and irinotecan) treatment [90], particularly in patients previously treated with irinotecan. Particularly notable was the observation that for three of the patients previously treated with irinotecan the PFS duration was significantly longer following CPX-1 treatment than was observed with the prior treatment with an irinotecan-containing regimen.

31.5.2.2 Phase II Clinical Trials of CPX-1

In view of the high level of disease control observed in the phase I trial as well as the positive results obtained in colorectal patients regardless of prior irinotecan exposure, CPX-1 was evaluated in colorectal cancer patients in a phase II setting [91]. A dose of 210 units/m^2 was administered biweekly to patients that were either irinotecan naïve (Arm A, 26 patients) or irinotecan refractory (Arm B, 33 patients). The independently audited PFS was followed for each patient. In both arms, CPX-1 exceeded the historical PFS performance of current therapies as reported from large phase III trials of current second-line (irinotecan-naïve receiving FOLFIRI) and third-line (irinotecan-refractory receiving best supportive care) therapies. For CPX-1 in second line, the PFS of irinotecan-naïve colorectal cancer patients compared favorably with that reported by Tournigard et al. [90] for second-line FOLFIRI treatment of colorectal cancer patients that progressed after FOLFOX (folinic acid with 5-FU and oxaliplatin) treatment. The median PFS, response rate, and overall disease control rate for CPX-1 were all greater than achieved for FOLFIRI [90]. Similar results were obtained in the irinotecan refractory arm. Although no confirmed PRs were achieved in this patient population, the proportion of patients benefiting from CPX-1 treatment and the duration of tumor growth delay were similar to the documented response of irinotecan refractory patients to the approved agent panitumumab [92]. Specifically, 20% of patients treated with CPX-1 exhibited PFS values of greater than 6 months compared to 15% reported previously for patients treated with panitumumab.

31.6
CombiPlex Formulations of Hydrophobic Agents

A strength of the CombiPlex ratiometric dosing platform is the inherent adaptability of the delivery vehicle that can be applied to achieve coordinated pharmacokinetics and maintain synergistic drug ratios *in vivo*. Above, we demonstrated the marked improvements in antitumor efficacy that can be achieved by fixing synergistic drug ratios through encapsulation of two drugs within a single liposome. These delivery systems have been shown to be capable of maintaining drug/drug ratios of disparate classes of drugs (e.g., topoisomerase I isomerase inhibitors (irinotecan), antimetabolites (floxuridine, cytarabine), and anthracycline antibiotics (daunorubicin)). We have also described applying the singly formulated strategy to achieve ratiometric dosing of reactive agents such as cisplatin and irinotecan formulated in separate vehicles. Each example discussed above involved liposomal encapsulation of hydrophilic drugs – a task to which liposomes are ideally suited. Recently, we demonstrated that the CombiPlex approach can also be used with hydrophobic drugs, such as the taxanes. Such drugs are typically difficult to stably encapsulate within a liposome, therefore amphipathic copolymer nanoparticles were used as the drug carrier. In this section, we describe the use of a novel nanoparticle approach to deliver combinations containing highly hydrophobic drugs such as paclitaxel, in which the properties of the prodrug and not the active agent dictate the *in vivo* release rate from the nanoparticle.

31.6.1
Nanoparticle CombiPlex Formulations for Delivering Drug Combinations Containing Hydrophobic Agents

While liposomes are well suited for delivering drugs that are water soluble or amphipathic, agents that are strongly hydrophobic present significant formulation challenges, particularly in the context of controlling drug release rates and *in vivo* pharmacokinetic properties. This is due to the fact that although hydrophobic drugs can often be incorporated into the bilayer membrane of liposomes with suitable stability properties as an injectable pharmaceutical, such drugs tend to exchange out of the liposomes very rapidly when the formulation is injected *in vivo*. For example, when a liposome formulation of paclitaxel was injected into rats, the earliest plasma drug concentration analyzed indicated that over 90% of the drug was eliminated in less than 1 h postadministration [93]. Such rapid drug release precludes the application of ratiometric dosing for drugs such as taxanes. This is particularly germane if one considers the coordinated delivery of very hydrophobic drugs with agents that are very water soluble, such as gemcitabine – a drug that is currently used in combination with paclitaxel for the treatment of breast cancer [94].

Many attempts to increase the circulation lifetime of hydrophobic drugs such as taxanes and nonamphipathic camptothecins [95, 96] have conjugated these agents to highly water-soluble polymers such as PEG [97–99], polypeptides [100–102], and polylactides [103]. However, another approach taken has been to conjugate all agents, both hydrophobic and hydrophilic, to extremely hydrophobic hydrocarbon anchors via linkers capable of regenerating the parent drug upon hydrolysis [104]. Mixing such hydrophobic prodrugs with appropriate amounts of amphipathic surface stabilizing agents (e.g., block copolymers comprised of hydrophobic and hydrophilic PEG sections) leads to the spontaneous formation of nanoscale (20–100 nm) solid core nanoparticles [105, 106]. The rationale of this strategy is that making all drugs sufficiently hydrophobic will allow their pharmacokinetic properties to be dictated by the distribution properties of the nanoparticle as well as the hydrolysis kinetics of the linker chemistry rather than the hydrophobic/hydrophilic partitioning properties of the parent drugs in order to maintain synergistic drug ratios *in vivo*.

This technology platform was iteratively optimized by testing the relationship of anchor hydrophobicity and linker lability with pharmacokinetic and efficacy properties using paclitaxel as a model compound. Hydrophobic paclitaxel prodrugs with varying linker and lipid anchor constructs were formulated into 20–30 nm diameter nanoparticles stabilized using 1-palmitoyl-2-oleyl-sn-glycero-phosphatidylcholine (POPC) and polystyrene–PEG block copolymers. These formulations were evaluated for plasma drug elimination kinetics after intravenous administration to mice in order to determine the influence of linker lability and anchor hydrophobicity on drug circulation lifetime [104]. Paclitaxel linked to a very hydrophobic tocopherol anchor via a succinate linker demonstrated slow drug elimination kinetics that were dictated predominantly by the intact nanoparticle as revealed by labeling the particle with radioactive nonmetabolizable cholesterylhexadecyl ether (CHE) where the prodrug/particle ratio remained constant over 24 h. This formulation, however, exhibited negligible efficacy against HT-29 solid tumor xenografts, which indicated the need to maintain bioavailability of the parent drug in order to obtain significant *in vivo* antitumor activity. This was accomplished by conjugating paclitaxel to hydrophobic anchors via the more labile diglycolate linker. Increased bioavailability was observed for these prodrug constructs and the drug plasma elimination kinetics could be systematically varied by altering the hydrophobicity of the lipid anchor. As shown in Figure 31.8, paclitaxel conjugated to oleyl alcohol displayed very rapid plasma elimination kinetics (only 10% of injected dose remaining after 4 h), whereas unsaturated C22 : 0 and cholesterol anchors provided increased circulation longevity with 20–30% of the administered prodrug remaining in the plasma 24 h after injection [104]. The rate of paclitaxel/prodrug release from the nanoparticles could be determined by normalizing plasma drug levels to circulating nanoparticle concentration (as determined by radiolabeled CHE content). This revealed that parent drug release half-lives increased from 1 to 2 h for unsaturated and saturated

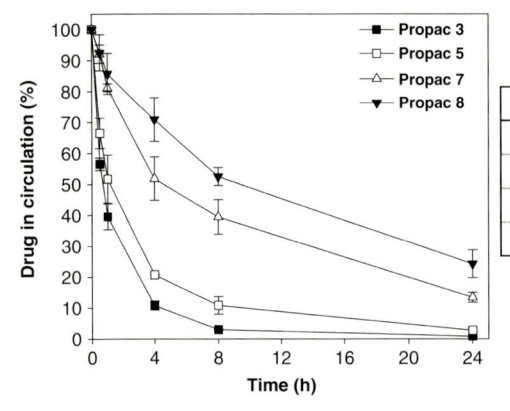

Produrg	Anchor	Release halflife
Propac3	C18:1	1 h
Propac5	C18:0	2 h
Propac7	C22:0	12 h
Propac8	Cholesterol	24 h

Figure 31.8 Elimination of paclitaxel prodrugs (Propac) formulated as 1 : 1 : 2 (w/w) prodrug/POPC/PEG2000-*b*-polystyrene3000 (2kPS3k) formulations and administered intravenously to athymic nude Foxn1^{nu} mice at 7 mg/kg ($n = 3$/timepoint, error bars represent standard deviation). Plasma release half-lives of the prodrugs were determined by subtracting the plasma elimination rate of radiolabeled nanoparticles from the observed plasma elimination profiles of each prodrug, as described in the text. CX:Y refers to the length of the carbon chain anchor (X) and degree of unsaturation (Y) of the lipophilic anchor. (Adapted from [104, 107].)

C18 lipid anchors to 12–24 h for the more hydrophobic C22:0 and cholesterol anchors, respectively.

The effect of linker chemistry and anchor hydrophobicity prodrug pharmacokinetic behavior was correlated with *in vivo* therapeutic activity against HT-29 human colorectal cancer solid tumor xenografts. This was completed by comparing the tumor growth inhibition properties of various nanoparticles after intravenous administration at the same dose based on paclitaxel molar equivalents and at lower dose levels to facilitate differentiation of therapeutic activity. Only diglycolate-linked prodrugs, not those that possessed the succinate linker, exhibited significant antitumor activity. Within the diglycolate series, increasing the hydrophobicity of the lipid anchor (from C18 : 1 up to C22 : 0) markedly increased tumor growth inhibition. Full dose-escalation efficacy studies comparing the most active C22 : 0 (Propac7) and cholesterol (Propac8) paclitaxel prodrug nanoparticles to conventional Taxol® were then completed to determine the maximum therapeutic improvement achievable for the nanoparticle formulation when both drugs were dosed at MTD. Propac8 nanoparticles were able to achieve a significant proportion of complete tumor regression and tumor regrowth was delayed approximately 6 weeks beyond that achieved for the Taxol-treated group. It is also important to note that pilot studies have provided evidence that these nanoparticles accumulate and remain in tumor tissue for prolonged periods of time due to the enhanced penetration and retention (EPR) effects associated with small particulate drug delivery vehicles [107].

Once the relationship between linker/anchor construct and therapeutic efficacy was established, application of this nanoparticle technology to coformulate

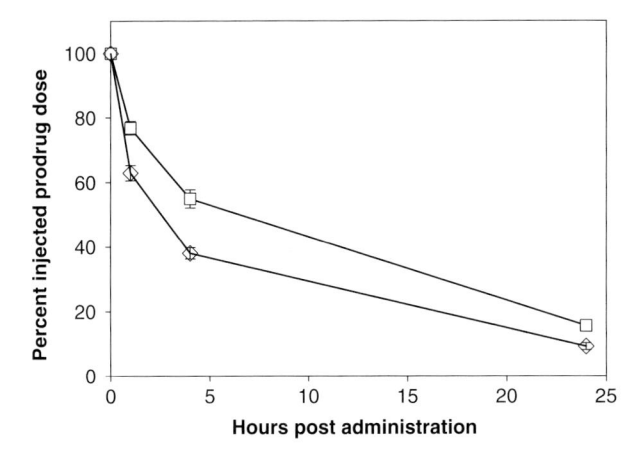

Figure 31.9 Plasma elimination of Propac7 (□) and Progem12 (◇) prodrugs coformulated as Propac/Progem/POPC/PEG2000-b-polystyrene3000 (2kPS3k) (4 : 1 : 2 : 8 w/w). Error bars represent standard deviation. (Adapted from data presented in [104].)

combinations of agents that were hydrophobic (paclitaxel) and hydrophilic (gemcitabine) was investigated. For gemcitabine, single aliphatic anchors were insufficiently hydrophobic to retain the prodrug in nanoparticles for extended times. However, conjugating gemcitabine to diacyl glycerol (C18 : 0, Progem12) enabled the prodrug to be stably incorporated into nanoparticles and when coformulated with paclitaxel conjugated via a diglycolate linker to a C22 : 0 anchor (Propac7), the two prodrugs exhibited coordinated pharmacokinetics and maintenance of the formulated paclitaxel/gemcitabine ratio after intravenous administration (Figure 31.9). These results demonstrate that the hydrophobic prodrug-based nanoparticle approach is capable of coordinating the pharmacokinetics and maintaining synergistic ratios of agents that would otherwise be unsuitable for coformulation in liposomes or passively incorporated nanoparticles. This technology therefore expands the scope of drug combinations that can be evaluated for the benefits of drug delivery vehicle-based ratiometric dosing.

31.7
Conclusions

The systematic analysis of anticancer drug combinations for drug ratio-dependent synergy *in vitro* has uncovered a previously unrecognized parameter that may impact the ultimate effectiveness of combination chemotherapy regimens in treating cancer. Increasing evidence indicates that many drug combinations exhibit antagonism at specific ratios which suggests that many existing chemotherapy cocktails may, in fact, be less efficacious than expected based on additive activity. While this represents a potential shortcoming for conventional chemotherapy cocktails, the ability to control drug ratios *in vivo* through the use of nanoscale drug delivery vehicles provides the opportunity to exploit this phenomenon by locking in synergistic drug ratios while avoiding antagonistic ones. The use of liposomes and hydrophobic produg nanoparticles to coordinate the pharmacokinetics of coformulated drugs and maintain synergistic drug ratios *in vivo* opens the possibility to prospectively exploit *in vitro* informatics on drug ratio dependency for improved therapeutic outcomes. Preclinical and early clinical evidence obtained for synergistic, fixed-ratio drug combinations indicates that this may indeed be achievable.

References

1. Frei, E. III and Freireich, E.J. (1964) Leukemia. *Sci. Am.*, **210**, 88–96.
2. Freireich, E.J. and Frei, E. III (1964) Recent advances in acute leukemia. *Prog. Hematol.*, **27**, 187–202.
3. Frei, E. III (1991) in *Synergism and Antagonism in Chemotherapy* (eds T. Chou and D. Rideout), Academic Press, San Diego, CA, pp. 103–108.
4. Cunningham, D., Humblet, Y., Siena, S., Khayat, D., Bleiberg, H., Santoro, A., Bets, D., Mueser, M., Harstrick, A., Verslype, C., Chau, I., and Van Cutsem, E. (2004) Cetuximab monotherapy and cetuximab plus irinotecan in irinotecan-refractory metastatic colorectal cancer. *N. Engl. J. Med.*, **351**, 337–345.
5. Shah, M.H., Varker, K.A., Collamore, M., Zwiebel, J.A., Coit, D., Kelsen, D., and Chung, K.Y. (2009) G3139 (Genasense) in patients with advanced merkel cell carcinoma. *Am. J. Clin. Oncol.*, **32**, 174–179.
6. Tolcher, A.W., Chi, K., Kuhn, J., Gleave, M., Patnaik, A., Takimoto, C., Schwartz, G., Thompson, I., Berg, K., D'Aloisio, S., Murray, N., Frankel, S.R., Izbicka, E., and Rowinsky, E. (2005) A phase II, pharmacokinetic, and biological correlative study of oblimersen sodium and docetaxel in patients with hormone-refractory prostate cancer. *Clin. Cancer Res.*, **11**, 3854–3861.
7. Giantonio, B.J., Catalano, P.J., Meropol, N.J., O'Dwyer, P.J., Mitchell, E.P., Alberts, S.R., Schwartz, M.A., and Benson, A.B. III (2007) Bevacizumab in combination with oxaliplatin, fluorouracil, and leucovorin (FOLFOX4) for previously treated metastatic colorectal cancer: results from the Eastern Cooperative Oncology Group study E3200. *J. Clin. Oncol.*, **25**, 1539–1544.
8. Bokemeyer, C., Bondarenko, I., Makhson, A., Hartmann, J.T., Aparicio, J., de Braud, F., Donea, S., Ludwing, H., Schuch, G., Stroh, C., Loos, A.H., Zubel, A., and Koralewski, P. (2009) Fluorouracil, leucovorin, and oxaliplatin with and without cetuximab in the first-line treatment of metastatic colorectal cancer. *J. Clin. Oncol.*, **27**, 663–671.
9. Van Cutsem, E., Kohne, C.H., Hitre, E., Zaluski, J., Chang Chien, C.R., Makhson, A., D'Haens, G., Pinter, T., Lim, R., Bodoky, G., Roh, J.K., Folprecht, G., Ruff, P., Stroh, C., Tejpar, S., Schlichting, M., Nippgen, J., and Rougier, P. (2009) Cetuximab and chemotherapy as initial treatment for metastatic colorectal cancer. *N. Engl. J. Med.*, **360**, 1408–1417.
10. Oakervee, H.E., Popat, R., Curry, N., Smith, P., Morris, C., Drake, M., Agrawal, S., Stec, J., Schenkein, D., Esseltine, D.-L., and Cavenagh, J.D. (2005) PAD combination therapy (PS-341/bortezomib, doxorubicin and dexamethasone) for previously untreated patients with multiple myeloma. *Br. J. Haematol.*, **129**, 755–762.
11. Geyer, C.E., Forster, J., Lindquist, D., Chan, S., Romieu, C.G., Pienkowski, T., Jagiello-Gruszfeld, A., Crown, J., Chan, A., Kaufman, B., Skarlos, D., Campone, M., Davidson, N., Berger, M., Oliva, C., Rubin, S.D., Stein, S., and Cameron, D. (2006) Lapatinib plus capecitabine for HER-positive advanced breast cancer. *N. Engl. J. Med.*, **355**, 2733–2743.
12. Gatzemeier, U., Pluzanska, A., Szczesna, A., Kaukel, E., Roubec, J., De Rosa, F., Milnowski, J.,

Karnicka-Mlodkowski, H., Pesek, M., Serwatowski, P., Ramlau, R., Janaskova, T., Vansteenkiste, J., Strausz, J., Manikhas, G.M., and Von Pawl, J. (2007) Phase III study of erlotinib in combination with cisplatin and gemcitabine in advanced non-small-cell lung cancer: the Tarceva lung cancer investigation trial. *J. Clin. Oncol.*, **25**, 1545–1552.

13. Moore, M.J., Goldstein, D., Hamm, J., Figer, A., Hecht, J.R., Gallinger, S., Au, H.J., Murawa, P., Walde, D., Wolff, R.A., Campos, D., Lim, R., Ding, K., Clark, G., Voskoglou-Nomikos, T., Ptasynski, M., and Parulekar, W. (2007) Erlotinib plus gemcitabine compared with gemcitabine alone in patients with advanced pancreatic cancer: a phase III trial of the National Cancer Institute of Canada Clinical Trials Group. *J. Clin. Oncol.*, **25**, 1960–1966.

14. Erler, J.T. and Lindling, R. (2010) Network-based drugs and biomarkers. *J. Pathol.*, **220**, 290–296.

15. Borisy, A.A., Elliot, P.J., Hurst, N.W., Lee, M.S., Lehar, J., Price, E.R., Serbedzija, G., Zimmermann, G.R., Foley, M.A., Stockwell, B.R., and Keith, C.T. (2003) Systematic discovery of multicomponent therapeutics. *Proc. Natl. Acad. Sci. USA*, **100**, 7977–7982.

16. Keith, C.T., Borisy, A.A., and Stockwell, B.R. (2005) Multicomponent therapeutics for networked systems. *Nat. Rev. Drug Discov.*, **4**, 1–8.

17. Lehar, J., Zimmermann, G.R., Krueger, A.S., Molnar, R.A., Ledell, J.T., Heilbut, A.M., Short, G.F. III, Giusti, L.C., Nolan, G.P., Magid, O.A., Lee, M.S., Borisy, A.A., Stockwell, B.R., and Keith, C.T. (2007) Chemical combination effects predict connectivity in biological systems. *Mol. Syst. Biol.*, **3**, 1–14.

18. Lee, M.S., Johansen, L., Zhang, Y., Wilson, A., Keegan, M., Avery, W., Elliott, P., Borisy, A.A., and Keith, C.T. (2007) The novel combination of chlorpromazine and pentamidine exerts synergistic antiproliferative effects through dual mitotic action. *Cancer Res.*, **67**, 11359–11365.

19. Dancey, J.E. and Chen, H.X. (2006) Strategies for optimizing combinations of molecularly targeted anticancer agents. *Nat. Rev. Drug Discov.*, **5**, 649–659.

20. Chou, T.C. (2008) Preclinical versus clinical drug combination studies. *Leuk. Lymphoma*, **49**, 2059–2080.

21. Greco, W.R., Bravo, G., and Parsons, J.C. (1995) The search for synergy: a critical review from a response surface perspective. *Pharmacol. Rev.*, **47**, 331–385.

22. Harasym, T.O., Liboiron, B.D., and Mayer, L.D. (2010) Drug ratio-dependent antagonism: a new category of multidrug resistance and strategies for its circumvention. *Methods Mol. Biol.* **596**, 291–323.

23. Chou, T.C. (1991) in *Synergism and Antagonism in Chemotherapy* (eds T.C. Chou and D.C. Rideout), Academic Press, New York, pp. 61–102.

24. Chou, T.C. (2006) Theoretical basis, experimental design, and computerized simulation of synergsim and antagonism in drug combination studies. *Pharmacol. Rev.*, **58**, 621–681.

25. Chou, T.C. and Talalay, P. (1984) Quantitative analysis of dose-effect relationships: the combined effects of multiple drugs or enzyme inhibitors. *Adv. Enzyme Regul.*, **22**, 27–55.

26. Loewe, S. (1953) The problem of synergism and antagonism of combined drugs. *Arzneim. Forsch.*, **3**, 285–290.

27. Prichard, M.N. and Shipman, C. Jr. (1990) A three dimensional model to analyze drug–drug interactions (review). *Antiviral Res.*, **14**, 181–206.

28. Gore, S.D. (2005) Combination therapy with DNA methyltransferase inhibitors in hematologic malignancies. *Nat. Clin. Pract. Oncol.*, **2**, S30–S35.

29. Plimack, E.R., Kantarjian, H.M., and Issa, J.P. (2007) Decitabine and its role in the treatment of hematopoietic malignancies. *Leuk. Lymphoma*, **48**, 1472–1481.

30. Harasym, T.O., Tardi, P.G., Johnstone, S.A., Mayer, L.D., Bally, M.B., and Janoff, A.S. (2007) Fixed drug ratio liposome formulations of combination cancer therapeutics in *Liposome Technology*, Interactions of Liposomes with Biological Milieu, vol. III , 3rd edn (ed.

G. Gregoriadis), Informa Healthcare, New York, pp. 25–46.

31. Mayer, L.D., Harasym, T.O., Tardi, P.G., Harasym, N.L., Shew, C.R., Johnstone, S.A., Ramsay, E.C., Bally, M.B., and Janoff, A.S. (2006) Ratiometric dosing of anticancer drug combinations: controlling drug ratios after systemic administration regulates therapeutic activity in tumor-bearing mice. *Mol. Cancer Ther.*, **5**, 1854–1863.

32. Pavillard, V., Kherfellah, D., Richard, S., Robert, J., and Montaudon, D. (2001) Effects of the combination of camptothecin and doxorubicin or etoposide on rat glioma cells and camptothecin-resistant variants. *Br. J. Cancer*, **85**, 1077–1083.

33. Swaffar, D.S., Ang, C.Y., Desai, P.B., Rosenthal, G.A., Thomas, D.A., Crooks, P.A., and John, W.J. (1995) Combination therapy with 5-fluorouracil and L-canavanine: *in vitro* and *in vivo* studies. *Anti-Cancer Drugs*, **6**, 586–593.

34. Johnston, J.S., Johnson, A., Gan, Y., Wientjes, M.G., and Au, J.L. (2003) Synergy between 3′-azido-3′-deoxythymideine and paclitaxel in human pharynx FaDu cells. *Pharm. Res.*, **20**, 957–961.

35. Tardi, P.G., Dos Santos, N., Harasym, T.O., Johnstone, S.A., Zisman, N., Tsang, A.W., Bermudes, D.G., and Mayer, L.D. (2009) Drug ratio-dependent antitumor activity of irinotecan and cisplatin combinations *in vitro* and *in vivo*. *Mol. Cancer Ther.*, **8**, 2266–2275.

36. Engblom, P., Rantanen, V., Kulmala, J., Helenius, H., and Grenman, S. (1999) Additive and supra-additive cytotoxicity of cisplatin-taxane combinations in ovarian carcinoma cell lines. *Br. J. Cancer*, **79**, 286–292.

37. Raitanen, M., Rantanen, V., Kulmala, J., Helenius, H., Grenman, R., and Grenman, S. (2002) Supra-additive effect with concurrent paclitaxel and cisplatin in vulvar squamous cell carcinoma in vitro. *Int. J. Cancer*, **100**, 238–243.

38. Adams, D.J., Sandvold, M.L., Myhren, F., Jacobsen, T.F., Giles, F., and Rizzieri, D.A. (2008) Anti proliferative activity of ELACY (CP-4055) in combination with cloretazine (VNP40101M), idarubicin, gemcitabine, irinotecan and topetecan in human leukemia and lymphoma cells. *Leuk. Lymphoma*, **49**, 786–797.

39. Tardi, P.G., Johnstone, S.A., Harasym, N.L., Xie, S., Harasym, T.O., Zisman, N., Harvie, P., Bermudes, D., and Mayer, L.D. (2009) In vivo maintenance of synergistic cytarabine/daunorubicin ratios greatly enhances therapeutic efficacy. *Leuk. Res.*, **33**, 129–139.

40. Xu, J.M., Azzariti, A., Colucci, G., and Paradiso, A. (2003) The effect of gefitinib (Iressa, ZD1839) in combinatin with oxaliplatin is schedule-dependent in colon cancer cell lines. *Cancer Chemother. Pharmacol*, **52**, 442–448.

41. Shanks, R.H., Rizzieri, D.A., Flowers, J.L., Colvin, O.M., and Adams, D.J., (2005) Preclinical evidence of gemcitabine combination regimens for application in acute myeloid leukemia. *Clin. Cancer Res.*, **11**, 4225–4233.

42. Aung, T.T., Davis, M.A., Ensminger, W.D., and Lawrence, T.S., (2000) Interaction between gemcitabine and mitomycin-C in vitro. *Cancer Chemother. Pharmacol.*, **45**, 38–42.

43. Harasym, T.O., Tardi, P.G., Harasym, N.L., Harvie, P., Johnstone, S.A., and Mayer, L.D. (2007) Increased preclinical efficacy of irinotecan and floxuridine coencapsulated inside liposomes is associated with tumor delivery of synergistic drug ratios. *Oncol. Res.*, **16**, 361–374.

44. Kanzawa, F., Koizumi, F., Koh, Y., Nakamura, T., Tatsumi, Y., Fukumoto, H., Saijo, N., Yoshioka, T., Nishio, K., (2001) In vitro synergistic interactions between the cisplatin analogue nedaplatin and the DNA topoisomerase I inhibitor irinotecan and the mechanism of this interactions. *Clin. Cancer Res.*, **7**, 202–209.

45. Mercalli, A., Sordi, V., Formicola, R., Dandrea, M., Beghelli, S., Scarpa, A., Di Carlo, V., Reni, M., Piemonti, L., (2007) A preclinical evaluation of pemetrexed and irinotecan combination as second-line chemotherapy in pancreatic cancer. *Br. J. Cancer*, **96**, 1358–1367.

46. Lammers, T., Subr, V., Ulbrich, K., Peschke, P., Huber, P.E., Hennink, W.E., and Storm, G. (2009) Simultaneous delivery of doxorubicin and

gemcitatine to tumors *in vivo* using prototypic polymeric drug carriers. *Biomaterials*, **30**, 3466–3475.

47. Na, H.S., Lim, Y.K., Jeong, Y.I., Lee, H.S., Lim, Y.J., Kang, M.S., Cho, C.S., and Lee, H.C. (2010) Combination antitumor effects of micelle-loaded anticancer drugs in a CT-26 murine colorectal carcinoma model. *Int. J. Pharm.*, **383**, 192–200.

48. Wu, J., Lu, Y., Lee, A., Pan, X., Yang, X., Zhao, X., and Lee, R.J. (2007) Reversal of multidrug resistance by transferrin-conjugated liposomes co-encapsulating doxorubicin and verapamil. *J. Pharm. Pharm. Sci.*, **10**, 350–357.

49. Wang, J., Goh, B., Lu, W., Zhang, Q., Chang, A., Liu, X.Y., Tan, T.M.C., and Lee, H. (2005) *In vitro* cytotoxicity of stealth liposomes co-encapsulating doxorubicin and verapamil on doxorubicin-resistant tumour cells. *Biol. Pharm. Bull.*, **28**, 822–828.

50. Abraham, S.A., McKenzie, C., Masin, D., Ng, R., Harasym, T.O., Mayer, L.D., and Bally, M.B. (2004) *In vitro* and *in vivo* characterization of doxorubicin and vincristine coencapsulated within liposomes through use of transition metal ion complexation and pH gradient loading. *Clin. Cancer Res.*, **10**, 728–738.

51. Zhao, X., Wu, J., Muthusamy, N., Byrd, J.C., and Lee, R.J. (2008) Liposomal coencapsulated fludarabine and mitoxantrone for lymphoproliferative disorder treatment. *J. Pharm. Sci.*, **97**, 1508–1518.

52. Li, X., Lu, W.L., Liang, G.W., Ruan, G.R., Hong, H.Y., Long, C., Zhang, Y.T., Liu, Y., Wang, J.C., Zhang, X., and Zhang, Q. (2006) Effect of stealthy liposomal topotecan plus amlodipine on the multidrug-resistant leukaemia cells *in vitro* and xenograft in mice. *Eur. J. Clin. Invest.*, **36**, 409–418.

53. Du, J., Lu, W.L., Ying, X., Liu, Y., Du, P., Tian, W., Men, Y., Guo, J., Zhang, Y., Li, R.J., Zhou, J., Lou, J.N., Wang, J.C., Zhang, X., and Zhang, Q. (2009) Dual-targeting topotecan liposomes modified with tamoxifen and wheat germ agglutinin significantly improve drug transport across the blood–brain barrier and survival of brain tumor-bearing animals. *Mol. Pharm.*, **6**, 905–917.

54. Song, X., Zhao, Y., Hou, S., Xu, F., Zhao, R., He, J., Cai, Z., Li, Y., and Chen, Q. (2008) Dual agents loaded PLGA nanoparticles: systematic study of particle size and drug entrapment efficiency. *Eur. J. Pharm. Biopharm.*, **69**, 445–453.

55. Liu, X.Y., Lu, W.L., Guo, J., Du, J., Li, T., Wu, J.W., Wang, G.L., Wang, J.C., Zhang, X., and Zhang, Q. (2008) A potential target associated with both breast cancer and cancer stem cells: a combination therapy for eradication of breast cancer using vinorelbine stealthy liposomes plus parthenolide stealthy liposomes. *J. Control. Release*, **129**, 18–25.

56. Webb, M.S., Saxon, D., Wong, F.M., Lim, H.J., Wang, Z., Bally, M.B., Choi, L.S., Cullis, P.R., and Mayer, L.D. (1998) Comparison of different hydrophobic anchors conjugated to poly(ethyleneglycol): effects on the pharmacokinetics of liposomal vincristine. *Biochim. Biophys. Acta*, **1372**, 272–282.

57. Saxon, D., Mayer, L.D., and Bally, M.B. (1999) Liposomal anticancer drugs as agents to be used in combination with other anticancer agents: studies on a liposomal formulation with two encapsulated drugs. *J. Liposome Res.*, **9**, 507–522.

58. Tardi, P.G., Gallagher, R.C., Johnstone, S., Harasym, N., Webb, M., Bally, M.B., and Mayer, L.D. (2007) Coencapsulation of irinotecan and floxuridine into low cholesterol-containing liposomes that coordinate drug release *in vivo*. *Biochim. Biophys. Acta*, **1768**, 678–687.

59. Devalapally, H., Duan, Z., Seiden, M.V., and Amiji, M.M., (2007) Paclitaxel and ceramide co-administration in biodegradable polymeric nanoparticulate delivery system to overcome drug resistance in ovarian cancer. *Int. J. Cancer*, **121**, 1830–1838.

60. Ganta, S. and Amiji, M. (2009) Codadministration of paclitaxel and curcumin in nanoemulsion formulations to overcome multidrug resistance in tumor cells. *Mol. Pharmaceut*, **6**, 928–939.

61. Dicko, A., Frazier, A.A., Liboiron, B.D., Hinderliter, A., Ellena, J.F., Xie, X., Cho, C., Weber, T., Tardi, P.G., Cabral-Lilly, D., Cafiso, D.S., and Mayer, L.D. (2008) Intra and inter-molecular interactions dictate the aggregation state of irinotecan co-encapsulated with floxuridine inside liposomes. *Pharm. Res.*, **25**, 1702–1713.
62. Drummond, D.C., Noble, C.O., Hayes, M.E., Park, J.W., and Kirpotin, D.B. (2008) Pharmacokinetics and *in vivo* drug release rates in liposomal nanocarrier development. *J. Pharm. Sci.*, **97**, 4696–4740.
63. Johnston, M.J., Semple, S.C., Klimuk, S.K., Edwards, K., Eisenhardt, M.L., Leng, E.C., Karlsson, G., Yanko, D., and Cullis, P.R. (2006) Therapeutically optimized rates of drug release can be achieved by varying the drug-to-lipid ratio in liposomal vincristine formulations. *Biochim. Biophys. Acta*, **1758**, 55–64.
64. Lasic, D.D. and Martin, F.J. (1995) *Stealth Liposomes*, CRC Press, Boca Raton, FL.
65. Ganta, S. and Amiji, M. (2009) Coadministration of paclitaxel and curcumin in nanoemulsion formulations to overcome multidrug resistance in tumor cells. *Mol. Pharm.*, **6**, 928–939.
66. McCauley, D.L. (1992) Treatment of adult acute leukemia. *Clin. Pharm.*, **11**, 767–796.
67. Dicko, A., Kwak, S., Frazier, A.A., Mayer, L.D., and Liboiron, B.D. (2010) Biophysical characterization of a liposomal formulation of cytarabine and daunorubicin. *Int. J. Pharm.*, **391**, 248–259.
68. Berger, N.A. and Eichhorn, G.L. (1971) Interaction of metal ions with polynucleotides and related compounds XIV: nuclear magnetic resonance studies of the binding of copper(II) to adenine nucleotides. *Biochemistry*, **10**, 1847–1857.
69. Chao, Y.H. and Kearns, D.R. (1977) Magnetic resonance studies of copper(II) interaction with nucleosides and nucleotides. *J. Am. Chem. Soc.*, **99**, 6425–6534.
70. Greenaway, F.T. and Dabrowiack, J.C. (1982) The binding of copper ions to daunomycin and adriamycin. *J. Inorg. Biochem.*, **16**, 91–107.
71. Bayne, W.F., Mayer, L.D., and Swenson, C. (2009) Pharmacokinetics of CPX-351 (cytarabine/daunorubicin HCl) liposome injection in the mouse. *J. Pharm. Sci.*, **98**, 2540–2548.
72. Janoff, A., Louie, A., Swenson, C., Cabral-Lilly, D., Batist, G., Harasym, T., Tardi, P., Chiarella, M., and Mayer, L. (2006) Ratiometric dosing of anticancer drug combinations. *Mol. Cancer Ther.*, **5**, 1854–1863.
73. Lim, W.-S., Tardi, P.G., Dos Santos, N., Xie, X., Fan, M., Liboiron, B.D., Huang, X., Harasym, T.O., Bermudes, D., and Mayer, L.D. (2010) Leukemia-selective uptake and cytotoxicity of CPX-351, a synergistic fixed-ratio cytarabine:daunorubicin formulation, in bone marrow xenografts. *Leuk. Res.*, **34**, 1214–1223.
74. Kim, P., Gerhard, G., Harasym, T.O., Lim, W.-S., Zisman, N., Mayer, L.D., and Hogge, D.E. (2009) Improved selectivity against acute myeloid leukemia (AML) blasts over normal hematopoietic progenitors for cytarabine/daunorubicin delivered as CPX-351 liposome injection. *Blood*, **114**, 2071.
75. Mayer, L.D., Lim, W.-S., Dos Santos, N., Xie, S., Hopkins, A., Huang, R., Wilkins, L., Kelly, S., Bermudes, D., Harasym, T., and Tardi, P. (2008) Synergistic cytarabine:daunorubicin ratios delivered by CPX-351 to human leukemia xenografts is associated with liposome-mediated bone marrow drug accumulation, intracellular delivery of encapsulated agents to leukemia cells, and increased efficacy. *Blood*, **112**, 942.
76. Khayat, D., Gil-Delgado, M., Antoine, E.C., Coeffic, D., Benhammouda, A., Grapin, J.P., and Bastian, G. (1998) European experience with irinotecan plus fluorouracil/folinic acid or mitomycin. *Oncology*, **12**, 64–67.
77. Saltz, L.B., Cox, J.V., Blanke, C., Rosen, L.S., Fehrenbacher, L., Moore, M.J., Maroun, J.A., Ackland, S.P., Locker, P.K., Pirotta, N., Elfring, G.L., and Miller, L.L. (2000) Irinotecan plus fluororuracil and leucovorin for metastatic

colorectal cancer. *N. Engl. J. Med.*, **343**, 905–914.

78. Reitemeier, R.J., Moertel, C.G., and Hahn, R.G. (1965) Comparison of 5-fluorouracil and 5-fluoro-2′-deoxyuridine in treatment of patients with advanced adenocarcinoma of colon or rectum. *Cancer Chemother. Rep.*, **44**, 39–43.

79. Mayer, L.D. and Janoff, A.S (2007) Optimizing combination chemotherapy by controlling drug ratios. *Mol. Interv*, **7**, 216–223.

80. Evans, W.K., Shepherd, F.A., Feld, R., Osoba, D., Dang, P., and Deboer, G. (1985) VP-16 and cisplatin as first-line therapy for small-cell lung cancer. *J. Clin. Oncol.*, **3**, 1471–1477.

81. Termogt, J.M., Groenewegen, G., Pluim, D., Maliepaard, M., Tibben, M.M., Huisman, A., Ten Bokkel Huinink, W.W., Schot, M., Welbank, H., Voest, E.E., Beijnen, J.H., and Schellens, J.H.M. (2002) Phase 1 and pharmacokinetic study of SPI-77, a liposomal encapsulated dosage form of cisplatin. *Cancer Chemother. Pharmacol.*, **49**, 201–210.

82. Vail, D.M., Kurzman, I.D., Glawe, P.C., O'Brien, M.G., Chun, R., Garrett, L.D., Obradovich, J.E., Fred, R.M. III, Khanna, C., Colbern, G.T., and Working, P.K. (2002) STEALTH liposome-encapsulated cisplatin (SPI-77) versus carboplatin as adjuvant therapy for spontaneously arising osteosarcoma (OSA) in the dog: a randomized multicenter clinical trial. *Cancer Chemother. Pharmacol.*, **50**, 131–136.

83. White, S.C., Lorigan, P., Margison, G.P., Margison, J.M., Martin, F.J., Thatcher, N., Anderson, H., and Ranson, M. (2006) Phase 2 study of SPI-77 (sterically stabilized liposomal cisplatin) in advanced non-small-cell lung cancer. *Br. J. Cancer*, **95**, 822–828.

84. Bandak, S., Goren, D., Horowitz, A., Tzemach, D., and Gabizon, A. (1999) Pharmacological studies of cisplatin encapsulated in long-circulating liposomes in mouse tumor models. *Anti-Cancer Drugs*, **10**, 911–920.

85. Feldman, E., Lancet, J., Kolitz, J.E., Asatiani, E., Swenson, C., Mayer, L., Janoff, A., and Louie, A. (2007) Phase 1 study of a liposomal carrier (CPX-351) containing an optimized, synergistic, fixed molar ratio of cytarabine and daunorubicin in advanced leukemias and myelodysplastic syndromes. *Blood*, **110**, 990.

86. Feldman, E., Lancet, J., Kolitz, J.E., Asatiani, E., Mayer, L., and Louie, A. (2008) Phase 1 study of a liposomal carrier (CPX-351) containing a synergistic, fixed molar ratio of cytarabine (Ara-C) and daunorubicin (DNR) in advanced leukemias. *Blood*, **112**, 2984.

87. Estey, E., Kornblau, S., Pierce, S., Kantarjian, H.M., Beran, M., and Keatin, M. (1996) A stratification system for evaluating and selecting therapies in patients with relapsed or primary refractory acute myelogenous leukemia. *Blood*, **88**, 756.

88. Lancet, J., Feldman, E., Cortes, J., Hogge, D., Kovacsovics, T., Tallman, M., Damon, L., Solomon, S., Kolitz, J., Komrokji, R., Chiarella, M., and Louie, A. (2009) Phase 2b randomized study of CPX-351 vs. conventional cytarabine + daunorubicin in newly diagnosed AML patients aged 60–75: safety report. *Blood*, **114**, 2033.

89. Batist, G., Gelmon, K.A., Chi, K.N., Miller, W.H., Chia, S.K.L., Mayer, L.D., Swenson, C.E., Janoff, A.S., and Louie, A.C. Jr. (2009) Safety, pharmacokinetics, and efficacy of CPX-1 liposome injection in patients with advanced solid tumors. *Clin. Cancer Res.*, **15**, 692–700.

90. Tournigand, C., Andre, T., Achille, E., Lledo, G., Flesh, M., Mery-Migard, D., Quinaux, E., Couteau, C., Buyse, M., Ganem, G., Landi, B., Colin, P., Louvet, C., and de Gramont, A. (2004) FOLFIRI followed by FOLFOX6 or the reverse sequence in advanced colorectal cancer: a randomized GERCOR study. *J. Clin. Oncol.*, **22**, 1–9.

91. Batist, G., Sawyer, M.B., Gabrail, N., Christiansen, N., Marshall, J., Spigel, D., and Louie, A. (2008) A multi-center, phase 2 study of CPX-1 liposome injection in patients with advanced colorectal cancer. *J. Clin. Oncol.*, **28**, 4108.

92. Giusti, R.M., Ahstri, K.A., Cohen, M.H., Keegan, P., and Pazdur, R. (2007)

FDA drug approval summary: panitumumab (Vectibix™). *Oncologist*, **12**, 577–583.

93. Guo, W., Johnson, J.L., Khan, S., Ahmad, A., and Ahmad, I. (2005) Paclitaxel quantification in mouse plasma and tissues containing liposome-entrapped paclitaxel by liquid chromatography-tandem mass spectrometry: application to a pharmacokinetics study. *Anal. Biochem.*, **336**, 213–220.

94. Albain, K.S., Nag, S.M., Calderillo-Ruiz, G., Jordaan, J.P., Llombart, A.C., Pluzanska, A., Rolski, J., Melemed, A.S., Reyes-Vidal, J.M., Sekhon, J.S., Simms, L., and O'Shaughnessy, J. (2008) Gemcitabine plus paclitaxel versus paclitaxel monotherapy in patients with metastatic breast cancer and prior anthracycline treatment. *J. Clin. Oncol.*, **26**, 3950–3957.

95. Hu, X. and Jing, X. (2009) Biodegradable amphiphilic polymer–drug conjugate micelles. *Expert Opin. Drug Deliv.*, **6**, 1079–1090.

96. Kratz, F., Abu Ajaj, K., and Warnecke, A. (2007) Anticancer carrier-linked prodrugs in clinical trials. *Expert Opin. Invest. Drugs*, **16**, 1037–1058.

97. Fleming, A.B., Haverstick, K., and Saltzman, W.M. (2004) *In vitro* cytotoxicity and *in vivo* distribution after direct delivery of PEG–camptothecin conjugates to the rat brain. *Bioconjug. Chem.*, **15**, 1364–1375.

98. Gopin, A., Ebner, S., Attali, B., and Shabat, D. (2006) Enzymatic activation of second-generation dendritic prodrugs: conjugation of self-immolative dendrimers with poly(ethylene glycol) via click chemistry. *Bioconjug. Chem.*, **17**, 1432–1440.

99. Yu, D., Peng, P., Dharap, S.S., Wang, Y., Mehlig, M., Chandna, P., Zhao, H., Filpula, D., Yang, K., Borowski, V., Borchard, G., Zhang, Z., and Minko, T. (2005) Antitumor activity of poly(ethylene glycol)–camptothecin conjugate: the inhibition of tumor growth *in vivo*. *J. Control. Release*, **110**, 90–102.

100. Cavallaro, G., Licciardi, M., Caliceti, P., Salmaso, S., and Giammona, G. (2004) Synthesis, physico-chemical and biological characterization of a paclitaxel macromolecular prodrug. *Eur. J. Pharm. Biopharm.*, **58**, 151–159.

101. Singer, J.W., Bhatt, R., Tulinsky, J., Buhler, K.R., Heasley, E., Klein, P., and de Vries, P. (2001) Water-soluble poly-(L-glutamic acid)–Gly–camptothecin conjugates enhance camptothecin stability and efficacy *in vivo*. *J. Control. Release*, **74**, 243–247.

102. Veronese, M.L., Flaherty, K., Kramer, A., Konkle, B.A., Morgan, M., Stevenson, J.P., and O'Dwyer, P.J. (2005) Phase I study of the novel taxane CT-2103 in patients with advanced solid tumors. *Cancer Chemother. Pharmacol.*, **55**, 497–501.

103. Tong, R., Yala, L., Fan, T.M., and Cheng, J. (2010) The formulation of aptamer-coated paclitaxel–polylactide nanoconjugates and their targeting to cancer cells. *Biomaterials*, **31**, 3043–3053.

104. Ansell, S.M., Johnstone, S.A., Tardi, P.G., Lo, L., Xie, S., Shu, Y., Harasym, T.O., Harasym, N.L., Williams, L., Bermudes, D., Liboiron, B.D., Saad, W., Prud'homme, R.K., and Mayer, L.D. (2008) Modulating the therapeutic activity of nanoparticle delivered paclitaxel by manipulating the hydrophobicity of prodrug conjugates. *J. Med. Chem.*, **51**, 3288–3296.

105. Johnson, B.K. and Prud'homme, R.K. (2003) Flash nanoprecipitation of organic actives and block copolymers using a confined impinging jets mixer. *Aust. J. Chem.*, **56**, 1021–1024.

106. Johnson, B.K. and Prud'homme, R.K. (2003) Mechanism for rapid self-assembly of block copolymer nanoparticles. *Phys. Rev. Lett.*, **91**, 118302.

107. Ansell, S.M., Johnstone, S.A., Tardi, P.G., Lo, L., Beck, J., Xie, S., Bermudes, D., Prud'homme, R.K., and Mayer, L.D. (2008) Development of highly efficacious hydrophobic paclitaxel prodrugs delivered in nanoparticles for fixed-ratio drug combination applications. American Association for Cancer Research Meeting, Washington, DC, abstract 5734.

Polymer-Based Systems

Drug Delivery in Oncology: From Basic Research to Cancer Therapy, First Edition.
Edited by Felix Kratz, Peter Senter, and Henning Steinhagen.
© 2012 Wiley-VCH Verlag GmbH & Co. KGaA. Published 2012 by Wiley-VCH Verlag GmbH & Co. KGaA.

32
Micellar Structures as Drug Delivery Systems

Nobuhiro Nishiyama, Horacio Cabral, and Kazunori Kataoka

32.1
Introduction

Block copolymers, which are composed of two or more covalently-linked polymers with different physical and chemical properties, self-assemble into highly ordered nanoarchitectures such as spherical micelles (polymeric micelles), cylindrical micelles (worm- or filo-micelle), and polymer vesicles (polymersomes) in aqueous media (Figure 32.1) [1]. In the past two decades, these polymer assemblies, especially polymeric micelles, have been demonstrated to be useful as drug vehicles, because they possess several advantages, such as (i) applicability to various therapeutic agents, including hydrophobic substances, metal complexes, nucleic acids, and proteins, (ii) ease of physical loading drugs without chemical modifications, (iii) simplicity of micelle preparation, (iv) high drug loading capacity, and (v) controlled drug release [2–4]. These properties can be modulated and optimized by engineering the constituent block copolymers. Furthermore, the polymer assemblies can show prolonged circulation after systemic administration, since the drug-loaded core is surrounded by the palisade of dense water-soluble and biocompatible polymers such as poly(ethylene glycol) (PEG). Such long-circulating polymer assemblies have an opportunity to accumulate in cancerous tissues due to the vascular hyperpermeability and impaired lymphatic drainage, which is termed the enhanced permeability and retention (EPR) effect [5], when the dimensions of the assemblies are smaller than the vascular cutoff size [6]. Based on such superior properties, micellar structures have gained increasing popularity as drug vehicles and several formulations incorporating anticancer agents are currently in clinical trials [7, 8]. Recent advances in micellar structures and their molecular payload (cargo) in clinical and preclinical study are summarized in Table 32.1.

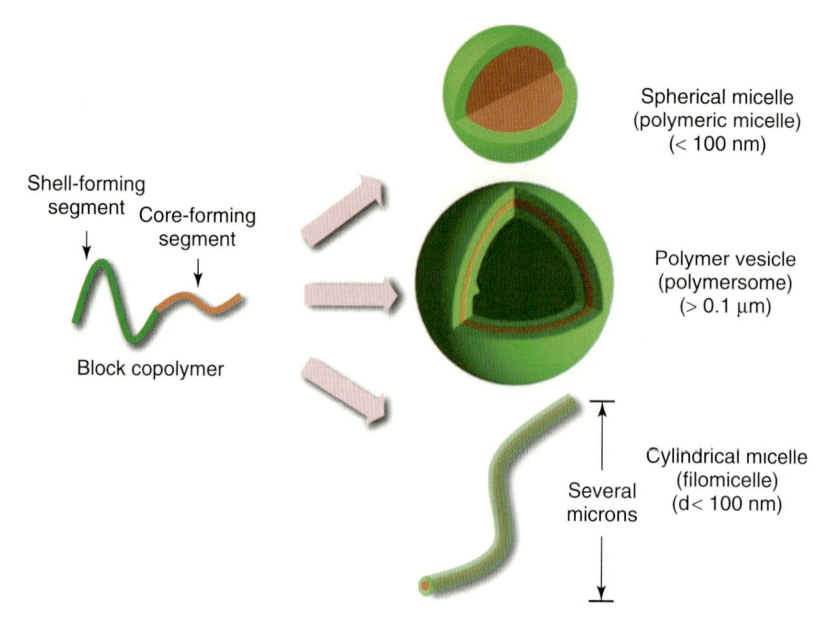

Figure 32.1 Highly ordered nanoarchitectures – spherical micelles (polymeric micelles), polymer vesicles (polymersomes), and cylindrical micelles (filo-micelles), formed through the self-assembly of block copolymers.

32.2
Rationale and Recent Advances in Micellar Structures as Drug Delivery Systems

32.2.1
Smart Polymeric Micelles for Site-Specific Drug Delivery

Smart polymeric micelles for site-specific drug delivery and their functions in cancer cell are illustrated in Figures 32.2 and 32.3, respectively. The rational design of block copolymers to construct smart polymeric micelles is described as follows.

Recently, there has been a strong incentive to develop polymeric micelles that can function in response to specific environments to cancerous tissues. It is known that the pH in the tumor microenvironment decreases to 6.6–6.8 depending on the distance from blood vessels, because anaerobic glycolysis is facilitated due to the limited oxygen supply [16]. Also, the endosomes and lysosomes in the cells produce acidic environments with a pH of 5.0–6.0. Therefore, acidic pH is a useful chemical stimulus for designing environmentally sensitive polymeric micelles. The acidic pH-sensitive polymeric micelles are assumed to minimize drug leakage during blood circulation, thereby ensuring safety in clinical use.

pH-sensitive polymeric micelles can be constructed by the use of an acid-labile bond between the drug and the carrier polymer. Although various acid-labile

Table 32.1 Recent advances in micellar structures and their molecular payload (cargo) in clinical and preclinical study.

Name	Payload	Polymer	Company	Progress	References
NK911	doxorubicin	PEG–P(Asp)–doxorubicin conjugate	Nippon Kayaku, Co., Japan	phase II	[9]
SP-1049C	doxorubicin	PEO–PPO–PEO	Supratek Pharma, Inc., Canada	phase II	[10]
Paxceed™	paclitaxel	PEG–PDLLA	Angiotech Pharmaceuticals, Inc., Canada	phase I/II	–
Genexol-PM	paclitaxel	PEG–PDLLA	Samyang Corp., South Korea	Approved in South Korea	[11]
NK105	paclitaxel	PEG–PAPB	Nippon Kayaku, Co., Japan	phase II	[12]
NK012	SN-38	PEG–P(Glu)–SN-38 conjugate	Nippon Kayaku, Co., Japan	phase II	[13]
NC-6004	cisplatin	PEG–P(Glu)	Nanocarrier, Co., Japan	phase II	[14]
NC-4016	oxaliplatin	PEG–P(Glu)	Nanocarrier, Co., Japan	phase I	[15]

P(Asp), poly(aspartic acid); PEO, poly(ethylene oxide); PPO, poly(propylene oxide); PDLLA, poly(D,L-lactic acid); PAPB, polyaspartate modified with 4-phenyl-butanol; P(Glu), poly(glutamic acid).

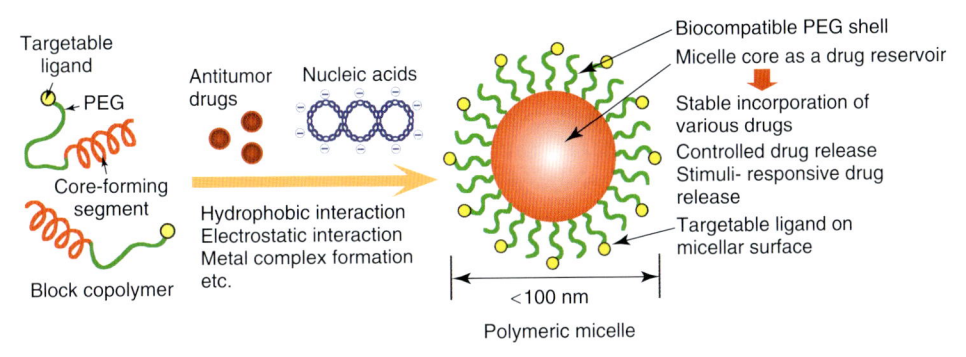

Figure 32.2 Polymeric micelles as versatile nanocarriers for site-specific delivery of antitumor drugs and nucleic acids.

polymer–drug linkages have been proposed, the hydrazone bond appears to be particularly useful for acidic pH-induced drug release [17, 18]. Since the stability of this bond is in an equilibrium, the cleavage of the bond occurs over a wide range of pH and the rate of the cleavage is affected by the proton concentration. Importantly, although cleavage of the hydrazone bond can be induced by dilution,

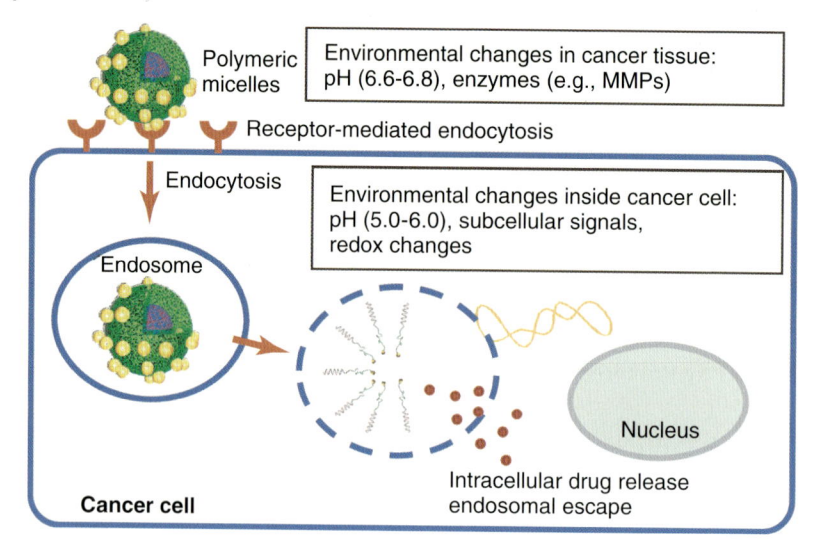

Figure 32.3 Functions of smart polymeric micelles responding to environmental changes in cancer tissue and cell.

the micellar structures prevent it because the environments in the micellar core are not affected by dilution. Nevertheless, the micellar structures can maintain the pH sensitivity of the drug–polymer linker, since the proton can access the nanoscaled micellar core. These properties are clearly advantageous in comparison with other formulations such as polymer–drug conjugates and liposomes.

pH-sensitive polymeric micelles can also be formed by block copolymers, of which the protonation alters by the decrease in pH. For example, PEG-*b*-poly(L-histidine) copolymers act as amphiphilic copolymers to form polymeric micelles around the physiological pH (7.4). Under endo/lysosomal acidic pH conditions, however, these micelles dissociate due to substantial protonation of the poly(L-histidine) segment, leading to accelerated release of the loaded drug [19, 20]. The pH sensitivity of the micellar structures can be optimized by mixing PEG-*b*-poly(L-histidine) with pH-insensitive amphiphilic copolymers such as PEG-*b*-poly(L-lactic acid) [19].

In addition to the proton concentration, the tumor-specific enzymes and intracellular signals in cancer cells can be utilized for site-specific drug delivery. Several matrix metalloproteinases (MMPs), such as MMP-2 and MMP-9, are known to be overexpressed in the tumor tissue; therefore, the substrate peptides for MMPs are used as linkers of polymer–drug conjugation [21]. A number of protein kinases or phosphatases overexpressed in cancer cells are also available for designing enzymatically activated polymeric micelles. When synthetic polymers with a low critical solution temperature (LCST) are modified with the substrate peptides, phosphorylation or dephosphorylation of the target sequence might trigger a change in the LCST, inducing a dramatic change in the solubility of the polymers [22].

Thus, polymeric micelles containing such polymers alter their conformation to activate the loaded drugs responding to the activity of specific protein kinases or phosphatases in the cell.

Further improvement in the selectivity to the target tissue can be achieved by the modification of polymeric micelles with targetable ligands (i.e., active targeting). Targetable ligands include small molecules [19, 23, 24], carbohydrates [25], peptide [26], growth factors [27], and antibodies [28] with a high affinity to surface markers of the target cells. The use of specific ligands to cancer cells may not affect the accumulation behavior of polymeric micelles in the tumor, because the micelles need to extravasate to the tumor tissue prior to reaching cancer cells. Nevertheless, the tumor-specific ligands should contribute to local retention in the tumor and also promote cellular internalization through receptor-mediated endocytosis. It is reported that folate-conjugated micelles remarkably lowered the *in vitro* and *in vivo* effective doses of antitumor agents in folate-binding protein-overexpressing cancer cells compared with nontargeted micelles, although both micelles showed similar biodistribution [24]. Also, folate-conjugated micelles have been demonstrated to overcome multidrug resistance in cancer cells [19]. Presumably, targetable polymeric micelles may bypass the drug efflux pumps (P-glycoprotein) overexpressed on the plasma membrane of cancer cells through the active cellular internalization induced by the ligand–receptor interaction. Alternatively, the ligands specifically binding to vascular endothelial cells can be introduced to the surface of polymeric micelles. The recent advances in *in vivo* phage display technique facilitates the discovery of specific peptides to the vascular endothelium in each organ and tissue (vascular mapping) [29]. Targeting vascular endothelium cannot only increase the accumulation level at the target site, but also facilitate transport across the vascular wall even at organs or tissues where nanocarriers hardly accumulate by the EPR effect (tissue-specific delivery). In this regard, conjugation with a monoclonal antibody specific to lung caveolae enabled nanoparticles to target rat lungs after intravenous injection and undergo rapid sequential transcytosis to reach the alveolar air space [30, 31]. Surprisingly, more than 80% of injected antibodies accumulated at the target site within 30 min, which is in a marked contrast with the passive targeting that can achieve less than 10% accumulation at the tumor site after 24 or 48 h. Caveolae-mediated transcellular delivery is expected to overcome anatomical barriers such as the blood–brain barrier. Recently, the iRGD peptide (CRGDK/RGPD/EC), which was identified by *in vivo* phage display, has been demonstrated to target the tumor vasculature by its specific binding to α_v integrins, and then induce the transcytosis initiated by interaction between proteolytically truncated iRGD peptide (CRGDK/R) and neuropilin-1 [32, 33]. Therefore, the modification with iRGD peptide resulted in more than 3-fold higher accumulation of nanoparticles including polymeric micelles in a tumor-specific manner compared with nontargeted nanoparticles [32]. Such multifunctional peptides are promising candidates for the targetable ligands to construct smart polymeric micelles.

32.2.2
Polyion Complex Micelles for Gene and siRNA Delivery

Genes and small interfering RNA (siRNA) hold great promise for the treatment of intractable diseases such as genetic disorders, degenerative diseases, infections, and malignancies. The efficient gene and siRNA vectors should be a key to the practical use of such nucleic acids medicine. In this regard, nonviral synthetic vectors composed of cationic polymers, termed polyplexes, are attractive alternatives to viral vectors with potential risks of immunogenicity and mutagenicity due to the safety for clinical use, simplicity of preparation, and easy large-scale production. Polyion complex (PIC) micelles, which are formed through the electrostatic interaction between nucleic acids and oppositely charged PEG-b-polycation copolymers, have attracted increasing attention as nonviral vectors [34, 35]. PEG-b-polycation copolymers such as PEG-b-poly(L-lysine) have the ability to mask the negative charge of nucleic acids and condense them into small particles (less than 100 nm), which are suitable for cellular internalization, while protecting nucleic acids from hydrolytic and enzymatic degradations [36]. The characteristic core–shell structure of PIC micelles with a dense PEG shell provides excellent biocompatibility with remarkably reduced nonspecific adhesion of biological components such as serum proteins and blood cells. Eventually, the cellular uptake and transfection efficiency of PIC micelles are not hampered by incubation with serum. When intravenously injected to mice, PIC micelles show a longer residence in circulation compared with cationic polyplexes [37]. Nevertheless, the circulation period of PIC polyplex micelles (half-life less than 5 min) is still much shorter than that of polymeric micelles from amphiphilic copolymers (half-life more than 10 h). To improve the micellar structures even under harsh *in vivo* conditions, cross-linkers having thiol groups or hydrophobic moieties such as cholesterol derivatives were introduced into PEG-b-polycation copolymers [38–40]. The disulfide cross-linking is quite stable under extracellular conditions, while being cleaved in the cytoplasm due to 50–1000 times higher glutathione concentration inside the cells [38, 39]. Eventually, disulfide cross-linked PIC micelles showed further prolonged circulation with approximately 2–3 times longer half-lives compared with non-cross-linked micelles, without compromising the transfection ability. Alternatively, the modification of PEG-b-polycation with hydrophobic moieties can also improve the stability of PIC micelles through the hydrophobic interaction. It is worth mentioning that the introduction of a single cholesteryl group to the distal end of the polycation segment remarkably stabilized the micellar structure, achieving prolonged circulation and *in vivo* gene transfection [40].

In addition to the circulating property after systemic administration, micellar structures have several advantages as nonviral vectors. (i) PIC micelles should be safer vectors compared with cationic polyplexes. Generally, cationic polyplexes interact with negatively charged cellular membranes leading to cytotoxicity, and induce unfavorable biological reactions, such as platelet activation and cytokine production [41]. The PEG palisade of PIC micelles might weaken or prevent such polycation-derived cell death [42] and biological reactions [43]. We previously reported that the transfection to rabbit carotid artery with cationic polyplexes induced vessel occlusion by thrombus, while that by PIC micelles showing appreciable gene transfer without any vessel occlusion [43]. (ii) PIC micelles might possess higher tissue penetrability than cationic polyplexes. We demonstrated that PIC micelles show facilitated percolation and well-distributed transfection in both *in vitro* multicellular tumor spheroid models and solid tumors after intratumoral injection, whereas cationic polyplexes exhibit limited percolation and localized transfection [44]. The PEG palisade might prevent aggregation of polyplexes under physiological conditions and mask the cationic nature of the core polyplexes, preventing nonspecific interaction with serum proteins and extracellular matrices. Such prevention of aggregate formation and reduced interaction with biological components may contribute to the facilitated percolation of the polyplexes into the tumor tissue.

One of the major limitations of nonviral vectors is a relatively lower transfection efficiency compared with viral vectors. Generally, polyplex systems are internalized by endocytosis, followed by localization in endosomal and lysosomal compartments. Therefore, the polyplexes must escape from these compartments into the cytoplasm to circumvent hydrolytic and enzymatic degradation of nucleic acids. Thus, endosomal escape is a key to efficient gene and siRNA transfection. In this regard, several polycations with pK_a values in the range of physiological and endosomal pH, such as polyethylenimine [45], have been demonstrated to facilitate endosomal escape. This phenomenon is explained by the hypothetic "proton sponge effect" [45], where the protonation of polycations in the endosomal compartment causes osmotic swelling of the endosome, leading to disruption of the endosomal membrane and subsequent release of therapeutic cargo into the cytoplasm. We have recently reported that poly(N-(N-(2-aminoethyl)-2-aminoethyl)aspartamide) (PAsp(DET)) with different protonation states at neutral and acidic pH shows efficient endosomal escape [46, 47], because this polymer might exhibit minimal membrane destabilization at pH 7.4, but a remarkable membrane destabilizing effect at pH 5.5 [47]. However, PIC micelles from PEG-*b*-PAsp(DET) showed much a lower transfection efficiency compared with counterpart PAsp(DET) polyplexes [48, 49], since the interaction between polycations and cellular membranes may be essential to the destabilization of the endosomal membrane. These results motivated us to design PEG-SS-polycations, where PEG and polycations are tandemly connected through the disulfide linkage, to construct PEG-detachable PIC micelles [49]. Indeed, PEG-detachable PIC micelles from PEG-SS-PAsp(DET) displayed considerable enhancement in terms of transfection efficiency. Thus, PEGylation of the polyplexes may improve the biocompatibility for *in vivo* use but impair the membrane-destabilizing ability essential to the efficient transfection; however, such a PEG dilemma can be solved by designing PEG-detachable systems.

The transfection efficiency of PIC micelles is further improved by the introduction of ligand molecules on their surface. The ligand molecules not only improve cellular uptake of nonviral vectors, but also alter their subcellular trafficking pathways through receptor-mediated endocytosis. Clathrin-dependent endocytosis (Figure 32.4) – the most frequent internalization pathway – might transport

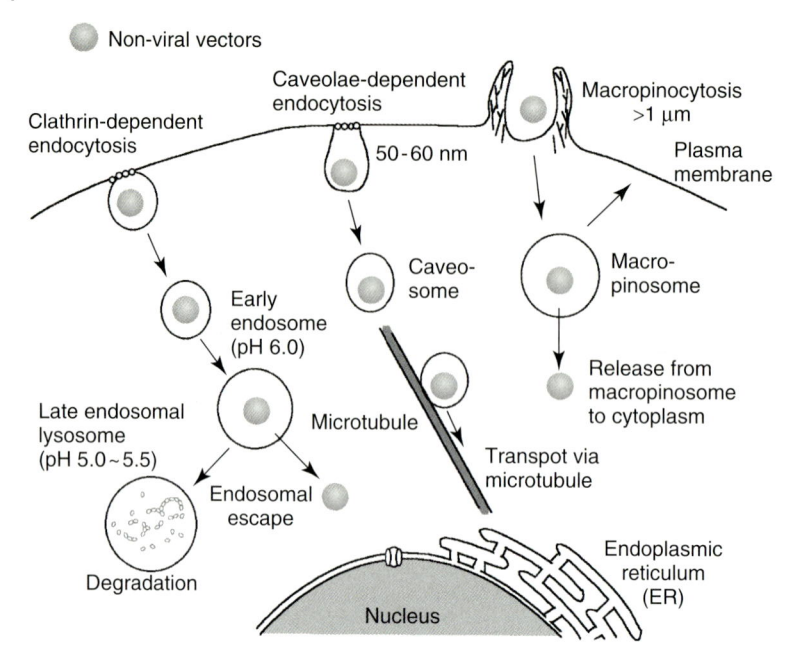

Figure 32.4 Internalization and subcellular trafficking pathways of nonviral vectors directed to efficient transfection.

nonviral vectors to acidic vesicular organelles such as the late endosome and lysosome; therefore, the endosomal escaping function is essential to successful transfection [50]. Caveolae/lipid-raft-dependent endocytosis (Figure 32.4) might deliver nonviral vectors to the caveosome with neutral pH; therefore, the vectors are not exposed to harsh endo/lysosomal acidic conditions [51]. Furthermore, the caveosome is suggested to directly reach the endoplasmic reticulum [52], facilitating nuclear transport of nonviral vectors [53]. We previously reported that PIC micelles modified with the cyclic RGD peptide, which specifically binds to $\alpha_v\beta_3$ and $\alpha_v\beta_5$ integrins overexpressed in proliferating endothelial cells and cancer cells, were internalized through caveolae-dependent endocytosis, resulting in enhanced gene transfection [54, 55]. Macropinocytosis (Figure 32.4), which is induced by several types of growth factors, is also suggested to facilitate the intracellular delivery of nonviral vectors [56]. The macropinosome, which is characterized by a relatively large size (more than 1 μm) and weakly acidic conditions, possesses more leaky membrane structures compared with the endosome and lysosome; therefore, nonviral vectors are believed to easily escape from the macropinosome to the cytoplasm [57].

32.2.3
Other Block Copolymer Assemblies

As described in Section 32.1, block copolymers self-assemble into other highly ordered nanoarchitectures such as cylindrical micelles (worm- or filo-micelle) [58] and polymer vesicles (polymersomes) [1, 59]. Among them, polymersomes have received considerable attention as drug vehicles. Polymersomes can incorporate hydrophobic substances into the vesicle bilayers and encapsulate hydrophilic compounds, including nucleic acids and proteins. Compared with vesicles from phospholipids (liposomes), polymersomes have a robust membrane structure, but chemical versatility to engineer their properties as drug vehicles. After intravenous administration, polymersomes display a longer circulation period (half-life more than 24 h) compared with polymeric micelles [1], because larger particles have few opportunities to extravasate in several organs (e.g., sinusoidal capillaries in the liver have a cutoff size of 100 nm). Owing to such outstanding properties, increasing attention has been paid on the construction of polymersomes with smart functionalities.

The most important challenge is the controlled drug release from polymersomes. The use of PEG-b-polyesters such as PEG-b-poly(lactic acid) and PEG-b-poly(ε-caprolactone) enables sustained release of the contents via hydrolytic degradation of polyester blocks [60, 61]. This degradation can be accelerated under endo/lysosomal acidic pH conditions and might induce morphological transitions from polymersomes to micellar structures, facilitating drug release. Alternatively, smart polymersomes are constructed from block copolymers that can respond to external stimuli such as light [62], temperature [63], pH [64], and redox changes [65, 66]. For example, polymersomes composed of PEG-b-poly(propylene-sulfide)-b-PEG triblock copolymers can release their contents responding to oxidizing environments at the inflammatory sites or in the endo/lysosomal compartments through destabilization of the vesicle structure due to the oxidation-mediated transitions of poly(propylene-sulfide) to more polar poly(sulfoxides) and poly(sulfones) [66]. Another challenge is the efficient intracellular delivery of polymersomes. The modification of polymersomes with ligand molecules might facilitate their cellular internalization and enable the control of their subcellular trafficking. In this regard, polymersomes from poly(L-arginine)-b-poly(L-leucine) copolymers have been demonstrated to exhibit effective cellular internalization, because the shell of poly(L-arginine) segments may trigger transport via macropinocytosis [67], which is similar to protein-transduction domains [68]. One of the most expected applications of polymersomes should be the delivery of nucleic acids and proteins. Until now, there have been several studies regarding polymersomes for the delivery of plasmid DNA [69], siRNA [70], and proteins [71]; however, their biological properties should be further improved for practical use. The introduction of smart functionalities should be a key to successful polymersome-mediated delivery of such bioactive materials.

Recently, we have reported a novel class of polymersomes formed by simple mixing of water-soluble and oppositely charged block copolymers (a set of block aniomers and block catiomers), termed "PICsomes" [72–76]. Compared with conventional vesicles including liposomes, PICsomes possess several advantages as drug vehicles, such as simple preparation without organic solvents and easy encapsulation of water-soluble compounds [73, 76]. Also, PICsomes consist of PIC membranes sandwiched between outer and inner PEG layers, thereby showing semipermeability [73, 75, 76]. Therefore, the bioactive enzymes encapsulated into PICsomes can react the low-molecular-weight substrates, while exhibiting the resistance to protease-mediated degradation [73]. These properties suggest the utility of PICsomes as chemical reactors used under harsh *in vivo* conditions, and applications might include artificial red blood cells [77] and enzyme prodrug therapy [78]. Furthermore, we have recently succeeded in the preparation of nanoscaled PICsomes (Nano-PICsomes), of which the size can be precisely controlled in the range between 100 and 400 nm by simply changing the concentration of constituent block copolymers [76]. Cross-linking of the PIC membranes by cross-linking reagents stabilizes the structure of Nano-PICsomes even against freeze-drying and centrifugation treatment, while enabling tuning of the membrane permeability for controlled drug release [76]. Similarly to polymersomes, Nano-PICsomes have been demonstrated to show extraordinarily prolonged blood circulation, exceeding that of polymeric micelles [76].

32.2.4
Theranostic Nanodevices

Recently, increasing attention has been paid to theranostic nanodevices. A "theranostic" is defined as an integrated nanotherapeutic system, which can diagnose, deliver targeted therapy, and monitor the response to therapy [79–81]. In this regard, polymeric micelles should be ideal nanocarriers because they can incorporate multiple agents (i.e., imaging and therapeutic agents). Theranostic nanodevices can visualize their biodistribution and tumor accumulation in a real-time manner, allowing prediction of the efficacy and side-effects for successful and safe cancer therapy. Also, theranostic nanodevices can allow us to follow the therapeutic response in each cancer patient and realize early feedback of the treatment efficacy to optimize the treatment protocol for eradication of malignancies (i.e., report of efficacy). That is, theranostic nanodevices enable targeted cancer therapy customized to each patient. Furthermore, theranostic nanodevices might be useful for contrast enhancement during imaging-guided surgery to detect the surgical margin of small tumors or metastatic lesions and to map sentinel lymph nodes, because they might selectively and effectively accumulate in malignant tissues due to the EPR effect.

Recently, we have developed theranostic micelles incorporating both a platinous antitumor drug and a clinically approved magnetic resonance imaging (MRI) contrast agent, gadolinium (III)-diethylenetriaminepentaacetic acid (Gd-DTPA) complex (Figure 32.5) [82]. MRI possesses superior contrast resolution enabling us to detect and characterize noncontour deforming lesions of malignancies, and allowing us to predict the therapeutic efficacy and the prognosis in cancer patients. In our study, the theranostic micelles achieved clear detection of cancerous lesions in the abdominal cavity in an orthotopic human pancreatic cancer xenograft model by MRI [82]. Also, these theranostic micelles showed a strong antitumor activity against pancreatic cancers without any serious toxicity, of which the treatment

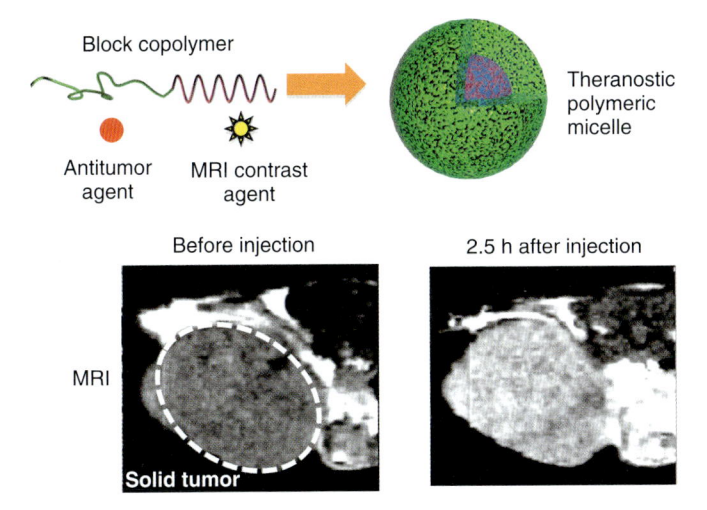

Figure 32.5 Theranostic polymeric micelles incorporating antitumor agents and MRI contrast agents, which allow simultaneous imaging and therapy of malignant tumors. Intravenous administration of theranostic micelles resulted in remarkable contrast enhancement selectively in solid tumors in T_1-weighted MRI [82].

processes were successfully visualized by MRI enhanced by theranostic micelles [82]. These results seem to be clinically important because the diagnosis and treatment of pancreatic cancer has been considered to be the most difficult among digestive cancers. Thus, theranostic micelles are expected to improve the effectiveness and safety of cancer targeting therapy.

32.3
Conclusions and Perspectives

We have reviewed recent progress in research on block copolymer assemblies as drug vehicles for cancer-targeting therapy. These assemblies incorporate various therapeutic and imaging agents, and smart functions, such as environmental sensitivity and specific tissue targetability, can be integrated to them by engineering the constituent block copolymers. Polymeric micelles have been demonstrated to show effectiveness against malignant tumors intractable by other treatments, including pancreatic tumors, and are expected to be approved for practical use in the near future. One of the most important issues in the development of polymeric micelles is the organelle-specific delivery of bioactive materials such as siRNA. On the other hand, polymersomes are emerging nanocarriers with extraordinary properties exceeding polymeric micelles, such as remarkably prolonged blood circulation (i.e., super-stealth property) and easy incorporation of water-soluble compounds, including quantum dots. These nanocarriers are expected to be theranostic nanodevices, which can diagnose, deliver targeted therapy, and monitor the response to therapy. In the near future, it will be feasible to construct smart polymeric micelles with integrated multifunctions to achieve not only controlled disposition at the tissue and cell level, but also sensing, processing, and operation at the subcellular level. Such multifunctional micellar nanodevices can be regarded as an artificial virus and will contribute to advanced medicine as well as basic science as a tool to realize *in situ* molecular biology in living animals.

References

1. Discher, D.E. and Eisenberg, A. (2002) Polymer vesicles. *Science*, **297**, 967–973.
2. Kataoka, K., Kwon, G.S., Yokoyama, M., Okano, T., and Sakurai, Y. (1993) Block copolymer micelles as vehicles for drug delivery. *J. Control. Release*, **24**, 119–132.
3. Kataoka, K., Harada, A., and Nagasaki, Y. (2001) Block copolymer micelles for drug delivery: design, characterization and biological significance. *Adv. Drug Deliv. Rev.*, **47**, 113–131.
4. Nishiyama, N. and Kataoka, K. (2006) Current state, achievements, and future prospects of polymeric micelles as nanocarriers for drug and gene delivery. *Pharmacol. Ther.*, **112**, 630–648.
5. Matsumura, Y. and Maeda, H. (1986) A new concept for macromolecular therapeutics in cancer chemotherapy: mechanism of tumoritropic accumulation of proteins and the antitumor agent Smancs. *Cancer Res.*, **46**, 6387–6392.
6. Hobbs, S.K., Monsky, W.L., Yuan, F., Roberts, W.G., Griffith, L., Torchilin, V.P., and Jain, R.K. (1998) Regulation of transport pathways in tumor vessels: role of tumor type and microenvironment. *Proc. Natl. Acad. Sci. USA*, **95**, 4607–4612.
7. Aliabadi, H.M. and Lavasanifar, A. (2006) Polymeric micelles for drug delivery. *Expert Opin. Drug Deliv.*, **3**, 139–162.
8. Matsumura, Y. and Kataoka, K. (2009) Preclinical and clinical studies of anticancer agent-incorporating polymer micelles. *Cancer Sci.*, **100**, 572–579.
9. Matsumura, Y., Hamaguchi, T., Ura, T., Muro, K., Yamada, Y., Shimada, Y., Shirao, K., Okusaka, T., Ueno, H., Ikeda, M., and Watanabe, N. (2004) Phase I clinical trial and pharmacokinetic evaluation of NK911, a micelle-encapsulated doxorubicin. *Br. J. Cancer*, **91**, 1775–1781.
10. Danson, S., Ferry, D., Alakhov, V., Margison, J., Kerr, D., Jowle, D., Brampton, M., Halbert, G., and Ranson, M. (2004) Phase I dose escalation and pharmacokinetic study of pluronic polymer-bound doxorubicin (SP1049C) in patients with advanced cancer. *Br. J. Cancer*, **90**, 2085–2091.
11. Kim, T.Y., Kim, D.W., Chung, J.Y., Shin, S.G., Kim, S.C., Heo, D.S., Kim, N.K., and Bang, Y.J. (2004) Phase I and pharmacokinetic study of Genexol-PM, a cremophor-free, polymeric micelle-formulated paclitaxel, in patients with advanced malignancies. *Clin. Cancer Res.*, **10**, 3708–3016.
12. Hamaguchi, T., Matsumura, Y., Suzuki, M., Shimizu, K., Goda, R., Nakamura, I., Nakatomi, I., Yokoyama, M., Kataoka, K., and Kakizoe, T. (2005) NK105, a paclitaxel-incorporating micellar nanoparticle formulation, can extend *in vivo* antitumour activity and reduce the neurotoxicity of paclitaxel. *Br. J. Cancer*, **92**, 1240–1246.
13. Hamaguchi, T., Doi, T., Eguchi-Nakajima, T., Kato, K., Yamada, Y., Shimada, Y., Fuse, N., Ohtsu, A., Matsumoto, S., Takanashi, M., and Matsumura, Y. (2010) Phase I study of NK012, a novel SN-38-incorporating micellar nanoparticle, in adult patients with solid tumors. *Clin. Cancer Res.*, **16**, 5058–5066.
14. Nishiyama, N., Okazaki, S., Cabral, H., Miyamoto, M., Kato, Y., Sugiyama, Y.,

Nishio, K., Matsumura, Y., and Kataoka, K. (2003) Novel cisplatin-incorporated polymeric micelles can eradicate solid tumors in mice. *Cancer Res.*, **63**, 8977–8983.

15. Cabral, H., Nishiyama, N., and Kataoka, K. (2007) Optimization of (1,2-diamino-cyclohexane)platinum(II)-loaded polymeric micelles directed to improved tumor targeting and enhanced antitumor activity. *J. Control. Release*, **121**, 146–155.

16. Jain, R.K. (2001) Delivery of molecular and cellular medicine to solid tumors. *Adv. Drug Deliv. Rev.*, **46**, 149–168.

17. Bae, Y., Fukushima, S., Harada, A., and Kataoka, K. (2003) Design of environment-sensitive supramolecular assemblies for intracellular drug delivery: polymeric micelles that are responsive to intracellular pH change. *Angew. Chem. Int. Ed.*, **42**, 4640–4643.

18. Bae, Y., Nishiyama, N., Fukushima, S., Koyama, H., Matsumura, Y., and Kataoka, K. (2005) Preparation and biological characterization of polymeric micelle drug carriers with intracellular pH-triggered drug release property: tumor permeability, controlled subcellular drug distribution, and enhanced *in vivo* antitumor efficacy. *Bioconjug. Chem.*, **16**, 122–130.

19. Lee, E.S., Na, K., and Bae, Y.H. (2005) Doxorubicin loaded pH-sensitive polymeric micelles for reversal of resistant MCF-7 tumor. *J. Control. Release*, **103**, 405–418.

20. Lee, E.S., Gao, Z., and Bae, Y.H. (2008) Recent progress in tumor pH targeting nanotechnology. *J. Control. Release*, **132**, 164–170.

21. Lee, G.Y., Park, K., Kim, S.Y., and Byun, Y. (2007) MMPs-specific PEGylated peptide DOX conjugate micelles that contain free doxorubicin. *Eur. J. Pharm. Biopharm.*, **67**, 646–654.

22. Katayama, Y., Sonoda, T., and Maeda, M. (2001) A polymer micelle responding to the protein kinase A signal. *Macromolecules*, **34**, 8569–8573.

23. Bae, Y., Jang, W.-D., Nishiyama, N., Fukushima, S., and Kataoka, K. (2005) Multifunctional polymeric micelles with folate-mediated cancer cell targeting and pH-triggered drug releasing properties for active intracellular drug delivery. *Mol. BioSyst.*, **1**, 242–250.

24. Bae, Y., Nishiyama, N., and Kataoka, K. (2007) *In vivo* antitumor activity of the folate-conjugated pH-sensitive polymeric micelle selectively releasing adriamycin in the intracellular acidic compartments. *Bioconjug. Chem.*, **18**, 1131–1139.

25. Nagasaki, Y., Yasugi, K., Yamamoto, Y., Harada, A., and Kataoka, K. (2001) Sugar-installed block copolymer micelles: their preparation and specific interaction with lectin molecules. *Biomacromolecules*, **2**, 1067–1070.

26. Nasongkla, N., Shuai, X., Ai, H., Weinberg, B.D., Pink, J., Boothman, D.A., and Gao, J. (2004) cRGD-functionalized polymer micelles for targeted doxorubicin delivery. *Angew. Chem. Int. Ed.*, **43**, 6323–6327.

27. Zeng, F., Lee, H., and Allen, C. (2006) Epidermal growth factor-conjugated poly(ethylene glycol)-*block*-poly(δ-valerolactone) copolymer micelles for targeted delivery of chemotherapeutics. *Bioconjug. Chem.*, **17**, 399–409.

28. Torchilin, V.P., Lukyanov, A.N., Gao, Z., and Papahadjopoulos-Sternberg, B. (2003) Immunomicelles: targeted pharmaceutical carriers for poorly soluble drugs. *Proc. Natl. Acad. Sci. USA*, **100**, 6039–6044.

29. Arap, W., Kolonin, M.G., Trepel, M., Lahdenranta, J., Cardó-Vila, M., Giordano, R.J., Mintz, P.J., Ardelt, P.U., Yao, V.J., Vidal, C.I., Chen, L., Flamm, A., Valtanen, H., Weavind, L.M., Hicks, M.E., Pollock, R.E., Botz, G.H., Bucana, C.D., Koivunen, E., Cahill, D., Troncoso, P., Baggerly, K.A., Pentz, R.D., Do, K.-A., Logothetis, C.J., and Pasqualini, R. (2002) Steps toward mapping the human vasculature by phage display. *Nat. Med.*, **8**, 121–127.

30. McIntosh, D.P., Tan, X.-Y., Oh, P., and Schnitzer, J.E. (2002) Targeting endothelium and its dynamic caveolae for tissue-specific transcytosis *in vivo*: a pathway to overcome cell barriers to drug and gene delivery. *Proc. Natl. Acad. Sci. USA*, **99**, 1996–2001.

31. Oh, P., Borgström, P., Witkiewicz, H., Li, Y., Borgström, B.J., Chrastina, A., Iwata, K., Zinn, K.R., Baldwin, R., Testa, J.E., and Schnitzer, J.E. (2007) Live dynamic imaging of caveolae pumping targeted antibody rapidly and specifically across endothelium in the lung. *Nat. Biotechnol.*, **25**, 327–337.

32. Sugahara, K.N., Teesalu, T., Karmali, P.P., Kotamraju, V.R., Agemy, L., Girard, O.M., Hanahan, D., Mattrey, R.F., and Ruoslahti1, E. (2009) Tissue-penetrating delivery of compounds and nanoparticles into tumors. *Cancer Cell*, **16**, 510–520.

33. Feron, O. (2010) Tumor-penetrating peptides: a shift from magic bullets to magic guns. *Sci. Transl. Med.*, **2**, 1–5.

34. Harada, A. and Kataoka, K. (1995) Formation of polyion complex micelles in aqueous milieu from a pair of oppositely-charged block copolymers with poly(ethylene glycol) segments. *Macromolecules*, **28**, 5294–5299.

35. Katayose, S. and Kataoka, K. (1997) Water-soluble polyion complex associates of DNA and poly(ethylene glycol)–poly(L-lysine) block copolymer. *Bioconjug. Chem.*, **8**, 702–707.

36. Itaka, K., Yamauchi, K., Harada, A., Nakamura, K., Kawaguchi, H., and Kataoka, K. (2003) Polyion complex micelles from plasmid DNA and poly(ethylene glycol)–poly(L-lysine) block copolymer as serum-tolerable polyplex system: physiological properties of micelles relevant to gene transfection efficiency. *Biomaterials*, **24**, 4495–4506.

37. Harada-Shiba, M., Yamauchi, K., Harada, A., Takamisawa, I., Shimokado, K., and Kataoka, K. (2002) Polyion complex micelles as vectors in gene therapy – pharmacokinetics and *in vivo* gene transfer. *Gene Ther.*, **9**, 407–414.

38. Miyata, K., Kakizawa, Y., Nishiyama, N., Harada, A., Yamasaki, Y., Koyama, H., and Kataoka, K. (2004) Block catiomer polyplexes with regulated densities of charge and disulfide cross-linking directed to enhance gene expression. *J. Am. Chem. Soc.*, **126**, 2355–2361.

39. Oba, M., Vachutinsky, Y., Miyata, K., Kano, M.R., Ikeda, S., Nishiyama, N., Itaka, K., Miyazono, K., Koyama, H., and Kataoka, K. (2010) Antiangiogenic gene therapy of solid tumor by systemic injection of polyplex micelles loading plasmid DNA encoding soluble Flt-1. *Mol. Pharmacol.*, **7**, 501–509.

40. Oba, M., Miyata, K., Osada, K., Christie, R.J., Sanjoh, M., Li, W., Fukushima, S., Ishii, T., Kano, M.R., Nishiyama, N., Koyama, H., and Kataoka, K. (2010) Polyplex micelles prepared from ω-cholesteryl PEG-polycation block copolymers for systemic gene delivery. *Biomaterials*, **32**, 652–663.

41. Itaka, K., Ishii, T., Hasegawa, Y., and Kataoka, K. (2010) Biodegradable polyamino acid-based polycations as safe and effective gene carrier minimizing cumulative toxicity. *Biomaterials*, **31**, 3707–3714.

42. Han, M., Bae, Y., Nishiyama, N., Miyata, K., Oba, M., and Kataoka, K. (2007) Transfection study using multicellular tumor spheroids for screening non-viral polymeric gene vectors with low cytotoxicity and high transfection efficiencies. *J. Control. Release*, **121**, 38–48.

43. Akagi, D., Oba, M., Koyama, H., Nishiyama, N., Fukushima, S., Miyata, T., Nagawa, H., and Kataoka, K. (2008) Biocompatible micellar nanovectors achieve efficient gene transfer to vascular lesions without cytotoxicity and thrombus formation gene transfer to vascular lesions. *Gene Ther.*, **14**, 1029–1038.

44. Han, M., Oba, M., Nishiyama, N., Kano, M.R., Kizaka-Kondoh, S., and Kataoka, K. (2009) Enhanced percolation and gene expression in tumor hypoxia by PEGylated polyplex micelles. *Mol. Ther.*, **17**, 1404–1410.

45. Boussif, O., Lezoualc'h, F., Zanta, M.A., Mergny, M.D., Scherman, D., Demeneix, B., and Behr, J.P. (1995) Versatile vector for gene and oligonucleotide transfer into cells in culture and *in vivo*: polyethylenimine. *Proc. Natl. Acad. Sci. USA*, **92**, 7297–7301.

46. Kanayama, N., Fukushima, S., Nishiyama, N., Itaka, K., Jang, W.-D., Miyata, K., Yamasaki, Y., Chung, U.-I., and Kataoka, K. (2006) A PEG-based biocompatible block catiomer with high buffering capacity for the construction

of polyplex micelles showing efficient gene transfer toward primary cells. *ChemMedChem*, **1**, 439–444.
47. Miyata, K., Oba, M., Nakanishi, M., Fukushima, S., Yamasaki, Y., Koyama, H., Nishiyama, N., and Kataoka, K. (2008) Polyplexes from poly(aspartamide) bearing 1,2-diaminoethane side chains induce pH-selective, endosomal membrane destabilization with amplified transfection and negligible cytotoxicity. *J. Am. Chem. Soc.*, **130**, 16287–16294.
48. Han, M., Bae, Y., Nishiyama, N., Miyata, K., Oba, M., and Kataoka, K. (2007) Transfection study of using multicellular tumor spheroids for screening non-viral polymeric gene vectors with low cytotoxicity and high transfection efficiencies. *J. Control. Release*, **121**, 38–48.
49. Takae, S., Miyata, K., Oba, M., Ishii, T., Nishiyama, N., Itaka, K., Yamasaki, Y., Koyama, H., and Kataoka, K. (2008) PEG-detachable polyplex micelles based on disulfide-linked block catiomers as bioresponsive nonviral gene vectors. *J. Am. Chem. Soc.*, **130**, 6001–6009.
50. Khalil, I.A., Kogure, K., Akita, H., and Harashima, H. (2006) Uptake pathways and subsequent intracellular trafficking in nonviral gene delivery. *Pharmacol. Rev.*, **58**, 32–45.
51. Pelkmans, L., Kartenbeck, J., and Helenius, A. (2001) Caveolar endocytosis of simian virus 40 reveals a new two-step vesicular-transport pathway to the ER. *Nat. Cell Biol.*, **3**, 473–483.
52. Mineo, C. and Anderson, R.G. (2001) Potocytosis. *Histochem. Cell Biol.*, **116**, 109–118.
53. Rejman, J., Bragonzi, A., and Conese, M. (2005) Role of clathrin- and caveolae-mediated endocytosis in gene transfer mediated by lipo- and polyplexes. *Mol. Ther.*, **12**, 468–474.
54. Oba, M., Fukushima, S., Kanayama, N., Aoyagi, K., Nishiyama, N., Koyama, H., and Kataoka, K. (2007) Cyclic RGD peptide-conjugated polyplex micelles as a targetable gene delivery system directed to cells possessing alphavbeta3 and alphavbeta5 integrins. *Bioconjug. Chem.*, **18**, 1415–1423.
55. Oba, M., Aoyagi, K., Miyata, K., Matsumoto, Y., Itaka, K., Nishiyama, N., Yamasaki, Y., Koyama, H., and Kataoka, K. (2008) Polyplex micelles with cyclic RGD peptide ligands and disulfide cross-links directing to the enhanced transfection via controlled intracellular trafficking. *Mol. Pharmacol.*, **5**, 1080–1092.
56. Swanson, J.A. and Watts, C. (1995) Macropinocytosis. *Trends Cell Biol.*, **5**, 424–428.
57. Khalil, I.A., Kogure, K., Futaki, S., and Harashima, H. (2006) High density of octaarginine stimulates macropinocytosis leading to efficient intracellular trafficking for gene expression. *J. Biol. Chem.*, **281**, 3544–3551.
58. Geng, Y., Dalhaimer, P., Cai, S.S., Tsai, R., Tewari, M., Minko, T., and Discher, D.E. (2007) Shape effects of filaments versus spherical particles in flow and drug delivery. *Nat. Nanotechnol.*, **2**, 249–255.
59. Christian, D.A., Cai, S., Bowen, D.M., Kim, Y., Pajerowski, J.D., and Discher, D.E. (2009) Polymersome carriers: from self-assembly to siRNA and protein therapeutics. *Eur. J. Pharm. Biopharm.*, **71**, 463–474.
60. Ahmed, F. and Discher, D.E. (2004) Self-porating polymersomes of PEG–PLA and PEG–PCL: hydrolysis-triggered controlled release vesicles. *J. Control. Release*, **96**, 37–53.
61. Ghoroghchian, P.P., Li, G.Z., Levine, D.H., Davis, K.P., Bates, F.S., Hammer, D.A., and Therien, M.J. (2006) Bioresorbable vesicles formed through spontaneous self-assembly of amphiphilic poly(ethylene oxide)-*block*-polycaprolactone. *Macromolecules*, **39**, 1673–1675.
62. Jiang, Y.G., Wang, Y.P., Ma, N., Wang, Z.Q., Smet, M., and Zhang, X. (2007) Reversible selforganization of a UV-responsive PEG-terminated malachite green derivative: vesicle formation and photoinduced disassembly. *Langmuir*, **23**, 4029–4034.
63. Qin, S.H., Geng, Y., Discher, D.E., and Yang, S. (2006) Temperature-controlled assembly and release from polymer vesicles of poly(ethylene oxide)-*block*-poly

(N-isopropylacrylamide). *Adv. Mater.*, **18**, 2905.

64. Borchert, U., Lipprandt, U., Bilang, M., Kimpfler, A., Rank, A., Peschka-Suss, R., Schubert, R., Lindner, P., and Forster, S. (2006) pH-induced release from P2VP–PEO block copolymer vesicles. *Langmuir*, **22**, 5843–5847.
65. Cerritelli, S., Velluto, D., and Hubbell, J.A. (2007) PEG-SS-PPS: reduction-sensitive disulfide block copolymer vesicles for intracellular drug delivery. *Biomacromolecules*, **8**, 1966–1972.
66. Napoli, A., Valentini, M., Tirelli, N., Muller, M., and Hubbell, J.A. (2004) Oxidation-responsive polymeric vesicles. *Nat. Mater.*, **3**, 183–189.
67. Holowka, E.P., Sun, V.Z., Kamei, D.T., and Deming, T.J. (2007) Polyarginine segments in block copolypeptides drive both vesicular assembly and intracellular delivery. *Nat. Mater.*, **6**, 52–57.
68. Wadia, J.S., Stan, R.V., and Dowdy, S.F. (2004) Transducible TAT-HA fusogenic peptide enhances escape of TAT-fusion proteins after lipid raft macropinocytosis. *Nat. Med.*, **10**, 310–315.
69. Korobko, A.V., Backendorf, C., and van der Maarel, J.R.C. (2006) Plasmid DNA encapsulation within cationic diblock copolymer vesicles for gene delivery. *J. Phys. Chem. B*, **110**, 14550–14556.
70. Kim, Y., Tewari, M., Pajerowski, J.D., Cai, S., Sen, S., Williams, J., Sirsi, S., Lutz, G., and Discher, D.E. (2009) Polymersome delivery of siRNA and antisense oligonucleotides. *J. Control. Release*, **134**, 132–140.
71. Arifin, D.R. and Palmer, A.F. (2005) Polymersome encapsulated hemoglobin: a novel type of oxygen carrier. *Biomacromolecules*, **6**, 2172–2181.
72. Koide, A., Kishimura, A., Osada, K., Jang, W.-D., Yamasaki, Y., and Kataoka, K. (2006) Semipermeable polymer vesicle (PICsome) self-assembled in aqueous medium from a pair of oppositely charged block copolymers: physiologically stable micro-/nanocontainers of water-soluble macromolecules. *J. Am. Chem. Soc.*, **128**, 5988–5989.
73. Kishimura, A., Koide, A., Osada, K., Yamasaki, Y., and Kataoka, K. (2007) Encapsulation of myoglobin in PEGylated polyion complex vesicles made from a pair of oppositely charged block ionomers: a physiologically available oxygen carrier. *Angew. Chem. Int. Ed.*, **46**, 6085–6088.
74. Dong, W.-F., Kishimura, A., Anraku, Y., Chuanoi, S., and Kataoka, K. (2009) Monodispersed polymeric nanocapsules: spontaneous evolution and morphology transition from reducible hetero-PEG PICmicelles by controlled degradation. *J. Am. Chem. Soc.*, **131**, 3804–3805.
75. Kishimura, A., Liamsuwan, S., Matsuda, H., Dong, W.-F., Osada, K., Yamasaki, Y., and Kataoka, K. (2009) pH-Dependent permeability change and reversible structural transition of PEGylated polyion complex vesicles (PICsomes) in aqueous media. *Soft Matter*, **5**, 529–532.
76. Anraku, Y., Kishimura, A., Oba, M., Yamasaki, Y., and Kataoka, K. (2010) Spontaneous formation of nanosized unilamellar polyion complex vesicles with tunable size and properties. *J. Am. Chem. Soc.*, **132**, 1631–1636.
77. Spahn, D.R. (2000) Current status of artificial oxygen carriers. *Adv. Drug Deliv. Rev.*, **40**, 143–151.
78. Sherwood, R.F. (1996) Advanced drug delivery reviews: enzyme prodrug therapy. *Adv. Drug Deliv. Rev.*, **22**, 269–288.
79. McCarthy, J.R., Jaffer, F.A., and Weissleder, R. (2006) A macrophage-targeted theranostic nanoparticle for biomedical applications. *Small*, **2**, 983–987.
80. Pan, D., Caruthers, S.D., Hu, G., Senpan, A., Scott, M.J., Gaffney, P.J., Wickline, S.A., and Lanza, G.M. (2008) Ligand-directed nanobialys as theranostic agent for drug delivery and manganese-based magnetic resonance imaging of vascular targets. *J. Am. Chem. Soc.*, **130**, 9186–9187.
81. Nasongkla, N., Bey, E., Ren, J., Ai, H., Khemtong, C., Guthi, J.S., Chin, S.F., Sherry, A.D., Boothman, D.A., and Gao, J. (2006) Multifunctional polymeric micelles as cancer-targeted, MRI-ultrasensitive drug delivery systems. *Nano Lett.*, **6**, 2427–2430.

82. Kaida, S., Cabral, H., Kumagai, M., Kishimura, A., Terada, Y., Sekino, M., Nishiyama, N., Tani, T., and Kataoka, K. (2010) Visible-drug delivery by supra-molecular nanocarriers directing to single-platformed diagnosis and therapy of pancreatic tumor model. *Cancer Res.*, **70**, 7031–7041.

33
Tailor-Made Hydrogels for Tumor Delivery

Sungwon Kim and Kinam Park

33.1
Introduction

Use of cross-linked hydrophilic polymers, now called "hydrogels," for biological applications was first introduced more than half a century ago [1]. Since that time, hydrogels have been used as a major component of controlled drug delivery formulations. The drug release from a hydrogel is mainly controlled by two mechanisms – diffusion of drug molecules and swelling of the hydrogel network [2, 3]. Recent advances in hydrogel technology have allowed manipulation of hydrogel properties in such a way that drug diffusion and hydrogel swelling can be controlled, and thus also drug release kinetics. For example, hydrogel swelling and drug diffusion may not occur actively until the hydrogel is triggered by environmental factors.

One of the most widely used applications of hydrogels has been cancer treatment. Clinical therapeutic interventions include surgery, radiotherapy, chemotherapy, immunotherapy, and a combination of these. Hydrogels play an important role in all of these therapeutic methods. In surgery, for example, hydrogels are used as an osmotic tissue expander after cancer ablative procedures [4, 5]. In other therapeutic systems, hydrogels contain at least one active pharmaceutical ingredient to obtain a therapeutic effect. Many excellent reviews have summarized the state-of-the-art technologies on cancer therapy using hydrogels. Those publications are, however, too focused on a specific method or system to provide an overview of hydrogel-based cancer therapy. The goal of this chapter, therefore, is to present a summary of the aspects of materials and therapeutic mechanisms for the purpose of providing a comprehensive understanding of hydrogel systems for cancer treatment.

33.2
Rationale for Hydrogel-Based Cancer Therapy

A hydrogel is a physically and/or chemically cross-linked polymer network that absorbs a large quantity of water without dissolution. The hydrophilic nature is one of the best advantages of hydrogels for *in vivo* applications, because a hydrophilic surface attracts water molecules more than other biological components, especially proteins [6]. The hydrophilic nature can also be considered a drawback in controlling drug release. Almost one-third of therapeutic drugs, including most anticancer drugs, are poorly soluble in water [7], so that the loading capacity of hydrophobic drugs is significantly limited. Moreover, hydrogels hardly achieve a sustained release profile of small-molecule drugs for a prolonged period because of the presence of microscopic spaces between polymer chains. Another problem in using hydrogels for cancer therapy has been the nonbiodegradability of most synthetic acrylic polymers. In a practical sense, it is highly desirable to have hydrogels degraded and cleared after implantation or injection to avoid invasive surgical procedures.

Successful development of hydrogel formulations for cancer therapy requires proper exploitation of the hydrogel properties. Since hydrogels are hydrophilic, holding water in their structures, loading of hydrophobic drugs is difficult. On the other hand, hydrogels provide an excellent matrix to formulate protein drugs, which can be easily denatured when exposed to organic solvents. In addition to protein drugs, genes, small interfering RNAs (siRNAs), and other biomacromolecules can be easily formulated into hydrogels. For controlled release of small molecules from a hydrogel formulation, they can be chemically grafted onto the polymer backbone. Hydrogel prodrugs allow efficient drug loading and easy control of drug release profiles using biodegradable spacers.

Development of novel hydrogel platforms has opened new opportunities for cancer therapy. Many biodegradable polymers are now available as hydrogels. *In situ* gelation technology has facilitated injectable formulations of anticancer drugs without surgical implantation procedures. Hydrogel microbeads have been used for sustained drug delivery or for embolization application since the beginning of hydrogel-based formulations. Recent advances in nanotechnology, however, have allowed the development of nanosized hydrogels ("nanogels") and composite hydrogels containing inorganic materials. Hydrogel systems with different materials and new drug delivery mechanisms make the hydrogels more useful and versatile in drug delivery.

33.3
Examples

33.3.1
Materials and Biodegradability

Conventional hydrogels are usually produced from acrylic copolymers, such as poly(hydroxyethyl methacrylate) (PHEMA) copolymers, or from natural polymers, such as gelatin and alginate. Recent hydrogel-based cancer therapy has moved toward using degradable polymers and making smaller hydrogels such as nanogels. Table 33.1 lists some representative polymers utilized to make hydrogels. Proteins and DNAs are easily degraded in the body by numerous enzymes. Polysaccharides are degradable because of the hydrolyzable backbones. Biodegradation has been an important issue in the drug delivery field, along with biocompatibility. Most

Table 33.1 Polymers for hydrogel networks.

Source	Degradability		Advantages	Disadvantages
	Nondegradable	Degradable		
Natural		proteins: gelatin, SELP; peptides; polysaccharide: dextran, chitosan, alginate, agarose, hyaluronic acid; DNA	mostly biodegradable	limited solvent system; difficulty in chemical modification
Synthetic	Pluronics; PHEMA copolymers; PNiPAAm copolymers; other acrylic copolymers	PEG-b-polyester; polyphosphazene	monomer versatility; various physical property; tunable drug release profile; well-established chemistry	low biocompatibility
Advantages	secured hydrogel integrity after administration	no need for ablation after administration		
Disadvantages	normal implantation and surgical ablation; reactive chemicals for cross-linking.	multiple mechanisms of biodegradation		

nondegradable polymers are produced from reactive chemicals, including vinyl groups and free radical initiators. *In situ* gelation is a convenient method to form a gel from an injectable formulation. For *in situ* gelation based on free radical polymerization rather than on physical cross-linking methods, toxicity derived from monomers and initiators should be carefully considered. Although many natural polymers take advantage of biodegradability, most natural polymers are limited in their chemical modification due to lack of appropriate solvent systems other than water. Also, degradation *in vivo* is governed by multiple factors, so that prediction of drug release from a hydrogel needs to be evaluated by taking many parameters into consideration [8]. In other words, the swelling property and mesh size of a hydrogel can be changed by degradation, and those chemically controlled events significantly modulate the drug release profile. Figure 33.1a shows drug release mechanisms of chemically cross-linked hydrogels and Figure 33.1b presents a simple concept of physical cross-linking to form a hydrogel.

Although hydrogels have played an important role in cancer therapy, there still exist some limitations. Table 33.2 shows recently developed hydrogel-based

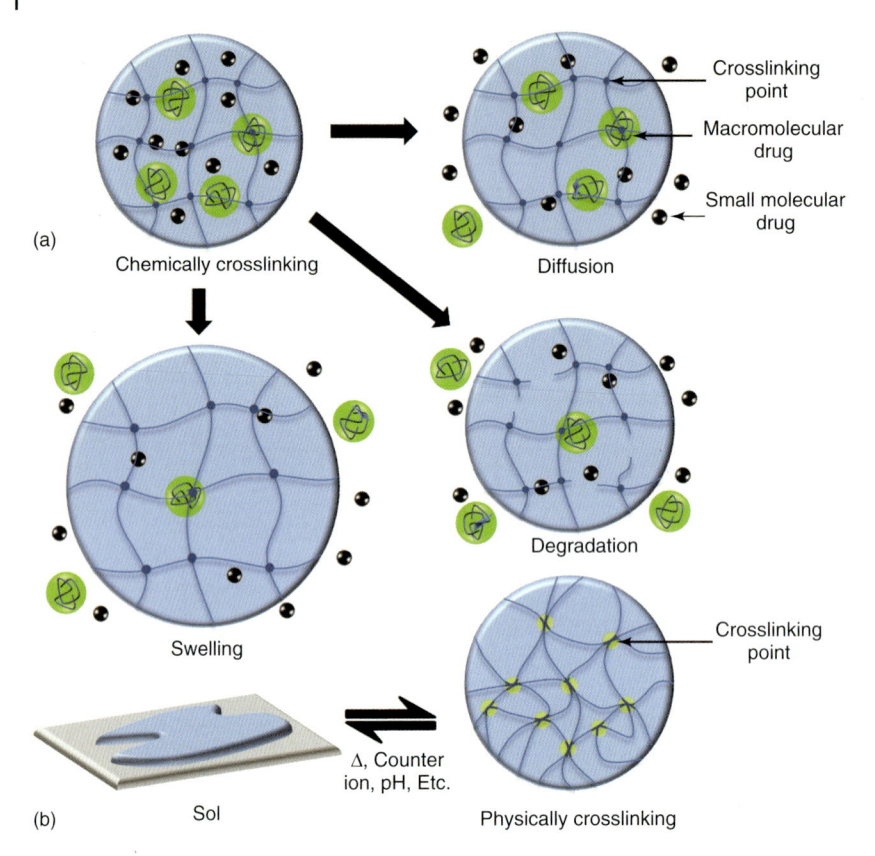

Figure 33.1 Hydrogels are formed either by chemical cross-linking or by physical cross-linking. (a) Hydrogels have at least three mechanisms to release drugs. For example, a chemically cross-linked hydrogel liberates drugs by diffusion, swelling, and degradation. (b) Physical cross-linking typically shows a sol–gel phase transition. Change in temperature, counterion species, or pH determines the physical phase.

drug delivery systems to treat cancer. It is noticeable that a broad range of therapeutic mechanisms is possible for hydrogel systems. Although there are various administration routes, intravenous injection has hardly been performed with hydrogel formulations. Moreover, many experiments were carried out by implantation of precured hydrogels. Localized applications of therapeutic drugs might reduce the systemic toxicity, but drug delivery to solid tumors of recognizable size is not possible to most of cancer patients.

Many interesting physical and chemical properties of hydrogel-based drug delivery systems have resulted from smart polymers. Smart (or stimuli-sensitive) polymers change their physical and/or chemical properties in response to environmental stimuli, such as temperature, pH, ion species, and biomolecules [45]. Although some natural polymers, such as gelatin, alginate, or chitosan, show stimuli sensitivity, most smart polymers have been synthesized from well-designed synthetic monomers to have fine control of the sensitivity. Recent advances in smart

Table 33.2 Examples of hydrogel formulations recently developed for cancer therapy.

Method	Polymer	Drug	Administration	References
Chemo- and immunotherapy				
Small-molecule drugs	cross-linked gelatin	cisplatin	s.c. implantation	[9]
	cross-linked PEG hydrogel	TPT-liposome	i.v. injection	[10]
	N-trimethyl chitosan/DPO	CPT	s.c. injection	[11]
	cross-linked chitosan	PTX	s.c. injection	[12]
	chitosan/DPO	DOX	p.t. injection	[13]
	chitosan/β-glycerophosphate	PTX	i.t. injection	[14]
	Pluronic F127	ibuprofen[a]	*in vitro*	[15]
	polyphosphazene	PTX	i.p. injection	[16]
	OSM-*b*-PCLA-*b*-PEG-*b*-PCLA-*b*-OSM	PTX	s.c. injection	[17]
	PEG-*b*-PCL-*b*-PEG	5-FU	i.p. injection	[18]
	P(HEMA-*co*-DMHA)	DOX, VLB, CsA	s.c. implantation	[19, 20]
Prodrugs	PLGA-*b*-PEG-*b*-PLGA	PEGylated CPT	i.d. implantation	[21]
	DOX–polyphosphazene	DOX–polyphosphazene	i.t. injection	[22, 23]
	DOX–chitosan	DOX–chitosan	i.t. injection	[24]
	cross-linked HA–BP	cross-linked HA–BP	*in vitro*	[25]
Protein/peptide drugs	P(HEMA-*co*-HPMA-*co*-TMPMA)	histrelin acetate	s.c. implantation	[26]
	gelatin	IL-12	s.c. injection	[27]
	polycarbophil	GM-CSF	i.t. injection	[28]
	alginate/chitosan	GOD	*in vitro*	[29]
	gelatin	PEGylated catalase	s.c. implantation	[30]
		ED-catalase	i.p. implantation	[31]
Drug combination	chitosan	GM-CSF + DOX or cisplatin or CTX	i.t. injection	[32]
	chitosan	vaccinia virus vaccine + DOX	i.t. injection	[33]
Gene and cell delivery				
Genes/siRNAs	chitosan/DPO	pPEDF	p.t. injection	[34]
	alginate, cross-linked alginate, collagen	siRNA to silence GFP[b]	*in vitro*	[35]
	SELP	pRL-CMV[b]	i.t. injection	[36]
	SELP	adenovirus expressing[b] GFP	i.t. injection	[36, 37]

(*continued overleaf*)

Table 33.2 (continued)

Method	Polymer	Drug	Administration	References
Cells/viruses	alginate + collagen + PLL	myoblast secreting angiostatin	i.p. implantation	[38]
	agarose	macrophage	in vitro	[39]
Radiotherapy				
Radiochemotherapy	alginate	^{188}Re + cisplatin	i.t. injection	[40]
Physical methods				
Embolization	PHEMA	DOX	p.t. injection	[41]
	PMMA		p.t. injection	[42]
	dextran		i.a. injection	[43]
Thermal therapy	alginate, chitosan/β-glycerophosphate, Poloxamer 407	SPION	i.t. injection	[44]

^{a}To reduce inflammation-induced cancer cell migration.
^{b}Reporter systems.
BP, bisphosphonate; CsA, cyclosporine A; DMHA, N,O-dimethacryloyl-hydroxyamine; DPO, dipotassium orthophosphate; ED, ethylenediamine; FGF-2, fibroblast growth factor-2; 5-FU, 5-fluorouracil; HA, hyaluronan; i.a., intra-arterial; i.d., intradermal; i.p., intraperitoneal; i.t., intratumoral; i.v., intravenous; OSM, sulfamethazine oligomer; PCL, poly(ε-caprolactone); PCLA, poly(ε-caprolactone-*co*-lactic acid); PLGA, poly(lactic-*co*-glycolic acid); PLL, poly(L-lysine); pRL-CMV, *Renilla* luciferase-coding plasmid with cytomegalovirus enhancer; p.t., peritumoral; PVA, poly(vinyl alcohol); s.c., subcutaneous; TMPMA, trimethylolpropane trimethylmethacrylate; TPT, topotecan (water-soluble CPT analog); VLB, vinblastine sulfate. See text for other abbreviations.

hydrogel systems have made hydrogels smarter. Additional stimuli (e.g., enzymes, redox states, etc.) can now be applied to change the physicochemical properties of polymers. More smart polymers are now available by integrating controlled polymerization chemistry, combinatorial chemistry, and genetic engineering. For example, genetic engineering allows more options of smart polymers and hydrogels with good biodegradability by tailor-made protein structures [46, 47].

33.3.2
Injectable Formulations

Hydrogel-based drug delivery systems can be divided into the macro, micro, and nano systems. As shown in Figure 33.2, the macroscopic precured hydrogel system can be implanted as a depot by surgery or as an *in situ* gel-forming hydrogel system by injection. The microparticle systems are typically used for embolism-mediated cancer therapy. The nanogels are expected to be accumulated at a tumor tissue by the enhanced permeation and retention (EPR) effect through leaky blood vessels (see Chapter 3). Among them, injectable formulations are much more advantageous because no surgery is necessary. In particular, *in situ* gelation methods and nanogel formulations have been recently highlighted, which will be briefly discussed here.

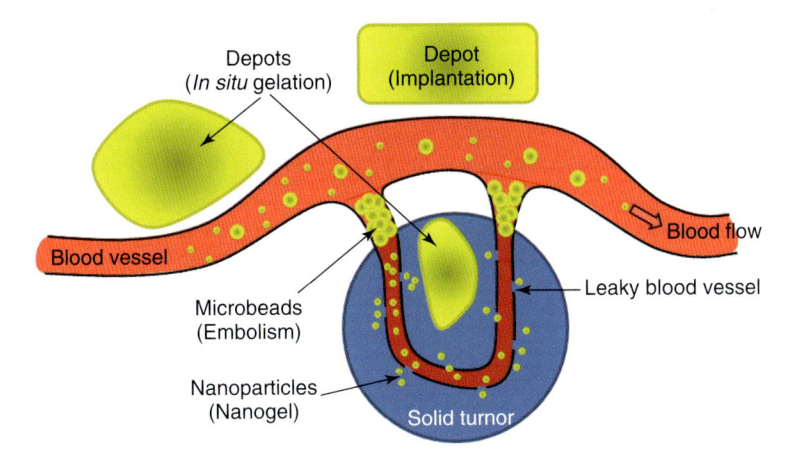

Figure 33.2 Examples of hydrogel-based drug delivery systems for cancer therapy.

33.3.2.1 *In Situ* Gelation

In situ gelation is a technique to inject polymer solutions that can subsequently form a gel inside the body. Hydrogels are produced by either chemical or physical cross-linking. In chemical cross-linking systems, vinyl groups are utilized for photopolymerization [48]. However, chemical cross-linking of acrylic monomers is not a desirable method if biodegradability is not guaranteed. As a unique example, chemical cross-linking can be accomplished by enzymatic activity. Davis *et al.* produced genetically engineered proteins with repeating peptide blocks containing lysine and glutamine [49]. Those proteins could be cross-linked by treating transglutaminase that forms a chemical bond between lysine and glutamine.

Many hydrogels based on *in situ* gelation utilize physical cross-linking method such as thermosensitive gelation or ionic complex. Poly(*N*-isopropylacrylamide) (PNiPAAm, Figure 33.3) is a representative polymer possessing a temperature-dependent sol–gel phase transition property [50]. Nondegradability of PNiPAAm,

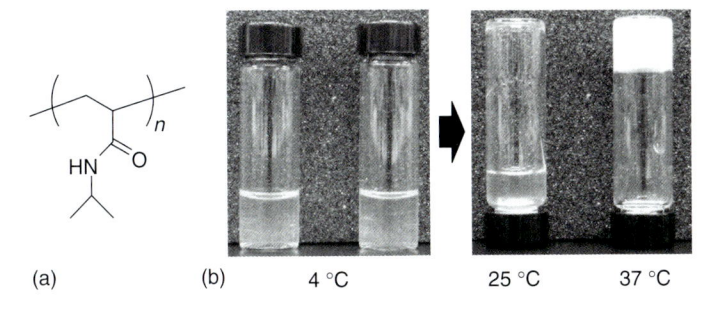

Figure 33.3 (a) Chemical structure of PNiPAAm. (b) At 4 °C, PNiPAAm (5% w/v in water) is a clear solution, which turns into a hydrogel by elevating the temperature above 32 °C. Therefore, PNiPAAm is a sol phase at room temperature (25 °C), while a gel phase at body temperature (37 °C).

however, still limits its clinical applications. Hence, researchers have developed several polymer systems possessing thermosensitivity as well as biodegradability. Block copolymers of poly(ethylene glycol) (PEG) and polyesters spontaneously generate a micelle structure in water, so that hydrophobic drugs can be incorporated into the micelle core. Moreover, those polymers have thermosensitivity depending on the molecular weight of each block and block length ratio [51]. Biodegradable polyphosphazene [52] and chitosan neutralized by β-glycerol phosphate or dipotassium orthophosphate [53] also have good biocompatibility and sufficient thermosensitivity to be used for a hydrogel formulation formed by *in situ* gelation.

33.3.2.2 Nanogels

A "nanogel" is a nanoparticle that has a physically or chemically cross-linked core. Typically, macroscopic hydrogels swell by absorbing a large quantity of water and shrink upon drying, which explain the major mechanism of drug release. Most nanogels, however, hardly show a significant swelling/shrinking property, especially to release drugs. However, the size of nanogels in water, which is usually determined by the hydrodynamic diameter measured by dynamic light scattering, can be significantly reduced after drying. The polymer micelle has also been categorized as a nanogel because of its cross-linking in the core and the hydrophilic outer shell [54, 55]. Since the field of nanogels is still evolving, a clear definition of a nanogel has not yet been established and, for that reason, examples of nanogel formulations are excluded in Table 33.2.

Nanogels for drug delivery take advantage of various properties of nanoparticles. These include injectability of formulation, escape from the reticuloendothelial system (RES), prolonged circulation time, enhanced EPR effect, and so on. Many nanogels have been produced by self-assembly of amphiphilic polymers. One of advantages of self-assembled nanoparticles is their capability of drug loading in the hydrophobic core. Various nanogels built from polysaccharides, such as pullulan [56], curdlan [57], chitosan [58], or chondroitin sulfate [59], have been extensively developed to deliver small-molecule and macromolecule drugs. (It is important to understand that natural polymers are degradable, but not necessarily in the human body because of the lack of specific enzymes for specific polysaccharides.) Physical assembly of nanogels can also be obtained by using thermosensitivity. Pluronic® types [60], copolymers of PEG and polyester, and copolymers of acrylamide [61] have been used to produce nanogels and to deliver small-molecule drugs to cancer. Smart polymers can be used not only to build a self-assembled nanogel, but also to specifically localize drugs only at tumor sites [62]. For example, a pH-sensitive nanogel containing histidine moieties showed pH-dependent drug release to tumor cells [63]. It is considered that the extracellular environment of solid tumors has a slightly lower pH than the physiological condition. When a pH-sensitive nanogel is accumulated at tumor tissue, drugs will be immediately released if the smart polymer of the nanogel is sensitive enough to recognize such a small change of pH. Nanogel systems have been modified with ligands, such as folate [56] or the RGD peptide sequence [62], that can interact with receptors on the tumor cell surface. Nanogel systems with surface-grafted ligands may interact with the target cell better once they are delivered to the surface of target cells.

33.3.3
Therapeutic Mechanisms

33.3.3.1 Small-Molecule Drugs

Hydrogels are versatile in cancer therapy as shown in Figure 33.4. Some examples of recently studied hydrogel formulations to treat cancer are listed in Table 33.2. Most hydrogel formulations have been developed to deliver small-molecule anticancer drugs, such as paclitaxel (PTX) [12, 14, 16, 17, 64], doxorubicin (DOX) [13, 19, 20], and camptothecin (CPT) [11]. To load drugs into a hydrogel, it is important to select a cross-linking method and control cross-linking density. For example, chitosan is a hydrophilic natural polymer forming a gel at high pH. Various cross-linking methods have been studied, which include photo-cross-linking of chemically modified chitosan by UV irradiation or physical cross-linking by changing pH or temperature [53]. Among those methods, temperature-induced gelation may be the most practical approach. BST-Gel™ (BioSyntech) is a unique platform of thermosensitive chitosan hydrogel. Chitosan aqueous solution in 0.1 M acetic acid containing β-glycerophosphate becomes a hydrogel at elevated temperature, typically from 4 to 37 °C [65]. *In situ* gelation of chitosan via pH change necessitates a low pH less than 5–6 and such a low pH may cause side-effects after injection. The pH range where the chitosan/β-glycerophosphate is able to have a complete sol–gel transition temperature is close to the physiological pH. On the other hand, chemical cross-linking can be done only when chitosan is modified to have polymerizable groups. For instance, a lactose-conjugating chitosan is cross-linkable by UV irradiation in the presence of azide [66]. One advantage of the modified chitosan is the improved solubility in a neutral aqueous solution due to the hydrophilic lactose. However, it should be further clarified how safe the reactive species of azide is and how to remove residual azide.

The major problem of hydrogel systems delivering small-molecule drugs is that most anticancer drugs are hydrophobic. Hydrogels possessing little or no hydrophobic moiety have a difficulty with drug loading without use of organic solvent. For instance, PTX is a well-known anticancer drug with poor solubility in water. The log P value (octanol/water partition coefficient) is 3.98 and the aqueous solubility is 0.3 µg/ml [67]. To load PTX into a hydrogel such as chitosan gel, Ruel-Gariépy *et al.* directly poured sterilized chitosan solution into γ-irradiated PTX powder [14]. They did not clarify whether the heterogeneity in PTX particle size has any influence on the drug release profile. In other study, Obara *et al.* loaded a Taxol® formulation into chitosan hydrogel [12]. As the toxicity of Cremophor EL® is well known, it will be a key issue whether the local toxicity is tolerable or not after treatment. To overcome those issues, it was attempted to load drug nanocolloids into hydrogel. In this preliminary study, CPT was manufactured to generate nanoparticles 30–50 nm in diameter [11]. The nanoparticles were sterilizable by

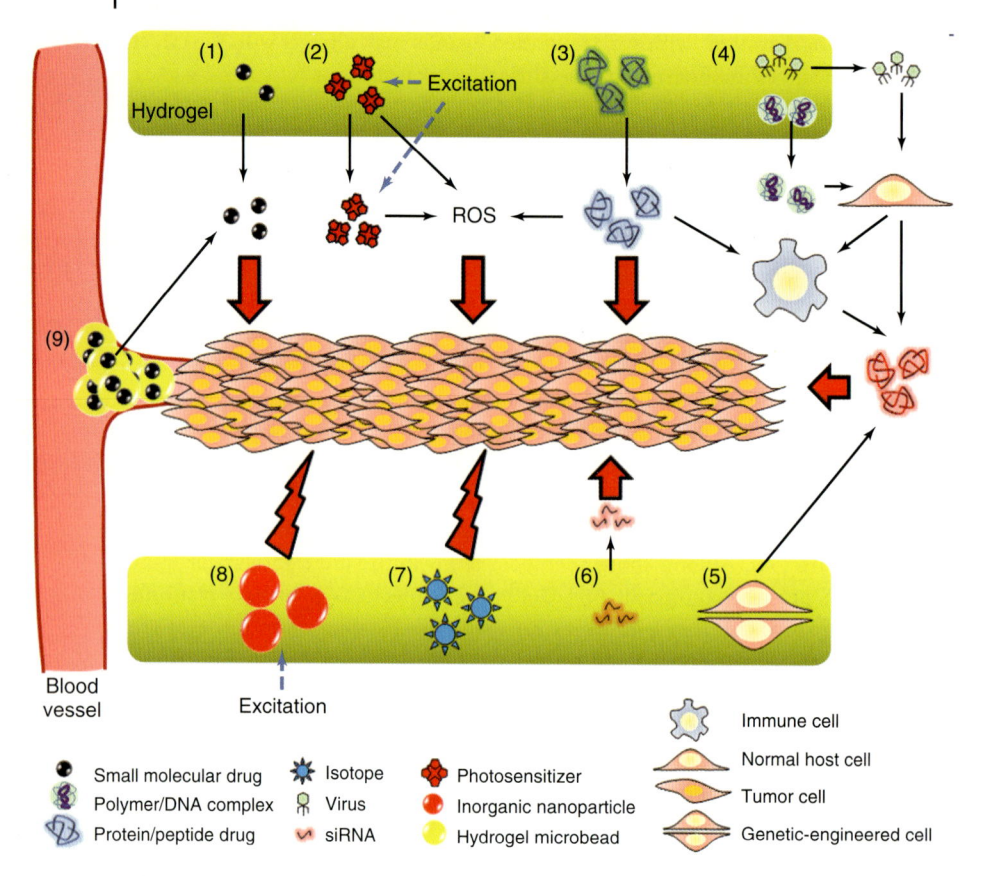

Figure 33.4 Therapeutic mechanisms of hydrogel-based anticancer drug delivery systems. (1) Small-molecule drugs induce tumor cell death or inhibit cell growth. In the prodrug approach, small drugs are chemically conjugated to polymer backbones, which are released by cleavage of chemical bond. (2) Photosensitizers in PDT generate ROS as well as singlet oxygen. (3) Macromolecule drugs directly control the tumor cell viability, modulate the host immune system, or generate ROS to kill tumor cells. (4) Viral or nonviral gene delivery method is used to produce protein/peptide drugs. (5) Genetically engineered cells also produce therapeutic proteins. (6) siRNAs are translocated inside tumor cells to control tumor cell growth and proliferation. (7) Isotopes generate radiation to eliminate tumor cells. (8) Inorganic nanoparticles such as GNPs or SPIONs produce heat for thermotherapy. (9) Embolic microbeads are also able to release anticancer agents for chemoembolism therapy.

simple filtration instead of irradiation and were more predictable in terms of drug release kinetics.

A simple and conventional way to load drug into a hydrogel is the absorption method. As chemically cross-linked hydrogels are not dissolved in organic solvent, a dried gel can be swollen in a solution of drug and water-miscible solvent, followed by drying to remove the solvent [19, 20]. Drug release primarily depends on the drug diffusion rate and the hydrogel swelling rate (Figure 33.1a). The mesh size of a typical hydrogel is around 1.5–7 nm, which may exert no interference for diffusion of small molecules [68]. Therefore, small-molecule drugs can be easily absorbed into hydrogel and also rapidly diffuse out from the gel. In this case, Fick's law and other empirical equations are applicable [8]. Usually, a polymer consisting of the hydrogel undergoes a phase transition from a glassy to a rubbery state, and thus the rate of polymer relaxation affecting the diffusion of drug molecules plays a key role in drug release [8].

Several methods have been developed to obtain an improved control on drug release, such as control of mesh size, drug size, and drug–polymer conjugation [69]. The mesh size can be further reduced by formation of an interpenetrating polymer network (IPN). Cross-linking density and physical properties of the monomer/polymer control the mesh size. However, it is almost impossible to inject an IPN hydrogel, so that surgical implantation (or oral administration for cancer in the gastrointestinal tract) is the only method for application. The control of the drug size means incorporation of drug-containing particles into hydrogels, which are designed to delay drug release until particle degradation or disintegration occurs. Microparticles [70], nanoparticles [71], or liposomes [10] containing anticancer agents have been loaded into hydrogels and successfully showed sustained drug release profiles. In addition to particle systems, the ligand–drug complex can extend the duration of drug release. The best example is cyclodextrin that has amphiphilicity [72].

The prodrug approach has been a useful tool to deliver poorly soluble drugs [73]. In polymeric prodrugs, drugs are conjugated to a polymer backbone via degradable linkers such as ester bonds or polypeptide spacers. Rihova et al. conjugated DOX to a copolymer of N-(2-hydroxypropyl)methacrylamide (HPMA) using a Gly–Phe–Leu–Gly peptide linker [74]. It was found that the antitumor activity of prodrug-type DOX against mouse T-cell lymphoma was proportional to the degradation time and DOX dose. The hydrogel significantly increased the administered DOX dose without any toxicity issue, but HPMA is a nondegradable acrylic polymer. Therefore, surgical removal should be followed when the hydrogel becomes nonfunctional after DOX consumption. Hydrogels made of biodegradable polymers will be much more beneficial in this aspect. In a recent study, Chun et al. used a polyphosphazene hydrogel to deliver DOX [22, 23]. Polyphosphazene is a biodegradable polymer having a sol–gel phase transition depending on temperature. Chemical conjugation of DOX to polyphosphazene extended DOX release to more than 1 month and showed good antitumoral activity superior to free DOX (Figure 33.5). The toxicity of the polyphosphazene systems, however, has not been established. TransCon™ (Asendis Pharma) is a good example of a commercially available prodrug-type hydrogel. The TransCon technology employs biodegradable linkers to conjugate small-molecule and macromolecule drugs to biodegradable polymers such as PEG or albumin. The albumin-based hydrogel is a particularly promising platform because it is injectable intravenously.

Small-molecule drugs are generally hydrophobic, but not always. There are many hydrophilic drugs with good anticancer activity. Those drugs have no problem with administration, because intravenous injection as a solution form is possible. Issues

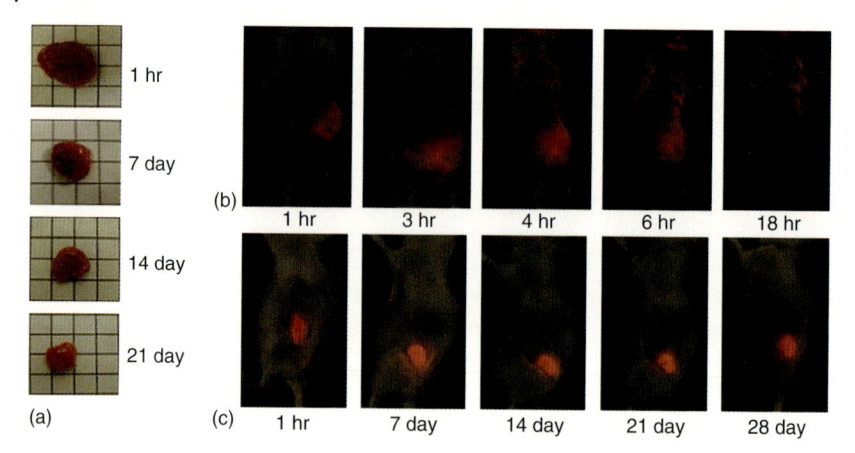

Figure 33.5 Prolonged antitumoral activity of DOX-conjugating polyphosphazene might be due to sustained release of free DOX by hydrolysis. (a) Mass loss of intratumorally injected polyphosphazene–DOX conjugate with time. (b) Free DOX intratumorally injected completely disappeared within 1 day, while the polymer–DOX conjugate still remained at the tumor tissue even 28 days after injection. (Reproduced with permission from [22]. © 2009 Elsevier.)

occur when injected drugs show systemic toxicity, fast clearance rate, and poor biodistribution to cancerous tissue. In this case, other drug delivery systems such as nanoparticles will be useful, but hydrogels are also applicable. Cisplatin – an excellent anticancer agent – is very hydrophilic (log $P = -2.53$), but provokes severe neurotoxicity after systemic administration [75]. When a gelatin hydrogel loaded with cisplatin was intratumorally injected into tumor-bearing mice, no side-effects (hemotoxicity in this study) were observed with an improved survival rate [9]. Absorption of cisplatin by the hydrogel seems to be stabilized by coordination bonding between cisplatin and some amino acids such as phenylalanine, histidine, or aspartic acid. Casolaro et al. prepared polymers based on N-acryloyl-L-phenylalanine to load and release cisplatin [76]. Although an initial burst was observed, hydrogels showed a sustained release profile over 1 week in vitro. Tauro et al. introduced a peptide into a PEG hydrogel that can be hydrolyzed by matrix metalloproteinase (MMP)-9 overexpressed at tumor tissues and also contains aspartic acids [77]. Cisplatin that was expected to be complexed with aspartic acid was rapidly released by treatment of MMP-9. It was reported that a simple blend of PNiPAAm and chitosan was able to significantly extend cisplatin release [78].

33.3.3.2 Protein and Peptide Drugs

A hydrogel is the best carrier to deliver protein and peptide drugs in terms of protein stability due to its hydrophilic nature. Loss of protein stability that is often caused by a water/organic interface during formulation processes results in a poor therapeutic effect and also immunogenicity [79]. However, hydrogels may be too hydrophilic to control the release of hydrophilic drugs. To control the release rate of macromolecule drugs, several methods have been developed, which are almost

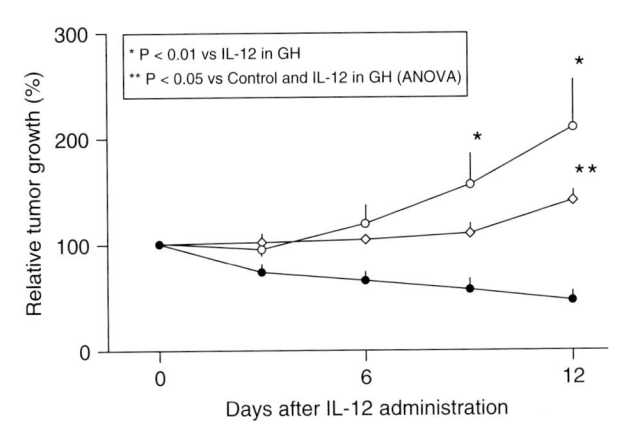

Figure 33.6 Relative antitumoral activity of IL-12 incorporated in gelatin hydrogel. A single dose of 500 ng IL-12/mouse (closed circles) or double dose of 250 ng/mouse (open diamonds) was subcutaneously injected to mice bearing mouse colon carcinoma cells (CMT-93). In comparison with the control group (open circles), the single-dose formulation effectively regressed tumor volume. (Reproduced with permission from [27]. © 2003 Springer.)

the same as used for small-molecule drugs. It is obvious that macromolecule drugs have a larger molecular weight than small-molecule drugs, so that cross-linking density or mesh size can be an important parameter to control the drug release rate [80]. However, cross-linked hydrogels should be implanted to work on tumor therapy. For this reason, only limited studies using hydrogels have been performed for cancer therapy.

There exist many protein or peptide drugs to treat cancer, which include toxins, cytokines, chemokines, enzymes, and hormones [81]. Toxins directly suppress or kill tumor cells, while cytokines, chemokines, enzymes, and hormones modulate local physiological environments to do so. For example, diphtheria toxin is a good protein drug candidate for cancer therapy, which directly inhibits protein synthesis and induces cellular apoptosis. It was found that growth of most human cancer cells is inhibited by diphtheria toxin [82]. However, normal cells can also be affected by the toxin. Since using hydrogel drug localization at a tumor tissue is relatively difficult, targeted delivery strategies have been employed to deliver toxins rather than hydrogel systems. On the other hand, cytokines act on specific receptors, so that hydrogel-based cytokine delivery has been considered as a promising regime to treat cancer. Interleukin (IL)-2 and -12 enhance antitumoral activity of natural killer cells and cytotoxic T-cells [83]. It was observed that the IL-12 loaded in a gelatin hydrogel significantly enhanced tumor regression effects on a mouse model bearing colon carcinoma cells compared with a solution formulation (Figure 33.6) [27]. A sustained release profile of IL-12 from the hydrogel might be attributed to the improved antitumoral activity. Similarly, granulocyte-macrophage colony-stimulating factor (GM-CSF) provokes a local physiological environment to suppress tumor cell growth. GM-CSF recruits macrophages, dendritic cells, and monocytes, and increases their cytotoxicity [84]. A GM-CSF formulation in

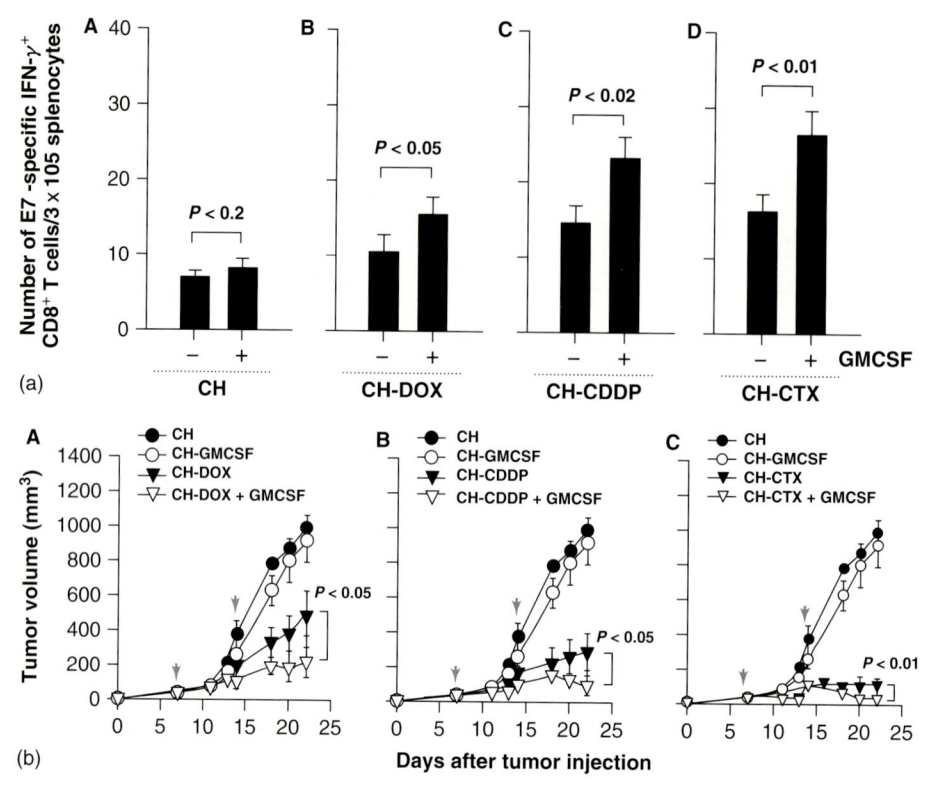

Figure 33.7 (a) Induction of E7-specific CD8+ T-cell immune response after treating chitosan hydrogel (CH; A) and chitosan hydrogels containing DOX (B), cisplatin (C), or CTX (D). Immune activity was much enhanced by addition of GM-CSF, but the combination of CTX and GM-CSF was superior. However, the order of immune activation (CTX > cisplatin > DOX) was not changed regardless of adding GM-CSF. IFN, interferon. (b) Antitumoral activity of various formulations in terms of tumor volume change. Hydrogels were intratumorally injected (twice in week 1 and 2 after tumor inoculation, arrows) into mice bearing murine TC-1 cervical cancer cells. Extent of antitumoral activity followed the order of immune induction. (Reproduced with permission from [32]. © 2009 Springer.)

a polycarbophil polymer gel showed that the protein drug was stable for at least 1 week without loss of dendritic cell recruitment function [28]. Furthermore, GM-CSF that was coloaded with DOX, cisplatin, or cyclophosphamide (CTX) in a chitosan hydrogel synergistically improved antitumoral activity of those drugs via strengthened T-cell-mediated immunity (Figure 33.7) [32].

Enzymes used to treat cancer can be divided into two types: (i) those that activate an anticancer prodrug at the tumor site and (ii) those that modulate the pathophysiological environment of the tumor tissue. Hydrogel-based therapy has been preferably attempted with the latter type of enzymes, including catalase and superoxide dismutase (SOD) to remove reactive oxygen species (ROS). ROS induce many negative issues in the body and, especially, prompt tumor progression [85].

Hyoudou et al. showed that a hydrogel loading PEGylated catalases significantly reduced pulmonary metastasis of B16-BL6 melanoma cells [30]. The same group confirmed that cationized catalase of ethylenediamine-conjugated catalase was retained in an acidic gelatin hydrogel for up to 2 weeks with suppression of tumor cell growth [31]. Li et al. loaded SOD in a thermosensitive hydrogel to remove ROS of inflammatory tissues [86]. On the contrary, Liu et al. delivered glucose oxidase (GOD) to the tumor site [29]. It is well known that GOD generates hydrogen peroxide (a kind of ROS) by metabolizing glucose. They found that ROS produced by GOD encapsulated in alginate/chitosan hydrogel microparticles increased cytotoxicity of tumor cells. Treatment with intracellular antioxidant enzyme inhibitors greatly enhanced tumor cell cytotoxicity. SOD plays a role to remove ROS and modulate local inflammation around tumor tissues, while GOD directly delivers ROS to tumor tissues. Those proof-of-concept studies should be carefully reproduced because inflammation, tumor metastasis, and the role of ROS in the biological environment are hardly defined in a simple manner.

Hydrogels have been extensively used to deliver various growth factors for tissue engineering and peptide hormones such as insulin and human growth hormone. Application to cancer therapy has been limited, but successful. Prostate cancer is a hormone-dependent disease and androgen plays a pivotal role to maintain pathophysiology of the cancer. Administration of a gonadotropin-releasing hormone (GnRH) agonist is known to suppress androgen production. Vantas® (Endo Pharmaceuticals) is a US Food and Drug Administration-approved formulation of histrelin (a GnRH agonist), in which, to sustain release of histrelin, a hydrogel consisting of a PHEMA is used as a reservoir. In clinical studies, Vantas showed complete suppression of testosterone and luteinizing hormone, resulting in a long-term androgen withdrawal (Figure 33.8) [26]. Surgical removal of the hydrogel implant resulted in a rapid increase of testosterone and luteinizing hormone [87].

33.3.3.3 Gene and siRNA Delivery

Delivery of protein/peptide drugs can be accomplished in three ways, as shown in Figure 33.3. One method is to deliver specific genes that can either deteriorate tumor cell viability or enhance immunity to kill tumor cells [88]. A couple of hydrogel-based gene delivery systems have been developed. To prevent metastasis of osteosarcoma, Ta et al. delivered a plasmid DNA encoding pigment epithelium-derived factor (PEDF) that creates a natural barrier to progression of tumor cells (Figure 33.9) [34]. Chitosan neutralized by dipotassium phosphate was used as a matrix. The main mechanism of plasmid DNA release was degradation of the hydrogel. A therapeutic effect, however, could be obtained only when the PEDF gene expression was assisted by an anticancer drug, DOX. According to this result, gene delivery to cancer seems to have a marginal or synergistic effect in combination with chemotherapy.

Hydrogels provide a unique property in gene therapy. Systemic administration of DNA/polymer complexes in nonviral gene delivery and engineered viruses in viral gene delivery has been hindered by a major problem – systemic toxicity. It is most desirable if a designated gene is expressed only at or around cancerous tissue. Although nanogels consisting of plasmid DNA and cationized polymer

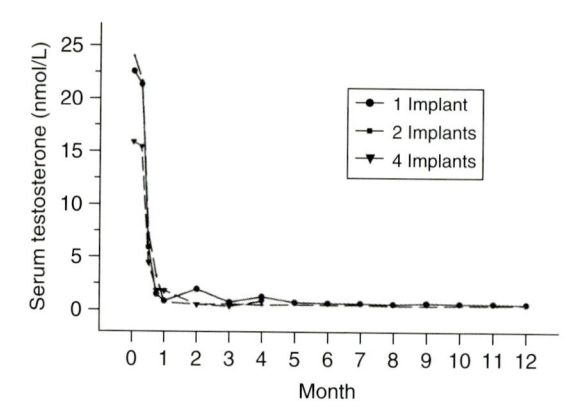

Figure 33.8 Serum testosterone level of patients with prostate cancer who received one, two, or four hydrogel implant(s) containing histrelin. After rapid decrease for 1 month, the basal level of serum testosterone was maintained for up to 1 year after implantation. (Reproduced with permission from [26]. © 2001 Elsevier.)

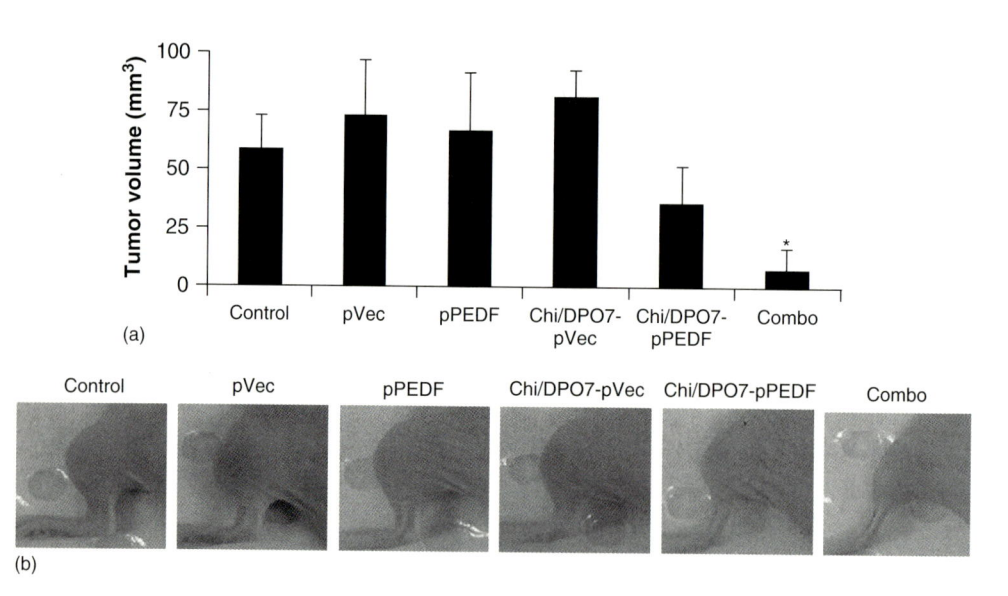

Figure 33.9 (a) Measured tumor volume when tumor-bearing mice (SaOS-2 cells with Matrigel) were intratibially treated by plasmid vector (pVec), plasmid expressing PEDF (pPEDF), chitosan hydrogels (Chi/DPO7) containing pVec or pPEDF, and Chi/DPO7 hydrogel containing pPEDF and DOX (Combo). (b) Chi/DPO7 hydrogel containing gene and anticancer agents clearly regressed the tumor mass. (Reproduced with permission from [34]. © 2009 Elsevier.)

have primarily focused on targeted delivery, systemic toxicity is more serious than for small-molecule anticancer agents. DNA continuously expresses a protein for a certain period of time while small-molecule drugs are cleared within several days. Hydrogel-based systems are able to provide a sustained release of therapeutic genes only at local tissues. Also, viral vectors carrying engineered DNA can be loaded in a hydrogel to reduce the risk of systemic toxicity. Megeed et al. developed a unique hydrogel system based on silk-elastinlike protein (SELP) polymer [36]. They loaded plasmid DNAs as well as genetically engineered viruses into the hydrogel in order to transfect cancer cells. In vitro study showed that release of plasmid DNA and virus was sustained for more than 1 month [37].

Instead of gene expression, hydrogel systems are useful to silence specific genes inducing tumorigenesis. RNA interference has been focused on as a promising strategy to treat various diseases, including cancer. Usually, siRNAs are employed to inhibit gene expression via suppressing protein synthesis at the level of mRNA. As a proof-of-concept study, Krebs et al. delivered siRNA to Green Fluorescent Protein (GFP)-expressing cancer cells using a hydrogel consisting of alginate, photo-cross-linkable alginate, and collagen [35]. Likewise with DNA delivery, siRNA release from a hydrogel can be highly localized at an injection or implantation site with a sustained release profile, so that systemic toxicity can be significantly reduced.

33.3.3.4 Cell Delivery

Hydrogels have also played a critical role in cell-based drug delivery. Living cells have been loaded and encapsulated in a hydrogel matrix to continuously release a certain protein or peptide drug. Cells secrete hormones required to normalize physiological function, such as insulin, neurotropic factors, or growth factors [89]. To treat cancer, Wang et al. attempted to deliver macrophages entrapped in an agarose hydrogel. It was found that macrophages activated by lipopolysaccharide to express antitumoral cytokines such as tumor necrosis factor-α survived up to 2–3 months. In other study, Li et al. engineered myoblasts to produce angiostatin – a potential protein drug to prevent neovascularization and subsequently to inhibit tumor cell growth (Figure 33.10) [38, 90]. They employed a conventional microencapsulation technology based on the layer-by-layer coating of hydrogel microspheres. Alginate and poly(L-lysine) were used to encapsulate myoblasts expressing angiostatin, which reduced tumor volume up to 80% in 21 days after implantation.

33.3.3.5 Photodynamic Therapy

In photodynamic therapy (PDT), photosensitizers that are delivered to tumor tissue generate cytotoxic singlet oxygen and ROS by external irradiation. By controlling irradiation power and area, cancer therapy can, in theory, be accomplished without any systemic toxicity. However, photosensitizers are generally poorly soluble and their systemic circulation often induces skin necrosis due to natural light, so that a drug carrier is required. Hydrogels suggested a possible solution to solve those problems. Bae and Na prepared a polysaccharide-based nanogel to deliver photosensitizers [91]. The nanogel was spontaneously generated in water

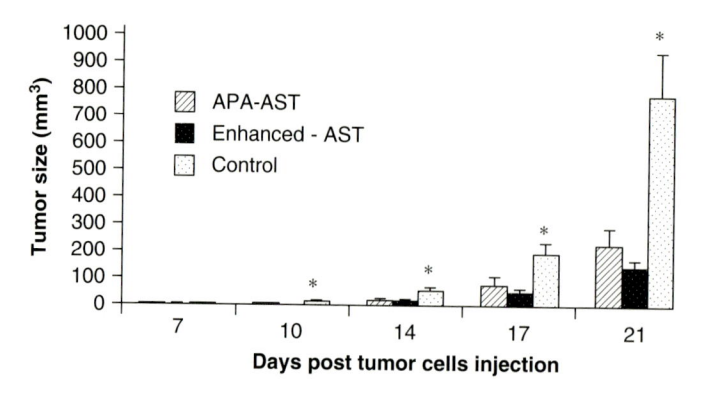

Figure 33.10 Antitumoral activity of angiostatin-secreting myoblast (AST) cells that were encapsulated in alginate–poly(L-lysine)–alginate (APA) microcapsules. After inoculation of B16-F0/neu tumor cells into mice, APA-AST capsules were intratumorally injected. In enhanced APA-AST microcapsules, basic fibroblast growth factor (bFGF), insulin-like growth factor-2 (IGF-2), and collagen were coencapsulated with AST cells. (Reproduced with permission from [38]. © 2006 Wiley.)

from a pullulan derivative conjugating tumor-targeting moieties (folate) and a photosensitizers (Pheo-A). *In vivo* imaging was conducted to observe location of intravenously injected nanogel. Trace of the nanogel was monitored up to 3 weeks after injection, which was due to the internalization of nanoparticles mediated by the folate receptor. In another study, they utilized hydrophobicity of the photosensitizer to make a nanogel [92]. Partially acetylated hyaluronic acid conjugating Pheo-A successfully generated a nanogel in water based on the hydrophobic effect between photosensitizers on the polysaccharide. Confocal laser microscopy revealed that the hydrogels were localized inside tumor cells via hyaluronic acid-mediated endocytosis. Although there are only few studies with no *in vivo* antitumoral activity, PDT is a promising method to treat solid tumors. Specific localization of photosensitizers at tumor tissues will be a key issue.

33.3.3.6 Radiotherapy

Radiotherapy is a popular method to treat cancer and almost 60% of cancer patients have been treated up to now. However, hydrogel-based radiation therapy has not been used widely in recent years. This may be due to the invasive nature and long half-life of isotopes such as ^{125}I. A recent study of hydrogel application to radiotherapy was combined with chemotherapy [40]. The alginate hydrogel bead loaded with ^{188}Re as well as cisplatin showed successful tumor suppression in a mouse model bearing mammary tumor cells up to 35 days, while ^{188}Re or cisplatin alone was not fully able to achieve antitumoral activity (Figure 33.11).

33.3.3.7 Thermotherapy

Hyperthermia at local cancerous tissue induces tumor cell apoptosis and tumor shrinkage [93]. The key issue is how to specifically generate heat only at tumor tissue. Hydrogels, especially nanogels containing inorganic nanoparticles, have suggested

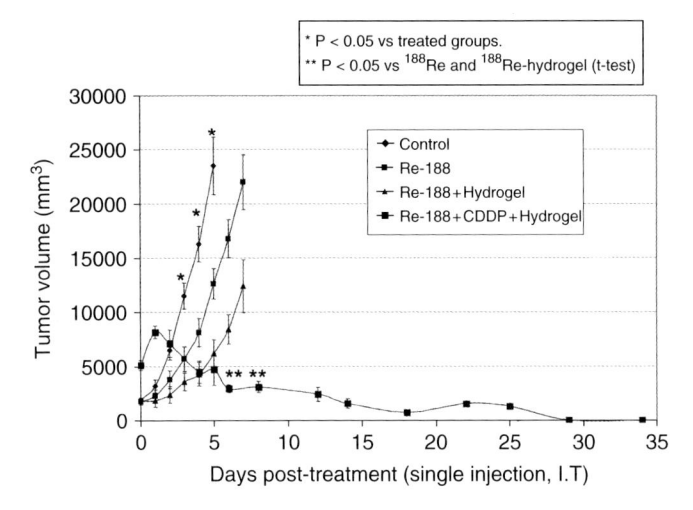

Figure 33.11 Hydrogel formulation containing both ^{188}Re and cisplatin (CDDP) almost completely suppressed tumor growth in 35 days after intratumoral (I.T.) injection into mice bearing RBA CRL-1747 rat breast cancer cells. (Reproduced with permission from [40]. © 2005 Springer.)

a clue for local hyperthermia. Gold nanoparticles (GNPs) are able to generate heat energy induced by irradiation of a external laser. Nakamura et al. entrapped PEGylated GNPs in poly(2-(N,N-diethylamino)ethyl methacrylate) nanogels [94]. It was found that viability of HeLa cells was significantly deteriorated by irradiation with an Ar$^+$ laser. Superparamagnetic iron oxide nanoparticles (SPIONs) have been utilized to enhance contrast during nuclear magnetic resonance imaging. Recently, it was suggested that SPIONs are useful for cancer thermotherapy. Le Renard et al. used various formulations consisting of chitosan, Poloxamer 407, alginate, poly(ethylene-co-vinyl alcohol), polyurethane, and cellulose acetates to load SPIONs and to conduct thermotherapy in vivo [44]. After intratumoral injection, those formulations were monitored in terms of gelation and the effect of magnetically induced thermotherapy. It was found that at least 20% SPIONs were required to achieve effective thermotherapy.

33.3.3.8 Embolization

Particle embolization has been used to treat many pathological issues, including cancer. Many microbeads of hydrogel-forming polymers, such as poly(vinyl alcohol), gelatin, dextran, poly(methyl methacrylate), and PHEMA, have been developed [41–43]. As most nontoxic hydrogel materials have been already developed for embolization material, only a few new reports have been produced during the past decade. For cancer therapy, embolization has been frequently combined with chemotherapy (chemoembolization) in order to maximize the therapeutic effect. Horák et al. reported that the dose of a chemotherapeutic agent, DOX, could be significantly reduced (around 10-fold) when DOX was used with embolic PHEMA beads [41]. It is expected that well-established chemoembolization in combination with imaging agents may provide a unique opportunity for imaging-guided therapy.

33.4
Conclusions and Perspectives

Through the years many hydrogel systems have been developed for cancer therapy. Recent systems preferably use biodegradable polymers. Many biodegradable polymers are now available, including degradable synthetic polymers as well as natural polymers and their chemically modified derivatives. Drug release from conventional hydrogel systems is primarily based on hydrogel swelling and drug diffusion through the polymer network. Biodegradable hydrogels have another mechanism of chemically controlled drug release. The *in situ* gelation method takes advantage of avoiding surgical implantation. Physical cross-linking methods do not use any reactive chemicals, so that chemical-derived toxicity can be reduced. For this reason, smart polymers have played an important role in the *in situ* gelation method. Smart hydrogels are also a useful tool in modulating or fine-tuning drug release profiles. Nanogels – another injectable formulation based on hydrogels – can deliver various drugs to cancerous tissues by their prolonged circulation time and the EPR effect.

Advances in anticancer therapy using hydrogels have been accelerated by the development of new materials as well as new applications of existing materials. Although efforts have been made to overcome cancer by developing an effective formulation of anticancer agents, only a limited number of hydrogel formulations have been used in clinical applications. As shown in Table 33.2, most anticancer hydrogel formulations are applicable only for local administration. Chemically cross-linked hydrogels often have a predefined shape (i.e., a disk) so that they are not injectable and a surgical implantation procedure should be conducted for therapy. Two injectable formulations were introduced previously: *in situ*-forming hydrogels and nanogels. However, even a hydrogel having a sol–gel phase transition is not always injectable via the intravenous route. The reason is shown in Figure 33.3. A polymer solution containing anticancer agents would rapidly turn into a hydrogel within a few minutes after injection. To achieve an intravenously injectable formulation, polymers conjugating drug molecules should be specifically accumulated only at the tumor tissue and then cross-linked there by external or internal triggering. Therefore, reducing the size of a hydrogel (i.e., a nanogel) will be a promising method in the future. Recent technology allows chemical modification, smart polymers, and targeting ligands to nanogels in order to maximize anticancer efficacy. However, more add-ons inevitably generate more variables, which need to be carefully examined before considering them for clinical applications.

Research on hydrogel systems for drug delivery must be continued to improve existing formulations. Application of hydrogel systems to other fields is also important for effective cancer therapy. Hydrogels can be used for bioimaging, biosensors, and cancer modeling as well. A nanogel containing an imaging probe is a handy tool to observe pharmacokinetics, biodistribution, RES uptake, and targeting efficiency [95–100]. Various imaging modalities are now available to image those nanogels or hydrogels depending on the conjugated or loaded imaging probes. Better understanding of the *in vivo* fate of hydrogels will lead to well-designed and effective drug delivery systems. Many biosensors constructed from hydrogels [101, 102] have been developed to monitor metabolic changes or detect and amplify cancer-related biomarkers. Tissue engineering research using hydrogels has resulted in the construction of *in vitro* models of solid tumors, which include the angiogenic ability of tumor cells [103] and three-dimensional tissue models for various cancer cells [26, 104]. Hydrogels have been and will continue to be a valuable tool for developing pharmaceutical formulations to treat cancer as well as for studying the fundamental aspects of cancer.

References

1. Wichterle, O. and Lim, D. (1960) Hydrophilic gels for biological use. *Nature*, **185**, 117–118.
2. Kim, S.W., Bae, Y.H., and Okano, T. (1992) Hydrogels – swelling, drug loading, and release. *Pharm. Res.*, **9**, 283–290.
3. Kou, J.H., Amidon, G.L., and Lee, P.I. (1988) pH-dependent swelling and solute diffusion characteristics of poly(hydroxyethyl methacrylate-*co*-methacrylic acid) hydrogels. *Pharm. Res.*, **5**, 592–597.
4. Berge, S.J., Wiese, K.G., von Lindern, J.J., Niederhagen, B., Appel, T., and Reich, R.H. (2001) Tissue expansion using osmotically active hydrogel systems for direct closure of the donor defect of the radial forearm flap. *Plast. Reconstr. Surg.*, **108**, 1–5.
5. Obdeijn, M.C., Nicolai, J.P., and Werker, P.M. (2009) The osmotic tissue expander: a three-year clinical experience. *J. Plast. Reconstr. Aesthet. Surg.*, **62**, 1219–1222.
6. Andrade, J.D. and Hlady, V. (1986) Protein adsorption and materials biocompatibility – a tutorial review and suggested hypotheses. *Adv. Polym. Sci.*, **79**, 1–63.
7. Lipinski, C.A. (2000) Drug-like properties and the causes of poor solubility and poor permeability. *J. Pharmacol. Toxicol. Method*, **44**, 235–249.
8. Lin, C.C. and Metters, A.T. (2006) Hydrogels in controlled release formulations: network design and mathematical modeling. *Adv. Drug. Deliv. Rev.*, **58**, 1379–1408.
9. Konishi, M., Tabata, Y., Kariya, M., Suzuki, A., Mandai, M., Nanbu, K., Takakura, K., and Fujii, S. (2003) *In vivo* anti-tumor effect through the controlled release of cisplatin from biodegradable gelatin hydrogel. *J. Control. Release*, **92**, 301–313.
10. Lalloo, A., Chao, P., Hu, P., Stein, S., and Sinko, P.J. (2006) Pharmacokinetic and pharmacodynamic evaluation of a novel *in situ* forming poly(ethylene glycol)-based hydrogel for the controlled delivery of the camptothecins. *J. Control. Release*, **112**, 333–342.
11. Li, X., Kong, X., Zhang, J., Wang, Y., Shi, S., Guo, G., Luo, F., Zhao, X., Wei, Y., and Qian, Z. (2011) A novel composite hydrogel based on chitosan and inorganic phosphate for local drug delivery of camptothecin nanocolloids. *J. Pharm. Sci.*, **100**, 232–241.
12. Obara, K., Ishihara, M., Ozeki, Y., Ishizuka, T., Hayashi, T., Nakamura, S., Saito, Y., Yura, H., Matsui, T., Hattori, H., Takase, B., Kikuchi, M., and Maehara, T. (2005) Controlled release of paclitaxel from photocrosslinked chitosan hydrogels

and its subsequent effect on subcutaneous tumor growth in mice. *J. Control. Release*, **110**, 79–89.

13. Ta, H.T., Dass, C.R., Larson, I., Choong, P.F., and Dunstan, D.E. (2009) A chitosan–dipotassium orthophosphate hydrogel for the delivery of doxorubicin in the treatment of osteosarcoma. *Biomaterials*, **30**, 3605–3613.

14. Ruel-Gariepy, E., Shive, M., Bichara, A., Berrada, M., Le Garrec, D., Chenite, A., and Leroux, J.C. (2004) A thermosensitive chitosan-based hydrogel for the local delivery of paclitaxel. *Eur. J. Pharm. Biopharm.*, **57**, 53–63.

15. Redpath, M., Marques, C.M., Dibden, C., Waddon, A., Lalla, R., and Macneil, S. (2009) Ibuprofen and hydrogel-released ibuprofen in the reduction of inflammation-induced migration in melanoma cells. *Br. J. Dermatol.*, **161**, 25–33.

16. Kwak, M.K., Hur, K., Yu, J.E., Han, T.S., Yanagihara, K., Kim, W.H., Lee, S.M., Song, S.C., and Yang, H.K. (2010) Suppression of *in vivo* tumor growth by using a biodegradable thermosensitive hydrogel polymer containing chemotherapeutic agent. *Invest. New Drugs*, **28**, 284–290.

17. Shim, W.S., Kim, J.H., Kim, K., Kim, Y.S., Park, R.W., Kim, I.S., Kwon, I.C., and Lee, D.S. (2007) pH- and temperature-sensitive, injectable, biodegradable block copolymer hydrogels as carriers for paclitaxel. *Int. J. Pharm.*, **331**, 11–18.

18. Wang, Y., Gong, C., Yang, L., Wu, Q., Shi, S., Shi, H., Qian, Z., and Wei, Y. (2010) 5-FU-hydrogel inhibits colorectal peritoneal carcinomatosis and tumor growth in mice. *BMC Cancer*, **10**, 402.

19. St'astny, M., Plocova, D., Etrych, T., Kovar, M., Ulbrich, K., and Rihova, B. (2002) HPMA-hydrogels containing cytostatic drugs. Kinetics of the drug release and *in vivo* efficacy. *J. Control. Release*, **81**, 101–111.

20. St'astny, M., Plocova, D., Etrych, T., Ulbrich, K., and Rihova, B. (2002) HPMA-hydrogels result in prolonged delivery of anticancer drugs and are a promising tool for the treatment of sensitive and multidrug resistant leukaemia. *Eur. J. Cancer*, **38**, 602–608.

21. Yu, L., Chang, G.T., Zhang, H., and Ding, J.D. (2008) Injectable block copolymer hydrogels for sustained release of a PEGylated drug. *Int. J. Pharm.*, **348**, 95–106.

22. Chun, C., Lee, S.M., Kim, C.W., Hong, K.Y., Kim, S.Y., Yang, H.K., and Song, S.C. (2009) Doxorubicin–polyphosphazene conjugate hydrogels for locally controlled delivery of cancer therapeutics. *Biomaterials*, **30**, 4752–4762.

23. Al-Abd, A.M., Hong, K.Y., Song, S.C., and Kuh, H.J. (2010) Pharmacokinetics of doxorubicin after intratumoral injection using a thermosensitive hydrogel in tumor-bearing mice. *J. Control. Release*, **142**, 101–107.

24. Cho, Y.I., Park, S., Jeong, S.Y., and Yoo, H.S. (2009) *In vivo* and *in vitro* anti-cancer activity of thermo-sensitive and photo-crosslinkable doxorubicin hydrogels composed of chitosan–doxorubicin conjugates. *Eur. J. Pharm. Biopharm.*, **73**, 59–65.

25. Varghese, O.P., Sun, W., Hilborn, J., and Ossipov, D.A. (2009) *In situ* cross-linkable high molecular weight hyaluronan–bisphosphonate conjugate for localized delivery and cell-specific targeting: a hydrogel linked prodrug approach. *J. Am. Chem. Soc.*, **131**, 8781–8783.

26. Schlegel, P.N., Kuzma, P., Frick, J., Farkas, A., Gomahr, A., Spitz, I., Chertin, B., Mack, D., Jungwirth, A., King, P., Nash, H., Bardin, C.W., and Moo-Young, A. (2001) Effective long-term androgen suppression in men with prostate cancer using a hydrogel implant with the GnRH agonist histrelin. *Urology*, **58**, 578–582.

27. Liu, L., Sakaguchi, T., Kanda, T., Hitomi, J., Tabata, Y., and Hatakeyama, K. (2003) Delivery of interleukin-12 in gelatin hydrogels effectively suppresses development of transplanted colonal carcinoma in mice. *Cancer Chemother. Pharmacol.*, **51**, 53–57.

28. Hubert, P., Evrard, B., Maillard, C., Franzen-Detrooz, E., Delattre, L., Foidart, J.M., Noel, A., Boniver, J., and Delvenne, P. (2004) Delivery of granulocyte-macrophage colony-stimulating factor in bioadhesive hydrogel stimulates migration of dendritic cells in models of human papillomavirus-associated (pre)neoplastic epithelial lesions. *Antimicrob. Agents Chemother.*, **48**, 4342–4348.

29. Liu, Q., Shuhendler, A., Cheng, J., Rauth, A.M., O'Brien, P., and Wu, X.Y. (2010) Cytotoxicity and mechanism of action of a new ROS-generating microsphere formulation for circumventing multidrug resistance in breast cancer cells. *Breast Cancer Res. Treat.*, **121**, 323–333.

30. Hyoudou, K., Nishikawa, M., Ikemura, M., Kobayashi, Y., Mendelsohn, A., Miyazaki, N., Tabata, Y., Yamashita, F., and Hashida, M. (2009) Prevention of pulmonary metastasis from subcutaneous tumors by binary system-based sustained delivery of catalase. *J. Control. Release*, **137**, 110–115.

31. Hyoudou, K., Nishikawa, M., Ikemura, M., Kobayashi, Y., Mendelsohn, A., Miyazaki, N., Tabata, Y., Yamashita, F., and Hashida, M. (2007) Cationized catalase-loaded hydrogel for growth inhibition of peritoneally disseminated tumor cells. *J. Control. Release*, **122**, 151–158.

32. Seo, S.H., Han, H.D., Noh, K.H., Kim, T.W., and Son, S.W. (2009) Chitosan hydrogel containing GMCSF and a cancer drug exerts synergistic anti-tumor effects via the induction of CD8$^+$ T cell-mediated anti-tumor immunity. *Clin. Exp. Metastasis*, **26**, 179–187.

33. Han, H.D., Song, C.K., Park, Y.S., Noh, K.H., Kim, J.H., Hwang, Y., Kim, T.W., and Shin, B.C. (2008) A chitosan hydrogel-based cancer drug delivery system exhibits synergistic antitumor effects by combining with a vaccinia viral vaccine. *Int. J. Pharm.*, **350**, 27–34.

34. Ta, H.T., Dass, C.R., Larson, I., Choong, P.F., and Dunstan, D.E. (2009) A chitosan hydrogel delivery system for osteosarcoma gene therapy with pigment epithelium-derived factor combined with chemotherapy. *Biomaterials*, **30**, 4815–4823.

35. Krebs, M.D., Jeon, O., and Alsberg, E. (2009) Localized and sustained delivery of silencing RNA from macroscopic biopolymer hydrogels. *J. Am. Chem. Soc.*, **131**, 9204–9206.

36. Megeed, Z., Haider, M., Li, D., O'Malley Jr., B.W., Cappello, J., and Ghandehari, H. (2004) *In vitro* and *in vivo* evaluation of recombinant silk-elastinlike hydrogels for cancer gene therapy. *J. Control. Release*, **94**, 433–445.

37. Hatefi, A., Cappello, J., and Ghandehari, H. (2007) Adenoviral gene delivery to solid tumors by recombinant silk-elastinlike protein polymers. *Pharm. Res.*, **24**, 773–779.

38. Li, A.A., Shen, F., Zhang, T., Cirone, P., Potter, M., and Chang, P.L. (2006) Enhancement of myoblast microencapsulation for gene therapy. *J. Biomed. Mater. Res. B*, **77**, 296–306.

39. Wang, C., Adrianus, G.N., Sheng, N., Toh, S., Gong, Y., and Wang, D.A. (2009) *In vitro* performance of an injectable hydrogel/microsphere based immunocyte delivery system for localised anti-tumour activity. *Biomaterials*, **30**, 6986–6995.

40. Azhdarinia, A., Yang, D.J., Yu, D.F., Mendez, R., Oh, C., Kohanim, S., Bryant, J., and Kim, E.E. (2005) Regional radiochemotherapy using *in situ* hydrogel. *Pharm. Res.*, **22**, 776–783.

41. Horak, D., Guseinov, E., Vishnevskii, V., Adamyan, A., Kokov, L., Tsvirkun, V., Tchjao, A., Titova, M., Skuba, N., Trostenyuk, N., and Gumargalieva, K. (2000) Targeted chemoembolization of tumors with poly(2-hydroxyethyl methacrylate) particles. *J. Biomed. Mater. Res.*, **51**, 184–190.

42. Phadke, R.V., Venkatesh, S.K., Kumar, S., Tandon, V., Pandey, R., Tyagi, I., Jain, V.K., and Chhabra, D.K. (2002) Embolization of cranial/spinal tumours and vascular malformations with hydrogel microspheres. An experience of 69 cases. *Acta Radiol.*, **43**, 15–20.

43. van Es, R.J., Nijsen, J.F., Dullens, H.F., Kicken, M., van der Bilt, A., Hennink, W., Koole, R., and Slootweg, P.J. (2001) Tumour embolization of the Vx2 rabbit head and neck cancer model with dextran hydrogel and holmium–poly (L-lactic acid) microspheres: a radionuclide and histological pilot study. *J. Craniomaxillofac. Surg.*, **29**, 289–297.
44. Le Renard, P.E., Jordan, O., Faes, A., Petri-Fink, A., Hofmann, H., Rufenacht, D., Bosman, F., Buchegger, F., and Doelker, E. (2010) The *in vivo* performance of magnetic particle-loaded injectable, *in situ* gelling, carriers for the delivery of local hyperthermia. *Biomaterials*, **31**, 691–705.
45. Chaterji, S., Kwon, I.K., and Park, K. (2007) Smart polymeric gels: redefining the limits of biomedical devices. *Prog. Polym. Sci.*, **32**, 1083–1122.
46. Banta, S., Wheeldon, I.R., and Blenner, M. (2010) Protein engineering in the development of functional hydrogels. *Annu. Rev. Biomed. Eng.*, **12**, 167–186.
47. Ehrick, J.D., Deo, S.K., Browning, T.W., Bachas, L.G., Madou, M.J., and Daunert, S. (2005) Genetically engineered protein in hydrogels tailors stimuli-responsive characteristics. *Nat. Mater.*, **4**, 298–302.
48. Burkoth, A.K. and Anseth, K.S. (2000) A review of photocrosslinked polyanhydrides: *in situ* forming degradable networks. *Biomaterials*, **21**, 2395–2404.
49. Davis, N.E., Ding, S., Forster, R.E., Pinkas, D.M., and Barron, A.E. (2010) Modular enzymatically crosslinked protein polymer hydrogels for *in situ* gelation. *Biomaterials*, **31**, 7288–7297.
50. Jeong, B., Kim, S.W., and Bae, Y.H. (2002) Thermosensitive sol–gel reversible hydrogels. *Adv. Drug Deliv. Rev.*, **54**, 37–51.
51. Nguyen, K.T., Shukla, K.P., Moctezuma, M., Braden, A.R., Zhou, J., Hu, Z., and Tang, L. (2009) Studies of the cellular uptake of hydrogel nanospheres and microspheres by phagocytes, vascular endothelial cells, and smooth muscle cells. *J. Biomed. Mater. Res. A*, **88**, 1022–1030.
52. Lakshmi, S., Katti, D.S., and Laurencin, C.T. (2003) Biodegradable polyphosphazenes for drug delivery applications. *Adv. Drug Deliv. Rev.*, **55**, 467–482.
53. Ta, H.T., Dass, C.R., and Dunstan, D.E. (2008) Injectable chitosan hydrogels for localised cancer therapy. *J. Control. Release*, **126**, 205–216.
54. Shidhaye, S., Lotlikar, V., Malke, S., and Kadam, V. (2008) Nanogel engineered polymeric micelles for drug delivery. *Curr. Drug Ther.*, **3**, 209–217.
55. Hamidi, M., Azadi, A., and Rafiei, P. (2008) Hydrogel nanoparticles in drug delivery. *Adv. Drug Deliv. Rev.*, **60**, 1638–1649.
56. Kim, S., Park, K.M., Ko, J.Y., Kwon, I.C., Cho, H.G., Kang, D., Yu, I.T., Kim, K., and Na, K. (2008) Minimalism in fabrication of self-organized nanogels holding both anti-cancer drug and targeting moiety. *Colloids Surf. B*, **63**, 55–63.
57. Na, K., Park, K.H., Kim, S.W., and Bae, Y.H. (2000) Self-assembled hydrogel nanoparticles from curdlan derivatives: characterization, anti-cancer drug release and interaction with a hepatoma cell line (HepG2). *J. Control. Release*, **69**, 225–236.
58. Oh, N.M., Oh, K.T., Baik, H.J., Lee, B.R., Lee, A.H., Youn, Y.S., and Lee, E.S. (2010) A self-organized 3-diethylaminopropyl-bearing glycol chitosan nanogel for tumor acidic pH targeting: *in vitro* evaluation. *Colloids Surf. B*, **78**, 120–126.
59. Park, W., Park, S.J., and Na, K. (2010) Potential of self-organizing nanogel with acetylated chondroitin sulfate as an anti-cancer drug carrier. *Colloids Surf. B*, **79**, 501–508.
60. Huang, S.J., Sun, S.L., Feng, T.H., Sung, K.H., Lui, W.L., and Wang, L.F. (2009) Folate-mediated chondroitin sulfate–Pluronic 127 nanogels as a drug carrier. *Eur. J. Pharm. Sci.*, **38**, 64–73.
61. Ray, D., Mohapatra, D.K., Mohapatra, R.K., Mohanta, G.P., and Sahoo, P.K. (2008) Synthesis and colon-specific drug delivery of a poly(acrylic acid-*co*-acrylamide)/MBA nanosized

hydrogel. *J. Biomater. Sci. Polym. Ed.*, **19**, 1487–1502.
62. Oishi, M. and Nagasaki, Y. (2010) Stimuli-responsive smart nanogels for cancer diagnostics and therapy. *Nanomedicine*, **5**, 451–468.
63. Na, K., Lee, E.S., and Bae, Y.H. (2007) Self-organized nanogels responding to tumor extracellular pH: pH-dependent drug release and *in vitro* cytotoxicity against MCF-7 cells. *Bioconjug. Chem.*, **18**, 1568–1574.
64. Yu, J., Lee, H.J., Hur, K., Kwak, M.K., Han, T.S., Kim, W.H., Song, S.C., Yanagihara, K., and Yang, H.K. (2010) The antitumor effect of a thermosensitive polymeric hydrogel containing paclitaxel in a peritoneal carcinomatosis model. *Invest. New Drugs*, Epub ahead of print. DOI: 10.1007/s10637-010-9499-y.
65. Cho, J., Heuzey, M.C., Begin, A., and Carreau, P.J. (2005) Physical gelation of chitosan in the presence of beta-glycerophosphate: the effect of temperature. *Biomacromolecules*, **6**, 3267–3275.
66. Ishihara, M., Obara, K., Nakamura, S., Fujita, M., Masuoka, K., Kanatani, Y., Takase, B., Hattori, H., Morimoto, Y., Maehara, T., and Kikuchi, M. (2006) Chitosan hydrogel as a drug delivery carrier to control angiogenesis. *J. Artif. Organs*, **9**, 8–16.
67. Kim, J.Y., Kim, S., Papp, M., Park, K., and Pinal, R. (2010) Hydrotropic solubilization of poorly water-soluble drugs. *J. Pharm. Sci.*, **99**, 3953–3965.
68. Cruise, G.M., Scharp, D.S., and Hubbell, J.A. (1998) Characterization of permeability and network structure of interfacially photopolymerized poly(ethylene glycol) diacrylate hydrogels. *Biomaterials*, **19**, 1287–1294.
69. Hoare, T.R. and Kohane, D.S. (2008) Hydrogels in drug delivery: progress and challenges. *Polymer*, **49**, 1993–2007.
70. Ranganath, S.H., Kee, I., Krantz, W.B., Chow, P.K., and Wang, C.H. (2009) Hydrogel matrix entrapping PLGA–paclitaxel microspheres: drug delivery with near zero-order release and implantability advantages for malignant brain tumour chemotherapy. *Pharm. Res.*, **26**, 2101–2114.
71. Fang, F., Gong, C., Qian, Z., Zhang, X., Gou, M., You, C., Zhou, L., Liu, J., Zhang, Y., Guo, G., Gu, Y., Luo, F., Chen, L., Zhao, X., and Wei, Y. (2009) Honokiol nanoparticles in thermosensitive hydrogel: therapeutic effects on malignant pleural effusion. *ACS Nano*, **3**, 4080–4088.
72. Davis, M.E. and Brewster, M.E. (2004) Cyclodextrin-based pharmaceutics: past, present and future. *Nat. Rev. Drug Discov.*, **3**, 1023–1035.
73. Stella, V.J. and Nti-Addae, K.W. (2007) Prodrug strategies to overcome poor water solubility. *Adv. Drug Deliv. Rev.*, **59**, 677–694.
74. Rihova, B., Srogl, J., Jelinkova, M., Hovorka, O., Buresova, M., Subr, V., and Ulbrich, K. (1997) HPMA-based biodegradable hydrogels containing different forms of doxorubicin. Antitumor effects and biocompatibility. *Ann. NY Acad. Sci.*, **831**, 57–71.
75. Screnci, D., McKeage, M.J., Galettis, P., Hambley, T.W., Palmer, B.D., and Baguley, B.C. (2000) Relationships between hydrophobicity, reactivity, accumulation and peripheral nerve toxicity of a series of platinum drugs. *Br. J. Cancer*, **82**, 966–972.
76. Casolaro, M., Cini, R., Del Bello, B., Ferrali, M., and Maellaro, E. (2009) Cisplatin/hydrogel complex in cancer therapy. *Biomacromolecules*, **10**, 944–949.
77. Tauro, J.R. and Gemeinhart, R.A. (2005) Matrix metalloprotease triggered delivery of cancer chemotherapeutics from hydrogel matrixes. *Bioconjug. Chem.*, **16**, 1133–1139.
78. Fang, J.Y., Chen, J.P., Leu, Y.L., and Hu, J.W. (2008) The delivery of platinum drugs from thermosensitive hydrogels containing different ratios of chitosan. *Drug Deliv.*, **15**, 235–243.
79. Ye, M., Kim, S., and Park, K. (2010) Issues in long-term protein delivery using biodegradable microparticles. *J. Control. Release*, **146**, 241–260.
80. Mellott, M.B., Searcy, K., and Pishko, M.V. (2001) Release of protein

81. Lu, Y., Yang, J., and Sega, E. (2006) Issues related to targeted delivery of proteins and peptides. *AAPS J.*, **8**, E466–E478.
82. Zhang, Y., Schulte, W., Pink, D., Phipps, K., Zijlstra, A., Lewis, J.D., and Waisman, D.M. (2010) Sensitivity of cancer cells to truncated diphtheria toxin. *PLoS ONE*, **5**, e10498.
83. Kikuchi, T., Joki, T., Abe, T., and Ohno, T. (1999) Antitumor activity of killer cells stimulated with both interleukin-2 and interleukin-12 on mouse glioma cells. *J. Immunother.*, **22**, 245–250.
84. Hamilton, J.A. (2002) GM-CSF in inflammation and autoimmunity. *Trends Immunol.*, **23**, 403–408.
85. Wu, W.S. (2006) The signaling mechanism of ROS in tumor progression. *Cancer Metastasis Rev.*, **25**, 695–705.
86. Li, Z., Wang, F., Roy, S., Sen, C.K., and Guan, J. (2009) Injectable, highly flexible, and thermosensitive hydrogels capable of delivering superoxide dismutase. *Biomacromolecules*, **10**, 3306–3316.
87. Fridmans, A., Chertin, B., Koulikov, D., Lindenberg, T., Gelber, H., Leiter, C., Farkas, A., and Spitz, I.M. (2005) Reversibility of androgen deprivation therapy in patients with prostate cancer. *J. Urol.*, **173**, 784–789.
88. Vile, R.G., Russell, S.J., and Lemoine, N.R. (2000) Cancer gene therapy: hard lessons and new courses. *Gene Ther.*, **7**, 2–8.
89. Schmidt, J.J., Rowley, J., and Kong, H.J. (2008) Hydrogels used for cell-based drug delivery. *J. Biomed. Mater. Res. A*, **87**, 1113–1122.
90. Matsumoto, G. and Shindo, J. (2001) Cancer therapy by gene therapy with angiostatin. *Drugs Today*, **37**, 815–821.
91. Bae, B.C. and Na, K. (2010) Self-quenching polysaccharide-based nanogels of pullulan/folate–photosensitizer conjugates for photodynamic therapy. *Biomaterials*, **31**, 6325–6335.
92. Li, F., Bae, B.C., and Na, K. (2010) Acetylated hyaluronic acid/photosensitizer conjugate for the preparation of nanogels with controllable phototoxicity: synthesis, characterization, autophotoquenching properties, and in vitro phototoxicity against HeLa cells. *Bioconjug. Chem.*, **21**, 1312–1320.
93. Hildebrandt, B., Wust, P., Ahlers, O., Dieing, A., Sreenivasa, G., Kerner, T., Felix, R., and Riess, H. (2002) The cellular and molecular basis of hyperthermia. *Crit. Rev. Oncol. Hematol.*, **43**, 33–56.
94. Nakamura, T., Tamura, A., Murotani, H., Oishi, M., Jinji, Y., Matsuishi, K., and Nagasaki, Y. (2010) Large payloads of gold nanoparticles into the polyamine network core of stimuli-responsive PEGylated nanogels for selective and noninvasive cancer photothermal therapy. *Nanoscale*, **2**, 739–746.
95. Yang, Z., Leon, J., Martin, M., Harder, J.W., Zhang, R., Liang, D., Lu, W., Tian, M., Gelovani, J.G., Qiao, A., and Li, C. (2009) Pharmacokinetics and biodistribution of near-infrared fluorescence polymeric nanoparticles. *Nanotechnology*, **20**, 165101.
96. Zhang, J., Chen, H., Xu, L., and Gu, Y. (2008) The targeted behavior of thermally responsive nanohydrogel evaluated by NIR system in mouse model. *J. Control. Release*, **131**, 34–40.
97. Wang, J., Loh, K.P., Wang, Z., Yan, Y., Zhong, Y., Xu, Q.H., and Ho, P.C. (2009) Fluorescent nanogel of arsenic sulfide nanoclusters. *Angew. Chem. Int. Ed. Engl.*, **48**, 6282–6285.
98. Gaur, U., Sahoo, S.K., De, T.K., Ghosh, P.C., Maitra, A., and Ghosh, P.K. (2000) Biodistribution of fluoresceinated dextran using novel nanoparticles evading reticuloendothelial system. *Int. J. Pharm.*, **202**, 1–10.
99. Mitra, S., Gaur, U., Ghosh, P.C., and Maitra, A.N. (2001) Tumour targeted delivery of encapsulated dextran–doxorubicin conjugate using chitosan nanoparticles as carrier. *J. Control. Release*, **74**, 317–323.

100. Wu, W., Shen, J., Banerjee, P., and Zhou, S. (2010) Core-shell hybrid nanogels for integration of optical temperature-sensing, targeted tumor cell imaging, and combined chemo-photothermal treatment. *Biomaterials*, **31**, 7555–7566.
101. Bhardwaj, U., Papadimitrakopoulos, F., and Burgess, D.J. (2008) A review of the development of a vehicle for localized and controlled drug delivery for implantable biosensors. *J. Diabetes Sci. Technol.*, **2**, 1016–1029.
102. Huang, H., Qi, Z., Deng, L., Zhou, G., Kajiyama, T., and Kambara, H. (2009) Highly sensitive mutation detection based on digital amplification coupled with hydrogel bead-array. *Chem. Commun.*, 4094–4096.
103. Fischbach, C., Kong, H.J., Hsiong, S.X., Evangelista, M.B., Yuen, W., and Mooney, D.J. (2009) Cancer cell angiogenic capability is regulated by 3D culture and integrin engagement. *Proc. Natl. Acad. Sci. USA*, **106**, 399–404.
104. Xu, X. and Prestwich, G.D. (2010) Inhibition of tumor growth and angiogenesis by a lysophosphatidic acid antagonist in an engineered three-dimensional lung cancer xenograft model. *Cancer*, **116**, 1739–1750.

34
pH-Triggered Micelles for Tumor Delivery

Haiqing Yin and You Han Bae

34.1
Introduction

Among various cancer therapies, chemotherapy is one of the major treatment modalities, along with debulking surgery. Although anticancer agents may be locally administered, many cancerous tissues can only be reached through the systemic administration of agents. Despite the discovery and development of a spectrum of anticancer drugs for the treatment of cancers, their clinical outcomes have been disappointing [1]. This is often due to severe side-effects as a result of their exposure to other cell types before reaching the tumor cells [2]. Poor bioavailability, lack of tumor selectivity, and recurrence of cancers with intrinsic or acquired drug resistance [3] have also decreased the therapeutic efficacy of the drugs.

Since it was found that colloidal carriers in the nanometer size range are able to escape the vasculature through abnormally leaky tumor blood vessels and are subsequently retained in the tumor tissue due to a lack of effective tumor lymphatic drainage [4], also known as the enhanced permeability and retention (EPR) effect (see Chapter 3), nanocarrier-mediated delivery has emerged as a successful strategy to enhance delivery of therapeutics and imaging agents to tumors. As a typical kind of supermolecular self-assembly formed in aqueous solutions from amphiphilic polymers, micelles have been receiving increased attention as potential drug carriers due to their nanoscale size and the ability to encapsulate hydrophobic drugs [5–8].

The ultimate goal of controlled drug delivery is to achieve a desired therapeutic concentration at the targeting site while the drug concentrations at other tissues are kept at safe levels. This challenge has motivated the development of various stimulus-responsive micelle systems that are designed to release their payload in a controlled manner upon arrival at the target site in response to a specific external or internal stimulus, such as pH, temperature, light, magnetic field, redox-potential, and so on. Among all the stimuli, change in the acidity (pH) is a particularly useful environmental stimulus for tumor delivery owing to various pH gradients that exist in both normal and pathophysiological states, as shown in Table 34.1. For example,

Table 34.1 pH variations in different tissues and subcellular organelles.

Tissues/subcellular organelles	pH
Normal tissue intracellular	7.2
Blood and normal tissue extracellular	7.4
Tumor extracellular	average 6.8, mostly lower than 7.2
Tumor intracellular	7.2
Early endosome	6.5–6.0
Late endosome	6.0–5.0
Lysosome	5.0–4.5

it is known that interstitial fluid in tumors tends to have a lower pH than in normal tissues [9–12]. pH changes are also encountered when the carriers are internalized via endocytotic pathways, where pH can drop to as low as 6.5–5.0 in endosomes and 5.0–4.5 in lysosomes [13, 14]. All the above pH discrepancies can be used as an internal signal to direct the response of the drug carriers to selectively release the loaded anticancer agents within tumor tissue or inside tumor cells.

In this chapter, features and causes of tumor extracellular acidity are first introduced. Thereafter, general approaches to construct pH-sensitive polymeric micelle carriers are addressed, followed by a comprehensive review of recent advances in the development of pH-sensitive micelles for tumor-targeted drug delivery. Finally, a perspective toward potential pharmaceutical products is envisaged. Interested readers are also encouraged to refer to other review articles [15–18].

34.2
Tumor Extracellular Acidity

The same as the blood pH, the extracellular pH (pH_e) of normal tissue is typically kept at pH 7.4 while their intracellular pH (pH_i) at 7.2. However, evidence accumulated over the past 50 years has consistently shown that human tumor pH_e is substantially lower than the pH_e of normal tissue [9–12]. One early study conducted by Thistlethwaite et al. [19] revealed that the average value of 53 tumor pH readings from 14 human tumors was 6.81 as measured by needle-type microelectrodes even though there was a relatively wide distribution in tumor pH values, ranging between 5.55 and 7.69. Similar low pH profiles were also reported in human tumor xenografts in mice (Figure 34.1a). Recent studies using noninvasive technologies such as ^{19}F-, ^{31}P-, or ^{1}H-magnetic resonance spectroscopy further verified such consistently low pH_e [20, 21]. In fact, more than 80% of all reported tumor pH_e values taken in human and animal solid tumors (via either invasive or noninvasive methods) were below pH 7.2 [22–25].

Figure 34.2 indicates the correlative factors that affect pH_i and pH_e in normal and tumor tissue. A major cause of tumor acidity is thought to be the greater

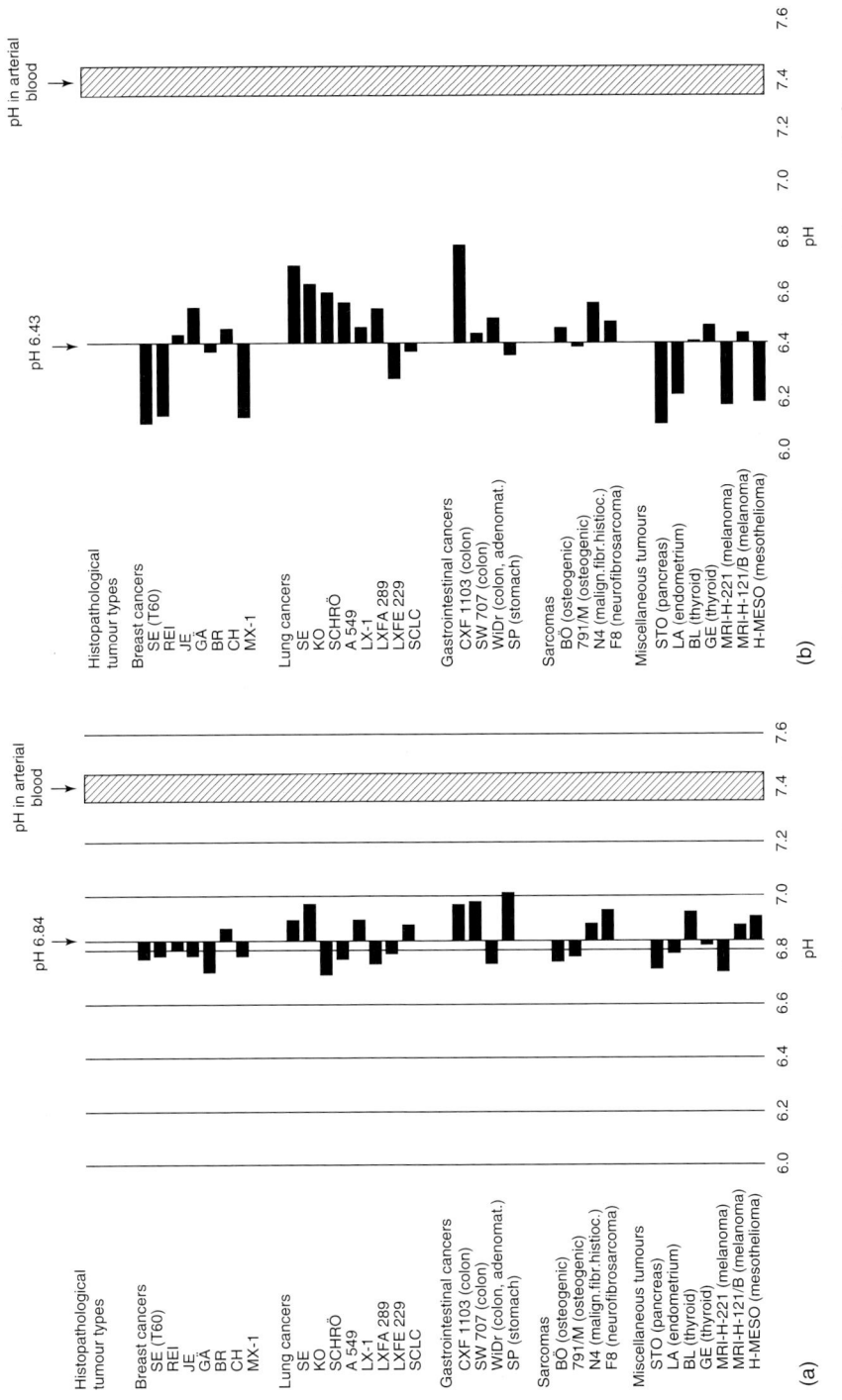

Figure 34.1 (a) pH in human tumor xenografts. pH 6.84 indicates the average value of all single-point measurements recorded in a total of 268 xenografts. Black bars indicate the difference between the average value and the mean pH of individual tumor xenografts. (b) pH following glucose-mediated stimulation of aerobic glycolysis. pH measurements were performed at 4 h after the plasma glucose concentration was raised to 30 ± 3 mm [22].

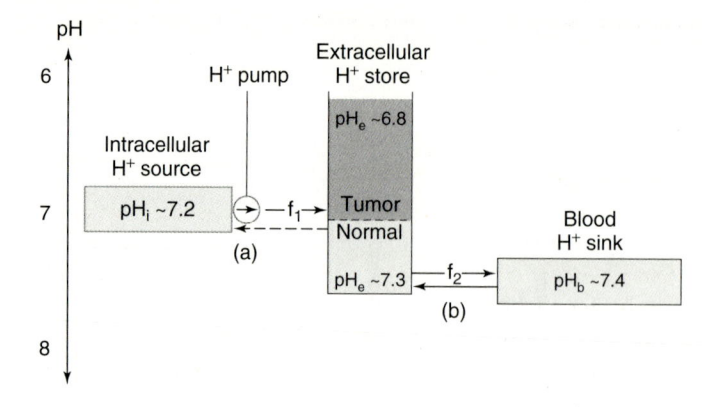

Figure 34.2 Factors affecting pH$_i$ and pH$_e$ in normal and tumor tissue. H$^+$ produced by metabolism is pumped from the intracellular compartment into the interstitial compartment and subsequently flows into the blood. At steady state, the flow (f) of H$^+$ between the compartments is equal ($f_1 = f_2$). The increased interstitial acidity of tumor cells could be caused by (a) an increase in H$^+$ pumping or (b) an increase in resistance induced by altered gene expression at the interstitial/vascular interface [30].

production of lactic acid in tumor cells through the glycolysis pathway, even under aerobic conditions [12]. One direct consequence of the high glycolytic rate in tumors is the increased glucose transport and consumption that forms the biological basis for positron emission tomography (PET) using the glucose analog tracer ^{18}F-fluorodeoxyglucose (^{18}F-FDG) [26]. ^{18}F-FDG uptake imaged by PET has confirmed substantially increased glucose uptake in the vast majority of primary and metastatic tumors when compared with normal tissue [27, 28]. It has been further established that the excess hydrogen ions produced are excreted from the cell via hydrogen ion pumps, such that the intracellular environment is maintained at a more physiologically normal pH [29]. The disorganized vasculature of tumors, poor lymphatic drainage, and elevated interstitial pressure lead to the inefficient washout of the acidic products, and further contribute to the development of the chronically acidic extracellular environment [30]. Recent work suggests the pH$_e$ of solid tumors may be independently regulated *in vivo* [31] and other metabolic pathways may also contribute to the acid production [32, 33]. An acidic extracellular environment can confer survival and growth advantages of tumor cells by facilitating extracellular matrix breakdown as well as tumor migration and invasion [34]. Low pH$_e$ has also been associated with tumorigenic transformation and induction of the expression of cell growth factors and proteases [30]. The above facts indicate the acidic pH$_e$ may not be just a consequence of tumor metabolism, but rather an intrinsic part of the tumor phenotype. Additionally, it is found that tumor pH$_e$ can be further reduced upon intravenous administration of glucose as a result of more accelerated glycolysis [22, 35] (Figure 34.1b).

34.3
General Approaches to Construct pH-Sensitive Polymeric Micelles for Tumor Delivery

Amphiphilic block copolymers of the AB type are generally used to fabricate polymeric micelles, where "A" represents a hydrophilic block and "B" represents a hydrophobic block. A typical spherical micelle possesses a core–shell structure of 20–200 nm in diameter in which water-hating (hydrophobic) ends of the individual polymers (unimers) are held together by hydrophobic interactions to make the core and water-loving (hydrophilic) ends make the corona (shell) [36]. Poly(ethylene glycol) (PEG) is most commonly used as the hydrophilic segment due to its good biocompatibility and minimum interactions with serum proteins to prolong circulation time *in vivo* by avoiding the reticuloendothelial system [37]. For intravenously injected drug carriers, the normal physiological pH (7.4) is maintained during their systemic circulation, while a more acidic environment is encountered either in the tumor extracellular matrix following passive accumulation via the EPR effect or in the endocytic compartments of tumor cells. Therefore, it is not difficult to consider that a pH-responsive micelle carrier designed for tumor delivery should be stable at pH 7.4, but it is able to undergo some kind of structural transformation at lower pH to trigger drug release or/and enhance drug uptake into the tumor cells. Two major approaches can be applied to endow the micelles formed from an AB diblock polymer with such suitable pH sensitivity (Figure 34.3):

1) The A or B block has "titratable" groups. Typical polymers of this type are polyacids or polybases. Polyacids are generally polymers that have pendant weak acidic groups like carboxylic acid, while polybases are polymers that have pendant weak basic groups like secondary or tertiary amine groups. pH-triggered micelle transformation is basically attributed to ionization (protonation or deprotonation) of the pendant groups, which turns the molecules from soluble to insoluble or vice versa. For example, micelles formed from a amphiphilic copolymer of PEG-*b*-poly(L-histidine) were found to gradually dissociate below pH 7.4 due to the protonation of imidazole groups that turned the poly(L-histidine) block from hydrophobic to hydrophilic [38]. Due to the nature of fast protonation/deprotonation rate in water, this type of polymers can enable a rapid structural transition of the micelles and lead to quick drug release upon a small pH change; therefore, they have been widely exploited for pH-triggered drug delivery.

2) The polymer bears acid-cleavable linkages. Dependent on the linkage location, different acid-labile bonds can be positioned either in the main-chain, at the side-chain, or at the terminal of the core-forming block. On the other hand, dependent on the different triggering mechanisms, these polymers can be further divided into three subcategories: (i) attach the drug molecule to the polymer via acid-cleavable linkages like hydrazone and *cis*-acotinyl [39] so that drug release can be induced by direct linkage cleavage; (ii) incorporate acid-sensitive hydrophobic linkages like acetal [40] onto the polymer backbone so that detachment of the linkage provides sufficient structural change of

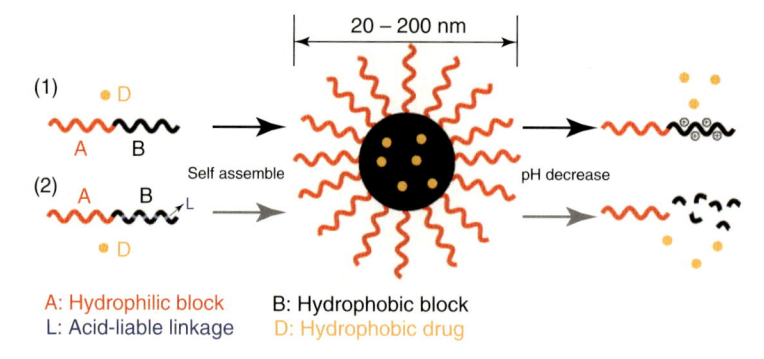

Figure 34.3 Representative approaches to construct pH-sensitive micelles for tumor delivery. The AB diblock polymer bears either (1) titratable groups or (2) acid-labile linkages. Anticancer drug can be encapsulated into the micelle core at pH 7.4, while drug release is triggered at lower pH due to dissociation of the micelles.

the micelles to trigger drug release; (iii) simply construct the core-forming segment with acid-degradable polymers such as poly(α-hydroxy esters) and poly(*ortho*-esters) [41], in which case the polymer backbone can be entirely disintegrated into monomers under an acidic condition. For all the above subcategories relatively lower pH (below pH 5) is usually required to ensure quick linkage cleavage when compared to the first approach, therefore the second approach is more frequently applied for intracellular delivery where more acidic conditions can be encountered in certain subcellular organelles.

34.4
Recent Development in pH-Sensitive Micelles for Tumor-Targeted Drug Delivery

In the past decade, great efforts have been made to develop pH-sensitive polymeric micelles for tumor-targeted drug delivery. Table 34.1 summarizes a selection of these studies that represent the pioneering work and the latest advances in this area. By utilizing the aforementioned approaches in designing pH-sensitive polymers, a variety of targeting strategies have been explored and they will be introduced below.

34.4.1
pH-Triggered Drug Release

34.4.1.1 Tumor Extracellular pH (pH$_e$)-Triggered Drug Release
Although it is recognized that malignant tissue generally has a more acidic environment than normal tissue, there are considerable variations in tumor pH$_e$ values, and the average distinction between tumor pH$_e$ and physiological pH could range from -0.4 to -0.8 pH units [29]. In order to utilize the acidic tumor pH$_e$ as

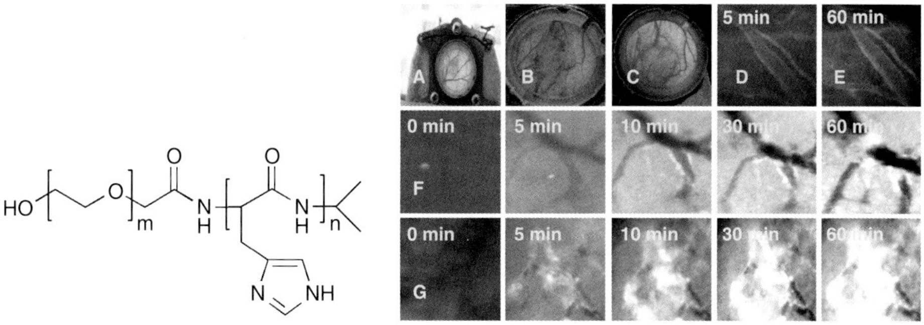

34.4 Recent Development in pH-Sensitive Micelles for Tumor-Targeted Drug Delivery

Figure 34.4 (a) Chemical structure of poly(L-histidine)-b-PEG. (b) mouse dorsal skinfold window chamber made of two symmetrical titanium frames. A tumor piece was inoculated into the *nu/nu* mouse window chamber (A). After implanting the MDA 213 breast cancer tumor piece, tumor blood vessels were growing in the window chamber on day 1 (B) and day 15 (C). Normal blood vessel images after intravenous injection of DOX-loaded pH-sensitive micelles at 5 and 60 min are shown in (D) and (E), respectively. The tumor blood vessels after intravenous injection of DOX-loaded pH-insensitive and pH-sensitive micelles during a 60-min period were present in rows (F) and (G), respectively. The bright color is from DOX fluorescence [18].

an internal signal to trigger drug release, the micelle carrier must be highly pH sensitive so as to be able to distinguish the difference in pH value of less than 1 pH unit.

Based on the scaffold of histidine-derived polymers, the Bae group at the University of Utah was one of the few research teams that first explored pH-sensitive polymeric micelles for tumor pH_e targeting [38, 71, 72]. The imidazole ring of a polyhistidine polymer has a lone pair of electrons on the unsaturated nitrogen that endow it an amphoteric property. A pH-sensitive diblock copolymer of poly(L-histidine) ($M_n \sim$ 5 kDa)-b-PEG ($M_n =$ 2 kDa) (Figure 34.4a) was found to exhibit a pK_b value of around 7.0 and a buffering pH region from 5.5 to 8.0 [38]. Micelles constructed from poly(L-histidine)-b-PEG were about 110 nm in size at pH 8.0 and began to dissociate below pH 7.4. In order to lower the transition pH value to the more acidic tumor pH_e, another biodegradable polymer, poly(L-lactic acid) ($M_n \sim$ 3 kDa)-b-PEG ($M_n =$ 2 kDa) (PLLA-b-PEG) was blended with poly(L-histidine)-b-PEG to form mixed micelles. In particular, the micelles composed of 25 wt% PLLA-b-PEG were quite stable above pH 7.0, but underwent destabilization as pH decreased below 6.8 [71]. An anticancer drug, doxorubicin (DOX), was successfully incorporated into the mixed micelles with a high loading content (around 20 wt%) and loading efficiency (around 90%). Little drug leakage was detected above pH 7.4 in the *in vitro* study, but a remarkably accelerated drug release was observed below pH 6.8 [72]. When drug-loaded micelles were tested in MDA 231 breast tumor-bearing mice using a skinfold window chamber model [18], the visualized intensity of DOX fluorescence carried by the pH-sensitive micelles was significantly more intense and spread in the tumor site more than that carried

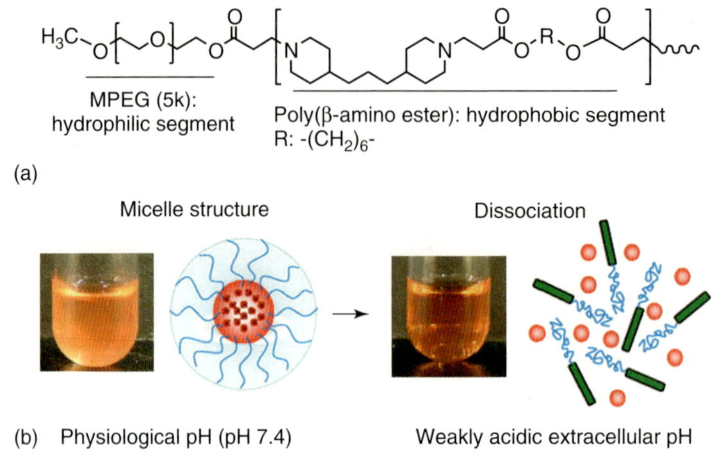

Figure 34.5 (a) Structure of MPEG–HPAE block copolymer. (b) DOX-loaded MPEG–HPAE micelles under physiological pH were completely dissociated and rapidly released DOX at weakly acidic pH environments [53].

by a control pH-insensitive PLLA-*b*-PEG micelle, indicating the enhanced drug delivery to tumors for the pH-sensitive micelles (Figure 34.4b).

Another type of poly(β-amino esters) (HPAE) polymers developed by Langer *et al.* [73] was also found to be feasible for tumor pH$_e$ targeting because of its pH-responsive tertiary amine with a pK_b of about 6.5. In particular, Lee *et al.* synthesized a series of amphiphilic methyl ether PEG-*b*-HPAE (MPEG–HPAE) diblock polymers to fabricate polymeric micelles and they showed sharp pH-dependent micellization–demicellization transitions at the acidic extracellular pH of tumor cells (pH 6.8–7.2) [74]. DOX could be efficiently loaded into the MPEG–HPAE micelles and under the *in vitro* conditions the DOX-loaded polymeric micelles showed rapid release of DOX from the micelles in weakly acidic environments (pH 6.4), but very slow release under physiological conditions (pH 7.4) (Figure 34.5). Moreover, intravenously injected DOX-loaded micelle formulations notably suppressed tumor growth and also prolonged survival of the B16F10 tumor-bearing mice compared with free DOX (Figure 34.6) [53].

34.4.1.2 Endocytic pH-Triggered Drug Release

It has already been proved by strong evidence that polymeric micelles can be captured from extracellular fluid and internalized by cells via an endocytic pathway [75]. This process normally involves three principle successive compartments (i.e., early endosomes, late endosomes, and lysosomes) and a gradual decrease in pH value from around 6.5 to 4.5 is encountered (Table 34.2) due to the presence of vacuolar type H$^+$-ATPase (V-ATPase) to actively transfer protons across the membranes of endocytic organelles [76]. Compared to tumor pH$_e$, the more acidic environment of endocytic compartments allows utilization of more diverse pH-sensitive systems for intracellular delivery.

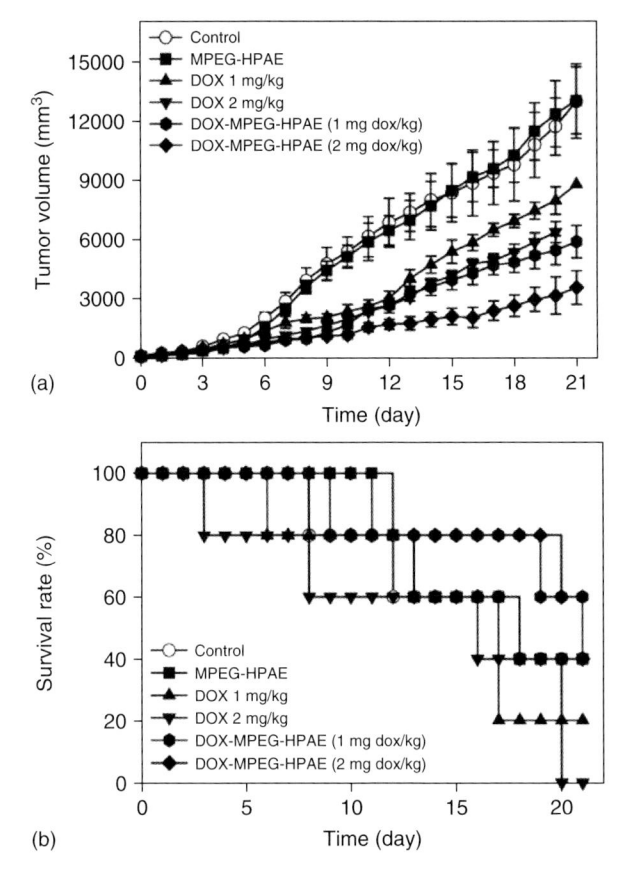

Figure 34.6 Antitumor effects of MPEG–HPAE micelles, DOX, and DOX–MPEG–HPAE micelles. (a) Tumor growth of B16F10 tumor-bearing mice (1 × 10^6 cells/mouse, n = 5) treated with normal saline (○), MPEG–HPAE (■), DOX at 1 mg/kg (▲) and 2 mg/kg (▼), or DOX–MPEG–HPAE at 1 mg DOX/kg (●), and 2 mg DOX/kg (♦). (b) Survival rates of tumor-bearing mice [53].

Since it was found the hydrazone derivatives of DOX are stable under neutral pH conditions, but are able to undergo fast hydrolysis to release free active DOX below pH 5 [77], the acid-sensitive hydrazone linkage has been widely exploited in micelle-mediated drug delivery [39, 64–66]. The group of Park has demonstrated the first approach by attaching DOX to the end of a micelle-forming copolymer with an acid-sensitive hydrazone linkage [39] (Figure 34.7). It was found the hydrazone linkage was readily cleaved to generate intact DOX at pH 5, resulting in a faster drug release than at pH 7.0. The DOX-conjugated micelles were more potent in cell cytotoxicity than free DOX, suggesting that they were more easily taken up within cells with concomitant rapid release of cleaved DOX into the cytoplasm from acidic late endosomes/lysosomes. In a later study carried out by Kataoka et al. [64], DOX was attached to the side-chain of the core-forming segment via the hydrazone bond.

Table 34.2 Overview of pH-sensitive polymeric micelles for tumor-targeted drug delivery.

Polymers	pH-sensitive components	Responses to lower pH	Delivery strategies	Anticancer drugs	In vivo tumor models	References
Poly(L-histidine)-b-PEG and PLLA-b-PEG–folate	polyhistidine	protonation of polybase	(i) folate receptor-mediated endocytosis; (ii) tumor pH_e and endocytic pH-triggered drug release; (iii) polyhistidine-mediated endosomal escape	DOX	BALB/c nu/nu mice bearing human breast MCF-7, MCF-7/DOX^R, and ovarian A2780/DOXR xenografts	[42–45]
Poly(L-histidine-co-phenylalanine)-b-PEG and PLLA-b-PEG–folate	poly(His-co-Phe)	protonation of polybase	(i) folate receptor-mediated endocytosis; (ii) early endosomal pH-triggered drug release; (iii) polyhistidine-mediated endosomal escape	DOX	BALB/c nu/nu mice bearing human ovarian A2780/DOX^R xenografts	[46, 47]
Poly(L-histidine)-b-PEG and PLLA-b-PEG-b-poly(L-histidine)-biotin/ PLLA-b-PEG-b-poly(L-histidine)–TAT	polyhistidine	protonation of polybase	(i) TAT/biotin-mediated active uptake; (ii) early endosomal pH-triggered drug release; (iii) polyhistidine-mediated endosomal escape	DOX	BALB/c nu/nu mice bearing human breast MCF-7, lung A549, epidermoid KB, and MDR A2780/AD xenografts	[48, 49]

Folate–BSA cross-linked PEG-b-poly(L-histidine-co-phenylalanine)	poly(His-co-Phe)	protonation of polybase	(i) folate receptor-mediated endocytosis; (ii) early endosomal pH-triggered drug release; (iii) polyhistidine-mediated endosomal escape; (iv) virus-mimetic multiple infectious cycles	DOX	NA	[50]
PLLA-b-PEG–TAT and poly(methacryloyl sulfadimethoxine)-b-PEG/poly(L-cystine bisamide-g-sulfadiazine)-b-PEG	polysulfonamide	deprotonation of polyacid	TAT-mediated active internalization	DOX	NA	[51, 52]
MPEG-b-HPAE	poly(β-amino ester)	protonation of polybase	tumor pH_e-triggered drug release	DOX/paclitaxel	male C57BL/6 mice bearing murine melanoma B16F10 xenografts	[53, 54]
Folate–poly(2-(methacryloyloxy)ethyl phosphoryl choline)-b-poly(2-(diisopropylamino)ethyl methacrylate)	poly(2-(diisopropylamino)ethyl methacrylate)	protonation of polybase	(i) folate receptor-mediated endocytosis; (ii) endocytic pH-triggered drug release	tamoxifen/paclitaxel	NA	[55, 56]

(continued overleaf)

Table 34.2 (continued)

Polymers	pH-sensitive components	Responses to lower pH	Delivery strategies	Anticancer drugs	In vivo tumor models	References
poly(N^ε-(3-diethylamino)propyl isothiocyanato-L-lysine)-b-PEG-b-PLL	poly(N^ε-(3-diethylamino)propyl isothiocyanato-L-lysine)	protonation of polybase	tumor pH_e-triggered drug release	DOX	NA	[57]
Stearic acid-grafted chitosan oligosaccharide PLL-b-poly(2-ethyl-2-oxazoline)-b-PLL	chitosan oligosaccharide poly(2-ethyl-2-oxazoline)	protonation of polybase hydrogen bond formation	endocytic pH-triggered drug release endocytic pH-triggered drug release	DOX DOX	NA NA	[58] [59]
P(NIPAm-co-MAA)-g-PLA, methoxy PEG-b-PLA, galactosamine–PEG–PLA, and fluorescein isothiocyanate–PEG–PLA	P(NIPAm-co-MAA)	hydrogen bond formation	(i) asialoglycoprotein-mediated endocytosis; (ii) endocytic pH-triggered drug release	DOX	NA	[60, 61]
Folate-conjugated P(NIPAAm-co-DMAAm-co-AMA)-b-PUA	P(NIPAAm-co-DMAAm-co-AMA)	hydrogen bond formation	(i) folate receptor-mediated endocytosis; (ii) endocytic pH-triggered drug release	DOX	BALB/c mice bearing murine breast 4T1 xenografts	[62]
PEG benzoic-imine-C18	benzoic-imine	linkage cleavage	(i) tumor pH_e-triggered surface charge conversion; (ii) endocytic pH-triggered drug release	DOX	NA	[63]

System	Linkage	Mechanism	Drug	Model	Ref.
DOX-Hz-PLLA-b-PEG/ DOX-cis-acotinyl-PLLA-b-PEG	hydrazone or cis-acotinyl	linkage cleavage	endocytic pH-triggered drug release	DOX	NA	[39]
PEG-b-poly (aspartate hydrazone adriamycin)	hydrazone	linkage cleavage	endocytic pH-triggered drug release	DOX	SPF CDF1 nude mice bearing murine colon 26 (C26) xenografts	[64, 65]
PEG-b-poly(allyl glycidyl ether- Hz-DOX)	hydrazone	linkage cleavage	endocytic pH-triggered drug release	DOX	NA	[66]
RGD4C-PEG-b-P(CL-Hyd-DOX)	hydrazone	linkage cleavage	(i) integrin ($\alpha_v\beta_3$)-mediated endocytosis; (ii) endocytic pH- triggered drug release	DOX	SCID mice bearing human breast drug-sensitive MDA-435/LCC6^{WT} and resistant MDA-435/LCC6MDR xenografts	[67]
PEG-[G-3]-polyester-carbamate-acetal	cyclic acetal	linkage cleavage	endocytic pH-triggered drug release	DOX	NA	[68]
Poly(hydroxyethyl acrylate)-b-poly(n-butyl acrylate) with core cross-linked by di(2-acryloyloxy ethoxy)-(4-hydroxyphenyl) methane	di(2-acryloyloxy ethoxy)-(4-hydroxyphenyl) methane	linkage cleavage	endocytic pH-triggered drug release	DOX	NA	[69]
PEG-b-PTMBPEC/PEG-b-poly(4-methoxybenzylidene-pentaerythritol carbonate)	cyclic acetal	linkage cleavage	endocytic pH-triggered drug release	DOX/ paclitaxel	NA	[70]

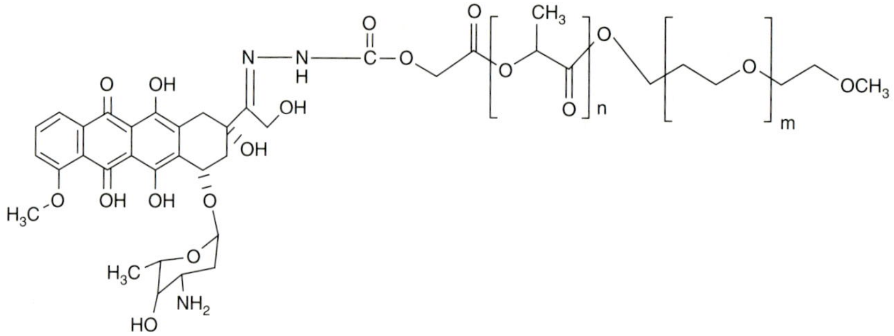

Figure 34.7 Doxorubicin conjugated to the terminal end of PEO-*b*-PLLA by a hydrazone linkage [39].

A biodistribution study revealed a minimal leakage of free drug into circulation and a selective accumulation in solid tumors where it was released from the carrier upon intracellular uptake via endocytosis [65].

Employing acid-labile linkages in the core-forming polymeric block is another strategy for pH-triggered intracellular delivery. Compared to the above polymer–drug conjugate approach, this approach can be applied more generally to different drugs without modifying the linkage. The acid-labile acetals were first exploited by Frechet *et al.* by attaching hydrophobic trimethoxybenzylidene acetals on the periphery of a PEG–dendritic polyester copolymer [68]. Hydrolysis of the acetals at mildly acidic pH (pH 5) was designed to reveal polar groups on the core-forming block, thus changing its solubility, disrupting the micelle, and triggering drug release. *In vitro* studies in MDA-MB-231 breast cancer cells revealed that the encapsulated DOX is located in intracellular organelles in contrast to free DOX, which is localized in the cell nucleus after 24 h. In another study by Bulmus *et al.*, micelles were prepared from poly(hydroxyethyl acrylate)-*b*-poly(*n*-butyl acrylate) with the core cross-linked by a divinyl cross-linker having acetal bonds [69]. High DOX loading capacities (60 wt%) were obtained and hydrolysis of less than half of the cross-links in the core was found to be sufficient to release DOX faster at pH 5 compared to neutral pH. Inspired by the above works, Zhong *et al.* synthesized a novel acid-labile polycarbonate hydrophobe using the monomer of 2,4,6-trimethoxybenzylidene-pentaerythritol carbonate (TMBPEC) [70]. As illustrated in Figure 34.8, the acetals of the micelles formed from PEG-*b*-PTMBPEC, while stable at pH 7.4, are prone to rapid hydrolysis at mildly acidic pH of 4.0 and 5.0 with a half-life of 1 and 6.5 h, respectively. Both paclitaxel and DOX could be efficiently encapsulated into the micelles, and the *in vitro* release studies showed a significantly faster drug release at mildly acidic pH of 4.0 and 5.0, compared to physiological pH.

It has been further demonstrated that when combined with other tumor-specific targeting strategies (such as receptor-mediated endocytosis), polymeric micelles bearing an endocytic pH-triggered release mechanism are able to realize a more

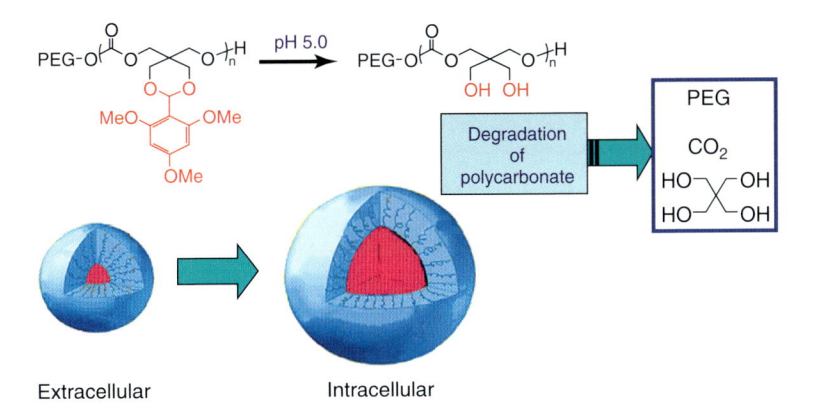

Figure 34.8 pH-responsive biodegradable micelles. The micelles are sufficiently stable at neutral pH, while rapid acetal hydrolysis takes place at mildly acidic pHs, resulting in swollen particles. Finally, biodegradation of hydroxy polycarbonate occurs [70].

efficient intracellular delivery. These multifunctional systems will be introduced in Section 34.4.3.

34.4.2
Tumor pH$_e$-Triggered Modulation of Micelle Surface Functionality

In addition to enabling custom-designed drug release profiles, pH-sensitive polymers may also be used to modulate the surface functionality of micelles. Such systems can be designed to activate their surface functionality only in response to the slightly acidic tumor pH$_e$ so as to realize tumor-specific uptake while avoiding nonspecific interactions with normal cells.

34.4.2.1 pH$_e$-Triggered Conversion of Micelle Surface Charge
Yang et al. developed an amphiphilic polymer by inserting an acid benzoic-imine linker between PEG and the core-forming block [63]. While stable at physiological pH, the partial hydrolysis of the imine bond at tumor pH (6.8) converted the surface charge of the micelle from neutral to positive due to the generation of amino groups and therefore remarkably facilitates the cellular uptake of the loaded DOX through electrostatic attractions between the micelle and the negatively charged cell membrane.

34.4.2.2 pH$_e$-Triggered Exposure of Cell Penetrating Peptide (TAT)
The peptide (GRKKRRQRRRPQ) derived from the transactivator of transcription (TAT) of HIV is one of the nonspecific cell-penetrating peptides and it is able to overcome the lipophilic barrier of the cellular membranes, and deliver large molecules and even small particles inside the cell for their biological actions [78]. It was found TAT-mediated cytoplasmic uptake of drug conjugates can deliver the

cargo directly at the periphery of the nucleus, avoiding the endocytotic pathway [79]. A major hurdle in using TAT for drug delivery is its nonspecificity [80], as it can basically interact with any cell.

The first attempt to control TAT exposure on the micelle surface was by Torchilin et al. [81]. Micelles were prepared by mixing MPEG750–phosphatidylethanolamine (PE), TAT–PE, rhodamine–PE, and MPEG2000-Hz-PE, where the acid-labile hydrazone bond was inserted between PEG and PE. Under normal pH values (pH 7.4–8.0), TAT function on the surface of micelles was "shielded" by the long protecting PEG chain. However, upon brief incubation (15–30 min) at lower pH values (pH 5.0–6.0), the micelles lost their protective PEG shell because of acidic hydrolysis of PEG-Hz-PE and acquired the ability to be effectively internalized by cells via the exposed TAT moieties.

Recently, a novel TAT-conjugated polymeric micelle system was developed by Bae et al. using pH-sensitive polysulfonamides to control the exposure of TAT via a shielding/deshielding mechanism [51]. The delivery system consisted of two components: (i) a polymeric micelle constructed from the TAT-conjugated PLLA-b-PEG copolymer and (ii) an ultra pH-sensitive diblock copolymer of poly(methacryloyl sulfadimethoxine) (PSD) and PEG (PSD-b-PEG) (pK_b value around 7.0). At normal blood pH, the negatively charged PSD-b-PEG is complexed with the cationic TAT-conjugated micelle by electrostatic interactions to realize the shielding purpose and only PEG is exposed to the outside, which could make the carrier long-circulating; when the system experiences a decrease in pH (near tumor), sulfonamide loses charge and detaches, thus exposing TAT for interaction with tumor cells (Figure 34.9). The significantly higher uptake of the micelles at pH 6.6 compared to pH 7.4 from the results of flow cytometry and confocal microscopy clearly demonstrated the shielding/deshielding mechanism. Later, a biodegradable poly(L-cystine bisamide-g-sulfadiazine)-b-PEG (PCBS-b-PEG) polymer was applied to replace the nondegradable PSD-b-PEG to reduce the toxicity and DOX was encapsulated into the micelles [52]. The drug-loaded formulation showed minimal cytotoxicity against human breast MCF-7 cells above pH 7.4 due to the shielding of the PCBS-b-PEG polymer, whereas significantly high cytotoxicity was observed between pH 6.8 and 6.0 as a result of enhanced cellular uptake of the TAT-exposed micelles. More recently, another pH-triggered TAT exposure by a pop-up mechanism was also developed and will be introduced in the Section 34.4.3.3.

34.4.3
Beyond pH-Triggered Drug Release – Multifunctional pH-Sensitive Micelles

Despite great success in developing various novel pH-responsive micelles that are able to release anticancer drugs in a controlled manner, significantly lower or delayed cytotoxic responses of the encapsulated drugs against cancer cells are often observed when compared to free drugs [59, 65, 82]. This is because micelles with a PEGylated surface are normally internalized into the cell through nonspecific fluid-phase pinocytosis, which results in a slower internalization and lower retention in comparison to diffusion of free hydrophobic agents [83, 84]. To

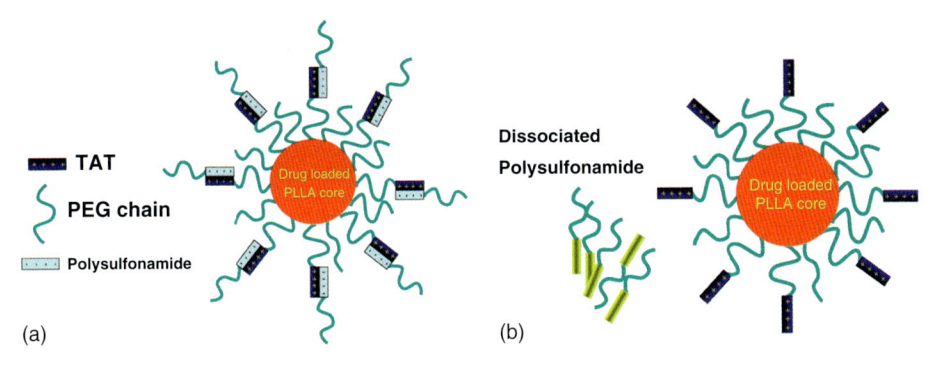

34.4 Recent Development in pH-Sensitive Micelles for Tumor-Targeted Drug Delivery

Figure 34.9 Schematic models for the proposed drug delivery system with controllable TAT exposure via a shielding/deshielding mechanism. (a) At normal blood pH the sulfonamide is negatively charged and shields the TAT on the micelle by electrostatic interaction. Only PEG is exposed to the outside, which could make the carrier-long circulating. (b) When the system experiences a decrease in pH (near tumor) sulfonamide loses its negative charge and detaches, thus exposing TAT for interaction with tumor cells [51].

overcome this limitation, multifunctional pH-sensitive micelles have been further proposed that are enabled to selectively bind, rapidly internalize, and effectively remain in tumor cells.

34.4.3.1 Synergy of Receptor-Mediated Endocytosis and Endocytic pH-Triggered Drug Release

A common approach toward construction of multifunctional pH-sensitive micelles is to decorate the micelle surface with high-affinity ligands such as antibodies, small organic molecules, carbohydrates, or aptamers that can actively bind the specific receptors on tumor cell membranes [85]. This not only promotes tumor-specific binding and association of the micelle carriers, but also facilitates the entry of micelles via a faster and more efficient internalization process, called receptor-mediated endocytosis [86]. Although the intracellular trafficking of micelles is also dependent on other factors such as the micelle size and shape as well as the cell type [87, 88], a number of studies have demonstrated that the synergy of receptor-mediated endocytosis and pH-triggered drug release is able to significantly improve intracellular drug bioavailability.

Among various targeting ligands, the receptor for folic acid is most studied as it is overexpressed in many types of cancers including malignancies of ovarian, breast, brain, kidney, and lung [89]. Folate receptor-mediated endocytosis followed by an endocytic pH-triggered drug release has been proved to notably increase the intracellular delivery of anticancer drugs [55, 56, 62, 90]. Yang *et al.* synthesized a micelle-forming copolymer of poly(*N*-isopropylacrylamide-*co*-*N*,*N*-dimethylacrylamide-*co*-2-aminoethyl methacrylate)-*b*-poly(10-undecenoic acid) (P(NIPAAm-*co*-DMAAm-*co*-AMA)-*b*-PUA) with folate conjugated to AMA (Figure 34.10a) [62]. The DOX-loaded micelles were stable in phosphate-buffered saline (pH 7.4) at 37 °C, but in an acidic environment the micelle shell was

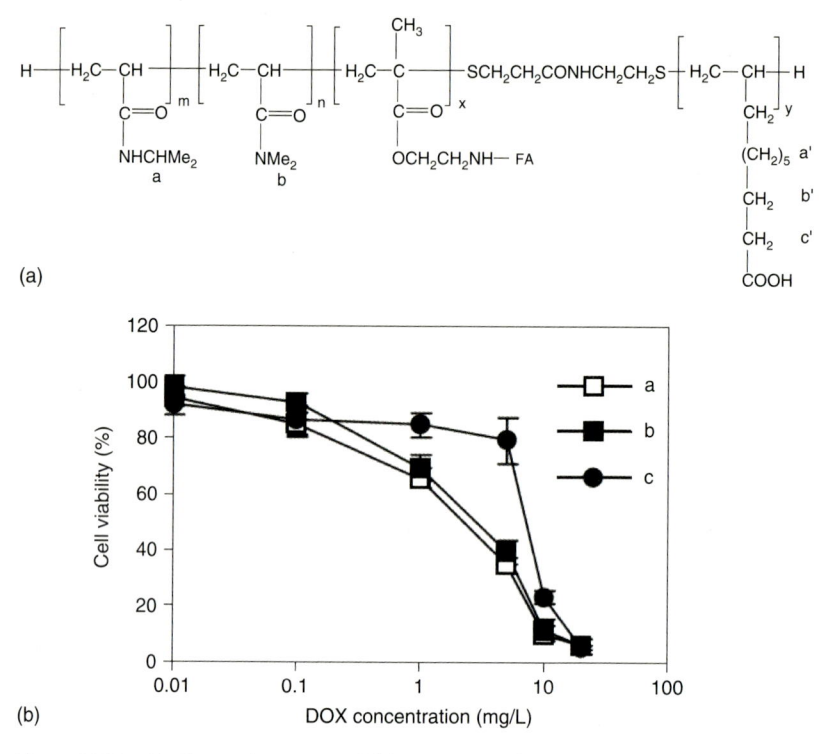

Figure 34.10 (a) Chemical structure of folate-conjugated P(NIPAAm-co-DMAAm-co-AMA)-b-PUA. (b) Viability of 4T1 cells after incubation with DOX (a), DOX-loaded folate-conjugated micelles (b), and unfunctionalized micelles (c), at 37 °C for 48 h [62].

converted from hydrophilic to hydrophobic due to the formation of hydrogen bonds in the P(NIPAAm-co-DMAAm-co-AMA) segment. The loss of hydrophilicity/hydrophobicity balance of the micelles eventually resulted in the deformation of the core–shell structure, releasing the enclosed drug molecules. An increase uptake of the drug-loaded micelles with folate by 4T1 cells (mouse breast cancer) compared to the DOX-loaded micelles without folate as well as free drug was confirmed by confocal microscopy and, in turn, significantly higher cytotoxicity toward the cancer cells was also observed with the IC_{50} value even slightly lower than that of free DOX (Figure 34.10b).

In addition to folate, other targeting ligands have also been studied [61, 67, 91]. Employing a similar release mechanism to the above study, Hsiue et al. developed a series of pH-responsive polylactide-g-poly(N-isopropylacrylamide-co-methacrylic acid) (PLA-g-P(NIPAm-co-MAA)) polymers [60]. Multifunctional micelles were prepared from PLA-g-P(NIPAm-co-MAA), mPEG-b-PLA, and two functionalized diblock copolymers–galactosamine–PEG–PLA, and fluorescein isothiocyanate–PEG–PLA – in which the galactose residue serves as the targeting moiety to

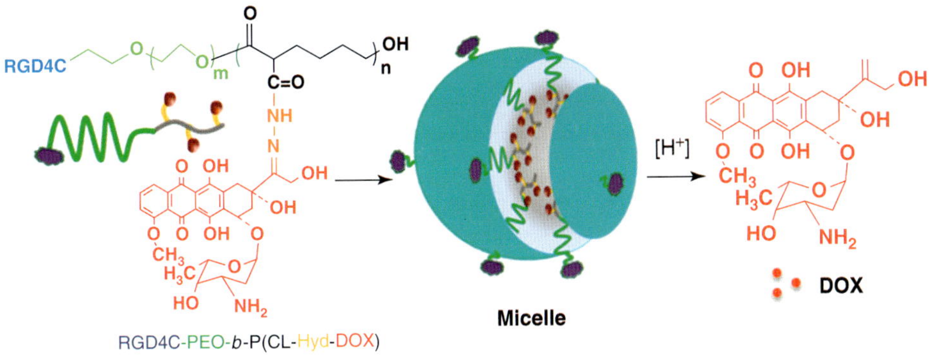

Figure 34.11 Schematic representation of RGD4C micelles containing hydrazone-linked DOX [67].

specifically bind with the asialoglycoprotein of HepG2 cells (hepatocellular carcinoma) [61]. From the drug release study, a change in pH from pH 7.4 to 5.0 can cause the release of a significant quantity of loaded DOX from the micelles. Drug-loaded micelles had high cytotoxicity against the HepG2 cells with a similar IC_{50} value to free DOX after 72 h of incubation, whereas the cytotoxic effect was abolished in the presence of 150 mM free galactose, supporting the active entry of the micelles via the asialoglycoprotein receptor-mediated endocytosis pathway. Lavasanifar et al. prepared poly(ethylene oxide)-b-poly(ε-caprolactone) (PEO-b-PCL) micelles decorated with an RGD-containing peptide, RGD4C, which strongly binds to integrin $\alpha_v\beta_3$ overexpressed on certain cancer cells (such as human breast cancer MDA-435) [67]. DOX was then conjugated to the PCL core using the pH-sensitive hydrazone bonds to obtain RGD4C-PEO-b-P(CL-Hyd-DOX) (Figure 34.11). In MDA-435/LCC6^{WT} cells, a better cytotoxic response than free drug was achieved using RGD4C-PEO-b-P(CL-Hyd-DOX), which is correlated with a higher cellular uptake and preferential nuclear accumulation of DOX. In vivo studies showed the lifespan of animals xenografted with MDA-435/LCC6^{WT} and treated with the integrin $\alpha_v\beta_3$-targeted micelles was significantly longer (44.8 days) than other groups (33, 35.7, and 33.3 days for saline, free DOX- and acetal-PEO-b-P(CL-Hyd-DOX)-treated animals, respectively) (Figure 34.12a). The targeted pH-sensitive micelles were also as effective as free DOX in animals xenografted in terms of inhibiting tumor growth after 25-day treatment (Figure 34.12b).

34.4.3.2 Overcoming Multidrug Resistance

Most anticancer drugs work at the subcellular level to kill cancerous cells by inhibiting cell division or DNA synthesis, or by causing direct damage to the DNA. However, their therapeutic efficacy against cancer cells is often compromised due to the intrinsic or acquired resistance to the drugs. The most common reason for acquisition of resistance to a broad range of anticancer drugs, known as "multidrug resistance" (MDR), is expression of one or more energy-dependent transporters

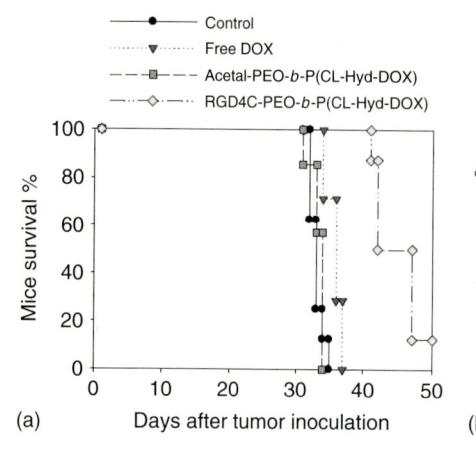

Figure 34.12 (a) Kaplan–Meier survival curve of SCID mice bearing MDA-435/LCC6^{WT} solid tumor after receiving different treatments. (b) Tumor size changes of the treated mice bearing MDA-435/LCC6^{WT} tumors. *$P < 0.05$, free DOX and RGD4C micelles versus other groups. Treatment was initiated on established 0.1-cm^3 tumors (i.e., day 12 after tumor inoculation). These tumor-bearing mice were treated with 50 mg/week of DOX equivalent (2.5 mg DOX/kg) by tail vein injection every seventh day for four doses (days 1, 7, 14, and 21) [67].

(e.g., P-glycoprotein, MDR-associated protein, and breast cancer resistance protein) on the membranes that detect and eject anticancer drugs from cells [92]. Other mechanisms of resistance including insensitivity to drug-induced apoptosis and induction of drug-detoxifying mechanisms also play an important role [93].

The challenge of MDR has motivated great interest in developing novel carrier-mediated drug delivery that can bypass or overcome the above drug resistance mechanisms. To fulfill this task, a desirable drug carrier should be endowed with at least two characteristics: (i) it should be able to effectively transport the drug across the membrane of tumor cells, bypassing various drug efflux transporters, and (ii) it should be able to release significantly high doses of drug into the cytosol and the target site of action to overcome other drug resistance factors. The first characteristic can be realized by functionalizing the micelle surface with tumor-specific targeting ligands to take advantage of receptor-mediated endocytosis. Following active internalization, an endocytic pH-triggered release mechanism can induce the accumulation of free drug molecules in the endosomes. However, the endosomal membrane still remains as a barrier before the drug can reach its cytoplasmic target, as the formed early endosomes will either be recycled back to the plasma membrane via exocytosis or mature into late endosomes and finally fuse with lysosomes where sensitive drug molecules are subject to harsh degradation. Endosomolytic polymers have thus been proposed with the ability to disrupt endosomal membranes and help the drug escape endosomes via the so-called "proton sponge" mechanism [94]. The amphoteric groups in such polymers can become protonated in the acidic environment of endosomes, accompanied by the influx of Cl$^-$ ions to maintain overall electroneutrality. It is assumed that both the influx and swelling induce an increased osmotic pressure, and thus a destabilization of the endosome, eventually resulting in the escape of the vector [94]. Such endosome-disrupting property can be found in many imidazole-containing polymers [95], including polyhistidine-based polymers [45]. In the past few years, the Bae group has made significant progress in overcoming MDR using multifunctional polyhistidine-based pH-sensitive micelles.

The first generation of folate receptor-targeted pH-sensitive micelles was fabricated from a mixture of two block copolymers of poly(L-histidine)-*b*-PEG–folate (75 wt%) and PLLA-*b*-PEG–folate (25 wt%) [43–45]. Following DOX encapsulation, the system showed much higher cytotoxicity against drug-resistant MCF-7 human breast cancer cells (MCF-7/DOX^R) (20% viability) compared to free DOX and non-targeted micelles (85–90% viability) at the same equivalent concentration of drug (10 µg/ml) [43]. *In vivo* evaluation of tumor regression was carried out in a mouse model bearing MCF-7/DOX^R xenografts [43]. The accumulated drug level of targeted micelles in solid tumors was 20 times higher than free DOX group and 3 times higher than the nontargeted group. Correspondingly, the tumor volumes of mice treated with targeted micelles were significantly less than control groups treated with free DOX or nontargeted ones. One drawback of the system is the partial drug leakage from the micelles in the extracellular matrix of tumors due to a relatively low pK_b value (around 7) of polyhistidine [38, 42]. To prevent micelle destabilization before internalization, another pH-insensitive amino acid (i.e., phenylalanine) was copolymerized with histidine to further increase the pK_b value [96].

The second generation of folate receptor-targeted micelles was designed consisting of poly(His-*co*-Phe(16 mol%))-*b*-PEG (80 wt%) and PLLA-*b*-PEG–folate (20 wt%) [46]. *In vitro* study showed that little DOX content (around 25%) was leaked at pH 6.5, but the majority (more than 80%) was released at pH 6.0 within 12 h, indicating the system is highly desirable for early endosomal pH targeting. The drug-loaded formulation can efficiently kill DOX-resistant ovarian carcinoma cells (A2780/DOX^R), whereas free DOX and control groups of nontargeted pH-sensitive micelles and targeted insensitive micelles only showed little cytotoxicity at the same equivalent drug concentration (10 µg/ml). The *in vivo* biodistribution study using a near-IR fluorescence imaging method in tumor-xenografted mice showed remarkably higher fluorescence intensity was observed in the xenograft tumor after intravenous injection of the folate receptor-targeted pH-sensitive micelles labeled by near-IR fluorophore Cy5.5 when compared to the group of folate receptor-targeted pH-insensitive micelles and such distinct fluorescence intensity was maintained for up to 12 h (Figure 34.13), which further supported the long circulation and tumor-selective accumulation of the pH-sensitive micelles. The tumor growth inhibition experiments revealed that the formulation can effectively suppress the growth of existing MDR tumors in mice for at least 50 days by three intravenous injections at a 3-day interval and a dose of 10 mg of DOX/kg (Figure 34.14). The success in defeating MDR was justified by a comprehensive strategy combining active internalization via folate receptor-mediated endocytosis, early endosomal pH-triggered drug release, and poly(L-histidine)-mediated endosomal disruption, as illustrated in Figure 34.15.

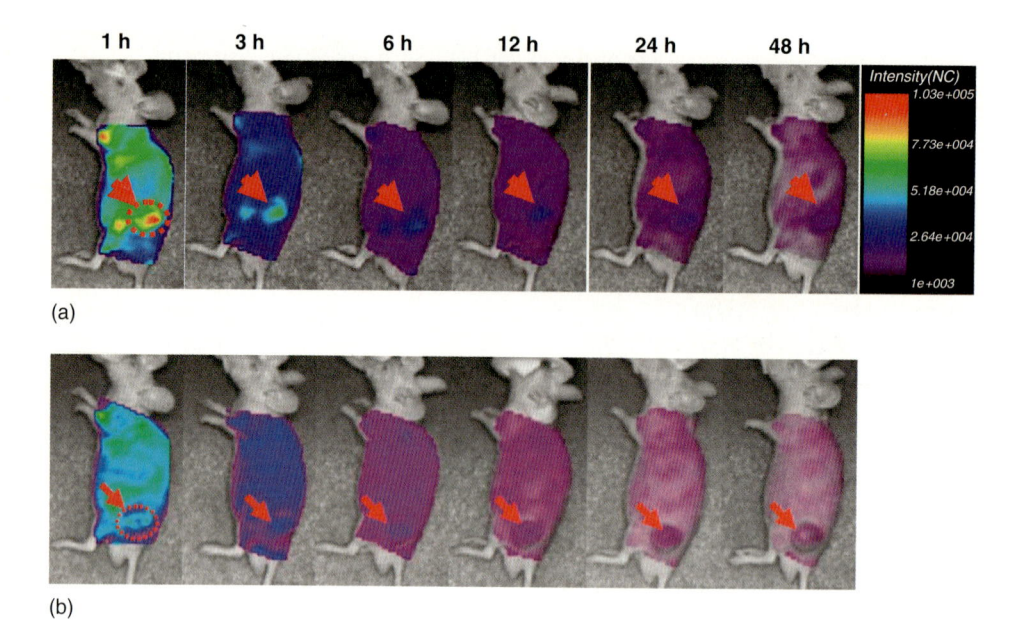

Figure 34.13 *In vivo* optical fluorescence imaging of KB tumor xenografted athymic nude mice following intravenous injection of (a) folate-conjugated pH-sensitive micelles and (b) folate-conjugated pH insensitive micelles. Arrows specifies the location of tumor [45, 47].

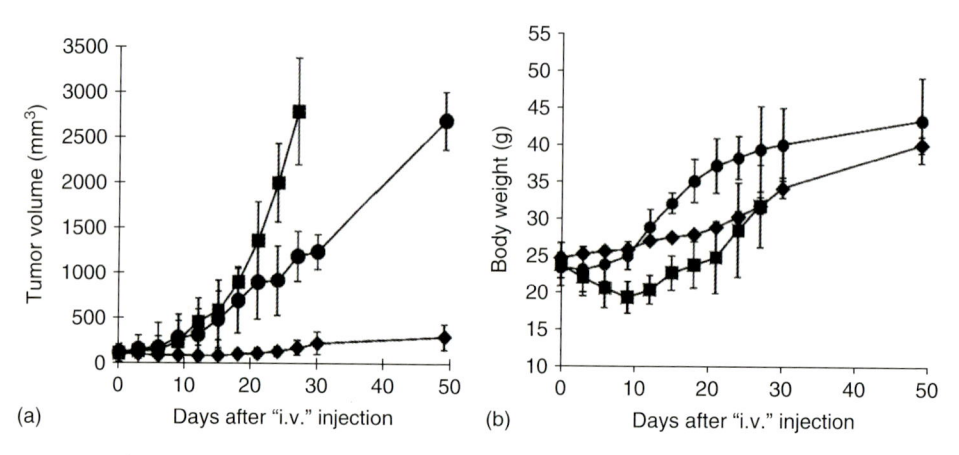

Figure 34.14 (a) *In vivo* tumor growth inhibition test and (b) body weight change of subcutaneous ovarian A2780/DOX^R xenografted BALB/c nude mice ($n = 7$): 10 mg/kg of DOX equivalent dose was injected as several formulations including free DOX in phosphate-buffered saline (■), folate-conjugated pH-insensitive micelles, and (●) folate-conjugated pH-sensitive micelles (♦). Three intravenous injections were made on days 0, 3, and 6 [47].

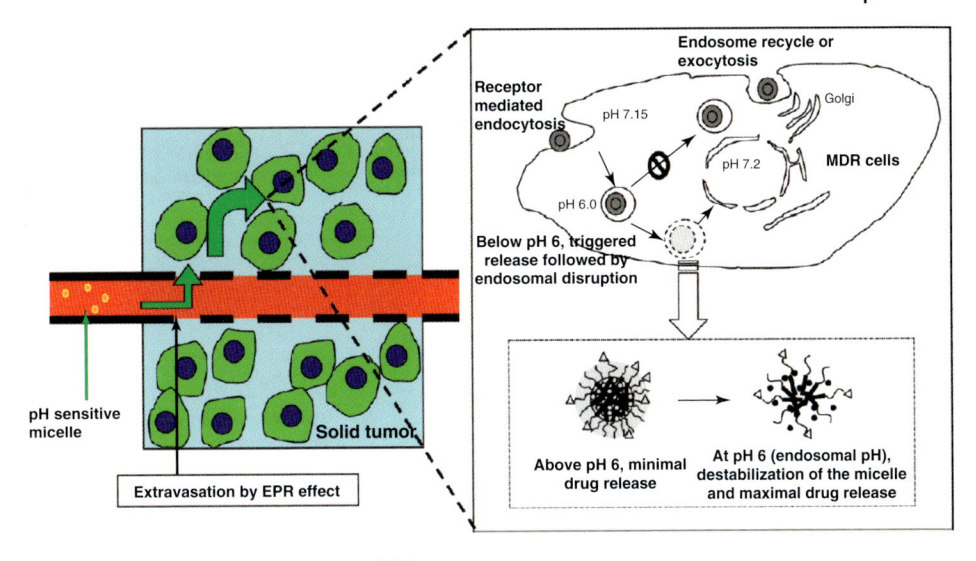

34.4 Recent Development in pH-Sensitive Micelles for Tumor-Targeted Drug Delivery

Figure 34.15 Schematic mechanism of folate receptor-targeted pH-sensitive micelles after intravenous injection [47].

34.4.3.3 TAT-Functionalized Micelles with a Pop-Up Mechanism for Versatile Tumor Targeting

It has been argued that one potential serious problem in employing specific receptors for tumor-directed targeting is the actually rather heterogeneous distribution of these receptors in tumors [97], which may result in unpredictable therapeutic efficacies or even cause the therapy to be ineffective. In attempt to address this issue, the Bae group have proposed a new strategy utilizing pH-sensitive micelles functionalized with nonspecific endogenous ligands or viral cell-penetrating peptides via a controlled pop-up mechanism [48, 49]. The concept was first tested with a nonspecific ligand, biotin, in pH-sensitive micelles consisting of poly(L-histidine) ($M_n \sim 5$ kDa)-b-PEG and PLLA-b-PEG-b-poly(L-histidine) ($M_n \sim 1$ kDa)–biotin [48]. As shown in Figure 34.16, under physiological conditions, the hydrophobic interfacial poly(L-histidine) causes the PEG chain to bend and bury biotin inside the hydrophilic shell. As the pH is lowered below pH 7.0 (tumor pH$_e$), the micelle core still remains stable, but the increased ionization degree of the interfacial poly(L-histidine) segment tends to stretch and expose the biotin out of the PEG shell due to an increased hydrophilicity, which facilitates biotin receptor-mediated endocytosis. As the pH is further lowered below 6.5 (endosomal pH), the micelle destabilizes due to the protonation of the core-forming poly(L-histidine) segment, resulting in enhanced drug release and endosomal membrane disruption. The efficient cytosolic drug release by the pop-up mechanism was further supported by enhanced cell cytotoxicity of the DOX-loaded micelles against MCF-7 cells at tumor acidic pH.

In the latest work, biotin was replace by a nonspecific cell-penetrating peptide, TAT, to construct the micelles of poly(L-histidine)-b-PEG and

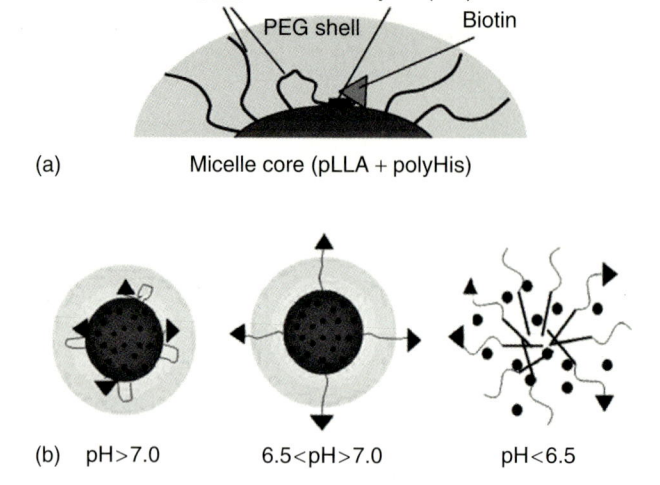

Figure 34.16 (a) Schematic diagram depicting the central concept of pH-induced vitamin repositioning on the micelle. (b) While above pH 7.0, biotin that is anchored on the micelle core via a pH-sensitive molecular chain actuator (poly(L-histidine)) is shielded by the PEG shell of the micelle; biotin is exposed on the micelle surface (6.5 < pH < 7.0) and can interact with cells, which facilitates biotin receptor-mediated endocytosis. When the pH is further lowered (pH < 6.5), the micelle destabilizes, resulting in enhanced drug release [48].

PLLA-*b*-PEG-*b*-poly(L-histidine) ($M_n \sim 2$ kDa)–TAT (Figure 34.17a) [49]. The pH-dependent micelle uptake by MCF-7 cells showed 70-fold increased micelle cellular uptake at pH 6.8 compared to pH 7.4 (Figure 34.17b). This observation is correlated with the exposure of TAT on the micelle surface at tumor pH_e to facilitate active macropinocytosis, which is known as a receptor-independent form of endocytosis [98]. Combined with the following processes of endosomal pH-triggered release and poly(L-histidine)-mediated endosomal membrane disruption, the system is able to deliver high doses of drug in the cytosol and its target site. Following DOX encapsulation, *in vivo* efficacies of the TAT pop-up pH-sensitive micelles (PHSM$^{\text{pop-upTAT}}$) were tested in mice bearing a number of wide-type and drug-resistant tumor xenografts, including drug-resistant human ovarian tumor A2780/AD, drug-sensitive human breast tumor MCF-7, and human lung tumor A549. All the tumor xenografts were significantly regressed in size by three injections at a dose of DOX equivalent to 10 mg/kg body weight per injection at 3-day intervals (Figure 34.18), while minimum weight loss was observed. Thus, this approach is very promising to serve as a general strategy for solid tumor targeting regardless of tumor types and heterogeneities.

34.4.3.4 Virus-Mimetic Cross-Linked Micelles (Nanogels) for Maximal Drug Efficacy

Many leading edge studies in this field have been dedicated to improving the efficiency of drug delivery into the cytosol of tumor cells. An important fact that is often neglected is that the endocytosis pathway usually proceeds only in a time

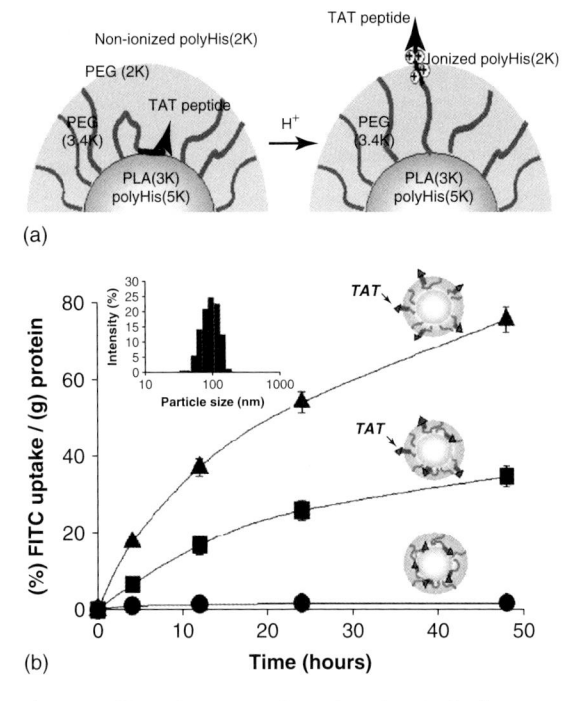

Figure 34.17 pH sensitivity for polymeric micelle drug targeting of drug-sensitive tumors. (a) Schematic representation of the acid-induced pop-up targeting mechanism for the peptide-conjugated micelle corona. (b) Cellular uptake of the micelles in cultured MCF-7 cells [49].

frame of minutes to an hour [86]. However, for many systems designed for cytosolic delivery [55, 61, 64, 67–70], the *in vitro* results indicated it took more than several hours or even up to 1 day to release most of the encapsulated drug at endocytic pH. If a carrier cannot quickly deliver its cargo into the cytosol with the short frame of endocytosis it will be exposed to the harsh lysosomal environment or be exocytosed, which will probably lead to compromised therapeutic efficacy. It still remains as a great challenge that the balance has to be finely controlled between the stability of drug-loaded micelles during the *in vivo* circulation and their prompt response to the acidic subcellular compartments in tumor cells. A recent study carried out by the Bae group offered another feasible strategy toward this problem [50]. A novel nanogel system was prepared by cross-linking the hydrophilic shell of the pH-sensitive poly(His-*co*-Phe)-*b*-PEG micelles with bovine serum albumin (BSA) and it was further conjugated with folate. These nanogels are colloidally stable at neutral pH, but swell substantially at endosomal pH (below pH 6.5), resulting in the faster release rate of the encapsulated DOX (Figure 34.19a). More importantly, they are able to release the anticancer agent in a pH-triggered pulsatile fashion owing to their reversible swelling/deswelling transitions (Figure 34.19b). Following folate-mediated endocytosis, the swelling of the nanogels together with

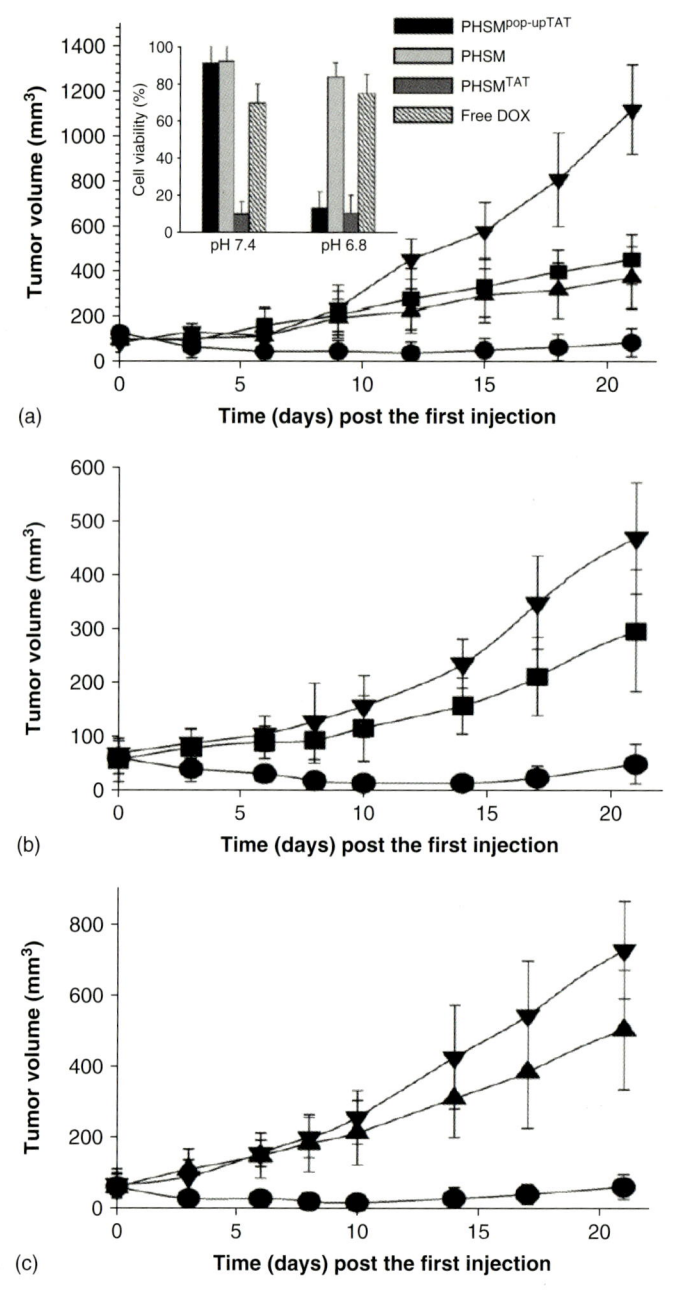

Figure 34.18 In vivo efficacies of DOX-loaded PHSM[pop-upTAT] (●) against (a) A2780/AD, (b) MCF-7 ($n = 4$), and (c) A549 tumor xenografts. DOX equivalent of 10 mg/kg body weight was intravenously injected 3 times (days 0, 3, and 6 post the first injection) to the mice ($n = 4$). Formulations of PHSM (■), PHSM[TAT] (▲), and free DOX (▼) were used as the control ($n = 4$). The inset in (a) shows corresponding in vitro cytotoxicities against A2780/AD cells of the four formulations at DOX equivalent concentration of 1 μg/ml for 48 h ($n = 9$) [49].

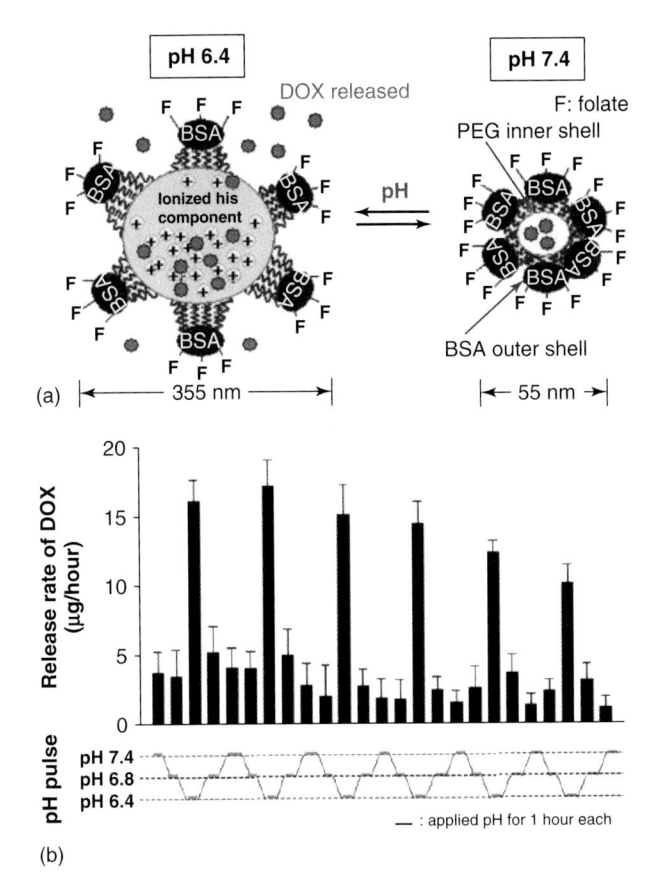

Figure 34.19 (a) Protonation of histidine moieties in nanogels at lower pH results in swelling of the nanogel core, triggering DOX release, while the opposite pH increase leads to reversible deswelling. (b) Pulsatile release pattern of DOX from the nanogels as a result of swelling/deswelling transitions in response to a change in environmental pH [50].

the buffering effect of poly(L-histidine) is able to disrupt the endosomal membranes, thereby facilitating the transfer of the released DOX to the cytoplasm where the nanogels shrink again to their original size, imparting further release of DOX. The released DOX induces apoptosis that allows the nanogels, still containing sufficient amounts of DOX, to be taken up by the neighboring cells. In this case, the nanogels may "infect" several cells in a similar way to biological viruses and thus have high potential of maximizing drug efficacy in tumor treatment.

34.5
Conclusions and Perspective

Currently, a number of polymeric micelles for anticancer therapy are being tested in clinical trials, such as NK012, NK105, and Genexol®-PM [99]. However, no micelle formulation bearing a pH-triggered release mechanism has ever reached this stage so far. In fact, pH-sensitive micelles share some common bottlenecks toward commercialization with other nanoparticle-based therapeutics, including lack of reproducibility from batch to batch, scalability issues, high fabrication costs, and issues of biocompatibility and toxicity, among others [100]. Despite the above challenges, many innovative drug formulations based on pH-sensitive micelles have been demonstrated to have many advantages over conventional therapeutics, and especially multifunctional pH-sensitive micelles have huge potential to maximize drug bioavailability and/or overcome drug resistance. More efforts still need to be made to gain a better understanding of the precise molecular targets and *in vivo* fates of the delivered micelle carriers. The developing imaging technologies will also greatly advance improvement of the current systems and the development of new formulations. The authors hold a strong belief that revolutionary chemotherapeutic products will eventually be generated from pH-sensitive micelles in the future.

References

1. Rothenberg, M.L., Carbone, D.P., and Johnson, D.H. (2003) Improving the evaluation of new cancer treatments: challenges and opportunities. *Nat. Rev. Cancer*, **3**, 303–309.
2. Carelle, N., Piotto, E., Bellanger, A., Germanaud, J., Thuillier, A., and Khayat, D. (2002) Changing patient perceptions of the side effects of cancer chemotherapy. *Cancer*, **95**, 155–163.
3. Higgins, C.F. (2007) Multiple molecular mechanisms for multidrug resistance transporters. *Nature*, **446**, 749–757.
4. Matsumura, Y. and Maeda, H. (1986) A new concept for macromolecular therapeutics in cancer chemotherapy: mechanism of tumoritropic accumulation of proteins and the antitumor agent smancs. *Cancer Res.*, **46**, 6387–6392.
5. Torchilin, V.P. (2007) Micellar nanocarriers: pharmaceutical perspectives. *Pharm. Res.*, **24**, 1–16.
6. Kataoka, K., Harada, A., and Nagasaki, Y. (2001) Block copolymer micelles for drug delivery: design, characterization and biological significance. *Adv. Drug Deliv. Rev.*, **47**, 113–131.
7. Lavasanifar, A., Samuel, J., and Kwon, G.S. (2002) Poly(ethylene oxide)-*block*-poly (L-amino acid) micelles for drug delivery. *Adv. Drug Deliv. Rev.*, **54**, 169–190.
8. Kabanov, A.V., Batrakova, E.V., and Alakhov, V.Y. (2002) Pluronic block copolymers as novel polymer therapeutics for drug and gene delivery. *J. Control. Release*, **82**, 189–212.
9. Vaupel, P., Kallinowski, F., and Okunieff, P. (1989) Blood flow, oxygen and nutrient supply, and metabolic microenvironment of human tumors: a review. *Cancer Res.*, **49**, 6449–6465.
10. Wike-Hooley, J.L., Haveman, J., and Reinhold, H.S. (1984) The relevance of tumour pH to the treatment of malignant disease. *Radiother. Oncol.*, **2**, 343–366.
11. Engin, K., Leeper, D.B., Cater, J.R., Thistlethwaite, A.J., Tupchong, L., and McFarlane, J.D. (1995) Extracellular pH distribution in human tumours. *Int. J. Hyperthermia*, **11**, 211–216.
12. Tannock, I.F. and Rotin, D. (1989) Acid pH in tumors and its potential for therapeutic exploitation. *Cancer Res.*, **49**, 4373–4384.
13. Grabe, M. and Oster, G. (2001) Regulation of organelle acidity. *J. Gen. Physiol.*, **117**, 329–344.
14. Watson, P., Jones, A.T., and Stephens, D.J. (2005) Intracellular trafficking

pathways and drug delivery: fluorescence imaging of living and fixed cells. *Adv. Drug Deliv. Rev.*, **57**, 43–61.

15. Gillies, E.R. and Frechet, J.M.J. (2004) Development of acid-sensitive copolymer micelles for drug delivery. *Pure Appl. Chem.*, **76**, 1295–1307.

16. Rapoport, N. (2007) Physical stimuli-responsive polymeric micelles for anti-cancer drug delivery. *Prog. Polym. Sci.*, **32**, 962–990.

17. Oh, K.T., Yin, H.Q., Lee, E.S., and Bae, Y.H. (2007) Polymeric nanovehicles for anticancer drugs with triggering release mechanisms. *J. Mater. Chem.*, **17**, 3987–4001.

18. Lee, E.S., Gao, Z., and Bae, Y.H. (2008) Recent progress in tumor pH targeting nanotechnology. *J. Control. Release*, **132**, 164–170.

19. Thistlethwaite, A.J., Leeper, D.B., Moylan, D.J. III, and Nerlinger, R.E. (1985) pH distribution in human tumors. *Int. J. Radiat. Oncol. Biol. Phys.*, **11**, 1647–1652.

20. Ojugo, A.S., McSheehy, P.M., McIntyre, D.J., McCoy, C., Stubbs, M., Leach, M.O., Judson, I.R., and Griffiths, J.R. (1999) Measurement of the extracellular pH of solid tumours in mice by magnetic resonance spectroscopy: a comparison of exogenous ^{19}F and ^{31}P probes. *NMR Biomed.*, **12**, 495–504.

21. van Sluis, R., Bhujwalla, Z.M., Raghunand, N., Ballesteros, P., Alvarez, J., Cerdan, S., Galons, J.P., and Gillies, R.J. (1999) In vivo imaging of extracellular pH using ^{1}H MRSI. *Magn. Reson. Med.*, **41**, 743–750.

22. Volk, T., Jahde, E., Fortmeyer, H.P., Glusenkamp, K.H., and Rajewsky, M.F. (1993) pH in human tumour xenografts: effect of intravenous administration of glucose. *Br. J. Cancer*, **68**, 492–500.

23. Stubbs, M., Rodrigues, L., Howe, F.A., Wang, J., Jeong, K.S., Veech, R.L., and Griffiths, J.R. (1994) Metabolic consequences of a reversed pH gradient in rat tumors. *Cancer Res.*, **54**, 4011–4016.

24. Gillies, R.J., Raghunand, N., Garcia-Martin, M.L., and Gatenby, R.A. (2004) pH imaging. A review of pH measurement methods and applications in cancers. *IEEE Eng. Med. Biol. Mag.*, **23**, 57–64.

25. Leeper, D.B., Engin, K., Thistlethwaite, A.J., Hitchon, H.D., Dover, J.D., Li, D.J., and Tupchong, L. (1994) Human tumor extracellular pH as a function of blood glucose concentration. *Int. J. Radiat. Oncol. Biol. Phys.*, **28**, 935–943.

26. Gatenby, R.A. and Gillies, R.J. (2004) Why do cancers have high aerobic glycolysis? *Nat. Rev. Cancer*, **4**, 891–899.

27. Di Chiro, G., Hatazawa, J., Katz, D.A., Rizzoli, H.V., and De Michele, D.J. (1987) Glucose utilization by intracranial meningiomas as an index of tumor aggressivity and probability of recurrence: a PET study. *Radiology*, **164**, 521–526.

28. Hawkins, R.A., Hoh, C., Glaspy, J., Choi, Y., Dahlbom, M., Rege, S., Messa, C., Nietszche, E., Hoffman, E., Seeger, L. et al. (1992) The role of positron emission tomography in oncology and other whole-body applications. *Semin. Nucl. Med.*, **22**, 268–284.

29. Gerweck, L.E. and Seetharaman, K. (1996) Cellular pH gradient in tumor versus normal tissue: potential exploitation for the treatment of cancer. *Cancer Res.*, **56**, 1194–1198.

30. Stubbs, M., McSheehy, P.M., Griffiths, J.R., and Bashford, C.L. (2000) Causes and consequences of tumour acidity and implications for treatment. *Mol. Med. Today*, **6**, 15–19.

31. Stubbs, M., McSheehy, P.M., and Griffiths, J.R. (1999) Causes and consequences of acidic pH in tumors: a magnetic resonance study. *Adv. Enzyme Regul.*, **39**, 13–30.

32. Newell, K., Franchi, A., Pouyssegur, J., and Tannock, I. (1993) Studies with glycolysis-deficient cells suggest that production of lactic acid is not the only cause of tumor acidity. *Proc. Natl. Acad. Sci. USA*, **90**, 1127–1131.

33. Yamagata, M., Hasuda, K., Stamato, T., and Tannock, I.F. (1998) The contribution of lactic acid to acidification of tumours: studies of variant cells

lacking lactate dehydrogenase. *Br. J. Cancer*, **77**, 1726–1731.
34. Martinez-Zaguilan, R., Seftor, E.A., Seftor, R.E., Chu, Y.W., Gillies, R.J., and Hendrix, M.J. (1996) Acidic pH enhances the invasive behavior of human melanoma cells. *Clin. Exp. Metastasis*, **14**, 176–186.
35. Naeslund, J. and Swenson, K.E. (1953) Investigations on the pH of malignant tumors in mice and humans after the administration of glucose. *Acta Obstet. Gynecol. Scand.*, **32**, 359–367.
36. Torchilin, V.P. (2001) Structure and design of polymeric surfactant-based drug delivery systems. *J. Control. Release*, **73**, 137–172.
37. Klibanov, A.L., Maruyama, K., Torchilin, V.P., and Huang, L. (1990) Amphipathic polyethyleneglycols effectively prolong the circulation time of liposomes. *FEBS Lett.*, **268**, 235–237.
38. Lee, E.S., Shin, H.J., Na, K., and Bae, Y.H. (2003) Poly (L-histidine)–PEG block copolymer micelles and pH-induced destabilization. *J. Control. Release*, **90**, 363–374.
39. Yoo, H.S., Lee, E.A., and Park, T.G. (2002) Doxorubicin-conjugated biodegradable polymeric micelles having acid-cleavable linkages. *J. Control. Release*, **82**, 17–27.
40. Gillies, E.R., Goodwin, A.P., and Frechet, J.M.J. (2004) Acetals as pH-sensitive linkages for drug delivery. *Bioconjug. Chem.*, **15**, 1254–1263.
41. Gaucher, G., Marchessault, R.H., and Leroux, J.C. (2010) Polyester-based micelles and nanoparticles for the parenteral delivery of taxanes. *J. Control. Release*, **143**, 2–12.
42. Lee, E.S., Na, K., and Bae, Y.H. (2003) Polymeric micelle for tumor pH and folate-mediated targeting. *J. Control. Release*, **91**, 103–113.
43. Lee, E.S., Na, K., and Bae, Y.H. (2005) Doxorubicin loaded pH-sensitive polymeric micelles for reversal of resistant MCF-7 tumor. *J. Control. Release*, **103**, 405–418.
44. Mohajer, G., Lee, E.S., and Bae, Y.H. (2007) Enhanced intercellular retention activity of novel pH-sensitive polymeric micelles in wild and multidrug resistant MCF-7 cells. *Pharm. Res.*, **24**, 1618–1627.
45. Kim, D., Lee, E.S., Park, K., Kwon, I.C., and Bae, Y.H. (2008) Doxorubicin loaded pH-sensitive micelle: antitumoral efficacy against ovarian A2780/DOX^R tumor. *Pharm. Res.*, **25**, 2074–2082.
46. Kim, D., Lee, E.S., Oh, K.T., Gao, Z.G., and Bae, Y.H. (2008) Doxorubicin-loaded polymeric micelle overcomes multidrug resistance of cancer by double-targeting folate receptor and early endosomal pH. *Small*, **4**, 2043–2050.
47. Kim, D., Gao, Z.G., Lee, E.S., and Bae, Y.H. (2009) *In vivo* evaluation of doxorubicin-loaded polymeric micelles targeting folate receptors and early endosomal pH in drug-resistant ovarian cancer. *Mol. Pharm.*, **6**, 1353–1362.
48. Lee, E.S., Na, K., and Bae, Y.H. (2005) Super pH-sensitive multifunctional polymeric micelle. *Nano Lett.*, **5**, 325–329.
49. Lee, E.S., Gao, Z., Kim, D., Park, K., Kwon, I.C., and Bae, Y.H. (2008) Super pH-sensitive multifunctional polymeric micelle for tumor pH$_e$ specific TAT exposure and multidrug resistance. *J. Control. Release*, **129**, 228–236.
50. Lee, E.S., Kim, D., Youn, Y.S., Oh, K.T., and Bae, Y.H. (2008) A virus-mimetic nanogel vehicle. *Angew. Chem. Int. Ed.*, **47**, 2418–2421.
51. Sethuraman, V.A. and Bae, Y.H. (2007) TAT peptide-based micelle system for potential active targeting of anti-cancer agents to acidic solid tumors. *J. Control. Release*, **118**, 216–224.
52. Sethuraman, V.A., Lee, M.C., and Bae, Y.H. (2008) A biodegradable pH-sensitive micelle system for targeting acidic solid tumors. *Pharm. Res.*, **25**, 657–666.
53. Ko, J., Park, K., Kim, Y.S., Kim, M.S., Han, J.K., Kim, K., Park, R.W., Kim, I.S., Song, H.K., Lee, D.S., and Kwon, I.C. (2007) Tumoral acidic extracellular pH targeting of pH-responsive MPEG–poly(beta-amino ester) block copolymer micelles for cancer therapy. *J. Control. Release*, **123**, 109–115.

54. Han, J.K., Kim, M.S., Lee, D.S., Kim, Y.S., Park, R.W., Kim, K., and Kwon, I.C. (2009) Evaluation of the anti-tumor effects of paclitaxel-encapsulated pH-sensitive micelles. *Macromol. Res.*, **17**, 99–103.
55. Licciardi, M., Giammona, G., Du, J.Z., Armes, S.P., Tang, Y.Q., and Lewis, A.L. (2006) New folate-functionalized biocompatible block copolymer micelles as potential anti-cancer drug delivery systems. *Polymer*, **47**, 2946–2955.
56. Licciardi, M., Craparo, E.F., Giammona, G., Armes, S.P., Tang, Y., and Lewis, A.L. (2008) *in vitro* biological evaluation of folate-functionalized block copolymer micelles for selective anti-cancer drug delivery. *Macromol. Biosci.*, **8**, 615–626.
57. Oh, K.T., Oh, Y.T., Oh, N.M., Kim, K., Lee, D.H., and Lee, E.S. (2009) A smart flower-like polymeric micelle for pH-triggered anticancer drug release. *Int. J. Pharm.*, **375**, 163–169.
58. Ye, Y.Q., Yang, F.L., Hu, F.Q., Du, Y.Z., Yuan, H., and Yu, H.Y. (2008) Core-modified chitosan-based polymeric micelles for controlled release of doxorubicin. *Int. J. Pharm.*, **352**, 294–301.
59. Wang, C.H. and Hsiue, G.H. (2005) Polymeric micelles with a pH-responsive structure as intracellular drug carriers. *J. Control. Release*, **108**, 140–149.
60. Lo, C.L., Lin, K.M., and Hsiue, G.H. (2005) Preparation and characterization of intelligent core-shell nanoparticles based on poly (D,L-lactide)-g-poly (N-isopropyl acrylamide-co-methacrylic acid). *J. Control. Release*, **104**, 477–488.
61. Huang, C.K., Lo, C.L., Chen, H.H., and Hsiue, G.H. (2007) Multifunctional micelles for cancer cell targeting, distribution imaging, and anticancer drug delivery. *Adv. Funct. Mater.*, **17**, 2291–2297.
62. Liu, S.Q., Wiradharma, N., Gao, S.J., Tong, Y.W., and Yang, Y.Y. (2007) Bio-functional micelles self-assembled from a folate-conjugated block copolymer for targeted intracellular delivery of anticancer drugs. *Biomaterials*, **28**, 1423–1433.
63. Ding, C.X., Gu, J.X., Qu, X.Z., and Yang, Z.Z. (2009) Preparation of multifunctional drug carrier for tumor-specific uptake and enhanced intracellular delivery through the conjugation of weak acid labile linker. *Bioconjug. Chem.*, **20**, 1163–1170.
64. Bae, Y., Fukushima, S., Harada, A., and Kataoka, K. (2003) Design of environment-sensitive supramolecular assemblies for intracellular drug delivery: polymeric micelles that are responsive to intracellular pH change. *Angew. Chem. Int. Ed.*, **42**, 4640–4643.
65. Bae, Y., Nishiyama, N., Fukushima, S., Koyama, H., Yasuhiro, M., and Kataoka, K. (2005) Preparation and biological characterization of polymeric micelle drug carriers with intracellular pH-triggered drug release property: tumor permeability, controlled subcellular drug distribution, and enhanced *in vivo* antitumor efficacy. *Bioconjug. Chem.*, **16**, 122–130.
66. Hruby, M., Konak, C., and Ulbrich, K. (2005) Polymeric micellar pH-sensitive drug delivery system for doxorubicin. *J. Control. Release*, **103**, 137–148.
67. Xiong, X.B., Ma, Z., Lai, R., and Lavasanifar, A. (2010) The therapeutic response to multifunctional polymeric nano-conjugates in the targeted cellular and subcellular delivery of doxorubicin. *Biomaterials*, **31**, 757–768.
68. Gillies, E.R. and Frechet, J.M. (2005) pH-responsive copolymer assemblies for controlled release of doxorubicin. *Bioconjug. Chem.*, **16**, 361–368.
69. Chan, Y., Wong, T., Byrne, F., Kavallaris, M., and Bulmus, V. (2008) Acid-labile core cross-linked micelles for pH-triggered release of antitumor drugs. *Biomacromolecules*, **9**, 1826–1836.
70. Chen, W., Meng, F., Li, F., Ji, S.J., and Zhong, Z. (2009) pH-responsive biodegradable micelles based on acid-labile polycarbonate hydrophobe: synthesis and triggered drug release. *Biomacromolecules*, **10**, 1727–1735.
71. Yin, H.Q., Lee, E.S., Kim, D., Lee, K.H., Oh, K.T., and Bae, Y.H. (2008) Physicochemical characteristics of pH-sensitive poly

(L-histidine)-*b*-poly (ethylene glycol)/poly (L-lactide)-*b*-poly(ethylene glycol) mixed micelles. *J. Control. Release*, **126**, 130–138.

72. Yin, H. and Bae, Y.H. (2009) Physicochemical aspects of doxorubicin-loaded pH-sensitive polymeric micelle formulations from a mixture of poly (L-histidine)-*b*-poly(ethylene glycol)/poly (L-lactide)-*b*-poly(ethylene glycol). *Eur. J. Pharm. Biopharm.*, **71**, 223–230.

73. Lynn, D.M. and Langer, R. (2000) Degradable poly(beta-amino esters): synthesis, characterization, and self-assembly with plasmid DNA. *J. Am. Chem. Soc.*, **122**, 10761–10768.

74. Kim, M.S., Hwang, S.J., Han, J.K., Choi, E.K., Park, H.J., Kim, J.S., and Lee, D.S. (2006) pH-responsive PEG-poly(beta-amino ester) block copolymer micelles with a sharp transition. *Macromol. Rapid Commun.*, **27**, 447–451.

75. Luo, L., Tam, J., Maysinger, D., and Eisenberg, A. (2002) Cellular internalization of poly(ethylene oxide)-*b*-poly(epsilon-caprolactone) diblock copolymer micelles. *Bioconjug. Chem.*, **13**, 1259–1265.

76. Mellman, I., Fuchs, R., and Helenius, A. (1986) Acidification of the endocytic and exocytic pathways. *Annu. Rev. Biochem.*, **55**, 663–700.

77. Kaneko, T., Willner, D., Monkovic, I., Knipe, J.O., Braslawsky, G.R., Greenfield, R.S., and Vyas, D.M. (1991) New hydrazone derivatives of adriamycin and their immunoconjugates – a correlation between acid stability and cytotoxicity. *Bioconjug. Chem.*, **2**, 133–141.

78. Rapoport, M. and Lorberboum-Galski, H. (2009) TAT-based drug delivery system – new directions in protein delivery for new hopes? *Expert Opin. Drug Deliv.*, **6**, 453–463.

79. Nori, A., Jensen, K.D., Tijerina, M., Kopeckova, P., and Kopecek, J. (2003) Subcellular trafficking of HPMA copolymer–Tat conjugates in human ovarian carcinoma cells. *J. Control. Release*, **91**, 53–59.

80. Vives, E., Richard, J.P., Rispal, C., and Lebleu, B. (2003) TAT peptide internalization: seeking the mechanism of entry. *Curr. Protein Pept. Sci.*, **4**, 125–132.

81. Sawant, R.M., Hurley, J.P., Salmaso, S., Kale, A., Tolcheva, E., Levchenko, T.S., and Torchilin, V.P. (2006) "SMART" drug delivery systems: double-targeted pH-responsive pharmaceutical nanocarriers. *Bioconjug. Chem.*, **17**, 943–949.

82. Lo, C.L., Lin, K.M., Huang, C.K., and Hsiue, G.H. (2006) Self-assembly of a micelle structure from graft and diblock copolymers: an example of overcoming the limitations of polyions in drug delivery. *Adv. Funct. Mater.*, **16**, 2309–2316.

83. Allen, C., Yu, Y.S., Eisenberg, A., and Maysinger, D. (1999) Cellular internalization of PCL20-*b*-PEO44 block copolymer micelles. *Biochim. Biophys. Acta*, **1421**, 32–38.

84. Rapoport, N., Marin, A., Luo, Y., Prestwich, G.D., and Muniruzzaman, M.D. (2002) Intracellular uptake and trafficking of pluronic micelles in drug-sensitive and MDR cells: effect on the intracellular drug localization. *J. Pharm. Sci.*, **91**, 157–170.

85. Sutton, D., Nasongkla, N., Blanco, E., and Gao, J.M. (2007) Functionalized micellar systems for cancer targeted drug delivery. *Pharm. Res.*, **24**, 1029–1046.

86. Bareford, L.M. and Swaan, P.W. (2007) Endocytic mechanisms for targeted drug delivery. *Adv. Drug Deliv. Rev.*, **59**, 748–758.

87. Jiang, W., Kim, B.Y.S., Rutka, J.T., and Chan, W.C.W. (2008) Nanoparticle-mediated cellular response is size-dependent. *Nat. Nanotechnol.*, **3**, 145–150.

88. Sahay, G., Alakhova, D.Y., and Kabanov, A.V. (2010) Endocytosis of nanomedicines. *J. Control. Release*, **145**, 182–195.

89. Weitman, S.D., Weinberg, A.G., Coney, L.R., Zurawski, V.R., Jennings, D.S., and Kamen, B.A. (1992) Cellular localization of the folate receptor: potential role in drug toxicity and folate homeostasis. *Cancer Res.*, **52**, 6708–6711.

90. Bae, Y., Nishiyama, N., and Kataoka, K. (2007) *In vivo* antitumor activity of the folate-conjugated pH-sensitive polymeric micelle selectively releasing adriamycin in the intracellular acidic compartments. *Bioconjug. Chem.*, **18**, 1131–1139.
91. Wu, X.L., Kim, J.H., Koo, H., Bae, S.M., Shin, H., Kim, M.S., Lee, B.H., Park, R.W., Kim, I.S., Choi, K., Kwon, I.C., Kim, K., and Lee, D.S. (2010) Tumor-targeting peptide conjugated pH-responsive micelles as a potential drug carrier for cancer therapy. *Bioconjug. Chem.*, **21**, 208–213.
92. Borst, P., Evers, R., Kool, M., and Wijnholds, J. (1999) The multidrug resistance protein family. *Biochim. Biophys. Acta*, **1461**, 347–357.
93. Gottesman, M.M. (2002) Mechanisms of cancer drug resistance. *Ann. Rev. Med.*, **53**, 615–627.
94. Behr, J.P. (1997) The proton sponge: a trick to enter cells the viruses did not exploit. *Chimia*, **51**, 34–36.
95. Pack, D.W., Putnam, D., and Langer, R. (2000) Design of imidazole-containing endosomolytic biopolymers for gene delivery. *Biotechnol. Bioeng.*, **67**, 217–223.
96. Kim, G.M., Bae, Y.H., and Jo, W.H. (2005) pH-induced micelle formation of poly(histidine-*co*-phenylalanine)-*block*-poly(ethylene glycol) in aqueous media. *Macromol. Biosci.*, **5**, 1118–1124.
97. Bae, Y.H. (2009) Drug targeting and tumor heterogeneity. *J. Control. Release*, **133**, 2–3.
98. Kaplan, I.M., Wadia, J.S., and Dowdy, S.F. (2005) Cationic TAT peptide transduction domain enters cells by macropinocytosis. *J. Control. Release*, **102**, 247–253.
99. Matsumura, Y. and Kataoka, K. (2009) Preclinical and clinical studies of anticancer agent-incorporating polymer micelles. *Cancer Sci.*, **100**, 572–579.
100. Bawa, R. (2008) Nanoparticle-based therapeutics in humans: a survey. *Nanotechnol. Law Bus.*, **5**, 135–155.

35
Albumin–Drug Nanoparticles
Neil Desai

35.1
Introduction

In recent years, the field of oncology has witnessed a tremendous explosion of novel anticancer therapies. Potential treatment choices include a wide range of cytotoxic and targeted small-molecule agents, antibodies, and various nucleic acid- and peptide/protein-based drugs. However, the efficient and safe delivery of these therapeutic compounds remains a serious challenge for the pharmaceutical industry. The formulation of many hydrophobic drugs requires toxic solvents and surfactants, which often impair drug distribution and are associated with severe side-effects. For example, the conventional formulation of the hydrophobic chemotherapeutic agent paclitaxel (Taxol®; Bristol-Myers Squibb) contains a high concentration of Cremophor-EL® (polyethoxylated castor oil; BASF), which is associated with significant toxicities, including peripheral neuropathy and potential fatal hypersensitivity reactions that require premedication [1, 2]. In addition, Cremophor sequesters paclitaxel in micelles, which prolongs the systemic exposure and increases drug toxicity [3]. The delivery of macromolecules such as proteins and nucleic acids also presents a largely unmet need. The extremely small size of nanoparticles confers them with unique physical and chemical properties. Albumin is a versatile carrier for different kinds of hydrophobic and charged molecules, and thus a suitable candidate for nanoparticle delivery system.

35.2
Rationale for Using Albumin Nanoparticles for Drug Delivery

Human serum albumin (HSA) is the most abundant protein in plasma and constitutes approximately 60% of total plasma protein. Albumin plays an important physiological role in regulating plasma volume by increasing osmotic pressure in the vascular compartment. The half-life of albumin is calculated to be 19 days. During its lifetime, an albumin molecule will normally make 15 trips to the extravascular space through transcytosis (discussed in detail below) and returns to

Drug Delivery in Oncology: From Basic Research to Cancer Therapy, First Edition.
Edited by Felix Kratz, Peter Senter, and Henning Steinhagen.
© 2012 Wiley-VCH Verlag GmbH & Co. KGaA. Published 2012 by Wiley-VCH Verlag GmbH & Co. KGaA.

the circulation through the lymphatic system [4]. Albumin binds to and transports a wide range of molecules, including bilirubin, free fatty acids, hydrophobic vitamins, hormones, and metal ions (copper, nickel, calcium, and zinc), as well as many acidic and hydrophobic drugs [5]. For example, albumin is able to bind the drug paclitaxel at more than six sites with different affinities and with positive cooperativity [6]. Based on Scatchard plots, Paal *et al.* calculated that paclitaxel binds to albumin both specifically ($K_{sp} = 1.7 \times 10^6$ M^{-1}) and nonspecifically ($K_{nonsp} = 8.2 \times 10^4$ M^{-1}) [6]. Interestingly, the binding of paclitaxel to albumin is strongly inhibited by commonly used surfactants, including Cremophor EL, Tween 80, and TPGS (tocopheryl poly(ethylene glycol) (PEG) 1000 succinate) at clinically relevant concentrations, with IC$_{50}$s of 0.009, 0.003, and 0.008% (v/v), respectively [7]. Therefore, paclitaxel and other hydrophobic drugs formulated with surfactants often cannot take advantage of serum albumin as a drug carrier. Additionally, Makriyannis *et al.* have demonstrated that albumin can facilitate the diffusion of lipophilic drugs into the membrane lipid bilayer [8]. It was determined that the diffusion of the highly lipophilic drug Δ8-tetrahydrocannabinol into multilamellar dimyristoylphosphatidylcholine membranes was increased 5-fold in the presence of bovine serum albumin (BSA).

Another key character of albumin is that it is highly accumulated by various proliferating tumors, and is used as a major energy and nitrogen source through endocytosis and lysosomal degradation, with the resulting amino acids used in *de novo* protein synthesis [9]. Following injection, the dye Evans Blue binds to circulating albumin and enters subcutaneously growing tumors within a few hours [10]. Stehl *et al.* have shown that there is high tumor uptake rate of albumin with more than 25% of a single dose of radiolabeled albumin accumulated in a Walker 256 carcinosarcoma *in vivo* within 3 days [9]. The blood vessels of proliferating tumors are leaky due to structural defects and high permeability, which allows albumin and other macromolecules to extravasate into tumors, but not into normal tissue. The lack of proper lymphatic drainage in tumors reduced the clearance of albumin and other molecules with molecular weight greater than 40 kDa [11]. In addition to the "enhanced permeability and retention" effect of the tumor microenvironment, recent studies have identified active albumin transport mechanisms. The transcytosis of albumin across the endothelial barrier is facilitated by the binding to the gp60 receptor and caveolar transport [12]. The 60-kDa glycoprotein gp60, also known as albondin, is located on the endothelial cell surface that binds to native albumin with a high affinity in the nanomolar range [12]. Albumin binding induces gp60 clustering and association with caveolar-scaffolding protein caveolin-1. Activation of caveolin-1 induces the activation of tyrosine kinase Src, which stimulates the phosphorylation of gp60, caveolin-1, and the GTPase dynamin-2, leading to caveolar fission [13]. The plasmalemmal vesicles carrying both gp60-bound and fluid-phase albumin migrate from the apical to basal membrane, and release their contents by exocytosis into the subendothelial space. Depletion of cell surface gp60 by prolonged exposure to gp60 antibody reduces the albumin uptake by 85%, demonstrating the importance of the gp60 pathway in albumin transport [13]. Interestingly, Wang *et al.* reported that BSA-coated nanoparticles up to 100 nm in diameter could be internalized by endothelial cells via caveolae-mediated endocytosis [14]. The caveolae-mediated nanoparticle uptake process requires albumin coating, demonstrating the feasibility of drug delivery by albumin nanoparticles across the endothelium of blood vessels using the natural albumin transport pathway.

Upon entering the tumor interstitium, the accumulation of albumin is possibly facilitated by SPARC (secreted protein, acidic and rich in cysteine, also known as osteonectin and BM 40), an albumin-binding protein with significant homology to gp60 [15]. SPARC was first identified as a 43-kDa secreted matricellular glycoprotein with high binding affinity to albumin [16]. Trieu *et al.* demonstrated by solid-phase binding assay that the albumin/SPARC binding was saturable and specific with an estimated K_d of 700 µM, which is similar to the physiological concentration of albumin in plasma [17]. A key modulator of extracellular matrix proliferation and cell migration, overexpression of SPARC is associated with increased tumor invasion, metastasis, and poor prognosis in multiple tumor types [18]. Trieu *et al.* further revealed the association of albumin and SPARC in tumor cells and xenografts [19]. In cultured MX-1 breast tumor cells, immunofluorescence and confocal microscopy revealed that fluorescein isocyanate-conjugated albumin colocalized with SPARC and was rapidly taken up by MX-1 cells in a lysosome-independent manner. Immunohistochemical staining of the MX-1 tumor xenograft showed SPARC to be colocalized with albumin and detected at high levels adjacent to areas of necrosis, consistent with previous research showing that SPARC expression in tumors is enhanced by hypoxia and acidity [20].

The preferential accumulation of albumin in tumors, combined with its long half-life and great biocompatibility, makes albumin an ideal carrier for delivering anticancer therapeutics. Strategies for the delivery of peptides and proteins using soluble albumin include conjugation, physical binding, and the creation of albumin fusion proteins [10]. Small-molecule anticancer agents can be directly conjugated to albumin or modified into albumin-binding prodrugs. Soluble albumin conjugates have been developed for methotrexate and doxorubicin [10]. The pharmacokinetic profile, stability, solubility, and drug targeting of these therapeutics are improved with albumin-mediated delivery. With the recent advances in nanotechnology, there are compelling reasons to take the further step to combine the unique and desirable properties of albumin and nanoparticles to create albumin nanoparticle drug delivery platforms.

35.3
Examples of Albumin-Based Nanoparticles

Over the years, numerous albumin-based nanoparticles have been developed in the laboratory. There are many variations in the process, composition, and characteristics among the different albumin nanoparticles. These albumin nanoparticles can be categorized into different groups based on whether or not the drug is covalently linked to albumin and whether or not the albumin is cross-linked into a matrix

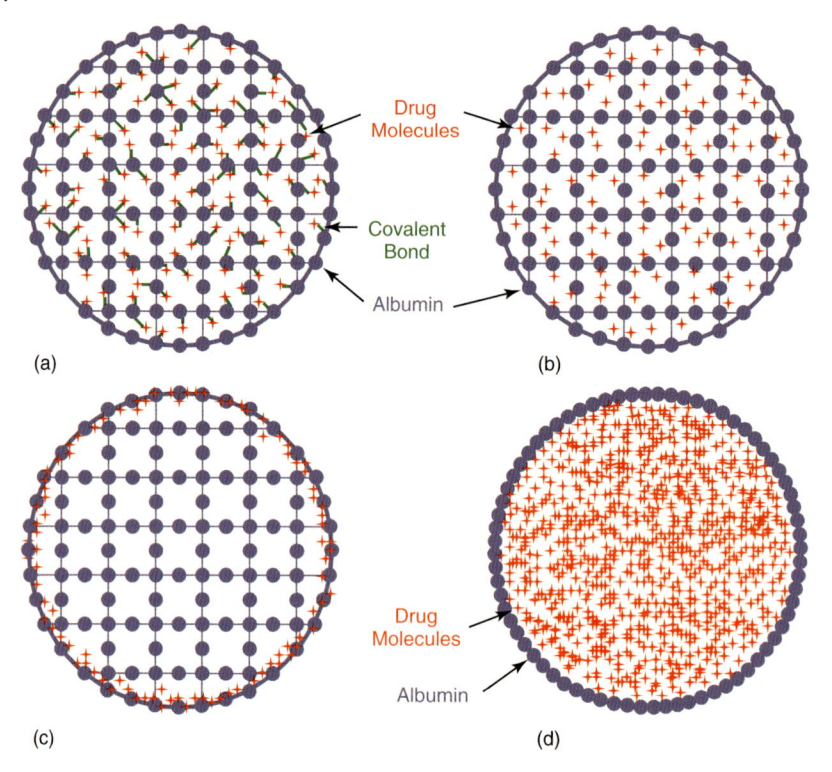

Figure 35.1 Schematics of different albumin nanoparticles. (a) Cross-linked matrix of albumin with drug molecules covalently attached; (b) cross-linked matrix of albumin with drug molecules noncovalently entrapped; (c) cross-linked matrix of albumin with drug molecules noncovalently absorbed on surface; and (d) *nab* technology-based nanoparticles with albumin coated on a core formed by hydrophobic drug molecules.

or gel (Figure 35.1). The majority of reported albumin nanoparticles involve a cross-linking procedure using glutaraldehyde or other cross-linking agents during nanoparticle formation, resulting in a cross-linked albumin matrix that entraps the drug of interest, with the payload being chemically conjugated to the albumin nanoparticles or physically entrapped within the cross-linked albumin matrix. These nanoparticles will initially remain intact in circulation, requiring enzymatic degradation of albumin for sustained drug release. On the other hand, some nanoparticles are prepared without cross-linking of the albumin matrix or without the drug being covalently linked to albumin. For example, *nab*™ (nanoparticle albumin bound) technology creates albumin nanoparticles without the addition of external cross-linking agents but by coating the drug of interest. The nanoparticles consist of drug coated with a layer of albumin, with the payload noncovalently bound to albumin via hydrophobic interaction, which allows for rapid bioavailability and tissue distribution (Figure 35.2). Alternatively, drugs can be absorbed onto the surface of preformed albumin nanoparticles.

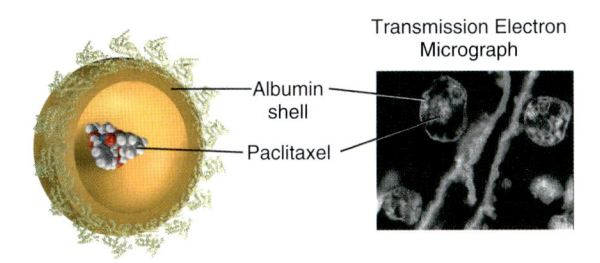

Figure 35.2 Structural illustration and transmission electron micrograph of *nab*-paclitaxel nanoparticles showing drugs encapsulated in the albumin shell.

The preparation of most albumin nanoparticles involves a cross-linking process. For example, Müller *et al.* used an emulsion cross-linking method using glutaraldehyde with ultrasound and static mixing as homogenization steps to produce albumin particles in the sub-200-nm range with a narrow size distribution [21]. Lin *et al.* used a surfactant-free pH-coacervation method by adding acetone dropwise to an aqueous HSA solution (pH 7–9) and subsequent cross-linking with glutaraldehyde [22]. The albumin nanoparticles had a diameter around 100 nm and were stable in both phosphate-buffered saline (PBS) and rat serum, but degraded rapidly over 6 h when incubated in PBS solution containing trypsin. Langer *et al.* further optimized the process with a desolvation method with ethanol as desolvating agent followed by glutaraldehyde cross-linking [23]. A particle size between 200 and 300 nm was reproducibly achieved at pH 8.0 and above, and the albumin nanoparticles were degradable by pepsin and cathepsin B, trypsin, proteinase K, and protease [24]. In contrast, the albumin nanoparticles produced with *nab* technology involve no addition of cross-linking agents. The drug and albumin are not covalently linked, but rather associated through hydrophobic interactions [15]. As a result, the *nab* nanoparticles are not immunogenic, as demonstrated clinically by the absence of hypersensitivity reactions even without corticosteroid premedication [25]. The *nab* nanoparticle typically has a size of less than 200 nm with a high negative ζ potential, and due to steric stabilization by albumin, is readily dispersible and stable in saline after reconstitution at high concentrations. The *nab* nanoparticles can rapidly dissolve in circulation upon infusion, releasing soluble albumin–drug complexes with size similar to native albumin [26].

Attempts have also been made to modify albumin nanoparticles to provide them with additional functionality. Weber *et al.* introduced thiol groups onto the surface of cross-linked HSA nanoparticles with several methods, including by the reaction with dithiothreitol or 2-iminothiolane, by quenching reactive aldehyde residues with cystaminium dichloride, or by coupling L-cysteine and cystaminium dichloride with the aqueous carbodiimide reaction [27]. The introduced thiol groups were relatively stable with a half-life of 28.2 days, which can serve as targets for the covalent linkage of drugs and proteins to the nanoparticle surface using sulfhydryl-reactive cross-linkers. Zhang *et al.* modified BSA nanoparticle surfaces by electrostatic adsorption of cationic polyethylenimine (PEI) [28]. The PEI concentration used for nanoparticle coating efficiently controlled the release of the bone-inducing growth factor bone morphogenetic protein-2 (BMP-2).

Other modifications aim to enhance the targeting of albumin nanoparticles to specific organs. The blood–brain barrier (BBB) is a major obstacle for drug delivery to the central nervous system (CNS). Roser *et al.* adjusted the surface charges on albumin nanoparticles by the covalent coupling of different primary amines [29]. *In vitro*, albumin particles with a neutral ζ potential showed a reduced phagocytic uptake by macrophages compared with charged particles, especially those positively charged. However, no differences in blood circulation times and organ accumulation were observed in rats *in vivo*. In contrast, unlike native albumin ($pI \sim 4$), cationized albumin with additional amines ($pI > 8$) prepared by cationization with hexamethylenediamine rapidly binds to and is endocytosed by isolated bovine brain capillaries, and quickly enters cerebrospinal fluid from blood [30]. For brain drug delivery, Lu *et al.* generated cationic BSA (cationic bovine serum albumin CBSA) from BSA by cationization with ethylenediamine followed by thiolation. CBSA was covalently conjugated with the maleimide function group distal of PEG to create CBSA-conjugated PEG– poly(lactide) (PLA) nanoparticles with a mean diameter around 100 nm [31]. The transendothelial permeability of the CBSA nanoparticles is 7.76-fold higher than that of native control BSA nanoparticles, allowing the CBSA nanoparticles to preferentially transport across BBB with little toxicities. Kreuter *et al.* used another approach for brain drug delivery by covalently attaching apolipoprotein E3, A-I, and B-100 to HSA nanoparticles with the NHS-PEG-Mal 3400 linker [32]. Intravenous administration of modified albumin nanoparticles carrying antinociceptive agent loperamide yielded considerable effects, whereas the loperamide solution achieved no effect, demonstrating the feasibility of this system for drug delivery to the CNS. For liver targeting, Li *et al.* prepared BSA nanoparticles encapsulating water-soluble drug sodium ferulate (SF-BSA nanoparticles) by a desolvation procedure and subsequent glutaraldehyde cross-linking of the BSA wall material [33]. The obtained spherical nanoparticles were negatively charged, and had a narrow size distribution between 100 and 200 nm. Following intravenous injection into mice, SF-BSA nanoparticles showed a much higher drug distribution into liver and a lower drug concentration in other tissues compared with SF solution, suggesting albumin nanoparticles might be a suitable platform for hepatic targeted drug delivery. Mao *et al.* modified the surface of BSA nanoparticles by conjugating glycyrrhizin to the surface reactive amino groups with sodium periodate oxidization [34]. The resulting glycyrrhizin-conjugated BSA nanoparticles had an average diameter of 77 nm. Facilitated by internalization via glycyrrhizin binding sites on the surface of rat hepatocytes, the uptake amount of glycyrrhizin-conjugated BSA nanoparticles was 4.43-fold higher than that of BSA nanoparticles.

The albumin nanoparticles described above share some common characteristics, including high biocompatibility, low toxicity, and good stability. Combined with potential mechanisms that preferentially target albumin and albumin nanoparticles to tumors, there is a strong rationale to utilize albumin nanoparticles as delivery vehicles for anticancer therapies. While there has been extensive laboratory research on albumin-based nanoparticles, currently only drugs based on the *nab* technology platform (developed by Abraxis BioScience/Celgene, Los Angeles, CA) have successfully reached clinical testing and gained market approval. Summarized below are numerous preclinical and clinical studies with albumin-based nanoparticles in the field of oncology.

35.3.1
In Vitro and Animal Studies with Albumin-Based Nanoparticles

35.3.1.1 Delivery of Hydrophobic Small-Molecule Drugs Using *nab* Technology

As the first example of *nab* technology, *nab*-paclitaxel is the most extensively studied albumin nanoparticle-based drug. The size distribution of *nab*-paclitaxel nanoparticles in solution was narrow with a mean particle size of 130 nm as determined by dynamic laser light scattering [26]. Transmission electron microscopy and cryo-transmission electron microscopy images revealed that the nanoparticles were spherical and highly monodispersed with sizes well below 200 nm (Figure 35.3). The nanoparticles had a high negative ζ potential of -31 mV, contributing to their stability in suspension along with steric stabilization provided by the albumin molecules. X-ray powder diffraction revealed that paclitaxel within the nanoparticles is noncrystalline and amorphous [26], making the drug readily bioavailable without the time lag needed to dissolve crystalline paclitaxel as observed for nanocrystals [35]. Reconstituted to 5 mg/ml with 0.9% (w/v) sodium chloride solution, *nab*-paclitaxel nanoparticles are stable at room temperature for several days. No nanoparticles were observed in pig blood samples collected at any timepoints following intravenous administration of high doses of *nab*-paclitaxel at 300 mg/m^2 (equivalent to the maximum tolerated dose (MTD) in humans) or 900 mg/m^2, demonstrating a rapid dissolution time of the nanoparticles in the circulation [26]. The nanoparticles dissolve rapidly into soluble albumin-bound paclitaxel complexes with a size very similar to that of endogenous albumin molecules in blood [26]. The albumin–paclitaxel complexes can potentially utilize the natural gp60/caveolae-mediated albumin transport pathway and potential association with tumoral SPARC to achieve enhanced drug targeting to tumors (Figure 35.4).

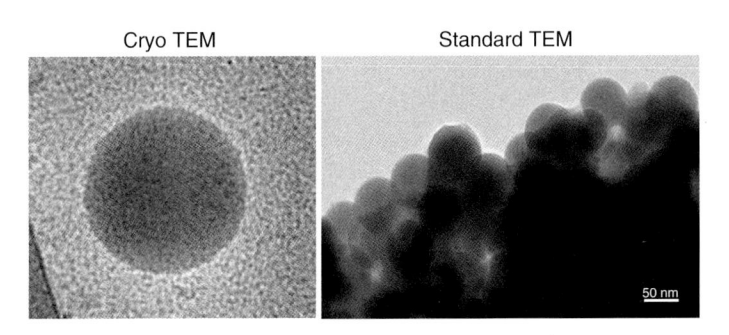

Figure 35.3 Transmission electron micrographs of *nab*-paclitaxel nanoparticles.

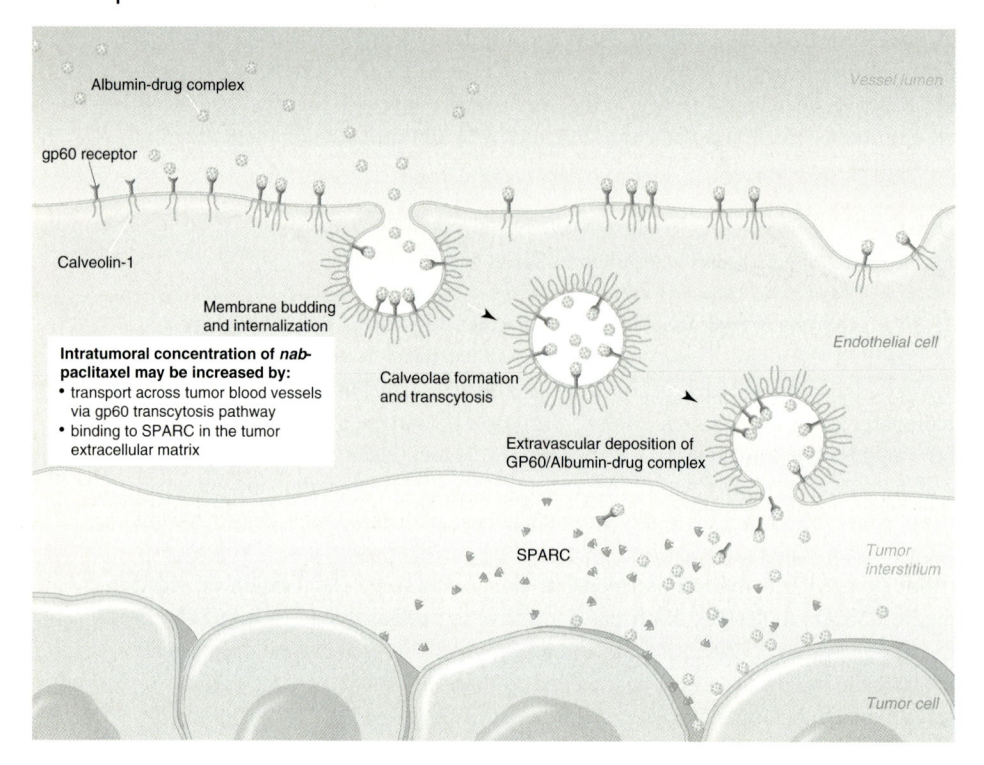

Figure 35.4 Mechanisms for the transport and accumulation of *nab*-paclitaxel in tumors [36]. The transcytosis of albumin-bound paclitaxel across the endothelial barrier is facilitated by the binding to the gp60 receptor and caveolar transport. In the tumor interstitial space, albumin–paclitaxel complexes bind to SPARC and are rapidly internalized in tumor cells via a nonlysosomal pathway.

Desai *et al.* have shown that compared with Cremophor-based paclitaxel (Taxol), the *nab*-paclitaxel formulation increased the endothelial binding of paclitaxel by 9.9-fold ($P < 0.0001$) and the transport of paclitaxel across microvessel endothelial cell monolayers by 4.2-fold ($P < 0.0001$) [7]. The enhanced paclitaxel transcytosis was completely abolished by caveolar disrupting agent methyl-β-cyclodextrin, demonstrating that caveolae is required for the major transport mechanism (Figure 35.5a). In MX-1 tumor xenografts, intravenously administered *nab*-paclitaxel achieved 33% higher intratumoral paclitaxel concentration than equal dose of Taxol (Figure 35.5b) [7]. Rapid accumulation of fluorescent *nab*-paclitaxel nanoparticles in tumors was observed following intravenous injection (Figure 35.6).

In preclinical animal models, *nab*-paclitaxel as a single agent displayed superior antitumor activity compared with currently available taxane treatments. The elimination of toxic solvent Cremophor allows *nab*-paclitaxel to have a higher MTD than Taxol in mice (30 versus 13.4 mg/kg, qd × 5) [7]. In nude mice bearing human tumor xenografts (H522: lung; MX-1: breast; SKOV-3: ovarian; PC-3: prostate; and HT29: colon), *nab*-paclitaxel treatment at MTD resulted in more

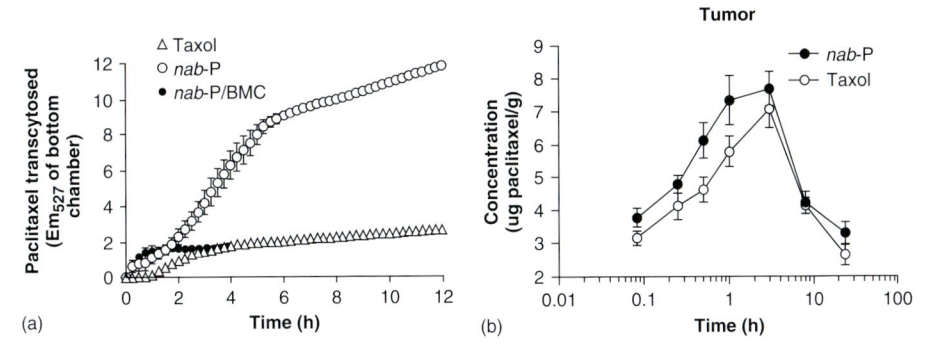

Figure 35.5 Enhanced tumor penetration and accumulation by *nab*-paclitaxel. (a) Transcytosis of paclitaxel across an endothelial cell monolayer increased 4.2-fold in *nab*-paclitaxel (ABI-007) compared with Cremophor-paclitaxel (Taxol, $P < 0.0001$). The enhanced transcytosis by *nab*-paclitaxel was inhibited by methyl-β-cyclodextrin (BMC), a known inhibitor of gp60/caveolar transport. (b) Intratumor paclitaxel concentrations following equal doses of Cremophor-paclitaxel and *nab*-paclitaxel in MX-1 tumor-bearing nude mice.

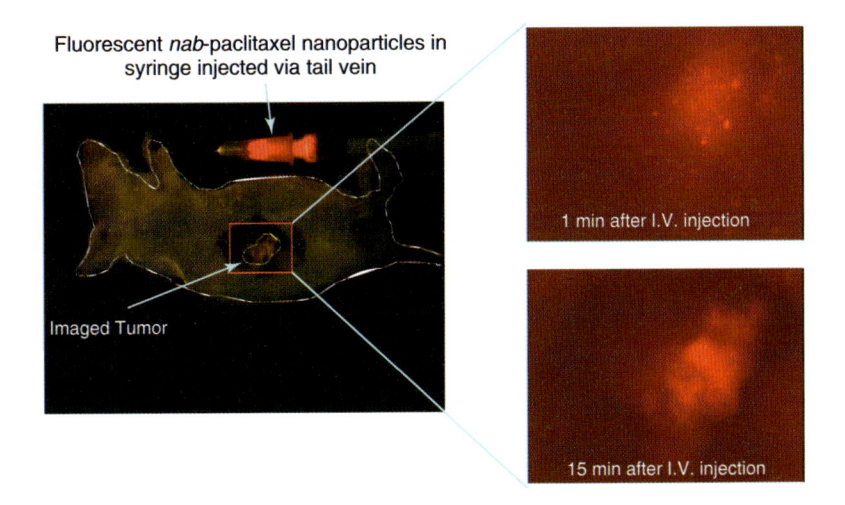

Figure 35.6 Rapid tumor accumulation by *nab*-paclitaxel. *nab*-Paclitaxel nanoparticles containing fluorescent-labeled paclitaxel were injected via the tail vein into tumor-bearing mice. Imaging was performed under a mercury lamp with 500- to 550-nm bandpass excitation.

complete regressions, longer time to recurrence, longer tumor doubling time, and prolonged survival compared with Taxol at MTD (Figure 35.7) [7]. Desai *et al.* further demonstrated that *nab*-paclitaxel at sub-MTD was significantly more effective than polysorbate-based docetaxel (Taxotere®; Sanofi Aventis, Bridgewater, NJ) at its MTD of 15 mg/kg, q4d × 3 in multiple xenograft models including LX-1

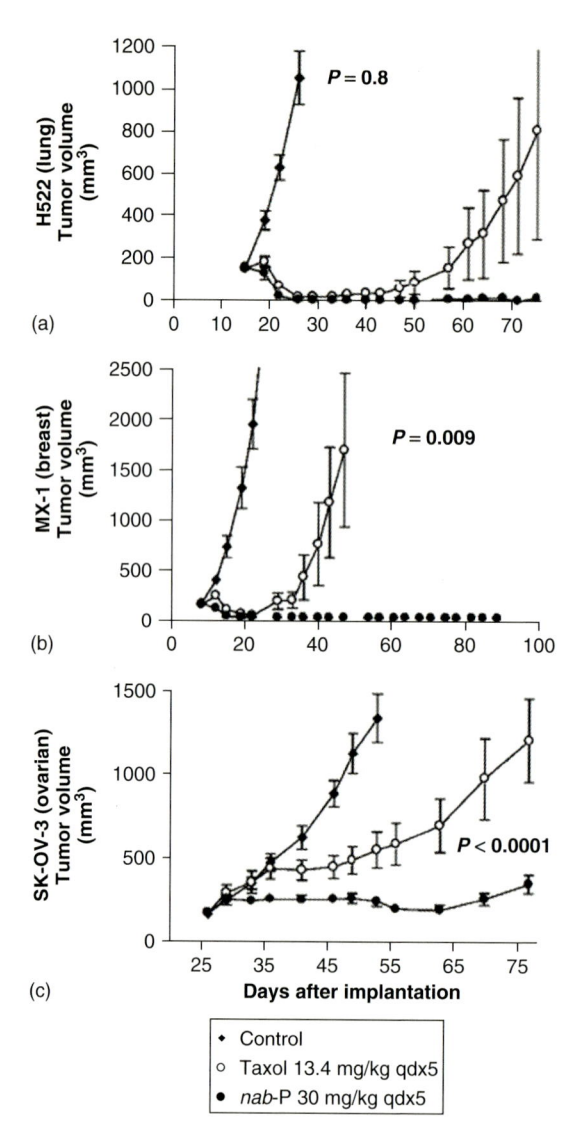

Figure 35.7 Treatment with *nab*-paclitaxel (30 mg/kg, qd × 5) demonstrated superior antitumor activity compared with equitoxic doses of Cremophor-paclitaxel, Taxol (13.4 mg/kg, qd × 5), in three mouse tumor xenografts: (a) H522 (lung tumor xenograft), (b) MX-1 (breast tumor xenograft), and (c) SKOV-3 (ovarian tumor xenograft).

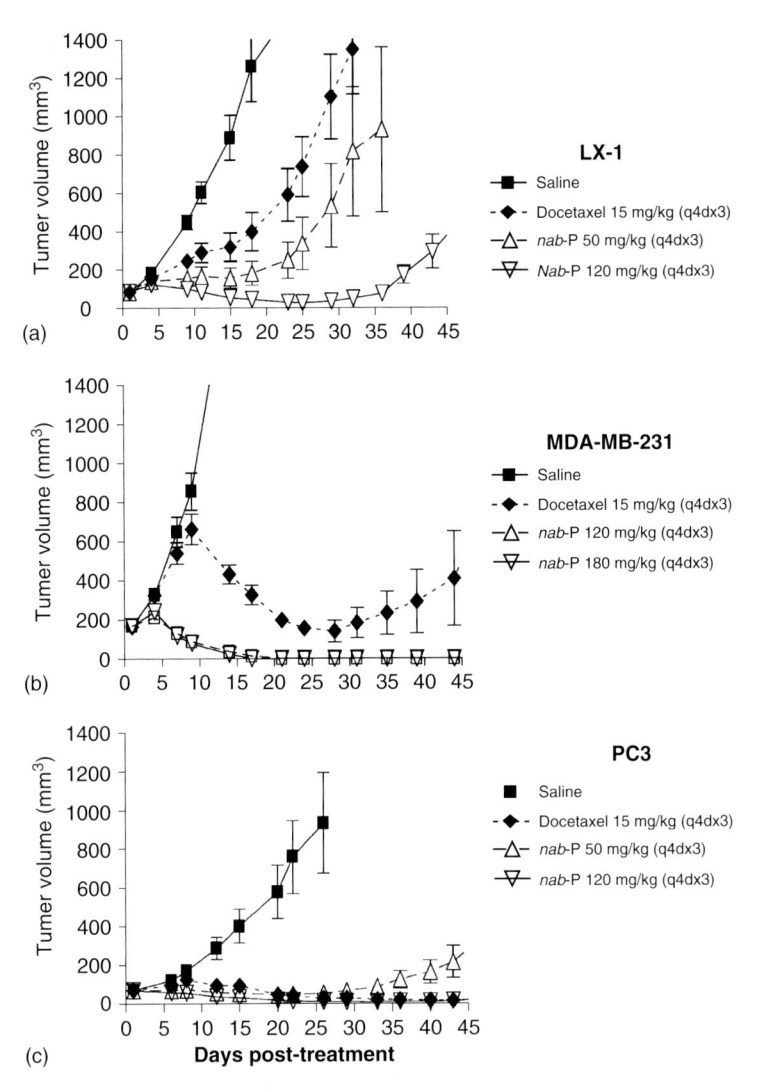

Figure 35.8 Efficacy of *nab*-paclitaxel compared with polysorbate-based docetaxel Taxotere' in three human tumor xenografts. *nab*-Paclitaxel at sub-MTD was significantly more effective than polysorbate-based docetaxel at its MTD of 15 mg/kg, q4d × 3 in (a) LX-1 (lung), (b) MDA-MB-231 (breast), and (c) PC-3 (prostate) tumor models.

(lung), MDA-MB-231 (breast), and PC-3 (prostate) tumors (Figure 35.8) [37]. In another study investigating the potential mechanism of action and transport of *nab*-paclitaxel, the SPARC-overexpressing xenograft PC-3/SP exhibited enhanced response to *nab*-paclitaxel with 97% tumor growth inhibition (TGI) compared with wild-type PC-3 xenograft with 84% TGI ($P < 0.0001$, analysis of variance)

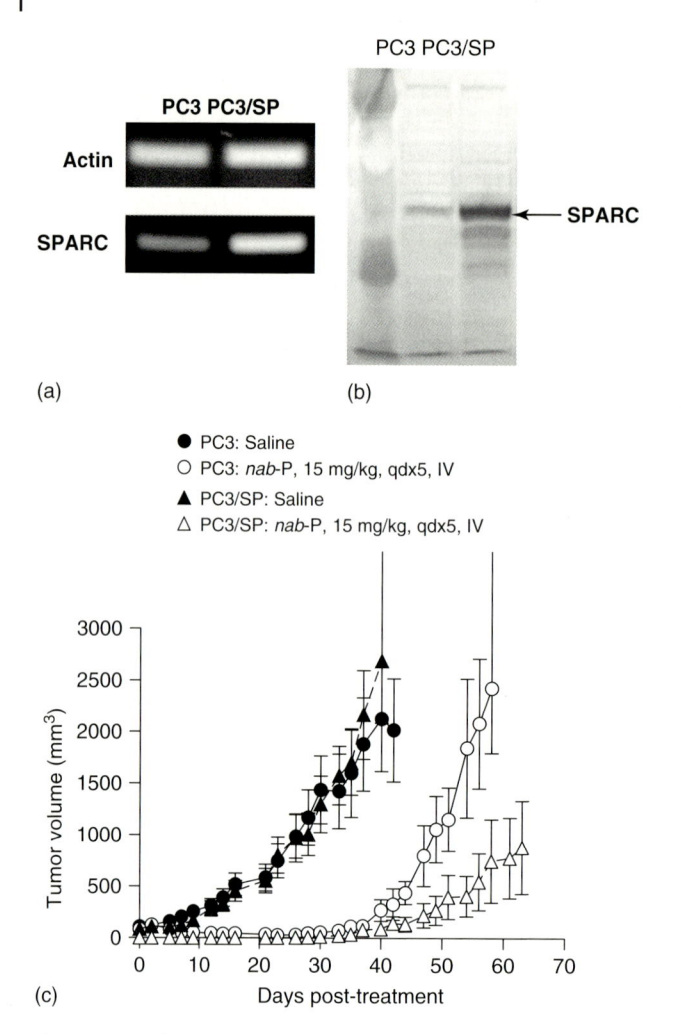

Figure 35.9 The SPARC-overexpressing tumor xenograft PC-3/SP exhibited greater sensitivity to *nab*-paclitaxel than the parental human prostate cancer PC-3 tumor. (a) Overexpression of SPARC in PC-3/SP as confirmed by reverse transcription polymerase chain reaction. (b) Overexpression of SPARC in PC-3/SP as confirmed by Western blot. (c) Treatment with *nab*-paclitaxel resulted in stronger tumor suppression in PC-3/SP than in PC-3 tumor xenografts.

[17], suggesting the potential role of SPARC in facilitating the accumulation of albumin-bound drugs (Figure 35.9).

Preclinical studies also tested the combination of *nab*-paclitaxel with a broad range of other anticancer therapies. Wiedenmann *et al.* demonstrated that *nab*-paclitaxel acted as a radiosensitizer to enhance the antitumor effect of radiation and might be used in taxane-based chemoradiotherapy [38]. Volk *et al.* showed that vascular endothelial growth factor-A protected cultured MDA-MB-231 tumor cells against *nab*-paclitaxel cytotoxicity, whereas bevacizumab (Avastin®; Genentech, South San Francisco, CA), a monoclonal antibody (mAb) against VEGF-A, enhanced the cytotoxic effect of the drug. *In vivo* studies have shown that bevacizumab could inhibit the reactionary angiogenesis of tumors in response to *nab*-paclitaxel treatment [39]. In athymic mice bearing luciferase-tagged, well-established MDA-MB-231 tumors, compared with monotherapies, the combination of *nab*-paclitaxel and bevacizumab resulted in strong TGI and more complete regressions, and significantly reduced the incidence of lymphatic and pulmonary metastases. More recently, Maitra *et al.* [40, 41] showed that against pancreatic cancer xenografts, combination of *nab*-paclitaxel with gemcitabine doubled the response rate of either agent alone. Compared with gemcitabine alone, addition of *nab*-paclitaxel effectively eliminated or depleted the fibrotic stroma and increased tumor vascularization in pancreatic cancer, resulting in 3.7-fold higher intratumoral gemcitabine concentration for the combination versus gemcitabine alone.

In addition to *nab*-paclitaxel, the *nab* technology platform has been employed to deliver other hydrophobic drugs, including the taxane drug *nab*-docetaxel (ABI-008), mTOR (mammalian target of rapamycin) inhibitor *nab*-rapamycin (ABI-009), heat-shock protein 90 inhibitor *nab*-17AAG (ABI-010), tubulin polymerization/topoisomerase I dual inhibitor *nab*-5404 (ABI-011), and a novel taxane *nab*-CY196 (ABI-013). The efficacy of these drugs as a single agent has been demonstrated in preclinical studies in multiple tumor xenograft models (Figure 35.10).

Combination studies with some of the *nab* drugs have also shown promising efficacy and synergy (Figure 35.11). For example, Cirstea *et al.* demonstrated that mutual suppression of mTOR by *nab*-rapamycin and phosphatidylinositol/AKT by perifosine resulted in synergistic cytotoxicity and TGI in the MM1S multiple myeloma mouse xenograft model [42]. In the HER2-positive H358 lung xenograft model, the combination of *nab*-17AAG with *nab*-paclitaxel and trastuzumab (Herceptin®) demonstrated synergy of the triple combination. In the HT29 colon xenograft model, the combination of *nab*-5404 and bevacizumab (Avastin) showed remarkable synergy, with the combination exhibiting significantly better antitumor activity than either Avastin or ABI-011 alone. These *nab* technology-based drugs are currently at different stages of clinical and preclinical development (Figure 35.12).

35.3.1.2 Other Albumin Nanoparticles Carrying Small Molecules

In addition to drugs formulated with *nab* technology, many other labs have experimented with the delivery of hydrophobic small-molecule anticancer drugs using albumin nanoparticles. Maghsoudi *et al.* used ethanol desolvation followed by glutaraldehyde cross-linking to prepare 5-fluorouracil (5-FU)-loaded BSA nanoparticles, which displayed a mean diameter and ζ potential of 210 nm and -31.7 mV, respectively [43]. The 5-FU–BSA nanoparticles in suspension maintained constant release of drug for 20 h. Yi *et al.* used emulsion solidification method to prepare an oral formulation of 5-FU sodium alginate ^{125}I-BSA nanoparticles, which had a mean diameter of 166 nm and released 84.0% of the drug in suspension within 72 h [44]. Following oral administration to rats, the nanoparticles mainly distributed in the liver, spleen, lungs, and kidneys. Arbos *et al.* prepared

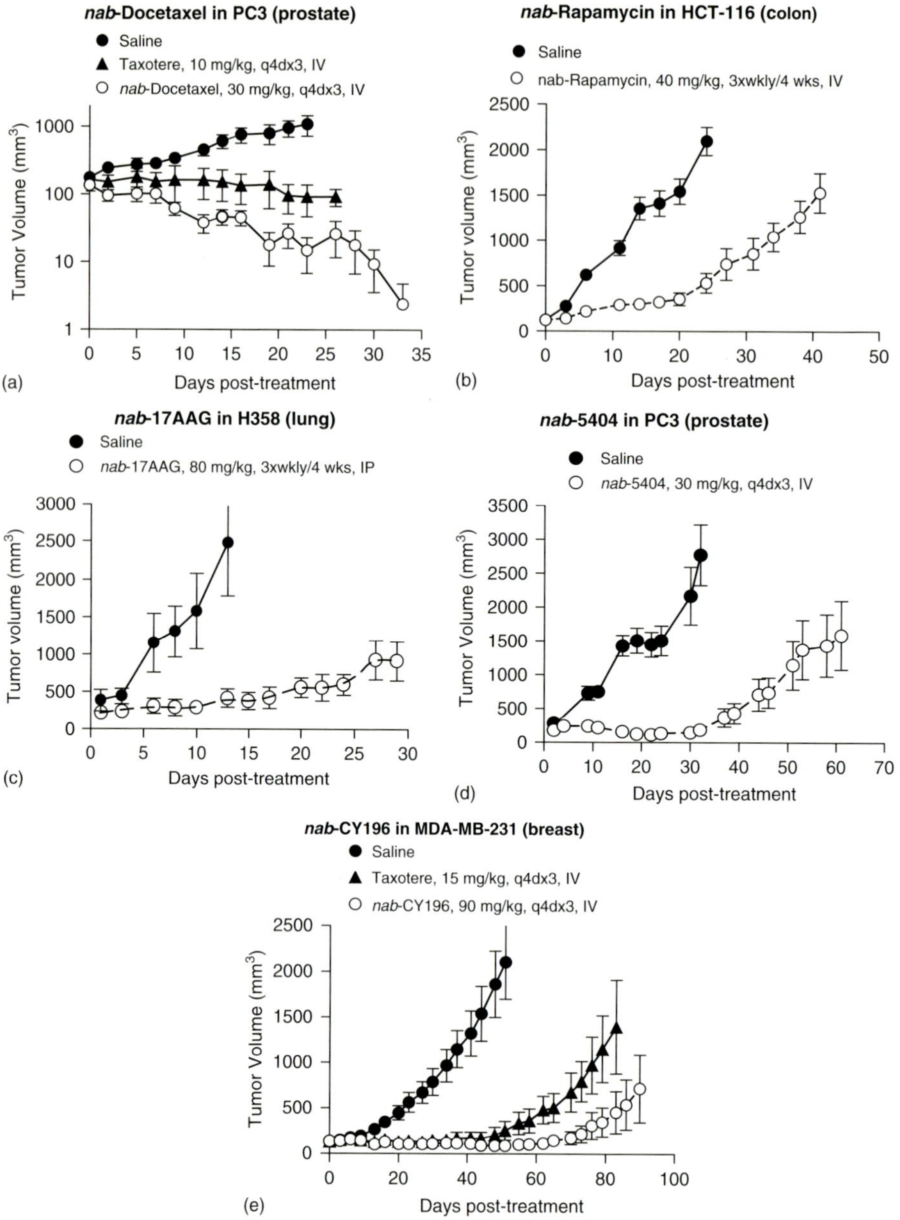

Figure 35.10 Drugs based on *nab* technology demonstrated antitumor activity as single agents in different tumor xenograft models. (a) *nab*-Docetaxel in PC-3 prostate tumors; (b) *nab*-rapamycin in HCT-116 colon tumors; (c) *nab*-17AAG in H358 lung tumors; (d) *nab*-5404 in PC-3 prostate tumors; and (e) *nab*-CY196 in MDA-MB-231 breast tumors.

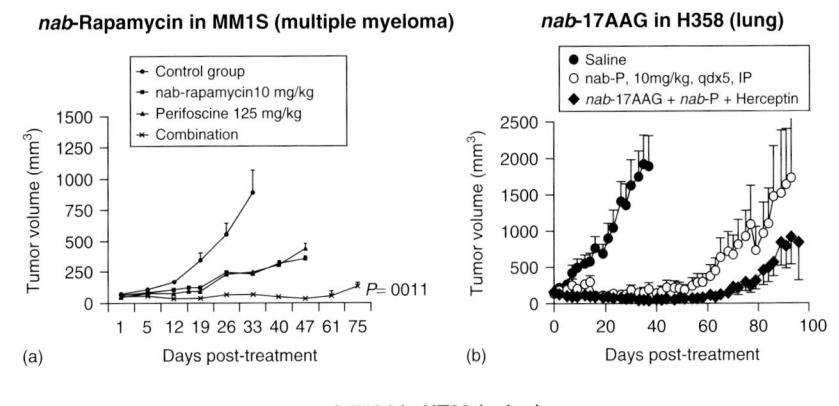

Figure 35.11 Combination of *nab* technology-based drugs with other anticancer therapeutics. (a) *nab*-Rapamycin and perifosine combination therapy triggered more potent inhibition of MM1S multiple myeloma tumor growth than *nab*-rapamycin or perifosine alone ($P \leq 0.0011$). (b) Combination of *nab*-17AAG with *nab*-paclitaxel and trastuzumab (Herceptin) demonstrated synergy in the HER2-positive H358 lung xenograft model. (c) Combination of *nab*-5404 with bevacizumab demonstrated strong synergy in the HT29 colon xenograft model compared with either agent alone ($P = 0.028$ versus bevacizumab; $P = 0.003$ versus ABI-011).

poly(methylvinylether-*co*-maleic anhydride) nanoparticles coated with BSA encapsulating 5-fluorouridine (FURD) [45]. The BSA nanoparticles showed a tropism for the stomach. Following oral administration, FURD bioavailability when loaded in BSA nanoparticles was 79%, significantly higher than the bioavailability of 21% for nanoparticles without albumin. Dreis *et al.* prepared HSA nanoparticles by a desolvation and glutaraldehyde cross-linking method, and loaded doxorubicin by adsorption to the surfaces of preformed nanoparticles or by incorporation into the particle matrix during nanoparticle preparation [46]. The doxorubicin–HSA nanoparticles had a size range between 150 and 500 nm with a drug-loading efficiency of 70–95%. The nanoparticles displayed stronger inhibition of cell viability compared with doxorubicin solution in two different neuroblastoma cell lines. Pereverzeva *et al.* also demonstrated that compared to the free drug, doxorubicin

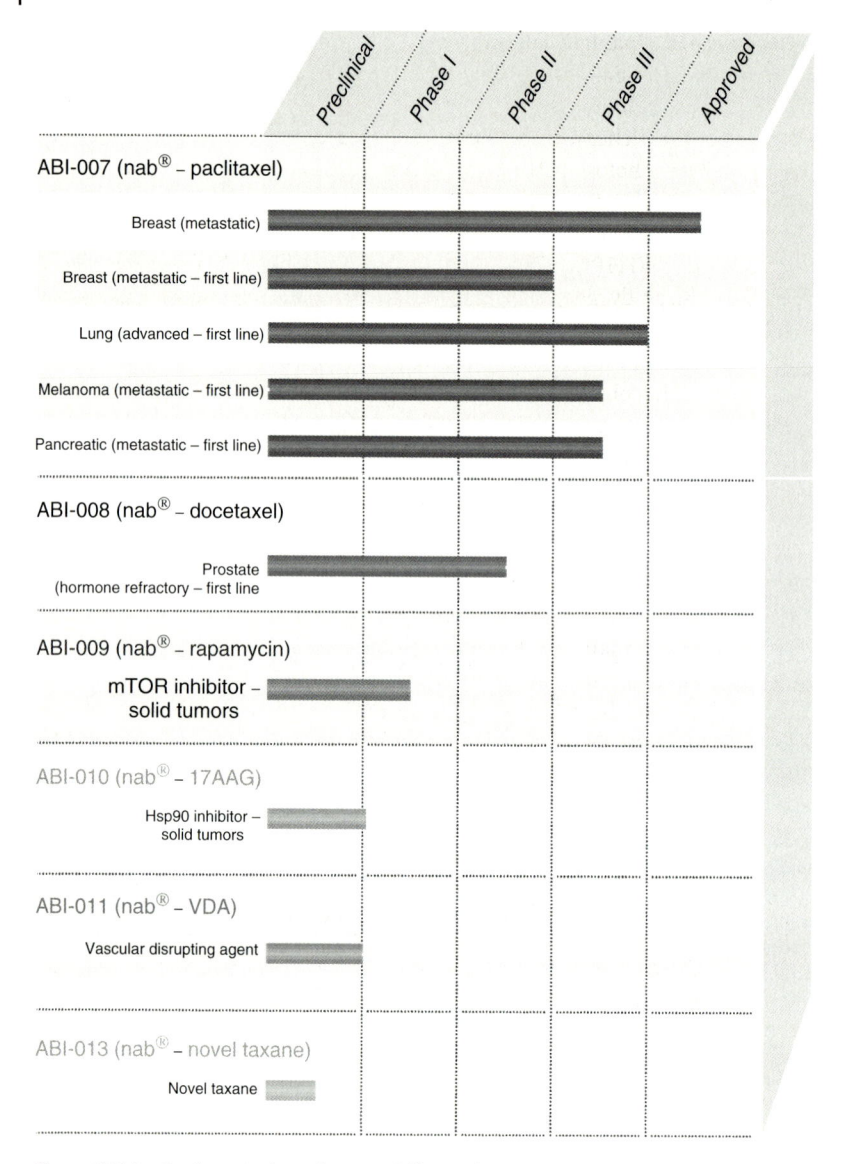

Figure 35.12 Product pipeline showing different development stages for current *nab* technology-based drugs.

bound to HSA nanoparticles coated with polysorbate 80 had favorable toxicological profiles with a considerably reduced cardio- and testicular toxicity [47]. Yadav *et al.* prepared albumin nanoparticles loaded with paclitaxel using the emulsion-solvent evaporation technique [48]. Esmaeili *et al.* chemically conjugated docetael with HSA via a succinic spacer [49]. The docetaxel–HSA nanoparticles had a size of 90–110 nm and showed enhanced solubility, and significantly higher cytotoxicity against T47D and SKOV-3 tumor cells. Two hours following injection into BALB/c mice, docetaxel–HSA nanoparticles maintained 6- to 7-fold higher docetaxel plasma level with 16.2% of initial dose remaining in plasma, compared to Taxotere with 2.5% of initial dose still in plasma.

In addition to these chemotherapeutic agents, albumin nanoparticles have been utilized to deliver photosensitizers in photodynamic therapy against tumors. Wacker et al. prepared HSA nanoparticles carrying photosensitizers 5,10,15,20-tetrakis(m-hydroxyphenyl)porphyrine (mTHPP) and 5,10,15,20-tetrakis(m-hydroxyphenyl)chlorin (mTHPC) [50]. The mTHPP- and mTHPC-loaded HSA nanoparticles efficiently generated singlet oxygen when incubated with Jurkat cells, indicating the release of photosensitizer molecules from the nanoparticles within the cells. Chen et al. loaded photosensitizer pheophorbide onto preformed 100 and 40% glutaraldehyde cross-linked HSA nanoparticles through noncovalent drug adsorption to prepare pheophorbide–HSA nanoparticles PHSA100 and PHSA40 [51]. These nanoparticles were effectively taken up by Jurkat cells and showed strong phototoxicity as the result of nanoparticle decomposition in the cellular lysosomes.

Previous studies have also tested the effect of additional targeting moieties and modifications to further enhance the specific tumor targeting of albumin nanoparticles. Sheng et al. chemically coupled a mAb BDI-1 against bladder carcinoma to albumin nanoparticle containing adriamycin [52], which showed strong cytotoxicity in in vitro assays against bladder cancer cells (EJ) while having no effect on nontargeted human colon carcinoma cells (Lovo). Wagner et al. reported the covalent conjugation of the anti-α_v integrin mAb DI17E6 to doxorubicin–HSA nanoparticles [53]. Expression of $\alpha_v\beta_3$ integrin is enhanced in various tumor types. Doxorubicin–HSA nanoparticles were prepared with desolvation and glutaraldehyde cross-linking method, modified to obtain sulfhydryl-reactive nanoparticles, and reacted with thiolated antibodies. In in vitro assays, the antibody-conjugated nanoparticles demonstrated increased cellular uptake and cytotoxicity in $\alpha_v\beta_3$ integrin-positive melanoma cells (Figure 35.13). Karmali et al. coupled tumor-homing peptides to nab-paclitaxel nanoparticles through their cysteine sulfhydryl group using a sulfo-SMCC cross-linker [54]. The CREKA peptide binds to clotted plasma proteins present in interstitial tissue and vessel walls of tumors, whereas the cyclic LyP-1 (CGNKRTRGC) peptide targets p32 or gC1qR receptor overexpressed on the surface of tumor lymphatics, tumor cells, and a subset of myeloid cells. When injected intravenously into mice bearing MDA-MB-435 human cancer xenografts, fluorescein-labeled CREKA- and LyP-1-nab-paclitaxel nanoparticles showed enhanced tumor targeting. LyP-1-nab-paclitaxel produced a significant inhibition of tumor growth compared with untargeted nab-paclitaxel ($P = 0.013$), demonstrating the effective targeting of nanoparticles into tumor blood vessels and extravascular tumor tissues. To deliver chemotherapy across BBB for treatment of glioma, Lu et al. incorporated aclarubicin (ACL) into cationic albumin-conjugated PEGylated nanoparticles (CBSA-NP-ACL) [55]. Following intravenous administration into rats with intracranially implanted C6 glioma, fluorescent 6-coumarin-labeled CBSA-NPs were shown to preferentially accumulate in tumor mass, and CBSA-NP-ACL displayed higher tumor drug concentration and retention than NP-ACL and ACL

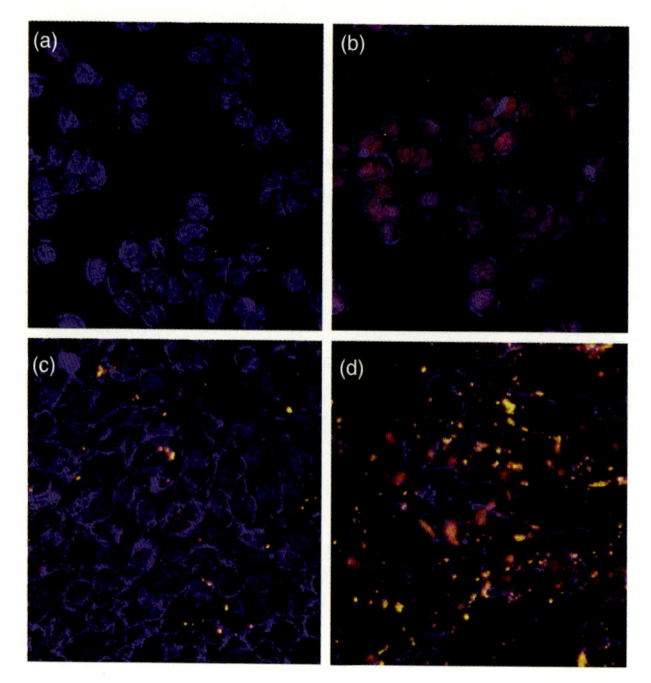

Figure 35.13 Cellular uptake and intracellular distribution of albumin nanoparticles by confocal laser scanning microscopy in melanoma cells expressing $α_vβ_3$ integrin [53]. Autofluorescence of the nanoparticles (green); autofluorescence of doxorubicin (red); cell membranes stained with concanavalin A AlexaFluor® 350 (blue). (a) Control, cells without nanoparticles, (b) incubation of the cells with free doxorubicin, (c) incubation of the cells with the nonspecific nanoparticles (NP-Dox-IgG), and (d) incubation of the $α_vβ_3$-positive cells with the specific nanoparticles carrying anti-$α_v$ integrin mAb DI17E6 (NP-Dox-DI17E6).

solution. Further, CBSA-NP-ACL treatment resulted in a significant increase of median survival time compared with that of animals receiving saline, NP-ACL, and ACL solution. CBSA-NP-ACL also showed reduced toxicity to liver, kidney, and heart, and had no effect on tight junction in BBB coculture.

Besides the above anticancer chemotherapies, albumin nanoparticles are used as a solvent-free platform for intravenous delivery of other small molecules, such as the antiviral drug ganciclovir [56], anesthetic drug propofol [57], bisphosphate antiosteoporosis drug alendronate [58], antifungal drug itraconazole [59], and the brain-targeting delivery of antipsychotic drug sulpiride [60]. These examples clearly demonstrate the usefulness of albumin nanoparticles as drug delivery vehicles in indications beyond oncology.

35.3.1.3 Albumin Nanoparticle Delivery of Oligonucleotides and Proteins

In addition to small-molecule drugs, albumin nanoparticles have been shown to be effective in delivering macromolecules such as oligonucleotides and proteins. Mayer *et al.* prepared by self-assembly oligonucleotide-protamine-albumin nanoparticles [61]. Interestingly, while nanoparticles prepared with protamine free base had diameters around 200 nm, substitution with protamine sulfate leads to dramatic reduction in nanoparticle size to around 40 nm in diameter with otherwise unchanged properties. The nanoparticles were stable and efficiently taken up by cells, and readily released oligodeoxynucleotides and the more stable phosphorothioates. Arnedo *et al.* prepared albumin nanoparticles carrying phosphodiester and phosphorothioate oligonucleotides using a coacervation process and cross-linking with glutaraldehyde [62, 63]. The oligonucleotides were either absorbed onto preformed albumin nanoparticles or incorporated into the particle matrix prior to the formation of nanoparticles. However, only the oligonucleotide incorporated into the nanoparticle matrix was protected against enzymatic degradation with its released controlled by the albumin degradation. Antisense oligonucleotides carried by albumin nanoparticles showed improved nuclear presence and increased antiviral activity in MRC-5 fibroblasts infected with human cytomegalovirus.

More specifically, the feasibility of delivering antisense oligonucleotides as anticancer therapy has been demonstrated in several studies. Wartlick *et al.* incorporated antisense oligonucleotides into the matrix of HSA nanoparticles by desolvation and glutaraldehyde cross-linking procedure [64]. The oligonucleotide loading increased with longer chain length and the use of a phosphorothioate backbone. Different tumor cell lines all showed a significant cellular uptake of HSA nanoparticles, with no cytotoxic effect observed up to 5000 µg/ml of control HSA nanoparticles. The cross-linking step was identified as a crucial parameter for biodegradability and drug release of the nanoparticles, as lower amounts of glutaraldehyde produced nanoparticles that rapidly degraded intracellularly, leading to a significant accumulation of antisense oligonucleotides in cytosol of tumor cells. Spankuch *et al.* further proved the specific downregulation of tumor target with the delivery of antisense oligonucleotides by albumin nanoparticles [65]. Thiolated anti-HER2 mAb trastuzumab was coupled to glutaraldehyde-cross-linked albumin nanoparticles carrying antisense oligonucleotides against polo-like kinase 1 (Plk1), an early trigger of G_2/M transition that is overexpressed in many tumor types. Antibody-conjugated nanoparticles showed a specific targeting to HER2-positive BT-474 cells with cellular uptake by receptor-mediated endocytosis and intracellular oligonucleotide release, resulting in a significant reduction of Plk1 mRNA and protein expression, and increased activation of caspase-3/7. This is the first report demonstrating tumor-targeting albumin nanoparticles as a promising carrier for antisense oligonucleotides and may reduce their off-target effects.

As a protein-based delivery system, albumin nanoparticles can be adapted to deliver peptides and proteins, either by conjugation or absorption. Zhang *et al.* delivered BMP-2 absorbed to PEI-coated albumin nanoparticles for *in vivo* bone induction [28]. Such systems may prove to be useful as a platform for peptide and protein therapeutics against tumors.

35.3.2
Clinical Studies with Albumin-Based Nanoparticles

So far, *nab*-paclitaxel is the only albumin nanoparticle-based anticancer drug extensively studied in multiple clinical trials. First approved by the US Food and Drug Administration in January 2005 for the treatment of breast cancer after a failure of combination chemotherapy for metastatic disease or a relapse within 6 months of adjuvant chemotherapy, *nab*-paclitaxel is recognized as the first nanotechnology-based drug on the market and has since been approved in 41 countries around the world.

In a phase I trial with 19 patients with solid tumors, the lower toxicities of *nab*-paclitaxel allowed the administration of 70% higher dose than the approved dose of Cremophor-based paclitaxel (300 versus 175 mg/m^2, q3w) over a shorter infusion time (30 min versus 3 h), without the need for corticosteroid premedication [25]. *nab*-Paclitaxel displayed linear pharmacokinetics over the dose range of 135–300 mg/m^2, in contrast with the nonlinear pharmacokinetics observed with Taxol in previous studies. In a comparative pharmacokinetic study of *nab*-paclitaxel (260 mg/m^2 intravenously over 30 min, q3w) and Taxol (175 mg/m^2 intravenously over 3 h, q3w) in 27 patients with solid tumors, *nab*-paclitaxel displayed significantly higher rate of clearance (21.13 versus 14.76 l/h/m^2, $P = 0.048$) and volume of distribution (663.8 versus. 433.4 l/m^2, $P = 0.040$) compared with Taxol [66]. The improved pharmacokinetic profile of *nab*-paclitaxel over Taxol is potentially due to the sequestration of paclitaxel in micelles by Cremophor, which delays the paclitaxel distribution for Taxol [67]. The drug bioavailability is also significantly higher with *nab*-paclitaxel. In a randomized crossover pharmacokinetic study in patients with solid tumors, the mean fraction of unbound paclitaxel was considerably higher with *nab*-paclitaxel compared with Taxol (0.063 ± 0.021 versus 0.024 ± 0.009; $P < 0.001$). Combined with higher dose and shorter infusion time, the maximal concentration of unbound paclitaxel after *nab*-paclitaxel administration was 10-fold higher than Taxol (1283.7 ± 532.17 versus 121.79 ± 39.62 ng/ml) [68].

In a randomized phase III study in 460 patients with metastatic breast cancer [69], compared with Taxol at 175 mg/m^2 q3w, *nab*-paclitaxel administered at 260 mg/m^2 q3w had statistically significantly higher response rates (33 versus 19%, $P = 0.001$; Figure 35.14), longer time to tumor progression (5.3 versus 3.9 months, $P = 0.006$), and increased survival in the subset of patients receiving second-line or greater treatment (12.9 versus 10.7 months, $P = 0.024$; Figure 35.15). The incidence of grade 4 neutropenia with *nab*-paclitaxel was significantly lower than in the Taxol group (9 versus 22%, $P = 0.001$). No severe hypersensitivity reactions occurred with *nab*-paclitaxel treatment despite the lack of premedication. Grade 3 neuropathy was higher for *nab*-paclitaxel (10 versus 2%, $P = 0.001$) due to the approximately 50% higher dosage, but was easily managed and improved quickly. Overall, the phase III study demonstrated that *nab*-paclitaxel has improved antitumor activity and is well tolerated compared with Taxol. These results were further supported by results from an open-label study of 210 Chinese patients with metastatic breast cancer, which suggested that *nab*-paclitaxel (260 mg/m^2 intravenously over 30 min, q3w) provided

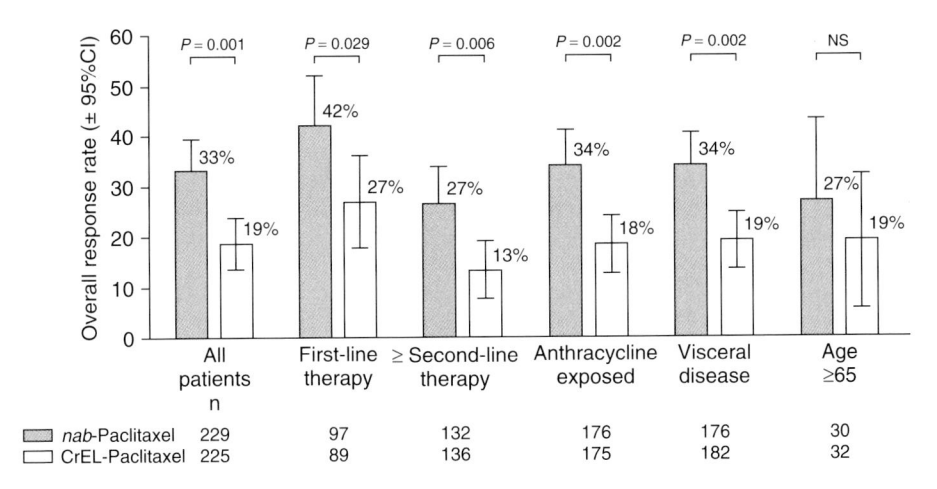

Figure 35.14 nab-Paclitaxel was approved in January 2005 for use in patients with metastatic breast cancer who have failed combination therapy. Phase III trial comparing 3-week cycles of either nab-paclitaxel 260 mg/m^2 intravenously without premedication ($n = 229$) or Cremophor-paclitaxel 175 mg/m^2 intravenously with premedication ($n = 225$) demonstrated improved clinical response with nab-paclitaxel.

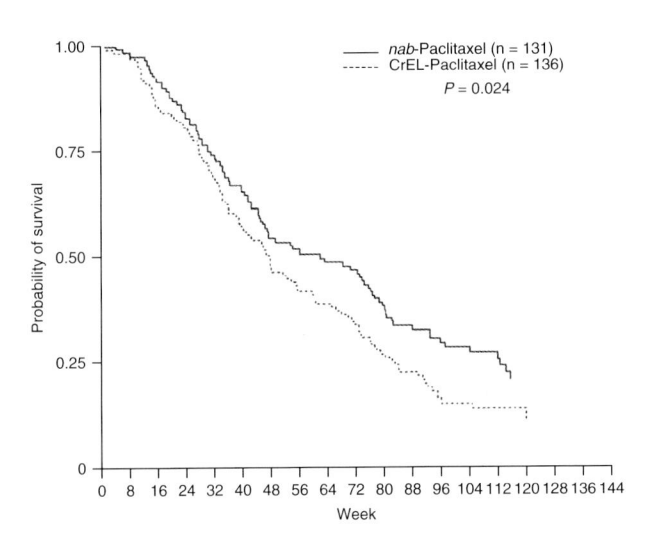

Figure 35.15 Survival advantage in patients with metastatic breast cancer who received greater than or equal to second-line therapy of nab-paclitaxel (median: 12.9 months) versus Cremophor-paclitaxel (median: 10.7 months, $P = 0.024$) [69].

higher response rates and longer time to tumor progression without increased toxicity compared with Taxol (175 mg/m^2 intravenously over 3 h, q3w) [70].

nab-Paclitaxel has also exhibited improved clinical efficacy over polysorbate-based docetaxel (Taxotere). In a randomized phase II clinical trial of first-line treatment of 300 patients with metastatic breast cancer [71], independent radiologist assessment showed that nab-paclitaxel at 150 mg/m^2 weekly resulted in significantly longer progression-free survival (PFS) compared with Taxotere at 100 mg/m^2, q3w (median 12.9 versus 7.5 months; $P = 0.0065$), and nab-paclitaxel at 100 mg/m^2 weekly also significantly prolonged PFS (more than 5 months) compared with docetaxel (median 12.8 versus 7.5 months). Overall, all doses of nab-paclitaxel displayed a very favorable safety and toxicity profile compared with docetaxel.

In addition to breast cancer, nab-paclitaxel is also being investigated for treatment of other tumor types, including non-small-cell lung cancer (NSCLC), pancreatic cancer, and melanoma. In a recent phase III trial with advanced NSCLC [72], patients were randomized to received nab-paclitaxel (100 mg/m^2, qw) in combination with carboplatin (area under curve 6, q3w) (nab-PC group, $n = 521$), or Taxol (200 mg/m^2, q3w)/carboplatin combination (PC group, $n = 531$). The nab-PC group showed an overall response rate (ORR) superior to the PC group by independent radiological review (33 versus 25%, $P = 0.005$), a 31% improvement (1.31 response ratio; 95% confidence interval: 1.08, 1.59).

nab-Paclitaxel has also shown potential efficacy against pancreatic cancer. In a phase I/II study in patients with metastatic pancreatic cancer [73], the combination of nab-paclitaxel 125 mg/m^2 and gemcitabine 1000 mg/m^2 on days 1, 8, and 15 of an every-28-day cycle ($n = 44$) resulted in impressive clinical activity with a disease

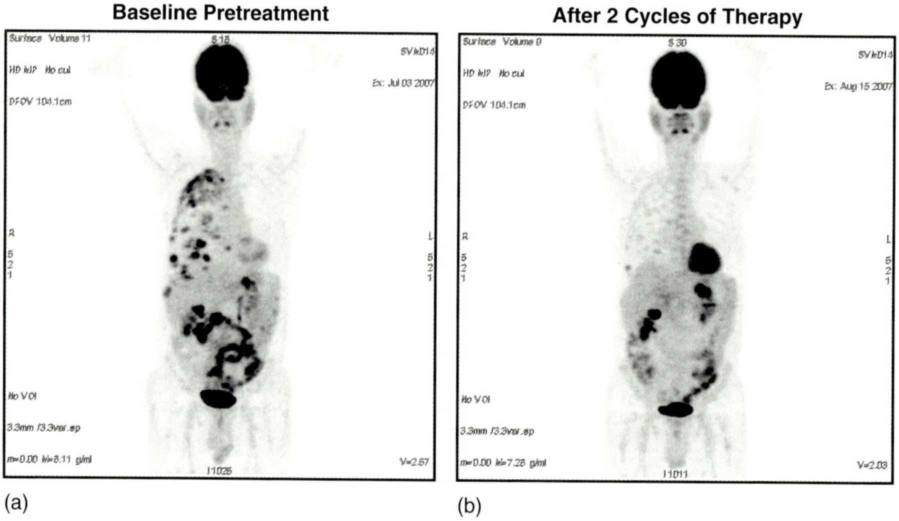

Figure 35.16 Rapid response of metastatic pancreatic cancer to nab-paclitaxel/gemcitabine combination detected by PET scans in phase I/II trial [73].

control rate of 80% (independent radiologist assessment), 8.0 months of median PFS, and 12.2 months of median overall survival. Impressive and rapid responses in these pancreatic cancer patients were observed via PET scans (Figure 35.16). Efficacy of this combination is being tested in an ongoing phase III trial in patients with advanced pancreatic cancer.

Clinical studies have suggested that SPARC may be an important part of the mechanism of action for *nab*-paclitaxel and may contribute to its improved clinical efficacy. In a retrospective analysis of 16 head and neck cancer patients, response to *nab*-paclitaxel was higher for SPARC-positive patients (10/12, 83%) than SPARC-negative patients (1/4, 25%). The SPARC-negative patients exhibited significantly lower response than the ORR among all 60 patients enrolled in the study (1/4, 25 versus 45/60, 75%, $P < 0.05$) [74]. In the phase I/II study in patients with metastatic pancreatic cancer treated with *nab*-paclitaxel and gemcitabine [73], higher overall SPARC levels across all tumor components correlated with

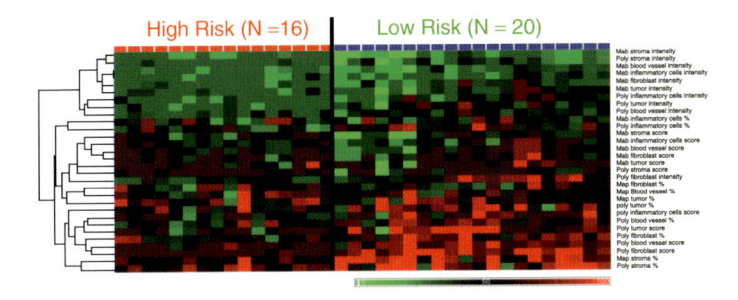

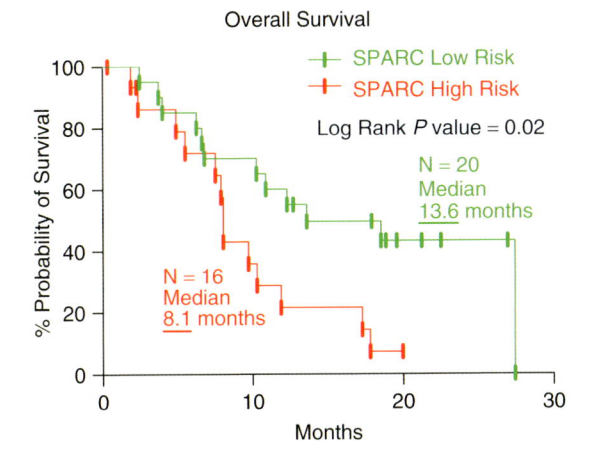

Figure 35.17 Higher overall SPARC levels across all tumor components correlated with improved survival in metastatic pancreatic cancer patients treated with *nab*-paclitaxel and gemcitabine. SPARC immunohistochemistry-based microenvironment signature distinguished a low-risk group with higher SPARC expression ($n = 20$) from a high-risk group ($n = 16$; median survival 13.6 versus 8.1 months, $P = 0.02$) [73].

improved survival. The SPARC immunohistochemistry-based microenvironment signature distinguished a low-risk group with higher SPARC expression ($n = 20$) from a high-risk group ($n = 16$; median survival 13.6 versus 8.1 months, $P = 0.02$; Figure 35.17). The potential of SPARC as a predictive biomarker for clinical response to *nab*-paclitaxel is currently being investigated in several large clinical studies.

35.4
Conclusions and Perspectives

A great variety of albumin nanoparticles have been developed to deliver both small-molecule and macromolecule anticancer therapies. Drug loading and nanoparticle properties can be controlled during preparation by adjusting various parameters, including drug and protein concentrations, pH, and amount of cross-linker. Most albumin nanoparticles involve glutaraldehyde cross-linking, which results in the drug being incorporated into a cross-linked albumin matrix [43, 46, 62, 64, 65]. In contrast, *nab* nanoparticles consist of drug coated with a layer of albumin through noncovalent hydrophobic interaction [15]. Other nanoparticles have drugs noncovalently absorbed onto the surface of preformed albumin nanoparticles [46, 51, 62].

Albumin nanoparticles are usually readily water dispersible without any solvent and surfactant. Loading of therapeutics onto albumin nanoparticles may increase solubility and stability, diminish toxicity, improve tissue distribution and pharmacokinetic profile, enhance tumor targeting, and potentially overcome drug resistance. As a versatile drug delivery platform, albumin nanoparticles can be modified to carry different kinds of therapeutic agents and additional targeting moieties that may be suited for specific indications. The great potential of this system is demonstrated by the clinical success of *nab*-paclitaxel. Albumin nanoparticles can provide powerful tools in the fight against cancer. The future may see more types of albumin nanoparticles move from laboratory concepts into clinical applications.

Acknowledgments

Dr. Shihe Hou's expert editorial and writing assistance of this manuscript is greatly appreciated. The author would like to thank Dr. Raffit Hassan of the National Cancer Institute for kindly granting permission to include his illustration of transport mechanisms for albumin-bound drugs in this chapter.

References

1. Gelderblom, H., Verweij, J., Nooter, K., and Sparreboom, A. (2001) Cremophor EL: the drawbacks and advantages of vehicle selection for drug formulation. *Eur. J. Cancer*, **37**, 1590–1598.
2. Weiss, R.B., Donehower, R.C., Wiernik, P.H., Ohnuma, T., Gralla, R.J., Trump,

D.L., Baker, J.R. Jr., Van Echo, D.A., Von Hoff, D.D., and Leyland-Jones, B. (1990) Hypersensitivity reactions from taxol. *J. Clin. Oncol.*, **8**, 1263–1268.

3. van Zuylen, L., Verweij, J., and Sparreboom, A. (2001) Role of formulation vehicles in taxane pharmacology. *Invest. New Drugs*, **19**, 125–141.

4. John, T.A., Vogel, S.M., Tiruppathi, C., Malik, A.B., and Minshall, R.D. (2003) Quantitative analysis of albumin uptake and transport in the rat microvessel endothelial monolayer. *Am. J. Physiol.*, **284**, L187–L196.

5. Herve, F., Urien, S., Albengres, E., Duche, J.C., and Tillement, J.P. (1994) Drug binding in plasma. A summary of recent trends in the study of drug and hormone binding. *Clin. Pharmacokinet.*, **26**, 44–58.

6. Paal, K., Muller, J., and Hegedus, L. (2001) High affinity binding of paclitaxel to human serum albumin. *Eur. J. Biochem.*, **268**, 2187–2191.

7. Desai, N., Trieu, V., Yao, Z., Louie, L., Ci, S., Yang, A., Tao, C., De, T., Beals, B., Dykes, D., Noker, P., Yao, R., Labao, E., Hawkins, M., and Soon-Shiong, P. (2006) Increased antitumor activity, intratumor paclitaxel concentrations, and endothelial cell transport of Cremophor-free, albumin-bound paclitaxel, ABI-007, compared with Cremophor-based paclitaxel. *Clin. Cancer Res.*, **12**, 1317–1324.

8. Makriyannis, A., Guo, J., and Tian, X. (2005) Albumin enhances the diffusion of lipophilic drugs into the membrane bilayer. *Life Sci.*, **77**, 1605–1611.

9. Stehle, G., Sinn, H., Wunder, A., Schrenk, H.H., Stewart, J.C., Hartung, G., Maier-Borst, W., and Heene, D.L. (1997) Plasma protein (albumin) catabolism by the tumor itself – implications for tumor metabolism and the genesis of cachexia. *Crit. Rev. Oncol. Hematol.*, **26**, 77–100.

10. Kratz, F. (2008) Albumin as a drug carrier: design of prodrugs, drug conjugates and nanoparticles. *J Control. Release*, **132**, 171–183.

11. Maeda, H., Sawa, T., and Konno, T. (2001) Mechanism of tumor-targeted delivery of macromolecular drugs, including the EPR effect in solid tumor and clinical overview of the prototype polymeric drug SMANCS. *J Control. Release*, **74**, 47–61.

12. Schnitzer, J.E. (1992) gp60 is an albumin-binding glycoprotein expressed by continuous endothelium involved in albumin transcytosis. *Am. J. Physiol.*, **262**, H246–H254.

13. Tiruppathi, C., Song, W., Bergenfeldt, M., Sass, P., and Malik, A.B. (1997) Gp60 activation mediates albumin transcytosis in endothelial cells by tyrosine kinase-dependent pathway. *J. Biol. Chem.*, **272**, 25968–25975.

14. Wang, Z., Tiruppathi, C., Minshall, R.D., and Malik, A.B. (2009) Size and dynamics of caveolae studied using nanoparticles in living endothelial cells. *ACS Nano*, **3**, 4110–4116.

15. Hawkins, M.J., Soon-Shiong, P., and Desai, N. (2008) Protein nanoparticles as drug carriers in clinical medicine. *Adv. Drug Deliv. Rev.*, **60**, 876–885.

16. Sage, H., Johnson, C., and Bornstein, P. (1984) Characterization of a novel serum albumin-binding glycoprotein secreted by endothelial cells in culture. *J. Biol. Chem.*, **259**, 3993–4007.

17. Trieu, V., Hwang, J., and Desai, N. (2007) Nanoparticle albumin-bound (nab) technology may enhance antitumor activity via targeting of SPARC protein. New Targets and Delivery System for Cancer Diagnosis and Treatment, San Diego, CA, abstract 53.

18. Podhajcer, O.L., Benedetti, L.G., Girotti, M.R., Prada, F., Salvatierra, E., and Llera, A.S. (2008) The role of the matricellular protein SPARC in the dynamic interaction between the tumor and the host. *Cancer Metastasis Rev.*, **27**, 523–537.

19. Trieu, V., Frankel, T., Labao, E., Soon-Shiong, P., and Desai, N. (2005) SPARC expression in breast tumors may correlate to increased tumor distribution of nanoparticle albumin-bound paclitaxel (ABI-007) vs taxol. American Association for Cancer Research Annual Meeting, Anaheim, CA, abstract 5584.

20. Koukourakis, M.I., Giatromanolaki, A., Brekken, R.A., Sivridis, E.,

Gatter, K.C., Harris, A.L., and Sage, E.H. (2003) Enhanced expression of SPARC/osteonectin in the tumor-associated stroma of non-small cell lung cancer is correlated with markers of hypoxia/acidity and with poor prognosis of patients. *Cancer Res.*, **63**, 5376–5380.

21. Muller, B.G., Leuenberger, H., and Kissel, T. (1996) Albumin nanospheres as carriers for passive drug targeting: an optimized manufacturing technique. *Pharm. Res.*, **13**, 32–37.

22. Lin, W., Coombes, A.G., Davies, M.C., Davis, S.S., and Illum, L. (1993) Preparation of sub-100 nm human serum albumin nanospheres using a pH-coacervation method. *J. Drug Target.*, **1**, 237–243.

23. Langer, K., Balthasar, S., Vogel, V., Dinauer, N., von Briesen, H., and Schubert, D. (2003) Optimization of the preparation process for human serum albumin (HSA) nanoparticles. *Int. J. Pharm.*, **257**, 169–180.

24. Langer, K., Anhorn, M.G., Steinhauser, I., Dreis, S., Celebi, D., Schrickel, N., Faust, S., and Vogel, V. (2008) Human serum albumin (HSA) nanoparticles: reproducibility of preparation process and kinetics of enzymatic degradation. *Int. J. Pharm.*, **347**, 109–117.

25. Ibrahim, N.K., Desai, N., Legha, S., Soon-Shiong, P., Theriault, R.L., Rivera, E., Esmaeli, B., Ring, S.E., Bedikian, A., Hortobagyi, G.N., and Ellerhorst, J.A. (2002) Phase I and pharmacokinetic study of ABI-007, a Cremophor-free, protein-stabilized, nanoparticle formulation of paclitaxel, *Clin. Cancer Res.*, **8**, 1038–1044.

26. Desai, N., De, T., Ci, S., Louie, L., and Trieu, V. (2008) Characterization and *in vitro/in vivo* dissolution of *nab*-paclitaxel nanoparticles. American Association for Cancer Research Annual Meeting, San Diego, CA, abstract 5624.

27. Weber, C., Reiss, S., and Langer, K. (2000) Preparation of surface modified protein nanoparticles by introduction of sulfhydryl groups. *Int. J. Pharm.*, **211**, 67–78.

28. Zhang, S., Wang, G., Lin, X., Chatzinikolaidou, M., Jennissen, H.P., Laub, M., and Uludag, H. (2008) Polyethylenimine-coated albumin nanoparticles for BMP-2 delivery. *Biotechnol. Prog.*, **24**, 945–956.

29. Roser, M., Fischer, D., and Kissel, T. (1998) Surface-modified biodegradable albumin nano- and microspheres. II: effect of surface charges on *in vitro* phagocytosis and biodistribution in rats. *Eur. J. Pharm. Biopharm.*, **46**, 255–263.

30. Kumagai, A.K., Eisenberg, J.B., and Pardridge, W.M. (1987) Absorptive-mediated endocytosis of cationized albumin and a beta-endorphin-cationized albumin chimeric peptide by isolated brain capillaries. Model system of blood–brain barrier transport. *J. Biol. Chem.*, **262**, 15214–15219.

31. Lu, W., Tan, Y.Z., Hu, K.L., and Jiang, X.G. (2005) Cationic albumin conjugated pegylated nanoparticle with its transcytosis ability and little toxicity against blood–brain barrier. *Int. J. Pharm.*, **295**, 247–260.

32. Kreuter, J., Hekmatara, T., Dreis, S., Vogel, T., Gelperina, S., and Langer, K. (2007) Covalent attachment of apolipoprotein A-I and apolipoprotein B-100 to albumin nanoparticles enables drug transport into the brain. *J. Control. Release*, **118**, 54–58.

33. Li, F.Q., Su, H., Wang, J., Liu, J.Y., Zhu, Q.G., Fei, Y.B., Pan, Y.H., and Hu, J.H. (2008) Preparation and characterization of sodium ferulate entrapped bovine serum albumin nanoparticles for liver targeting. *Int. J. Pharm.*, **349**, 274–282.

34. Mao, S.J., Hou, S.X., He, R., Zhang, L.K., Wei, D.P., Bi, Y.Q., and Jin, H. (2005) Uptake of albumin nanoparticle surface modified with glycyrrhizin by primary cultured rat hepatocytes. *World J. Gastroenterol.*, **11**, 3075–3079.

35. Merisko-Liversidge, E., Sarpotdar, P., Bruno, J., Hajj, S., Wei, L., Peltier, N., Rake, J., Shaw, J.M., Pugh, S., Polin, L., Jones, J., Corbett, T., Cooper, E., and Liversidge, G.G. (1996) Formulation and antitumor activity evaluation of nanocrystalline suspensions of poorly soluble anticancer drugs. *Pharm. Res.*, **13**, 272–278.

36. Hassan, R. (2010) Optimizing care in advanced lung cancer, American Society of Clinical Oncology Annual Meeting, Chicago, IL.
37. Desai, N., Trieu, V., Hwang, L., Wu, R., Hawkins, M.J., Soon-Shiong, P., and Gradishar, W. (2007) HER2 and SPARC status in tumors play an important role in the relative effectiveness of nanoparticle albumin-bound (nab) paclitaxel versus polysorbate-based docetaxel. 30th Annual San Antonio Breast Cancer Symposium, San Antonio, TX, abstract 2013.
38. Wiedenmann, N., Valdecanas, D., Hunter, N., Hyde, S., Buchholz, T.A., Milas, L., and Mason, K.A. (2007) 130-nm albumin-bound paclitaxel enhances tumor radiocurability and therapeutic gain. *Clin. Cancer Res.*, **13**, 1868–1874.
39. Volk, L.D., Flister, M., Bivens, C.M., Stutzman, A., Desai, N., Trieu, V., and Ran, S. (2008) *nab*-Paclitaxel efficacy in the orthotopic model of human breast cancer is significantly enhanced by concurrent anti-vascular endothelial growth factor a therapy. *Neoplasia*, **10**, 613–623.
40. Maitra, A., Rajeshkumar, N.V., Rudek, M., Garrido-Laguna, I., Laheru, D., Iglesias, J., Desai, N., Von Hoff, D.D., and Hidalgo, M. (2009) nab®-Paclitaxel targets tumor stroma and results, combined with gemcitabine, in high efficacy against pancreatic cancer models. AACR–NCI–EORTC International Conference on Molecular Targets and Cancer Therapeutics, Boston, MA, abstract C246.
41. Garber, K. (2010) Stromal depletion goes on trial in pancreatic cancer. *J. Natl. Cancer Inst.*, **102**, 448–450.
42. Cirstea, D., Hideshima, T., Rodig, S., Santo, L., Pozzi, S., Vallet, S., Ikeda, H., Perrone, G., Gorgun, G., Patel, K., Desai, N., Sportelli, P., Kapoor, S., Vali, S., Mukherjee, S., Munshi, N.C., Anderson, K.C., and Raje, N. (2010) Dual inhibition of Akt/mammalian target of rapamycin pathway by nanoparticle albumin-bound-rapamycin and perifosine induces antitumor activity in multiple myeloma. *Mol. Cancer Ther.*, **9**, 963–975.
43. Maghsoudi, A., Shojaosadati, S.A., and Farahani, E.V. (2008) 5-Fluorouracil-loaded BSA nanoparticles: formulation optimization and *in vitro* release study. *AAPS PharmSciTech*, **9**, 1092–1096.
44. Yi, Y.M., Yang, T.Y., and Pan, W.M. (1999) Preparation and distribution of 5-fluorouracil ^{125}I sodium alginate–bovine serum albumin nanoparticles. *World J. Gastroenterol.*, **5**, 57–60.
45. Arbos, P., Campanero, M.A., Arangoa, M.A., and Irache, J.M. (2004) Nanoparticles with specific bioadhesive properties to circumvent the pre-systemic degradation of fluorinated pyrimidines. *J. Control. Release*, **96**, 55–65.
46. Dreis, S., Rothweiler, F., Michaelis, M., Cinatl, J. Jr., Kreuter, J., and Langer, K. (2007) Preparation, characterisation and maintenance of drug efficacy of doxorubicin-loaded human serum albumin (HSA) nanoparticles. *Int. J. Pharm.*, **341**, 207–214.
47. Pereverzeva, E., Treschalin, I., Bodyagin, D., Maksimenko, O., Langer, K., Dreis, S., Asmussen, B., Kreuter, J., and Gelperina, S. (2007) Influence of the formulation on the tolerance profile of nanoparticle-bound doxorubicin in healthy rats: focus on cardio- and testicular toxicity. *Int. J. Pharm.*, **337**, 346–356.
48. Yadav, A.A. and Vadali, S. (2008) Preparation of water-soluble albumin loaded paclitaxil nanoparticles using emulsion-solvent evaporation technique. *Curr. Bioact. Comp.*, **4**, 51–55.
49. Esmaeili, F., Dinarvand, R., Ghahremani, M.H., Amini, M., Rouhani, H., Sepehri, N., Ostad, S.N., and Atyabi, F. (2008) Docetaxel–albumin conjugates: preparation, *in vitro* evaluation and biodistribution studies. *J. Pharm. Sci.*, **98**, 2718–2730.
50. Wacker, M., Chen, K., Preuss, A., Possemeyer, K., Roeder, B., and Langer, K. (2010) Photosensitizer loaded HSA nanoparticles. I: preparation and photophysical properties. *Int. J. Pharm.*, **393**, 253–262.
51. Chen, K., Preuss, A., Hackbarth, S., Wacker, M., Langer, K., and Roder, B.

(2009) Novel photosensitizer–protein nanoparticles for photodynamic therapy: photophysical characterization and *in vitro* investigations. *J. Photochem. Photobiol. B*, **96**, 66–74.

52. Sheng, J., Samten, B.K., Xie, S.S., and Wei, S.L. (1995) Study on the specific killing activity of albumin nanoparticles containing adriamycin targeted by monoclonal antibody BDI-1 to human bladder cancer cells. *Yao Xue Xue Bao*, **30**, 706–710.

53. Wagner, S., Rothweiler, F., Anhorn, M.G., Sauer, D., Riemann, I., Weiss, E.C., Katsen-Globa, A., Michaelis, M., Cinatl, J. Jr., Schwartz, D., Kreuter, J., von Briesen, H., and Langer, K. (2010) Enhanced drug targeting by attachment of an anti alpha$_v$ integrin antibody to doxorubicin loaded human serum albumin nanoparticles. *Biomaterials*, **31**, 2388–2398.

54. Karmali, P.P., Kotamraju, V.R., Kastantin, M., Black, M., Missirlis, D., Tirrell, M., and Ruoslahti, E. (2009) Targeting of albumin-embedded paclitaxel nanoparticles to tumors. *Nanomedicine*, **5**, 73–82.

55. Lu, W., Wan, J., Zhang, Q., She, Z., and Jiang, X. (2007) Aclarubicin-loaded cationic albumin-conjugated pegylated nanoparticle for glioma chemotherapy in rats. *Int. J. Cancer*, **120**, 420–431.

56. Merodio, M., Arnedo, A., Renedo, M.J., and Irache, J.M. (2001) Ganciclovir-loaded albumin nanoparticles: characterization and *in vitro* release properties. *Eur. J. Pharm. Sci.*, **12**, 251–259.

57. Naguib, M., Baker, M.T., Gregerson, M., Desai, N., and Trieu, V. (2003) Potency of albumin-stabilized propofol formulations containing low and no oil. American Society of Anesthesiologists Meeting, San Francisco, CA, abstract.

58. Markovsky, E., Koroukhov, N., and Golomb, G. (2007) Additive-free albumin nanoparticles of alendronate for attenuating inflammation through monocyte inhibition. *Nanomedicine*, **2**, 545–553.

59. Chen, W., Gu, B., Wang, H., Pan, J., Lu, W., and Hou, H. (2008) Development and evaluation of novel itraconazole-loaded intravenous nanoparticles. *Int. J. Pharm.*, **362**, 133–140.

60. Parikh, T., Bommana, M.M., and Squillante, E. III (2009) Efficacy of surface charge in targeting pegylated nanoparticles of sulpiride to the brain. *Eur. J. Pharm. Biopharm.*, **74**, 442–450.

61. Mayer, G., Vogel, V., Weyermann, J., Lochmann, D., van den Broek, J.A., Tziatzios, C., Haase, W., Wouters, D., Schubert, U.S., Zimmer, A., Kreuter, J., and Schubert, D. (2005) Oligonucleotide–protamine–albumin nanoparticles: protamine sulfate causes drastic size reduction. *J. Control. Release*, **106**, 181–187.

62. Arnedo, A., Espuelas, S., and Irache, J.M. (2002) Albumin nanoparticles as carriers for a phosphodiester oligonucleotide. *Int. J. Pharm.*, **244**, 59–72.

63. Arnedo, A., Irache, J.M., Merodio, M., and Espuelas Millan, M.S. (2004) Albumin nanoparticles improved the stability, nuclear accumulation and anticytomegaloviral activity of a phosphodiester oligonucleotide. *J. Control. Release*, **94**, 217–227.

64. Wartlick, H., Spankuch-Schmitt, B., Strebhardt, K., Kreuter, J., and Langer, K. (2004) Tumour cell delivery of antisense oligonuclceotides by human serum albumin nanoparticles. *J. Control. Release*, **96**, 483–495.

65. Spankuch, B., Steinhauser, I., Wartlick, H., Kurunci-Csacsko, E., Strebhardt, K.I., and Langer, K. (2008) Downregulation of Plk1 expression by receptor-mediated uptake of antisense oligonucleotide-loaded nanoparticles. *Neoplasia*, **10**, 223–234.

66. Sparreboom, A., Scripture, C.D., Trieu, V., Williams, P.J., De, T., Yang, A., Beals, B., Figg, W.D., Hawkins, M., and Desai, N. (2005) Comparative preclinical and clinical pharmacokinetics of a cremophor-free, nanoparticle albumin-bound paclitaxel (ABI-007) and paclitaxel formulated in Cremophor (Taxol). *Clin. Cancer Res.*, **11**, 4136–4143.

67. Sparreboom, A., van Zuylen, L., Brouwer, E., Loos, W.J., de Bruijn, P., Gelderblom, H., Pillay, M., Nooter, K., Stoter, G., and Verweij, J. (1999)

Cremophor EL-mediated alteration of paclitaxel distribution in human blood: clinical pharmacokinetic implications. *Cancer Res.*, **59**, 1454–1457.

68. Gardner, E.R., Dahut, W.L., Scripture, C.D., Jones, J., Aragon-Ching, J.B., Desai, N., Hawkins, M.J., Sparreboom, A., and Figg, W.D. (2008) Randomized crossover pharmacokinetic study of solvent-based paclitaxel and *nab*-paclitaxel. *Clin. Cancer Res.*, **14**, 4200–4205.

69. Gradishar, W.J., Tjulandin, S., Davidson, N., Shaw, H., Desai, N., Bhar, P., Hawkins, M., and O'Shaughnessy, J. (2005) Phase III trial of nanoparticle albumin-bound paclitaxel compared with polyethylated castor oil-based paclitaxel in women with breast cancer. *J. Clin. Oncol.*, **23**, 7794–7803.

70. Guan, Z., Feng, F., Li, Q.L., Jiang, Z., Shen, Z., Yu, S., Feng, J., Huang, J., Yao, Z., and Hawkins, M.J. (2007) Randomized study comparing *nab*-paclitaxel with solvent-based paclitaxel in Chinese patients (pts) with metastatic breast cancer (MBC), American Society of Clinical Oncology Annual Meeting, Chicago, IL, abstract 1038.

71. Gradishar, W.J., Krasnojon, D., Cheporov, S., Makhson, A.N., Manikhas, G.M., Clawson, A., and Bhar, P. (2009) Significantly longer progression-free survival with *nab*-paclitaxel compared with docetaxel as first-line therapy for metastatic breast cancer. *J. Clin. Oncol.*, **27**, 3611–3619.

72. Socinski, M.A., Vinnichenko, I., Okamoto, I., Hon, J.K., and Hirsh, V. (2010) Results of a randomized, phase 3 trial of *nab*-paclitaxel (nab-P) and carboplatin (C) compared with cremophor-based paclitaxel (P) and carboplatin as first-line therapy in advanced non-small cell lung cancer (NSCLC). American Society of Clinical Oncology Annual Meeting, Chicago, IL, abstract LBA7511.

73. Von Hoff, D.D., Ramanathan, R., Borad, M., Laheru, D., Smith, L., Wood, T., Korn, R., Desai, N., Iglesias, J., and Hidalgo, M. (2009) SPARC correlation with response to gemcitabine (G) plus *nab*-paclitaxel (nab-P) in patients with advanced metastatic pancreatic cancer: A phase I/II study. American Society of Clinical Oncology Annual Meeting, Orlando, FL, abstract 4525.

74. Desai, N., Trieu, V., Damascelli, B., and Soon-Shiong, P. (2009) SPARC expression correlates with tumor response to albumin-bound paclitaxel in head and neck cancer patients. *Transl. Oncol.*, **2**, 59–64.

36
Carbon Nanotubes

David A. Scheinberg, Carlos H. Villa, Freddy Escorcia, and Michael R. McDevitt

36.1
Introduction

Among numerous nanomaterials available as potential scaffolds or carriers for the development of a new generation of cancer therapeutics, carbon nanotubes (CNTs), including single-wall CNTs (SWNTs) and multiwall CNTs (MWNTs), stand out with unusual features that distinguish them from other possible carriers (Table 36.1). CNTs are rolled graphene cylinders, composed of 100% carbon with very large aspect ratios (length/width) (Figure 36.1). Typical SWNTs have diameters of 1–2 nm and lengths of 50–5000 nm, yielding aspect ratios of 50–5000 and remarkable properties that we will describe below that are a direct consequence of this high aspect ratio. In SWNTs, 100% of the atoms are on the surface and, due to the shape, the surface area is extremely extensive relative to the mass, providing an opportunity to append hundreds of ligands per tube, as compared to less than a dozen for an antibody. Moreover, we will describe that CNTs are also chemically inert, biochemically stable, and nonimmunogenic; importantly, when nanoscale CNTs are soluble at pharmacological doses, they appear to be nontoxic in animals. Furthermore, CNTs are often rapidly internalized into target cells, thereby efficiently delivering their cargo inside. Finally, CNTs display unusual electronic, thermal, and optical properties, making future uses in biomedical sensors, reporters, or even simple circuits possible.

In this chapter, we discuss the properties of CNTs and how they can be utilized in cancer therapy, including the first applications in animals testing their functions. We describe their chemical properties and interactions with cells and tissues. The effects of size, shape, and charge are discussed. Potential ligands, targeting agents, cargo, and uses as imaging agents are evaluated. The limited knowledge about the pharmacology and toxicology of CNTs will be described and the consequences of this on pathways to drug development of CNT-based agents will be illuminated.

While many of the unusual properties of CNTs make them interesting and possibly highly useful as cancer therapeutics, these features also generate new hurdles to overcome before successful therapeutics can be approved. There are

Drug Delivery in Oncology: From Basic Research to Cancer Therapy, First Edition.
Edited by Felix Kratz, Peter Senter, and Henning Steinhagen.
© 2012 Wiley-VCH Verlag GmbH & Co. KGaA. Published 2012 by Wiley-VCH Verlag GmbH & Co. KGaA.

Table 36.1 Interesting properties of CNTs.

Feature	Comment
Very high aspect ratios of 50–1000 : 1	confers unusual clearance properties; penetrate or enter cells rapidly for cargo delivery
More than 100 available carbon atoms per nanometer length	allows multivalency and multifunctionality
Chemical and biochemical stability; relatively inert	long-lived *in vivo*; may be issue for toxicity; lysosomes may degrade
Pure carbon structure	hydrophobic; requires functionalization to solubilize and disperse
Electronically active; absorbs near-IR and radiofrequency	may allow sensors to be developed; thermoablation strategies possible
Nonimmunogenic	will not be easily neutralized by the immune system

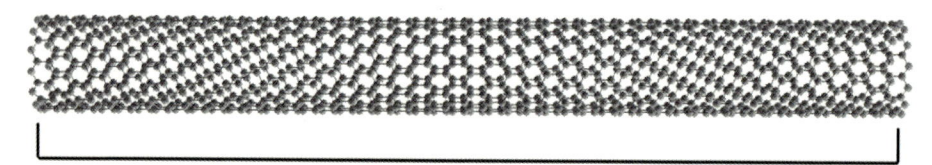

Length - 10nm
Diam - 1nm
Carbons - 1222
Bonds - 1820

Figure 36.1 Schematic of the structure of a SWNT.

already a number of successful nanomaterial-based drugs in trials and approved by the US Food and Drug Administration (FDA). Each offers distinct features that may be specifically useful in different tumor systems. Here, we try to present the arguments for and against the use of CNTs in cancer therapy.

36.1.1
Chemistry of CNTs for Biologic Applications

SWNTs and MWNTs can be produced through several methods such as high-pressure carbon monoxide conversion, chemical vapor deposition, plasma arc methods, or the use of cobalt/molybdenum catalysts, among several others. In most preparations, the resulting product is a polydisperse mixture of both metallic and semiconducting species of several diameters and lengths. Recent technological advances have enabled improved purification of nanotubes by length, diameter, and chirality separation. Regardless of the method of production or purification, pristine CNTs are insoluble in most organic or aqueous solvents. For applications in biologic environments, both SWNTs and MWNTs require further chemical modifications to render the nanotubes dispersible in aqueous media, and an array of strategies has been developed [1–5]. Adequate dispersion of nanotubes is necessary to ensure that nanotube solutions are free of large aggregates or bundles of nanotubes, which have been associated with induction of inflammatory pathways and ultimately toxicity [6] (see more details below). Indeed, adequate dispersion and individualization is one of the key predictors of biocompatibility of nanotubes [7], and can significantly impact their pharmacologic behavior, including pharmacokinetics, biodistribution, and cellular uptake. Recent data suggest that adequately functionalized CNTs can be nontoxic, biocompatible agents for drug delivery applications [8].

The chemistry used to render nanotubes dispersible in aqueous media usually falls into two broad categories – covalent and noncovalent approaches. Covalent approaches functionalize the nanotubes either on their side-walls or at defect sites containing sp^3 hybridized carbons (such as open nanotube ends) [9]. Covalent approaches serve to provide highly stable linkages, but can also significantly alter the spectroscopic and electronic properties of the nanotube material [10]. Noncovalent approaches typically use an amphiphilic molecule such as surfactants, DNA, or proteins in order to strongly adsorb a hydrophilic structure that allows for interactions with water molecules to disperse the material. Another class of nanotube chemistry, which is not directed toward solubilization or dispersion, involves filling of the interior cavities of the nanotubes, known as "endohedral filling." In biologic applications, this type of chemistry has been used to load paramagnetic gadolinium atoms into nanotube defect sites, which leads to greatly enhanced relaxivity. Ultimately, chemical approaches will depend on the biologic application of the nanotubes as a therapeutic or diagnostic device.

After functionalization of CNTs, the materials can be characterized through an array of techniques [11]. Microscopic approaches such as transmission electron microscopy or atomic force microscopy provide high-resolution images of the material, allowing qualitative description of nanotube length and purity. However, microscopic techniques are limited by their ability to sample only tiny fractions of the material and are also prone to artifacts of sample preparation, making it difficult to describe how the nanotubes exist in aqueous solutions. Spectroscopic techniques include near-IR spectroscopy and Raman spectroscopy. Near-IR spectroscopy can provide important information about nanotube purity and chirality due to the unique van Hove transition peaks characteristic of CNTs. Such spectroscopic features are highly disrupted by covalent modification of nanotube side-walls, so their utility may be limited in such materials. Raman spectroscopy remains one of the most widely used techniques for nanotube characterization. The Raman spectrum of CNTs has several highly characteristic features, including a strong peak at around 1600 cm^{-1} (the G-band), radial breathing mode peaks at around 100–300 cm^{-1}, and what is known as the "disorder" band at around 1200 cm^{-1}. The combination of these peaks allows for delineation of the degree of chemical modification or structure integrity, nanotube dispersion, and nanotube diameter. The highly characteristic G-band can even be exploited in medical imaging applications [12].

36.1.2
Covalent Modifications of Nanotubes

Covalent modification can be classified as either side-wall or defect-site covalent modifications. Side-wall covalent modification can be accomplished through halogenation, addition of radicals, and cycloadditions, among many other techniques. For biologic applications the most common approach has been the cycloaddition of azomethine ylides [10], sometimes referred to as the Prato reaction (Figure 36.2). This reaction offers a versatile set of functional groups that can be bound to the nanotubes. By adding hydrophilic ethylene glycol chains terminated with a primary amine, this approach has produced highly aqueous compatible nanotubes with minimal toxicity and a high propensity for cellular uptake. In this approach, the incorporated primary amine serves as a versatile chemical handle for attachment of a wide array of molecules, including radioisotopes [13], whole proteins [14], short peptides [15, 16], and oligonucleotides (ODNs). One drawback of covalent side-wall modification is the loss or reduction of characteristic electronic properties due to disruption of the π-electron network that can alter the nanotubes' spectroscopic properties. The other major class of covalent nanotube functionalization is addition to defect sites, which are present predominantly at open nanotube ends. These defect sites are often oxidized to yield carboxylic acid moieties that can be readily modified through amidation or, less frequently, esterification. Amidation is often performed through activation of the carboxylic acid groups with carbodiimides, which can then be directly reacted with primary amines or indirectly through a succinimidyl ester intermediate. The groups attached in this way are often hydrophilic polymers such as long poly(ethylene glycol)s (PEGs) that provide the hydrophilicity necessary for dispersion [17]. The PEG-derivatized nanotubes produced in this approach have also demonstrated good biocompatibility and aqueous solubility, and groups have also attached a range of biologically active species.

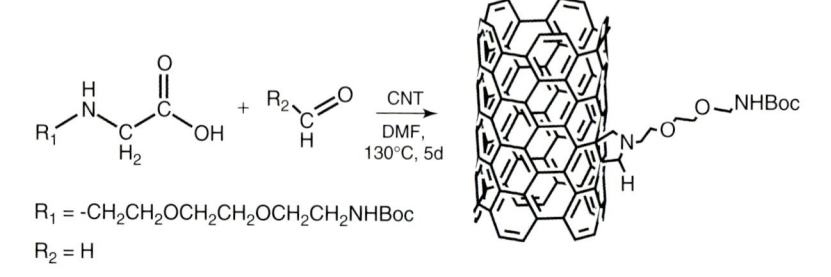

R_1 = -$CH_2CH_2OCH_2CH_2OCH_2CH_2NHBoc$
R_2 = H

Figure 36.2 Schematic of the covalent side-wall reaction of a SWNT. DMF, dimethylformamide; 5d, 5 days.

36.1.3
Noncovalent Modifications

Noncovalent approaches are characterized by strong adsorption of amphiphilic molecules onto nanotube surfaces. The hydrophobic anchor that adsorbs molecules onto the nanotube side-wall can be an aromatic species, such as pyrenes, or aliphatic carbon chains. Most commonly, phospholipid surfactants terminated with PEG chains have been used for adequate functionalization of CNTs [18, 19]. These approaches preserve the inherent electronic and spectroscopic properties of nanotubes, and are useful for applications that take advantage of these unique properties, such as Raman or optoacoustic imaging [20]. The phospholipid surfactant can be derivatized with a range of species including biological macromolecules [18, 21] and small-molecule drugs [22, 23]. While there is a strong hydrophobic interaction of hydrocarbons or aromatic species with the nanotube, in some cases there is some evidence that in the protein-rich environment of biologic organisms, these molecules can be rapidly displaced by hydrophobic protein sequences [24]. It is also important to distinguish between noncovalent approaches that use strongly bound specific functionalization agents versus suspension of pristine nanotubes in surfactants or detergents, which are likely to be less stable.

36.2
Arming of CNTs

The extremely high surface area of CNTs allows for simultaneous decoration, via covalent or noncovalent modification, with multiple types and numbers of targeting, imaging, and therapeutic moieties, yielding both multivalency and multifunctionality. These properties make nanotubes promising candidates for developing tumor-targeted therapies (Table 36.2).

Two general approaches to tumor targeting exist: passive and active. Passive targeting takes advantage of the enhanced permeability and retention (EPR) effect, which results in higher accumulation of macromolecules (above 40 kDa) in tumors due to aberrant, leaky vasculature [30, 31]. Passively targeted, long circulating nanotubes have been used to improve therapeutic efficacy of noncovalently appended chemotherapeutics [23].

In contrast, active targeting employs small molecules, peptides, or antibodies that take advantage of overexpressed receptors or proteins on transformed cells to home in on tumors. Many tumor-targeting moieties have been explored with the goal of causing specific accumulation on nanotubes at tumor sites. Monoclonal antibodies (mAbs) have been covalently conjugated to SWNTs for *in vivo* targeting of CD20, which is overexpressed in Burkitt lymphoma cells, and to carcinogenic embryonic antigen (CEA)-expressing colon cancer cells *in vitro* [14, 25]. The RGD peptide has been used to target nanotubes to tumor neovasculature, while other groups used peptides to help elicit an immunological response against tumor-associated proteins [32–34]. Epidermal growth factor (EGF) has

Table 36.2 Selected CNT constructs for cancer therapy.

Experiment type	Type of modification	Targeting ligand	Therapeutic	References
In vitro	covalent (target ligand); noncovalent (drug on side-wall)	anti-CEA mAb	doxorubicin	[25]
In vitro and in vivo	covalent (side-wall)	anti-CD20 mAb	^{225}Ac	[14]
In vitro and in vivo	covalent (ends)	EGF	paclitaxel	[26]
In vivo	noncovalent	peptide	paclitaxel	[23]
In vitro	covalent (side-wall)	folate	Pt(IV)	
In vitro	noncovalent (side-wall)	folate	doxorubicin	[27]
In vitro	covalent (side-wall)	–	methotrexate	[28]
In vivo	covalent	anti-CD22 mAb	thermolysis	[29]

also been coupled to nanotubes to target tumors overexpressing EGF receptor, notably squamous cell cancers, while folate-nanotube constructs have been used to take advantage of folate receptor overexpression in rapidly dividing cells [26, 27].

In addition to achieving tumor targeting, nanotube constructs require a therapeutic component in order to have antitumor effects. Consequently, nanotubes have been coupled to various existing chemotherapeutic drugs including cisplatin, paclitaxel, methotrexate, doxorubicin, camptothecin, as well as therapeutic radioisotopes [17, 22, 25–28]. Tumor cell gene silencing via nanotube-associated small interfering RNA delivery has also been explored [21, 35]. Nanotubes also have the *intrinsic* ability to emit heat upon introduction of a high-power external radiofrequency. This property has been exploited to cause local tissue heating at tumor sites, resulting in tumor thermolysis [29, 36]. Much of this work, however, has been done *in vitro* or with intratumoral injections and systemically administered *in vivo* targeting studies are still needed.

36.2.1
Interactions with Cells and Tissues

For a wide range of functionalized nanotubes, studies have observed rapid and robust internalization into cultured cells. While some nanotube materials have entered cells primarily through endocytosis [19], others have demonstrated energy-independent internalization and have proposed that the hydrophobic nature of the nanotube surface allows for penetration of the cell membrane [37]. How the mechanism of uptake depends on the functionalization remains unclear. The rapid internalization of nanotube materials has prompted their application in intracellular delivery of biologic cargos, such as gene silencing ODNs, peptides, and cytotoxins. Interestingly, the fate within cells also depends on functionalization, with endosomal, cytoplasmic [18, 37] as well as nuclear accumulation having been observed [38, 39]. The length of CNTs may also have a significant impact on cellular processing and trafficking [40]. The interaction of CNTs with whole tissues and organisms has only recently been explored, with diverse and surprising characteristics having been observed. For example, the biodistribution of CNTs appears to be highly dependent on the chemistry used to render the nanotubes dispersible in injection compatible formulations. Noncovalently modified CNTs that have long hydrophilic chains attached to their surface can resist protein opsonization and strong reticuloendothelial system (RES) uptake, allowing for long circulation and eventual hepatobiliary elimination [41]. This allows for long circulation times and has been exploited for prolonged delivery of chemotherapeutics in animal models [23]. In contrast, covalently modified CNTs, which are believed to be highly individualized, have rapid renal elimination [42]. Interestingly, this renal elimination appears to occur through filtration processes despite the high molecular weight of CNTs species [39, 43]. It is apparently the highly anisotropic geometry of nanotubes that allows for their alignment with flow that allows for longitudinal filtration. Such results demonstrate the necessity to reconsider models that have been derived through assumptions of globular or spherical geometries when attempting to apply them to CNTs.

36.2.2
Immunologic Responses

Several groups have studied the effect of CNTs on the activation of immunologic effector cells [44, 45]. Studies have demonstrated that pristine CNTs without functionalization have a propensity to trigger strong inflammatory responses with production of an array of inflammatory cytokines. Such nanotubes are often highly hydrophobic aggregates and trigger the formation of long-lived granulomas in animal models. However, with highly functionalized materials, CNTs were seen to be immunologically inert, with little toxicity and activation of immune cells [46]. The tendency of nanotubes to be internalized by a variety of cell types, including immune effectors, has led to investigation of their use in vaccine strategies. The nanoscale lengths and diameters and anisotropic geometry of nanotubes poses interesting questions in this regard, as these properties are known to affect the immunologic responses in particle-based vaccines [47]. When immunogenic proteins or peptides are attached to nanotubes, this may enhance the adaptive immune response to the appended antigens. There remains some debate about the activation of complement by nanotubes and this may also be a mechanism through which nanotubes can induce inflammatory responses [48].

36.2.3
Biodegradability and Biologic Persistence

Due to their high chemical stability and unusual physical characteristics, CNTs were initially thought to be highly persistent in biologic systems and incapable of biodegradation by human cells. However, recent evidence suggests that CNTs may indeed be susceptible to oxidation and breakdown by human myeloperoxidases [49]. In addition, in studying the long-term fate of CNTs in animal models, several groups have shown that nearly all of the injected dose is ultimately eliminated by either hepatobiliary or renal mechanisms. The potential biodegradability and ability to be eliminated through normal processes suggests that properly functionalized CNTs can potentially be safely implemented as therapeutic agents.

36.3
Toxicity of CNTs

Perhaps more than any other nanomaterial, CNTs have been labeled as potentially toxic when proposed for therapeutic uses [6, 49–51]. These conclusions are largely based on assumptions stemming from their high aspect ratio and chemical durability, thus likening them to asbestos (when they are clearly different), and on data obtained from study of insoluble and inhaled CNTs (which would not be the form or route of therapeutic CNTs designed to treat cancer). Indeed, the data published on the toxicity of soluble CNTs, given systemically at pharmacologic doses, show that these molecules appear to be relatively safe [7, 8, 52, 53]. More systematic studies of proposed CNT-based agents are clearly needed to confirm these early findings. This is especially important as large-scale production of SWNTs is advancing for nonmedical applications and may enter the environment or into workers inadvertently [49].

The potential toxicities of CNTs will be highly dependent on their size, solubility, appended moieties, and route of administration. In many applications, the CNTs will also serve as a scaffold or carrier of cytotoxic agents, targeting ligands, imaging agents, and the various linkers between the CNTs and the appended moiety. Therefore, potential toxicities also include the effects of these agents as well. Since the attachment of ligands to the CNTs may significantly alter the pharmacokinetics properties of the CNT, such as changing the plasma half-life, clearance mode, entry into cells, and biodistribution into normal tissues, and because the attachment will also change the pharmacokinetics of the cytotoxic agents in various similar ways, it will not be simple to predict the extent or types of toxicities of the final construct based solely on the toxicities of the components. For example, the attachment of a short-lived small-molecule anticancer agent may dramatically increase its plasma half-life, while at the same time reduce its penetration into a normal tissue and change its primary mode of clearance from renal to hepatic. Interestingly, complexing of potently cytotoxic agents with nanomaterials can often favorably affect the toxicity of the drug, making it more effective by allowing higher doses or a better therapeutic index. Widely used examples are Abraxane®, a nanoparticulate formulation of paclitaxel, and Doxil®, a liposomal form of doxorubicin.

A second consideration of particular relevance to the development of cancer therapeutics with CNTs is the tolerance of the patients and the treating physician to potential toxicities. Development and use of cancer therapeutics differs substantially from the same processes in nonmalignant diseases because the drugs are always used in patients with lethal diseases for which curative therapies are generally unavailable. Moreover, with the exception of a few recent additions to the anticancer armamentarium, nearly all FDA-approved cancer drugs have significant, often life-threatening adverse effects at doses equivalent to or modestly higher than the approved dose, leaving these drugs with low therapeutic indices. These affects typically include neutropenia and thrombocytopenia, which can lead to infections and bleeding, but may also include severe diarrhea, renal dysfunction, neurologic damage, pulmonary toxicity, severe rash, or even significant local reactions if the drug is extravasated at the site of injection. As a consequence of this context and history, both patients and physicians are willing to use experimental anticancer drugs at all levels of development, even if there is a risk of severe toxicity, up to and including death. These risks are reduced, but not eliminated, by careful dose-finding and safety studies prior to FDA approval, and for many widely used anticancer agents, the risk of dying from an adverse event related to the drug, and not the disease, is still present.

A final consideration, which is probably most particular to CNTs, is that CNTs are also under investigation for a large number of nonbiomedical applications such as in structural materials and electronics. As a consequence of expectations that large quantities of CNTs will be needed, many orders of magnitude greater than for medical uses, environmental concerns have been raised. This is partly due to the relatively nondegradable nature of the materials, which may suggest that once in the environment, such as soil or water, these materials may persist indefinitely [54]. These concerns are important, but not especially relevant to the anticancer applications discussed here. Interestingly, a recent report has described a peroxidase capable of degrading CNTs [55]. A more relevant concern is the potential pulmonary toxicity to manufacturers of CNTs who may inhale insoluble or aggregated products accidently or in low levels in a factory setting. These concerns have sparked the most controversy in the field and as such we will address them here, even though inhalation of insoluble CNTs is not directly relevant to proposed anticancer applications. However, the biology of inhaled CNTs may provide important clues to potential biomedical processes to be aware of in the development of CNTs as drugs.

Insoluble CNTs are similar to common soot and can cause a number of inflammatory reactions in the lung tissue [56, 57]. Inflammatory processes stimulated by insoluble CNTs have also been widely documented *in vitro* with tissue culture [58]. *In vitro*, various inflammatory cytokines are released [59, 60], cell death pathways (apoptosis) can be activated [61], and CNTs are often incorporated into cells [39, 62]. In the lung, inhaled CNTs, and in the peritoneum, suspended CNTs, can cause granuloma formation and scarring, leading some investigators to compare CNTs to asbestos [6, 51]. However, some studies do not confirm these findings [63]. Toxicity in many studies may also be related to the residual presence of the metal catalysts [49].

The last issue of granuloma formation is a primary concern and recent studies have now attempted to define it better [6, 64]. In one study, four types of insoluble

CNTs (50 µg) with diameters of 15–160 nm and lengths from 1000 to 56 000 nm were introduced into the peritoneal cavity of mice and compared to the effects of short and long amosite asbestos. Only the largest of CNTs samples (mean greater than 84 nm wide by 13 000 nm long) caused inflammation or granulomas [6]. Shorter samples containing fibers as long as 20 000 nm caused little inflammation. Even insoluble CNTs fibers of the nanoscale caused minimal damage. More reassuring is that these toxic CNTs samples were insoluble, in addition to being microscale and not nanoscale.

To address the question of whether it was the large aspect ratio or insolubility of CNTs that caused inflammation, another study was conducted in which dispersed CNTs were compared with aggregated CNTs for pathology in the lung after inhalation [64]. The study was designed to specifically address the toxicity of dispersed CNTs injected into mice intratracheally. This study involved CNTs that were solubilized using methods that did not covalently attach the solubilizing agent to the tube, thus allowing the possibility that the CNTs could become insoluble at some point *in vivo* and change its properties. In this study, dispersed SWNTs of dimensions 1×500 nm in Pluronic® detergent were compared to 2500-nm particulate matter air pollution and asbestos. The dispersed SWNTs produced minimal inflammation in the lung and no granulomas. In contrast, aggregated SWNTs and asbestos caused inflammation. In addition, the nanoscale dispersed CNTs were cleared from the lung by macrophages and were gone by 90 days.

There have been a limited number of studies of soluble CNTs used intravenously and these have not reported significant toxicity [8, 13, 52]. A study in mice of noncovalently PEG-modified, dispersed CNTs injected intravenously at large doses (50–150 mg) and examined for a number of clinical and laboratory parameters did not show significant changes in blood counts, chemistries, weight, survival, behavior, or cardiovascular pathology [8].

A second study used suprapharmacologic doses (up to 1000 mg/kg) administered orally and intraperitoneally. Three types of CNTs were compared: ultrashort (1×20–80 nm), purified (1×1000–2000 nm), and raw (similar to the previous form but still containing iron catalysts) [53]. All these preparations were suspensions of particles. Oral administration was safe. After intraperitoneal dosing there was persistence of the CNTs in tissues and at high doses aggregation of particles within cells, but minimal toxicity. Despite caveats with all of these investigations, none of these studies documented significant toxicity of short CNTs at feasible pharmacologic doses as measured by extensive histochemistry, clinical parameters, and survival.

In a commentary [51], the limitations of drawing conclusions about the link between CNTs and mesothelioma were outlined. These included the observations that the route of administration, the lack of solubility, the geometry of presentation, the use of a mesothelioma-susceptible inbred mouse model, the lack of evidence for long-term biopersistence, and the use of limited and different types of CNTs, all of which may have affected the results. If the proximate causes of sustained inflammation, granuloma formation, and carcinogenicity are due to "frustrated phagocytosis," then study of insoluble, long CNTs may not be appropriate for assessing the risks. In addition to the evidence that peroxidases in the environment may be able to degrade CNTs, a new report shows that neutrophil peroxidase and hydrogen peroxide can also rapidly degrade short CNTs after engulfment, thereby lessening the fears of persistence with the body of dispersed, or soluble, shorter CNTs [65, 66].

Indeed, in recent studies with CNTs solubilized and functionalized in various ways, toxicity to live cells in culture was minimal [25, 44, 67] and PEGylation also reduced toxicity [25, 35, 46]. Methods to assess the impact of functionalization are underway [68] by use of combinatorial approaches to modify CNT surfaces.

36.3.1
Pharmacokinetic Issues

Nanomaterials such as CNTs exhibit unique intrinsic chemical, physical, electronic, thermal, and optical properties, and can be chemically modified (e.g., with biological targeting ligands, and magnetic, radioactive, fluorescent, and chemotherapeutic moieties) to exhibit additional extrinsic properties. The key medicinal functions for these CNT constructs would be (i) specific targeting to a disease site, (ii) the ability to report information on the way to and from the site, (iii) the ability to deliver a therapeutic or reporting "cargo" to the site, and (iv) tolerability by the host. Utilization of the CNTs as a scaffold to combine several of these functions would be of particular interest especially if the sum of the individual components confers unique properties different than the individual parts. The initial steps in developing a CNT-based construct to perform these functions are: (i) the design, synthesis, purification, and thorough physicochemical characterization; (ii) determination of the pharmacokinetics profile; and (iii) evaluation of tolerability (toxicity and immunogenicity) by the host.

There are several generalized strategies used to deploy CNTs for *in vivo* application: (i) *pristine* CNTs that have no surface modification; (ii) *coated* CNTs that have been noncovalently modified with physisorbed atoms, PEGylated molecules, surfactants, or ODNs; (iii) *covalently modified* CNTs that have had some fraction of their sp^2 carbon surface-scaffold modified by chemical functionalization; and (iv) the CNT *encapsulation* strategy wherein the cargo is loaded inside the CNT cylinder. Typically the goal in all of these strategies is to employ the CNTs as a platform or an active constituent for executing some extrinsic or intrinsic imaging and/or therapeutic application.

Determining the pharmacokinetics profile of a CNT construct involves examining the absorption, distribution, metabolism, and excretion (ADME) *in vivo*. These four pharmacokinetics factors and the administered dosage determine the concentration of a drug at its sites of action and thus the intensity of its effects as a function of time [69]. Therefore, one of the most important questions to ask initially when developing a CNT-based construct for medical use *in vivo* is the following: "What is the pharmacokinetics profile of the CNT construct in an animal model?" If possible, these experiments can be performed using classic tracer methodology [70]. Briefly, the construct must be pure and well characterized [71], and the tracer moiety should be stable and not alter the overall pharmacokinetics profile of the parent material *in vivo*. Given the complexity of many CNT-based constructs, relevant control experiments must be performed; sufficiently large numbers of test subjects employed; data collected at early, middle, and late timepoints; and pertinent auxiliary data regarding the nature of the construct and its interaction with the host (i.e., tolerability) collected and evaluated. Initially, experiments should be done in both naïve (disease-free) and disease-bearing model animals to determine the normal pharmacokinetics profile. It is important to understand the pharmacokinetics of the nanomaterial in both systems.

36.3.1.1 Absorption

There has been debate and concern regarding the development of CNT nanomaterials [72, 73]. In particular, the potential for CNT absorption as it relates to toxicity is a primary concern. These novel materials have nanometer-range dimensions and may have very different specific physical or chemical interactions with their environment that are substantially different from those of bulk materials of the same composition [49]. While the high-aspect-ratio nanoscale CNT dimensions permit them to exhibit exceptional physical strength and reactivity, as well as unique thermal, electronic, and optical properties, it is always possible that undesirable harmful interactions with biological systems and the environment may result and render them potentially toxic. Pharmacokinetics absorption studies are quite important when evaluating the safe and responsible use of raw CNTs in efforts to avoid exposure via inhalation, ingestion, or skin absorption by the manufacturing workforce when handling large quantities of material or from the uncontrolled release into the environment. Preventing absorption by these routes can be controlled by appropriately engineered barriers and ventilation such as protective respiratory measures and attire, as well as implementation of training and safety protocols. Environmentally responsible regulatory mandates could be enabled and enforced to manage disposal of bulk quantities used in devices. Medical interventions that integrate CNTs into the drug design will be handled under current Good Manufacturing Practice conditions and their disposal highly regulated. Thus far, the literature has reported that raw, unfunctionalized, insoluble CNTs form large aggregates and are potentially toxic *in vivo* [6, 49, 74]. On the other hand, functionalized and solubilized CNTs have been observed to be nontoxic and well tolerated by the host animal model *in vivo* [8, 37, 46, 75]. The reasons for this differential toxicity include the aggregation state and purity of the CNTs as well as issues related to their distribution, metabolism, and excretion (see below). In cases where a therapeutic CNT drug construct is being designed and evaluated, the appended cargo (e.g., ^{225}Ac [76] or doxorubicin [77]) may be extremely cytotoxic in order to eradicate the diseased tissue. The establishment of principles to characterize and evaluate procedures to ensure safe manufacture and use of nanomaterials is required and should be an achievable goal [71].

36.3.1.2 Distribution

The systematic development of CNT-based constructs for medical application will depend greatly upon the key pharmacokinetics issue of distribution *in vivo* (i.e., biodistribution). Initially, an understanding of the biodistribution of prototype CNTs constructs in naïve animal models (see discussion above) will serve as a guide. As constructs are developed and modifications implemented the biodistribution may vary (Figure 36.3), necessitating further biodistribution investigations. It is important to know the (i) kinetics for the material to accumulate in the desired location, (ii) what the off-target tissue sites of accumulation are, and (iii) how clearance is affected in animal models of disease. The development path to translate any drug, especially such novel agents as CNTs, begins in the animal model and that data is extrapolated to predict biodistribution in man.

In vivo CNT biodistribution data in animal models has begun to appear over the past few years, and some general trends regarding the distribution and functionalization state of the construct have been observed. Cherukuri and Weisman examined individualized *pristine* SWNT, solubilized in the surfactant Pluronic F-108, in a rabbit model and monitored biodistribution through the intrinsic CNTs near-IR fluorescence using *ex vivo* spectroscopy and microscopy techniques [78]. Their data indicated that serum proteins rapidly displaced the synthetic surfactant molecules that coated the CNTs within seconds following intravenous administration. The SWNT concentration in the blood serum decreased exponentially with

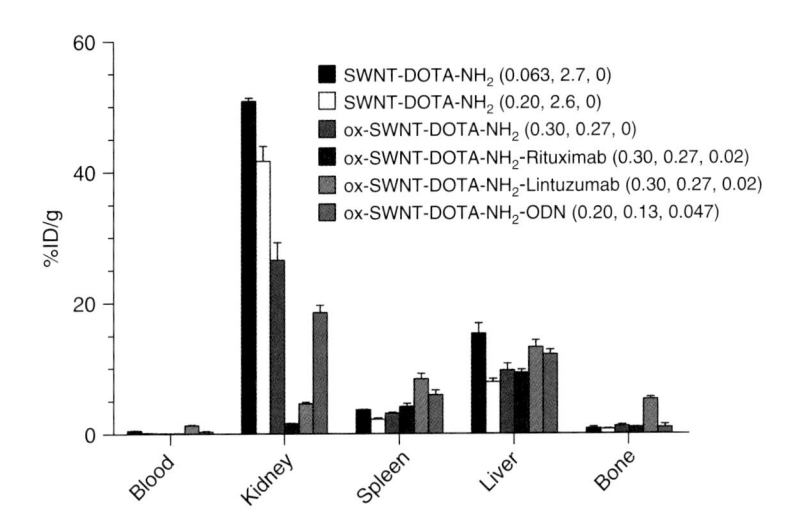

Figure 36.3 Comparative biodistribution data (mean ± SD %ID/g values) at 24 h after intravenous administration of several different *covalently modified* SWNT constructs in naïve, non-tumor-bearing mice. (The three values reported in parentheses in the key indicate the mmol of amine, DOTA, or IgG (or ODN) per gram of SWNT, respectively.) SWNTs that were acid-treated are indicated with the "ox-" prefix. Lintuzumab is an anti-CD33 IgG and rituximab is an anti-CD20 IgG(24). ODN indicates a phosphorothiolate backbone-modified ODN sequence.

a $t_{1/2} = 1.0 \pm 0.1$ h and at 1 day after intravenous administration a significant concentration of SWNTs was observed only in the liver [78].

The biodistribution of PEG-*coated* SWNTs was investigated in mouse models of disease [32] using positron emission tomographic (PET) imaging to follow the biodistribution of the radiolabel *in vivo*. It was found that SWNTs that were functionalized with PEG phospholipids were stable *in vivo*. The length of the PEG chain length had an effect on the biodistribution and blood clearance times. However, despite the PEG coating, there was significant RES uptake as evidenced by 20–40% of the injected dose per gram of the radiolabel in the liver. Approximately 3% of the radiolabel was found in the tumor using a SWNT s coated with PEG chains that were linked to an RGD peptide targeting the $\alpha_v\beta_3$ integrin. Selective uptake in tumor may also be driven by the EPR effect [30]. The intrinsic Raman spectral signature of SWNTs was used to directly probe the presence of nanotubes in several mouse tissues *ex vivo*. Again, a high liver uptake was noted with SWNTs that were only functionalized with physisorbed cargoes coated onto the CNT and there was no evidence of renal excretion noted.

Various solubilizing moieties, imaging and therapeutic cargoes, and/or targeting ligands have been directly attached to the CNT scaffold by modification of some percentage of the surface sp^2 carbon atoms in *covalently modified* CNT. There are a number of different chemical approaches to perform these functional modifications [79] but the 1,3-dipolar cycloaddition modification of CNTs pioneered by Prato and Bianco [3, 79] has perhaps been the most widely applied; this chemistry generates an azomethine ylide *in situ* that reacts with carbon–carbon double bonds [80] on the CNT surface to yield an appended pyrolidine. Approximately one primary amine can be appended for every 95 carbons [13] using this chemistry and that primary amine can be further used as a starting point to perform additional conjugation reactions under rather mild conditions with a wide variety of reactants with interesting extrinsic imaging capabilities. This chemistry works equally well with both amine- and 1,4,7,10-tetraazacyclododecane-1,4,7,10-tetraacetic acid (DOTA) chelate-functionalized prototype SWNT (Figure 36.4a and b) and MWNT (Figure 36.4c and d) precursors, and has yielded very similar distribution and blood compartment clearance results. These constructs were quite water soluble (approaching 20 g/l) and were well dispersed, and were purified by traditional gel-permeation or reverse-phase chromatography methods [13, 14, 33, 39]. It has been reported that radiolabeled prototype CNTs have minimal kidney, liver, and spleen accumulation, rapidly clear the blood compartment, and are also rapidly renally excreted [13, 14, 33, 39, 42, 43, 81, 82]. These constructs have also been multifunctionalized with radionuclides and mAbs (IgG), and have been shown to target disseminated lymphoma in a mouse model of disease [14]. A potential drawback with the *covalently modified* SWNTs constructs is that disruption of the sp^2 carbon scaffold reduces the effectiveness of the unique intrinsic (e.g., electronic, thermal, and optical) properties. However, the azomethine ylide chemistry can be adapted to MWNTs, modifying only the outer CNT scaffold while leaving the inner CNT scaffold unmodified and still in possession of the unique intrinsic properties. This

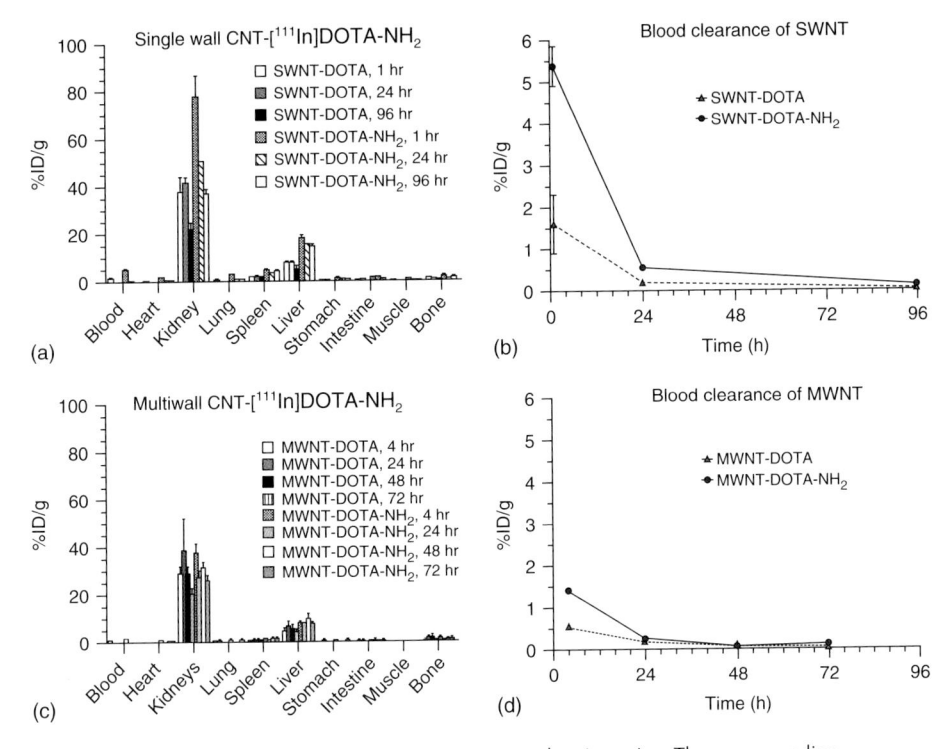

Figure 36.4 Biodistribution data (mean ± SD %ID/g values) following intravenous administration of two different amine and DOTA (a) *covalently modified* SWNT and (c) MWNT constructs in naïve, non-tumor-bearing mice. The corresponding blood compartment clearance of radioactivity of the same two amine and DOTA (b) *covalently modified* SWNT and (d) MWNT constructs as a function of time.

particular covalent modification methodology has yielded very stable complexes *in vivo* when conventional bioconjugation linkages are employed [39].

36.3.1.3 Metabolism

Biotransformation of CNTs by *in vivo* metabolic processes will be important with unstable, noncovalently assembled, and biodegradable materials. Recently, there have been several reports that described the enzymatic degradation of individualized CNTs *in vitro* and *in vivo* [55, 66, 83]. This is an interesting and potentially important aspect in the development of CNT drug constructs as the heretofore unanticipated enzymatic degradation of these nanomaterials has now been demonstrated. While the uptake of pristine SWNTs ($d \sim 1$ nm and $L \sim 1000$ nm) suspended in Pluronic F-108 by cultured mouse peritoneal macrophage-like cells was studied and reported using the intrinsic near-IR fluorescence [24], it was surprising that CNTs could undergo degradation by neutrophils and professional phagocytes given the exceptional mechanical strength of CNTs and the necessity to perform many of the preliminary covalent modification reactions under rather harsh conditions. These are rather new findings and should lead to further interesting studies.

36.3.1.4 Excretion

The primary routes of elimination of CNTs from the body are via the kidneys, liver, and skin in the urine, feces, and perspiration, and from the blood by breast milk [72]. Renal elimination [84] is perhaps the most preferred route [85], especially if the CNT agent is to be used in an imaging (see below) or therapeutic application. The *pristine* and *coated* CNTs materials seem to prefer the slower hepatobiliary route and exhibit little to no renal clearance.

Covalently modified CNT, on the other hand, seem to favor the renal elimination and do exhibit some small amount of hepatobiliary clearance. Both *covalently modified* MCNT and SWNT constructs have been found in the urine within a few minutes of intravenous administration in animal models [39, 42, 43]. Recently, the mechanism of elimination of *covalently modified* SWNTs constructs has been reported and involves the rapid ($t_{1/2} = 6$ min) glomerular filtration with a small amount of concomitant transient reabsorption in the proximal tubule [39]. Further, the CNT construct in the urine was fully characterized and was found to be excreted intact. No damage to the glomerular filtration apparatus or kidney toxicity was noted. This is a surprising and useful finding as this high-aspect-ratio (300 : 1), high-molecular-weight CNT construct (around 500 kDa) was able to align with flow and transit the filtration slit diaphragm as if it were a small molecule. Understanding the biophysics of clearance of these novel CNT materials via the glomerular filter helps further the design criteria of potentially new medicinally useful constructs.

36.3.2 Imaging Modalities

CNT-based nanomaterials are ideally suited scaffolds to incorporate features (intrinsic or extrinsic moieties) to report information and may afford significant increases in signal-to-noise relative to conventional imaging molecules [86–88]. Furthermore, they can be designed to possess multimodal means to report information by having combinations of tracer features (e.g., fluorescence, magnetic, and/or radionuclidic) [86–89]. Individually, these conventional imaging techniques have pros and cons: radionuclides yield high sensitivity, but suffer low spatial resolution; fluorescent labels may provide good spatial resolution *in vitro*, but are difficult to quantify *in vivo* because of signal attenuation in tissue and high background autofluorescence noise; magnetic particles offer high resolution and good contrast, but are not very sensitive. However, when used in combination, these different modalities can be built into a single cancer targeting CNT construct to simultaneously report distribution data to and at the disease site, targeting information, and clearance data *in vivo*, and could also be used to report cellular and perhaps subcellular location of the CNT–drug construct in a biopsied sample *ex vivo*. This global and local tissue and cellular imaging paradigm has been utilized to investigate the mechanism of renal clearance of SWNTs. Another potential advantage of CNTs, based upon their aspect ratio and surface area relative to smaller targeting scaffolds (e.g., peptides and proteins) would be the potential to incorporate multiple copies of fluorophores, chromophores, Gd(III), FeO, and/or radionuclides, thus leading to amplification of signal-to-noise relative to conventional imaging agents.

The pharmacokinetics profile of the *covalently modified* CNTs would suggest this platform as a good candidate to develop imaging agents. They have been functionalized with a variety of radionuclide and fluorescent imaging modalities [13, 14, 33, 39, 42, 43, 81, 82], and have been demonstrated to be targeted to tumor [33] and monomeric vascular endothelial cadherin (VE-cadh$_m$) [90], a tumor vascular epitope (see Figure 36.5a–c). They have minimal off-target accumulation, are rapidly cleared from the blood compartment, and can be rapidly renally excreted [39, 42, 43]. These agents have been administered safely and were well tolerated by the host. The rapid blood compartment clearance is especially useful if the desired target can be rapidly accessed and marked with the construct. In an ideal situation, a CNT construct loaded with a sensitive tracer can be administered, target, and bind,

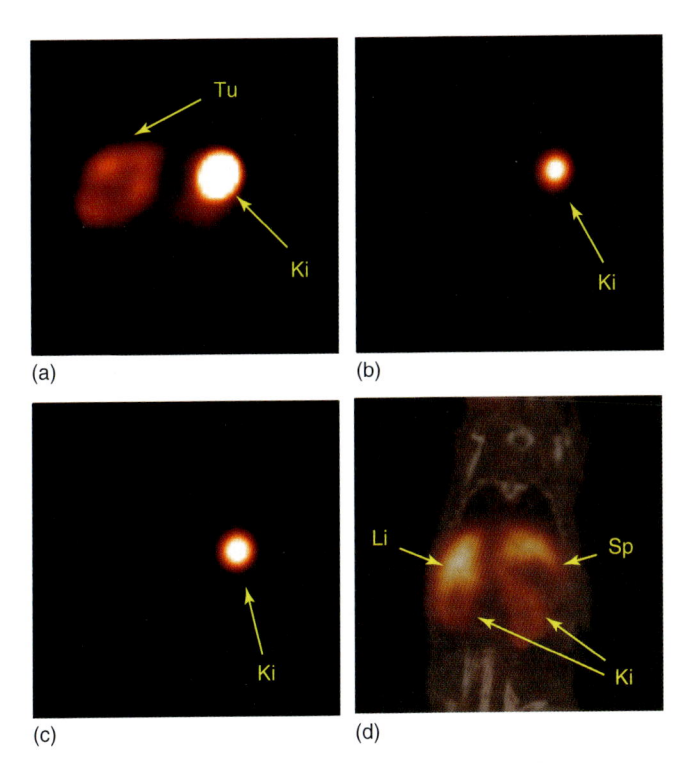

Figure 36.5 PET transverse images of three representative subcutaneous LS174t tumored-mice that received an intravenous injection of (a) SWNT-(^{89}Zr-DFO)(E4G10), (b) low-specific-activity ^{89}Zr-DFO-SWNT-E4G10 (competitive inhibition/blocking control experiment), and (c) nonspecific control construct SWNT-(^{89}Zr-DFO)(anti-KLH) recorded at 24 h postinjection. DFO, desferrioxamine B chelate; E4G10, specific anti-VE-cadh$_m$ IgG; anti-KLH, isotype control anti-keyhole limpet hemocyanin IgG). (d) Fused PET and computed tomography images at 3 h postinjection of ^{86}Y-CNT prototype construct in a naïve mouse model showing a coronal image of one representative animal. Tu, tumor; Ki, kidney; Li, liver; Sp, spleen.

while untargeted CNTs is rapidly (within 1–2 h) cleared. Compared to IgG-based imaging agents, which typically have clearance half-lives on the order of days, the CNTs would provide excellent contrast to perform imaging on the same day as administration.

Studies utilizing PET radionuclides as the imaging component of the CNTs [13, 33, 39] have been very useful in evaluating distribution and clearance in animal models (see Figure 36.5d). PET is extremely sensitive and a variety of radionuclides can be selected to optimize chemistry and half-life [91, 92]. Magnetic resonance imaging (MRI) CNTs agents have been reported using the *encapsulation* strategy with loading and confinement of Gd(III) clusters within ultrashort SWNTs (US-tubes). The Gd(III)@US-tube species were linear superparamagnetic molecular magnets with MRI efficacies 40–90 times greater than any Gd(III)-based contrast agent in current clinical use [93]. Emerging methodologies that base the imaging on an intrinsic CNT property are being evaluated. Noninvasive Raman microscopy was used to evaluate tumor targeting and localization of RGD-modified SWNTs in mice [94]. The near-IR photoluminescence of phospholipid–PEG-*coated* SWNTs produced imaging agents that were both bright and biocompatible *in vivo*. Deep tissue penetration and low background autofluorescence was observed, and permitted high-resolution intravital microscopic imaging of tumor vessels [95]. Photoacoustic imaging may overcome problems in optical imaging regarding resolution and signal attenuation while still maintaining high-contrast. Using *coated*-SWNTs technology, a novel photoacoustic contrast agent, (indocyanine green dye)-(PEG-RGD)-SWNT, was developed. This contrast agent was administered intravenously to tumor-bearing mice and showed significantly higher signal in the tumor than in mice given an untargeted control contrast agent. The specific agent yielded a 300-fold higher photoacoustic contrast in living tissues with subnanomolar sensitivities [96]. The design and synthesis of CNTs with targeting, reporting, and therapeutic capabilities that possess an acceptable pharmacokinetics and tolerability profile will determine the ultimate utility of these species in medical imaging and theranostic applications.

36.4
Conclusions

As one of the newest and most unusual nanomaterials to be developed, CNTs offer both interesting opportunities as drug carriers, as well as challenges for their development. Their biochemical and chemical inertness makes modification difficult and biodegradation slow, which in turn may raise issues of biopersistence and possible toxicities. At the same time, these are useful properties of *in vivo* carriers as they are not seen by the immune system or readily degraded. Their large surface area and aspect ratio allows the appending of large numbers of ligands, and imaging and cytotoxic agents, thereby offering the potential for highly potent and multifunctional probes and drugs. The structure, most interestingly, allows for modifications that can result in rapid renal clearance – a feature that is useful in cancer drug development. Finally, their unusual electrochemical properties (conduction of electricity, and absorption of radiation and near-IR with resulting heating) may open new avenues to direct detection and therapy of tumors. Preclinical development of CNTs has only recently begun and it is too early to predict how these promising new materials will ultimately be used.

References

1. Tasis, D., Tagmatarchis, N., Bianco, A., and Prato, M. (2006) Chemistry of carbon nanotubes. *Chem. Rev.*, **106**, 1105–1136.
2. Sun, Y.-P., Fu, K., Lin, Y., and Huang, W. (2002) Functionalized carbon nanotubes: properties and applications. *Acc. Chem. Res.*, **35**, 1096–1104.
3. Georgakilas, V., Tagmatarchis, N., Pantarotto, D., Bianco, A., Briand, J., and Prato, M. (2002) Amino acid functionalisation of water soluble carbon nanotubes. *Chem. Commun.*, 3050–3051.
4. Liu, Z., Sun, X., Nakayama-Ratchford, N., and Dai, H. (2007) Supramolecular chemistry on water-soluble carbon nanotubes for drug loading and delivery. *ACS Nano*, **1**, 50–56.
5. Tasis, D., Tagmatarchis, N., Georgakilas, V., and Prato, M. (2003) Soluble carbon nanotubes. *Chemistry*, **17**, 4000–4008.
6. Poland, C.A., Duffin, R., Kinloch, I. *et al.* (2008) Carbon nanotubes introduced into the abdominal cavity of mice show asbestos-like pathogenicity in a pilot study. *Nat. Nanotechnol.*, **3**, 423–428.
7. Mutlu, Gk.M., Budinger, G.R.S., Green, A.A. *et al.* (2010) Biocompatible nanoscale dispersion of single-walled carbon nanotubes minimizes *in vivo* pulmonary toxicity. *Nano Lett.*, **10**, 1664–1670.
8. Schipper, M.L., Nakayama-Ratchford, N., Davis, C.R. *et al.* (2008) A pilot toxicology study of single-walled carbon nanotubes in a small sample of mice. *Nat. Nanotechnol.*, **4**, 216–221.
9. Banerjee, S. (2005) Covalent surface chemistry of single-walled carbon nanotubes. *Adv. Mater.*, **17**, 17–29.
10. Georgakilas, V., Kordatos, K., Prato, M., Guldi, D., Holzinger, M., and Hirsch, A. (2002) Organic functionalization of carbon nanotubes. *J. Am. Chem. Soc.*, **124**, 760–761.
11. Itkis, M., Perea, D., Jung, R., Niyogi, S., and Haddon, R. (2005) Comparison of analytical techniques for purity evaluation of single-walled carbon nanotubes. *J. Am. Chem. Soc.*, **127**, 3439–3448.
12. Keren, S., Zavaleta, C., Cheng, Z., de la Zerda, A., Gheysens, O., and Gambhir, S.S. (2008) Noninvasive molecular imaging of small living subjects using Raman spectroscopy. *Proc. Natl. Acad. Sci. USA*, **105**, 5844–5849.
13. McDevitt, M.R., Chattopadhyay, D., Jaggi, J.S. *et al.* (2007) PET imaging of soluble yttrium-86-labeled carbon nanotubes in mice. *PLoS ONE*, **2**, e907.
14. McDevitt, M.R., Chattopadhyay, D., Kappel, B.J. *et al.* (2007) Tumor targeting with antibody-functionalized, radiolabeled carbon nanotubes. *J. Nucl. Med.*, **48**, 1180–1189.
15. Pantarotto, D., Partidos, C.D., Graff, R. *et al.* (2003) Synthesis, structural characterization, and immunological properties of carbon nanotubes functionalized with peptides. *J. Am. Chem. Soc.*, **125**, 6160–6164.
16. Herrero, M.A., Toma, F.M., Al-Jamal, K.T. *et al.* (2009) Synthesis and characterization of a carbon nanotube-dendron series for efficient siRNA delivery. *J. Am. Chem. Soc.*, **131**, 9843–9848.
17. Wu, W., Li, R., Bian, X. *et al.* (2009) Covalently combining carbon nanotubes with anticancer agent: preparation and antitumor activity. *ACS Nano*, **3**, 2740–2750.
18. Kam, N. and Dai, H. (2005) Carbon nanotubes as intracellular protein transporters: generality and biological functionality. *J. Am. Chem. Soc.*, **127**, 6021–6026.

19. Kam, N., O'Connell, M., Wisdom, J., and Dai, H. (2005) Carbon nanotubes as multifunctional biological transporters and near-infrared agents for selective cancer cell destruction. *Proc. Natl. Acad. Sci. USA*, **102**, 11600–11605.
20. De La Zerda, A., Zavaleta, C., Keren, S. *et al.* (2008) Carbon nanotubes as photoacoustic molecular imaging agents in living mice. *Nat. Nanotechnol.*, **3**, 557–562.
21. Liu, Z., Winters, M., Holodniy, M., and Dai, H. (2007) siRNA delivery into human T cells and primary cells with carbon-nanotube transporters. *Angew. Chem. Int. Ed.*, **46**, 2023–2027.
22. Dhar, S., Liu, Z., Thomale, J., Dai, H., and Lippard, S. (2008) Targeted single-wall carbon nanotube-mediated Pt(IV) prodrug delivery using folate as a homing device. *J. Am. Chem. Soc.*, **130**, 11467–11476.
23. Liu, Z., Chen, K., Davis, C. *et al.* (2008) Drug delivery with carbon nanotubes for *in vivo* cancer treatment. *Cancer Res.*, **68**, 6652–6660.
24. Cherukuri, P., Bachilo, S.M., Litovsky, S.H., and Weisman, R.B. (2004) Near-infrared fluorescence microscopy of single-walled carbon nanotubes in phagocytic cells. *J. Am. Chem. Soc.*, **126**, 15638–15639.
25. Heister, E., Neves, V., Tîlmaciu, C. *et al.* (2009) Triple functionalisation of single-walled carbon nanotubes with doxorubicin, a monoclonal antibody, and a fluorescent marker for targeted cancer therapy. *Carbon*, **47**, 2152–2160.
26. Bhirde, A.A., Patel, V., Gavard, J. *et al.* (2009) Targeted killing of cancer cells *in vivo* and *in vitro* with EGF-directed carbon nanotube-based drug delivery. *ACS Nano*, **3**, 307–316.
27. Zhang, X., Meng, L., Lu, Q., Fei, Z., and Dyson, P.J. (2009) Targeted delivery and controlled release of doxorubicin to cancer cells using modified single wall carbon nanotubes. *Biomaterials*, **30**, 6041–6047.
28. Pastorin, G., Wu, W., Wieckowski, S. *et al.* (2006) Double functionalization of carbon nanotubes for multimodal drug delivery. *Chem. Commun.*, 1182–1184.
29. Marches, R., Chakravarty, P., Musselman, I.H. *et al.* (2009) Specific thermal ablation of tumor cells using single-walled carbon nanotubes targeted by covalently-coupled monoclonal antibodies. *Int. J. Cancer*, **125**, 2970–2977.
30. Matsumura, Y. and Maeda, H. (1986) A new concept for macromolecular therapeutics in cancer chemotherapy: mechanism of tumoritropic accumulation of proteins and the antitumor agent smancs. *Cancer Res.*, **46**, 6387–6392.
31. Yuan, F., Dellian, M., Fukumura, D. *et al.* (1995) Vascular permeability in a human tumor xenograft: molecular size dependence and cutoff size. *Cancer Res.*, **55**, 3752–3756.
32. Liu, Z., Cai, W., He, L. *et al.* (2007) *In vivo* biodistribution and highly efficient tumour targeting of carbon nanotubes in mice. *Nat. Nanotechnol.*, **2**, 47–52.
33. Villa, C.H., McDevitt, M.R., Escorcia, F.E. *et al.* (2008) Synthesis and biodistribution of oligonucleotide-functionalized, tumor-targetable carbon nanotubes. *Nano Lett.*, **8**, 4221–4228.
34. Pantarotto, D., Partidos, C.D., Hoebeke, J. *et al.* (2003) Immunization with peptide-functionalized carbon nanotubes enhances virus-specific neutralizing antibody responses. *Chem. Biol.*, **10**, 961–966.
35. Zhang, Z.H., Yang, X.Y., Zhang, Y. *et al.* (2006) Delivery of telomerase reverse transcriptase small interfering RNA in complex with positively charged single-walled carbon nanotubes suppresses tumor growth. *Clin. Cancer Res.*, **12**, 4933–4939.
36. Gannon, C.J., Cherukuri, P., Yakobson, B.I. *et al.* (2007) Carbon nanotube-enhanced thermal destruction of cancer cells in a noninvasive radiofrequency field. *Cancer*, **110**, 2654–2665.
37. Kostarelos, K., Lacerda, L., Pastorin, G. *et al.* (2007) Cellular uptake of functionalized carbon nanotubes is independent of functional group and cell type. *Nat. Nanotechnol.*, **2**, 108–113.
38. Cheng, J., Fernando, K.A., Veca, L.M. *et al.* (2008) Reversible accumulation

of PEGylated single-walled nanotubes in the mammalian nucleus. *ACS Nano*, **2**, 2085–2094.
39. Ruggiero, A., Villa, C.H., Bander, E. et al. (2010) Paradoxical glomerular filtration of carbon nanotubes. *Proc. Natl. Acad. Sci. USA*, **107**, 12369–12374.
40. Jin, H., Heller, D.A., Sharma, R., and Strano, M.S. (2009) Size-dependent cellular uptake and expulsion of single-walled carbon nanotubes: single particle tracking and a generic uptake model for nanoparticles. *ACS Nano*, **3**, 149–158.
41. Liu, Z., Davis, C., Cai, W., He, L., Chen, X., and Dai, H. (2008) Circulation and long-term fate of functionalized, biocompatible single-walled carbon nanotubes in mice probed by Raman spectroscopy. *Proc. Natl. Acad. Sci. USA*, **105**, 1410–1415.
42. Singh, R., Pantarotto, D., Lacerda, L. et al. (2006) Tissue biodistribution and blood clearance rates of intravenously administered carbon nanotube radiotracers. *Proc. Natl. Acad. Sci. USA*, **103**, 3357–3362.
43. Lacerda, L., Herrero, M.A., Venner, K., Bianco, A., Prato, M., and Kostarelos, K. (2008) Carbon-nanotube shape and individualization critical for renal excretion. *Small*, **4**, 1130–1132.
44. Porter, A.E., Gass, M., Bendall, J.S. et al. (2009) Uptake of noncytotoxic acid-treated single-walled carbon nanotubes into the cytoplasm of human macrophage cells. *ACS Nano*, **3**, 1485–1492.
45. Konduru, N.V., Tyurina, Y.Y., Feng, W. et al. (2009) Phosphatidylserine targets single-walled carbon nanotubes to professional phagocytes *in vitro* and *in vivo*. *PLoS ONE*, **4**, e4398.
46. Dumortier, H., Lacotte, S., Pastorin, G. et al. (2006) Functionalized carbon nanotubes are non-cytotoxic and preserve the functionality of primary immune cells. *Nano Lett.*, **6**, 1522–1528.
47. Fifis, T., Gamvrellis, A., Crimeen-Irwin, B. et al. (2004) Size-dependent immunogenicity: therapeutic and protective properties of nano-vaccines against tumors. *J. Immunol.*, **173**, 3148–3154.
48. Moghimi, S.M. and Hunter, A.C. (2010) Complement monitoring of carbon nanotubes. *Nat. Nanotechnol.*, **5**, 382; author reply 383.
49. Shvedova, A.A. and Kagan, V.E. (2010) The role of nanotoxicology in realizing the "helping without harm" paradigm of nanomedicine: lessons from studies of pulmonary effects of single-walled carbon nanotubes. *J. Intern. Med.*, **173**, 106–118.
50. De Jong, W.H. and Borm, P.J. (2008) Drug delivery and nanoparticles: applications and hazards. *Int. J. Nanomed.*, **3**, 133–149.
51. Kane, A.B. and Hurt, R.H. (2008) The asbestos analogy revisited. *Nat. Nanotechnol.*, **3**, 328.
52. Lacerda, L., Bianco, A., Prato, M., and Kostarelos, K. (2006) Carbon nanotubes as nanomedicines: from toxicology to pharmacology. *Adv. Drug Deliv. Rev.*, **58**, 1460–1470.
53. Kolosnjaj-Tabi, J., Hartman, K.B., Boudjemaa, S. et al. (2010) In vivo behavior of large doses of ultrashort and full-length single-walled carbon nanotubes after oral and intraperitoneal administration to Swiss mice. *ACS Nano*, **4**, 1481–1492.
54. Boxall, A.B., Tiede, K., and Chaudhry, Q. (2007) Engineered nanomaterials in soils and water: how do they behave and could they pose a risk to human health? *Nanomedicine*, **2**, 919–927.
55. Allen, B.L., Kotchey, G.P., Chen, Y. et al. (2009) Mechanistic investigations of horseradish peroxidase-catalyzed degradation of single-walled carbon nanotubes. *J. Am. Chem. Soc.*, **131**, 17194–17205.
56. Lam, C.W., James, J.T., McCluskey, R., Arepalli, S., and Hunter, R.L. (2006) A review of carbon nanotube toxicity and assessment of potential occupational and environmental health risks. *Crit. Rev. Toxicol.*, **36**, 189–217.
57. Magrez, A., Kasas, S., Salicio, V. et al. (2006) Cellular toxicity of carbon-based nanomaterials. *Nano Lett.*, **6**, 1121–1125.
58. Reddy, A., Reddy, Y., Krishna, D., and Himabindu V. (2010) Multi wall carbon nanotubes induce oxidative stress and

cytotoxicity in human embryonic kidney (HEK293) cells. *Toxicology*, **272**, 11–16.
59. Hamad, I., Christy Hunter, A., Rutt, K.J., Liu, Z., Dai, H., and Moein Moghimi, S. (2008) Complement activation by PEGylated single-walled carbon nanotubes is independent of C1q and alternative pathway turnover. *Mol. Immunol.*, **45**, 3797–3803.
60. Ryman-Rasmussen, J.P., Tewksbury, E.W., Moss, O.R., Cesta, M.F., Wong, B.A., and Bonner, J.C. (2008) Inhaled multi-walled carbon nanotubes potentiate airway fibrosis in murine allergic asthma. *Am. J. Respir. Cell Mol. Biol.*, **40**, 349–358.
61. Elgrabli, D., Abella-Gallart, S., Robidel, F., Rogerieux, F., Boczkowski, J., and Lacroix, G. (2008) Induction of apoptosis and absence of inflammation in rat lung after intratracheal instillation of multiwalled carbon nanotubes. *Toxicology*, **253**, 131–136.
62. Simon-Deckers, A., Gouget, B., Mayne-L'hermite, M., Herlin-Boime, N., Reynaud, C., and Carriere, M. (2008) In vitro investigation of oxide nanoparticle and carbon nanotube toxicity and intracellular accumulation in A549 human pneumocytes. *Toxicology*, **253**, 137–146.
63. Muller, J., Delos, M., Panin, N., Rabolli, V., Huaux, F., and Lison, D. (2009) Absence of carcinogenic response to multiwall carbon nanotubes in a 2-year bioassay in the peritoneal cavity of the rat. *Toxicol. Sci.*, **110**, 442–448.
64. Mutlu, Gk.M., Budinger, G.R.S., Green, A.A. et al. (2010) Biocompatible nanoscale dispersion of single-walled carbon nanotubes minimizes in vivo pulmonary toxicity. *Nano Lett.*, **10**, 1664–1670.
65. Kagan, V.E., Bayir, H., and Shvedova, A.A. (2005) Nanomedicine and nanotoxicology: two sides of the same coin. *Nanomedicine*, **1**, 313–316.
66. Kagan, V.E., Konduru, N.V., Feng, W. et al. (2010) Carbon nanotubes degraded by neutrophil myeloperoxidase induce less pulmonary inflammation. *Nat. Nanotechnol.*, **5**, 354–359.
67. Alpatova, A.L., Shan, W., Babica, P. et al. (2010) Single-walled carbon nanotubes dispersed in aqueous media via non-covalent functionalization: effect of dispersant on the stability, cytotoxicity, and epigenetic toxicity of nanotube suspensions. *Water Res.*, **44**, 505–520.
68. Zhang, Q., Zhou, H., and Yan, B. (2010) Reducing nanotube cytotoxicity using a nano-combinatorial library approach. *Methods Mol. Biol.*, **625**, 95–107.
69. Goodman, LS and Gilman, A (eds) (1985) *The Pharmacological Basis of Therapeutics*, 7th edn, Macmillan, New York.
70. Wilson, B.J. (ed.) (1966) *The Radiochemical Manual*, 2nd edn, The Radiochemical Centre, Amersham.
71. Hall, J.B., Dobrovolskaia, M.A., Patri, A.K., and McNeil, S.E. (2007) Characterization of nanoparticles for therapeutics. *Nanomedicine*, **2**, 789–803.
72. Hagens, W.I., Oomen, A.G., de Jong, W.H., Cassee, F.R., and Sips, A.J.A.M. (2007) What do we (need to) know about the kinetic properties of nanoparticles in the body? *Regul. Toxicol. Pharmacol.*, **49**, 217–229.
73. Nel, A., Xia, T., Madler, L., and Li, N. (2006) Toxic potential of materials at the nanolevel. *Science*, **311**, 622–627.
74. Kisin, E.R., Murray, A.R., Keane, M.J. et al. (2007) Single-walled carbon nanotubes: geno- and cytotoxic effects in lung fibroblast V79 cells. *J. Toxicol. Environ. Health A*, **70**, 2071–2079.
75. Sayes, C.M., Liang, F., Hudson, J.L. et al. (2006) Functionalization density dependence of single-walled carbon nanotubes cytotoxicity in vitro. *Toxicol. Lett.*, **16**, 135–142.
76. McDevitt, M.R., Ma, D., Lai, L.T. et al. (2001) Tumor therapy with targeted atomic nanogenerators. *Science*, **294**, 1537–1540.
77. Liu, Z., Fan, A.C., Rakhra, K. et al. (2009) Supramolecular stacking of doxorubicin on carbon nanotubes for in vivo cancer therapy. *Angew. Chem. Int. Ed. Engl.*, **48**, 7668–7672.
78. Cherukuri, P., Gannon, C.J., Leeuw, T.K. et al. (2006) Mammalian pharmacokinetics of carbon nanotubes

using intrinsic near-infrared fluorescence. *Proc. Natl. Acad. Sci. USA*, **103**, 18882–18886.
79. Singh, P., Campidelli, S., Giordani, S., Bonifazi, D., Bianco, A., and Prato, M. (2009) Organic functionalisation and characterisation of single-walled carbon nanotubes. *Chem. Soc. Rev.*, **38**, 2214–2230.
80. Tsuge, O., Kanemasa, S., Ohe, M., and Takenaka, S. (1987) Simple generation of nonstabilized azomethine ylides through decarboxylative condensation of alpha-amino acids with carbonly compounds via 5-exazolidinone intermediates. *Bull. Chem. Soc. Jpn.*, **60**, 4079–4089.
81. Lacerda, L., Soundararajan, A., and Singh, R. (2008) Dynamic imaging of functionalized multi-walled carbon nanotube systemic circulation and urinary excretion. *Adv. Mater.*, **20**, 225–230.
82. Lacerda, L., Ali-Boucetta, H., Herrero, M.A. et al. (2008) Tissue histology and physiology following intravenous administration of different types of functionalized multiwalled carbon nanotubes. *Nanomedicine*, **3**, 149–161.
83. Allen, B.L., Kichambare, P.D., Gou, P. et al. (2008) Biodegradation of single-walled carbon nanotubes through enzymatic catalysis. *Nano Lett.*, **8**, 3899–3903.
84. Birkett, D. (1992) Clearance of drugs by the kidneys. *Aust. Prescriber*, **15**, 16–19.
85. Longmire, M., Choyke, P.L., and Kobayashi, H. (2008) Clearance properties of nano-sized particles and molecules as imaging agents: considerations and caveats. *Nanomedicine*, **3**, 703–717.
86. Kostarelos, K., Bianco, A., and Prato, M. (2009) Promises, facts and challenges for carbon nanotubes in imaging and therapeutics. *Nat. Nanotechnol.*, **4**, 627–633.
87. Escorcia, F.E., McDevitt, M.R., Villa, C.H., and Scheinberg, D.A. (2007) Targeted nanomaterials for radiotherapy. *Nanomedicine*, **2**, 805–815.
88. Scheinberg, D.A., Villa, C.H., Escorcia, F.E., and McDevitt M.R. (2010) Conscripts of the infinite armada: systemic cancer therapy using nanomaterials. *Nat. Rev. Clin. Oncol.*, **7**, 266–276.
89. Cai, W. and Chen, X. (2008) Multimodality molecular imaging of tumor angiogenesis. *J. Nucl. Med.*, **49**, 113S–128S.
90. May, C., Doody, J.F., Abdullah, R. et al. (2005) Identification of a transiently exposed VE-cadherin epitope that allows for specific targeting of an antibody to the tumor neovasculature. *Blood*, **105**, 4337–4344.
91. von Schulthess, G.K., Steinert H., and Hany, T.F. (2006) Integrated PET/CT: current applications and future directions. *Radiology*, **238**, 405–422.
92. Zanzonico, P. (2004) Positron emission tomography: a review of basic principles, scanner design and performance, and current systems. *Semin. Nucl. Med.*, **34**, 87–111.
93. Sitharaman, B., Kissell, K.R., and Hartman, K.B. (2005) Superparamagnetic gadonanotubes are high-performance MRI contrast agents. *Chem. Commun.*, 3915–3917.
94. Zavaleta, C., de la Zerda, A., Liu, Z. et al. (2008) Noninvasive Raman spectroscopy in living mice for evaluation of tumor targeting with carbon nanotubes. *Nano Lett.*, **8**, 2800–2805.
95. Welsher, K., Liu, Z., Sherlock, S.P. et al. (2009) A route to brightly fluorescent carbon nanotubes for near-infrared imaging in mice. *Nat. Nanotechnol.*, **4**, 773–780.
96. de la Zerda, A., Liu, Z., Bodapati, S. et al. (2010) Ultrahigh sensitivity carbon nanotube agents for photoacoustic molecular imaging in living mice. *Nano Lett.*, **10**, 2168–2172.

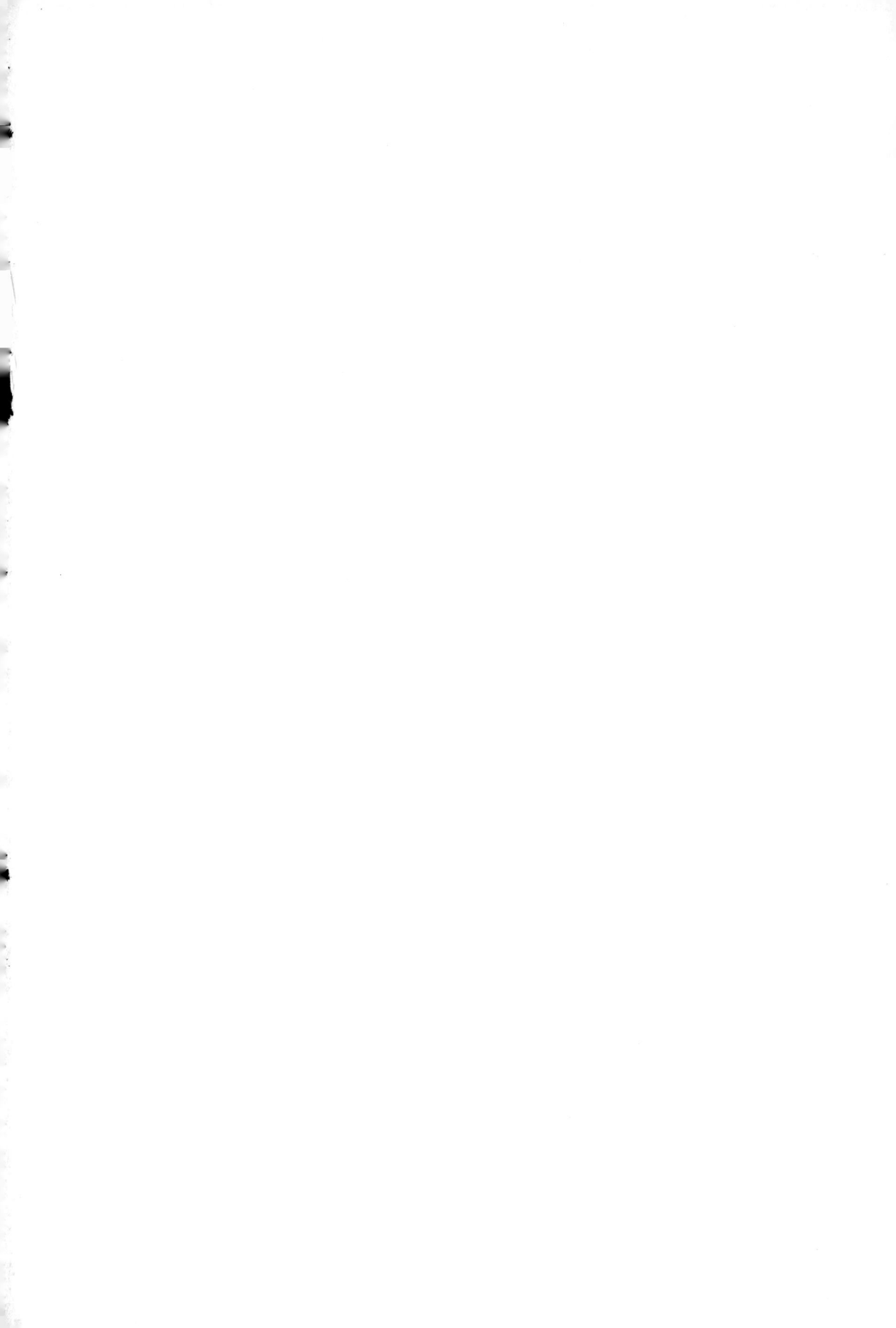